P9-CQU-943

The Life Extension Foundation's

Disease Prevention and Treatment

Expanded Fourth Edition

The Life Extension Foundation's

Disease
Prevention
and
Treatment

Scientific Protocols that Integrate
Mainstream and Alternative Medicine

Expanded Fourth Edition

*Based Upon Thousands of Research Studies
and the Clinical Experience of Physicians
Around the World*

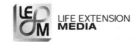

Editorial Staff
Editor: Melanie Segala
Research Associate: Amber Needham
Assistant Editors: Carolyn Lea
Dawn Davis
Page Design & Production
Publication Services
Cover Design
Jonathan Pennell

LIFE EXTENSION DISEASE PREVENTION AND TREATMENT, 4th edition, 2003. Copyright ©1997, 1998, 2000, 2003 Life Extension Media. All rights reserved. Printed in the United States. No part of this publication may be reproduced, stored in a retrieval system, or transmitted in any form by any means, electronic, mechanical, photocopying, recording, or otherwise, without prior written permission of the publisher.

This information (and any accompanying printed material) is not intended to replace the attention or advice of a physician or other healthcare professional. Anyone who wishes to embark on any dietary, drug, exercise, or other lifestyle change intended to prevent or treat a specific disease or condition should first consult with and seek clearance from a qualified healthcare professional.

The information published in the protocols is only as current as the day the manuscript was sent to the printer. This protocol raises many issues that are subject to change as new data emerge. None of our suggested protocol regimens can guarantee a cure.

Life Extension books may be purchased for personal, educational, business, or sales promotional use. For information, please write: Life Extension, P.O. Box 229120, Hollywood, Florida 33022-9120.

Web site: www.lef.org

1-800-544-4440

Library of Congress Control Number: 2003103297

FOURTH EDITION

ISBN 0-9658777-5-2

BRIDGING THE GAP BETWEEN SCIENCE AND MEDICINE
Preface

We live in a world where medical discoveries have become routine events. The sheer volume of new findings, however, has overwhelmed practicing physicians. The result is that people are dying needlessly, even though therapies to prevent or treat their diseases already exist.

The purpose of this book is to provide lifesaving information that is often overlooked by the medical establishment. Our mission has been to translate diverse scientific findings into therapeutic protocols that can be understood by the lay public.

It is important that the reader knows how this book came into being. In the 1970s, we began to uncover information that could be used to alleviate suffering and prevent death. Conveying this information to those with health problems often resulted in significant improvements in their condition.

As we delved deeper into scientific literature, it became clear that many people were dying from medical ignorance. This startling revelation did not go totally unnoticed. A growing number of individuals began to ask us for help when confronted with difficult-to-treat disorders. As more cases were presented to us, we came to the realization that a lethal communication gap exists between scientists and practicing physicians.

Marvelous discoveries are published in prestigious medical journals today, yet little of this information is utilized to save lives. It is as if an impenetrable barrier separates scientific solutions from those in critical need of this knowledge. The objective of this book is to break down the walls of ignorance and apathy that are the underlying causes of most human suffering and death.

RESISTANCE TO CHANGE

A review of past medical discoveries reveals how excruciatingly slowly the medical establishment adopts novel concepts. Even simple methods to improve medical quality often meet with fierce resistance.

A classic example of this occurred when a young Hungarian doctor named Ignatz Semmelweis discovered that a contagious disease was being transmitted to hospital patients because medical personnel failed to wash their hands.

In the 19th century, tens of thousands of women died every year from puerperal sepsis (childbed fever). The reason for this epidemic was that doctors were performing autopsies and then conducting vaginal exams with their hands covered with decomposing necrotic tissue. Dr. Semmelweis observed that women who used midwives instead of doctors had low rates of childbed fever. To test these observations, Semmelweis implemented a policy in his department that required doctors to wash their hands with disinfectant prior to attending patients. Mortality rates from childbed fever immediately declined from 18.3% to 1.3%.

When Semmelweis published his meticulous findings about the importance of hand washing, the medical community reacted with hostility or dismissal. The prevailing belief at the time was that childbed fever is caused by bad air. After strident attempts to persuade skeptics, Semmelweis was committed to an insane asylum where he died at age 42, possibly from beatings by asylum guards.

Why Hospitals Can Endanger Your Health

Regrettably, 137 years after Dr. Semmelweis's demise, hospital care remains abysmal. The best way to describe the modern hospital setting is to compare the service they render to what you would expect at a hotel. Just imagine checking into a hotel and being told the following:

1. You will check in at our convenience and be placed in a room of our choosing.

2. You will be disturbed at our convenience.

3. You will be fed at our convenience with whatever food we choose to give you.

4. You will share your room and bathroom with one or more total strangers who are sick and may be dying.

5. You will be expected to go to sleep at a time of our choosing. The door to your room will be left open so that you will be exposed to noise, light, and passing medical personnel throughout the night. These distractions will intensify early in the morning, which will awaken you.

6. You will be exposed to many harmful bacteria, which could lead to an antibiotic-resistant infection that might kill you.

7. In the event you experience difficulties while staying with us, we will respond to your calls for help at our convenience.

8. We don't know how much money we will charge you because we don't yet know how many doctors will examine you, what tests and procedures will be performed on you, and how long you will remain in the hospital.

9. Even though you may be curious as to why we keep sticking needles in you, strapping you onto machines, putting fluids in you, giving you enemas, and inducing other discomforts, we are not obligated to inform you of our reasons for these procedures.

10. You cannot check out of the hospital until you we pull all the needles, catheters, and other intrusive objects out of you, give you permission to leave, and force you to sign all kinds of papers.

If these ten rules sound worse than prison, in many respects they are! At least most of those in prison are in reasonably good health. People entering hospitals are often critically ill, yet they are given medieval-style care that sometimes exacerbates their illness, causes them to contract new diseases, and induces needless mortality.

What would never be tolerated at a hotel is considered standard hospital practice. In today's quasi-socialist system of healthcare, a hotel guest is treated far better than a wealthy individual checking into a hospital.

A Leading Cause of Death

The word "iatrogenic" is defined as illness that occurs as a result of a diagnostic or treatment procedure. The term is also used to describe problems occurring as the result of "exposure to the environment of a health care facility."

Iatrogenic illness is a leading cause of death in the United States. Large numbers of hospitalized Americans, for instance, die from the effects of malnutrition. This problem has been documented in medical journals, but many physicians continue to ignore obvious signs that their patients are starving to death. The archaic state of most hospitals directly causes seriously ill people to lose their appetite.

The goal of this book is to keep you out of the hospital. For those who must be hospitalized, we provide critical information about innovative therapies and ways of preventing harmful side effects that will help you get out alive and healthy.

ACCESS TO SCIENTIFIC PIONEERS

How many forward-thinking individuals like Dr. Semmelweis exist today? The answer is more than in any previous era. The challenge is in finding those who possess exceptional degrees of compassion, competence, and willingness to apply new discoveries.

Over the past three decades, we have been privileged to interact with scientific pioneers who have developed novel solutions for preventing and treating degenerative disease. Their methods are based upon reviewing thousands of published scientific papers, interacting with innovative doctors throughout the world, and making their own professional observations.

Medical history documents that discoveries are not made by bureaucratic committees. Instead, it is the individual with an insatiable desire for knowledge who innovates by thinking beyond prevailing dogmatic principles.

This book represents a compilation of work by individuals who are passionate about ending today's epidemic of unnecessary disease and death.

THE NEED TO STAY INFORMED

The majority of human suffering and premature death is avoidable. It is imperative that individuals be the front line soldiers in protecting their own health. Physicians attend to dozens of patients every day. One cannot expect a typical doctor to devote all the time needed to provide each patient with optimal individualized treatment. It is up to patients and their caregivers to fill this critical void.

In order to treat any serious disease in optimal fashion, a myriad of details have to be implemented precisely. You should not rely solely on physicians to prescribe and carry out treatment protocols. Patients need to gain a thorough understanding of their health status and the various treatment options open to them, so they can work effectively with their physician(s).

We cannot overemphasize the importance of educating yourself about any disorders that may affect you, including the aging process. Well-informed patients are more likely to survive longer than naive patients. Even if you are fortunate enough to find a brilliant physician, you should still learn everything about your disease and the treatments being prescribed. What you don't know could kill you!

There has never been a time in history when so many medical breakthroughs *have not* been implemented by clinical practitioners. It is not the intention of this book to replace the advice or attention of a physician or other health care professional. Instead, our objective is to help educate *both* patients and physicians about the latest, most scientific methods of preventing and treating diseases and premature aging.

Saul Kent and William Faloon
The Life Extension Foundation
June 2003

ACKNOWLEDGMENT

It is impossible to thank all of the dedicated physicians, scientists, and brilliant Life Extension members who contributed to this monumental work. Any attempt to provide a complete list of names would invariably leave out many who voluntarily provided research findings that represent essential elements of these protocols. A common attribute of the people who contributed to this book is an insatiable passion for knowledge relating to biological mechanisms. It is this infinite curiosity that motivates these individuals to relentlessly educate themselves about new methods of preventing and treating disease.

History describes medical pioneers who share common traits with the people who contributed to this book. One such inquisitive mind was Antony van Leeuwenhoek. An unlikely scientist, van Leeuwenhoek was a tradesman who received no university degrees. This would normally have excluded him from the scientific community. Yet with skill, diligence, endless curiosity, and an open mind free of dogma, van Leeuwenhoek succeeded in making some of the most important discoveries in the history of biology. Van Leewenhoek discovered bacteria, sperm cells, blood cells, microscopic nematodes and rotifers, and much more. His research was widely circulated and opened up an entire world of microscopic life to the awareness of scientists.

What distinguished van Leewenhoek was his curiosity to observe almost anything that could be placed under his lenses and his care in describing what he saw. Although van Leeuwenhoek could not draw well, he hired an illustrator to prepare drawings of the things he saw to accompany his written descriptions. In 1673, van Leeuwenhoek began writing letters to the Royal Society of London, describing what he had seen with his microscopes. For the next 50 years, van Leeuwenhoek corresponded with the Royal Society and his letters were eagerly awaited by scientists fascinated by what was found to exist in the microscopic world.

Seven years before his death, van Leeuwenhoek wrote the following to explain why he devoted his life to making discoveries and disseminating his findings to the world:

> . . . my work, which I've done for a long time, was not pursued in order to gain the praise I now enjoy, but chiefly from a craving after knowledge, which I notice resides in me more than in most other men. And therewithal, whenever I found out anything remarkable, I have thought it my duty to put down my discovery on paper, so that all ingenious people might be informed thereof.
>
> Antony van Leeuwenhoek
> Letter of June 12, 1716

While many contributors to this book are highly credentialed physicians and scientists, they share Leewenhoek's craving for knowledge and desire to pass on their findings to their fellow man.

The innovative methods contained in this book stem from the desire to inform those in need about lifesaving medical discoveries. The Life Extension Foundation has been privileged to be the recipient of knowledge from contributors throughout the world who are humanitarians and scientific geniuses.

A BIT OF MEDICAL HISTORY

A cursory reading of medical history reveals startling examples of scientific discoveries that were suppressed by whatever "establishment" ruled the day. Rejecting new ideas has long been a common medical ideology, and those who fell ill suffered horrendous deaths as a result.

One example of a medical breakthrough ignored by the medical mainstream was the development of the smallpox vaccine. Smallpox was mankind's worst scourge, killing a larger percentage of previous populations than any other disease.

In 1789, a British doctor named Edward Jenner performed an experiment that laid the foundation for the eradication of smallpox. Jenner tested this hypothesis by inoculating his own son with material obtained from a cowpox lesion. Six weeks later, his son proved resistant when challenged with material from a smallpox lesion. The principle of immunization was thus established. This is an epic story when you realize that Edward Jenner's young son would likely have died if Jenner were wrong.

Putting his son's life on the line was only the first challenge Jenner faced in convincing the world to accept his new idea. An article sent to the Royal Medical Society in 1796 describing 13 successfully vaccinated persons was rejected. Jenner was forced to pay the costs of publishing his own treatise in 1798, but it was not well received. Jenner's work was subjected to fierce criticism by the medical profession. Some physicians were opposed to any new ideas, while others had financial interests in less-effective forms of smallpox treatment. Jenner endured severe abuse from the press, religious groups, and the medical establishment. In today's regulated legal environment, Jenner almost certainly would have been jailed for practicing "unapproved" medicine.

Millions died of smallpox while medical authorities suppressed Jenner's lifesaving discovery. Regrettably, the same situation exists today *vis-à-vis* today's lethal diseases. Doctors routinely overlook novel therapies that have shown efficacy in published scientific studies. The result is that people die while potentially effective therapies wait to be accepted by the medical establishment or the FDA.

THE DELAY IN RECOGNIZING PENICILLIN

There are people alive today who remember the carnage inflicted by bacterial infections such as tuberculosis, diphtheria, rheumatic fever, cholera, syphilis, and pneumonia. Before the advent of antibiotics, agonizing deaths from bacterial infections were commonplace, especially in children.

In 1928, Dr. Alexander Fleming discovered penicillin. His work was published the very next year in the *British Journal of Experimental Pathology.* Nevertheless, the medical profession did not begin treating humans with this lifesaving therapy until 1941, and the general population did not gain access to penicillin until 1946.

Millions of people suffered and died from bacterial diseases at a time when penicillin had already been discovered and published in a respected medical journal. For 18 years, people could only watch helplessly as their loved ones suffered and died from diseases that penicillin could have cured.

Dr. Fleming and two other scientists who assisted in making sufficient quantities of penicillin to save human lives were awarded a Nobel Prize in 1945.

LETHAL DANGERS OF RADIOACTIVE FALLOUT COVERED UP

A U.S. government study released in the year 2002 says that radioactive fallout from nuclear weapons testing has caused at least 15,000 cancer deaths in the United States. This report was prepared as a joint effort by the *National Cancer Institute* and *Centers for Disease Control and Prevention.* Here is a chilling revelation from this report based on above-ground tests that took place between 1951 and 1962:

> "Any person living in the contiguous United States since 1951 has been exposed to radioactive fallout, and all organs and tissues of the body have received some radiation exposure."

For decades, the federal government contended that radioactive fallout from nuclear testing was harmless. Government propaganda films in the 1950s even showed American children playing in fresh radioactive ash to demonstrate that it was as "safe as snow."

Linus Pauling knew in the 1950s that radioactive fallout would cause cancer and other diseases in humans. Pauling joined with Albert Einstein and five others to form the Emergency Committee of Atomic Scientists. Their mission was to inform the public about the dangerous consequences that nuclear weapons and nuclear testing held for civilization.

In 1957, Pauling wrote a scientific appeal petition calling for a nuclear test ban treaty and distributed it throughout the scientific community. He soon gathered over 9,000 signatures from 49 countries including 2,000 American scientists. In 1958, Pauling presented the petition to the Secretary General of the United Nations, announcing that it represented the general consensus of the world's scientists and their plea for a ban on future nuclear testing.

Pauling gave hundreds of lectures against nuclear weapons testing and war. Unfortunately, he toured during a time of heightened Cold War suspicions and was marked a Communist supporter. The federal government refused to give Pauling a passport, thus denying him the opportunity to attend international scientific conventions. Pauling was twice subpoenaed to appear before congressional committees investigating anti-American activities to declare that he was not a Communist. On October 11, 1960 Pauling was threatened to be held in contempt of Congress because he refused to reveal the names of those who helped circulate his petition to ban nuclear testing.

Despite unrelenting governmental oppression, Pauling remained undaunted and continued his crusade by writing a draft resolution for a nuclear test ban treaty. He sent letters and copies of his resolution to both President Kennedy and Premier Khrushchev. The two superpowers eventually agreed on a limited test ban treaty—one that was strikingly similar to Pauling's. The treaty went into effect on October 10th, 1963: the very day it was announced that Pauling was to receive his second Nobel Prize.

By disseminating his knowledge about the lethal dangers of radioactive fallout, Pauling became a target of government harassment, persecution in the press, and charges of working for the enemy. He could have been jailed for refusing to provide Congress with the names of those involved in gathering more than 9,000 signatures for the scientific petition to ban above-ground nuclear testing.

We now know that the government knew about the effects of above-ground nuclear testing, but covered them up. In the 1950s for example, government officials notified suppliers of photographic film of expected fallout patterns so they could protect their film, but did not share the information with milk producers. Many children drank this radioactive contaminated milk. Forty-five years ago, Dr. Linus Pauling formulated a public health response to eradicate the problem caused by above-ground nuclear testing, but the federal government chose instead to persecute this brilliant scientist so that the practice of raining radioactive fallout throughout the United States could continue.

As is too often the case, when the government makes a criminal accusation against a political dissident (in this case, Linus Pauling), history later shows that it was the government itself that was involved in the sinister activities. What could be more anti-American than inflicting cancer on 15,000 innocent people?

MODERN DAY BLOODLETTING

When the oxygen-carrying capacity of the blood is impaired (i.e., anemia), people with reduced blood flow to any organ, such as those with coronary artery disease, are at a greater risk for infirmity and death. Cancer cells thrive in a low oxygen environment and even borderline anemia predicts higher mortality.

One study looking at elderly hospitalized heart attack patients found that those who were severely anemic were 78% more likely to die over a 30-day period, while those who were moderately anemic were 52% more likely to die. There was no increase in mortality in patients who were not significantly anemic.

Anemia can be detected by routine blood tests, yet busy doctors often accept anemia as a normal state in aged people and fail to treat it. Anemia is common in cancer patients. Conventional cancer therapies such as chemotherapy, radiation, and testosterone blockade often induce anemia. Elevated levels of inflammatory cytokines seen in cancer patients also suppress red blood cell formation.

The importance of avoiding anemia is well established in the scientific literature. One study systematically reviewed the effect of anemia on survival in cancer patients. The results showed that cancer patients who were anemic had a 65% increase in mortality. Despite this data, most oncologists fail to adequately treat for anemia.

Anemia is a strong predictor of early death in the elderly. Anemic individuals, ages 70–79, are 28% more likely to die over a five-year time period. Anemic people, ages 80–89, are 34% more likely to die, while those of age 90–99 are 48% more likely to die over a five-year period.

Two centuries ago, doctors treated sick people by draining their blood (bloodletting). This bloodletting resulted in severe anemia. Based on what we now know, those who could afford the bloodletting procedure died much sooner than those who avoided doctors. Medicine has not changed much over the past 200 years. Most physicians still do not take anemia seriously and this treatable disorder still claims a large number of needless victims each year.

WE CANNOT FORGET THE PAST, OR WE MAY HAVE TO RELIVE IT

Those with new ideas often face fierce attack by the medical establishment and the federal government. An example was the announcement that human embryonic stem cells had been produced and that there was an opportunity to cure many of today's lethal diseases.

You would think that the scientist who made this remarkable discovery, Dr. Mike West, would be proclaimed a hero. Instead, government leaders immediately vowed to pass new laws to make it a crime to create embryonic stem cells for therapeutic cloning purposes.

The concern of the Life Extension Foundation is that only a precious few brilliant minds like Edward Jenner, Alexander Fleming, Linus Pauling, and Mike West are ever born. When Linus Pauling stated that radioactive fallout caused cancer in humans, he was ridiculed, persecuted, and almost incarcerated. Pauling has now been proven right. This vindication does nothing for the 15,000 Americans who have perished from radioactive fallout-induced cancer.

Today, there are pockets of exceptional intelligence that are stifled by bureaucratic red tape. In order to create the scientific renaissance needed to radically extend the healthy human lifespan, the barriers that suppress implementation of new ideas must be broken down.

This book is dedicated to eradicating the ignorance that is causing humans to suffer and die from diseases that may already have cures, or at least palliative therapies. Almost every therapy discussed in this book has been documented extensively by peer-reviewed, published studies from the most prestigious medical journals in the world. Despite this scientific evidence, the medical establishment largely ignores these therapies.

"Each progressive spirit is opposed by a thousand mediocre minds appointed to guard the past."

-- Maurice Maeterlinck

MEDICAL ADVISORY BOARD

Gustavo Tovar Baez, M.D., operates the Life Extension Clinic in Caracas, Venezuela. He is the first physician in Caracas to specialize in anti-aging medicine.

Stephen A. Barnes, M.D., is a surgical oncologist who received his training at Johns Hopkins Hospital. Dr. Barnes has dedicated his life to the surgical care of cancer victims, and encourages patients to incorporate alternative therapies in their treatment.

Sam Baxas, M.D., head of the Baxamed Medical Center for Youth Restoration in Basel, Switzerland, has developed cell therapy and growth hormone therapies for a variety of diseases, including Parkinson's disease and arthritis.

Ricardo Bernales, M.D., is a general practitioner in Chicago who focuses on allergies, bronchial asthma, and immunodeficiency, and is a board-certified pediatrician.

Thomas F. Crais, M.D., F.A.C.S., a board-certified plastic surgeon, is medical director of the microsurgical research and training lab, Southern Baptist Hospital, in New Orleans.

Martin Dayton, M.D., D.O., practices at the Sunny Isles Medical Center in North Miami Beach, FL. His focus is on nutrition, aging, chelation therapy, holistic medicine, and oxidative medicine.

Arnold Fox, M.D., is an internist and cardiologist in Beverly Hills, CA, specializing in anti-aging medicine using nutritional and hormone therapies. He is the Dean of the Anti-Aging Concentration (School) of the University of Integrated Studies.

Carmen Fusco, M.S., R.N., C.N.S., is a research scientist and clinical nutritionist in New York City who has lectured about and written numerous articles on the biochemical approach to the prevention of aging and degenerative diseases.

Miguelangelo Gonzalez, M.D., is a certified plastic and reconstructive surgeon at the Miguelangelo Plastic Surgery Clinic, Cabo San Lucas, Baja California Sur, Mexico.

Garry F. Gordon, M.D., D.O., Payson, AZ, researches alternative medical approaches for medical problems unresponsive to traditional therapies. He is president of the International College of Advanced Longevity Medicine.

Richard Heifetz, M.D., is a board-certified anesthesiologist in Santa Rosa, CA, specializing in the delivery of anesthesia for office-based plastic or cosmetic surgery, chelation therapy, and pain management.

Maurice D. Marholin, D.O., D.C., fellow in nutrition under a grant from the National Cancer Institute, practices integrative medicine with a nutrition-based focus in Lake Wales, FL.

Philip Lee Miller, M.D., is Founder and Medical Director of the Los Gatos Longevity Institute in Los Gatos, California. His practice is dedicated to Anti-Aging Medicine focusing on bio-identical natural hormone replacement, nutritional medicine, complex lipid disorders, and stress management. He is a Diplomat of the American Board of Anti-Aging Medicine.

Michele G. Morrow, D.O., F.A.A.F.P., is a board-certified family physician who has successfully merged mainstream with alternative medicine by using functional medicine concepts and natural approaches with traditional modalities in her own private practice in Hollywood and Pembroke Pines, Florida. Dr. Morrow is an accomplished clinician, medical researcher, author and lecturer.

Herbert Pardell, DO, F.A.A.I.M., practices internal medicine at the Emerald Hills Medical Center in Hollywood, FL, and specializes in anti-aging, chelation, hormone replacement, and complementary medicine. He is a medical director of the Life Extension Foundation.

Lambert Titus K. Parker, M.D., practices internal medicine at Schuyler Hospital in Montour Falls, NY, and is the director of the clinic's intensive care unit.

Ross Pelton, R.Ph., Ph.D., C.C.N., is Director of Nutrition and Anti-Aging Research for Intramedicine, Inc. He also writes and teaches continuing education courses for health professionals on a wide variety of health topics. Dr. Pelton has authored six books.

ADDITIONAL NUTRIENTS TO ENHANCE SKIN HEALTH

Water is vital to the health of our bodies. Almost all biological reactions require water. Water is needed to deliver and utilize nutrients in every organ system of the body. Health professionals advise drinking eight 8-oz. glasses of water a day for several reasons. Water improves circulation by making blood less sticky and opening blood vessels. It is virtually necessary to digest food. Without adequate hydration, the body cannot effectively flush waste and disease-causing toxins from the body. Water is also needed to maintain proper functioning of protein structures and connective tissue in the body.

Other nutrients with skin-supporting qualities include fiber-rich foods, beta carotene, vitamin C, calcium, selenium, silica, the B vitamins, biotin, essential fatty acids, olive oil, cod liver oil, linseed oil, and all of the amino acids (Michaelsson et al. 1977a,b,c; Weimar et al. 1978; Kligman et al. 1981; Thomas et al. 1982; Michaelsson et al. 1984; Ruiz-Maldonado 1998).

Herbal Therapies

Some herbs are known for their abilities to heal the skin, soothe inflammation, and relieve itching. Chinese herbalists also recommend echinacea, calendula, tea tree oil, and goldenseal tincture or blue flag (works well with echinacea). Drinking a tea made from nettles and cleavers tincture may be effective.

If emotional stress is a possible contributing factor in your acne, relax with a cup of lavender or chamomile tea. A steaming facial treatment with these herbs 2 or 3 times a week may also help.

CAUTION Never use any herbal preparation on a newborn without consulting your doctor.

Natural Topical Products

In response to recommendations from herbalists and dermatologists, as well as requests from acne patients, manufacturers have created special products that use herbs and other natural substances to treat acne (Epstein 2000). A search of the Web will result in literally hundreds of sites that offer natural products for skin care and the treatment of acne. These products range from facial scrubs and moisturizers to antiseptics and facial masks.

Lipoic acid in particular can help heal acne scars. Lipoic acid activates a transcription factor known as AP-1, which leads to the production of enzymes called metalloproteinases. These enzymes digest the damaged collagen, thus helping erase wrinkles and even scars. At the same time, lipoic acid helps cells produce more energy in the mitochondria, thus making more energy available for healing (Greenwell 2001).

The following list includes natural ingredients found alone or in combination in various topical treatments for acne:

- Skin healing: Gels are available containing one or more of the following ingredients: lipoic acid, carnosine, dimethylaminoethanol (DMAE), collagen, protein, and vitamins C, E, and A. These ingredients will help repair damaged tissue and fight free radical damage.

- Inflammation and redness: Creams are available that contain chamomile, cat's claw, and geranium extract to reduce inflammation from infection or irritating topical medications.

- Cleansers: Facial washes may contain fruit and vegetable extracts, such as lemon, apricot, and cucumber, and herbal extracts such as ginseng, green tea, and ginkgo, for deep pore cleansing.

- Antibacterial/antifungal: tea tree oil, echinacea, and white willow bark are antiseptics that can kill microbes responsible for certain outbreaks.

- Astringents: witch hazel, herbal extracts, citrus seed extracts, and calendula can help remove excess facial oil.

- Facial masks: Seaweed extract and bentonite clay (a combination of montmorillonite and volcanic ash that is highly absorbent) will pull oils and toxins from the skin.

At-home Care of the Skin

- Wash your face *gently* with unscented, oil-free cleansers, and keep your skin clean. Remember: Acne is not caused by dirt, and scrubbing an inflamed skin condition only makes acne worse.

- Control the urge to squeeze, scratch, or pick at pimples; let them drain when they are ready.

- Try products that contain benzoyl peroxide for mild to moderate acne.

- Do not overexpose acne to sunlight; do so only in moderation. Exposure to the sun may make acne worse and increase your chance for developing skin cancer.

- Young men with moderate to severe acne should use a new razor blade every time they shave to lessen the risk of infection.

- Young men should avoid alcohol-based aftershaves; instead, use herbal alternatives that include essential oils of lavender, chamomile, or tea tree oil.

PREVENTION

Because of the association of acne with fluctuating hormone levels and the possible link to genetic influences, many doctors believe there is no way to prevent it. Although accepted wisdom is that neither good hygiene, nor diet can prevent acne outbreaks, dietary and nutritional recommendations may be helpful. Good general hygiene and sensible skin care are especially important for adolescents. The basics include a daily bath or shower and face- and hand-washing with an unscented or mild antibacterial soap. It is best for teenage girls not to use cosmetics regularly. Despite advertising claims to the contrary, few if any commercial skin medications have any beneficial effect on acne.

 ## SUMMARY

1. Avoid the sun. Overexposure to the sun can worsen acne.

2. Use only hypoallergenic, oil-free cosmetics. Use cosmetics sparingly.

3. Eliminate foods that are high in fat, hormones, and iodine.

4. Oral and topical antibiotics help prevent new blemishes by killing bacteria and breaking down sebum into FFA. Prescription-strength antibiotics must be obtained from a physician. However, lesser strengths are available as over-the-counter preparations from any pharmacy.

5. Chromium can improve glucose tolerance and potentially improve an acne condition. One 200 mcg capsule of chromium taken 2–3 times daily is suggested.

6. Lipoic acid has beneficial healing qualities for acne scars. Take 1–2 250-mg capsules of Super Alpha-Lipoic Acid w/Biotin. Persons with glucose intolerance should consider taking 2–4 capsules.

7. Take zinc, 50 mg daily, to reduce inflammation and aid in healing damaged skin.

8. Take vitamin B6, 50–100 mg daily, to aid in hormone metabolism.

9. Take vitamin B5 (pantothenic acid), 2000–10,000 mg daily, in divided doses with meals.

10. Take MSM, 2000–3000 mg daily, to detoxify skin.

11. Take vitamin E, 400 IU daily, for its antioxidant properties. Make sure you are consuming enough gamma tocopherol when taking alpha tocopherol vitamin E supplements.

12. Take vitamin A, less than 30,000 IU daily, to reduce sebum production. Some doctors believe that no more than 5000 IU of supplemental vitamin A should be taken a day. Pregnant women should only take vitamin A under the supervision of their obstetrician.

13. Several topically applied products contain vitamins, herbs, and other natural substances that will nourish the skin while treating an existing condition.

14. Consult a medical professional if acne does not respond to self-treatment. Your doctor may consider several drug therapies including Retin-A, Accutane, or Propecia.

 ## FOR MORE INFORMATION

Contact the American Academy of Dermatology, (202)842-3555.

PRODUCT AVAILABILITY

Chromium, zinc (methionate), Complete B-Complex, pantothenic acid (vitamin B5 powder and caps), vitamin B6 caps, alpha and gamma vitamin E succinate, Super Alpha Lipoic Acid w/Biotin, MSM, and the Life Extension multi-nutrient formula, may be ordered by calling (800)544-4440 or by ordering on line at www.lef.org.

Adrenal Disease

The adrenals are two crescent-shaped glands that sit on top of each kidney. The adrenal glands secrete hormones directly into the bloodstream. They are divided anatomically and functionally into two main parts: the medulla (middle) and the cortex (rind) (Clayman 1989). Additionally, each division of an adrenal gland consists of internal layers that produce different hormones.

The inner part, or adrenal medulla, manufactures epinephrine and norepinephrine, also known as adrenaline and noradrenaline. These hormones are the "fight or flight" hormones that are released in life-or-death situations. Their release increases heart rate, blood pressure, and diverts more blood to the brain, heart, and skeletal muscles. This is important when discussing stress.

The adrenal cortex surrounds the adrenal medulla and responds to a different type of stress. This is where the steroid hormones are made. These include cortisone, hydrocortisone, testosterone, estrogen, 17-hydroxy-keto-steroids, DHEA, pregnenolone, aldosterone, androstene-dione, progesterone, and some other intermediate hormones. Many of these hormones are also made elsewhere in the body, but aldosterone, cortisone, and hydrocortisone are made only in the adrenal glands.

The hormone aldosterone, together with the kidneys, regulates the balance of sodium and potassium in the body. This regulation is critical to many physiological function, including the ability to react to stress, maintain fluid balance, and regulate blood pressure.

Two disorders often associated with impaired function of the adrenal glands are Addison's disease and Cushing's syndrome.

ADDISON'S DISEASE: ADRENAL INSUFFICIENCY

Addison's disease is a profound chronic adrenal failure caused by damage or disease of the adrenal gland, resulting in a deficiency of cortisol. This disease is sometimes called chronic adrenal insufficiency or hypocortisolism. The most important job of cortisol is to help the body respond to stress. Among its other vital tasks, cortisol is partly responsible for:

- Maintaining blood pressure and cardiovascular function
- Balancing the effects of insulin in breaking down sugar for energy
- Slowing the immune system's inflammatory response
- Regulating the metabolism of proteins, carbohydrates, and fats

Addison's disease is characterized by muscle weakness, reduced blood sugar, nausea, loss of appetite, weight loss, and low blood pressure, which can impact the act of standing, causing dizziness or fainting. Skin changes also are common in Addison's disease, with areas of hyperpigmentation or dark tanning that are mostly visible on scars, skin folds, toes, lips, mucous membranes, and pressure points, such as the elbows, knees, and knuckles.

CUSHING'S SYNDROME: OVERPRODUCTION OF CORTISOL

The overproduction of cortisol by the adrenal glands leads to Cushing's syndrome (Clayman 1989). Cushing's syndrome also results when glucocorticoid drug hormones (such as hydrocortisone, prednisone, methylprednisolone, or dexamethasone) are taken in excess for a prolonged period of time. These steroid hormones are often used to treat inflammatory-related illnesses such as asthma, rheumatoid arthritis, systemic lupus erythematosus, and some allergies.

The overproduction of cortisol in the adrenal glands can happen in two ways. A pituitary tumor could be producing too much ACTH (adrenocorticotropic hormone, produced by the pituitary gland), stimulating the adrenals to grow and to produce too much cortisol, or a

Adrenal Glands

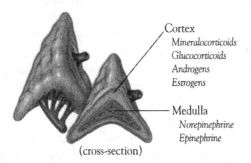

Cortex
Mineralocorticoids
Glucocorticoids
Androgens
Estrogens

Medulla
Norepinephrine
Epinephrine

(cross-section)

An adrenal gland curves over the top of each kidney. The adrenal gland is composed of two separate endocrine glands: the adrenal cortex and the adrenal medulla, each performing a different action. (Anatomical Chart Company 2002®, Lippincott Williams, & Wilkins.)

benign or malignant tumor outside the pituitary such as in the lung, thymus gland, pancreas, or other organs can produce too much ACTH. The pituitary form is classically called Cushing's disease.

Cushing's syndrome is characterized by central obesity; sparing of the arms and legs (thin extremities); a round, reddish moon face; buffalo hump; and a protuberant abdomen. Many people with Cushing's syndrome experience severe fatigue, weak muscles, ulcers, thin skin, high blood pressure, and high blood sugar. Irritability, anxiety, and depression are also very common. Women with Cushing's syndrome will usually have excess hair growth (hirsutism) on their face, necks, chests, abdomens, and thighs. Their menstrual periods may become irregular or stop. Men may have decreased fertility and desire for sex.

ADRENAL FATIGUE

Constant stress and poor nutrition can weaken the adrenal glands. When stress continues over prolonged periods of time, the adrenal glands can deplete the body's hormonal and energy reserves, and the glands may either shrink in size or hypertrophy (enlarge). The overproduction of adrenal hormones caused by prolonged stress can weaken the immune system and inhibit the production of white blood cells that protect the body against foreign invaders (in particular lymphocytes and lymph node function). Adrenal dysfunction can disrupt the body's blood sugar metabolism, causing weakness, fatigue, and a feeling of being run down. It can also interfere with normal sleep rhythms and produce a wakeful, unrelaxing sleep state, making a person feel worn out even after a full night's sleep.

If a person succumbs easily to allergies and infections, feels constantly drained and exhausted, and experiences low blood sugar and blood pressure, the culprit may be weak adrenals. Adrenal insufficiency is sometimes linked to chronic fatigue. In some fatigued patients, thyroid problems may overlap adrenal problems. In these cases, the status of the adrenal glands and the thyroid gland must be assessed. The appropriate treatment should be undertaken only after this determination is made. If adrenal fatigue is suspected, the patient should be evaluated by a physician with experience in recognizing and treating adrenal fatigue and issues of the relative Addisonian state. It is very important to make sure that full-blown Addison's disease is not the problem, since it must be treated vigorously (Ehlert et al. 2001; Tsigos et al. 2002). In most communities, a qualified internist or internal medicine subspecialist will begin the investigation.

DIAGNOSIS

If disturbed adrenal function is suspected, the levels of hormones such as hydrocortisone, aldosterone, epinephrine, and ACTH may be measured in blood, plasma, and urine. There are also tests (by injection) to measure the effects of substances that normally modify the production of a specific hormone. One test is called the ACTH challenge test. When ACTH is injected, there should be an increase in adrenal hormone output. If this does not happen, adrenal fatigue is probable. These tests are also helpful in localizing the underlying cause of a particular disorder (e.g., to distinguish between Cushing's syndrome caused by an adrenal tumor from that caused by pituitary disease). Conversely, a very high potency corticosteroid (dexamethasone) can be used to assess the suppressability of cortisone production in Cushing's syndrome.

If disease of the adrenal glands is suspected, imaging studies (abdominal x-ray, MRI, CT scan, arteriography, radionuclide scanning, and IV scanning of the position of kidneys using an IV dye) may show the presence of adrenal calcification, a tumor, atrophy, or the overgrowth of a gland.

Factors that May be Overlooked in Diagnosis

Cortisone is produced mainly in a reversible reaction from cortisol; it is also secreted in small amounts from the adrenal cortex. The term hydrocortisone refers to both naturally produced cortisone and the pharmaceutical preparation used to treat various inflammatory disorders. Naturally produced hydrocortisone is a glucocorticoid, meaning that it helps to regulate normal blood glucose concentration by converting amino acids and fatty acids to glucose, when needed, in a process called *gluconeogenesis*.

Synthetic hydrocortisone drugs (corticosteroids) became available in the late 1940s and were heralded as a miraculous treatment for rheumatoid arthritis due to their suppression of the immune system. However, it did not take long to learn that there was a serious price to pay for chronic corticosteroid use. People taking synthetic hydrocortisone developed many symptoms and physical abnormalities such as the symptoms of Cushing's syndrome, resulting from the body's overexposure to corticosteroids.

As a result of these adverse reactions, an often irrational approach developed in the medical community to the question of relative adrenal function. A person who has total failure of the adrenal glands is said to have Addison's disease even though low steroid levels can also be caused by failure of the hypothalamus tand pituitary areas of the brain. In this case, the adrenal glands still function. In the case of Cushing's syndrome, the disease may manifest due to physical abnormality or as the result of corticosteroid use.

When a physician evaluates a patient relying solely upon laboratory data, the patient is considered either normal or having Addison's disease or Cushing's syndrome. There may be no analysis of other contributing factors. This protocol is directed only at the function of the adrenal glands. However, just as in thyroid dysfunction (see the Thyroid Deficiency protocol), normal laboratory tests do not exclude what some physicians refer to as adrenal fatigue (or relative Cushing's or Addisonian states).

The association of impaired immune function and the administration of synthetic corticosteroids have blurred an important fact. Decreased levels of corticosteroids also impair immune function. What further complicates the matter is the fact that it is now thought that the continual overproduction of cortisol, not in the range that would produce Cushing's syndrome, contributes to immune suppression, atherosclerosis, brain cell injury, and accelerated aging.

DRUG TREATMENTS

Addison's Disease

Adrenal Cortical Extract

A few physicians recommend adrenal cortical extract (ACE), which contains all the corticosteroids in the proper proportions. ACE used to be widely available in this country, but at the present time it is not. Complementary physicians may have had experience with it. At times of increased stress, the addition of adrenal glandulars may be advisable but must be monitored carefully. Long-term use is not recommended and is likely hazardous. (The FDA removed all products containing adrenal cortex from market in 1997 due to concerns regarding contamination.)

Hydrocortisone

Cortisol is usually replaced orally with hydrocortisone tablets. The doses of this medication are adjusted to meet the needs of individual patients. During a critical stage, when blood pressure and blood sugar are dangerously low and potassium levels are high, therapy can involve the injection of hydrocortisone, saline, and dextrose.

Cushing's Syndrome

Treatment of Cushing's syndrome will depend upon the cause of the disorder. If the disorder is caused by long-term corticosteroid use, the drug must be slowly decreased and the patient weaned under medical

supervision. If it is caused by a pituitary or adrenal tumor, surgery is necessary to remove it. In Cushing's syndrome caused by an ectopic ACTH-secreting tumor, the tumor is resected. For a year after cessation of high-dose corticosteroid therapy, even minor illnesses can cause a full-blown Addisonian collapse. If the tumor is malignant and has metastasized and resection is not possible, treatment may include a combination of chemotherapy, immunotherapy, and radiation therapy.

Drugs such as ketoconazole, aminoglutethimide, or metyrapone may also be given to suppress cortisol metabolism and secretion. The European drug KH3 (the active ingredient is procaine), which can block some of the cell-damaging effects of cortisol and help protect against cortisol toxicity, is beneficial for Cushing's disease. KH3 has been also known for its beneficial effects in aging and depressed people (Cohen et al. 1974; Hall et al. 1983). A suggestion would be to take 1–2 KH3 capsules in the morning on an empty stomach and 1–2 KH3 capsules in mid-afternoon, also on an empty stomach.

NATURAL SUPPLEMENTS TO TREAT ADDISONIAN STATES

DHEA

Aging and diseases associated with aging can cause a decline in critical hormones produced by the adrenal glands. Pregnenolone is converted into crucial antiaging hormones such as dehydroepiandrosterone (DHEA), estrogen, progesterone, and testosterone. DHEA supplementation may help to partly rectify hormone imbalances caused by age-induced adrenal insufficiency.

An article in the journal Clinical Endocrinology described a study of the effect of oral DHEA replacement therapy in women with Addison's disease (Gebre-Medhin et al. 2000). The researchers found that DHEA and DHEA-sulfate (DHEA-S) levels were restored to normal in those patients receiving 50 mg of DHEA, whereas the DHEA-S level was slightly above the normal reference value in those receiving 200 mg of DHEA. Circulating levels of androgens (androstenedione, testosterone, and testosterone/SHBG ratio) were normalized in all patients. No serious side effects were seen, but some of the patients experienced increased apocrine sweat secretion (apocrine glands are in the armpit, anal, genital, and breast areas and produce a strong odor), itchy scalp, and acne, all of which were reversed when DHEA was discontinued. The authors concluded that a daily replacement dose of 50 mg of DHEA results in near physiological levels of DHEA,

DHEA-S, androstenedione, and testosterone in women with Addison's disease without severe side effects (Gebre-Medhin et al. 2000).

Another article described a randomized, double-blind study in which 39 patients with Addison's disease received 50 mg of oral DHEA daily for 12 weeks (Hunt et al. 2000). After DHEA treatment, levels of DHEA-S and delta-4-androstenedione rose from subnormal to within the adult physiological range. Total testosterone increased from subnormal to low normal with a fall in serum sex hormone-binding globulin in females, but with no change in either parameter in males. In both sexes, psychological assessment showed significant enhancement of self-esteem with a tendency for improved overall well-being. Mood and fatigue also improved significantly, with benefit being evident in the evenings. The authors concluded that DHEA replacement corrects this steroid deficiency effectively and improves some aspects of psychological function. These positive effects, in the absence of significant adverse events, suggest a role for DHEA replacement therapy in the treatment of Addison's disease. Studies suggest that low DHEA-S might be a prognostic marker and a sign of exhausted adrenal glands (Hunt et al. 2000; Beishuizen et al. 2002). (*Before taking DHEA or pregnenolone, refer to the Foundation's precautions in the DHEA Replacement Therapy protocol and to the Autoimmune Diseases protocol for additional suggestions.*)

CAUTION Even mild Addison's disease requires expert physician intervention and supervision. Glucocorticoid and mineralocorticoid component drugs are prescribed for Addison's disease. Once cortisol levels are stabilized, the serum levels of DHEA should be evaluated to determine if DHEA replacement therapy is warranted. In the majority of cases, Addison's disease is caused by an autoimmune attack on the adrenal glands. DHEA has been shown to suppress inflammatory cytokines and thereby down-regulate autoimmune reactions in the body. In the past, infection, such as tuberculosis or meningitis, was the main cause.

Licorice

Licorice (*Glycyrrhiza glabra* and *Glycyrrhiza uralensis*) is grown in Europe and Asia. Licorice is a highly prized medicinal Chinese medicine. It is used in almost all of the Chinese patent herbal formulas. *Glycyrrhiza* may be taken in a variety of ways, including as a tea. It helps to reduce the amount of hydrocortisone broken down by the liver, thereby reducing the workload of the adrenal glands. Licorice is a well-loved candy for children, although most commercial brands no longer contain real licorice. Instead commercial

products use anise seed and sugar, which taste similar. It is best to stay with teas or supplements. Licorice was prescribed for Addison's disease until the 1930s. Licorice is also a demulcent (an oily substance that reduces irritation), which makes it soothing to the digestive tract. Deglycyrrhized licorice (DGL) is made by removing the glycyrrhizin. For the adrenal effects, only real licorice should be used, not DGL.

CAUTION Long-term use of licorice containing more than 1 gram of glycyrrhizin (the amount in approximately 10 grams of licorice root) daily can cause increased blood pressure and water retention (edema) (Schambelan 1994). High doses of licorice should only be taken under the care of a qualified health professional.

Pantothenic Acid

Pantothenic acid (vitamin B_5) activates the adrenal glands. It is a precursor of acetyl CoA (a part of the Krebs's cycle which produces cellular energy) and acetylcholine (a primary neurotransmitter). Pantothenic acid deficiency results in adrenal insufficiency, which is characterized by fatigue, headache, sleep disturbances, nausea, and abdominal discomfort (Tarasov et al. 1985; Smith et al. 1996; Murray et al. 1997).

L-Theanine

L-theanine is an amino acid found in green tea that produces a calming effect in the brain. It works by increasing gamma-aminobutyric acid (GABA) that is a relaxer and creates a sense of well-being. *L*-theanine may be taken to help modulate mood and relieve stress in many health conditions (Abe et al. 1995; Kobayashi et al. 1998; Juneja et al. 1999).

NATURAL SUPPLEMENTS TO TREAT CUSHING'S SYNDROME

DHEA

DHEA may help to protect against the overproduction of cortisol from the adrenal glands and enhance the immune system. This is an important factor since too much cortisol accelerates aging and causes immune system disorders. Studies show that DHEA deficiency may actually debilitate immune status (Wisniewski 1993; Morio et al. 1996).

Vitamin C

Studies show that vitamin C and aspirin can attenuate and influence cortisol, inducing an anti-inflammatory response to prolonged exercise and stress. Vitamin C has been shown to reduce the elevation of cortisol in response to heavy exercise. In human studies, 3000 mg of vitamin C daily mitigated a rise in blood pressure, cortisol, and subjective response to acute psychological stress (Peters et al. 2001a, 2001b; Brody et al. 2002).

Phosphatidylserine (PS)

Phosphatidylserine is a phospholipid that is a structural component of the biological membranes in animals and plants. In studies, supplemental PS has been shown to improve mood and blunt the release of cortisol in response to physical stress (Monteleone et al. 1990; Kelly 1999; Benton et al. 2001).

Melatonin

Melatonin is secreted by the pineal gland and functions to regulate circadian rhythm and induce sleep. Melatonin circadian secretion in patients with pituitary- or adrenal-dependent Cushing's syndrome was shown to be significantly lower compared to healthy control groups. Studies also have shown that nightly administration of 2 mg of melatonin increased the DHEA-S-cortisol ratio after 6 months of treatment (Soszynski et al. 1989; Bruls et al. 2000; Pawlikowski et al. 2002).

NATURAL SUPPLEMENTS TO TREAT ADRENAL FATIGUE

After an evaluation by a physician, if stress is determined to be the cause of adrenal fatigue, the first goal is to relieve the stressful situations as much as possible. Consider lifestyle changes, including diet modification and exercise. Limit the consumption of processed foods, and avoid alcohol and tobacco use because these substances put extra stress on the adrenal glands. Many supplements recommended for either Addison's disease or Cushing's syndrome may also be taken for general adrenal fatigue because they can help to support healthy adrenal function, reduce stress, and blunt the release of excess cortisol during stress. Consider the following:

Vitamin C, 3000 mg a day

DHEA, 50 mg a day

L-theanine, 100–400 mg a day

Pantothenic acid (vitamin B$_5$), 1500 mg a day

Melatonin, 300 mcg–6 mg (at bedtime)

Phosphatidylserine capsules, 300 mg a day

Licorice (*Glycyrrhiza glabra*), no more than 1000 mg of glycyrrhizin

DIET AND ADDISON'S DISEASE

A possible link between gluten sensitivity (celiac disease) and Addison's disease has been proposed. An article in the *Journal of Endocrinological Investigation* described a patient with celiac disease and multiple endocrine disorders, including autoimmune Addison's disease and hypothyroidism (Valentino et al. 1999). Over a 3-month period, on a gluten-free diet, the patient showed a marked clinical improvement accompanied by a progressive decrease in the need for thyroid and adrenal replacement therapies. After 6 months, the serum IgA anti-endomysium antibody test (used to confirm celiac disease) became negative. After 12 months, a new jejunal biopsy showed complete mucosal recovery. (The jejunum is the middle third of the small intestine.) After 18 months on a gluten-free diet, the antithyroid antibodies titer decreased significantly, and thyroid substitutive therapy was discontinued. The authors proposed a link between autoimmune endocrine disease and celiac disease, noting that celiac disease is one of the causes for the failure of substitute hormonal therapy in patients with autoimmune thyroid disease (Valentino et al. 1999).

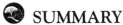 ## SUMMARY

According to the National Adrenal Diseases Foundation (Great Neck, NY), individuals who have Addison's disease as well as other diseases of the adrenal glands are often misdiagnosed or go for long, distressful periods without a correct diagnosis.

Symptoms of adrenal diseases often mirror those of chronic fatigue syndrome, including steadily worsening exhaustion, a loss of appetite, and weight loss. In Addison's disease, blood pressure is low and becomes even lower when the person stands, producing lightheadedness. Because of salt loss, a craving for salty foods is common. Darkened skin may appear as an inappropriate tan on a person who is ill (NADF 1998).

Cushing's disease is the symmetrical overproduction of cortisol by the adrenal glands. Cushing's syndrome is a constellation of signs and symptoms due to chronic overexposure to adrenal corticosteroids. Symptoms may include central obesity, wasting of the arms and legs (thin extremities), a reddish moon face, buffalo hump, a protuberant abdomen, and pigmented stretch marks (striae). Many people experience severe fatigue, weak muscles, high blood pressure, and high blood sugar. Irritability, anxiety, and depression are also common.

Adrenal fatigue can be caused by constant stress or poor nutrition, which can deplete and weaken the adrenal glands. There are many symptoms associated with this disorder, mostly fatigue and weakness. In some fatigued patients, thyroid problems overlap or are concomitant with adrenal problems.

- If you suspect that you have some form of adrenal disease, seek professional medical treatment from a physician.
- Identify and relieve sources of stress. Consider meditation or other stress-relieving exercises.
- Consider lifestyle changes such as diet and exercise.
- Obtain baseline corticosteroid, DHEA, and pregnenolone levels.
- Avoid smoking. Nicotine in tobacco initially raises cortisol levels, but chronic use results in low DHEA, testosterone, and progesterone levels.
- Consider laboratory testing for celiac disease (gluten sensitivity) and starting a gluten-free diet.
- If available, consider physician-administered injections of ACE (adrenal cortical extract) from a reliable source for 3–7 days.
- Hydrocortisone tablets (one of several forms available by prescription) may be taken up to 4 times daily for 3–7 days to treat Addison's disease (adrenal insufficiency). Physician supervision is mandatory.

The following natural supplements are recommended for Addison's disease:

1. DHEA, 50 mg daily and/or pregnenolone 50 mg daily, based on appropriate laboratory tests (*see the DHEA Replacement Therapy protocol for more information and precautions*).
2. Licorice tea or capsules to provide glycyrrhizin, no more than 1000 mg of glycyrrhizin should be taken in a given day and physician supervision is advised to guard against blood pressure increase and water retention.
3. Pantothenic acid (vitamin B$_5$), 1500 mg daily.
4. Vitamin C, 1000–3000 mg daily, in divided doses.
5. *L*-theanine may be taken to help modulate mood and relieve stress, one 100-mg capsule up to 4 times a day.
6. Phosphatidylserine, 100–300 mg daily.

The following natural supplements are recommended for Cushing's syndrome:

1. DHEA, 50 mg daily, or pregnenolone, 50 mg daily, based on appropriate laboratory tests (*see the DHEA Replacement Therapy protocol for more information and precautions*).
2. Vitamin C, 4000 mg daily, in divided doses.
3. One enterically coated aspirin tablet (325 mg). (Enteric coatings prevent the tablet from dissolving in the stomach.)
4. Phosphatidylserine, 300 mg daily.
5. Melatonin, 300 mcg–6 mg nightly.

Physician supervision is essential. To guard against underlying micronutrient deficiencies that could contribute to adrenal disease, take a high-potency multinutrient supplement such as Life Extension Mix (3 tablets 3 times a day).

 FOR MORE INFORMATION

Contact the American College for the Advancement of Medicine, (800) 532-3688, for a physician in your area who practices complementary medicine.

Contact the National Adrenal Diseases Foundation for support, information, and education for individuals who have Addison's disease as well as other diseases of the adrenal glands, (516) 487-4992.

 PRODUCT AVAILABILITY

DHEA and pregnenolone capsules, licorice capsules, pantothenic acid (vitamin B$_5$), vitamin C powder and capsules, phosphatidylserine (PS) capsules, melatonin, and *L*-theanine can be ordered by telephoning (800) 544-4440 or by ordering online at www.lef.org. ACE is not approved by the FDA for conventional use at this time.

Age-Associated Mental Impairment

An aging person often experiences a progressive decline in cognitive function. This typically begins with short-term memory loss and the inability to learn new information. Simple memory deficits, if not addressed, can worsen over time.

Numerous published studies indicate that brain aging can be controlled, at least in part. Some of these research findings demonstrate a *preventive* effect, whereas others show a benefit in *reversing* the neurological impairment caused by normal aging or by an age-related condition such as having had a stroke.

Conventional medicine has little to offer for people who notice a small decline in their memory or mental abilities. Often these changes are attributed to being a natural or inevitable part of growing old. Alternative physicians advocate that people should take responsibility for their own intellectual health as soon as possible, certainly before minor symptoms progress to a pathological illness.

This protocol has been designed specifically for persons who are experiencing age-associated mental impairment due either to aging itself or to an age-related disease. Fortunately, there are easy-to-follow lifestyle changes that can significantly help. Younger people, or parents who are concerned about possible cognitive deficits in their children, should consult the *Attention-Deficit Disorder protocol*.

WHAT CAUSES THE BRAIN TO AGE PREMATURELY?

Cognitive impairment has a variety of forms, including short-term memory loss, senility, and dementia. Dementia is a general term for diseases involving nerve cell deterioration. It is defined as a loss in at least two areas of complex behavior such as language, memory, visual and spatial abilities, and judgment that are severe enough to interfere with a person's daily living. Dementia, the most serious form of age-associated mental impairment, is often a slow, gradual process that may take months or even years to become noticeable. Symptoms vary depending on which areas of the brain are affected.

It is important to make a distinction between normal, age-associated mental impairment and conditions such as dementia that signal a *disease process*. Not all memory difficulties or cognitive complaints indicate the presence of Alzheimer's disease or other mental disorders. Many memory changes are temporary and are linked to environmental factors such as stress rather than to physiological (bodily) processes.

Neurological diseases such as dementia manifest most commonly in the elderly. The good news is that many of the underlying reasons for why people experience memory loss and other neurological disturbances are correctable. Any one or a combination of the following factors can cause age-associated cognitive dysfunction:

- The damaging effects of chronic inflammation causing injury to both cerebral blood vessels and neurons (brain cells).
- Changes in lifestyle and diet leading to nutrient deficiencies (e.g., many older people become deficient in critical nutrients).
- Hormonal imbalances and decreased levels of key hormones, especially DHEA, estrogen, testosterone, etc.
- Decreases in oxygen available to brain cells because of impaired circulation due to pathology (e.g., atherosclerosis or heart disease) or a lifetime of poor health habits (e.g., smoking, drinking, bad diet, or stress).
- Declining energy output of brain cells.
- Essential fatty acid deficiencies (the brain is composed almost entirely of fatty acids).
- The damaging effects of chronic free radical exposure.
- Adverse side effects from prescription medications.
- Elevated levels of MAO (monoamine oxidase).
- Reduced levels of neurotransmitters such as acetylcholine.

TAKE STEPS TO PRESERVE YOUR MENTAL FUNCTION

You do not have to remain helpless while your mental acuity deteriorates. Even taking relatively simple steps can help protect your brain cells from the negative effects of aging. If you already have a significant decline in cognitive function, there are still ways that may partially reverse these effects.

For instance, a study in the *Proceedings of the National Academy of Sciences* evaluated the effects of supplemental acetyl-L-carnitine and lipoic acid on the brains of old rats (Liu et al. 2002). Supplementation with acetyl-L-carnitine and lipoic acid resulted in improved memory. Electron microscopic studies in the hippocampus region of the brain showed that acetyl-L-carnitine and lipoic acid reversed age-associated mitochondrial structural decay. The conclusion of the scientists who conducted this study was that "these results suggest that feeding acetyl-L-carnitine and lipoic acid to old rats improves performance on memory tasks by lowering oxidative damage and improving mitochondrial function."

This study, published in one of the world's most respected scientific journals, confirms that age-associated cognitive impairment and mitochondrial structural dysfunction can be reversed. Acetyl-L-carnitine and lipoic acid are sold as expensive drugs in Europe, but are available as dietary supplements in the United States at a relatively low cost.

Protect Against Short-Term Memory Loss

The most commonly used memory-enhancing nutrients are precursors to the neurotransmitter "acetylcholine." Short-term memory function depends on acetylcholine acting as a signal to transmit messages between brain cells. Common acetylcholine precursors are various forms of choline and lecithin. Because acetylcholine helps brain cells to communicate with each other, it plays an important role in learning and memory.

An extensive review concerning the multiple effects of glyceryl-phosphorylcholine (GPC) appeared in the journal *Mechanisms of Ageing and Development* (Parnetti et al. 2001). The analysis covered 13 published clinical trials, which examined 4054 patients with various forms of brain disorders, including adult-onset cognitive dysfunction; Alzheimer's disease; stroke; and transient ischemic attack (TIA). Overall, the consistent finding was that "administration of GPC significantly improved patient clinical condition."

According to Parnetti et al. (2001), the effects of glyceryl-phosphorylcholine (GPC) were superior to the results observed in the placebo groups, especially with regard to cognitive disorders related to memory loss and attention deficit. They noted that the therapeutic benefits of GPC were superior to those of acetylcholine precursors used in the past, such as choline and lecithin. However, what most impressed the researchers were data indicating that GPC helps facilitate the functional recovery of patients who have experienced a stroke.

Brain aging is partially characterized by neurotransmitter deficiency, along with a structural deterioration of neurons and their connective transmission lines (axons and dendrites). Because research indicates that GPC may be of benefit in helping to prevent these pathological events, it may thus be possible to protect against underlying causes of brain aging while partially restoring cognitive function. Although sold as a prescription drug in European countries, GPC is available in the United States as a dietary supplement. Typical daily doses of GPC range from 600–1200 mg.

Brain Cell Energy Boosters

The brain requires a high level of energy to perform a myriad of functions. An effective memory-enhancing technique involves boosting the energy output of brain cells. In the aging process of the brain, there is a decline in the ability of neurons to take up glucose (primary fuel for the brain) and to produce energy. This decline in energy production not only causes memory and cognitive deficits, but also results in the accumulation of cellular debris, which eventually destroys brain cells. Senility is often diagnosed as a result of brain cell death that has been caused by accumulated cellular debris.

About 95% of cellular energy production occurs in the mitochondria, the cell's energy powerhouses. Many diseases of aging are increasingly being referred to as "mitochondrial disorders." Brain cells require a high level of energy metabolism to properly function. Acetyl-L-carnitine is a biologically active amino acid involved in the transport of fatty acids into the cell's mitochondria for the purpose of producing energy. Studies indicate that acetyl-L-carnitine can slow neurological aging. As discussed earlier in this protocol, supplemental acetyl-L-carnitine and lipoic acid have been shown to reverse certain parameters of brain aging in rats.

One of the most potent mitochondrial energizers is coenzyme Q_{10} (CoQ_{10}). When CoQ_{10} is orally administered, it is incorporated into the mitochondria of cells throughout the body where it facilitates and regulates the oxidation of fats and sugars into energy. Scientists have researched the effects of CoQ_{10}, discovering exciting findings. The following are highlights from a study in the *Proceedings of the National Academy of Sciences* (Matthews et al. 1998):

- When CoQ_{10} was administered to middle-aged and old rats, the level of CoQ_{10} increased by 10–40% in the cerebral cortex region of the brain. This increase was sufficient to restore the levels of CoQ_{10} to those seen in young animals.

- After only 2 months of CoQ_{10} supplementation, mitochondrial energy expenditure in the brain increased by 29% compared to the group that did not receive CoQ_{10}. The human equivalent dose of

CoQ_{10} to achieve these results was 100–200 mg daily.

- When a neurotoxin was administered, CoQ_{10} helped protect the striatal region of the brain where dopamine is produced against damage.

- When CoQ_{10} was administered to rats genetically bred to develop ALS (amyotrophic lateral sclerosis, or Lou Gehrig's disease), a significant increase in survival time was observed.

The conclusion by the scientists was that "CoQ10 can exert neuroprotective effects that might be useful in the treatment of neurodegenerative diseases."

This National Academy of Sciences study demonstrated that short-term supplementation with moderate amounts of CoQ_{10} produced profound anti-aging effects in the brain. Previous studies have shown that CoQ_{10} may protect the brain via several mechanisms, including reduction in free radical generation and protection from glutamate-induced excitotoxicity. The study documented that orally supplemented CoQ_{10} specifically enhanced metabolic energy levels of brain cells (Matthews et al. 1998).

Based on the types of brain cell injury that CoQ_{10} can provide protection from, the scientists suggested that CoQ_{10} might also be useful in the prevention or treatment of Huntington's disease and ALS. It was noted that, while vitamin E delays the onset of ALS in mice, it does not increase survival time. CoQ_{10} was suggested as a more effective treatment strategy for neurodegenerative disease than vitamin E because survival time was increased in mice treated with CoQ_{10} (Matthews et al. 1998).

CoQ_{10} might also be effective in the prevention and treatment of Parkinson's disease. One study reported that the brain cells of Parkinson's patients have a specific impairment that causes the disruption of healthy mitochondrial function. It is known that a "mitochondrial disorder" causes cells in the substantia nigra region of the brain to malfunction and die, thus creating a shortage of dopamine (Shults et al. 1997).

Another interesting finding was that CoQ_{10} levels in Parkinson's patients were 35% lower than age-matched controls. This deficit of CoQ_{10} caused a significant reduction in the activity of enzyme complexes that are critical to the mitochondrial function of brain cells affected by Parkinson's disease. An impressive study showed that high-dose CoQ_{10} supplementation slows the progression of Parkinson's disease by 44% (Shults et al. 2002).

The ramifications of these studies are significant. Parkinson's disease is becoming more prevalent as the human lifespan lengthens. The study by Shults et al. (2002) confirms the results of previous studies that Parkinson's disease may be related to CoQ_{10} deficiency. The conclusion of the scientists was that "the causes of Parkinson's disease are unknown. Evidence suggests that mitochondrial dysfunction and oxygen free radicals may be involved in its pathogenesis. The dual function of CoQ_{10} as a constituent of the mitochondrial electron transport chain and a potent antioxidant suggest that it has the potential to slow the progression of Parkinson's disease" (Shults et al. 2002). (See the *Parkinson's Disease protocol* for more information about this study.)

Levels of CoQ_{10} decrease with aging. This depletion is caused by *reduced synthesis* of CoQ_{10} in the human body along with *increased oxidation* of CoQ_{10} in the mitochondria. Therefore, a CoQ_{10} deficit results in the inactivation of enzymes needed for mitochondrial energy production, whereas supplementation with CoQ_{10} preserves mitochondrial function. Compared to the levels of CoQ_{10} present in young human adults, CoQ_{10} levels in older individuals are at only 50% of that of young adults, thus making CoQ_{10} an important nutrient supplement for aging persons.

The Brain Needs Essential Fatty Acids

The basic building blocks of our brain cells are essential fatty acids such as EPA and DHA from fish oil. These fatty acids are also used as fuel for brain metabolism and help control the chronic inflammatory processes involved in degenerative brain disorders.

When it comes to providing protection for the brain and encouraging overall brain health, DHA may be the more important fatty acid. Studies found that DHA supplementation significantly decreased the number of reference memory errors and working memory errors in aged male rats as well as in young rats (Gamoh et al. 1999, 2001).

Fish has long been referred to as "brain food," and scientific studies reveal that the oil of cold-water fish (high in omega-3 fatty acids such as DHA) functions via a variety of mechanisms to protect against common neurological impairments.

Hormone Deficiency Impairs Memory

The brain requires youthful levels of certain hormones to facilitate cell energy metabolism, maintain proper levels of acetylcholine, and protect brain cell membrane function. As a result, aging persons often require some hormone replacement to achieve the requisite levels.

DHEA (dehydroepiandrosterone) improves brain cell activity and enhances memory. The daily production of DHEA drops from 30 mg at age 20 to less than 6 mg at age 80. DHEA is naturally synthesized in abundance in young people from pregnenolone in the brain and the adrenal glands.

Current findings suggest that DHEA enhances memory by facilitating the induction of neural plasticity, a condition that permits the neurons (nerve cells of the brain) to change in order to record new memories. Studies have shown that DHEA not only improves memory deficits, but also relieves depression in older people and increases their perceived physical and psychological well-being. DHEA has been shown to help preserve youthful neurological function. DHEA also helps to maintain the ability of brain cells to store and retrieve information involved in short-term memory. (**Note:** Some persons should not take supplemental DHEA. For complete information about DHEA, refer to the DHEA Replacement Therapy and Precautions protocol.)

A thyroid hormone deficiency can also cause neurological disturbances that physicians often attribute to other health problems. Some symptoms caused by low thyroid hormone are poor concentration, memory disturbances, and depression. Many cases of thyroid deficiency are not diagnosed because of faulty laboratory blood reference ranges. For updated information about how to determine if you are thyroid hormone deficient, see the Thyroid Deficiency protocol elsewhere in this volume.

Female Hormones

An article in the journal Obstetrics and Gynecology evaluated 71 postmenopausal women relative to memory function: 28 were taking estrogen hormone replacement therapy. In those taking estrogen, there was significantly better verbal memory function (paragraph recall) than in those who were not (Kampen et al. 1994).

Another article in the journal Brain Research described an experiment using mice with surgically removed ovaries. The administration of both 17-beta-estradiol and estrone improved retention in a test of foot-shock avoidance in a T-maze. The authors concluded that these findings support the concept that estrogen improves memory by potentiating the activity of the cholinergic and glutamatergic systems (Farr et al. 2000).

The benefits of estrogen to the brain have long been known. However, the increased risk of breast cancer, heart attack, and other diseases associated with using estrogen drugs is motivating some women to change to DHEA (which converts to estrogen in the body) and, when necessary, to safer forms of estrogen such as estriol. For information about the optimal modulation of estrogen levels in aging women, refer to the Female Hormone Replacement Therapy protocol in this book.

Male Hormones

As men age, their levels of testosterone diminish significantly. Low levels of testosterone in men may contribute to memory impairment and increase vulnerability of the brain to Alzheimer's and related disorders.

One protective mechanism provided by testosterone is against Alzheimer's disease: brain cells are protected from a toxic peptide called beta-amyloid, which can accumulate in certain regions of an aging brain. Beta-amyloid has been implicated in the development of Alzheimer's disease. An article in Brain Research describes a study in which cultured neurons were exposed to beta-amyloid in the presence of testosterone. The resulting toxicity from beta-amyloid was significantly reduced by testosterone (Pike 2001).

Other researchers have discovered that testosterone decreases the secretion of harmful beta-amyloid and increases the secretion protective cell substances, indicating that testosterone supplementation in elderly men may be beneficial in the treatment of Alzheimer's (Godenough et al. 2000; Gouras et al. 2000).

Researchers in Oxford (England) found that lower levels of testosterone were present in men with Alzheimer's disease as opposed to controls (Hogervorst et al. 2001). The authors recommended further studies to determine whether low levels of total testosterone precede or follow the onset of Alzheimer's disease.

A consistent finding in the scientific literature is that testosterone replacement therapy produces an increased feeling of well-being. Low testosterone correlates with symptoms of depression and other psychological disorders (Moger 1980; Barrett-Connor et al. 1999; Rabkin et al. 1999; Schweiger et al. 1999; Seidman et al. 1999). Physicians can prescribe natural testosterone replacement therapies. A 12-month clinical trial using an FDA-approved natural testosterone drug (patch) resulted in a statistically significant reduction in the depression score (6.9 versus 3.9). Also noted were highly significant decreases in fatigue: from 79% before the patch to only 10% after 12 months (Androderm Testosterone Transdermal System 1997).

An article by Cherrier et al. (2001) described a randomized, double-blind, placebo-controlled study of 25 healthy volunteers aged 50–80 years. Participants received weekly intramuscular injections of either 100 mg testosterone enanthate or placebo (saline) for 6 weeks. Circulating total testosterone rose an average of 130% from baseline at week 3 and 116% at week 6 in the treatment group. Estradiol increased an average of 77% at week 3 and 73% at week 6 in the treatment group. The treatment group had significant improvements in cognition for spatial memory (recall of a walking route); spatial ability (block construction); and verbal memory (recall of a short story) compared with baseline and the placebo group. The results suggest that short-term testosterone administration enhances cognitive function in healthy older men (Cherrier et al. 2001).

However, it should be noted that sharp increases in estradiol are not good for men. What happens is that in response to the testosterone increase, the body converts (aromatizes) excess testosterone into estradiol (an estrogen). When a blood test reveals excess estradiol, the use of an aromatase-inhibiting drug such as Arimidex can block the rise in estradiol and thus enable the dose of testosterone to be reduced. Life Extension does not recommend testosterone injections. Natural testosterone patches, gels, or creams provide a consistent supply of testosterone through the skin and avoid the "spike" associated with testosterone injections. (For a complete explanation, refer to the *Male Hormone Modulation protocol*.)

According to Jonathan Wright, M.D. (co-author of *Maximize Your Vitality & Potency*), these effects have been reported in response to low testosterone levels (Wright et al. 1999):

- Loss of ability to concentrate
- Moodiness and emotionality
- Reduced intellectual agility
- Feeling weak
- Passive attitudes
- Reduced interest in surroundings

Testosterone replacement therapy in the aging male can provide considerable health benefits, but it is *critical* that proper blood tests are performed to guard against prostate cancer and estrogen overload. This requires the involvement of a knowledgeable physician. To obtain information about locating an enlightened physician in your area, log on to www.lef.org. Also refer to the *Male Hormone Modulation Therapy protocol* for an in-depth discussion.

Melatonin

Melatonin, a naturally occurring hormone produced in the brain's pineal gland, also enhances cognitive function. Melatonin is one of the body's most potent natural *antioxidants*, making it ideal to prevent age-related dementias such as Alzheimer's disease that are thought to be caused, or at least exacerbated, by a lifetime of free-radical damage.

Melatonin supplements easily enter the brain from the bloodstream. Melatonin is the primary regulator of brain cell synchronization (the body's internal clock) and is being researched as a possible treatment for various psychological conditions. Abnormally low levels of melatonin have also been discovered in patients who experience certain types of depression.

The suggested level of melatonin supplementation for enhancing neurological function in those over age 35 is 300 mcg to 3 mg a night, taken a half hour before going to bed (melatonin has a sedative effect). Those over age 50 can take up to 6 mg before bedtime.

The Brain Needs Vitamins

Vitamins can protect and enhance cognitive function. In particular, the B vitamins play an integral role in the functioning of the nervous system and help the brain synthesize chemicals that affect moods. A balanced complex of the B vitamins is essential for energy and for balancing hormone levels.

One study determined that low folate levels (a B vitamin) are not only associated with cognitive deficits, but that patients treated with folic acid for 60 days showed a significant improvement in both memory and attention efficiency (Fioravanti et al. 1997).

In a 6-year study to determine the relationship between nutritional status and cognitive performance in 137 elderly people, several significant associations were observed between cognition and vitamin status. Higher present and past intake of vitamins A, C, E, and B complex were significantly related to better performance on abstraction and visio-spatial tests (La Rue et al. 1997).

In addition to a direct effect, vitamins indirectly impact mental function by altering the levels of harmful or beneficial substances in the body. For instance, elevated homocysteine levels have been linked to heart disease and poorer cognitive function. Studies show that vitamin B_6 and folate taken at higher than recommended dosages reduced blood levels of homocysteine.

One study revealed that less-than-optimal levels of vitamin B_6, B_{12}, and folic acid lead to a deficiency of S-adenosylmethionine (SAMe). SAMe deficiency can cause depression, dementia, or demyelinating myelopathy (a degeneration of the nerves) (Abou-Saleh et al. 1986).

A typical American diet does not always provide enough essential vitamins. Because vitamin C and the B complex are water soluble and are rapidly excreted from the body, they must be replenished daily. Older persons are at greater risk for vitamin deficiency because they tend to not eat a variety of foods, although their requirements for certain vitamins such as B_6 are actually higher. Older persons may also have problems with efficient absorption of nutrients from food. Often even healthy older persons exhibit deficiencies in vitamin B_6, vitamin B_{12}, and folate, as well as zinc.

An article in the journal Psychopharmacology described a study of 76 elderly males who were given vitamin B_6 versus placebo in relation to memory function. The authors concluded that vitamin B_6 improves the storage and retrieval of information in the elderly patient (Deijen et al 1992).

Another article that appeared in the Annals of Internal Medicine reviewed vitamin B_{12} deficiency in the elderly population relative to memory impairment and neuropathy. The authors concluded that both memory problems and neuropathy have been treated successfully with vitamin B_{12} injections or supplementation (Carmel 1996).

Additionally, an article in the New England Journal of Medicine reviewed subclinical vitamin B_{12} deficiency and the resulting neurological symptoms. The author stated that many common difficulties, such as memory loss, muscle weakness, and parasthesias, might well be a product of vitamin B_{12} deficiency without accompanying macrocytosis or other clinical indicators (Lindenbaum et al. 1988).

Methylcobalamin is a coenzyme form of vitamin B that has been identified to protect against neurological disease associated with aging. The sublingual form of methylcobalamin is better absorbed because it does not become bound to food. Because most sources of B_{12} are from protein (meat products), vegetarian diets may be lacking in this vitamin.

Suppressing Free Radicals

Free radicals are atoms with unpaired electrons that can cause damage to cells by a process known as *oxidation*. Brain cells are particularly vulnerable to the effects of oxidation because of their high-energy production. The more energy a cell produces, the greater the number of damaging free radicals. The destructive effects of excess free radical activity have been implicated in many disease processes, including Alzheimer's disease and Parkinson's disease. Antioxidants neutralize free radicals and help prevent some of the damage associated with normal brain aging.

A study in the Journal of the American Geriatric Society compared groups of older people over time and at a given time with regard to antioxidant intake and memory performance. The study found that free recall, recognition, and vocabulary were significantly related to vitamin C and beta-carotene levels. The levels of these antioxidants were found to be significant predictors of cognitive function even after adjusting for possible confounding variables (Perrig et al. 1997).

For protection from the many types of free radicals to which it is vulnerable, the brain needs a wide variety of antioxidants.

To Protect the Cerebral Blood Flow

Vinpocetine

It is well established that normal aging results in a reduction of blood flow to the brain and a decrease in the metabolic activity of brain cells. Fortunately, there are dietary supplements and drugs that specifically enhance circulation to the brain.

Vinpocetine, an extract from the periwinkle plant, was introduced 24 years ago in Europe for the treatment of cerebrovascular disorders and symptoms related to senility. Since then, throughout the world, vinpocetine has been increasingly used in the treatment of cognitive deficits that are related to normal aging.

The biological actions of vinpocetine initially demonstrated that vinpocetine enhanced circulation and oxygen utilization in the brain; increased tolerance of the brain toward diminished blood flow; and inhibited abnormal platelet aggregation that can interfere with circulation or cause a stroke. Vinpocetine also enhances cyclic guanosine monophosphate (GMP) levels in the vascular smooth muscle, leading to reduced resistance of cerebral vessels and increased cerebral blood flow.

The effect of vinpocetine on memory functions was studied in 50 patients with disturbances of cerebral circulation. Improvement of cerebral circulation was observed after vinpocetine was administered. Blood flow was increased most markedly in the gray matter of the brain. After 1 month of vinpocetine treatment, improvement of memorizing capacity evaluated by psychological tests was recorded. Longer-term use was associated with alleviation or complete disappearance of symptoms of neurological deficit. No side effects attributable to the drug were observed. The physicians stated that vinpocetine was indicated in the treatment of ischemic disorders of the cerebral circulation, particularly in chronic vascular insufficiency (Hadjiev 1976).

Other studies also demonstrate that vinpocetine functions via several mechanisms to protect against the effects of brain aging. In a study to ascertain how vinpocetine boosts cognition, scientists measured the electrical firing effects in the neurons of anesthetized rats. The administration of vinpocetine produced a significant increase in the firing rate of neurons. The scientists also noted that the dose of vinpocetine used to increase electrical firing corresponded to the dose range that produced memory-enhancing effects. These results provided direct electrophysiological evidence that vinpocetine increases the activity of ascending noradrenergic pathways and that this effect can be related to the cognitive-enhancing characteristics of the compound (Gaal et al. 1990).

Additionally, vinpocetine has been shown to protect against oxidative damage from beta-amyloid, which may make it clinically useful for Alzheimer's disease (Pereira et al. 2000). Another study suggests that the antioxidant effect of vinpocetine might contribute to the protective role exerted by the drug in reducing neuronal damage (Santos et al. 2000).

The molecular evidence indicates that the neuroprotective action of vinpocetine is related to the ability to maintain brain cell electrical conductivity and to protect against damage caused by excessive intracellular release of calcium and sodium (Bonoczk et al. 2000; Solntseva et al. 2001).

In a double-blind clinical trial, vinpocetine was shown to effect significant improvement in elderly patients with chronic cerebral dysfunction: 42 patients received 10 mg of vinpocetine, three times a day for 30 days, and then they received 5 mg of vinpocetine, three times a day for 60 days. Placebo tablets were given to another 42 patients for the 90-day trial period. Patients taking vinpocetine scored consistently better in all evaluations of the effectiveness of treatment, including measurements on the Clinical Global Impression (CGI) scale, the Sandoz Clinical Assessment–Geriatric (SCAG) scale, and the Mini-Mental Status Questionnaire (MMSQ). There were no serious side effects related to the treatment drug (Balestreri et al. 1987).

In another double-blind study, 22 elderly patients with central nervous system degenerative disorders were treated with vinpocetine or placebo (Manconi et al. 1986). The patients received 10 mg of vinpocetine,

three times a day for 30 days; then they received 5 mg, three times a day for 60 days. Another 18 elderly patients were given matching placebo tablets for the 90-day trial. Vinpocetine-treated patients scored consistently better in all evaluations of the effectiveness of treatment, including measurements on the CGI and SCAG scales and the MMSQ. According to CGI assessments, severity of illness decreased in 73% of the patients in the vinpocetine group at day 30 and in 77% of patients at day 90. Improvement was seen in 77% and 87% of the patients at days 30 and 90, respectively. Patients also showed statistically significant improvement for all SCAG items (except for one) at days 30 and 90. The physicians rated the improvement in 59% of the vinpocetine-treated patients as "good" to "excellent." There were no serious side effects associated with the treatment drug (Manconi et al. 1986).

Vinpocetine safety and efficacy were demonstrated in a study of infants who experienced severe brain damage caused by birth trauma. In the infants treated with vinpocetine, vinpocetine caused a significant reduction or disappearance of seizures. The vinpocetine group also showed a decrease of the phenomena of intracranial hypertension and normalization of psychomotor development (Dutov et al. 1991).

The damaging effects of glutamate-induced excitotoxicity have been well established. A vitamin B_{12} metabolite called methylcobalamin has been shown to specifically protect against this type of neuronal injury. Vinpocetine has been documented to partially protect against excitotoxicity induced by a wide range of glutamate-related neurotoxins (Miyamoto et al. 1989; Erdo et al. 1990).

Ginkgo biloba

As previously stated, an inevitable consequence of aging is a reduced flow of blood to the brain. Common causes are chronic inflammation, arteriosclerosis, and increased blood "stickiness." The results of cerebral vascular disease can range from mild cognitive impairment to ischemic stroke. The third leading cause of death in the United States is stroke. Unfortunately, the effects of ischemic stroke result in many otherwise healthy people becoming institutionalized.

Ginkgo biloba extract has demonstrated specific mechanisms of action that counteract age-related vascular disorders. Human clinical studies show that ginkgo helps to slow down or restore cognitive dysfunction in those who have vascular dementia or Alzheimer's disease.

The first large-scale United States clinical study on ginkgo appeared in the *Journal of the American Medical*

Association (JAMA) (Lebars et al. 1997). This study demonstrated that, compared to placebo, ginkgo helped prevent short-term memory loss in patients with early diagnosed Alzheimer's disease. The researchers concluded that ginkgo improved cognitive performance and social functioning in these patients.

Ginkgo is a popular prescription drug in Europe and a dietary supplement in the United States. Hundreds of scientific studies demonstrate ginkgo's favorable effects in the human body. However, the primary benefit of ginkgo may be to help prevent the consequences of premature brain aging.

The brain depends on a steady supply of oxygen and glucose for proper functioning. It uses 20% of all the oxygen taken in through the lungs. Without enough oxygen, brain cells are irreparably damaged.

In a critical review of 40 clinical studies using ginkgo extract for "cerebral insufficiency" or age-related dementia, virtually all trials reported positive results (Kleijnen et al. 1992). The methodological quality of the eight most well-designed studies were found to be comparable to a U.S. Food and Drug Administration (FDA)–approved pharmaceutical used for the same indication.

In most of the studies [reviewed by Kleijnen et al. (1992)], a daily dose of 120–160 mg of ginkgo extract was given over a period of 4–12 weeks. Compared to the placebo group, significant improvement was observed in typical symptoms such as memory difficulties, confusion, fatigue, anxiety, dizziness, tinnitus, and headaches in the ginkgo extract group.

No serious side effects were reported in any of the assessed 40 trials, and the nonserious side effects were no different from those reported in patients treated with placebo (Kleijnen et al. 1992). This satisfying fact was also confirmed by the conclusion of DeFeudis et al. (2000) (in a summary of the ginkgo literature) that there is generally very little risk associated with products containing a properly standardized ginkgo extract.

In European studies, progressive degenerative dementia such as Alzheimer's disease has been treated with ginkgo extract. The results of these European trials were so impressive that the German government approved ginkgo biloba extract for treatment of dementia.

Free radicals are considered to be the reason for the excessive lipid peroxidation and cell damage observed in Alzheimer's disease (Cecchi et al. 2002). The main effect of ginkgo extract in these conditions appears to be related to its potent antioxidant properties. In a JAMA report, the efficacy and safety of ginkgo extract was tested on patients with Alzheimer's disease and multi-infarct dementia

(vascular) (Lebars et al. 1997). This 52-week, randomized, double-blind, placebo-controlled, multicenter study included 202 patients with mild to moderately severe cognitive impairment. The daily dose given was 120 mg. Measures of outcome included the Alzheimer's Disease Assessment Scale-Cognitive subscale (ADAS-Cog), the Geriatric Evaluation by Relative's Rating Instrument (GERRI), and the Clinical Global Impression of Change (CGIC).

Whereas the ginkgo group maintained its cognitive baseline over the year-long study and improved slightly in social functioning, the placebo group worsened over time in both aspects. The conclusion was that ginkgo appeared to be capable of stabilizing and *in a substantial number of cases* improving the cognitive performance and the social functioning of demented patients. This corresponds to a delay of 6 months to a year in the progression of the disease. Regarding the safety of ginkgo, there were no significant differences compared with placebo in either the number of patients reporting side effects or in the severity of these effects.

In a German double-blind, placebo-controlled study, Maurer et al. (1997) provided further support. In this study, 20 outpatients aged 50–80 and experiencing mild to moderate dementia of Alzheimer's type were treated with a daily dose of 240 mg of ginkgo extract for 3 months. Attention and memory performance of the patients (measured by SKT test) showed significant improvement after 3 months of treatment. The extract was well-tolerated with no adverse effects.

Ginkgo biloba has consistently shown that it can help protect against a variety of insults associated with restricted blood supply to the brain (cerebral vascular insufficiency). Ginkgo's three major pharmacological features are improving blood supply by dilating and toning blood vessels; reducing blood-clotting through antagonism of platelet-aggregating factor (PAF); and preventing membrane damage by means of its antioxidant activities.

Can Ginkgo Boost Memory in Healthy People?

While ginkgo has shown significant benefit in persons who already have neurological disease, there is a debate about the acute memory-boosting ability of ginkgo in healthy people. In a study that was widely publicized in the media, a group of healthy adults was given 40 mg of ginkgo extract three times a day or a placebo for 6 weeks. The results showed no difference in memory scores, self-reported perception, or rating by spouses, friends, and relatives after 6 weeks. The implication from the study is that ginkgo provides *no* short-term benefits in people with healthy cognitive function (Solomon et al. 2002).

However, this report contradicted a similar study conducted on healthy people who received 180 mg a day of ginkgo for 6 weeks (Mix et al. 2002). Compared to placebo, this study showed that ginkgo improved one memory score and significantly improved self-perception of memory. In this positive study, those who received ginkgo rated their overall ability to remember as "improved" compared to those receiving the placebo. This correlates well with previous studies indicating a potential short-term benefit to ginkgo supplementation.

It is known that ginkgo has improved clinical conditions in those diagnosed with severe neurological disease. Based on its multiple mechanisms of action, ginkgo may reduce the risk of developing senile dementia both of vascular and Alzheimer's types. Therefore, the question raised by the one negative study is whether ginkgo can help improve memory in healthy people. Most research shows a benefit, but the most important effect of ginkgo for healthy aging people may be in *preserving* cognitive function.

It should be pointed out that there is scientific support for memory enhancement even in young healthy people. Following just a single dose of 600 mg of ginkgo extract, a significant memory improvement was demonstrated in a randomized, double-blind, crossover study using Sternberg's memory scanning test. The effect lasted for several hours (Subhan et al. 1984). In a later study on healthy volunteers, Rigney et al. (1999) investigated the effects of ginkgo extract on memory and psychomotor function. In this randomized, double-blind, and placebo-controlled crossover study, 31 volunteers aged 30–59 years were given multiple doses of 50 or 100 mg; a single dose of 120 or 300 mg; or placebo during the day of testing. A psychometric test battery was administered before the first dose and at frequent intervals during the day until 11 hours after the last dose.

The results show that the memory-enhancing effect of ginkgo in healthy volunteers was most evident with the 120-mg dose; more apparent in the oldest age group of 50–59 years; and more pronounced for short-term memory than for other aspects of cognitive functioning. This study is interesting in that it showed that a single daily dose of 120 mg was more effective than smaller multiple doses given throughout the day (Rigney et al. 1999). In the negative study, 40 mg of ginkgo was given three times a day. Taking a 120-mg ginkgo capsule once a day (rather than dividing it into smaller 40-mg doses) might have yielded short-term memory improvement in the *JAMA* study.

Hundreds of scientific studies have confirmed ginkgo's beneficial effects on the human body. Because of its multiple mechanisms of action, ginkgo provides enormous potential protection against our most feared diseases. Aging humans have much to gain from using ginkgo biloba extract in a dose of 120 mg once a day as a preventive measure to help maintain neurological and circulatory health.

Therefore, that one study failed to show improved memory in healthy people who received 40 mg of ginkgo (three times a day) for only 6 weeks is not relevant to those seeking long-term anti-aging effects. The authors of the negative study acknowledge that higher doses of ginkgo or longer periods of exposure might produce the desired effects (Solomon et al. 2002).

To Protect Brain Cell Membranes

Phosphatidylserine

Because the health of brain cell membranes is crucial to neurological function, one of the reasons for the early popularity of lecithin was that it provided a wide range of "phospholipids" that are essential to cell membrane structure and function. However, newer extracts from soy provide a more concentrated means of protecting brain cell membranes. One of these is *phosphatidylserine*, which plays an important role in maintaining the integrity of brain cell membranes. The breakdown of brain cell membranes prevents glucose and other essential nutrients from entering the cell. By protecting the integrity of cell membranes, phosphatidylserine facilitates the efficient transport of energy-producing nutrients into cells, enhancing brain cell energy metabolism.

Abnormalities in the composition of phosphatidylserine have been found in patients with Alzheimer's disease (Corrigan et al. 1998). European studies have also shown enhancement in cognitive function when phosphatidylserine is administered to those in various stages of dementia.

Although it has been approved as a drug to treat senility in Europe, phosphatidylserine is sold as a dietary supplement in the United States. The typical daily dose for a healthy person is 100 mg, whereas those with cognitive impairment sometimes take 300 mg a day.

INNOVATIVE DRUG STRATEGIES

Piracetam

Piracetam is considered to be the "father" of nootropic drugs (cognitive enhancers). Piracetam has been shown to improve a series of mental activities, especially higher cortical functions. It can improve intelligence, concentration, memory, and creativity. Piracetam is a cyclic derivative (2-oxo-pyrrolidine acetamide) of the amino acid GABA (gamma amino butyric acid). Although GABA is an inhibitory neurotransmitter, piracetam does not appear to act in the same way.

In studies from the 1970s to the 1990s, piracetam was shown to

- Enhance memory, particularly when used in combination with choline (Bartus et al. 1981; Pragina et al. 1990; Senin et al. 1991)

- Increase attention and cognition (Gallai et al. 1991)

- Improve spatial learning (Canonico et al. 1991)

- Improve the use of glucose by the brain (Heiss et al. 1988, 1991)

- Improve brain circulation (Zykov 1992)

- Reduce lipofuscin (age pigment) buildup in the brain (Paula-Barbosa et al. 1991)

- Act as an antioxidant (Qian et al. 1992)

In animal experiments and in single photon emission computed tomography (SPECT) studies of patients with acute ischemic stroke, piracetam improved micro-circulation and neuronal metabolism and enhanced transmitter functions (Orgogozo 1998).

Another study found that piracetam provides neurological and functional protection from deficits resulting from a moderate or severe stroke when administered within a few days. This study noted that piracetam is well-tolerated and is effective when taken orally and that other treatments have very limited efficacy (Hitzenberger et al. 1998; Noble et al. 1998; Orgogozo 1998).

Research has demonstrated that piracetam's effect on circulation in the brain translates into improvements in aphasia (inability to speak) and level of consciousness, as well as fewer deaths (Poeck 1998).

A daily dose of 4800 mg of piracetam proved to be very effective in a double-blind study of 60 patients with post-concussional syndrome of 2–12 months' duration. After 8 weeks of treatment, piracetam significantly reduced the occurrence and severity of vertigo, headache, tiredness, decreased alertness, increased sweating, and neurasthenic symptoms (Hakkarainen et al. 1978).

A study showed that after 2 months of oral treatment with piracetam (2.4 g daily) in elderly human volunteers, SPECT imaging of the brain indicated a regional improvement in cerebral blood flow, particularly in the cerebellum. However, no beneficial effects with this drug were spontaneously reported (Dormehl et al. 1999).

Unfortunately, in the United States, piracetam has not been approved by the FDA for any use, despite its long track record and extensive clinical use in Europe. Therefore, piracetam is not available in the United States. Piracetam may be ordered from offshore pharmacies. The recommended dose of piracetam is 2400–4800 mg daily.

Hydergine

Hydergine was discovered in the 1940s and later approved by the FDA to treat individuals over age 60 who manifested signs or symptoms of mental incapacity. Unfortunately, when one study showed that Hydergine was not effective in treating Alzheimer's disease, United States physicians virtually stopped prescribing Hydergine, even though the drug was never approved for the treatment of Alzheimer's disease.

Hydergine remains a popular supplement among health-conscious people seeking to slow age-related mental decline. Studies have revealed several mechanisms by which Hydergine protects against brain aging:

- Increases blood supply and oxygen to the brain (Emmenegger et al. 1968)

- Enhances metabolism in brain cells (Emmenegger et al. 1968)

- Protects the brain from damage during periods of decreased or insufficient oxygen supply (Boismare et al. 1978)

- Slows the deposit of age pigment (lipofuscin) in the brain (Amenta et al. 1988)

- Prevents free radical damage to brain cells (Cahn et al. 1983)

- Increases intelligence, memory, learning, and recall (Ditch et al. 1971)

- Enhances the use of glucose by brain cells (Nagasawa et al. 1990)

- Normalizes the brain levels of serotonin (Markstein 1985)

- Increases superoxide dismutase (SOD) and catalase in the brain while decreasing toxic levels of monoamine oxidase (MAO) (Sozmen et al. 1998)

An article by Cover et al. (1996) discussed specific antibodies that bind to brain cell membranes and then target the cell for destruction and removal by the immune system.

Younger brains have significantly lower levels of these destructive antibodies compared to older brains. Hydergine-treated mice showed a reduction in these destructive antibodies, suggesting that middle-aged people who take Hydergine could retard the development of senile dementia caused by programmed immune destruction. The animals receiving Hydergine in middle age maintained healthy brain cell metabolic activities compared to the control group who did not receive Hydergine.

The scientists concluded that Hydergine therapy begun in middle age could protect against the initiation of the cascade that leads to Alzheimer's disease. The scientists emphasized that once the Alzheimer's disease cascade begins, Hydergine would be of little value because the brain cells have already been marked and targeted for immune destruction (Cover et al. 1996).

An article by Rosen (1975) described a double-blind study that evaluated the effectiveness of Hydergine versus papaverine in the treatment of selected symptoms associated with mental aging. After 12 weeks of treatment, ratings of overall clinical condition and global change showed that the 26 patients given Hydergine improved more than twice as much as the 27 patients given papaverine (Rosen 1975).

The Life Extension Foundation has long advocated the use of Hydergine to prevent the degenerative changes that lead to brain cell aging and Alzheimer's disease. Hydergine appears frequently in the scientific literature as therapy for a wide range of diseases ranging from asthma to stroke. Hydergine may be the most underutilized drug in the United States because of the one study that showed its failure to treat advanced Alzheimer's disease.

For middle-aged persons who have a family history of Alzheimer's disease, a daily dose of 10–20 mg of Hydergine is suggested. For middle-aged persons seeking to slow their rate of brain cell aging, a daily dose of 5–10 mg of Hydergine is suggested.

In 5% of people, Hydergine may induce mild nausea. However, for the remaining 95% for whom Hydergine does not cause nausea, 5-mg Hydergine tablets may be obtained from European suppliers, making taking high doses convenient and very economical.

Deprenyl

Another cause of brain aging is the elevation of an enzyme in the brain called monoamine oxidase (MAO). Monoamine oxidase A and B are the primary enzymes that degrade neurotransmitters in the central nervous system and peripheral tissues. Elevated MAO levels damage brain cells and are a specific cause of age-related neuronal deterioration. Too much MAO has also been shown to cause pathological disorders such as Parkinson's disease (Orru et al. 1999; Abell et al. 2000).

Low-dose deprenyl (selegiline) is thought to protect the brain from aging by specifically inhibiting monoamine oxidase B (MAO B) in the brain. Deprenyl was approved for use in Parkinson's disease in the 1980s and was often combined with L-dopa (levodopa). However, one study raised concerns about combining high doses of deprenyl (10 mg per day) with L-dopa due to an apparent increase in mortality in the deprenyl group (Lees 1995). The results of that paper were hotly debated and several flaws were found in the study design. Later studies showed clinical benefit with deprenyl without a decrease in mortality and no toxic effects, particularly when lower doses were used (5 mg per day or every other day) (LeWitt 1991; Shoulson 1992, 1998).

Deprenyl has long been recommended in very low doses (10 mg a week) as part of an overall anti-aging program because it has been shown to extend lifespan in animal studies. Deprenyl has also been shown to stimulate the efflux of norepinephrine, dopamine, and serotonin *in vitro* by a direct action on the hypothalamus. Some researchers are proposing that deprenyl may be considered as an alternative to levodopa for starting treatment in Parkinson's disease patients (Caracenia et al. 2001; Mohan Kumar et al. 2001).

Deprenyl has also been shown to induce rapid increases in nitric oxide (NO) production in brain tissue and cerebral blood vessels and also to protect the vascular endothelium from the toxic effects of amyloid-beta peptide (Thomas 2000). Another study showed that deprenyl protected cells from apoptosis induced by a neurotoxin, N-methyl(R)-salsolinol, and reactive oxygen species, and peroxynitrite (Naoi et al. 2000). Additionally, Zhu et al. (2000) showed that deprenyl significantly improved the cognitive function of rats after traumatic brain injury.

A study of 17 patients with Alzheimer's disease found that the Mini-Mental State Examination scores were significantly higher in those patients receiving selegiline (deprenyl) than in those receiving placebo (Alafuzoff et al. 2000). In India, another study of 32 patients with Parkinson's disease found a significant improvement in memory in patients treated with 10 mg a day of deprenyl as compared to placebo (Dixit et al. 1999).

Scientists who conducted lifespan studies using deprenyl have estimated the ideal dose to slow brain aging in humans to be about 1.5 mg daily. Because deprenyl is usually sold in 5-mg tablets and has a long-acting effect on the brain, most Life Extension members take a low dose of 5 mg of deprenyl twice a week.

However, Hydergine seems to be *more* effective when higher doses are used. European physicians often prescribe 4.5–20 mg daily of Hydergine without concern for toxicity. Persons seeking protection from neurological aging and wanting to boost cognitive function have used high-dose Hydergine and low-dose deprenyl together for more than 16 years. No adverse effects have been reported when using these two medications together.

CAUTION Care should be taken when administering dopamine to patients who have been using deprenyl (selegiline). One journal article noted a drastic increase in systolic blood pressure after a critically ill man using selegiline was given an infusion of dopamine (Rose et al. 2000).

Nimodipine

Nimodipine is particularly recommended for victims of head trauma. Nimodipine (brand name Nimotop) is a calcium channel blocker somewhat selective to the central nervous system. It prevents movement of calcium into the cells of blood vessels, thereby relaxing the vessels and increasing the supply of blood and oxygen. It dramatically improves cerebral blood flow.

Nimodipine is an FDA-approved drug that is used to prevent and treat problems caused by a blood vessel around the brain that has burst. But nimodipine has been ignored by most neurologists treating victims of stroke and other age-related neurological diseases.

An article by Pantoni et al. (2000a) described a 26-week, multinational, double-blind, placebo-controlled study of nimodipine in patients with multi-infarct dementia. This study failed to show a significant effect of nimodipine on cognitive, social, or global assessments. However, a lower incidence of cerebrovascular and cardiac events was observed in the nimodipine-treated patients in comparison with the placebo group. A subgroup analysis found that those patients with subcortical vascular dementia performed better on the majority of neuropsychological tests and functional scales in comparison with patients on placebo (Pantoni et al. 2000b). A recommended dose of nimodipine is 30 mg, three times daily.

Centrophenoxine

Centrophenoxine (meclofenoxate) is widely used in Europe in combination with piracetam to improve memory and enhance mental energy. Although Centrophenoxine is readily available in Europe, it is not sold in the United States. Centrophenoxine can be ordered from pharmacies in Europe.

Researchers have proposed several mechanisms for Centrophenoxine, including:

- Increasing activity of free radical scavengers, especially in brain and heart tissues (al-Zuhair et al. 1998)

- Providing antioxidant action, possibly due to the DMAE (dimethyl-amino-ethanol) it contains (Zs-Nagy 1989)

- Increasing acetylcholinesterase activity in the hippocampus and brain (Sharma et al. 1995)

- Decreasing the deposition of the age-pigment lipofuscin, which has been shown to cause neuronal damage (Patro et al. 1992)

- Inhibiting total MAO (monoamine oxidase), MAO-A and MAO-B, which has been shown to damage brain cells (Stancheva et al. 1988)

- Increasing the content of serotonin (5-HT), a key neurotransmitter that can be damaged by elevated MAO (Stancheva et al. 1988)

- Significantly increasing the fluidity of brain membranes, which can reverse the dehydration of nerve cells of older animals (Lustyik et al. 1985; Wood et al. 1986)

Centrophenoxine was shown to improve memory retention in aged rats in tests using the maze method for active avoidance with punishment reinforcement and the step-through method for passive avoidance with negative reinforcement. Centrophenoxine increased the number of responses to conditioned stimulus and strongly prolonged the time spent in the light chamber (a measure of improved retention) (Mosharrof et al. 1987).

A double-blind clinical trial of 50 patients with dementia examined the effects of 2 grams a day of Centrophenoxine for 8 weeks: 48% of the Centrophenoxine group displayed improvements in the memory functions versus 28% of the placebo group (Pek et al. 1989). Another study found that Centrophenoxine corrected the blood pressure drop when standing in 25 patients who had orthostatic hypotension due to brainstem ischemia (Stoica et al. 1991).

The recommended dose of Centrophenoxine is 250–1000 mg daily.

Other Factors to Consider

Lifestyle

Taking steps to improve one's overall health is highly recommended to help prevent or minimize age-associated mental impairment. For example, exercising regularly; not smoking; and monitoring blood cholesterol levels can reduce the risk of stroke and heart disease and keep arteries open, supplying the brain with essential oxygen and nutrients. Regular exercise improves some mental abilities by an average of 20–30%. Abstaining from alcohol or drug use, or minimizing it, can also help preserve mental function. Because most persons tend to eat less food as they age, the use of low-fat, nutrient-rich food is recommended. This type of diet will help prevent nutrient deficiencies, which can impair mental function as a result of physical illnesses. Eating large quantities of high antioxidant-containing fruits, especially berries (blueberries), may significantly provide protection from senility and many other age-related conditions. Mental exercise is another crucial lifestyle component. Forcing the memorization of dates, lists, and telephone numbers can help keep your mind sharp as you age. Engaging in activities that challenge acuity can also provide an "exercise" effect for your brain.

Guarding Against Prescription Drug Side Effects

Adverse side effects can result from either too high or too low doses of medications; unusual reactions to medications; or combinations of medications. It is especially common in the older population for individuals to be taking many different medications prescribed by different doctors, in addition to over-the-counter supplements. Be certain that your primary physician is aware of *all* prescription and nonprescription medications that you take.

Be Certain that You Are Not Anemic

A large number of aging people are anemic. Their physicians often fail to treat this condition because anemia is so common. Anemia represents a deficiency in the oxygen-carrying capacity of the blood. Blood should be tested annually. If there is any indication of even borderline anemia, seek medical assistance. For complete information about anemia, refer to the *Anemia protocol* in this book (also see Life Extension website at www.lef.org).

Keep Blood Pressure in the Low Normal Range

A 30-year study of male twins showed that elevated blood pressure in mid-life predisposed men to accelerated brain aging and an increased risk of stroke later in life. Men with even mildly elevated blood pressure 25 years before showed smaller brain volumes and more strokes compared to their twin brothers who did not have the elevation in blood pressure. This study in the journal *Stroke* emphasized the importance of aggressively treating elevated blood pressure even when it is not grossly abnormal (DeCarli et al. 1999). Refer to the *Hypertension protocol* in this book for information about natural methods of controlling blood pressure.

● SUMMARY

The brain is the center of personal identity that makes us uniquely human. Decline in brain function is the greatest fear most persons have when thinking about aging.

Age-associated mental impairment can range in severity from forgetfulness to senility to dementia. Age-associated mental impairment can be caused by a wide variety of specific disease processes, many of which are treatable. It can also result from normal brain aging. Whatever its form or cause, age-associated cognitive impairment does not need to be accepted as an inevitable consequence of growing older.

Behavioral modification such as participating in increased physical and mental activity and following a healthy diet can improve mental function both directly and indirectly by enhancing overall health.

Age-associated mental impairment can be treated safely and effectively with memory-enhancing nutrients, hormones, and drugs. These therapies improve cerebral circulation; boost brain cell metabolism; stabilize brain cell membranes; increase acetylcholine; provide structural building blocks to neurons; synchronize brain cell interaction; restore youthful hormone balance; suppress free radicals; and reduce chronic inflammatory processes.

The benefit of taking several different types of agents that protect and enhance neurological function is that these same agents can also *prevent* age-associated diseases from manifesting in *other* parts of the body. Nutrients such as coenzyme Q_{10}, acetyl-*L*-carnitine, and ginkgo, along with hormones such as DHEA, melatonin, and testosterone, can provide dramatic systemic anti-aging effects. A massive body of published scientific research indicates that one can take steps to boost cognitive function today, while simultaneously reducing the risk of Alzheimer's disease, stroke, and other degenerative brain diseases.

There is currently much debate as to whether mild cognitive decline or memory problems are a risk factor for developing more serious neurological disease, such as dementia or Alzheimer's disease. Some studies indicate that a significant percentage of elderly people complaining of mild cognitive impairment will go on to develop Alzheimer's disease. Clinical studies have been conducted in elderly people to see if the decline in cognitive function can be slowed and Alzheimer's disease can be postponed or prevented (Hanninen et al 1997; Richards et al. 1999; Grober et al. 2000; Collie et al. 2001; Goldman et al. 2001a; Goldstein et al. 2001; Petersen et al. 2001).

Perhaps the most important research paper published on age-associated memory impairment stated that memory decline is not a normal feature of aging. What the researchers found was that in persons with mild memory impairment, memory loss tended to progress, whereas persons who were healthy did not experience memory impairment as they aged (Goldman et al. 2001b).

If you have a neurological disorder such as cerebral vascular disease (stroke), Alzheimer's disease, Parkinson's disease, etc., refer to the in-depth protocols in this book that provide innovative treatment options that are often overlooked by conventional physicians.

The following are dietary supplements available in the United States that may benefit persons who have age-associated mental impairment:

1. Cognitex is a multi-ingredient formula providing nutrients such as vinpocetine, phosphatidylserine, glyceryl phosphorylcholine (GPC), and others discussed in this protocol. Three to six capsules of Cognitex daily are suggested.

2. Essential fatty acids such as DHA, GLA, and EPA are found in Super GLA/DHA. The recommended dose is six softgels daily of Super GLA/DHA, providing 1000 mg of DHA and 900 mg of GLA, along with 200–400 mg of EPA.

3. Ginkgo biloba extract, 120 mg daily.

4. Acetyl-*L*-carnitine, 2000 mg daily.

5. Coenzyme Q_{10}, 100–300 mg daily.

6. Super Alpha Lipoic Acid, 250–500 mg daily.

7. Life Extension Mix provides broad-spectrum, high-potency antioxidants, vitamins, and minerals. A suggested dose is three tablets, three times a day.

8. DHEA, 25–50 mg daily. Refer to the *DHEA Replacement Therapy protocol* before initiating DHEA or pregnenolone replacement.

9. Melatonin, 300 mcg to 3 mg nightly, a half hour before bedtime.

10. Phosphatidylserine (PS), 100–300 mg daily.

11. Vitamin B_{12} (preferably in the form of methylcobalamin), 1–40 mg daily.

Drugs and hormones requiring a prescription or that may be obtained from offshore pharmacies are:

1. Testosterone replacement, often indicated in aging males. Refer to the *Male Hormone Modulation protocol* in this book for complete details.

2. Estrogen replacement, often indicated in aging females. Increased risk of certain cancers and cardiovascular disease are of concern. Refer to the *Female Hormone Replacement protocol* for alternatives to estrogen drugs.

3. One or a combination of the following drugs may be considered:

- Piracetam, 2400–4800 mg daily.
- Centrophenoxine, 250–1000 mg daily.
- Hydergine, 5–20 mg daily.
- Deprenyl, one 5-mg tablet, two times weekly.
- Nimotop (nimodipine), 30 mg, three times daily.

Chronic inflammation inflicts devastating effects, particularly as humans grow older. The pathological consequences of inflammation are fully documented in the medical literature. For example, in Alzheimer's disease, an inflammatory cascade is involved in many of the destructive processes observed in the neurons of patients, including the formation of toxic beta-amyloid. As this toxic inflammatory process continues, the loss of functioning neurons is accelerated, first resulting in mild cognitive impairment. Many scientists believe that unchecked inflammation is an underlying culprit in the development of Alzheimer's disease.

Because chronic inflammation is so injurious to brain cells, aggressive steps should be taken to suppress the inflammatory cascade. Some of the supplements recommended in this protocol, such as Super GLA/DHA, ginkgo, DHEA, and Life Extension Mix, can significantly reduce chronic inflammatory processes. For more information about drugs and additional therapies that are available to suppress dangerous inflammatory components in blood, please refer to the *Inflammation (Chronic) protocol* in this book.

As you have learned from this protocol, there are *multiple* diverse factors involved in the development of cognitive impairment and senility. Therefore, the emphasis should be on incorporating as many supplements, hormones, and drugs as are feasible to guard against the mechanisms involved in neuro-degeneration. For example, while supplements that increase acetylcholine (such as GPC) have become popular agents to improve short-term memory, they do not suppress a chronic inflammatory state nor do they appreciably boost brain cell energy metabolism.

Therefore, to optimally protect your brain from the numerous insults incurred as a result of normal aging and environmental toxins, a multimodal approach is needed that includes the proper dose of the nutrients, hormones, and drugs discussed in this protocol.

☏ FOR MORE INFORMATION

Contact the National Institute on Aging, (800) 222-2225; the Alzheimer's Association, (800) 272-3900; and the National Institute of Neurological Disorders and Stroke, (800) 352-9424.

PRODUCT AVAILABILITY

Cognitex, Super GLA/DHA, ginkgo biloba, vinpocetine, acetyl-*L*-carnitine, coenzyme Q_{10}, alpha lipoic acid, Life Extension Mix (containing essential vitamins and minerals), DHEA, melatonin, methylcobalamin (vitamin B12), and phosphatidylserine are available by telephoning (800) 544-4440 or by ordering online at www.lef.org. Piracetam, high-dose Hydergine, and Centrophenoxine are available from overseas companies. A list of these companies can be obtained by calling (800) 226-2370. Testosterone patches, gels, or creams; estrogen drugs; and Hydergine, deprenyl, and nimodipine are available in the United States only by prescription.

Alcohol-Induced Hangover: Prevention

If you are reading this book, you are probably interested in life extension and antiaging concepts. Aging makes us increasingly vulnerable to alcohol-induced hangover, liver injury, and damage to the central nervous system. Because alcohol consumption produces toxic compounds and causes vitamin deficiencies, in the best of all possible worlds it would be better not to drink alcohol at all. For those who still want to drink, it is possible to do so more safely. The first piece of advice would be to drink only moderately and follow the preventive measures outlined in this protocol.

WARNING What follows is for those who choose to drink moderately. This advice is not for those who suffer from alcoholism. Simply put, an alcoholic has "lost the power of choice in drink" and is "without defense against the first drink." In short, an alcoholic *cannot* drink safely. The Foundation is all too aware that an alcoholic may easily misinterpret the following information as a license to drink. It is not. It is only for those who drink by choice and do so in moderation.

The consumption of alcohol results in the formation of two very toxic compounds, acetaldehyde and malondialdehyde. These compounds generate massive free-radical damage to cells throughout the body. The free-radical damage generated by these alcohol metabolites creates an effect in the body similar to that caused by radiation poisoning. That is the reason why people feel so sick the day after consuming too much alcohol. If the proper combination of antioxidants is taken at the time the alcohol is consumed or before the inebriated individual goes to bed, the hangover and much of the cellular damage caused by alcohol may be prevented.

Aging makes us increasingly vulnerable to alcohol-induced hangover, liver injury, and damage to the central nervous system. In the elderly, alcohol- and drug-induced injury are more common and more serious, and recovery is more difficult.

PROTECTING AGAINST HANGOVER AND CELLULAR DAMAGE

Nutrients that neutralize alcohol byproducts and protect cells against the damaging effects of alcohol include vitamin C, vitamin B_1, the amino acids S-allyl-cysteine and glutathione, vitamin E, and selenium (Sprince et al. 1975; Hell et al. 1976; Loguercio et al. 1993; van Zandwijk 1995; Marotta et al. 2001). There are several commercial preparations that can be taken at the time the alcohol is consumed or before bedtime to help prevent a hangover. One of these is called *Anti-Alcohol Antioxidants*. The ingredients in this formula will help prevent hangover while providing protection against the damaging byproducts of alcohol metabolism.

A study in the journal *Alcohol* showed how antioxidants could protect against brain damage. The study concluded by stating:

> Chronic pretreatment with vitamin E prevents alcohol-induced vascular injury and pathology in the brain (Altura et al. 1999).

Another study in the journal *Artery* confirmed a specific toxic metabolite of alcohol (acetaldehyde) and identified an antidote (*N*-acetyl-cysteine) (Vasdev et al. 1995). Here is an excerpt:

> All known pathways of ethanol metabolism result in the production of acetaldehyde, a highly reactive compound. *N*-acetyl cysteine, an analogue of the dietary amino acid cysteine, binds acetaldehyde, thus preventing its damaging effect on physiological proteins.

These findings should not surprise anyone who understands that the ingestion of alcohol inflicts massive free-radical damage throughout the body. When a person is exposed to a known toxic substance (such as alcohol), it makes sense to take an antidote (antioxidants) to provide at least partial protection against the short-term (hangover) and long-term (degenerative disease) effects.

Kyolic Garlic Formula 105

Another product that persons who drink alcohol may use is Kyolic Garlic Formula 105. Garlic contains S-allyl-cysteine, a neutralizer of acetaldehyde; this particular Kyolic-brand formula also contains vitamins C and E, beta-carotene, and selenium. Because the heavy consumption of alcohol produces many dele-terious effects within the body, including an increased risk of cancer, liver disease, and neurological disease, it is suggested that hangover-prevention formulas such as Kyolic Garlic Formula 105 and/or Anti-Alcohol Antioxidants be taken any time alcohol is consumed.

S-Adenosylmethionine (SAMe)

Free-radical damage is a major mechanism by which ethanol damages the liver. As has already been discussed, supplementing with the right antioxidants while consuming ethanol significantly reduces damage to cells throughout the body, including damage to the liver. Ethanol also damages the liver by depressing an enzyme required to convert methionine into S-adenosylmethionine (SAMe) (Mato et al. 1994). A deficiency of SAMe can predispose an alcoholic to develop liver cirrhosis. Alcohol-induced depletion of SAMe can be overcome by SAMe supplementation which restores hepatic SAMe levels and significantly reduces ethanol-induced liver injury (Lieber 1997; 2000a; 2000b; 2000c).

Supplementation with 400–800 mg of SAMe twice a day will help to protect the liver from damaging oxidation that may lead to further degenerative disease. For those who cannot afford SAMe, supplementation with 500 mg of trimethylglycine (TMG, also known as glycine betaine), 800 micrograms of folic acid, and 500 micrograms of vitamin B_{12}, taken twice a day, could help the liver to synthesize S-adenosylmethionine.

OTHER TREATMENTS

Probiotics

One of the reasons that 30% of alcoholics develop cirrhosis may be a leaky gastrointestinal system. According to research (Keshavarzian 1999), another factor might be a gut-derived endotoxin. This would suggest that the use of *probiotic substances* might aid in the prevention of cirrhosis or other liver damage. Probiotics are beneficial bacteria that help to recolonize the intestinal tract. Intestinal flora (bacteria) help our digestive system absorb nutrients and act as a protective barrier in keeping toxins out. Along with taking a probiotic formula, a supplement to nourish intestinal flora such as fructo-oligosaccharides (FOS) is recommended. FOS helps reduce the formation of toxic liver metabolites and therefore is beneficial to people with chronic liver problems.

Magnesium

Chronic alcohol consumption can constrict arteries in the brain and lead to neurological deficit (Thomson et al. 1988). Daily supplementation with 500–1500 mg of magnesium could help keep cerebral blood vessels open by blocking excess infiltration of calcium into endothelial cells.

Silibinin (Special Milk Thistle Extract)

Those who drink routinely might consider taking at least 500 mg a day of a special milk thistle extract called silibinin, which may have a protective effect on the liver (Flora et al. 1998). Silibinin is the most active constituent of silymarin. In Germany, silibinin is sold as a drug to treat liver diseases.

European Medications

European medications such as Picamilon (50 mg, three times a day) and Pyritinol (200 mg, three times a day) could help prevent and restore neurological function lost because of chronic ethanol intake. An expensive prescription drug called Nimotop (nimodipine), at the dose of 30 mg 3–4 times a day, can slowly repair central nervous system damage caused by excess alcohol intake.

PPC

Alcohol is most commonly associated with liver toxicity. The nutrients contained in Anti-Alcohol Antioxidants and other supplements discussed so far help to protect against hepatic injury. For those who consume large amounts of alcohol (i.e., binge drinkers), a supplement called polyenylphosphatidylcholine (PPC) is recommended prior to alcohol consumption. The administration of PPC has been shown to provide significant protection against certain forms of alcohol-induced liver injury in animals via several unique mechanisms (Aleynik et al. 1999; Lieber 1997, 2000a; 2000b; 2000c). PPC also reduces gastric irritation (Anand et al. 1999). PPC is the active ingredient in a product called HepatoPro. We suggest that four capsules of HepatoPro be taken prior to heavy alcohol consumption. For light alcohol consumption, two capsules of HepatoPro should be adequate. Each capsule of HepatoPro contains 900 mg of PPC.

THE ASTRONOMICAL COST OF HANGOVERS

A study in *Annals of Internal Medicine* compiled the enormous cost of lost productivity induced by hangovers (Wiese et al. 2000). Here is an excerpt from this study:

> The alcohol hangover is characterized by headache, tremulousness, nausea, diarrhea, and fatigue combined with decreased occupational, cognitive, or visual-spatial skill performance. In the United States, related absenteeism and poor job performance cost $148 billion annually (average annual cost per working adult, $2000). Although hangover is associated with alcoholism, most of its cost is incurred by the light-to-moderate drinker. Patients with hangover may pose substantial risk to themselves and others despite having a normal blood alcohol level. Hangover may also be an independent risk factor for cardiac death.

cognitively intact controls, subjects received either a tryptophan-free amino acid drink to induce acute tryptophan depletion, or a placebo drink containing a balanced mixture of amino acids. On each occasion, ratings of depressed mood were made at baseline and at 4 and 7 hours later, and the Modified Mini-Mental State was administered at baseline and 4 hours later. Patients with dementia of the Alzheimer type had a significantly lower mean score on the Modified Mini-Mental State after acute tryptophan depletion than after receiving placebo, while the comparison group showed no difference (Porter et al. 2000).

Adrenal Stress

The relationship between age-related memory loss and stress is central to the protocol used by Dharma Singh Khalsa. Excessive stress from a modern life causes the adrenal glands to secrete excessive amounts of cortisol, eventually leading to adrenal fatigue (Khalsa 1997).

DHEA

Alzheimer's disease patients with higher dehydroepiandrosterone (DHEA) levels did better on memory tests than those with lower DHEA levels (Carlson et al. 1999; Murialdo et al. 2000). Other data suggest that DHEA has a role in antioxidant status, Natural Killer (NK) cell immune function, and other immune functions. This study showed low DHEA was a risk factor for the development of Alzheimer's disease but did not show that replacing DHEA was of benefit. These studies still need to be done (Hillen et al. 2000).

A study of adrenal secretion in 23 healthy elderly subjects, 23 elderly demented patients and 10 healthy young subjects found a significant increase in cortisol levels during evening and nighttime in both groups of the aged subjects. In elderly subjects, particularly if demented, the mean serum dehydroepiandrosterone sulfate (DHEAs) levels throughout the 24-hour cycle were significantly lower than in young controls (Magri et al. 2000).

A cross-sectional study, called the Berlin Aging Study, found lower levels of DHEAs in cases that developed dementia of the Alzheimer type within 3 years as compared to matched controls (Hillen et al. 2000).

Inhibition of AGE Formation

Central to the process of forming advanced glycation end products (AGEs) is the presence of sugar (glucose) which is central to the diagnosis of both diabetes and insulin insensitivity (referred to as Syndrome X).

Appropriate lab tests would include the glucose tolerance test and insulin levels. Appropriate treatment is covered in the section on diabetes.

Vitamins B$_1$ and B$_6$

Derivatives of vitamins B$_1$ and B$_6$ (thiamine pyrophosphate and pyridoxamine) have been shown to decrease AGE formation (Booth et al. 1996; Booth et al. 1997).

Carnosine

Carnosine is a multifunctional dipeptide made from a combination of the amino acids beta-alanine and L-histidine. Meat is the main dietary source of carnosine. High doses of carnosine are necessary for therapeutic effect because the body naturally degrades carnosine with the enzyme carnosinase.

Copper and zinc are released during normal synaptic activity. However, in the presence of a mildly acidic environment which is a characteristic of Alzheimer's disease, they reduce to their ionic forms and become toxic to the nervous system. Research has shown that carnosine can buffer copper and zinc toxicity in the brain (Horning et al. 2000; Trombley et al. 2000).

Carnosine has also been shown, in vitro, to inhibit nonenzymic glycosylation and cross-linking of proteins induced by reactive aldehydes, including aldose and ketose sugars, certain triose glycolytic intermediates, and malondialdehyde (MDA, a lipid peroxidation product). Carnosine also inhibits formation of MDA-induced protein-associated advanced glycosylation end products (AGEs) and formation of DNA-protein cross-links induced by acetaldehyde and formaldehyde (Munch et al. 1997; Hipkiss 1998; Hipkiss et al. 1998; Preston et al. 1998).

Herbal Treatments

Huperzine A

Huperzine A is an alkaloid isolated from the Chinese herb *Huperzia serrata*. In experiments using rats, Huperzine A improved the decrease in acetylcholine activity in cortex and hippocampus (Cheng 1996; Tang 1996; Bai et al. 2000; Wang et al. 2000). A double-blind, multicenter study of Huperzine A was conducted in China. Fifty patients were given 0.2 mg Huperzine and 53 patients were given placebo for 8 weeks. About 58% (29/50) of patients treated with Huperzine showed improvements in their memory and cognitive and behavioral functions. The efficacy of Huperzine was better than placebo. No severe side effects were found (Xu et al. 1995).

- Hormone replacement therapy, preferably with natural forms of progesterone, testosterone, and estrogen.
- DHEA supplementation. The usual dose is 15–50 mg in females and 50–75 mg in males.

8. Innovative drug strategies can include the following

- Hydergine, 10–20 mg daily
- Piracetam, 2400–4800 mg daily
- Deprenyl, 5 mg, twice weekly

9. Drug-Supplement Interactions

- Ginkgo acts to thin the blood by reducing the ability of platelets (blood-clotting cells) to stick together. Care should be used when using ginkgo with other agents that thin the blood, such as heparin, warfarin, aspirin, and some NSAIDs (Harkness et al. 2000).
- Vitamin E has a long history of safe use. Vitamin E may add to the blood thinning effect of aspirin and cause an increased risk of bleeding. Care should be taken when taking aspirin with vitamin E (Harkness et al. 2000).
- Vitamin K directly counteracts the action of warfarin. Patients taking warfarin should seek qualified medical advice before taking vitamin K (Harkness et al. 2000).
- EPA and DHA have been shown to inhibit abnormal clotting in blood vessels. Care should be used with those taking anticoagulant medications such as warfarin.

10. The Life Extension Foundation has designed several products specifically for neurological support. These include:

- Cognitex contains phosphatidycholine, phosphatidylserine, vinpocetine, and pregnenolone. It is available with and without pregnenolone. Take 5 capsules in the morning and 5 in the evening.

- Chronoforte contains acetyl-*L*-carnitine, alphalipoic acid, carnosine, and zinc.
- CDP choline is a unique form of choline that readily passes through the blood-brain barrier directly into brain tissue where it enhances cerebral energy metabolism.
- Life Extension Foundation offers several forms of ginkgo biloba, including Super Ginkgo Extract, ginkgo with DMAE (DMAE-Ginkgo Caps), and ginkgo with phosphatidyl choline (PC-Ginkgo Caps).
- The Life Extension Mix has a wide variety of antioxidants, vitamins, and minerals.
- Essential Fatty Acids are available from several oils. Super GLA/DHA (also containing EPA) will help to control inflammation by balancing essential fatty acid intake.

 FOR MORE INFORMATION

Contact the Alzheimer's Association (800) 272-3900.

 PRODUCT AVAILABILITY

Life Extension Mix, Cognitex, Chronoforte, CDP choline, Super Ginkgo Extract, DMAE-Ginkgo Caps, PC-Ginkgo Caps, Super Carnosine, methylcobalamin lozenges, acetyl-*L*-carnitine, phosphatidylserine, lecithin granules, lecithin with B5 and BHA, Super CoQ10, TMG, SAMe, Super GLA/DHA, perilla oil, Super Max EPA, melatonin, DHEA, Natural Estrogen, pregnenolone, vinpocetine, Huperzine A, vitamin A, vitamin C, vitamin E, and vitamin K are available by phoning (800) 544-4440 or by ordering online at www.lef.org.

Piracetam and Hydergine (in high potencies) are available from overseas companies for personal use only. A list of these companies can be obtained by calling (800) 544-4440.

Amnesia

Amnesia is a term describing a group of disorders involving partial or total inability to remember past experiences. Memory can be divided into three major components: *immediate*, covering the past few seconds; *intermediate*, covering the duration from a few seconds past to a few days past; and *remote*, or long-term, extending further back in time. The more common types of amnesia occur after head trauma.

Retrograde Amnesia. Retrograde amnesia is the type of amnesia most people think of when they hear the term. People with retrograde amnesia find it hard to remember things that occurred prior to an incident in which they incurred damage to the head. Sometimes people never remember the seconds leading up to the incident.

Wernike-Korsakoff's Psychosis. Wernike-Korsakoff's psychosis is memory loss caused by extended alcohol abuse. This tends to be a progressive disorder and is usually accompanied by neurological problems, such as uncoordinated movements and loss of feeling in the fingers and toes.

Traumatic Amnesia. Traumatic amnesia is caused by brain damage from a hard blow to the head, such as in a car accident. It can lead to anything from a brief loss of consciousness to coma.

Infantile/Childhood Amnesia. Infantile/childhood amnesia refers to a person's inability to recall events from early childhood. Some say this type of amnesia could be linked to language development or the fact that some areas of the brain linked to memory were not fully mature.

Hysterical (Fugue) Amnesia. Hysterical (fugue) amnesia is usually triggered by a traumatic event that the person's mind is unable to properly handle. Usually, the memory slowly or suddenly returns a few days later, although memory of the trauma itself may remain incomplete.

AGING

Many aging persons gradually develop noticeable difficulties in memory: at first for names, then for events, and sometimes even occasionally for spatial relationships. This widely experienced, so-called benign type of forgetfulness bears no proven relationship to degenerative dementia, but may be a forewarning because some of the similarities are hard to overlook. Aside from severe head trauma, the most common causes of severe memory loss are degenerative dementia; brain anoxia (lack of oxygen) or ischemia (lack of blood); alcoholic nutritional disease; and various drug intoxications.

Transient global amnesia is the sudden appearance of severe, forgetful confusion lasting from as little as 30–60 minutes to as long as 12 hours or more. It is an unusual but not uncommon syndrome. During severe attacks, there is total disorientation except for one's identity, combined with a retrograde memory deficit that can extend back for several years, but which gradually resolves as the attack subsides. Patients generally have a rapid, total recovery; therefore no treatment is indicated. However, since this event may involve poor cerebral circulation due to atherosclerosis, further testing is indicated. If there is a personal or family history of cerebrovascular disease, it is suggested that the recommendations for atherosclerosis within the *Cardiovascular Disease protocol* be followed and consideration given to chelation therapy.

ALCOHOL ABUSE

Amnesia can also be caused by acute or long-term alcohol use. In particular, heavy alcohol consumption combined with poor diet and low intake of thiamine leads to a partially reversible syndrome called Wernicke-Korsakoff syndrome. Symptoms of confusion, ataxia of gait, and involuntary movement of the eye may be reversed by parenteral administration of thiamine. Even though only about 20% recover from the associated amnesia, some researchers believe that oral thiamine administered to alcoholics may act as a prophylactic (Cook 2000; Ambrose et al. 2001). In a report of a study of a 68-year-old man who had a slow onset of Wernicke-Korsakoff syndrome, the authors noted that an immediate high concentration of thiamine maintained wakefulness and level of consciousness (Kikuchi et al. 2000).

An interesting modality called cranio-electro-neuro-stimulation (CES) involves the passage of a low-voltage, low current (100 Hz) laterally between the ears. Studies have shown CES to be beneficial for treating the cognitive impairment associated with long-term alcohol use. However, CES is not indicated for the effects associated with Wernicke-Korsakoff syndrome.

MEDICATION SIDE EFFECTS

Benzodiazepines (Valium, Diazepam) are a class of drugs which are primarily used to treat anxiety and insomnia. Benodiazepines are one of the most commonly prescribed classes of drugs sold. One of the problems associated with long-term use of these drugs, particularly in the elderly, is memory loss. Because aging is inherently associated with some degree of increasing memory impairment and because the elderly population is prone to insomnia, prescribing benzodiazepines is inadvisable. In fact, benzodiazepines are specifically administered to patients prior to surgery because they cause anterograde amnesia. Patients who have not been given a benzodiazepine drug preoperatively have complained about remembering their surgery, which leads to lawsuits.

Adverse side effects, including amnesia-like symptoms, can also result from a too-high or too-low dosage of medications, an unusual reaction to medications, or from a combination of medications. In the older population, it is not uncommon for individuals to be taking many different medications that have been prescribed by several different physicians in addition to taking over-the-counter preparations. Be certain that your primary physician is aware of all prescription and nonprescription medications that you take.

TREATMENT STRATEGIES

European doctors prescribe the drugs piracetam and vasopressin to help people who have amnesia to recover their memories. Published studies show that the recovery of memory in amnesia patients can take from several hours to a few days when vasopressin or piracetam or both are used (Ostrovskaia et al. 1985; Rakhmankulova et al. 1985; van Wimersma Greidanus et al. 1986; Lenegre et al. 1988).

In studies spanning two decades, piracetam has been shown to enhance memory, particularly when used in combination with choline (Bartus et al. 1981; Pragina et al. 1990; Senin et al. 1991).

The recommended dosage of vasopressin is at least 16 IU a day, usually in the form of a nasal spray, although physicians may prescribe higher amounts to treat acute amnesia. A recommended dose of piracetam is 4800 mg daily until memory is restored.

Nimodipine is especially recommended for head trauma victims. Nimodipine (brand name Nimotop) is a calcium channel blocker specific to the central nervous system. It prevents movement of calcium into the cells of blood vessels, thereby relaxing the vessels and increasing the supply of blood and oxygen. It dramatically improves cerebral blood flow. Nimodipine is an FDA-approved drug used to prevent and treat problems caused by a burst blood vessel around the brain, but it has largely been ignored by most neurologists treating victims of stroke and other age-related neurological diseases.

NATURAL SUPPLEMENTS

Phosphatidylcholine

The most commonly used memory-enhancing nutrients are choline, lecithin, and phosphatidylcholine which are precursors to the chemical neurotransmitter acetylcholine that carries messages between brain cells. Because acetylcholine helps brain cells communicate with each other, it plays an important role in learning and memory. Acetylcholine deficiency can predispose a person to a wide range of neurological diseases, including Alzheimer's disease and stroke.

One study found that phosphatidylcholine administered with vitamin B_{12} improved the memory of rats in which brain damage had caused memory impairment (Masuda et al. 1998).

Ginkgo and Vitamin B_{12}

Ginkgo biloba and vitamin B_{12} may be helpful in treating memory loss. Extracts from Ginkgo biloba have been shown to thin the blood and improve blood flow to the brain, protect against free radicals, and improve memory. Ginkgo biloba is approved in Germany for the treatment of dementia. There are over 1200 published studies in the scientific literature on ginkgo biloba extract (Yoshikawa et al. 1999; DeFeudis et al. 2000; Diamond et al. 2000). In one study, patients with memory disturbances were supplemented with ginkgo biloba. Following ginkgo treatment, 15% of patients reported the total absence of memory disturbance symptoms and 62% reported that the remaining symptoms were mild to moderate (Enrique Gomez 1997).

An article by Carmel (1996) reviewed vitamin B_{12} deficiency in elderly persons relative to memory impairment and neuropathy. The authors concluded that both memory problems and neuropathy have been treated successfully with vitamin B_{12} injections or supplementation.

Lindenbaum et al. (1988) reviewed subclinical vitamin B_{12} deficiency and the resulting neurological symptoms. They stated that many common difficulties, such as memory loss, muscle weakness, and parasthesias, might well be a product of vitamin B_{12} deficiency.

Picamilon

Picamilon is a compound of niacin and the neurotransmitter GABA. The niacin in Picamilon acts as a nontoxic carrier molecule for GABA to make it easier for GABA to penetrate the blood-brain barrier and act within the brain. Picamilon improves circulation to the brain, thereby enhancing cognitive functioning. In Russian studies, Picamilon has been shown to improve cerebral blood flow and even to help treat brain trauma (Anon., two unpublished studies; Mirzoian et al. 1989; Phuaichenko et al. undated).

Hormones

Pregnenolone and DHEA improve brain cell activity and enhance memory. (Pregnenolone is converted into DHEA in the body.) DHEA is the most plentiful steroid hormone in the human body, but its exact function is unknown. What is known is that DHEA concentration plummets with age: its daily production drops from 30 mg at age 20 to less than 6 mg at age 80. DHEA is naturally synthesized in abundance in young people from pregnenolone in the brain and the adrenal glands. It is known to affect the excitability of neurons in the hippocampus, the part of the brain responsible for memory.

Findings suggest that DHEA enhances memory by facilitating the induction of neural plasticity, the condition that permits the neurons (nerve cells of the brain) to change in order to record new memories (Diamond et al. 1996). Studies have shown that DHEA not only improves memory deficits, but also relieves depression in older people and increases perceived physical and psychological well-being. DHEA has been shown to help preserve youthful neurological function (Morales et al. 1994; Wolkowitz et al. 1997). Together, pregnenolone and DHEA help to maintain the ability of brain cells to store and retrieve information in short-term memory (Mathis et al. 1999; Racchi et al. 2001; Vallee et al. 2001).

A study found that DHEA and 7-oxo-DHEA-acetate, which is formed from DHEA, completely reversed the memory deficit induced by an injection of scopolamine in young mice. Only 7-oxo-DHEA-acetate was effective, however, in similar tests on older mice (Shi et al. 2000). Pregnenolone initiates the memory storage process by stimulating the activity of an important molecule known as adenylate cyclase, which is needed to activate and regulate enzymes crucial to cellular energy production. Pregnenolone then regulates the sequential flow of calcium ions through the cell membrane. The pattern of calcium ion exchange may determine how memories are encoded by neurons.

Pregnenolone also modulates chemical reactions, calcium-protein binding, gene activation, protein turnover, and enzymatic reactions involved in the storage and retrieval of memory.

An article by Darnaudery et al. (2000) reported that pregnenolone sulfate increased acetylcholine release and enhanced spatial memory performance. Studies on rats showed that injections of pregnenolone into the brain caused a dose-dependent increase of acetylcholine output. The lower dose caused a short-term elevation (20 minutes) and the higher dose caused a long-term elevation (80 minutes). This study confirmed previous work suggesting that a modest increase in acetylcholine facilitates memory processes (Darnaudery et al. 2000).

A study investigated the possible relation between long-term depression and barbiturates/benzodiazepine-induced amnesia and attempted to determine the possible effect of pregnenolone sulfate on long-term depression. Results showed long-term depression was either blocked or reversed by pregnenolone sulfate at concentrations of 10 mcM. Thus, the prevention or reversal of this type of long-term depression by pregnenolone sulfate may suggest a clinical application of this agent in the management of amnesia or dementia (Akhondzadeh et al. 1998).

Additional agents which may be helpful can be found in the *Age-Associated Memory Impairment protocol.*

🌀 SUMMARY

1. Choline, lecithin, and phosphatidylcholine are best taken early in the day to maximize improvement in brain productivity throughout the day. Suggested dosage ranges are 1000–3000 mg a day of choline or 10,000 mg a day of lecithin. A popular way of obtaining several different forms of choline is a dietary supplement called Cognitex. Those with amnesia would take 12 Cognitex capsules a day until symptoms improved.

2. Both ginkgo biloba and vitamin B_{12} have been shown to improve memory.

   • Ginkgo, 120 mg a day.
   • Vitamin B_{12} in the form of methylcobalamin, one or more 5-mg lozenges daily.

3. Picamilon improves neuronal circulation, 100 mg 3 times daily.

4. Thiamine (vitamin B_1) is indicated for alcohol-induced memory loss, one 500-mg capsule daily with meals.

5. DHEA and pregnenolone are steroidal hormones that improve brain cell activity and improve memory. The suggested supplementation range for pregnenolone is 50–150 mg a day in 3 equal doses. The recommended dosage for DHEA is 25–50 mg a day. Women usually need less DHEA than men. DHEA is contraindicated in both men and women with hormone-related cancers. *Refer to the DHEA Replacement Therapy protocol before using pregnenolone or DHEA.*

6. Vasopressin, 16 IU a day (nasal spray) and/or piracetam in the dose of 4800 mg daily.

7. For alcoholic cognitive impairment and possibly for memory loss from other causes, cranio-electroneural stimulation (CES) 3 times a day for 45 minutes.

8. Chelation therapy is a procedure performed in a doctor's office. An infusion of the amino acid EDTA is given intravenously with a small needle to remove heavy metals or to improve circulation in vascular diseases. Chelation therapy may be considered for amnesia caused by atherosclerosis.

9. For head trauma victims, Nimotop in the dose of 30 mg 4 times daily.

 FOR MORE INFORMATION

Call the American College for the Advancement of Medicine, (800) 532-3688, for the location and phone number of a physician in your area who specializes in complementary medicine and has a familiarity with chelation therapy.

 PRODUCT AVAILABILITY

Cognitex (containing several forms of choline), lecithin granules, Choline Cooler powder, ginkgo biloba, methylcobalamin, vitamin B_1, DHEA, pregnenolone, and thiamine are available by phoning (800) 544-4440 or order online at www.lef.org. Vasopressin (Novartis) and Nimodiopine (Nimotop) are prescription medications. Piracetam is an unapproved drug that has to be ordered from offshore pharmacies.

Amyotrophic Lateral Sclerosis (ALS)

Amyotrophic lateral sclerosis: *a* "lack of," "myelin," *trophic* "nourishment," *lateralis* "side," *sklē rōsis* "hardening"

Amyotrophic lateral sclerosis (ALS) is also known as Lou Gehrig's disease. Lou Gehrig was one of baseball's greatest players and earned the nickname "Iron Horse" for his record of 2130 consecutive games. His outstanding career was ended by ALS.

ALS is a rapidly progressive neuromuscular disease caused by the destruction of nerve cells in the brain and spinal cord. This causes the loss of nervous control of voluntary muscles, resulting in the degeneration and atrophy of the muscles. Eventually the respiratory muscles are affected which leads to death from an inability to breathe.

Symptoms

ALS symptoms vary from one person to another according to which group of muscles is affected by the disease. Tripping, dropping things, abnormal fatigue in the arms and/or legs, slurred speech, difficulty in talking loudly, uncontrollable bouts of laughing or crying, and muscle cramps and twitches are all symptoms of ALS. The disease usually starts first in the hands and will cause problems in dressing, bathing, or other simple tasks. It may progress more on one side of the body and generally proceeds up the arm or leg. If it starts in the feet, walking will become difficult. ALS can also start in the throat, causing difficulty with swallowing.

People afflicted with ALS do not lose their ability to see, hear, touch, smell, or taste. The bladder, sexual drive and function, and muscles of the person's eyes are not affected. The disease does not affect the person's mind.

Epidemiology

Men make up the majority of those who contract ALS, although women also get the disease. Race, ethnicity, or socioeconomic boundaries make no difference as to who will come down with ALS. Most of those who get the disease are usually between the ages of 40 and 70, but people in their 20s and 30s can also get it. In most societies, there is an incidence of five in every 100,000 people (Fauci 1998; Onion 1998).

Course

The rate of progression of the symptoms of ALS varies for each person. The average life expectancy for a newly diagnosed person is 2–5 years, although improved medical care is resulting in longer life. ALS frequently takes its toll before being diagnosed, causing the people who have the disease to be significantly debilitated before they learn they have it.

CAUSES

There are three types of ALS: sporadic, familial, and Guamanian. The most common form is sporadic. A small number of cases are inherited genetic disorders (familial). A large number of cases, however, occur in Guam and other Pacific territories.

The familial type of ALS is caused by a genetic defect in superoxide dismutase, an antioxidant enzyme that continuously removes the highly toxic "superoxide" free radical. The causes of sporadic and Guamanian ALS are unknown. Several hypotheses have been proposed including:

- Glutamate toxicity
- Oxidative stress
- Mitochondrial dysfunction
- Autoimmune disease
- Infectious disease
- Toxic chemical exposure
- Exposure to heavy metals such as lead, mercury, aluminum, and manganese
- Calcium and magnesium deficiency
- Carbohydrate metabolism
- Growth factor deficiency

Glutamate Toxicity

Glutamate is the main excitatory neurotransmitter in the brain. It has been calculated that glutamate is responsible for 75% of excitatory neural transmissions. Glutamate is unique in that it can produce such marked stimulation that neurons die. It has been proposed that the neuronal damage following ischemia (deficiency of blood, for example, after a stroke) is due to the action of glutamate rather than a lack of oxygen (Ganong 1995).

ALS is highly linked with glutamate. One proposed mechanism is a defective glutamate transport system that permits neurotoxic levels to build up (Onion 1998). A study showed significant elevations (by about 70%) of plasma levels of glutamate in ALS patients as compared to controls (Plaitakis et al. 1993).

Oxidative Stress

Oxidative stress refers to a shift in the ratio of oxidants to antioxidants in the body. Free radicals are molecules that have an unpaired electron. Most free radicals react with molecules that contain oxygen to form reactive oxygen species, such as nitric oxide (NO), superoxide (O_2-), and hydroxyl (OH-). Free radical damage is associated with many degenerative conditions, including neurological disorders (Jenner 1994).

Antioxidants inhibit oxidation by free radicals. There are many types of antioxidants, including:

- Detoxification enzymes such as superoxide dismutase (SOD) catalase, glutathione peroxidase, and glutathione transferase
- Enzymes such as glutathione reductase, albumin, transferrin, ceruloplasmin, and metallothionein.
- Nutritional supplements including tocotrienols, coenzyme Q_{10}, vitamins C and E, lycopene, cysteine, glutathione, alpha lipoic acid, and melatonin.

Inflammation represents a major source of oxidants. Inflammation is often caused by bacterial or viral infections, toxic exposure, and aging-related cytokine changes. The continuous production of reactive oxidant species during chronic inflammation may deplete the store of antioxidants, eventually resulting in a spiral from health to disease (Jenner 1994).

Mitochondrial Dysfunction

Mitochondria are the power-generating units of the cell and are most abundant where energy-requiring processes take place (for example, in muscles). The outer membrane of the mitochondria is studded with oxidative enzymes that provide raw materials for the reactions occurring inside. In the interior, the citric acid cycle converts fats and carbohydrates into energy-releasing carbon dioxide. The energy produced by this reaction is used to form the high-energy phosphate bonds in adenosine triphosphate (ATP) in a process called oxidative phosphorylation. ATP is the principal energy source for both plants and animals. Mitochondrial DNA is transmitted genetically solely from the mother (Ganong 1995).

Mitochondrial dysfunction has been linked to neurodegenerative diseases (Beal 1996; Beal 1999b). Defects in mitochondrial DNA have also been proposed as a causative mechanism in sporadic ALS (Murphy et al. 1999; Beal 2000; Manfredi et al. 2000).

One study explored the role of mitochondrial dysfunction by transferring mitochondrial DNA from ALS subjects to normal human neuroblastoma cells (embryonic cells that form nervous tissue) with their mitochondrial DNA removed. The resulting hybrid cells exhibited abnormal electron transport chain functioning, increases in free radical scavenging enzyme activity, perturbed calcium homeostasis, and altered mitochondrial structure.

The nickname "Iron Horse" given to Lou Gehrig is quite appropriate. The energy forming process of oxidative phosphorylation relies heavily upon transferring electrons between several iron molecules that form the electron transport chain. The oxidative phosphorylation process also requires coenzyme Q_{10}, nicotinamide adenine dinucleotide (NAD), and flavin adenine dinucleotide (FAD). Niacin (vitamin B_3) is used to form NAD, and riboflavin (vitamin B_2) is used to form FAD.

Autoimmune Disease

Autoimmunity may play a role in ALS. In this disease, the immune system becomes confused and begins attacking tissues in the body. Under normal conditions, the body's immune system produces proteins called immunoglobulins which attach to their target antigen. An antigen is a substance that produces an immune response and is usually something foreign to the body. The immunoglobulins attach to and surround the target antigen, forming an antigen-antibody complex. This complex is then ingested by phagocytes, such as macrophages, in a process called phagocytosis.

In autoimmune disease, antibodies are produced that attach to the tissues of the body, instead of foreign substances. The following are examples of diseases with an autoimmune basis:

- In autoimmune hemolytic anemia, the body produces autoantibodies to red blood cell membrane proteins.
- In diabetes mellitus, autoantibodies are formed against insulin receptors.
- Graves's disease is associated with autoantibodies to thyroid stimulating hormone (TSH) receptors.
- Pernicious anemia can be caused when autoantibodies are formed against intrinsic factor which is needed for vitamin B_{12} absorption.

Researchers have proposed that ALS may have an autoimmune basis. The following are the bases for their hypotheses:

- Analyses of ALS patient sera have identified circulating antibodies secreted by denervated muscle. These antibodies inhibit the stimulation of the sprouting of axons, the long arms of neurons which conduct nervous impulses to other neurons throughout the body (Onion 1998).

- Researchers have found an immunoglobulin that affects the conductance of neuronal voltage-activated calcium channels which may induce an excessive release of glutamate from nerve endings (Onion 1998).

- Several studies of ALS patients found the presence of antibodies that interact with motor neurons (Pestronk et al. 1988a; Pestronk et al. 1988b; Pestronk et al. 1989; Niebroj-Dobosz et al. 1999).

- Immune complexes have been found in spinal cords of patients with ALS.

It has been proposed that T cells, activated microglia, and immunoglobulin G (IgG) within the spinal cord lesions may be the primary event that leads to tissue destruction in ALS.

The increased prevalence in Guam is associated with a decreased delayed hypersensitivity. The secondary response, which occurs with the second exposure to the antigen, is normally quicker and usually produces more antibodies than the primary response. The major reason for the enhanced secondary response is the formation of B memory cells during the primary response (Onion 1998). In an early study, a family history of thyroid disease was present in 19% of ALS patients, and an additional 21% of patients described family members with other possible autoimmune disorders. In 19% of the patients with ALS, either past or present thyroid disease was documented. Eleven of 47 additional patients with ALS had significant elevations of microsomal and/or thyroglobulin antibody levels (Appel et al. 1986).

Infectious Disease

ALS was once thought to be caused by persistent viral infection (Salazar-Grueso et al. 1995). This hypothesis fell out of favor when researchers could not isolate a single causative agent. Recently, however, many researchers are reconsidering infectious agents because many neurodegenerative disorders are associated with chronic infections, particularly latent viruses. Support for the continued investigation of infectious agents in ALS include the knowledge that:

- It is well-known that excess free radical activity is associated with chronic infection (Racek et al. 2001).

- Both Lyme disease and poliomyelitis have chronic states that resemble the symptoms of ALS (Garcia-Moreno et al. 1997).

- HIV infection is associated with a variety of neurological problems (Dalakas et al. 1988; Cruz Martinez et al. 1989).

- Tertiary syphilis affects the nervous system (neurosyphilis) causing tabes dorsalis, a syndrome marked by degeneration of the posterior columns and posterior roots and ganglia of the spinal cord.

Toxic Chemical Exposure

People with a history of exposure to agricultural chemicals, including fertilizers and pesticides used in gardening and lawn care, may be at twice the risk for developing ALS (Baker 1996; McGuire et al. 1997).

Chemicals foreign to the body are called xenobiotics. They include toluene, xylene, hexanes, benzene, trichloroethane, styrene, phytates, and pesticides. Most xenobiotics are lipophilic, which means that they are attracted to the fats (lipids) which make up cell membranes. Because the brain is full of lipids, xenobiotics are able to rapidly diffuse across cell membranes into the brain and cause neurological problems.

Many pesticides are specifically designed as neurotoxins (toxins that affect the nervous system). Pesticides are generally odorless and can cause progressive symptoms weeks after an exposure (Prazmo 1978; Ames et al. 1995; Keifer et al. 1997).

Xenobiotics are removed from the body by a process called detoxification, which takes place in two phases. Phase I takes place inside the cell and changes the toxic chemicals into less toxic forms by means of the chemical processes of oxidation, reduction, and hydrolysis. Phase II detoxification then attaches molecules such as glutathione, methionine, and sulfur compounds in a process called glucuronidation. The body is then able to excrete these modified toxins in stool, urine, or sweat.

The process of detoxification requires several nutritional cofactors including magnesium, zinc, and manganese. The glutathione, methionine, and sulfur molecules are a component in the Phase II detoxification process and are used up in the process. As the detoxification pathways become overloaded, any further toxic challenge, however slight, can cause symptoms. This is often referred to as chemical sensitivity.

Chemically sensitive people experience symptoms to a variety of chemical insults. Caffeine (the active component of coffee), aspirin, and acetaminophen (Tylenol) are often used to assess the functional capacity of the detoxification system. Alcohol is metabolized in Phase I by aldehyde dehydrogenase. Gasoline fumes, deodorizers, rubber, and solvents are sources of benzene. Trichloroethylene, if blocked from the normal Phase I pathway, will form a toxic secondary metabolite called chloral hydrate, the so-called "Mickey Finn," which causes disorientation and dizziness.

Toxic chemical exposure may be one reason why there is a higher incidence of ALS diagnosed in soldiers who participated in Operation Desert Storm. On April 6, 2000, the Associated Press reported that the Veterans Administration announced a year-long study to determine whether there is a higher incidence of Lou Gehrig's disease (ALS) among the veterans of the Gulf War. At least 28 Gulf veterans have been diagnosed with this deadly disease. Researchers are interested in locating other veterans, diagnosed with ALS or other motor neuron diseases, who were actively serving duty between August 2, 1990, and July 31, 1991, regardless of location. Those who did not go to the Persian Gulf will serve as part of the control group. Eligible veterans may call 1-877-342-5257 (Smith et al. 2000).

Heavy Metals

Because there are high numbers of ALS patients in Guam, Western New Guinea, and Japan, there is a theory that ALS might be caused by environmental problems. These areas have large amounts of heavy metals such as lead, mercury, and aluminum. These metals can poison the body and cause ALS symptoms (Conradi et al. 1976; Adams et al.1983; Armon et al. 1991).

Lead

Lead was used as an additive to gasoline and in many paints. Absorption of lead is enhanced by dietary deficiencies in calcium, iron, and zinc. Lead toxicity is most likely related to lead's affinity for cell membranes and mitochondria, where it interferes with several important enzymes.

In adults, systemic lead poisoning causes abdominal and joint pain, fatigue, anemia, and neurological symptoms, including headaches, irritability, peripheral motor neuropathy, short-term memory loss, and an inability to concentrate. Chronic subclinical lead exposure affects the kidneys, causing interstitial nephritis, renal tubular damage (with tubular inclusion bodies), hyperuricemia (with an increased risk of gout), and a decline in glomerular filtration rate and chronic renal failure. Armon et al. (1991) suggest that there may be an association between ALS in men and exposure to lead vapor.

Mercury

Mercury exposure is thought to occur from ingestion of contaminated fish (particularly tuna and swordfish, which can contain high levels of methyl mercury), inhalation of mercury vapor from dental amalgams, and possibly from drinking water contaminated by toxic waste sites.

Chronic mercury exposure produces a characteristic intention tremor and a constellation of findings, including excitability, memory loss, insomnia, timidity, and sometimes delirium. The neurotoxicity resulting from organic mercury exposure is characterized by paresthesia (an abnormal touch sensation often in the absence of external stimulus), impaired peripheral vision, hearing, taste, and smell, slurred speech, unsteadiness of gait and limbs, muscle weakness, irritability, memory loss, and depression. Dentists with occupational exposure to mercury score below normal on neurobehavioral tests of motor speed, visual scanning, verbal and visual memory, and visual-motor coordination (Harrison 1998).

ALS was diagnosed in one patient after accidental injection of mercury (Schwarz et al. 1996).

It is well-known that selenium decreases the toxicity of mercury in the human body. After measuring the mercury and selenium content in the hair of 13 ALS cases, one study concluded that mercury in the body with a low content of selenium may be one of the environmental factors involved in producing ALS (Mano et al. 1989; Khare et al. 1990; Mano et al. 1990).

Aluminum

High levels of aluminum are found in the delicate threads running through the cytoplasm of nerve cells (neurofibrillary tangles) in the cerebral cortex and hippocampus of patients with Alzheimer's disease. High levels of aluminum have also been found in the drinking water and soil of areas with an unusually high incidence of Alzheimer's disease (Harrison 1998).

Aluminum and calcium deposits were found in the neurons of patients with ALS from Guam (Garruto et al. 1985).

Manganese

Manganese toxicity can cause a syndrome similar to Parkinson's within 1–2 years, including gait disorders, postural instability, a masked, expressionless face, tremor, and psychiatric symptoms.

Manganese is emitted from the tail pipes of motor vehicles (Aschner 2000). Occupational exposure can occur in miners, dry-battery manufacturers, and arc welders (Harrison 1998).

A study showed that the nitrated manganese-SOD level was strikingly elevated in ALS patients. The authors also proposed that nitration of manganese SOD in cerebrospinal fluids is a marker for oxidative stress in neurodegenerative diseases (Aoyama et al. 2000).

Calcium and Magnesium Deficiency

It is proposed that chronic environment deficiencies of calcium and magnesium may result in increased intestinal absorption of toxic metals and lead to the mobilization of calcium and metals from the bone and the deposition of these elements in nervous tissue. This hypothesis, called metal-induced calcifying degeneration of central nervous system (CNS), has been supported by experimental studies using several animal species (Van den Bergh et al. 1977).

Low calcium/magnesium intake with excess amounts of aluminum and manganese are associated with the incidence of ALS in the Western Pacific. The authors conclude that the high incidence of ALS in the Western Pacific may be due to calcium/magnesium metabolism dysfunction, resulting in excess deposition of aluminum (Yasui et al. 1991a; Yasui et al. 1991b).

Carbohydrate Metabolism

Over the last 30 years glucose intolerance has been reported in a significant percentage of patients with ALS. Currently, a controversy exists in determining whether the carbohydrate abnormality is disease-specific or secondary to the decreased glucose utilization caused by muscle atrophy. One study showed that the glucose infusion rate, an estimate of *in vivo* insulin sensitivity, was significantly diminished in ALS patients compared to both normal and disease controls, which suggests that ALS may be associated with a dysfunction in carbohydrate metabolism (Van den Bergh et al. 1977; Nagano et al. 1979; Reyes et al. 1984).

Growth Factor Deficiency

A lack of trophic (growth) factors support has been hypothesized as a probable cause of ALS. Several growth factors have been identified, including insulin-like growth factor I (IGF-I), nerve growth factor (NGF), leukemia inhibitory factor (LIF), and ciliary neurotrophic factor (CNF). Specific information can be found about these growth factors in the *Drug Research section*.

DIFFERENTIAL DIAGNOSIS

Because the course of ALS is fatal within 3–5 years, a careful differential diagnosis is needed. The following should be considered (Harrison 1998):

- Physical causes such as compression of the cervical spinal cord
- Infectious diseases such as Lyme disease, post-poliomyelitis, HIV infection

- Enzyme disorders in SOD, hexosaminidase A, and alpha-glucosidase
- Other neurological diseases such as Pick's disease and Kennedy's syndrome
- Endocrine disorders including diabetic amyotrophy and thyrotoxicosis

Physical Causes

Compression of the Cervical Spinal Cord

An MRI of the head and cervical spine is usually ordered for patients with lower neurological disease to rule out compression of the spinal cord and impingement along the spinal nerves.

Infectious Diseases

Lyme Disease

The second and third stages of Lyme disease are associated with neurological changes that may cause an axonal, lower motor neuropathy. Lyme disease is caused by the bacterial spirochete (*Borrelia burgdorferi*) spread by a deer tick (*Ixodes dammini*). The first stage of Lyme disease is present with a fever, enlarged lymph glands, and a characteristic bulls-eye pattern around the bite (Hansel et al. 1995).

Post-Poliomyelitis

Polio is an *enterovirus*, a genus that preferentially inhabits the intestinal tract. Reactivation of a central nervous system polio infection (post-poliomyelitis) may cause a delayed deterioration of motor neurons and muscular atrophy, including difficulty in swallowing (dysphagia) from bulbar involvement. Bulbar involvement indicates that there is a malfunction in the medulla oblongata, a structure important for collections of nerve cells lying anterior to the cerebellum (Roos et al. 1980; Onion 1998).

HIV Infection

HIV infection is associated with extreme immune system dysfunction. HIV-1 proteins Tat and gp120 have been implicated in the pathogenesis of dementia associated with HIV infection (Jain et al. 2000).

Neurosyphilis

Tertiary syphilis is seen 3-4 years after the primary infection with the spirochete *Treponema pallidum*. It is often seen in AIDS patients. Tertiary syphilis usually presents with hypersensitivity reactions since few organisms are present. Tabes dorsalis is associated motor and sensory losses in the lower extremities which causes difficulties in coordination.

Enzyme Disorders

Superoxide Dismutase (SOD)

Familial ALS is an autosomal dominant genetic disorder. It is caused by a defect on the gene encoding SOD on chromosome 21 (SOD1).

Hexosaminidase A

Tay-Sachs disease and Sandhoff's disease are autosomal recessive genetic disorders resulting from a deficiency of hexosaminidase and the accumulation in lysosomes (small bodies in cells involved in the process of intracellular digestion) of GM2 gangliosides, particularly in the central nervous system. Motor weakness, progressive ataxia, and lower motor neuron symptoms predominate in the adult form. The patients often report clumsiness in childhood and motor weakness in adolescence. The diagnosis is established by visualizing cytoplasmic bodies by electron microscopy or by detecting reduced hexosaminidase-A activity in white blood cells (Eisen et al. 1987; Harrison 1998).

Alpha-Glucosidase

Accumulation of glycogen in lysosomes in Pompe's disease is due to deficiency of a specific enzyme, alpha-glucosidase. The juvenile form is characterized by progressive proximal muscle weakness, including impairment of respiratory function (Harrison 1998).

Other Neurological Diseases

Pick's Disease

Pick's disease exhibits a progressive atrophy of the frontal and temporal lobes of the brain. Swollen neurons called Pick cells and argentophilic (attracted to silver) neuronal inclusions known as Pick bodies affect the frontal and temporal cortical regions.

Kennedy's Syndrome

Kennedy's syndrome is an X-linked, lower motor neuron disorder in which progressive weakness and wasting of limb and bulbar muscles begins in males in adult life. Kennedy's syndrome is associated with androgen (testosterone) insensitivity, manifested by excessive growth of the male breasts (gynecomastia) and reduced fertility.

Endocrine Disorders

Diabetic Amyotrophy

Neuropathy is a common clinical manifestation associated with diabetes. The most common presentation is that of peripheral polyneuropathy which is also referred to as "stocking and glove neuropathy" due to the numbness and paresthesia of the hands and feet. Diabetic amyotrophy causes progressive muscle wasting, usually of the pelvic girdle and large muscles in the upper leg. Anorexia and depression may accompany amyotrophy.

Thyrotoxicosis

Thyrotoxicosis refers to the effects of excessive quantities of thyroid hormones in tissues found in patients with severe hyperthyroidism and Graves's disease. Symptoms include feeling hot and sweaty, palpitations, frequent diarrhea from impaired digestion of fats, and a prominent essential tremor.

ASSESSMENT

Neurologists use clinical tests such as blood testing, electromyograms (EMG), magnetic resonance imaging (MRI), CT scans, and nerve biopsies to establish a profile when diagnosing ALS. These profiles will eliminate other possibilities as to what the person might be suffering from. The following labs should be considered in the diagnosis of ALS:

- Lyme disease serology
- HIV testing
- Autoimmune panel
- Thyroid panel, including thyroid-stimulating hormone (TSH), T3 and T4
- Hormone panel, including testosterone, dehydro-epiandrosterone (DHEA) and pregnenolone
- Hexosaminidase A in urine warranted when adult Tay-Sachs is suspected
- Vitamin B_{12} levels also useful

After the diagnosis of ALS has been confirmed, additional lab tests can be used to identify the predominant etiology and thus direct appropriate treatment. Additional labs would include:

- A comprehensive detoxification profile
- Oxidative stress analysis
- Mineral analysis, including calcium, magnesium, copper, and zinc
- Toxin analysis, including heavy metals and chemicals
- Amino acid analysis

TREATMENT

Many things can be done to improve or maintain the lifestyle of a person who is suffering from the disease. First, the patient should continue his or her usual daily activities, stopping just before getting tired. Physicians often recommend specific exercises, such as breathing exercises and/or exercises to strengthen the muscles that are not affected with the disease. Foot braces, hand splints, or wheelchairs, combined with exercise, will enable the patient to remain independent for as long as possible.

Counseling can help to ease the mental anguish brought on by this disease. Family counseling can also be helpful to the person with ALS, as well as the family.

One of the side effects of this disease is uncontrolled muscle contractions or spasms. Physical therapy cannot restore normal muscle function but may help in preventing painful contractions of the muscles and in maintaining normal muscle strength and function. The physical therapist should show family members how to perform these exercises, so they can help maintain this therapy for the person with ALS.

Speech therapy may also be helpful in maintaining the person's ability to speak. Swallowing therapy is important as well, to assist with the problems of swallowing and drinking. This treatment helps prevent choking. It is recommended that the patient adopt a new head posture and positioning of the tongue. The patient should also change the consistency of the food to aid swallowing accordingly as the disease progresses.

Occupational therapy is also important. The therapist will come to the person's home and recommend where to move furniture to make it easier for the patient to move around his/her house. The therapist will also place kitchen appliances in areas where making meals will be easier. The occupational therapist will also bring devices that will help the person in making the telephone, computer, and other devices easier to use.

When the ability to breathe decreases, a respiratory therapist is needed to measure the breathing capacity. These tests should take place on a regular basis. To make breathing easier, the patient should not lie down immediately after eating. The patient should not eat large meals because they can increase abdominal pressure and prevent the diaphragm from expanding. When sleeping, the head should be elevated 15–30 degrees to keep the abdominal organs away from the diaphragm. When breathing capacity falls below 70%, noninvasive respiratory assistance should be provided. This involves a nasal mask connected to a mechanical ventilator. When the breathing capacity falls below 50%, a permanent hook-up to a ventilator should be considered.

MEDICATIONS

Various medications can be given to the patient as ALS progresses.

Baclofen (Lioresal)

Baclofen (Lioresal) is used to relieve stiffness in the limbs and throat. Patients with seizure disorder or impaired renal function should use caution. Serious adverse reactions include somnolence and stupor, cardiovascular collapse, seizures, and respiratory depression. Common adverse effects include headaches, dizziness, blurred vision, slurred speech, rash, weight gain, pruritus, constipation, and increased perspiration. Excessive dosing may lead to weakness. Baclofen may interact with alcohol, monoamine oxidase inhibitors (MAOI), narcotics, antipsychotics, tricyclic antidepressants, oral hypoglycemics, or insulin.

Tizanidine (Zanaflex)

Tizanidine (Zanaflex) is a centrally acting muscle relaxant. Zanaflex may interact with alcohol (to increase somnolence, stupor) and oral contraceptives (to decrease its clearance). Zanaflex can increase hypotensive effects when administered concurrently with diuretics. Elderly patients and patients with impaired renal function should use caution. Serious reactions include hallucinations, severe bradycardia, and liver toxicity. Common adverse effects include dryness of mouth, somnolence and sedation, dizziness, malaise, constipation, increased spasms, and hypotension.

Tricyclic Antidepressants

Tricyclic antidepressants may be used to control the production of excess saliva.

Rilutek (Riluzole)

Rilutek (Riluzole), the only FDA-approved drug to treat ALS, reduces the presynaptic release of glutamate. Riluzole is metabolized in the liver. It is contraindicated with active liver disease or elevated liver function tests (serum glutamic pyruvate transaminase [SGPT] or alanine aminotransferase [ALT] and glucose tolerance test [GTT]). Theophylline and caffeine may affect rate of elimination. Riluzole treatment may be associated with mild blood pressure elevation (Scelsa et al. 2000).

Unfortunately Riluzole, although described in medical journals as an effective treatment for ALS, provides almost no benefit and is associated with significant side effects in most patients. One journal noted, "It is often said that the benefits of riluzole are marginal but the side effects are major," One writer commented, "clearly, Riluzole does succeed at one important task. It allows treating physicians to end the day assured that they did something for the ALS patients they were treating since a prescription was written—an obligation was thus fulfilled" (Rowland 1996; Ludolph et al. 1999; Perlmutter 2000).

DRUG RESEARCH

Several drugs are being studied for treatment of ALS (Hurko et al. 2000). These include:

- N-methyl-D-aspartate (NMDA) receptor antagonists memantine and dextromethorphan

- Growth factors such as insulin-like growth factor-I, nerve growth factor, leukemia inhibiting factor, ciliary growth factor, pigment epithelium-derived factor, neurturin, and transforming growth factor-beta

- TR500, a glutathione-repleting agent

- Deprenyl, a selective monoamine oxidase B inhibitor

- Pimozide, a voltage-dependent calcium channel blocker

- Gabapentin, an antiseizure drug made from gamma-aminobutyric acid (GABA)

NMDA receptor antagonists

Memantine

Memantine is an NMDA receptor antagonist that has been approved for use in the treatment of dementia in Germany for more than 10 years. NMDA receptor antagonists have therapeutic potential in numerous CNS disorders. Memantine does not have the side effects common to other NMDA receptor antagonists such as dizocilpine (Parsons et al. 1999; Jain et al. 2000). Memantine will be available in the United States in 2004 pending FDA approval.

Dextromethorphan

Dextromethorphan is an NMDA receptor antagonist that is being explored for use in ALS. Preliminary studies, however, did not find positive effect (Askmark et al. 1993).

Growth Factors

Insulin-like Growth Factor I

Some authors have reported decreased IGF-I in patients with ALS (Eisen et al. 1993; Dore et al. 1996; Torres-Aleman et al. 1998). IGF-I receptors are present in the spinal cord where they mediate signal transduction via tyrosine kinase. IGF-I was found to prevent the loss of choline acetyltransferase activity in embryonic spinal cord cultures, as well as to reduce the programmed cell death of motor neurons in vivo during normal development or following axotomy or spinal transection. Clinical trials of recombinant human IGF-I have been initiated for patients with ALS (Lewis et al. 1993).

One study examined the cost effectiveness of treatment with recombinant human insulin-like growth factor I (rhIGF-I) in patients with ALS. They conclude that treatment with rhIGF-I is most cost effective in ALS patients who are either in earlier stages of the disease or progressing rapidly. The cost effectiveness of rhIGF-I therapy compares favorably with treatments for other chronic progressive diseases (Ackerman et al. 1999).

A double-blind, placebo-controlled, randomized study of 266 patients was conducted at eight centers in North America. The authors concluded that rhIGF-I slowed the progression of functional impairment and the decline in health-related quality of life in patients with ALS with no medically important adverse effects (Lange et al. 1996; Lai et al. 1997). A European placebo-controlled trial of IGF-I in ALS, however, showed no significant difference between treatment groups (Borasio et al. 1998).

Nerve Growth Factor

A moderate reduction in beta-nerve growth factor (beta-NGF) levels was seen in the serum of patients with ALS and multiple sclerosis. There was a statistically significant reduction in the patients who were carriers of Parkinson's disease and Huntington's disease (Lorigados et al. 1998).

Leukemia Inhibitory Factor

Leukemia inhibitory factor (LIF) was named after its effect on hemopoietic (blood-forming) cells. Studies have demonstrated a powerful effect of LIF in the survival of both motor and sensory neurons, while reducing denervation-induced muscle atrophy. LIF will also stimulate muscle regeneration in vivo when applied exogenously after injury. A human recombinant form of LIF (AM424) entered human clinical trials during 1998 (Kurek et al. 1998).

Ciliary Neurotrophic Factor

Ciliary neurotrophic factor is currently in clinical trials for the potential treatment of motor neuron disease or ALS (Lindsay 1994).

Pigment Epithelium-derived Factor

Pigment epithelium-derived factor (PEDF), a natural substance produced by the body, was located for the first time in the spinal cord and skeletal muscles of humans, monkeys, and rats. Previously, scientists believed that PEDF was found only in the pigmented layer of cells beneath the retina. Using slices of rat spinal cords kept alive in culture, PEDF showed a dramatic ability to protect cells from the toxic effects of threohydroxyaspartate (THA), a chemical that mimics the effects of ALS, causing slow death of motor neurons. The PEDF-treated sections showed a near normal neuron count compared with untreated cultures. According to Dr. Ralph Kuncl, who led the

Johns Hopkins research team, protection of the spinal cord nerves in culture by PEDF was nearly complete. He went on to state that ". . . If we had this same level of protection in patients with ALS, they'd experience slight muscle weakness at most." The effectiveness of PEDF will be tested next on transgenic mouse models.

Neurturin

The same research team reported on another natural compound known as neurturin, a neurotrophic substance that will stimulate regeneration of damaged nerve cells. Neurotrophic factors, including PEDF and neurturin, are believed to protect healthy cells from the damaging effects of glutamate, a neurotransmitter that gluts the spaces between motor nerve cells, causing over-stimulation and contributing to the progression of the disease. Although Riluzole mildly restrains the immediate release of glutamate, it provides minimal protection to motor neurons as do PEDF and neurturin. The researchers predict the development of an "ALS cocktail," drug combinations containing neurotrophic factors, "each working at a different point in the process" (Bilak et al. 1999).

TGF-Beta

In a commentary, Miller and Ragsdale of the University of Chicago discuss the function of transforming growth factor-beta (TGF-beta) in the programmed death, or apoptosis, of nerve cells. TGF-beta is part of a family of growth factors by the same name that are involved in many biological functions in all of the body's tissues, such as embryonic development, reproduction, and wound-healing (Miller et al. 2000).

In a study reported in the same issue, chick embryos were immunized to neutralize the three forms of TGF-beta during the restricted period of embryonic development in which 50% of the neurons that have formed experience apoptosis. Neuron death was halted in all of the cells that were destined to die, which included central nervous system motor neurons and peripheral nervous system autonomic neurons. It is possible that TGF-beta works only on those neurons that will die, acting in a way that permits rather than instructs the cells to die. In other circumstances TGF-betas may enhance neuron survival. Researchers, led by Krieglstein of the University of Saarland at Homburg, Germany, concluded that TGF-beta could function as a molecular switch, which determines the life and death of neurons (Krieglstein et al. 2000).

The authors of the commentary state that the findings may have important implication for diseases, such as ALS, which is characterized by the death of motor neurons and may involve programmed cell death. Spinal cord trauma may involve neuron death by apoptosis as well. The removal of TGF-betas may be able to reduce the death of neurons and prevent some of the disability associated with this and other conditions.

TR500

TR500, a glutathione-repleting agent, is being studied for use in ALS (Hurko et al. 2000).

Deprenyl

Deprenyl (Eldepryl, selegiline hydrochloride), a selective monoamine oxidase B inhibitor, is partially effective in Parkinson's disease and can slow the cognitive deterioration in Alzheimer's disease. Studies of its use in ALS, however, did not show any significant improvement (Kuhn et al. 1996; Lange et al. 1998). Deprenyl is available from offshore pharmacies for personal use only.

Orap (Pimozide)

Orap (pimozide) is a voltage-dependent calcium channel blocker that is being explored for use in ALS. One study showed a significant decrease of the index of progression of the disease in Pimozide-treated patients compared to selegiline and vitamin E. In a randomized trial 44 patients, diagnosed as either definite or possible ALS, were treated with 1 mg a day of Pimozide for 3–12 months. Statistical analysis showed a significant decrease of the index of progression of the disease in Pimozide-treated patients as compared to the others (Szczudlik et al. 1998).

Neurontin (Gabapentin)

Neurontin (Gabapentin) is derived from GABA. Gabapentin prevents seizures in a wide variety of models in animals, including generalized tonic-clonic and partial seizures. In vitro, Gabapentin modulates the action of the GABA synthetic enzyme, glutamic acid decarboxylase (GAD), and the glutamate synthesizing enzyme, branched-chain amino acid transaminase. Results with human and rat brain NMR spectroscopy indicate that Gabapentin increases GABA synthesis. In vitro, Gabapentin reduces the release of several monoamine neurotransmitters (Taylor 1997; Taylor et al. 1998).

Unfortunately gabapentin was found to provide no evidence of a beneficial effect on disease progression or symptoms in patients with ALS in a Phase III randomized double-blind placebo trial (Miller et al. 2001).

DIET

People suffering with ALS should avoid eating processed foods (foods with preservatives and artificial ingredients) and only eat fresh, natural foods. Fresh fruits and vegetables are good because they provide vitamins and antioxidants. Meat, fish, eggs, and cheese, which contain proteins used to build muscle and should also be consumed. Nutrient-dense foods should be eaten. These are foods a person can eat much less of to get adequate nutrition.

Monosodium Glutamate

Dietary intake of glutamate is associated with an increased risk of ALS (Nelson et al. 2000). Glutamate is found in monosodium glutamate (MSG), which occurs naturally in many foods. The following foods should be avoided:

Table 1: *Monosodium Glutamate Content in Food*

High	Roquefort cheese, parmesan cheese, soy sauce
Medium	Walnuts, fresh tomato juice, grape juice, peas, mushrooms, broccoli, tomatoes, oysters, corn, potatoes
Low	Chicken, fish (mackerel), beef, eggs, cow's milk

High	over 1000 mg/100 grams
Medium	100–1000 mg/100 grams
Low	1–99 mg/100 grams

Source: MSG Facts http://www.msginfo.com

Aspartate

Aspartate, another potent neurotoxin, should also be avoided in chronic neurologic disease. Aspartic acid is found in artificial sweeteners such as aspartame (NutraSweet).

NUTRITIONAL SUPPLEMENTS

Most of the research on nutritional supplements for ALS focuses on several areas:

- Protection against glutamate toxicity with vitamin B_{12} (methylcobalamin) and S-adenosylmethionine (SAMe)

- Antioxidants including *N*-acetyl-cysteine, vitamin C, vitamin E, tocotrienol (palm-oil derived), and alpha-lipoic acid

- Protection and regeneration of neurons with methylcobalamin, the proper balance of omega-3 and omega-6 essential fatty acids, acetyl-*L*-carnitine, pregnenolone, and DHEA

- Improving mitochondrial function with coenzyme Q_{10} and creatine

- Growth stimulation with human growth hormone and testosterone

- Mineral deficiencies of magnesium, calcium, and vitamin D

- Miscellaneous supplements including ginseng, branched-chain amino acids, Hydergine, vinpocetine, and trimethylglycine(TMG)

Protection Against Glutamate Toxicity

One cause of brain cell death is glutamate toxicity. Brain cells use glutamate as a neurotransmitter, but unfortunately glutamate is a double-edged sword in that it can also kill aging brain cells. The release of glutamate from the synapses is the usual means by which neurons communicate with each other. Effective communication means controlled release of glutamate at the right time to the right cells. However, when glutamate is released in excessive amounts, intercellular communication ceases. It is like replacing radio signals with x-rays. The flood of glutamate onto the receiving neurons drives them into hyperactivity, and the excessive activity leads to cellular degradation.

Methylcobalamin and SAMe

It may be possible to protect brain cells against glutamate toxicity by taking methylcobalamin supplements. A study demonstrated that chronic exposure of rat cortical neurons to methylcobalamin protected against glutamate-, aspartate-, and nitroprusside-induced neurotoxicity. This study also showed that SAMe protected against neurotoxicity (Akaike et al. 1993).

A combination of methylcobalamin and SAMe was used to protect against retinal brain cell toxicity caused by glutamate and nitroprusside. The mechanism by which methylcobalamin protected against neurotoxicity was postulated by the researchers to be enhancement of brain cell methylation. The scientists who conducted these studies emphasized that chronic exposure of methylcobalamin was necessary to protect against neurotoxicity (Kikuchi et al. 1997).

Based on its unique mechanisms of action, methylcobalamin could be effective in slowing the progression of diseases such as ALS. Because methylcobalamin is not a drug, there is little economic incentive to conduct expensive clinical studies. It may be a long time before we know just how effective this vitamin B_{12} analog is in

Anxiety and Stress

Anxiety: from Latin, *anxietas,* meaning distressed, pained.
Stress: from Middle English *stresse,* stress; short form of *destresse,* distress.

Anxiety and stress are two of the most common types of mental disorders in the United States. The National Institute of Mental Health reports that 19 million Americans per year are afflicted by these illnesses (Narrow et al. 1998). Frequently, they coexist with depression, eating disorders (obesity, bulimia, and anorexia), and substance abuse. In 1990, the direct and indirect costs of these debilitating conditions to the American economy were more than $46 billion. In Britain, the Office of National Statistics reported that approximately one in seven adults has some form of diagnosable mental disorder, with anxiety being the most commonly reported complaint. Conditions associated with anxiety and stress include depression, phobias, and chronic fatigue. Furthermore, accumulated stress and anxiety can predispose patients to medical conditions such as chronic headaches, hypertension, ulcers, and heart disease. Some physicians estimate that stress and anxiety may be a contributing factor in 90% of all illnesses.

ANXIETY DISORDERS

Anxiety disorders are illnesses that cause people to feel frightened and apprehensive for no apparent reason. These conditions are often related to the biological and psychological makeup of the individual and may be familial in nature. If untreated, these illnesses can significantly reduce productivity and inhibit a person's ability to function in daily life. There are five types of anxiety disorders. Many individuals may have more than one type, making then especially difficult to treat.

Women also tend to suffer from these illnesses more than men. Approximately twice as many females have panic disorder, post-traumatic stress disorder, generalized anxiety disorder, agoraphobia (fear of open places or public situations), and other specific phobias. About an equal number of men and women are diagnosed with obsessive-compulsive disorder (OCD) (Bourdon et al. 1988; Robins et al. 1991; Davidson 2000).

Panic Disorder

This disorder is characterized by repeated episodes of intense fear that appear suddenly, often without warning and with varying frequency. Symptoms of panic disorder include chest pains, heart palpitations, sweating palms, dizziness, shortness of breath, a sense of unreality, or an uncontrollable fear of death. Panic disorder affects between three and six million Americans and is twice as likely to occur in women. Onset may occur at any age but generally begins in early adulthood.

Obsessive-Compulsive Disorder (OCD)

OCD is characterized by anxious thoughts and uncontrollable ritualistic behavior: obsessions are the anxious thoughts and compulsions are the rituals used to dispel those thoughts. An example of an obsession would be cleanliness and fear of germs. The compulsion associated with this obsession would be excessive hand washing. No pleasure is derived from performing the rituals; rather, the rituals provide only temporary relief. OCD appears to afflict men and women equally, and approximately one in fifty people may experience some sort of obsessive-compulsive behavior. Onset is typically in early adulthood, although it may occur in childhood or adolescence.

Post-Traumatic Stress Disorder (PTSD)

Common in those who have served in combat, PTSD is a debilitating illness that can result from a traumatic event. Originally defined as battle fatigue or shell shock, this disorder can be precipitated by any traumatic life event such as a serious accident, crime victimization, and natural disasters. People diagnosed with PTSD may relive the event in nightmares or have disturbing recollections of it during waking hours. Ordinary events can trigger flashbacks that may result in a loss of reality, causing the person to believe the event is happening again. PTSD may occur at any age, and although the course of the illness is variable, it can become chronic.

Phobias

These are seemingly inexplicable fears that may be either specific or social in nature. Specific phobias are irrational fears of certain things or situations such as heights; certain animals; or closed-in places, which is known as claustrophobia. This type of phobia may affect one in ten people. Currently, there are no medications for specific phobias. Social phobias are an intense fear of humiliation in a public situation and may be characterized by a feeling of dread beginning weeks in advance of a social event.

Generalized Anxiety Disorder (GAD)

Similar to agoraphobia, which is a fear of open places, GAD is much more serious than the daily anxiety most people feel. It is chronic, excessive worrying about health, personal finances, work, and family. GAD is characterized by difficulty sleeping, trembling or twitching, lightheadedness, irritability, muscle tension, headaches, and other symptoms. Depression may accompany the anxiety. The onset of GAD is gradual, generally occurring in childhood or adolescence, although adult onset is not uncommon. GAD occurs more frequently in women and may be familial in nature.

STRESS

Stress is a psychological and physical response to the demands of daily life that exceed a person's ability to cope successfully. Stress is often characterized by fatigue, sleep disorders, irritability, and constant worrying. Depression often accompanies stress. The accumulated effects of stress may lead to more serious medical problems. Stress may be work-related or may stem from personal problems, such as divorce, family conflicts, or financial concerns. Often stress results from a combination of these.

Too much stress is not good and sustained stressors often cause adverse effects. There is ample evidence that living a highly stressful lifestyle damages the heart, raises blood pressure, and can contribute to digestive problems. Not surprisingly, stress can also be damaging to the brain, even leading to premature brain cell aging (Uno et al. 1994; Sapolsky 1996a, 1996b; Lombroso et al. 1998). Most people are familiar with the adrenaline rush response to an emergency. The heart pounds, the muscles constrict, and the lungs expand; and while this is happening, we are capable of greater than normal strength and speed. This response is the body's way of rescuing itself when faced with an emergency. We don't have to think about it to make it happen. It's automatic.

The same can be said of the stress response. Whether we're stuck in traffic, about to give a speech in front of a group, or sitting in the waiting room at a doctor's office, the human stress response happens automatically. The difference between the two is that the adrenaline response in an emergency starts and resolves itself quickly. The response to being stuck in traffic may not. The adrenal glands, located above the kidneys, secrete adrenaline until the emergency passes. Then the body returns to its normal function. However, the stress response is more complex and can last longer. Studies have shown that long-term,

chronic stress may cause neural damage (McEwen 1991, 1997, 1999, 2000; Uno et al. 1994; McEwen et al. 1997). Just as prolonged increased levels of adrenaline result in adverse physiological effects, it has been less appreciated that excessive stress can also compromise the nervous system. Lombroso et al. (1998) reviewed the mechanisms by which stress impaired and contributed to brain aging and cognitive impairment.

As stated earlier, physical stress and psychological stress set off a chain of events in the brain and body. Adrenaline is released for quick energy to the muscles. More importantly, a small part of the brain, the hypothalamus, sends a signal to the pituitary gland to start adding a hormone called corticotrophin into the bloodstream. In turn, corticotrophin tells the adrenal glands to release other stress hormones—the glucocorticoids.

In the short term, glucocorticoids are beneficial to the body. Glucocorticoids electrify the hippocampus—the part of the brain related to memory—helping you remember stressful encounters, so you can deal with a similar situation the next time it occurs. This sharpening of memory explains why so many people vividly remember where they were when a certain terrible events occurred, such as the Challenger explosion or John F. Kennedy's assassination. After glucocorticoids flood the bloodstream, the hippocampus signals the hypothalamus to stop releasing corticotrophins, ending the stress response.

However, in those individuals who repeatedly experience stress, this feedback loop degrades. Memory worsens, energy levels diminish, and other health problems emerge (McCraty et al. 1998). The stress response turns on, but does not automatically turn off. A few days of exposure to high levels of stress hormones can weaken hippocampal brain cells, leaving them more likely to die if oxygen is interrupted, such as in a stroke (Lombroso et al. 1998).

Weeks of exposure can wither connections between neurons. Studies on rats indicate that continued stress will eventually destroy brain cells in the hippocampus. The good news is that alterations in dendritic atrophy can return to normal when stress is removed (Sousa et al. 2000). The key is to learn how to deal with daily stress to allow the body to return to its normal state (McCraty et al. 1998).

CONVENTIONAL TREATMENTS FOR ANXIETY AND STRESS

Conventional treatments for anxiety and stress include psychotherapy and medication. There are two types of psychotherapy: behavioral therapy and cognitive-behavioral therapy. Behavioral therapy uses several techniques such as diaphragmatic breathing and exposure therapy. Diaphragmatic breathing teaches people how to control anxiety by taking slow, deep breaths. Exposure therapy gradually exposes people to whatever frightens them to help them cope with their fears. Cognitive-behavioral therapy. Modification of thinking patterns that control the thoughts and sensations accompanying anxiety is an integral part of this form of therapy.

Two behavioral techniques, "Cut-Thru" and "Heart Lock-In," are designed to teach the elimination of negative thoughts and to promote a sense of well-being. Research by McCraty et al. (1998) examined the effects of Cut-Thru and Heart Lock-In on healthy adults. These techniques have been designed to develop and maintain shifts in dispositional approach to stressors by changing a person's interpretive style, breaking negative thought loops, and eliminating unhealthy emotional patterns. Since it has been suggested that recurring negative emotional patterns may lead to adverse physiological effects and decreased general well-being through inappropriate activation of the autonomic nervous system and glucocorticoid secretion, the research of McCraty et al. examined the effects of Cut-Thru and Heart Lock-In techniques on emotions, stress, cortisol/DHEA levels, and autonomic nervous system balance in 45 (15 controls) healthy adults.

After 1 month, participants in the experimental group experienced an increase in positive emotions and a decrease in negative emotions. No significant changes were seen in the control group. The experimental group also experienced a 23% reduction in cortisol and a 100% increase in DHEA levels. McCraty et al. suggest that their study establishes that (1) interpretive styles associated with stress and negative emotions can be changed within a short period of time; (2) changed perspectives influence stress, emotions, and important physiological parameters; and (3) people have greater control over their overall health by controlling their conditioned emotional responses than previously thought.

Often-Prescribed Medications

Often psychotherapy is used in combination with medication. Antidepressants are frequently used in combination with behavioral therapy to mitigate anxiety and stress. The two major classes of antidepressants are selective serotonin reuptake inhibitors (SSRIs), such as Prozac, Zoloft, Paxil, and Luvox, and tricyclic depressants (TCAs), such as Elavil and Tofranil. These medications work by inhibiting the reuptake of neurotransmitters, such as serotonin, resulting in the accumulation of these neurotransmitters. Brain chemicals such as serotonin are thought to be low in conditions such as anxiety and depression. Preventing their reuptake by the nerve cells essentially increases the amount of available chemical. Monoamine oxidase (MAO) inhibitors are also used to treat anxiety and function much the same as SSRIs and TCAs. Antidepressants are among the most widely prescribed medications in the United States.

Less frequently, benzodiazepines such as Valium, Xanax and Serax, may be prescribed to treat anxiety, but they are highly addictive agents that can cause depression if overused. Worse than addiction is the tolerance effect that causes patients to take increasing quantities of the benzodiazepine until the drug stops working altogether. Tolerance to benzodiazepines can occur in as little as a few weeks. Withdrawal symptoms can include hyperanxiety, confusion, anorexia, shaking, memory loss, and reemergence of the original symptoms. There are alternatives to these medications. Doctors sometimes prescribe the beta-blocker propranolol (Inderal) or atenolol (Tenormin) to counter performance anxiety. It works by blocking certain actions of the sympathetic nervous system, the part of our chemical make-up that causes us to feel stress. This reduces sensations of anxiety such as racing pulse, speeding thoughts, hand tremors, and nervousness. Potential side effects include slow pulse (less than 50 beats per minute), drowsiness, fatigue, dry mouth, numbness or tingling of fingers or toes, dizziness, diarrhea, nausea, weakness, and cold hands and feet.

LIFESTYLE CHANGES

Diet

Eating a variety of whole foods will replenish nutrients essential to a healthy nervous system. Some people have hypoglycemia, which are bouts of low blood sugar that can feel much like an anxiety attack. Eating small frequent meals can help, as can avoiding simple sugars (like candy), which produce a blood sugar rush, followed by a nerve-racking bottoming out.

Avoid Stimulants

Many anxious people are sensitive to caffeine. Try to wean yourself off coffee, tea, and anything else containing caffeine, or switch to noncaffeinated varieties of these beverages. Chocolate and herb guarana also contain caffeine. Other stimulants will also produce unwanted anxiety, such as ephedra or ma huang. Avoid these substances unless directed by a physician.

Supplements

Deficiencies of many vitamins, minerals, amino acids, and fatty acids can imbalance the nervous system. You can take a high-quality multivitamin and mineral formula and consider adding a B-complex supplement along with extra calcium and magnesium at a one to one ratio. This will ensure you are getting enough of these essential nutrients you may not be receiving from your diet alone.

One daily tbsp of flaxseed oil can boost your essential fatty acids or you may choose encapsulated omega-3 oils.

Get Enough Sleep

Of course, this seems like common sense, but studies demonstrate that the consequences of not getting enough sleep are anxiety and irritability, along with a host of other unpleasant side effects. To cope with this, follow a few simple suggestions. The condition of insomnia is examined in great deal in the *Insomnia protocol* of this book. In summary, try to make your bedroom a place only for sleep. Do not read, eat, or watch TV in the bedroom. This will help train your body to prepare for sleep the moment you lie down. Also avoid stimulating activities before going to bed, like reading a book, or exercising. Some dietary supplements that are helpful in establishing sleep are melatonin and kava kava. And although alcohol is technically a depressant, it can greatly interfere with your sleep patterns. Avoid alcohol and cigarettes before going to bed.

Exercise Regularly

Exercising 10 minutes before bedtime is obviously not a good idea, but setting a time of day for regular physical activity is good for your body in many ways, including establishing a normal and healthy sleep pattern (Salmon 2001). It gets you out of your head, releases pent-up emotion, and afterward leaves your muscles toned and relaxed. Pick an activity that you enjoy, so that exercising becomes less of a chore and more of an enjoyment. Try walking, swimming, bicycling, jogging, yoga, tai-chi, skiing, and tennis; even golf burns calories. Interestingly, a study found that leisure-time physical activity buffered people against physical symptoms and anxiety associated with minor stress. What mattered wasn't the person's level of aerobic fitness, but simply the regular participation in an enjoyable physical activity (Carmack 1999). Another study found that although light-intensity exercise lowered anxiety, high-intensity exercise intensified feelings of anxiety (Katula et al. 1999). Some people feel it is necessary to work themselves practically to exhaustion while exercising, while the research indicates that light-impact exercise on a regular basis is actually more effective. As in all things, moderation is the key.

Take a Break

For some people, life tends to go nonstop. Find some way to give the body and mind a break. Light a candle, stare at the aquarium, play with your dog, go for a walk, smell a rose, soak in a warm bath, take a nap, or reward yourself with a massage—anything to break from the relentlessness of your routine.

Massage Therapy

This ancient practice relaxes the body, promotes circulation, and helps you identify and release tense muscles. When your muscles are relaxed, it's hard to maintain an anxious state of mind. In one study, 26 adults were given a chair massage, two times a week for five weeks. A control group simply relaxed in the chair, without receiving a massage. Compared to the control group, the massage group had reduced anxiety, decreased salivary cortisol levels (a measurement of stress), lowered job stress scores, increased EEG patterns consistent with relaxed alertness, and increased speed and accuracy on math tests (Field et al. 1996). Massage also reduces the anxiety, depression, and pain associated with premenstrual syndrome (Hernandez-Reif et al. 2000).

Aromatherapy

Studies on the use of aromatherapeutic massage show it has a mild, transient anxiety-reducing effect (Cook et al. 2000). Aromatherapeutic massage involves adding 10–12 drops of essential plant oil to 1 oz of carrier oil such as almond oil. Calming scents include lavender, neroli, lemon balm, chamomile, geranium, and clary sage. You can also add 10 drops of an essential oil to a warm bath. The benefits aren't sufficient to cure anxiety or stress alone, but regular massage is a good way to relax and reduce stress.

Center Your Mind

Meditation relaxes body, mind, and spirit. A variety of techniques can induce a meditative state: silently repeating a mantra or a prayer, gazing at a lit candle, or focusing on your breathing. Research confirms that two types of meditation can relieve anxiety: Transcendental Meditation (TM) and mindfulness. TM is a simple and effortless way to quiet the mind and deeply relax the body. In a nutshell, you sit in a comfortable position with eyes closed and silently repeat a mantra (a meaningless, simple sound). Ideally, do this for 15–20 minutes morning and evening. Research shows that other benefits of this type of meditation include reduction in blood pressure, pain, and insomnia.

In one study, a group of 83 African-Americans were assigned to learn (1) TM, (2) progressive muscle relaxation, or (3) cognitive behavioral strategies. At follow-up testing one year later, both the meditation and the progressive muscle relaxation groups showed significant increases in overall mental health and decreases in anxiety (Gaylord et al. 1989).

Mindfulness is an ancient Buddhist meditation practice with a goal of full awareness of the present moment, without becoming distracted by thoughts of the past or future. In theory, this sounds simple; in actuality, maintaining this state of mind requires effort and discipline. As noted earlier, the results of McCraty et al. (1998) suggest that people do have greater control over their overall health than previously recognized and that they can learn techniques to "reprogram" how they respond to situations so that they experience lower stress levels, fewer negative emotions, and an increased positive lifestyle. Kabat-Zinn (1990, 1994), author and the founder and director of the Stress Reduction Clinic at the University of Massachusetts Medical Center in Worcester, has conducted studies showing that mindfulness meditation can reduce stress and anxiety.

In 1992, he showed that a mindfulness meditation program reduced anxiety and panic in people with generalized anxiety disorder, panic disorder, and panic disorder with agoraphobia (Kabat-Zinn 1992). In 1995, Kabat-Zinn and colleagues followed up on this original group of 22 patients and found that the majority of them continued the meditation practice and that it had long-term benefits in reducing anxiety and panic attacks (Miller et al. 1995). Shapiro et al. (1998) found that mindfulness meditation reduced stress and anxiety among premedical and medical students.

Breathing

This is the one involuntary body function you can consciously control. The first step is to simply bring your breathing under control:

1. Exhale completely.
2. Then slowly take a deep breath in through your nose.
3. Expand your diaphragm/belly to bring air into the lower portion of your lungs.
4. As you gradually fill your lungs from bottom to top, expand your chest.
5. Lift your shoulders for a last bit of fresh air.

6. Then relax and let the air flow smoothly out of your body.
7. Pull in your stomach at the end to expel the last bit of stress.
8. Then begin another breath.

Allen Elkin, program director of New York's Stress Management and Counseling Center, recommends the following breathing technique for rapid relaxation:

> You take a deep breath, deeper than normal, and hold it in until you notice a little discomfort. At the same time, squeeze your thumb and first finger together (as if you were making the okay sign) for six or seven seconds. Then exhale slowly through your mouth, release the pressure in your fingers, and allow all your tension to drain out. Repeat these deep breaths three times to extend the relaxation. With each breath, allow your shoulders to droop, your jaw to drop and your body to relax.

Other Relaxation Techniques

Aside from meditation and massage therapy, experience and research show that listening to music, visual imagery (sitting quietly and imaging peaceful scenes), muscle relaxation, biofeedback, yoga, tai chi (a form of moving meditation), and even social support sessions can all decrease symptoms of stress and anxiety (Jin 1992; Field et al. 1997; Malathi et al. 1999).

NATURAL TREATMENTS FOR ANXIETY AND STRESS

Adapton

The active ingredient in Adapton is *Garum amoricum* extract, a class of unique polypeptides which act as precursors to endorphins and other neurotransmitters that exert a regulatory effect on the nervous system. This action improves the body's ability to adapt to mentally and physically stressful conditions. Adapton is widely used in Europe and Japan for the treatment of stress, anxiety, and depression. Some physicians in the United States are now prescribing its use in lieu of antidepressants. An extract of a deep sea fish, the garum, Adapton is a naturally occurring substance. It functions at the cellular level to increase energy efficiency, resulting in improved concentration, mood, and sleep while promoting a general sense of well-being. A number of European clinical trials document the beneficial effects of Adapton:

> Twenty patients with chronic, stress-related fatigue participated in a study in which they were given a placebo for 2 weeks, followed by a 2-week trial usage of

Adapton. Patients reported a 14% reduction in fatigue and a 4% reduction in the symptoms of anxiety and insomnia following the placebo trial period. After using Adapton for 2 weeks, patients reported a 51% decrease in fatigue, and the symptoms of anxiety improved by 65%. The results of the study indicated that Adapton was effective in the treatment of patients with chronic stress and fatigue.

In a study of 40 patients with chronic fatigue syndrome, Adapton was prescribed for a 2-week period. Using the Fatigue Study Group's criteria for the 10 functions that most accurately measure fatigue and depression, the results of the study showed that 50% of the participants reported beneficial effects from Adapton.

A study of 60 patients using garum extract reported three cases of mild side effects, including nervous irritation, heartburn, and diarrhea. No emotional stress or fatigue was reported, leading researchers to conclude that garum was a safe and effective treatment of anxiety and stress. Other beneficial effects included improved learning and enhanced electroencephalograph (EEG) readings.

Overall, Adapton benefits 90% of patients suffering from chronic stress and fatigue as compared with a 30% improvement rate in patients using placebos.

In Europe, hyperactive children with attention deficit disorder are being treated with Adapton rather than Ritalin, with positive results.

Overall, researchers in these European clinical trials reported that Adapton was well-tolerated, produced no major side effects, and had no apparent contraindications.

Adapton consists of a standardized dosage of polypeptides, which act as precursors to neurotransmitters and exert a regulatory effect on the nervous system, thereby improving the body's ability to adapt to mental and physical stress. Adapton contains an omega-3 essential fatty acid that enhances certain prostaglandins and prostacyclin, the chemical mediators that regulate major biological functions. These polypeptides are believed to contribute to the stress-relieving effects of Adapton. Adapton is a safe, effective, low-cost alternative to traditional antidepressant medications and may provide substantial beneficial effects to people suffering from chronic, stress-induced anxiety, fatigue, or depression. The recommended dosage of Adapton is 4 capsules taken in the morning on an empty stomach for 15 days. Thereafter, the dose is reduced to 2 capsules each morning. If complete relief of the symptoms occurs, Adapton may be discontinued and restarted if the symptoms return. There

is no toxicity involved in the daily use of Adapton. Some patients use 2–3 capsules of Adapton every other day and still report relief of their symptoms.

For people who suffer from panic attacks, the addition of a 10-mg dose of the cardiovascular medication propranolol can produce immediate results. Propranolol is a beta-adrenergic blocker that inhibits the overproduction of adrenaline during a panic attack. The low dose of propranolol required to produce this effect is well-tolerated by the majority of patients.

Reducing Cortisol Levels Naturally

In addition to Adapton, there are a number of other stress-reducing treatments currently available. One of these treatments is KH3, a European medication. KH3 mitigates the effects of the overproduction of cortisol, the adrenal hormone that can occur with anxiety and stress. The overproduction of cortisol has been shown to damage the immune system, arteries, and brain cells, and it may cause premature aging.

Suggested dosage: 1–2 tablets taken on an empty stomach in the morning and afternoon. KH3 should not be taken by people allergic to procaine (the active ingredient in the medication), is contraindicated for patients taking sulfa drugs, and should not be used by children or pregnant or lactating women. In addition to KH3, the hormones melatonin and dehydroepiandrosterone (DHEA) may also reduce and protect against the effects of cortisol. The recommended dose range of melatonin is from 500 mcg to 3 mg taken approximately one half hour before bedtime. DHEA should be taken in a dose of 25–50 mg a day.

CAUTION Prior to taking DHEA, refer to the *DHEA Replacement Therapy protocol.*

The Calming Effect of Theanine

Theanine is an amino acid found in tea that produces a calming effect on the brain (Yokogoshi et al. 1998b). It easily crosses the blood-brain barrier and exerts subtle changes in biochemistry that cause a tranquilizing effect. The production of GABA, the brain chemical known for its calming effect, is increased after taking theanine. Increased GABA can also put you in a better mood and create a sense of well-being. Dopamine, another brain chemical with mood-enhancing properties is also increased by theanine.

Japanese researchers have discovered that theanine is a caffeine antagonist, meaning that it offsets the "hyper" effect of caffeine (Kakuda et al. 2000). That is why many people will have a "soothing" cup of tea and not a soothing cup of coffee. Theanine does not cause drowsiness like kava kava, nor does it interfere with the ability to think clearly like prescription tranquilizers.

There is evidence that tea exerts far more than just a psychological effect. According to one study, drinking one or more cups of tea can almost halve the risk of heart attack (Sesso et al. 1999). Green tea contains a much higher concentration of theanine than other teas. Theanine has been proven to lower blood pressure (Abe et al. 1995; Yokogoshi et al. 1995; Yokogoshi et al. 1998a). It works through its GABA enhancing effects. Along with its calming effect on the brain, GABA also lowers blood pressure. Genetically hypertensive rats taking 2000 mg of theanine per kg of body weight each day showed significant reductions in blood pressure. Green tea extract contains a phytochemical known as GMA that also lowers blood pressure. Combining them may have significant effects. Theanine is now available in the United States as a dietary supplement.

Suggested dosage: The suggested dose of theanine to induce a state of relaxation is 100 mg. For those seeking a continuous mood elevating effect, 1 theanine capsule can be taken 4 times throughout the day.

Adaptogens: Herbs for Maintaining Energy and Coping with Stress

An adaptogen is a substance that helps the body deal with and recover from stress. By balancing various organ systems, herbal adaptogens also help us feel more vital and energetic. The following list highlights a few of the premiere adaptogenic herbs.

Asian Ginseng (Panax Ginseng) and American Ginseng (P. quinquefolius)

Asian and American Ginseng enhance immune function, lower blood sugar levels, reduce the risk of certain cancers, and improve adrenal function, physical performance, and mental alertness. "Ginseng is generally prescribed for conditions characterized by great weakness or conditions that are the result of great stress or strain," says Korngold (1991). Because ginseng can be stimulating, he finds it most appropriate for people over 40, whose "core energies have begun to decline."

One study found that when 12 menopausal women took 6 grams of Asian ginseng root a day for 30 days, they experienced significant reductions in anxiety, fatigue, insomnia, and depression. By the end of treatment, measurements for these symptoms were on par with an age-matched group of eight women who were not experiencing these menopausal symptoms. The treatment group also had reduced levels of the stress hormone cortisol, thus favorably altering the ratio of cortisol to DHEA (Tode et al. 1999).

Suggested dosage: For nonstandardized products, the usual dosage is up to four 500–600-mg capsules a day. For a product standardized to 5–7% ginsenosides, take 100 mg, 1–2 times a day. Brown (1996) recommends taking ginseng for 2–3 weeks, followed by a 1–2 week break, then repeat.

CAUTION Not recommended for pregnant or nursing women or people with high blood pressure. Don't take ginseng without medical supervision if you're on a blood-thinner such as warfarin or have diabetes (as your insulin dosage will need to be adjusted due to ginseng's ability to lower blood sugar). Discontinue use if ginseng produces ill effects such as an elevated blood pressure, hot flashes, insomnia, nervousness, or irritability. Combining ginseng with caffeine and other stimulants increases the risk of over-stimulation.

Eleuthero or Siberian Ginseng (Eleutherococcus Senticosus)

Eleuthero or Siberian ginseng has been used for 2000 years as a Chinese medicine for invigorating the Qi (vital energy) and promoting overall health. Although research in the former Soviet Union suggested that eleuthero improves athletic performance, preliminary research in the United States has failed to show significant benefit. It is said to sharpen mental alertness and help cope with stress. Compounds in eleuthero have been shown to have antioxidant, anticancer, cholesterol-lowering, immune-stimulating, radioprotective, anti-inflammatory, and fever-lowering properties (Davydov et al. 2000).

Suggested dosage: Twenty drops of tincture up to 3 times a day. Up to nine 400–500 mg capsules a day.

Reishi (Ganoderma Lucidum)

Reishi tones the immune system, supports nerve function, scavenges free radicals, protects the liver, and quells inflammation and allergies. According to Hobbs (1996), "Reishi has the unique ability among medicinal mushrooms to calm and support nerve function." In his practice, he recommends reishi to people with chronic stress, anxiety, or insomnia.

Suggested dosage: Reishi is available in capsules, tablets, syrups, and teas. Usual dosages are up to five 420-mg capsules a day; up to three 1 gram tablets up to 3 times a day; up to 2 tsp 2–3 times a day of tincture; or 1 tsp a day of the syrup.

Ashwaganda (Withania Somnifera)

Ashwaganda, also called Indian ginseng, has long been used by Ayurvedic practitioners as a rejuvenating tonic. A research review notes that this herb has anti-inflammatory, antitumor, antistress, antioxidant, immunomodulatory, and rejuvenating properties (Mishra et al. 2000). This data came largely from laboratory studies. Human studies on ashwaganda's stress-reducing ability have yet to be published in English-language journals. Douillard, an Ayurvedic physician in Boulder, CO, says his clinical experience is that this herb fortifies our ability to cope with stress, reduces anxiety, and also improves mental acuity, reaction time, and physical performance (Douillard et al. 2001).

Suggested dosage: Douillard recommends 500 mg 3 times a day of the powdered herb in tablets or capsules.

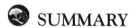 ## SUMMARY

Prescription antidepressants and other prescription medications for the treatment of anxiety-related disorders often produce unwanted side effects, have more contraindications, and may become habit forming in some cases. Alternatives to these treatments, such as Adapton, have proven to be safe and effective in the treatment of stress, anxiety, and fatigue. There are fewer reported side effects in those patients using natural substances such as Adapton, theanine, DHEA, and melatonin, and there may be greater long-term benefits involved. As with any medication, it is advisable to consult your physician prior to any treatment program.

1. Reduce environmental causes of stress as much as possible.

2. Behavioral modification techniques such as diaphragmatic breathing and exposure therapy may be beneficial.

3. Lifestyle changes that include dietary changes, exercise, and meditation can reduce symptoms of stress and anxiety.

4. A high-quality multivitamin and mineral formula such as Life Extension Mix for essential nutrients that may be missing from the diet, along with extra calcium and magnesium at a one to one ratio.

5. Adapton, 4 capsules in the morning on an empty stomach for 15 days; reduce to 2 capsules in the morning after 2 weeks.

6. For patients with panic attacks, the addition of 10 mg of propranolol or 25 mg atenolol in combination with Adapton may be highly effective.

7. Theanine, 100 mg daily to produce a calming effect or 400 mg (4 capsules) throughout the day for a mood-enhancing effect.

8. Melatonin, 300 mcg to 10 mg in the evening, one half hour prior to bedtime.

9. DHEA, 25–50 mg a day. (*Refer to DHEA Replacement Therapy protocol.*)

10. Ginseng may help relieve symptoms of stress and reduce cortisol levels; one or two 200-mg Sports Ginseng capsules daily are recommended.

11. Consider conventional medications such as SSRIs and tricyclic antidepressants if natural therapies fail to relieve symptoms.

 ### PRODUCT AVAILABILITY

Adapton, melatonin, DHEA, theanine, Life Extension Mix, Sports Ginseng, and calcium-magnesium formulas are available by calling (800) 544-4440 or ordering online at www.lef.org. Ask for a listing of offshore companies that sell KH3 to American citizens by mail for personal use.

Arthritis

The word arthritis literally means inflammation of the joint. Joints can become inflamed for many reasons, but most of us think of arthritis usually as one of two kinds: osteoarthritis or rheumatoid arthritis. These are two very distinct entities, and they are both a huge source of discomfort and disability. A significant amount of new research provides an understanding of both kinds of arthritis so that those who are afflicted may find relief.

The prevalence of arthritis and other rheumatic conditions in the United States is very high and is projected to rise as the population ages. Arthritis is a leading cause of disability among persons over age 64. In this protocol, you will learn about the underlying cause of most forms of arthritis and how you may be able to reverse these degenerative processes.

THE NORMAL JOINT

To understand diseases of the joint, we need to look at the normal healthy joint. Joints are held together by a joint capsule that is designed to allow smooth movement between adjacent bones. In the type of joint that is commonly affected by arthritic diseases (the highly movable joints), the bone ends are covered by articular cartilage over which the joint moves. A synovial membrane encloses the joint space itself. This thin membrane secretes synovial fluid that lubricates the space between the cartilage-covered, joint-forming bones. The cartilage contains no blood vessels or nerves and receives its nutrients by diffusion from the synovial fluid and from the bone.

Joint function depends on the health of the cartilage in the joint and the synovial membrane. Cartilage is a gel-like substance that acts as a shock absorber, essential for smooth and easy movement in the joint. Cartilage gets its elasticity from collagen fibers and its sponge-like quality from water, held together by a structure of big molecules called proteoglycans. Special cells (called chondrocytes) in the cartilage produce collagen and proteoglycans (Fassbender 1987). Joints can withstand enormous pressure by slowly releasing water from the cartilage.

As we age, the ability to restore and maintain a normal cartilage structure decreases. The activity of important repair enzymes is reduced, the water content diminished, and the joints become more prone to damage. Scientists are just now beginning to understand the specific mechanisms involved in the development of arthritis and how to effectively correct them.

Conventional medicine previously offered only symptomatic, temporary relief from chronic arthritic conditions. High doses of the nonsteroidal anti-inflammatory drugs (NSAIDs) are effective in reducing symptoms quickly but can cause side effects such as ulcers and gastrointestinal bleeding, and NSAIDs do not stop the progression of arthritis. In the long run, some antiarthritic drugs may actually worsen the condition by accelerating joint destruction.

However, in the last few years, research has brought hope to this dismal picture. New prescription drugs neutralize some of the inflammatory factors involved in joint cartilage destruction. Also, a compelling body of evidence shows that the proper combination of natural therapies such as fish and borage oils may work better than some of these prescription drugs. By taking advantage of this nutritional information, one can achieve not only symptomatic relief, but actually intervene at the root of the problem and help the body to rebuild functioning joints.

BIOCHEMICAL MECHANISMS OF ARTHRITIS

Inflammation is a living tissue response to mechanical, chemical, and immunological challenge. Normal aging often results in the excessive production of autoimmune factors that destroy joint cartilage and other tissues in the body. Suppressing these inflammatory factors is a critical component of an effective arthritis treatment program.

Inflammation is partially characterized by high levels of arachidonic acid products which are metabolized along two different enzymatic pathways: cyclooxygenase (COX) and lipoxygenase, leading to prostaglandin (PGE-2) and leukotriene (LTB4). Some physicians believe these are the most important mediators of inflammation (Srivastava et al. 1992). PGE2 and LTB4 play a crucial role in arthritis by causing resorption of bone, stimulating the secretion of collagen breakdown enzymes, and inhibiting the formation of proteoglycans—the building blocks of cartilage.

The destruction of cartilage and bone in both osteoarthritis (OA) and rheumatoid arthritis (RA) is related to the action of matrix enzymes (metalloproteinases), which include collagenases and stromelysins

Osteoarthritis

- Usually does NOT cause redness, warmth, or inflammation of joints
- Initially affects joints on one side of the body
- Does NOT cause a general feeling of sickness
- Usually develops slowly over many years

Rheumatoid Arthritis

- Redness, warmth, and swelling of joints
- Usually affects the same joint on both sides of the body
- Often causes a general feeling of sickness, fatigue, weight loss, and fever
- May develop suddenly, within weeks or months
- Usually begins between ages 25 and 50

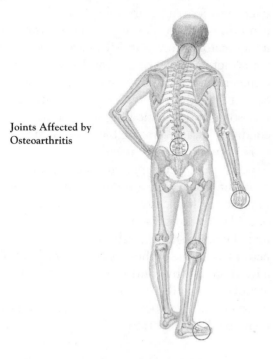

Joints Affected by Osteoarthritis

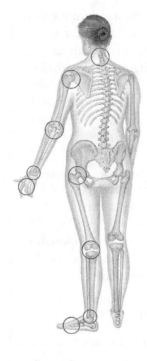

Joints Affected by Rheumatoid Arthritis

Comparison of symptoms of osteoarthritis vs. rheumatoid arthritis and joints typically affected. (Anatomical Chart Company 2002®, Lippincott Williams & Wilkins)

(Birkedal-Hansen et al. 1993; Hill et al. 1994). Some of these enzymes have pro-inflammatory characteristics and some have anti-inflammatory properties. The varying balance between these forces probably accounts for the variation in disease activity as it flares up and subsides. These enzymes are under the control of cytokines, such as interleukin 1 (IL-1b) and tumor necrosis factor-alpha (TNF-alpha), which are highly activated in RA and are elevated in the synovial membrane, the synovial fluid, and the cartilage of OA patients (Saklatvala 1986). Cytokines are proteins that carry messages between cells and regulate immunity and inflammation. In animal models, inhibition of TNF-alpha results in decreased inflammation, while inhibition of IL-1b effectively prevents cartilage destruction (Plows et al. 1995; Frye et al. 1996).

Health-conscious people should become familiar with pro-inflammatory cytokines because excess levels cause or contribute to many disease states. The following acronyms represent the most dangerous pro-inflammatory cytokines:

- Tumor necrosis factor alpha (TNF-*a*)

- Interleukin-6 (IL-6)

- Interleukin-beta (IL-1b)

Data from many studies confirm the important role of TNF-alpha in regulating production of both inflammatory and anti-inflammatory mediators in RA. Because of the demonstrated excess of pro-inflammatory cytokines, such as TNF-alpha, it was hypothesized that a blockade of TNF-alpha should be beneficial. Several experimental as well as clinical studies have been conducted with an anti-TNF-alpha antibody (Paulus et al. 1990). The results have confirmed that suppression of TNF-alpha is an effective treatment modality in treating RA. In addition to inhibiting TNF-alpha, it is also crucial to suppress excessive levels of PGE2, LTB4, IL-1, and IL-6. We now know how to suppress all of these pro-inflammatory factors that are involved in joint cartilage destruction.

CURRENT MEDICAL TREATMENT

The conventional treatment for both OA and RA has consisted of NSAIDs, including aspirin. Even stronger disease-modifying drugs such as corticosteroids, gold salts, and methotrexate are often prescribed for RA in an aggressive attempt to stop the development of the disease. These drugs are all aimed at alleviating pain and reducing inflammation. They can sometimes be effective, but more often, however, they prove unsatisfactory and many times intolerable due to toxicity. High-dose aspirin, for example, is effective, but it often causes gastric irritation and tinnitus (ringing in the ears) with the large dosages needed (Hubsher et al. 1979). Other NSAIDs may have an even greater risk for serious side effects, which limit their use. These treatments are only symptomatic because they do not act on the causes of arthritis and do not stop the progression of the disease. In fact, the opposite has shown to be true. It has been demonstrated in some studies that NSAIDs actually have an inhibitory effect on cartilage repair and accelerate cartilage destruction (Solomon 1973; Ronningen et al. 1979; Brooks et al. 1982; Newman et al.1985; Shield 1993).

How can it be that NSAIDs help relieve symptoms but facilitate cartilage destruction at the same time? NSAIDs exert their analgesic and anti-inflammatory effects through the inhibition of the enzyme COX. The discovery that two forms of COX (COX-1 and COX-2) exist has clarified the dual nature of NSAIDs (Needleman et al. 1979). While relieving pain and inflammation through COX-2 blockade, they also block, via COX-1, the biotransformation of arachidonic acid to substances that carry out various homeostatic (balancing) physiological functions, one of which is to protect the gastrointestinal mucosa and limit gastric acid output.

While NSAIDs inhibit PGE2 synthesis through a COX-2 blockade, they fail to influence the TNF-alpha and IL-1b activation of cartilage-destroying enzymes. NSAIDs also create what is known as a *leaky gut* that allows unwanted, partially digested protein products to enter the bloodstream via the intestine (Hollander 1999). These products can cause more inflammation and further activate an already over-stimulated immune response.

With this enhanced understanding of the underlying mechanisms for current medical treatment, researchers are now looking for new compounds that will relieve pain and inflammation and enhance the repair process in the joints without inhibiting important physiological functions. COX-2-specific inhibitors (e.g., Vioxx and Celebrex), are widely promoted,

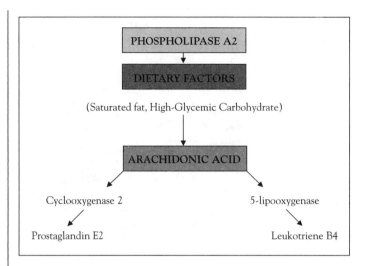

but they are showing similar side effects because they do not leave the COX-1 pathways totally unaffected. Another problem with COX-2 inhibitors is that while they block the formation of PGE2 from arachidonic acid, they do not adequately suppress the formation of LTB4 from arachidonic acid. In order to suppress both PGE2 and LTB4, it is necessary to inhibit their common precursor, which is arachidonic acid.

As can be seen from the chart, arachidonic acid converts to PGE2 by using the COX-2 enzyme. Arachidonic acid also converts to the pro-inflammatory cytokine LTB4 using the enzyme 5-lipoxygenase. Since drugs such as Celebrex only inhibit COX-2, they potentially leave more arachidonic acid available to convert to joint-destroying LTB4 (via the lipoxygenase pathway). Due to heavy marketing practices, Celebrex and Vioxx quickly became highly popular drugs. However, the FDA has written to both companies accusing them of minimizing side effects and over-promoting positive effects.

Celebrex could lead to bleeding in persons taking warfarin; serious gastrointestinal (GI) symptoms can occur without warning. Celebrex should not be used by persons allergic to sulfa, or by people who have an asthma attack upon taking aspirin. In addition, Celebrex and Vioxx are not for acute pain. We intentionally do not discuss these drugs in detail because of their toxicity potential.

A Partially Effective, But Cost-Prohibitive Drug

Enbrel is an FDA-approved drug that treats RA by suppressing the destructive cytokine, TNF-alpha. Enbrel is relatively safe, with the primary side effect being injection site reactions. Since TNF-alpha is needed to fight acute infectious disease, when one has a serious infection, Enbrel therapy is temporarily discontinued until the infection subsides.

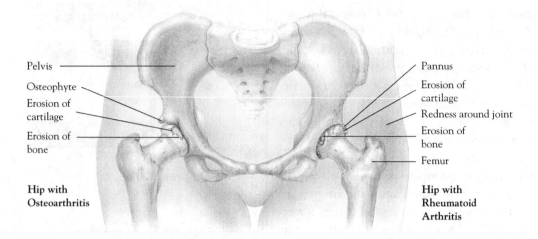

Pelvis
Osteophyte
Erosion of cartilage
Erosion of bone

**Hip with
Osteoarthritis**

Pannus
Erosion of cartilage
Redness around joint
Erosion of bone
Femur

**Hip with
Rheumatoid
Arthritis**

Warning Signs of Arthritis
- Pain in one or more joints
- Inabilty to move a joint normally
- Joint swelling sometimes

If you have any of these signs for more than
two weeks, contact your physician.

Illustration of bone and cartilage degeneration in the hip from osteoarthritis (left) and rheumatoid
arthritis (right). (Anatomical Chart Company 2002®, Lippincott Williams & Wilkins)

The high cost of Enbrel makes it prohibitive for most people (about $11,000 a year). It usually requires two visits every week to a physician's office for injections though some patients can administer their own injections at home. Many HMOs insist that arthritis patients use less costly COX-2 inhibiting drugs such as Celebrex or Vioxx in lieu of the more expensive Enbrel. COX-2 inhibiting drugs, however, are not as effective as Enbrel.

While Enbrel is only approved by the FDA for RA, it may also be effective in protecting against the cartilage destruction that occurs in OA. Both TNF-alpha and IL-1b have been shown to play a role in the cartilage destruction and inflammatory process characteristic of OA (Feldman et al. 2000). Even if one has insurance that will pay for Enbrel, a diagnosis of RA is still required for an insurance company to cover the cost of Enbrel. This means that those with OA face the prospect of both having to pay the $11,000 yearly out-of-pocket cost and locating a physician willing to prescribe Enbrel for an unapproved use, that is, the treatment of OA.

Enbrel has demonstrated impressive clinical results, but it only suppresses TNF-alpha. To adequately deal with the multiple processes involved in arthritic cartilage destruction, it is usually necessary to also reduce elevated levels of PGE2, LTB4, IL-1, IL-6, and TNF-alpha.

The Life Extension Foundation has identified safe methods to inhibit these multiple inflammatory factors involved in the arthritic process.

Following the Protocol

OA and RA have certain features in common, mainly inflammation. Because the inflammatory pathways are similar whatever the cause, some of the treatments will be similar for both forms of arthritis, whereas in some cases research has been more firmly dedicated to one kind or the other. In the protocol that follows, we have tried to be clear about dietary changes, drugs, hormones, and supplements that are being overlooked by conventional physicians.

CHRONIC INFLAMMATION...THE UNDERLYING VILLAIN

Chronic inflammation inflicts devastating effects, especially as we grow older. The pathological consequences of inflammation are fully documented in the medical literature (Licinio et al. 1999; Deon et al. 2001; Kanda 2001; Smith et al. 2001). Regrettably, the dangers of systemic inflammation continue to be ignored, even though proven ways exist to reverse this problem.

Many people join the Life Extension Foundation (LEF) because they suffer from the effects of various degenerative diseases. A common culprit found in these frail individuals is systemic inflammation.

Aging results in an increase of inflammatory cytokines (destructive cell-signaling chemicals) that contribute to many degenerative diseases. RA is a classic autoimmune disorder in which excess levels of cytokines such as TNF-alpha, IL-6, and IL-1b are known to cause or contribute to the inflammatory syndrome (Feldmann et al. 1996). Some of these same inflammatory factors can contribute to OA (Fernandes et al. 2002; Futani et al. 2002; Nishimura et al. 2002).

While chronic inflammation often symptomatically manifests as arthritis, it is also involved in diseases as diverse as atherosclerosis, heart valve dysfunction, congestive heart failure, Alzheimer's disease, and even cancer. In elderly people with multiple degenerative diseases, blood levels of C-reactive protein are often sharply elevated, indicating the presence of an underlying inflammatory disorder. When a cytokine blood profile is conducted in those with high C-reactive protein, we usually find excessive levels of one or more of the inflammatory factors (TNF-alpha, IL-6, IL-1b, and LTB4).

Scientists have identified dietary supplements and prescription drugs that can reduce levels of the pro-inflammatory cytokines. The docosahexaenoic acid (DHA) fraction of fish oil, for example, is the best documented supplement to suppress TNF-alpha, IL-6, IL-1b, and LTB4 (Khalfoun et al. 1997; Watanabe et al. 2000; Deon et al. 2001). Research studies in healthy humans and in persons with rheumatoid disease show that fish oil suppresses these dangerous inflammatory factors by up to 90% (James et al. 2000).

Other cytokine-lowering supplements are dehydroepiandrosterone (DHEA) (Daynes et al. 1993; Kipper-Galperin et al. 1999; Haden et al. 2000), vitamin K (Reddi et al. 1995; Weber 1997), gamma-linolenic acid (GLA) (Purasiri et al. 1994; Mancuso et al. 1997; Dirks et al. 1998; DeLuca et al. 1999), and nettle leaf extract (Teucher et al. 1996). Antioxidants (such as vitamin E and N-acetyl-cysteine) may also lower pro-inflammatory cytokines (Gosset et al. 1999; Devaraj et al. 2000) and protect against their toxic effects (Winrow et al. 1993; Horton et al. 2001; Langlois et al. 2001).

Prescription drugs such as Enbrel directly bind to TNF-alpha and block its interaction with TNF cell surface receptors. Enbrel has demonstrated significant clinical improvement in RA patients, as have high-dose fish oil supplements (Kremer 2000). There are no side-by-side comparison studies to determine whether fish oil or Enbrel is better.

WHEN CONVENTIONAL DRUGS ARE NOT ENOUGH

A problem identified by LEF is that high levels of TNF-alpha may persist even in people receiving Enbrel drug therapy. Even if Enbrel brings TNF-alpha down to a safe range, other inflammatory cytokines (such as IL-6 and IL-1b) may continue to wreak havoc throughout the body.

High levels of TNF-alpha are destructive to many vital tissues such as joint cartilage (e.g., RA) and heart muscle (e.g., congestive heart failure). Excess IL-6 and other inflammatory cytokines attack bone and cartilage and promote the formation of fibrinogen that can induce a heart attack or stroke via several established mechanisms (di Minno et al. 1992).

In order to prevent and treat the multiple diseases of aging, it is critical to keep these destructive immune chemicals (cytokines) in safe ranges. The chart found in the Summary section of this protocol relates the currently determined safe ranges of inflammatory factors as measured by blood levels.

Supplements such as DHA fish oil, nettle leaf extract, vitamin K, and DHEA have been shown to suppress the dangerous cytokines, TNF-alpha, IL-6, IL1b, and the pro-inflammatory eicosanoid LTB4. We discuss these supplements in detail later in this protocol. For those whose blood tests reveal persistently high inflammatory cytokine levels despite taking these supplements, a low-cost prescription drug may be of enormous benefit.

The generic name of this drug is pentoxifylline (PTX); the brand name is Trental. It was first used in Europe in 1972 and long ago came off patent (meaning it is not cost-prohibitive). PTX is prescribed to improve the flow properties of blood by decreasing its viscosity. It works by improving red blood cell flexibility, decreasing platelet aggregation, and reducing fibrinogen levels (Manrique et al. 1987; di Minno et al. 1992; de la Cruz et al. 1993; Gara 1993; Gaur et al. 1993). PTX has fallen out of favor because no drug company has the economic incentive to market it to physicians. PTX is primarily prescribed to patients with peripheral artery disease, although we believe it has potential efficacy in treating a wide range of diseases relating to chronic inflammation.

Numerous studies show that PTX is a potent inhibitor of TNF-alpha, IL-1b, IL-6, and other pro-inflammatory cytokines (Neuner et al. 1994; Blam et al. 2001; Pollice et al. 2001). A similar number of studies show that

DHA fish oil suppresses these same cytokines (De Caterina et al. 1998, 1999; Das et al. 2000; James et al. 2000; Kelley et al. 1999; Kremer 2000; Watanabe et al. 2000). In people suffering from the effects of a chronic disease involving elevated levels of the inflammatory cytokines, the daily administration of 800 mg of PTX or 1000–2000 mg of DHA fish oil could be of enormous benefit.

The first line of defense in protecting against excess pro-inflammatory cytokine activity is proper diet and use of appropriate cartilage-protecting supplements. We will discuss antiarthritic diets next. For arthritic patients who are unable to obtain relief via dietary modification and supplements, we suggest that PTX be considered as a cytokine-suppression therapy.

Why does your physician not tell you about PTX? The reason is that the FDA prohibits the companies that manufacture PTX from distributing off-label information about its potential antiarthritic benefits. Life Extension can provide this information because we do not sell PTX. Before taking PTX, refer to the precautions that we list at the end of this protocol.

Convincing a physician to prescribe PTX as an adjuvant therapy for arthritis can be difficult. That is why most people first choose to try natural therapies that have a proven track record of safety and efficacy.

THE IMPORTANCE OF ADDRESSING ALL THE INFLAMMATORY PATHWAYS

The body's inflammatory pathway has two branches, COX (cyclooxygenase) and LOX (lipoxygenase). Aspirin and other non-steroidal anti-inflammatory drugs (NSAIDs), long the mainstays of arthritis treatment, block COX in both its forms, COX-1 and COX-2. COX-2 produces prostaglandins, which are powerful triggers of pain and inflammation. However, COX-1 is necessary for stomach lining protection, so interfering with its activity can cause gastrointestinal disturbances ranging from simple discomfort to bleeding ulcers. For this reason the new COX-2 inhibitors, which block COX-2 with little effect on COX-1 are more desirable and more expensive.

Medications that block COX-2 and have little or no effect on COX-I include Celebrex, Vioxx, and Bextra. Although all three drugs work on the same COX-2 pathway, if one drug does not relieve the symptoms of inflammation, another might work for that particular individual. Therefore, it is worth a trial of switching from one COX-2 inhibiting agent to a different one under such circumstances. Although the new COX-2 inhibitors are marketed with emphasis on the advantage of not blocking the necessary COX-1 pathway, infrequent reports of gastrointestinal problems still exist from the use of these medications. An over-the-counter COX-2 inhibitor called Nexrutin provides a natural way to inhibit the COX-2 pathway. Curcumin also provides some COX-2 inhibition.

The LOX pathway produces leukotrienes. When only COX-2 is blocked, the LOX pathway still produces these potent mediators of inflammation and the condition may even be exacerbated by blocking only the inflammatory cascade of COX-2, thus allowing the LOX branch to accelerate the formation of leukotrienes.

The pharmaceutical industry is aware of this phenomenon and some companies have been working on the development of prescription medications that block both the COX-2 and the LOX pathways of inflammation. Thus far, they have not been able to bypass certain limiting barriers to the production of such a medication. The good news is that there exists a natural LOX inhibiting agent that can be combined with Nexrutine as well as with other compounds that block the pro-inflammatory cytokines. This LOX inhibitor is called boswellic acid or 5-loxin.

This is important since some researchers have found that COX-2 inhibition alone results in the exacerbation of the production of pro-inflammatory cytokines such as tumor necrosis factor alpha (TNF-alpha) and interleukin-1 beta (IL-1beta) which cause destructive damage to the joints. Now we can use this combination to block all three kinds of mediators of arthritic inflammation since the research emphasizes the importance of inhibiting the pro-inflammatory cytokines (specifically TNF-alpha and IL-1 beta) and the COX-2 and LOX pathways. The etiology of the inflammatory process makes sense now that we understand the biochemistry of these pathways. The mediators involved in inflammation need to be addressed at the same time in order to more effectively prevent and treat arthritic inflammation.

DIET AND INFLAMMATION

Dietary modification can help block common inflammatory pathways involved in cartilage destruction. One such pathway involves over-production of pro-

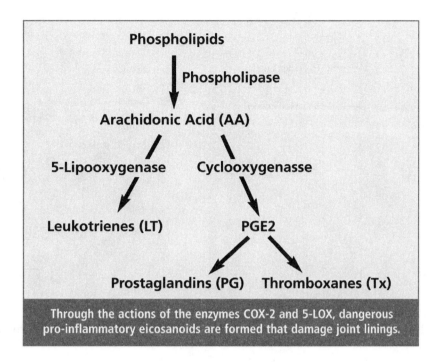

Phospholipids

↓ Phospholipase

Arachidonic Acid (AA)

5-Lipooxygenase   Cyclooxygenasse

↓   ↓

Leukotrienes (LT)   PGE2

↓   ↓

Prostaglandins (PG)   Thromboxanes (Tx)

Through the actions of the enzymes COX-2 and 5-LOX, dangerous pro-inflammatory eicosanoids are formed that damage joint linings.

inflammatory hormone-like messengers (such as PE2) and underproduction of anti-inflammatory messengers (such as PE1 and PE3).

Omega-3 fatty acids found in fish oil help to suppress the formation of undesirable PE2 and promote synthesis of beneficial PE3 (Kelley et al. 1985; Wanatabe et al. 2000). GLA induces the production of the anti-inflammatory PE1 (Das et al. 1989; Fan et al. 1997). Diet can significantly affect whether you have more of the beneficial prostaglandins (E1 and E3) as opposed to the pro-inflammatory PE2.

Since PE2 is a culprit in inflammation, reducing the consumption of foods that are high in omega-6 fatty acids (such as meat and egg yolks) and increasing omega-3 rich foods, such as salmon and other fish, can be beneficial. Limiting foods that convert to arachidonic acid can help reduce inflammation. Arachidonic acid is a precursor to both PE2 and the pro-inflammatory eicosanoid LTB4 (Brock et al. 1999). Another dietary factor that can lead to high levels of arachidonic acid is over-consumption of high-glycemic index carbohydrates that causes an excessive production of insulin (Kreisberg et al. 1983).

Foods that may contribute to chronic inflammation are foods with a high glycemic index (foods that digest quickly), such as fruit juices or rice cakes, foods heavy in polyunsaturated or saturated fats, and foods high in arachidonic acid. Some specific foods to avoid are

- Fatty cuts of red meat (high in saturated fats)
- Organ meats: liver, kidney, and so forth (high in arachidonic acid)
- Egg yolks (high in arachidonic acid)
- Pasta (high glycemic index)
- Juices (high glycemic index)
- Rice, especially rice cakes (high glycemic index)
- White bread (substitute whole grain breads such as rye or whole wheat)

Better choices are foods with a low glycemic index and foods that are heavy in monounsaturated fats. Some specific good foods are

- Salmon and other fish
- Oatmeal
- Fresh fruits and vegetables
- Olives and olive oil
- Peanuts and other nuts
- Whey proteins

Food and arthritis have long been connected in the field of alternative medicine. Many nonconventional practitioners think that fasting and attention to diet could cure arthritis. For some persons with arthritis, these relatively simple dietary changes may have a beneficial impact.

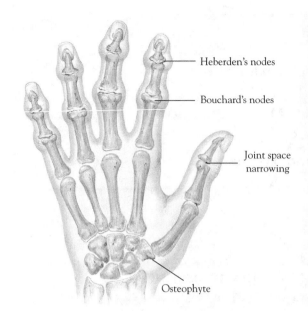

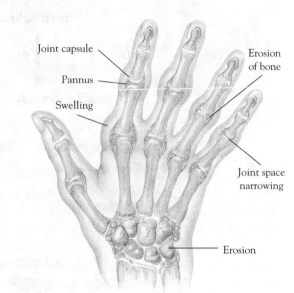

Hand and Wrist with Osteoarthritis   **Hand and Wrist with Rheumatoid Arthritis**

Degeneration of articular cartilage (covering joint ends of bones) is the characteristic feature of osteoarthritis. In rheumatoid arthritis, inflammation begins in the synovial membrane and spreads to cartilage and other tissue. (Anatomical Chart Company 2002®, Lippincott Williams & Wilkins)

For those who do not find effective relief from simple dietary changes, the addendum at the end of this protocol entitled *Food and Arthritis* discusses radical changes that can be made in the way one eats. We understand that many people will not be able to follow these kinds of aggressive changes in eating patterns. For persons with arthritis who are unable to substantially alter their diet, we next discuss specific natural approaches that have shown significant improvements in human clinical studies.

OSTEOARTHRITIS AND RHEUMATOID ARTHRITIS

While OA and RA are medically classified as different diseases, for the purposes of this protocol, the therapies for each are similar. Our primary treatment objective for either OA or RA is to suppress the known pro-inflammatory factors (PGE2, TNF-alpha, IL-1b, LTB4, and IL-6) through a combination of diet, dietary supplements, and, if necessary, certain prescription drugs.

OA is a disease mainly characterized by degeneration of the articular cartilage but these changes also involve the synovial membrane and the bone next to the cartilage. It is a gradual decay that most often affects the weight-bearing joints (knees, hips, and spinal

joints) and the joints of the hand. A breakdown of the cartilage matrix leads to cracks and ulcers and a thinning of the cartilage with a loss of shock absorption. The underlying bone starts to thicken as a response to the increasing stress, and bone spurs are formed. In the advanced phases of OA, an inflammatory reaction in the synovial membrane can be seen. This severe degeneration causes pain, swelling, deformation, and reduced range of motion. Because the joints of the hand and the large joints of the spine, hips, knees, and ankles are frequently involved, disability is significant. OA comes with the normal processes of aging and affects approximately 70–80% of the population over age 50. The onset is marked by stiffness, crackling joints, and pain. As it worsens, more pain and disability occur causing an enormous consumption of painkillers and anti-inflammatory drugs that many times have undesirable long-term effects.

RA is considered an autoimmune disease, characterized by chronic inflammation and thickening of the synovial lining in addition to cartilage destruction. In autoimmune diseases, the immune system attacks body tissues as if they were foreign invaders. The etiology and pathogenesis of RA is considered directly related to a chronic inflammatory syndrome. Contributing factors are thought to include food allergies, leaky gut syndrome, hereditary factors, and microbes.

Normal Right Knee

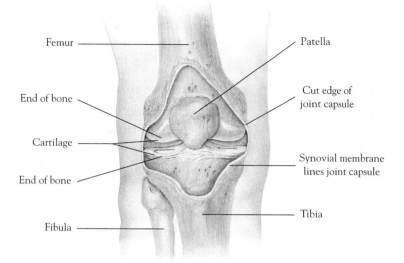

Femur

Patella

End of bone

Cut edge of
joint capsule

Cartilage

End of bone

Synovial membrane
lines joint capsule

Fibula

Tibia

Structural comparison of a normal right knee compared to a right knee damaged by
either osteoarthritis or rheumatoid arthritis. (Anatomical Chart Company 2002®,
Lippincott Williams & Wilkins)

Right Knee
with Osteoarthritis
Knee usually bends out

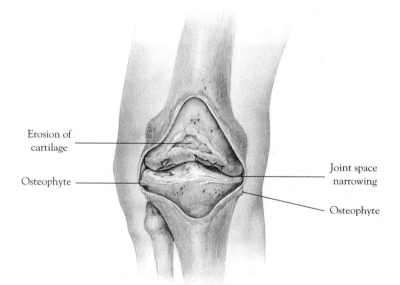

Erosion of
cartilage

Osteophyte

Joint space
narrowing

Osteophyte

Patella removed to visualize joint
(Anatomical Chart Company 2002®, Lippincott Williams & Wilkins)

Right Knee with
Rheumatoid Arthritis
Knee usually bends inward

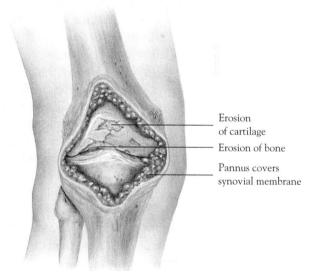

Erosion
of cartilage

Erosion of bone

Pannus covers
synovial membrane

Patella removed to visualize joint.
(Anatomical Chart Company 2002®, Lippincott Williams & Wilkins)

RA strikes women 3 times as often as men. The clinical picture varies from mild chronic joint inflammation with occasional flareups to painfully deformed joints. Involvement of the small joints of the hands and feet are often the key to the diagnosis. Low-grade fever, weight loss, and a general feeling of sickness, fatigue, and joint deformities and pain often accompany the disease. There can be anemia and other health problems that are a result of the underlying chronic inflammatory syndrome. Most sufferers (90%) have a positive rheumatoid factor in the serum.

Scientists have identified underlying factors involved in the pathology of both OA and RA. This published research has enabled novel natural therapies to be developed that work along multiple pathways. These natural agents have an extraordinary safety profile and a long track record of clinical success.

NATURAL THERAPIES

Nettle Leaf

As noted, TNF-alpha and IL-1b have been identified as factors in the destruction of cartilage in both OA and RA. Studies show that the blockade of these aberrant immune factors can produce therapeutic results. Nettle leaf has been shown to reduce TNF-alpha levels and IL-1b. Nettle leaf also inhibits the genetic transcription factor that activates TNF-alpha in synovial tissue.

Antiarthritic drugs are being developed to suppress TNF-alpha, but similar effects may be obtained safely today using nettle leaf. Please note that nettle leaf extract contains different phytochemicals than the nettle root extract used to treat benign prostate disease.

Nettle leaf is an herb that has a long tradition of use as an adjuvant remedy in the treatment of RA in Germany. Nettle leaf extract has been found to contain a variety of active compounds, such as COX and lipoxygenase inhibitors and substances that affect cytokine secretion (Obertreis et al. 1996; Teucher et al. 1996).

A placebo-controlled trial by Feldman et al. (1997) provided the first convincing evidence that blockade of a specific cytokine could be effective treatment in human autoimmune or inflammatory diseases. Interesting results with TNF-alpha blockade have also been achieved in trials conducted on Crohn's disease, sepsis, and HIV/AIDS. A placebo-controlled human trial showed that leaves of the nettle exhibited a potent effect in lowering TNF-alpha levels in arthritis patients.

Another study conducted on 40 patients suffering from acute arthritis compared the effects of 200 mg of a NSAID (diclofenac) with 50 mg of the NSAID in combination with 50 grams of stewed nettle leaf a day (Chrubasik et al. 1997). Total joint scores improved significantly in both groups by approximately 70%. The addition of nettle extract made possible a 75% dose reduction of the NSAID, while still retaining the same anti-inflammatory effect with reduced side effects. The nettle leaf extract clearly enhanced the anti-inflammatory effect of the NSAID.

Not only does nettle leaf reduce TNF-alpha levels, but it has recently been demonstrated that it does so by potently inhibiting the genetic transcription factor that activates TNF-alpha and IL-1b in synovial tissue (Riehemann et al. 1999). This pro-inflammatory transcription factor, known as nuclear factor-kappa-beta (NF-KB), is known to be elevated in chronic inflammatory diseases and is essential to activation of TNF-alpha. Nettle is thought to work by preventing degradation of the natural inhibitor of NF-KB in the body. It has also been shown that TNF-alpha activates NF-KB in synovial cells, leading to the suggestion that a cycle of cross-activation between TNF-alpha and NF-KB may sustain and amplify the disease process in RA (Jue et al. 1999).

A study on healthy volunteers showed the anti-inflammatory potential of nettle. Irritants were used to stimulate and increase the secretion of pro-inflammatory cytokines. When nettle extract was given simultaneously in a dose-dependent manner, TNF-alpha and IL-1b concentrations were significantly reduced (Obertreis et al. 1996).

Because nettle leaf works at the level of anti-inflammation, it could also be tried on OA, although no studies have specifically been done with it on that condition.

S-Adenosylmethionine (SAMe)

S-adenosylmethionine (SAMe) is the activated form of methionine. Because it has so many actions in different parts of the body, SAMe can have many health benefits that seem unrelated, but in fact all depend on SAMe.

A study was done on the effect of free radicals on RA. Researchers in The Netherlands discovered that the synovial fluid in RA patients contains nonfunctioning T-cells. The deficit is caused by a lack of IL-2, the cytokine crucial for T-cell activation. Free radicals are to blame, although all the science has not been worked out. However, researchers did find that N-acetyl-L-cysteine (NAC) restores T-cell activity (Maurice et al. 1997). (NAC naturally elevates the body's antioxidant, glutathione.)

Researchers theorize that SAMe, like NAC, protects synovial cells by reversing glutathione depletion. The reason researchers believe this, is that SAMe acts as a precursor to glutathione production (Lieber et al. 2002). (SAMe is naturally converted to cysteine in the body.) But in addition to its antioxidant protection, researchers believe SAMe has other important effects. It may protect synovial cells by blocking the enzymes that degrade cartilage. This would occur through its role in the polyamine pathway that leads to protein synthesis. It may also protect the important cartilage proteins and proteoglycans in the joint lining.

In a study published in the *British Journal of Rheumatology*, researchers demonstrated for the first time that SAMe reversed the effects of damage caused by TNF when added to cells at the same time as TNF (Gutierrez et al. 1997).

Almost all of the arthritis studies done with SAMe involve OA. In the test tube, SAMe increases the number of chondrocytes (cartilage cells) and proteoglycans (protein). This suggests that SAMe treatment may reverse the underlying process of OA by stimulating cartilage to grow (Barcelo et al. 1990; Kalbhen et al. 1990). The other main component of the joint is synovial fluid, which acts as a lubricant. The pro-inflammatory cytokine TNF-alpha has been found in the synovial fluid of people with RA, and it plays a role in bone and cartilage destruction (Bertolini et al. 1986). Until recently, scientists did not know the effects of SAMe on synovial fluid; it was discovered that SAMe reverses the damaging effects of TNF-alpha.

In 1987, the *American Journal of Medicine* published a series of articles on the use of SAMe for treating OA (as an example, see Tavoni et al. 1987). The SAMe provided for the studies was spread out among numerous physicians and clinics (in one case, 33 different medical centers). The studies confirmed that SAMe works as well as the most popular arthritis treatments on the market. The series is published under the title *Osteoarthritis: The Clinical Picture, Pathogenesis, and Management with studies on a New Therapeutic Agent, S-Adenosylmethionine.*

Many years earlier, studies had been done in Italy showing the benefits of SAMe. One of the studies involved approximately 22,000 patients. This large-scale trial lasted 2 months. Participants were not allowed to take any pain medication or other arthritis treatment during the study. Physicians found that patients taking SAMe improved steadily from the beginning. At the end of the study, about 80% of the subjects who took SAMe reported improvement: 70% of the subjects with the most severe knee pain improved significantly. Side effects were minimal, and only 2.3% of the group stopped taking it because it did not work. The most severe side effect reported was gastrointestinal upset.

In four double-blind studies, SAMe was compared either to placebo or to NSAIDs. SAMe was generally better tolerated than the NSAIDs (Glorioso et al. 1985; Maccagno et al. 1987; Vetter 1987; Domljan et al. 1989).

The latest study assessed the efficacy of SAMe against placebo and nonsteroidal anti-inflammatory drugs (NSAIDs) in the treatment of OA. The investigators looked at 13 different human clinical trials to assess pain scores, functional limitation, and adverse side effects. When compared with placebo, SAMe was more effective in reducing functional limitation. When compared against NSAIDs, SAMe worked as well as NSAIDs with far fewer adverse effects. The conclusion of the researchers was: "SAMe appears to be as effective as NSAIDs in reducing pain and improving functional limitation in patients with osteoarthritis without the adverse effects often associated with NSAID therapies." Those with OA often resort to NSAIDs that can induce serious long-term side effects. Even COX-2 inhibiting drugs have demonstrated more side effects than anticipated. SAMe has shown itself to not only alleviate arthritic pain and functional limitation, but to also rebuild joint cartilage (Soeken et al. 2002).

Nexrutine

Nexrutine is a natural anti-inflammatory ingredient that has a unique mechanism of action: it is a COX-2 gene expression inhibitor without COX-1 inhibition. It inhibits the gene expression of COX-2, rather than inhibiting the COX-2 enzyme directly, achieving a broader inhibition of pro-inflammatory processes and a faster onset of action. Absence of COX-1 activity should result in limited gastrointestinal irritation, a common side effect of many NSAIDs such as ibuprofen (Advil) and naprosyn (Aleve).

Nexrutine was tested and found to be a safe, effective, and rapid-acting dietary supplement which helps avoid or relieve the general aches and pains associated with physical activity or overexertion. Fifty-three subjects were treated with Nexrutine for 2 weeks. Based on preclinical studies, Nexrutine was evaluated to help avoid or relieve the general aches and pains associated with physical activity or overexertion such as sore joints, sore muscles, muscle aches and pains, and stiff joints. Post-trial analysis revealed that 79% of the participants reported this effect. The efficacy parameters for Nexrutine included the following: it eases soreness in joints and muscles, makes everyday activities more comfortable, relieves aching joints, and relieves muscle aches. Additionally, the subjects were comfortable using the product. No significant side effects were reported. The product was judged to be gentle on the stomach by 86% of the subjects.

Nexrutine was compared to naproxen in a classic animal model for inflammation-induced pain. Naproxen is a well-known and widely used over-the-counter anti-inflammatory. The results observed were more dramatic than anticipated. Nexrutine demonstrated faster onset of analgesia than naproxen in one study while maintaining the same duration of activity as naproxen in another study. Nexrutine was shown to provide rapid onset and an extended duration of pain relief.

An extensive literature review of the chemical constituents plus the use of the plant from which Nexrutine is extracted for hundreds of years suggests that this material is safe for its intended use. In addition, an acute toxicity study in rats (5 grams/kg) with 14-day observation revealed no untoward effects from Nexrutine. No side effects are expected at the recommended human dosage.

5-Loxin

Boswellic acid (5-Loxin) is the active component of the *Boswellia serrata* tree native to India. The aromatic gum resins from this tree have been used by practitioners of the Ayurvedic system of medicine to treat arthritis for centuries. Scientists have isolated the active component of *Boswellia serrata* and it is the only known natural preparation that inhibits the 5-LOX pathway of the inflammatory cascade.

Since this recent discovery, pharmaceutical companies have been vigorously trying to create a prescription medication that works in much the same way as 5-Loxin by inhibiting the chemical reaction that leads to the formation of pain and inflammation-producing leukotrienes from arachidonic acid (the precursor to the mediators of inflammation). Since present medications on the market target only the COX-1 and COX-2 pathways which are contributors to the arachidonic acid cascade, this natural 5-LOX inhibitor is particularly desirable for anyone who is suffering from the symptoms of arthritis. Recent research has strongly suggested that both the COX-2 and 5-LOX pathways should be inhibited to fight against arthritis and other inflammatory diseases (Dennis and Company Research 2002; Boileau et al. 2002; Safayhi et al. 1995).

Ginger

Ginger is an herb which has been used for centuries in Ayurdevic medicine to relieve the pain of arthritis although few studies are available to demonstrate its benefits. A Danish study of 56 people who had either arthritis or muscular discomfort reported that three-fourths of the arthritis sufferers experienced relief from their symptoms, while 100% of the people who had muscular achiness experienced relief from their painful symptoms. This was not a double-blinded random placebo controlled study and the population was small. However, if one considers that the herb has relieved the pain of arthritis for centuries in other cultures, this study becomes significant. The mechanism of action is believed to be due to the inhibition of prostaglandin and leukotriene synthesis but this hypothesis needs further investigation (Srivastava et al. 1992).

Glucosamine

Glucosamine is a naturally occurring substance in the body, synthesized by chondrocytes for the purpose of producing joint cartilage. In OA this synthesis is defective, and supplementation with glucosamine has proven to be useful. The body uses supplemented glucosamine to synthesize the proteoglycans and the water-binding glycosaminoglycans in the cartilage matrix. In addition to providing raw material, the presence of glucosamine seems to stimulate the chondrocytes in their production of these substances. Glucosamine also inhibits certain enzymes such as collagenase and phospholipase, which destroy the cartilage. By blocking pathogenic mechanisms that lead to articular degeneration, glucosamine delays the progression of the disease and relieves symptoms even for weeks after termination of the treatment. Among the natural therapies for OA, glucosamine sulfate is probably the best known. It is extensively used as a drug for OA in Europe and is readily available in health food stores in the United States.

Research into glucosamine began in the early 1980s. To date there have been many significant positive studies regarding this treatment for OA. Studies have been double-blind and frequently have compared glucosamine either to a placebo or to one of the NSAIDs such as ibuprofen or piroxicam. Studies have been done on intramuscular glucosamine sulfate as well as oral and IV forms.

Glucosamine has been almost totally free of side effects, particularly when compared to the NSAIDs. Rovati et al. (1994) compared 310 patients with knee OA by randomizing them into four groups, each of which received oral treatment with glucosamine sulfate, piroxicam, both drugs, or a placebo. While piroxicam had a similar efficacy at the start of treatment, it was less well tolerated, and its effect wore off quickly. This study followed patients for 90 days plus another 60 days after treatment. While 24% had adverse effects with piroxicam, only 15% had adverse effects with glucosamine (Rovati et al. 1994). In one well-designed study of 178 patients with OA of the knee, one group was treated for 4 weeks with glucosamine sulfate, 1500 mg daily, and the other group was treated with ibuprofen at 1200 mg a day. Again, glucosamine relieved the symptoms as effectively as ibuprofen and was significantly better tolerated than ibuprofen. The safety and tolerability of glucosamine can easily be explained by the fact that it is a physiological substance normally used by the body (Qui et al. 1998).

As with most natural remedies, the therapeutic effect of glucosamine is not immediate. It usually takes 1–8 weeks to appear. Once achieved, it tends to persist for a notable time even after discontinuation of the treatment. The probable reason for this is that glucosamine is incorporated into rebuilding the cartilage itself. One study has shown through electron microscopy of the articular cartilage that patients treated with glucosamine show a picture more similar to healthy cartilage than that of the placebo-treated cartilage of the control group (Drovanti et al. 1980).

Given the amount of available evidence, the comparisons with NSAIDs, and the number of positive double-blind, placebo-controlled studies, glucosamine sulfate should be used as a first natural choice for OA. Certainly the evidence prevails that it is at the very least equal in efficacy to NSAIDs and that it has much fewer side effects. In most studies, the dose has been 500 mg 3 times daily. At least one study suggests that the sulfate salt of glucosamine is also an important component and that other salts such as glucosamine hydrochloride may not work as well. Sulfate is an important mineral in building cartilage (Hoffer et al. 2001).

Chondroitin Sulfate

Chondroitin sulfate is a major component of cartilage. It is a very large molecule, composed of repeated units of glucosamine sulfate. Like glucosamine, chondroitin sulfate attracts water into the cartilage matrix and stimulates the production of cartilage. Likewise it has the ability to prevent enzymes from dissolving cartilage. Although the absorption of chondroitin sulfate is much lower than that of glucosamine (10–15% versus 90–98%), a few studies have shown very good results from long-term treatment with chondroitin sulfate, reducing pain and increasing range of motion.

Uebelhart et al. (1998) performed a year long, double-blind clinical study including 42 patients with OA, showing that chondroitin sulfate was well tolerated and significantly reduced pain and increased joint mobility. The patients were given 800 mg of chondroitin sulfate a day or placebo. These results confirm that oral chondroitin 4- and 6-sulfate is an effective and safe, slow-acting supplement for the treatment of knee OA. In addition, it may be able to stabilize the joint space width and to modulate bone and joint metabolism. This is the first preliminary demonstration

that chondroitin might influence the natural course of OA in humans.

In another double-blind study, 119 patients that had finger-joint OA were treated and then followed for 3 years (Verbruggen et al 1998). The chondroitin dosage was 400 mg 3 times daily. X-rays of the finger joints were carried out at the start and at yearly intervals. The number of patients that developed progression of the disease (i.e., decreased joint space and joint erosion) was significantly less in the group treated with chondroitin sulfate.

The improvement in walking time was studied in 80 patients with OA in the knee. In this double-blind study, the treatment period was 6 months and the chondroitin sulfate dosage was 400 mg twice daily. The minimum time to perform a 20 m walk showed a constant reduction of time only in the chondroitin group. Lower consumption of pain-killing drugs and excellent tolerability was also observed (Bucsi et al. 1998).

Glucosamine alone or in combination with chondroitin sulfate is more and more becoming recognized as the treatment of choice for OA, even in the United States. Its ability to actually repair and improve joint function in addition to providing pain relief gives it a significant advantage compared to conventional treatment.

Willow Bark

Salicylic acid, the basis of aspirin, was first prepared from willow bark by an Italian chemist in 1838. The name of the compound is derived from Salix, the Latin name for the willow genus. Aspirin, acetylsalicylic acid, is a synthetic form of salicylic acid. Willow bark is rich in salicin and related salicylates that metabolize into salicylic acid. Many plants, such as meadowsweet and wintergreen, also contain these compounds. They have a long tradition of use in Europe and have far fewer side effects than aspirin.

While aspirin has been shown to have a lowering effect on some of the pro-inflammatory factors, it can also *increase* LTB4, which is a major inflammation-promoting mediator. An interesting study compared the effect on pro-inflammatory substances of aspirin alone with a combination of low-dose aspirin and fish oil (Engstrom et al. 1997). The results showed that the combination of fish oil and low-dose aspirin has significantly more favorable effects on the pattern of pro- and anti-inflammatory factors than the aspirin alone. LTB4 increased 19% when aspirin was taken by itself but decreased 69% after intake of aspirin and fish oil together.

This makes sense based on the fact that aspirin inhibits COX-2, but not lipoxygenase. Remember that arachidonic acid is converted into PGE2 and

LTB4 by COX-2 and lipoxygenase, respectively. Since fish oil suppresses arachidonic acid levels, it reduces the precursor to both PGE2 and LTB4.

Omega-3-Oils (Omega-3-Fatty Acids)

It is established that dietary fatty acids determine the composition of lipids in the cell membranes which influence the production of prostaglandins and leukotrienes that regulate inflammation.

Omega-3 oils have been shown to suppress the production of PGE-2, which contributes to arthritis by degrading collagen needed for the cartilage that lines the joints. PGE-2 is also a pro-inflammatory prostaglandin that contributes to the arthritis inflammatory cascade. A large number of studies have confirmed the usefulness of omega-3 oils in relieving tender joints and morning stiffness, in some cases eliminating the need for NSAID medication. One study found that patients consuming fish oil which contains the omega-3-fatty acids EPA and DHA were able to significantly reduce their NSAID dose compared with a control group (Lau et al. 1993).

Omega-3 oils, such as fish oil and perilla and flaxseed oils, have the ability to suppress the production of inflammatory mediators and thereby influence the course of chronic inflammatory diseases such as RA (Kremer et al. 1985; Kremer et al. 1992). The advantage of taking fish oil is that the EPA and DHA type of omega-3-fatty acids is already in its active form compared to ALA omega-3-fatty acid in perilla and flaxseeds which have to be converted to the EPA and DHA by the liver in order to exert its anti-inflammatory activity.

An enteric-coated fish-oil preparation was used in a 1-year, double-blind study of 78 patients with inflammatory bowel disease. The absorption rate and tolerability was high with this preparation, and after 1 year, 59% of the fish-oil group remained in remission compared to 36% in the placebo group, indicating an anti-inflammatory effect (Belluzzi et al. 1996).

In other studies, dietary omega-3 oils have shown a suppressive effect on the production of the cytokines IL-1b, IL-6, and TNF-alpha, in addition to PGE2 and LTB4 (Caugey et al. 1996; James et al. 1997). When fish oil supplementation was given to RA patients, inflammatory arachidonic acid levels were reduced by 33% compared to presupplement values (Sperling et al. 1987), suggesting that an increase of dietary omega-3 oils can be complementary in treating RA.

A large number of publications from around the world have confirmed the usefulness of dietary supplementation with omega-3 oils in relieving tender joints and morning stiffness in patients with RA, in some cases eliminating the need for NSAID medication

(Kremer et al. 1995). Skoldstam et al. (1992) and Lau et al. (1993) found that patients consuming fish oil were able to significantly reduce their NSAID dose compared with a control group.

Of 12 published double-blind and placebo-controlled studies with a duration of 12–52 weeks, decreased joint tenderness was the most common favorable outcome reported. Fish oil supplementation significantly decreased the use of NSAIDs in the three studies in which NSAIDs were used. Unlike NSAID use, fish-oil consumption is not associated with GI toxicity. The results of the studies suggest that the effective dose of fish oil is approximately 3–6 grams a day. Higher dosages did not give better results (Robinson et al. 1989).

A study by James et al. (1997) emphasized the potential for increased efficacy of anti-inflammatory drugs when using omega-3 oils in the diet. It was observed that diets rich in omega-3 oils and low in omega-6 fats had a drug-sparing effect with decreased side effects. Drug toxicity is estimated to contribute 60% of the total cost of treating RA patients in the United States (Prashker et al. 1995). Use of omega-3 oils in the diet would appear to offer a simple, safe, and inexpensive way to reduce toxicity and side effects from OA and RA medications.

Antioxidants

Oxidative stress or free-radical damage is a factor of importance in the development of OA, just as it is a major cause of most chronic degenerative diseases as well as aging. There is also strong evidence that oxidative damage occurs in RA patients (Jikimoto et al. 2002). Increased oxidation of lipids (peroxidation) as well as depletion of ascorbate in serum and synovial fluid has been observed (Vijayalakshmi et al. 1997; Sakai et al. 1999). High doses of vitamin E, an antioxidant, are reported to diminish pain (Edmonds et al. 1997). Most importantly, TNF-alpha which plays a key role in RA and is a well-known cause of oxidative stress, is reduced by vitamin E.

Increased selenium was given over a period of 3 months to RA patients whose red blood cells showed significantly lower selenium levels than the normal populations. At the end of the 3 months, selenium levels were not restored despite supplementation higher than the RDA. However, the patients showed improvement with less tender or swollen joints and less morning stiffness. The patients using selenium needed less cortisone and NSAIDs than the control group. Laboratory indicators of inflammation were also reduced (Heinle et al. 1997).

In order to counteract free-radical damage, antioxidants are needed. A diet rich in vegetables and fruits is likely to add important antioxidants to the body. However, this may not always be enough. Vitamin C and vitamin E supplements have been studied and found to be important in the treatment of OA. Deficient vitamin C intake, which is common with elderly people, impairs the synthesis of collagen, the main protein of cartilage (Bates 1977). Studies on vitamin E have shown its ability to stimulate the production of cartilage components, such as glycosaminoglycans, as well as to inhibit the breakdown of cartilage.

Healthy food and a minimum of toxins may be more important for our health than we want to believe. The body strives to heal itself, whether it is a cut finger, a cold, or a damaged or inflamed joint. It makes sense to find ways to support the body with natural substances that the body can use in the healing process.

Recent research has provided us with new insights into the mechanisms of arthritis and has left us with a scientific understanding of how natural remedies work in harmony with the body rather than against it.

Gamma-Linolenic Acid (GLA)

GLA is a fatty acid found in evening primrose oil, borage oil, and black currant seed oil that has been used to suppress chronic inflammation. In the *Annals of Internal Medicine* (1993), the findings of a 24-week, double-blind, placebo-controlled trial with GLA derived from borage oil were reported. The patients receiving the borage oil experienced a 36% reduction in the number of tender joints, a 45% reduction in the tender joint score, a 41% reduction in the swollen joint score, and a 28% reduction in the swollen joint count. The placebo group showed no benefits (Leventhal et al. 1993).

A paper in the *British Journal of Rheumatology* (1994) reports the findings of a 24-week, double-blind, placebo-controlled trial in RA patients treated with black currant seed oil rich in GLA and alpha-linolenic acid. Patients receiving black currant seed oil showed reductions in the signs and symptoms of the disease. The placebo group showed no change in disease status. According to the researchers, the study showed that black currant seed oil is a potentially effective treatment for active RA. No adverse reactions were observed, although some people dropped out of the trial because of the size and number of capsules they were required to take (Leventhal et al. 1994).

In *Seminars in Arthritis and Rheumatism* (1995), there was a review of all published literature on the use of GLA for the treatment of RA. GLA reduced the effects of autoimmune disease on joint linings, although more research was needed to determine the ideal dose of GLA for arthritis (Rothman et al. 1995).

Methylsulfonylmethane (MSM)

MSM is a natural sulfur compound found in all living things. It should not to be confused with sulfur (sulfa) drugs or dimethyl sulfoxide (DMSO) to which some people are allergic. It is one of the most prominent compounds in our bodies after water and sodium. MSM has been shown to produce a multitude of actions including pain relief, reducing inflammation, dilating blood vessels and increasing blood flow, reducing muscle spasms, and promoting immune normalizing effects (Jacob et al. 1999). In a double-blind study of patients with degenerative joint disease, MSM was administered at a dose of 2250 mg daily. At the conclusion of the study, the overall improvement in pain of those taking MSM was 82% after 6 weeks (Lawrence 1998).

BLOCKING PLA2

Dietary factors can influence how much arachidonic acid is produced in the body. An enzyme that is needed to convert dietary factors into arachidonic acid is phospholipase A2 (PLA2). Arthritic pain and inflammation are the end result of a pathway known as the *arachidonic acid cascade*.

Researchers have been seeking agents that block the PLA2 enzyme in order to reduce the amount of arachidonic acid produced in the body. By suppressing PLA2 enzyme activity, arachidonic levels are reduced along with the pro-inflammatory compounds it generates, such as leukotrienes, thromboxanes, and PE2. Suppressing PLA2 enzyme activity interferes with the arachidonic acid cascade that is responsible for the chronic pain and tissue destruction seen in so many age-related diseases. High levels of PLA2 enzyme activity have been found in synovial tissue in the joint, and scientists have linked elevated levels of serum PLA2 to activity associated with RA (Vades et al. 1985). In fact, PLA2 has been found in a variety of human tissues, including platelets, cartilage cells known as chondrocytes, placenta, cartilage, peritoneal cells and peritoneal fluid, and the spleen (Vades et al. 1990).

Scientific studies have shown that inflammation that accompanies arthritis is directly linked to enzymatic actions. As can be seen from the chart at the top of the next page, the PLA2 enzyme increases arachidonic acid, which is then converted by enzymatic actions (COX-2, lipoxygenase, COX-1) into PE2, leukotrienes, and thromboxanes. In fact, the evidence has

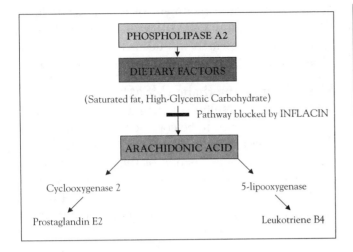

PHOSPHOLIPASE A2

DIETARY FACTORS

(Saturated fat, High-Glycemic Carbohydrate)

Pathway blocked by INFLACIN

ARACHIDONIC ACID

Cyclooxygenase 2   5-lipooxygenase

Prostaglandin E2   Leukotriene B4

demonstrated that excessive concentrations of extracellular PLA2 may initiate and spread inflammation and cause cellular damage. High activities of PLA2 have been identified in several inflammatory diseases, including RA and OA (Vades et al. 1985).

In their quest to find PLA2-inhibiting agents, scientists have discovered a group of compounds trademarked under the name Inflacin. When tested, these topically applied compounds alleviated pain associated with arthritis and increased joint mobility.

In a double-blind, patient-randomized, placebo-controlled, crossover clinical trial enrolling 30 participants, Inflacin was tested to evaluate its analgesic benefit when applying the topical cream to areas of the body affected by stiffness, soreness, and pain. These included hands, feet, knees, and shoulders and muscles of the neck, arms, legs, and back. Assessment tools used to measure changes in pain and handgrip strength included a visual analog scale (VAS) that recorded pain levels and a hydraulic hand dynamo meter that evaluated changes in handgrip strength. The VAS is a common assessment tool that accurately evaluates pain and stiffness based on

a ranking recorded on a 0–10 scale, with zero being no pain and 10 being very severe pain. Each assessment in the study was conducted 3 times using this method, and an average of three rankings was recorded as the value for that time point.

Assessments using the hydraulic hand dynamometer were recorded 3 times with each hand by holding the device at arm's length vertically. After initial assessments, the blinded investigator applied measured amounts of either Inflacin or placebo to affected areas. Subsequent assessments were then recorded at intervals of 5 minutes, 60 minutes, and 120 minutes.

Results of the study showed that Inflacin significantly reduced pain and stiffness after just one application of 2 grams. On average, Inflacin reduced pain by 45% (as compared to 15% in the placebo group) after one dose in the first 60 minutes of application. In several test subjects, researchers recorded a dramatic reduction of pain. In some subjects, a complete eradication of pain and almost total loss of stiffness occurred. Over the next 60 minutes, pain and stiffness returned among those in the placebo group, while subjects in the Inflacin group continued to experience a decrease in pain and stiffness. Moreover, subjects in the Inflacin group experienced an average increase in grip strength of 10% in both hands; grip strength did not improve in subjects using the placebo.

In the clinical test, Inflacin showed an immediate effect (within 5 minutes) of statistically reducing pain and stiffness (by as much as 72%, compared to 15% for the placebo in one subject). Inflacin was also shown to improve handgrip strength within 5 minutes, whereas the same improvements were not demonstrated among those using the placebo.

Data indicated that at every time point in the trial (at 5, 30, 60, and 120 minutes) Inflacin improved the pain score and performed better than the placebo in decreasing pain.

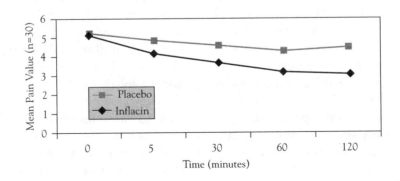

The overall conclusions drawn from the study indicate that in subjects with mild-to-moderate pain, Inflacin is an effective compound for reducing pain and stiffness and improving grip strength when applied topically. Despite some relief of pain and stiffness noted within the first 60 minutes among those in the placebo group, symptoms ultimately began to return. Additionally, subjects who used the placebo cream reported no improvement in handgrip strength (Keller 2002).

Inflacin's combination of active ingredients and unique delivery system makes it an effective anti-inflammatory topical analgesic. The patent-pending ingredient used to make Inflacin specifically inhibits certain enzyme systems that mediate a variety of physiological responses, including a cascade of biochemical reactions that help facilitate pain, fever, inflammation, and other functions. The resulting anti-inflammatory action is much more effective than that used in other marketed topical products that have a counterirritant mode of action but are only marginally effective at disguising the pain.

Copper Deficiency

Research suggests that people with RA tend toward copper deficiency. A study in the *Journal of Rheumatology* showed that patients with RA had low levels of several micronutrients, including copper, compared to the typical American diet (Kremer et al. 1996). Consequently, the authors suggested that "routine dietary supplementation with multivitamins and trace elements is appropriate in this population." A deficiency may also explain why copper, which is an anti-inflammatory agent, is useful in the treatment of RA and other inflammatory conditions. An early study in the *Journal of the American Medical Association* reported that copper supplementation surpassed aspirin in terms of anti-inflammatory action, boasting 130% of the activity of cortisone (Gordon et al. 1974).

Unlike other micronutrients that can be taken in large doses before reaching a toxicity threshold, a small amount of copper is all that it takes to perform its meticulous tasks that are so essential to human health. An excess of copper may encourage free-radical activity and subsequent oxidative damage at the cellular, tissue, and organ level (Dameron et al. 1998). Good dietary sources of copper include crabmeat, oysters, beans (such as kidney, pinto, and black beans), brown rice, potatoes, and spinach. Vitamin and mineral supplements containing trace amounts of copper will also ensure that proper levels are achieved.

Curcumin

Curcumin comes from a plant similar to ginger and is an anti-inflammatory that inhibits both COX-2 and LOX enzyme activity. In addition, curcumin interferes with NF-KB to stop autoimmune activation and lessen tissue destruction (Joe et al. 1997; Plummer et al. 1999).

Some studies revealed that users of curcumin supplements were not getting optimal benefits from the extract. The reason is that for curcumin to be effectively assimilated into the bloodstream, it must be combined with small amounts of piperine (a component of black pepper). Piperine has been shown to enhance the serum concentration, the extent of absorption, and the bioavailability of curcumin in both rats and humans with no adverse effects (Shoba et al. 1998).

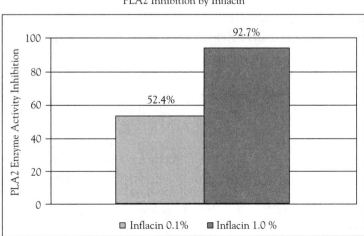

PLA2 Inhibition by Inflacin

AN INNOVATIVE ALTERNATIVE TO JOINT REPLACEMENT

When a joint threatens to deteriorate completely, orthopaedic surgeons can repair or replace it. However, replacement parts wear away or loosen over time and often need an additional operation (sometimes more). A novel method of treating degenerative cartilage diseases has been developed by an orthopaedic surgeon in Miami, FL, as a possible alternative to invasive procedures such as joint replacement.

The innovative procedure developed and patented by Dr. Allan Dunn involves the injection of human growth hormone directly into the affected joint spaces of the arthritic patient that, in turn, stimulates the growth of cartilage. The cartilage regrowth causes increased space between the ends of the bones, often up to 4 mL in volume, enough to ease pain and stiffness in the affected joint. Growth hormone also increases the production of collagen, the strong fibrous connective tissue that attaches cartilage to bone and provides a framework for the gelatinous matrix, the resilient part of cartilage.

IntraArticular Growth Hormone (IAGH) gives the body the cues it needs to set the cartilage growth process in motion. Stimulation of cartilage regeneration with growth hormone reproduces the same environment in which joint tissues grow during childhood. The IAGH procedure has been successfully used on hips, knees, ankles, shoulders, and elbows. (Dr. Allan Dunn may be reached at (888) 848-6534.)

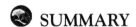 **SUMMARY**

Unlike toxic FDA-approved drugs, natural therapies and diet modification can often provide relief from chronic inflammation and pain. One of the most compelling reasons for using natural therapies in arthritic conditions is that while some drugs can cause cartilage destruction, natural therapies correct the underlying factors involved in arthritic cartilage degeneration. Natural therapies have been shown to work by the following mechanisms:

- Inhibiting COX-2
- Inhibition of the 5-LOX pathway
- Suppressing TNF-alpha, IL-1b, and IL-6
- Reducing production of LTB4
- Preventing the over-expression of NF-KB
- Inhibiting the formation of PE2
- Promoting the synthesis of proteoglycans and glycosaminoglycans in the joints

- Suppressing cartilage-destroying enzymes, collagenase and phospholipase
- Attracting water to the cartilage to enhance synovial lubrication

There are several different natural antiarthritic combinations that one may try to find the ideal program to suit their individual need. A convenient way of using several different natural approaches at once can be found in a product called ArthroPro. Some of the better-documented, cartilage-protection and inflammation-suppressing supplements are contained in each capsule of ArthroPro. The suggested dose for the first 3 months is two capsules of ArthroPro twice a day, with or without food. After 3-6 months, some persons may be able to reduce the dose by half. Each capsule provides the following ingredients:

- Nexrutine
- Nettle leaf extract (super concentrated)
- N-acetyl-D-Glucosamine
- Glucosamine sulfate
- Chondroitin sulfate
- Vitamin E
- 5-Loxin (boswellic acid)
- Ginger (powdered extract) (5% gingerols)

Note: *Persons who are allergic to aspirin may not be able to use ArthroPro because of the small amount of naturally derived aspirin contained in the willow bark extract.*

In addition to the 4 capsules a day of the AthroPro formula, persons with arthritis might want to use:

1. SAMe, 400–1200 mg a day; or MSM, 2000–3000 mg daily.

Based on data from published studies, 800–1200 mg of SAMe should be taken a day to start. If GI upset occurs, SAMe should be reduced by half, then gradually increased again. In a long-term study, patients were given 600 mg of SAMe a day for the first 2 weeks, then 400 mg daily. In other studies, patients were consistently given 1200 mg of SAMe from day one. People taking SAMe should experiment with the 400–1200 mg range to find the best dose for them. Several studies indicate that it may take several weeks or months for SAMe to achieve its full effect. SAMe is a substance that is naturally made in the body. No serious side effects have ever been reported with SAMe, even in high doses administered intravenously.

MSM has reduced inflammation and eased joint pain in some people with arthritis. Daily dosages of between 2000–3000 mg, and in severe cases up to 5000 mg daily, have been used without side effects. Since SAMe and MSM work via similar mechanisms, it may only be necessary to take one of the other to obtain desired benefits.

2. Gamma-linolenic acid (GLA): 800–1200 mg daily.

GLA is a fatty acid found in evening primrose oil, borage oil, and black currant seed that can suppress chronic inflammation by boosting production of the anti-inflammatory PE1. The most efficient way of obtaining high amounts of GLA is to use borage oil. Those taking ArthroPro may consider taking a borage oil supplement that provides 800–1200 mg a day of GLA.

3. Life Extension Mix: 9 tablets, 14 capsules, or 1 tbsp of powder daily.

Life Extension Mix is a multinutrient supplement containing pharmaceutical grade extracts from vegetable, fruits, herbs, and other food concentrates known for their potent antioxidant action. Life Extension Mix also provides a potent amount of N-acetyl-cysteine (NAC) and vitamin E. The proper amount (1 mg) of the anti-inflammatory agent copper is also included. Copper has been shown to be deficient in many people with RA. Life Extension Mix is available in three varieties: tablets (9 daily), capsules (12 daily), and powder (3 scoops daily).

If taking ArthroPro, GLA, SAMe (or MSM), and Life Extension Mix do not provide adequate relief from arthritis inflammation and pain, consider having your blood tested for markers of systemic inflammation (such as C-reactive protein). With the availability of cytokine blood profile tests, it is now possible to ascertain the underlying cause of chronic inflammatory disease. The appropriate drugs and additional nutrients can then be used to suppress the specific cytokines (such as TNF-alpha or IL-6) that are promoting the inflammatory cascade.

If a cytokine profile blood test reveals excess levels of the inflammatory factors TNF-alpha, IL-1b, IL-6 or LTB4, the following supplements are suggested:

1. High doses of the DHA fraction of fish oil. Some studies suggest that DHA works much better than the EPA fraction of fish oil in suppressing inflammatory cytokines. A product called Super GLA/DHA provides GLA along with a potent combination of DHA from fish oil. The suggested dose for those with elevated cytokines is 8 capsules a day of Super GLA/DHA.

2. DHEA, 15–75 mg a day (*refer to the DHEA Replacement Therapy protocol in this book for safety information*)

3. Vitamin K, 10 mg daily.

If these nutrients fail to lower pro-inflammatory cytokine levels to the safe ranges (as indicated on the following chart), then ask your physician to prescribe 800 mg daily of the drug pentoxifylline (PTX). PTX is a cytokine-suppressing drug that has been overlooked by most of the medical establishment. Supplements such as fish oil, nettle leaf, DHEA, and vitamin K possess mechanisms of suppressing inflammatory cytokines similarly to PTX, but some people may require PTX. There are no side-by-side comparisons to categorically state whether PTX or natural agents (such as DHA fish oil) work better.

For those who have arthritis that is not alleviated by diet modification and supplements, we recommend the cytokine profile blood test. Your own physician can do this, or you can inquire about it by calling (800) 208-3444. If the results of your cytokine test reveals excess levels of cytokines such as TNF-alpha and/or IL-1b, you may consider different combinations of supplements such as GLA, DHA, vitamin K, DHEA, and nettle leaf extract (contained in Arthro-Pro). If you have tried different combinations of these inflammatory-suppressing nutrients and blood tests show that you still have high levels of inflammatory cytokines, you should consider 800 mg daily of low-cost PTX or the higher-priced Enbrel.

For potential immediate relief of arthritis pain, consider applying Inflacin cream topically to arthritic areas of the body.

Inflammatory Cytokine Blood Reference Ranges

There are at least three different methods of testing blood levels of the pro-inflammatoray cytokines. Listed below are the standard reference ranges for each different type of test. To protect against arthritis and other diseases associated with chronic inflammation, people should be within or below these reference cytokine ranges. (Other blood testing laboratory methods may have different reference ranges.)

Proinflammatory	Optimal Range (pg/mL)			
Cytokine	LabCorp	ISI	DPC	Quest
TNF-a	< 8.1	10–50	0–8.1	0–25
IL-6	< 12.0	2–29	0–9.7	2–29
IL-1b	< 15.0	0–150	0–5	0–150
IL-8	< 32.0	10–80	.0–62	10–80

Note: The symbol "<" means less than.

Ask your doctor to prescribe these cytokine blood tests for you. You may also inquire about ordering these cytokine blood tests by calling (800) 208-3444.

One test that can help determine if your arthritis is a result of systemic inflammation is the inexpensive C-reactive protein (high-sensitivity) blood test (CRP-hs). If your C-reactive protein level is over 1.3 mg/L, this is an indication that you have an inflammatory event occurring in your body. Those with elevated CRP-hs levels (and who have arthritis) should consider using the supplement protocol and/or prescription drugs known to suppress elevated pro-inflammatory cytokines. Using the cytokine profile blood test will help monitor their progress.

A high-sensitivity C-reactive protein blood test may be ordered by calling (800) 208-3444. This test may also be obtained at your physician's office.

Pentoxifylline (PTX)

CAUTION PTX should not be used in persons with bleeding disorders such as those with recent cerebral or retinal hemorrhage (PDR 2001). Patients taking Coumadin should have more frequent monitoring (once a week is suggested) of prothrombin times and regular template bleeding time tests (White et al. 1989; Stigendal et al. 1999). Those who have other types of bleeding should receive frequent physician examinations. According to two studies, PTX should be avoided by Parkinson's patients (Godwin-Austen et al. 1980; Serrano-Duenas 2001).

It is important to note that the body uses TNF-alpha to acutely fight infections. If patients are showing any sign of infectious disease, drugs such as Enbrel (that inhibit the effects of TNF-alpha) are temporarily discontinued. A new FDA advisory states that patients should be tested and treated for inactive tuberculosis prior to therapy with another TNF-alpha inhibiting therapy (infliximab). Since PTX, fish oil, and nettle directly suppress TNF-alpha, perhaps these agents should be temporarily discontinued during the time when one has an active infection.

Refer to the *Chronic Inflammation protocol* in this book for further information.

 FOR MORE INFORMATION

Contact the Arthritis Foundation (800) 283-7800.

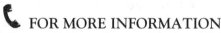 **PRODUCT AVAILABILITY**

ArthroPro, SAMe, Mega GLA, Mega EPA, Super GLA/DHA, DHEA, Glucosamine and Chondroitin capsules, MSM, vitamin K, vitamin E, Gamma E Tocopherol/Tocotrienols, Super Curcumin (with bioperine), Inflacin, nettle leaf extract, and Life Extension Mix are available by telephoning (800) 544-4440 or by ordering online at www.lef.org. Blood tests may be ordered by calling (800) 208-3444.

ADDENDUM: FOOD AND ARTHRITIS... AGGRESSIVE DIETARY STRATEGIES

Conventional research, particularly in the area of RA, but also in OA, has shown that in many cases the inflammation of arthritis can be significantly and positively affected by nutrition. The impact of diet on arthritis is almost certainly related to the strong connection between the intestinal lining, where food is absorbed, and the surrounding immune system structures known as gut-associated lymphoid tissue (GALT). Hunter (1991) first suggested in conventional medical literature that metabolic changes in the gut can cause the individual to react to the influence of gut bacteria and incomplete breakdown products of digestion on the immune system (Nenonen et al 1998). Buchanan et al. (1991), writing in the *British Journal of Rheumatology* commented: "There is evidence from several well documented case reports that occasional patients with rheumatoid arthritis (RA) may develop aggravation of their arthritis as a result of allergy to some ingredient in the diet. A variety of foodstuffs have been implicated including milk and milk products, corn..."

Five years later, a unique series of papers by Kjeldsen-Kragh and a number of coauthors in various rheumatology journals showed the effect of vegetarian diet in RA over a 2-year period (Kjeldsen-Kragh 1994a; 1994b; 1995a; 1995b; 1999). Overall, these papers demonstrate that not only do omnivores with RA improve with fasting and a subsequent vegetarian diet, but immune parameters, bowel bacterial balance, and several other markers of RA also change in a positive way. Furthermore, they identified a group of responders versus nonresponders to diet. About one-third of the total appears to be responders. Over the 2-year period, in which participants were allowed to return to a regular diet if they wished, compared with baseline, the improvements measured were significantly greater in the vegetarians who previously benefited from the diet (diet responders) than in diet nonresponders and omnivores. The beneficial effect could not be explained by patients' psychological characteristics, antibody activity against food antigens, or changes in concentrations of prostaglandin and leukotriene precursors. Dietary responders appear to make up about one-third of the population of RA studied in these papers.

Nenonen et al. (1998) tested the effects of an uncooked vegan diet, rich in lactobacilli (friendly gut bacteria), in RA patients randomized into diet and control groups. The results showed that this uncooked vegan diet, rich in lactobacilli, decreased subjective symptoms of RA (Neonen et al. 1998). They also found that large amounts of living lactobacilli consumed daily may have positive effects on objective measures of RA but that it was difficult for patients to stick to such a strict diet. They concluded that a vegan diet changes the fecal microbial flora in RA patients and changes in the fecal flora are associated with improvement in RA activity. Similar results were reported in the *British Journal of Rheumatology* (Peltonen et al. 1994).

An uncooked vegan diet consists of berries, fruits, vegetables, roots, and nuts, with germinated seeds and sprouts, which are rich sources of carotenoids, and vitamins C and E. Hanninen et al. (2000) demonstrated that the subjects eating this type of diet showed highly increased levels of alpha- and beta-carotenes, lycopene, and lutein in their blood. Also, the increases of vitamin C and vitamin E were statistically significant. Because the berry intake was threefold that of controls, the intake of antioxidant compounds such as quercetin and myricetin was much higher than in the omnivorous controls. RA patients subjectively benefited from the vegan diet rich in antioxidants, lactobacilli, and fiber, and this was also seen in objective measures (Hanninen et al. 2000).

Studies concerning OA and diet in peer-reviewed literature are lacking. Again, the fields of alternative and complementary medicine show significant benefit with nutritional and dietary changes for OA in clinical observation. As noted previously, peer-reviewed literature has shown that NSAIDs significantly alter intestinal permeability, increase inflammatory response, and cause a hyperimmune state. This is true not only for people with RA, but also OA.

Changing Your Diet

Life Extension Foundation supports nutritional change as a means of preventing or alleviating chronic disease. Nowhere is this more significant than in the case of arthritis, and it is suggested that significant nutritional change be made by persons who suffer from the effects of arthritis, in addition to the suggested supplementation. Although it is sometimes difficult to change dietary and eating habits around food intake, the significant benefits to be gained are worth the challenge. The following dietary changes are suggested as an initial start to combating arthritis. The elimination of common food allergens along with a shift in the types of fat in the diet is likely to bring fairly significant relief to those who are nutritional responders. This will apply both to RA and OA.

- Remove as many processed foods as possible from your diet. This means eliminating all sugar-containing foods and high-fat foods. Learn to read food labels effectively.

- Common food allergens include wheat, rye, oats, and barley (all of which contain a protein called gluten). Antigluten antibodies have been found in many people with RA. Other common allergens include corn, dairy, and red meats. Significant inflammation can also occur with the nightshade family foods: These are all types of peppers, potatoes, tomatoes, and eggplant. For at least the first 2 weeks it is suggested that these foods be removed.

- Avoid all citrus fruits for the first 2 weeks, then reintroduce as described.

- Drink plenty of filtered water. Fish (preferably the cold water variety: herring, mackerel, salmon, or tuna) or soy are the preferred proteins. Except for these examples, your diet can contain any vegetables and fruits. Sulfur-containing vegetables such as broccoli and cauliflower, cabbage, onion, and garlic are particularly good for detoxification. Depending upon the degree of toxic load your body is carrying, you can expect some detoxifying symptoms as those elements start to work their way out of your system. These symptoms usually start on day 2 or 3 but keep in mind that they usually begin to be resolved by day 4 or 5. Typical symptoms of detoxification during these initial days are mild-to-strong headaches and an increase in muscular aches and pains, weakness, light-headedness or a feeling that everything is happening in slow motion, plus a variety of intestinal symptoms, including loose bowels or cessation of bowel movements.

- By the end of the first week, you may begin to feel some relief from your symptoms of arthritis. If you do, you can be fairly sure that food is a significant contributor to your arthritic symptoms. If you do not have some relief after 2–3 weeks on this program, you may not be a dietary responder. Even if this is not the case, you will have now embarked upon a healthy diet anyway, so stay with it.

- You may begin to reintroduce the foods that you have eliminated: one new food every 3 days. You may develop symptoms of joint pain if you eat a food to which you are intolerant, usually within about 1–2 days. If this is the case, eliminate the food again. In any event, stay away from processed foods and a saturated high fat diet.

- You may find that you can reintroduce dairy and wheat without difficulties; however, these are two of the common foods that cause sensitivity.

- A maintenance diet should be those foods which you have found tolerable, with a focus on low-to-moderate fat, preferably from fish or flaxseed oil, and with an emphasis on high concentrations of fresh fruits and vegetables.

This is a simplified nutritional detoxification program. There are products on the market that will aid in detoxification. After removal of toxins, you should begin to replace any vitamins and minerals that may be deficient or ones that have been found in the research to benefit people with arthritis.

Asthma

Asthma: from the Greek word, *asthma*, meaning "difficult breathing"; now refers to constriction of the bronchi.

Asthma is a chronic inflammatory disorder of the airways characterized by episodes of wheezing, shortness of breath, chest tightness, racing heart, mucus production, flared nostrils, and cough. According to the Morbidity and Mortality Weekly Report (2001) asthma is among the most common chronic diseases in the United States, affecting approximately 10.2 million adults during 1996 (7.2% of adults residing in the United States report having asthma).

Asthma has been considered a rare disease in the elderly, but recent studies have shown that it is as common in the elderly as in the middle-aged (Quadrelli and Roncoroni 2001). Diagnosis of asthma is often overlooked in older patients and is more severe in this group.

Asthma is diagnosed using lung function tests such as spirometry and expiratory flow, as well as histamine challenge tests (histamine is the compound that causes runny nose, watery eyes, and itching). While asthma is usually fairly simple to diagnose, it is sometimes confused with chronic bronchitis and emphysema.

Physiology

Asthma, like so many diseases, is simply an adaptive biological response gone bad. According to evolutionary biologists, allergic and asthmatic responses evolved initially to protect us against parasitic organisms and for the expulsion of toxins via sneezing. Most natural toxins are highly allergenic. They cause swelling, heat, constriction of the muscles of the bronchi, and the release of fluid, which expel or dilute offending toxins. The resulting dilation of blood vessels lowers blood pressure and slows the dissemination of any by-products through the body. Some research suggests that people with allergies do not get cancer in allergenic tissues because of this heightened immune sensitivity to toxins (Profet 1991).

Asthma is closely tied to the immune system. In particular, a part of the immune system called humoral, or antibody based, immunity is overactive in people with asthma, while another part, called cell-mediated immunity is sluggish. Humoral immunity is controlled by cell-signaling chemicals called cytokines (e.g., IL-4, IL-5, IL-6), which turn on and turn off the activity of various cells (antibodies) of the immune system, such as mast cells, basophils, eosinophils, and B cells. Allergic antigens bind to mast cells and basophils. When the antigen-bound mast cells and basophils come into contact with another antibody known as immunoglobulin E (IgE), a hypersensitivity response occurs leading to inflammation and the resultant bronchoconstriction (Miller 2001).

PHARMACEUTICALS

The current pharmaceutical drugs used for asthma are bronchodilators and anti-inflammatory compounds. Short-acting beta-2 agonists are used for relief of acute symptoms and prevention of exercise-induced bronchospasm (EIB). Inhaled corticosteroids (very powerful anti-inflammatory compounds) are used in long-term control of asthma, and systemic corticosteroids are for quick control of asthma symptoms. Long-acting bronchodilators are also combined with anti-inflammatory medications for long-term control and nocturnal asthma. Sustained release theophylline is a mild bronchodilator used principally with inhaled corticosteroids for nocturnal asthma.

Leukotriene modifiers are an alternative to inhaled corticosteroids (Balachandran et al. 2001) that can cause several negative side effects. Oral glucocorticoids inhibit growth in children by blunting growth hormone (GH) secretion, decreasing insulin-like growth factor 1 activity, and inhibiting new collagen (protein) synthesis. Similarly, corticosteroids cause short-term growth suppression (Allen 2002). Corticosteroids also deplete the body of calcium, magnesium, potassium, and zinc and may lead to osteoporosis. These nutrients should be supplemented during long-term corticosteroid therapy.

New drugs with fewer side effects are being developed to treat asthma. The first selective anti-IgE therapy, a monoclonal anti-IgE antibody (omalizumab), binds with a receptor on IgE, reducing the amount of free IgE available to bind to antigen receptors on mast cells, basophils, and other cells involved in allergic responses. So far in trials, omalizumab controls allergic responses, reduces or eliminates the need for inhaled or oral corticosteroids, and has an excellent safety profile (Boushey 2001).

Hydergine is another useful drug for asthma. It works, like theophylline, by safely boosting intracellular levels of the messenger molecule cyclic adenosine monophosphate (cAMP) which can reduce bronchial constriction. The recommended dose of hydergine is 5–10 mg a day with food. (*For more information about the benefits of the drug hydergine, please refer to the Age-Associated Mental Impairment protocol.*)

Certain supplements can interact with asthma medications, so be cautious when combining the two. Ipriflavone can slow liver detoxification and thus raise blood levels of theophylline, giving you a longer period of stimulation than you expected. Be sure to consult with a health professional when combining supplements with asthma medications or attempting to reduce the use of pharmaceutical drugs.

Foods

Food allergies are a common cause of asthma, and effort should be made to eliminate allergenic foods from the diet. Baker and Ayres (2000) explain that the "role of food intolerance in asthma is well recognized and where food avoidance measures are instituted, considerable improvement in asthma symptoms and in reduction in drug therapy and hospital admissions can result."

Cereal grains, given their prevalence and evolutionary novelty, are among the biggest offenders. A high intake of cereals in the diet during early life causes IgE sensitization to cereals because allergens in cereals cross-react with proteins in grass pollen leading to pollen allergies (Armentia et al. 2001). Hypoallergenic, gluten-free flour suppresses gluten-caused allergic reactions. In rats fed a hypoallergenic flour after an allergen challenge, body weight remained the same, indicating no allergic reaction had occurred. (Watanabe et al. 2001). In addition, cereal grains and seeds are a major source of airborne asthma allergens including molds, fungi, insects such as mites, and insect droppings.

Other common allergenic food that can cause an asthma attack include nuts, chocolate, fish, tomatoes and other nightshade plants, cow milk, eggs, and cheese. Also be wary of food colorings, MSG, and aspirin. Hydrochloric acid and pancreatin supplements are useful if asthma attacks are related to food sensitivity. These help break down food proteins, minimizing allergic reactions.

Obesity and high intake of certain types of dietary fats are also associated with asthma. High caloric intake and the consumption of saturated fats are associated with asthma, while monounsaturated fats (such as olive oil) reduce risk of asthma (Huang and Pan 2001). People with high body mass (referred to as body mass index or BMI) are at a higher risk of asthma due to the added mass on their lungs and more active inflammatory mechanisms (von Mutius et al. 2001).

In general, asthma increases in industrialized societies due to worsening dietary habits. In one study in Saudi Arabia, people who ate at fast food restaurants and had the lowest intakes of vegetables, fiber, vitamin E, calcium, magnesium, and potassium had the highest risk of asthma (Hijazi et al. 2000). Another study in Taiwan revealed that high intake of meat (especially liver) and fat-rich foods were associated with asthma (Huang et al. 2001). Finally, another team of researchers has found that the risks of bronchial hyper-reactivity are increased seven fold among those with low intake of vitamin C, although the lowest intake of saturated fats gives a 10-fold protection. Furthermore, the risk of adult-onset asthma is increased five fold by the lowest intake of vitamin E (Seaton and Devereux 2000). All of these studies also cite urban location as a major risk factor for asthma.

Vitamins and Minerals

In addition to the above research on food groups and asthma, an increasing body of research supports the use of vitamin and mineral supplementation to prevent and control this disorder.

In a study of people age 16–50 carried out in London, researchers found that selenium protected against asthma and that the intake of this mineral has been declining in Britain (Shaheen et al. 2001). The decline in blood selenium concentration in the United Kingdom and other European Union countries may be leading to increased rates of asthma. Selenium helps to deregulate the inflammatory mediators in asthma (Brown and Arthur 2001). Magnesium intake is also related to asthma. With lower levels of intake, the incidence of allergies and asthma increases. A dose of 1000 mg a day of magnesium is recommended (Hijazi et al. 2000). Zinc is another helpful mineral in the fight against asthma (Miller 2001).

Leukotrienes are regulators of allergic and inflammatory reactions. In asthma and allergy patients, leukotrienes are overexpressed, leading to bronchial constriction and other respiratory reactions. Tocopherol (vitamin E) and tocopherol acetate inhibit the formation of leukotrienes, thus suppressing an antibody response (Centanni et al. 2001). Higher concentrations of vitamin E intake are also associated with lower blood IgE concentrations and a lower frequency of allergen sensitization (Fogarty et al. 2000).

Vitamin C levels in bronchoalveolar lavage fluid (BAL) are directly correlated to the levels in the blood and work to protect bronchial tissues from oxidative damage, which is one cause of asthma. Vitamin C also rids the body of excess histamine, which is a factor in asthma. A dose of several grams per day is recommended (Schock et al. 2001). Asthma patients have lower blood levels of vitamin C than people without this disease (Vural et al. 2000).

Supplementation with both N-acetyl-L-cysteine (NAC) and glutathione helps balance humoral and cell-mediated immunity by lowering levels of IL-4 and enhancing T-cell proliferation (Bengtsson et al. 2001). Glutathione binds with nitric oxide (NO), which increases airway inflammation and creates nitrosothiols (RS-Nos), which are related to insufficient oxygen reaching the blood (hypoxia) (Corradi et al. 2001). Glutathione, NAC, and other antioxidants also counter cellular oxidative damage, which occurs at high levels in asthma (Willis et al. 2001).

Plant Medicines

Herbs and plant products are extremely helpful for asthma. Michael Heinrich, at the Center for Pharmacognosy and Phytotherapy, School of Pharmacy, in London, discovered that a key target for asthma (as well as arthritis) is the nuclear factor kappa B (NF-kappaB) transduction pathway, which activates many inflammatory cytokines. Some well-known plant chemicals that target NF-kappaB include several phenolics such as curcumin (in curcumin), and flavonoids, such as silybin (in milk thistle) (Bremner and Heinrich 2002).

Other bioflavonoids are potent weapons against asthma. Researchers recently looked at the effects of lycopene on airway hyper-reactivity in patients with exercise-induced asthma (EIA). The researchers used 30 mg a day of lycopene and 7-minute exercise sessions. All patients given placebo showed a postexercise reduction of more than 15% in their forced expiratory volume (how much air you can blow out). After receiving a daily dose of 30 mg of lycopene for 1 week, 55% of patients were significantly protected against EIA (Neuman et al. 2000). Pycnogenol, a standardized extract of French maritime pine bark, rich in bioflavonoids, reduces asthmatic symptoms and circulating leukotrienes, and improves lung function in asthma patients (Rohdewald 2002). Finally, a diet enriched in isoflavones results in reduced antigen-induced eosinophilia (increase in eosinophils) in the lung in asthma patients (Regal et al. 2000). Eosinophils are white blood cells that may become overexpressed due to an allergic response.

The flavonoid quercetin helps reduce allergic reactions, asthma, and hay fever by preventing the release of histamine. By blocking the release of histamine rather than acting on histamine receptors on other cells, quercetin reduces allergic reactions more safely (no drowsiness) than many conventional drugs (Miller 2001).

Ginkgo leaf concentrated oral liquor (GLC) significantly reduces airway hyper-reactivity and improves clinical symptoms and pulmonary functions of asthma patients (Li et al. 1997). BN52021 (Ginkgolide B) an anti-inflammatory extract of ginkgo biloba inhibits platelet activating factor (PAF), which is important in the pathogenesis of asthma. Ginkgolide B also inhibits uneccessary immune activation in asthmatics (Mahmoud et al. 2000).

Other botanicals and plant products that can help asthma include licorice, Yerba mate, bee pollen, Ephedra, and American angelica.

- Licorice combats coughs and lung congestion. It works as a demulcent (soothing, coating agent) due to its high mucilage content which soothes irritated mucous membranes. It can be as effective as codeine, and safer, when used as a cough suppressant. It also works as an expectorant to help with coughs by increasing the secretion of the bronchial glands.

- Yerba mate helps relieve asthma and allergies by stimulating the adrenal glands to produce corticosteroids, which suppress inflammation and overactive immune responses to allergens. It also opens the respiratory passages to overcome asthma and allergy symptoms. Yerba mate's ability to relax muscles makes it useful for asthma since it dilates the bronchi (gas absorbers in your lungs).

- Bee pollen prevents onset of allergenic symptoms in asthmatics due to the presence of quercetin, which inhibits the release of histamine in the body.

- Ephedra has long been used by the Chinese to relieve bronchial spasms and treat asthma. Most species of Ephedra contain the adrenaline-like substances ephedrine and pseudoephedrine, which stimulate the sympathetic nervous system and help relieve asthma, cold, and allergy symptoms. Synthetic ephedrine compounds are widely used in over-the-counter cold remedies like Sudafed.

- American angelica has compounds that can relax the windpipe and thus may be beneficial for asthma. More exotic botanicals such as *Tylophora asthmatica*, *Boswellia serrata*, and *Petasites hybridus* are worth checking into as well (Miller 2001).

The Importance of Essential Fatty Acids

The increase in the prevalence of asthma has recently been linked to the altered consumption of polyunsaturated fatty acids (PUFAs). Western diets contain almost 10 times more linoleic acid (omega-6 fatty acids) than alpha-linoleic acid (omega-3 fatty acids) resulting in excess production of eicosanoids derived from arachidonic acid that increase levels of Th-2 immune cells, thus increasing the production of IgE. Omega-3 fatty acids help prevent an asthmatic response by limiting eicosanoid production (Kankaanpaa et al. 1999). Consumption of gamma linolenic acid (GLA) stimulates production of prostaglandin E1

(PGE1), which dilates the bronchioles and calms inflammation.

New Theories

One of the most fascinating new theories of the cause of asthma is the "hygiene hypothesis," which proposes that the relatively sterile environment present in industrialized Western countries and the reduced microbial exposure in early life, has contributed to the recent epidemic of asthma. The load of infectious agents, including respiratory viruses, encountered early in life is important for maturation of the immune system from a type 2 (humoral) bias at birth toward type 1 (cell mediated) responses, thus avoiding diseases such as asthma (Message and Johnston 2002). Lactobacillus, a type of beneficial intestinal bacteria that is effective in treatment of allergic inflammation and food allergy, has shown to prevent asthma when given to mothers prenatally or to infants postnatally (Kalliomaki et al. 2001).

Breastfeeding is important for asthma prevention. One study from Brazil confirmed that the low rate of asthma in that country is related to the number of breastfed infants. Children who were breastfed for more than 6 months had a lower risk of developing asthma than those who were not breastfed (Romieu et al. 2000). Similarly, in a study from Western Australia, a substantial reduction in risk of childhood asthma was uncovered if exclusive breastfeeding was continued for at least the first 4 months of life. Breast milk carries antibodies, which may contribute to increased immune function.

Babies are born with immature immune systems, and they need all the immunological properties and bioactive factors in their mother's milk for normal development, according to the researchers (Oddy 2000). Gamma-linolenic acid (GLA) and preformed di-hommo-gamma linolenic acid (DGLA) are found in human breast milk. GLA and DGLA are essential in the production of PGE1 prostaglandins, which are powerful anti-inflammatory compounds. Glycoprotein lactoferrin in breast milk builds immunity by competing for the iron necessary for pathogenic microorganisms to replicate.

Finally, a supercritical fluid (CO_2) extraction of freeze-dried New Zealand green-lipped mussel powder (Lyprinol) shows significant anti-inflammatory activity that may make it useful for asthma. Much of this activity is due to omega-3 fatty acids and natural antioxidants such as carotenoids. Lyprinol is extremely potent and can be used at doses 200 times less than plant or marine oils currently used for inflammation, such as flax and fish oils (Halpern 2000).

Mind Body Therapies

Asthma is intimately tied to socioeconomic status (SES) with poor neighborhoods and minorities suffering from much higher rates of this disease. Research shows that high rates of depression often occur with asthma in inner-city clinics (Nejtek et al. 2001). A large part of the reason for this association is the higher rates of stress experienced in these populations. Stress reducing therapies such as yoga, massage, biofeedback, and acupuncture can help prevent asthma and other diseases (Miller 2001). One type of acupuncture treatment called drug accupoint application is an effective technique against asthma, as is moxibustion (a treatment using topical applications of herbs and heat) (Lai et al. 2001).

Neurologically, people with asthma often suffer from an overactive parasympathetic nervous system, which conserves energy by constricting various systems in the body, slowing heart rate, lowering blood pressure, and triggering inflammation. People with asthma have weak adrenal glands and thus poor secretion of epinephrine and nor-epinephrine, chemicals that stimulate the sympathetic system and control inflammation. As a result, supplements that support adrenal function, such as licorice, are effective therapies for asthma.

Environmental Health

Asthma is intimately tied to environmental health factors. One recent study at the Harvard School of Public Health examined the effect of daily ambient air pollution on asthmatic children residing in eight urban areas of the United States, using data from the National Cooperative Inner-City Asthma Study. Daily air pollution concentrations were extracted from the Aerometric Information Retrieval System database from the Environment Protection Agency. The air pollutants examined included ozone, sulphur dioxide (SO_2), nitrogen dioxide (NO_2), and particles smaller than 10 microns (PM10). Peak expiratory flow rate was assessed, and each pollutant was associated with an increased incidence of morning symptoms. The researchers conclude: "This analysis supports previous findings that at levels below current USA air-quality standards, summer-air pollution is significantly related to symptoms and decreased pulmonary function among children with asthma" (Mortimer et al. 2002).

Another recent study found that ozone-induced bronchial hyperresponsiveness in adults with asthma can be controlled using dietary antioxidants (400 IU vitamin E and 500 mg vitamin C). The study used exposure at 0.12 ppm (parts per million) of ozone combined with moderate exercise along with 10-minute sulfur dioxide (0.10 ppm and 0.25 ppm) inhalation challenges (Trenga et al. 2001).

Innovative community responses to air pollution are dramatically reducing rates of asthma in urban environments. For example, in Boston one monitoring and warning system has cut rates of asthma caused by diesel buses and trucks signficantly and is providing the impetus for cleaner, alternative fuel transporation. (Loh et al. 2002).

🌀 SUMMARY

1. Although asthma prevalence continues to skyrocket due to declining nutrition and worsening air quality, numerous options exist for preventing this disorder using dietary and lifestyle strategies. Essential fatty acids: Omega-3 fatty acids found in fish oil and certain plant extracts can reduce inflammation by helping to dilate bronchioles and suppress inflammation. One or more of the following supplements may be considered:

   - Super GLA/DHA, 6 capsules daily
   - Lyprinol (derived from green lipped mussels), as directed
   - Flaxseed oil, 6 grams daily
   - Perilla oil, 6 grams daily

2. Probiotics: lactobacillus, a healthy digestive bacterium is an excellent probiotic for asthma.

   - LifeFlora, 6 capsules daily
   - NutraFlora, 3/4–1 tsp. daily

3. Enzymes: the enzymes pancreatine and hydrochloric acid can help in food-related asthma attacks (as directed).

4. Bioflavonoids, such as water-soluble quercetin, isoflavones, pycnogenol, and lycopene, may help improve lung function. Life Extension Mix and Life Extension Booster contain bioflavonoids and important antioxidants such as vitamin E, vitamin C, and selenium.

   - Life Extension Mix, 9 tablets daily
   - Life Extension Booster, 1 capsule daily

5. The herbs milk thistle (containing silybin) and turmeric (containing curcumin) help to inhibit inflammatory cytokines.

   - Silibinin Plus, 1 capsule twice daily
   - Super Curcumin w/Bioperine, 1 capsule daily

6. Corticosteroids taken to relieve asthmatic symptoms often deplete the body of vital minerals such as calcium, magnesium, potassium, and zinc. These minerals will be replenished by taking 6 capsules each night of a multimineral supplement like Bone Assure.

7. N-acetyl-L-cysteine, 600 mg/day and glutathione, 250–500 mg/day can lower IL-4 and enhance T-cell proliferation.

8. Certain herbs can soothe respiratory passages, act as an expectorant, and lessen mucous secretions.

   - Yerba mate, 5 drops of tincture daily
   - Licorice standardized extract, 200–600 mg daily, not to be taken for more than 6 weeks
   - American angelica, 1.5 grams of tincture daily

9. Ginkgo biloba can inhibit PAF and reduce airway hyperreactivity, 120 mg daily.

10. Bee pollen will help inhibit the release of histamine. Various formulations of bee pollen with ingredients such as propolis and royal jelly exist. Follow the manufacturer's dosing directions.

11. Foods: hypoallergenic foods such as gluten-free flour may help. Also be sure to choose foods high in potassium, such as fresh fruits and vegetables.

12. Drugs: Hydergine is useful at a dose of 5–10 mg once a day with food.

13. Exercise: Although improving lung function will help with symptoms, be cautious where you work out because exercising in cold or polluted air can aggravate asthma.

14. Mind-body: Yoga, massage, and biofeedback are useful. Acupuncture and moxibustion may help as well.

15. Environmental health: Be sure to obtain a high quality air filter. HEPA filters are especially useful for eliminating particulates from the air.

 PRODUCT AVAILABILITY

Life Extension Mix, Life Extension Booster, Super GLA/DHA, flaxseed oil, perilla oil, Udo's Choice, Life Flora, Nutra Flora, Super Ginkgo Extract, Silibinin Plus, NAC, Bone Assure, and Super Curcumin w/Bioperine are available by calling (800) 544-4440 or ordering online at www.lef.org.

Atherosclerosis (Coronary Artery Disease)

The most common form of heart disease is caused by atherosclerosis. It is generally referred to as coronary heart disease or hardening and/or thickening of the arteries. *Atherosclerosis* involves the slow buildup of deposits of fatty substances, cholesterol, body cellular waste products, calcium, and *fibrin* (a clotting material in the blood) in the inside lining of an artery. The buildup that results (referred to as *plaque*) can partially or totally block the flow of blood through the artery. This can lead to the formation of a blood clot (*thrombus*) on the surface of the plaque. If either of these events occurs and blocks the entire artery, a heart attack or stroke may result.

Atherosclerosis-related diseases are a leading cause of death and impairment in the United States, affecting over 60 million people. Additionally, *50% of Americans* have levels of cholesterol that place them at high risk for developing coronary artery disease. However, cholesterol is only one factor that causes the occlusion of arteries that is technically known as atherosclerosis.

The high mortality of atherosclerosis, the widespread suffering, and the huge economic impact demand integrated medical approaches and therapies. This protocol reflects that demand.

ETIOLOGY

Although the terms are used interchangeably, **athero**sclerosis (or "hardening of the arteries") is one type of **arterio**sclerosis. Arteriosclerosis is actually a generic term for a number of diseases in which the arterial wall becomes thickened and loses elasticity. The term atherosclerosis is derived from combining the Greek words *athero* (paste) and *sclerosis* (hardness). Atherosclerosis involves a process that causes a build-up of deposits on artery walls called plaque. Typically, the deposits occur in the *tunica intima* (the innermost layer of a blood vessel) of large and medium-sized arteries. The plaques contain fatty substances, cholesterol, cellular waste products, fibrin found in blood), and calcium.

Plaque can become large enough to partially or totally block the flow of blood through an artery. A build-up of plaque or a rupture occurring within the plaque can result in a blood clot. The dislodged plaque material can travel to other parts of the body (e.g., brain, heart, kidneys, and legs), resulting in serious injury to tissues and organ (AHA 2002b; NIH 2003; Washington University 2003), principally by blocking blood flow through smaller arteries.

Atherosclerosis is a progressive, complex disease often associated with the aging process, but for some it starts much earlier in life. One study found that healthy soldiers returning from World War II already had occluded arteries (22% occlusion) even though their average age was 22.1 years. Early signs of atherosclerosis have been identified in children.

Half of the children and siblings of individuals with diseased coronary arteries had signs of atherosclerosis, even though they had no symptoms of heart or vessel disease (Strong 1986; Pharmabiz 2001; AHA 2002b). This indicates that genetic factors play an important role, but as you will soon read, it is possible to modify many of these hereditary defects.

Atherosclerosis is a factor in several conditions including *coronary heart disease* (CHD), myocardial infarction (MI), angina pectoris, cerebral vascular disease (CVD), thrombotic stroke, transient ischemic attacks (TIAs), insufficient blood supply to lower limbs and feet (claudication), organ damage, and vascular complications of diabetes (NIH 2003). Because symptoms can be few or minor in the early stages, atherosclerosis is referred to as "the silent killer" because it can progress undetected for years, particularly in individuals who are at high risk for heart disease.

Elevated blood pressure is associated with many factors (obesity, lack of exercise, increased blood sugar, and cholesterol levels), but high blood pressure can also be an indication of atherosclerosis. Increases in blood pressure generally occur gradually, concurrent with signs of advancing atherosclerotic disease. A study of 18,682 healthy American males (age 40-84 years; follow-up of 11.7 years) confirmed that blood pressure readings of 140/90 or higher were a risk factor for cardiovascular disease (including stroke and cardiovascular death). Hypertension is a major cardiovascular risk factor and borderline, isolated, systolic hypertension deserves special attention as a cardiac risk factor. Systolic hypertension has greater prognostic significance than diastolic hypertension. It is now recognized that the effective treatment of systolic hypertension proportionally reduces cardiac risk (O'Donnell et al. 1997; Izzo 2000).

Note: *On May 21, 2003 the* Journal of the American Medical Association *provided new guidelines for hypertension management: (1) in individuals over 50 years of age, systolic blood pressure over 140 mmHg is a greater risk factor for cardiovascular disease than diastolic blood pressure; (2) beginning at 115/75 mmHg, risk of cardiovascular disease doubles with each increment of 20/10 mmHg; (3) individuals who have normal blood pressure at age 55 have a 90% lifetime risk for developing hypertension; (4) individuals with a systolic blood pressure 120 to 139 mmHg or a diastolic blood pressure 80 to 89 mmHg should be considered pre-hypertensive. To prevent cardiovascular disease, these individuals require lifestyle changes that promote health (Chobanian et al. 2003).*

Precisely what causes atherosclerosis is not known, but several theories have been proposed. Scientists think atherosclerosis begins with damage to the *endothelium* (the inner layer of an artery). Possible causes of damage to the arterial wall are free-radical reactions; elevated levels of oxidized serum cholesterol, triglycerides, *fibrinogen*, homocysteine, insulin; high blood pressure; obesity; chronic inflammation, lifestyle factors (physical inactivity and tobacco smoking); and diabetes (AHA 2002b).

FACTORS IN THE DEVELOPMENT OF ATHEROSCLEROSIS

Some controllable mechanisms that are involved in the development of atherosclerosis are: (1) homocysteine overload, (2) oxidation of *low density lipoprotein-cholesterol* (LDL-C), and (3) abnormal platelet aggregation; and (4) inflammation. This protocol will empower individuals, enabling them to positively impact the factors contributing to atherosclerosis.

There is evidence that dietary supplementation, combined with appropriate changes in lifestyle, diet, and an exercise program, can prevent or reverse cardiovascular disease (Oakley 1998). The conventional medical establishment has long questioned the benefits of vitamin supplementation, but now even the *American Medical Association* encourages the use of homocysteine-lowering vitamin supplements to reduce the risks of cardiovascular disease (McCully 1998).

The Life Extension Foundation recommends using four different approaches to reduce elevated homocysteine levels. One approach is to supply supplements such as folic acid, vitamin B_{12}, and *trimethylglycine* (TMG) to increase the *remethylation* of homocysteine

back to *methionine* The second approach employs the detoxification method using vitamin B_6 to enhance the transsulfuration pathway to convert homocysteine into cysteine, which can be used to synthesize such beneficial amino acids such as glutathione and taurine. The third approach entails addition to the diet of 'methylated nutrients', such as creatine and various choline-containing supplements. More than half of the body's *S-adenosylmethionine* (**SAMe**) is used to synthesize creatine alone (Devlin 2002), which generates most of the homocysteine that must be either remethylated or detoxified. The fourth approach is to cut down or eliminate ingestion of foods containing high amounts of methionine such as red meat.

Homocysteine

Overview of Metabolic Pathways

All homocysteine is derived from the essential amino acid methionine. Homocysteine is converted into cysteine, methionine, or SAMe (Bottiglieri 1996). SAMe donates *methyl groups* to form *creatine, phosphatidylcholine, carnitine*, and other compounds (Devlin 2002). These methylation reactions create homocysteine that must be (1) remethylated to methionine or (2) catabolized into *cysteine, glutathione*, and *taurine*. Homocysteine is mostly remethylated (Jacobs et al. 2001; Ratnam et al. 2002) with new methyl carbons supplied by folic acid.

Elevated homocysteine occurs in man with nutritional deficiencies in folic acid, vitamin B_{12} and vitamin B_6, particularly in the elderly or in those with these genetic defects. The prevalence of these genetic defects, associated with marginal B vitamin intake, indicates that homocysteine is a risk factor in cardiovascular disease (Guilland et al. 2003; Haynes 2002).

Elevated homocysteine is predominantly *remethylated* by 5-*methyl*tetrahydrofolic acid (5-MTHF) to resynthesize methionine (Finkelstein et al. 1984) using the enzyme *methionine synthase*. High levels of methionine decrease methionine synthase, the primary enzyme for remethylation of homocysteine.

Humans with cardiovascular disease showed a significantly higher plasma homocysteine and reduced TMG levels (Schwahn et al. 2003). Scientists have found that mice deficient in remethylation enzymes had high levels in liver of homocysteine with low levels of phosphocholine and TMG. These levels were restored to normal by supplemental TMG (Schwahn et al. 2003).

About 11% of Caucasians possess gene mutations of a key enzyme involved in remethylation of homocysteine and express mild homocysteine elevation that is normalized by folic acid (Wilcken et al.

1998). Additional genetic mutations to this enzyme and to methionine synthase occur in man (Rozen 2000). Hyperhomocysteinemia is common when any of three different enzymes are defective in man (Selhub 1999). A genetic deficiency of the enzyme that irreversibly catabolizes homocysteine that was found in 32 patients with endothelial cell and smooth muscle cell dysfunction and increased thrombogenesis was treated with high folic acid, vitamin B_6, and vitamin B_{12} (Wilcken et al. 1998). Fifteen of the patients were unresponsive to vitamin B_6 but were successfully treated with TMG. TMG is most effective if taken regularly (Dudman et al. 1996).

What is considered to be normal levels of homocysteine (5–15 micromoles/L) is subject to debate because there is a proportional relationship between the development of cardiovascular disease and homocysteine (Robinson et al. 1995). Specifically, all levels over 6.3 mcmol/L proportionally increased cardiovascular disease.

Methionine generates SAMe (Bottiglieri 1996), the principal provider of methyl groups for biosynthetic reactions. Half of SAMe is used to biosynthesize creatine (Finkelstein et al. 1984) predominantly in kidney, liver (Stead et al. 2001; Lee 1998), and perhaps brain (Silveri et al. 2003). Humans excrete 1.4 grams of creatinine in urine per day, mostly derived from creatine (Devlin 2002). Animals fed (0.3%) creatine showed inhibition of creatine biosynthesis at the gene level (McGuire et al. 1984). A human consuming 400 grams of food per day may only require 1 gram of creatine to inhibit creatine biosynthesis and cut in half production of homocysteine. Supplemental creatine diminishes the need for SAMe, reduces formation of homocysteine, and the need to remethylate homocysteine. Supplemental creatine for two weeks lowered homocysteine by 25% in rats (Stead et al. 2001). Human subjects taking 1600 mg of SAMe per day increased phosphocreatine in brain (Silveri et al. 2003). This increase of phosphocreatine suggests creatine biosynthesis was enhanced by SAMe.

The liver biosynthesizes phosphatidylcholine for export as lipoproteins. This is a major use of SAMe in liver for the biosynthesis of choline via methylation of phosphatidylethanolamine (Devlin 2002). This is a primary source of homocysteine and a therapeutic target for hyperhomocysteinemia (Noga et al. 2003). Animals showed "significant depression of [homocysteine remethylation] when choline plus creatine were infused" (Lobley et al. 1996).

Food Sources of Methionine and Homocysteine

Methionine is the only amino acid that creates homocysteine, therefore, individuals who eat foods high in methionine (red meat) and develop high serum levels of homocysteine might benefit from intake of additional vitamins that enhance remethylation of homocysteine including folate, vitamin B_{12}, and TMG, which detoxify dietary homocysteine (and methionine). Dietary intake of supplements containing creatine and phosphatidylcholine, CDP-choline, a-glycerylphosphorylcholine, and choline, reduces the demand for methylation reactions and lower levels of homocysteine. Vitamin B_6 facilitates homocysteine detoxification via the transsulfuration pathway.

Primary Genetic Defects in the Catabolism of Homocysteine

Elevated homocysteine can be very pronounced if there is a genetic defect in the transsulfuration pathway that affects the activity of the B_6-dependent enzyme, cystathionine-ß-synthase (Perry 1999; Guilland et al. 2003). High doses of vitamin B6 are often required to suppress excessive homocysteine accumulation. Cofactors derived from vitamin B_6 catalyze the catabolism of homocysteine via pathways of transsulfuration. During transsulfuration, homocysteine is converted to cysteine, taurine, and eventually, sulfate. The amount of vitamin B_6 required to lower homocysteine varies considerably among individuals, and varies according to the severity of certain clinical (and subclinical) genetic disorders related to the metabolism of this amino acid. Some of the enzyme mutations alter the binding coefficients for B_6, thus increasing the requirement of the enzyme for vitamin B_6.

Genetic deficiency of cystathionine-ß-synthase in 32 patients (with adversely affected endothelial cell and smooth muscle cell function, and increased thrombogenesis) was effectively treated with high dietary levels of vitamin B_6, vitamin B_{12}, and folic acid. Half of the patients, apparently with minimal enzyme function even at high levels of vitamin B_6, benefited by additional supplementation with TMG (Wilcken et al. 1998). This genetic deficiency is particularly troublesome because if residual function of the enzyme cannot be restored by vitamin B_6, then the elimination of excess homocysteine and methionine through the normal catabolic route is difficult. Dietary intake of methionine must be carefully controlled and excess amounts of methylating vitamins are needed to remethylate homocysteine.

Excessive doses of vitamin B_6 should not be taken if peripheral neuropathy results (following chronic dosages of 300-500 mg daily) (IM 1998; NIH 2001). Homocysteinemia can be monitored through blood tests to determine if supplemental B_6 is maintaining safe levels in homocysteine. Some individuals lack the enzyme pyridoxine phosphokinase that converts vitamin B_6 into its biologically active cofactor form, pyridoxal-5-phosphate (Ubbink et al. 1993). If low-cost vitamin B_6 (pyridoxine) supplements do not sufficiently lower homocysteine levels, then a higher-cost pyridoxal-5-phosphate supplement may be required. (Supplement recommendations are in the Summary section at the end of this protocol.)

How Does Homocysteine Contribute to Atherosclerosis?

Homocysteine often causes the initial lesions on arterial walls that enable accumulated LDL and fibrinogen to eventually obstruct blood flow. Homocysteine contributes to the oxidation of LDL, accumulation of arterial plaque, and subsequent vascular blockage. Homocysteine directly damages cells by promoting oxidative stress. Homocysteine also can cause abnormal arterial blood clots (thrombosis) that can completely block an artery. Even if cholesterol and triglyceride levels are not significantly elevated, homocysteine alone promotes atherosclerosis and thrombosis.

Consumption of remethylation-enhancing nutrients such as folic acid, TMG, and vitamin B_{12} provides one of the most readily available and effective anti-aging therapies presently known. Provision of methylated nutrients such as creatine and several choline derivatives might effectively diminish the formation of homocysteine in vivo, thereby reducing homocysteine levels by reducing its formation. Useful choline-containing supplements include phosphatidylcholine (lecithin), cytidine-5-diphosphocholine (CDP-choline), choline, and a-glycerolphosphorylcholine (α-GPC).

However, it is important to tailor the intake of remethylation-enhancing and methylated nutrients to each individual's biochemistry. The most effective method to assess your rate of remethylation is to measure homocysteine blood levels. Elevated serum homocysteine is a classic sign of deficient remethylation and/or the over-production of methylated biochemical intermediates, which is correctable by ensuring the proper intake of remethylation-enhancing and methylated nutrients such as folic acid, vitamin B_{12}, TMG; and creatine, CDP-phosphatidylcholine, phosphatidylcholine, α-glycerylphosphorylcholine, and choline.

Note: *Recommendations for lowering homocysteine levels have been published by the* Journal of the American Medical Association *(Tucker et al. 1996) and in the* New England Journal of Medicine *(Malinow et al. 1998). Conventional physicians have begun to recognize the etiology of homocysteine in heart attack and stroke. Many now recommend folic acid to lower homocysteine levels in patients with coronary artery disease (Verhoef et al. 1996). However, in most instances it requires more than just folic acid to adequately suppress elevated blood levels of homocysteine.*

The Homocysteine/Atherosclerosis Link is Not Novel

The dangers of homocysteine were recognized in the 1950s (McCully et al. 1999). The Foundation identified a role for homocysteine in cardiovascular disease in its November 1981 issue of *Life Extension Magazine* (pp. 85–86). Life Extension's position has been confirmed by numerous studies showing that homocysteine, like cholesterol, is strongly associated with risk of heart disease (Haynes 2002; Guilland et al. 2003). Findings suggest there is *no* safe "normal range" for homocysteine. While commercial laboratories state that normal homocysteine can range from 5–15 micromoles/L of plasma, epidemiological data has revealed that homocysteine levels above 6.3 cause a steep, progressive risk of heart attack. The risk for coronary artery disease rises with increasing plasma homocysteine regardless of age and sex (Robinson et al. 1995).

Based on results of very large, long-term studies, elevated levels of homocysteine are associated with cardiovascular disease risks including male gender, age, smoking, high blood pressure, elevated cholesterol levels, and lack of exercise (Nygard et al. 1995). The overall risk of coronary and other vascular disease was 2.2 times higher in subjects with plasma total homocysteine levels in the top fifth of the normal range compared to those in the bottom four-fifths. Overall risk was independent of other risk factors, but was notably higher in subjects who smoked or had high blood pressure (Graham et al. 1997). The risk of death after 4–5 years was proportional to the level of plasma total homocysteine (Nygard et al. 1997). 3.8% of the subjects in the group with the lowest levels (< 9 micromoles/L) had died compared to 25% in the group with the highest levels (> 15 micromoles/L).

The American Heart Association recognized the role of homocysteine in atherosclerosis by issuing an advisory statement emphasizing the importance of reducing homocysteine blood levels and screening high-risk individuals (e.g., senior subjects, individuals diagnosed with chronic renal failure, thromboembolic disease or hypothyroidism, and patients taking drugs such as L-dopa, methotrexate, and theophylline) (Malinow et al. 1999).

Homocysteine Testing: A Measurement of Risk for Atherosclerosis and Cardiovascular Disease

Plasma homocysteine levels were 11% higher in cases of myocardial infarction (MI), whereas dietary and plasma levels of vitamin B6 and folate were lower (Verhoef et al. 1996). This is further evidence that plasma homocysteine is an independent risk factor for MI and that folate was the most important determinant of plasma homocysteine, even in subjects with apparently adequate folate intake. Fasting total plasma homocysteine levels were a strong predictor of severe coronary artery atherosclerosis. These researchers found a significant correlation of homocysteine levels with increasing numbers of occluded arteries. This showed a positive association between plasma homocysteine levels and the risk of coronary atherosclerosis. This association existed over such a wide range of homocysteine levels that no level could be established below which the risk was not related to homocysteine levels (Verhoef et al. 1997).

Note: *"Post-load" blood levels of homocysteine can be measured after giving a "load" of oral methionine, the precursor of homocysteine. Each 10% increase in homocysteine levels carried with it a 10% increase in the risk of developing heart disease. A similar percentage increase in cholesterol levels represents a 20% increased risk for heart disease. A 1999 study by Verhoef et al. was important because of its size and that it showed a positive correlation of risk of atherosclerosis with both "fasting" homocysteine levels and "post-load" homocysteine levels). The study showed that: (1) fasting homocysteine levels were lower in women than in men, (2) homocysteine levels were associated with age in both sexes, including post-menopausal women, (3) homocysteine levels after a methionine load were higher in women than in men, (4) in pre-menopausal women, low circulating levels of vitamin B6 increased the risk of vascular disease by two- to three-fold, independent of homocysteine, and (5) in men, low folate levels increased the risk of cardiovascular disease by 50%. It was concluded that "elevation of plasma total homocysteine appears to be at least as strong a risk for vascular disease in women as men, even before menopause" (Verhoef et al. 1999).*

Do Not Be Misled

Individuals taking vitamin supplements often think they are protected from the lethal effects of homocysteine, but supplement users can have homocysteine levels far above the accepted safe level of 6.3–7.0 micromoles/L. The Life Extension Foundation discovered a flaw in conventional homocysteine-reduction therapy back in 1999. The findings of this original study published in *Life Extension* magazine showed that a significant percentage of people taking vitamin supplements still have dangerously elevated blood homocysteine (LEF 1999). Although folic acid, vitamin B_{12}, vitamin B_6, and TMG can lower homocysteine levels, it is difficult to know if a safe level of homocysteine is attained unless homocysteine levels are determined by blood testing.

Recommendation: Homocysteine blood testing should be done to establish a baseline as an indicator of present disease risk, and to monitor the effects of homocysteine-lowering supplements.

Oxidized LDL

LDL (or low-density lipoprotein) is often referred to as "bad cholesterol." LDL, however, is not cholesterol. LDL is combination of a fat and a protein that acts as a carrier for cholesterol and fats in the blood stream. Cholesterol, on the other hand, is a fat-like steroid alcohol. Both LDL and cholesterol participate in the atherosclerosis process.

High LDL levels are considered more dangerous than high total cholesterol. Not only is the *amount* of LDL in the bloodstream important, so is its size. LDL comes in three sizes. The smallest size is the most troublesome. Small LDLs penetrate the artery wall easier than large LDLs; so they are more easily trapped in the artery wall and participate in plaque buildup. The small, dense LDLs are more vulnerable to oxidation than larger LDL particles. When LDL is oxidized, it is more dangerous. Oxidation of LDL renders it "sticky" and facilitates its deposition on the internal lining of blood vessels. Oxidized LDL initiates and contributes to the development of atherosclerosis through the following steps (Lau 2001):

1. By direct cytotoxic actions on endothelial cells. (This induces endothelial injury and contributes to the pathogenesis of atherosclerosis).

2. By increasing chemotactic stimulus for monocytes. (These monocytes are attracted to the arterial intima where atherogenesis begins. Monocytes then differentiate into macrophages.)

3. By transforming macrophages into foam cells. (Production of foam cells is a starting point in atherogenesis but their presence is also typical for advanced atherosclerotic lesions, which are prone to rupture; producing clinical complications such as myocardial infarction and stroke) (Bobkova et al. 2003).

4. By enhancing the proliferation of various cell types, e.g., endothelial cells, monocytes, and smooth muscle cells. (Proliferation and migration of cells leads to a thickening within the intima (innermost) layer and a marked occlusion of the vessel).

Homocysteine is a significant factor in the oxidation process that results in atherosclerosis. Homocysteine damages the artery and then oxidizes cholesterol before cholesterol infiltrates the vessel. Hemochromatosis (iron overload) can also contribute to the oxidation of cholesterol. (Free iron oxidizes LDL, increasing the damage imposed upon the heart and vascular system through promotion of free radicals.)

Although oxidized LDL plays an important role in the etiology of arterial disease, evidence shows that even if oxidation of LDL is prevented, it might still be dangerous. The binding of C-reactive protein to non-oxidized LDL enhances *complement* activation (complement plays a pathogenetic role in promoting lesion progression) (Bhakdi et al. 1999). Elevated LDL, whether it is oxidized or not, can alter the ability of endothelial cells to release nitric oxide. Nitric oxide allows the arteries of the cardiovascular system to properly dilate (Feron et al. 1999; Sheehan 2003).

Guidelines recommend getting LDL below 100, but many are uncertain that lower is still better. One study targeted a level of 80 and concluded that the more rigorous treatment aggressively stopped arterial clogging (CTV 2003). Other findings showed benefits to reducing LDL in individuals with average serum cholesterol levels and no evidence of coronary heart disease (Marais 1998).

Abnormal Platelet Aggregation: An Important Player in Atherosclerosis

Platelets are small blood elements, but they play a major role in cardiovascular health. The primary role of platelets is to prevent bleeding by 'clotting' leaks in the vessel wall. Blood vessels with smooth interior walls enable platelets to flow over their surface. When a blood vessel is damaged, exposing the underlying collagen, the platelets adhere to cover the gap. Activated platelets do more than form a plug. They release potent vasoconstrictors such as serotonin and the powerful platelet aggregator thromboxane A2. Though this action is desirable in response to injury, it can have deleterious effects. Abnormal platelet stickiness increases atherosclerosis and further narrows the internal diameter of the artery, factors that predispose one to strokes and heart attacks (Braly 1985).

Fibrinogen

Fibrinogen is a blood protein that controls coagulation. In good health there are normal levels of fibrinogen and normal coagulation. When fibrinogen levels rise above normal there is an increased chance of abnormal blood clotting. If fibrinogen levels decrease below normal, a hemorrhage can result. Although the reference range used by most laboratories is 150-460 mg/dL, it is crucial to keep serum fibrinogen under 300 mg/dL, a level considered safe.

The coagulation of blood depends upon clotting factors that are activated following injury. A series of reactions produces a clot by converting fibrinogen to fibrin (a network of protein fibers that can trap blood cells and platelets), thus plugging the leak (Whiting 1989; Seeley et al. 1991; Kohler et al. 2000).

Fibrin provides a scaffold along which cells migrate and which can bind fibronectin. This stimulates cell migration, monocyte adhesion, and smooth muscle proliferation, further occluding the vessel. In advanced plaque, fibrin may also be involved in the tight binding of LDL-C and the accumulation of lipids (Smith 1986; Koenig 1999a).

Plaque is highly susceptible to breakage and clot formation. About 700,000 heart attacks and stroke deaths occur in the United States each year as a result of a blood clot obstructing the delivery of blood to the heart or brain. People with high levels of fibrinogen are more than twice as likely to die of a heart attack, but also from stroke (Wilhelmsen et al. 1984; Packard et al. 2000). Fibrinogen is a predictor of stroke, but the odds worsen with high blood pressure (Bots et al. 2002).

Fibrinogen promotes platelet aggregation (Koenig 1999b). Fibrinogen deposition at the vessel wall promotes platelet adhesion during ischemia (Massberg et al. 1999). Platelets are essential in sealing all vascular injuries. When the interior of the vessel is smooth, platelets are not activated; however, when traumatized, platelets are activated to plug the wound. Activated platelets release serotonin (a vasoconstrictor) and the platelet aggregator thromboxane A2, furthering clot formation (Braly 1985; Smith 1986; Ernst et al. 1993).

The Life Extension Foundation was the first research group to recognize the importance of assessing fibrinogen as an independent risk factor for cardiovascular disease, which was later corroborated (Ma et al. 1999). Individuals having heart attacks had significantly higher fibrinogen levels compared to healthy individuals. Several studies have shown a stronger association between cardiovascular deaths and fibrinogen levels than with cholesterol levels. Higher baseline levels of fibrinogen are predictive of a heart attack and the likelihood of sudden cardiac death. Coronary risk is low among patients with low fibrinogen concentrations despite increased serum cholesterol levels (Thompson 1995). Fibrinogen is directly associated with the risk of myocardial infarction (Acevedo et al. 2002; Bots et al. 2002; GSDL 2002).

High levels of homocysteine are toxic to the cardiovascular system. Part of this toxicity may result from the ability of homocysteine to block the natural breakdown of fibrinogen-derived fibrin by inhibiting the production of tissue plasminogen activator (t-PA) (Midorikawa et al. 2000). If fibrin cannot be digested by the enzymatic action of plasminogen, fibrin-containing clots accumulate, contributing to an increased incidence of heart attack and formation of larger plaques inside the arteries.

The *Therapeutic* section describes products with fibrinolytic and anti-platelet aggregating activity, such as aspirin, bromelain, curcumin, essential fatty acids, garlic, ginger, ginkgo biloba, green tea, gugulipid, niacin, pantethine, policosanol, proanthocyanidins, vitamin A, beta-carotene, vitamin C, and vitamin E. A novel drug approach to reduce excess fibrinogen is to take 400 mg of pentoxifylline twice daily. Vitamin C has been shown to break down excess fibrinogen (Bordia 1980).

Inflammation

Typically, the risk of developing heart disease is assessed by monitoring plasma levels of cholesterol and by routinely checking for high blood pressure. Newer risk factors including C-reactive protein (CRP) and fibrinogen are markers of systemic inflammation.

Fibrinogen and CRP are produced in the liver by pro-inflammatory cytokines called interleukin-1b, interleukin-6, and tumor necrosis factor alpha (TNF-α) (Ridker et al. 2000). Injury to the inner lining of the arterial vessels, or arteriosclerosis, plays an important role in the development of atherosclerosis, which is characterized by the build up of fatty deposits in the lining of arteries (Auer et al. 2002).

Research indicates that the presence in blood of indicators of inflammation are strong predictors for who will develop CHD or have a cardiac-related death (Lindahl et al. 2000; Packard et al. 2000; Radar 2000). CRP levels increase during systemic inflammation and tests to determine the levels of this protein in the blood can help assess the risk of cardiovascular

disease. Some evidence suggests that blood levels of CRP may be a stronger predictor of heart disease than levels of LDL-C (Ridker et al. 2002). High levels of CRP have predicted future coronary events in patients with stable CHD. Studies have shown that high CRP levels predict the risk of future heart attack, stroke, peripheral arterial disease and vascular death in people that have no other signs of cardiovascular disease (Ridker 2001; Ridker et al. 2000; Kuller et al. 1996; Mendall et al. 2000; Ridker et al. 1998). High CRP has also been associated with increased vascular events in people with acute ischemic heart disease, stable angina, and a history of heart attack (Ridker 2001).

If a person has an intermediate risk of cardiovascular disease, the American Heart Association recommends that a CRP test can be useful in predicting a future cardiovascular event or stroke. This information can help direct further evaluation and therapy. A person at high risk or who has established heart disease or stroke should be treated intensively regardless of CRP levels.

CRP rises several hundred-fold after tissue injury, but stays relatively stable in the absence of inflammation. Elevated CRP levels indicate a low-grade inflammation, including vascular disease (Pasceri et al. 2000). Responses to rising levels of CRP may include disruption of existing plaque resulting in a blood clot. There is significant improvement in predicting cardiac health when models include CRP testing. CRP levels can predict future coronary events in healthy individuals. Increased monocytes (white blood cells critical in early plaque development) and macrophages (mononuclear phagocytic cells capable of scavenging and ingesting dead tissue and degenerated cells) are present in atherosclerosis, particularly at points of plaque rupture. It appears that CRP and several other inflammatory markers may be elevated many years prior to a coronary event.

CRP acts upon blood vessels to activate adhesion molecules in endothelial cells: the intercellular adhesion molecule (ICAM-1) and the vascular cell adhesion molecule (VCAM-1). VCAM-1 is an early molecular marker of lesion-prone areas in response to experimental hypercholesterolemia. In humans, ICAM-1 and VCAM-I expression is increased in the endothelium of atherosclerotic plaque. CRP is involved in the inflammatory process and may be a target for the treatment of atherosclerosis (Pasceri et al. 2000; Biomedical Science 2001; Alvaro-Gonzalez et al. 2002).

CRP affects the activity of LDL, which contributes to the process of increasing atherogenesis. The cycle begins as stranded LDL is taken up by macrophages, becomes engorged with fats, and develops into foam cells, which explode and discharge their fats into the blood vessel walls. This recruits more macrophages to clean up the mess and the cycle repeats. CRP readies the LDL for uptake by the macrophages, initiating the sequence (Braley 1985; Zwaka et al. 2001). Higher levels of CRP increase the risk of stroke, heart attack, and peripheral vascular disease (Rifai et al. 2001a, b). Stroke patients with the highest CRP levels were 2-3 times more likely to die within a year than patients with low levels (DiNapoli et al. 2001).

Persistent CRP elevation following coronary stent implantation is predictive of restenosis (Gottsauner-Wolf et al. 2000). Patients requiring restenosis had increased CRP levels for over four days following the implant procedure, although their baseline CRP was normal at the time of restenosis.

Many of the newer risk factors are not standardized, yet some laboratories use a CRP reference range of 0.24-1.69 mg/L. Test results can be artificially high if there has been recent tissue injury, infection, or inflammation.

CRP levels decline following, DHEA, fish oil, pravastatin, vitamin C, vitamin E, and vitamin K supplementation (see the *Therapeutic* sections of this protocol and others in this book). Many nutrients and herbs with anti-inflammatory properties may maintain low CRP levels. Because CRP reduces vitamins A, C, E, carotenoids, zinc, and selenium, supplementation with these nutrients may contribution to better cardiovascular health when CRP levels are high.

Adding fish to your diet can help lower your risk of heart disease. Research indicates that fish oil supplements (1 gram per day) reduced the risk of cardiac deaths after 6–8 months in people who had a prior heart attack. Patients that took fish oil supplements had a 45% lower death rate than those who did not (Marchioli et al. 2002).

Supplements such as highly concentrated DHA derived from fish oil and the adrenal hormone, DHEA, suppress excess production of some of the dangerous cytokines. Interleukin-6 increases the risk of heart attack, even without the participation of CRP, which is otherwise released by interleukin-6 (Rader 2000).

Low Testosterone = Increased Heart Attack Risk

The influence of sex hormones, especially testosterone, on coronary artery disease in men has been relatively ignored (Brewer Science Library 2003). Men with CHD have lower concentrations of testosterone than men with normal heart health (Wu et al. 1993; Channer et al. 2003). Hypogonadism, characterized by low testosterone levels, is twice as common in men with heart disease (Brewer Science Library 2003). Low testosterone is associated with high LDL, low HDL, high triglycerides, and high blood pressure. Administration of testosterone dilates blood vessels (Channer et al. 2003), improves exercise tolerance, and reduces angina in men with CHD (English et al. 2000). Low testosterone in older men may promote atherosclerosis and explain the higher incidence of CHD.

Although heart disease continues to be an epidemic, you can take a number of steps to lower your risk of developing the condition. Besides checking your cholesterol and blood pressure, have your blood assayed for CRP, homocysteine, fibrinogen, and free testosterone. Exercise naturally lowers the risk of stroke by lowering blood pressure, but also lowers levels of CRP that are an important measure of systemic inflammation (Szymanski et al. 1994; Ford 2002).

The most recent study showed that low free testosterone is an independent risk factor for developing aggressive coronary artery disease (Philips et al. 2004).

THE BENEFITS OF NUTRIENT SUPPLEMENTATION

B Vitamins (Homocysteine Lowering Nutrients)

Landmark studies, part of the large Framingham Heart Study started in 1948 demonstrated that high plasma levels of homocysteine and low levels of folic acid and vitamin B6 are associated with increased narrowing of the carotid arteries (Selhub et al. 1995). Numerous studies have reported positive outcomes following the use of B vitamins for reduction of homocysteine. Healthy men with moderate hyperhomocysteinemia had lower concentrations of vitamins B6, B12, and folic acid (25.0%, 56.8%, and 59.1%, respectively). Daily supplementation with these vitamins normalized elevated plasma homocysteine levels within 6 weeks, indicating that moderate vitamin therapy is an efficient and cost-effective method of controlling elevated homocysteine (Ubbink et al. 1993).

Patients and normal volunteers, with or without elevated homocysteine levels (>16 micromoles/L) that received multivitamin supplements showed normalized plasma homocysteine levels, if these levels were initially high, and lower homocysteine levels even if their homocysteine levels were normal. Supplementation with 500 mcg of folic acid led to a substantial reduction of blood homocysteine levels in all populations (den Heijer et al. 1998).

Patients were treated daily with placebo, folic acid (650 mcg), vitamin B_{12} (400 mcg), vitamin B_6 (10 mg), or a combination of the three vitamins for 6 weeks. Folic acid supplementation reduced plasma homocysteine concentrations by 42%; vitamin B_{12} lowered homocysteine by 15%; but vitamin B_6 (in this low dose) caused no significant changes. The combination of all three vitamins reduced homocysteine by 50%. "Folate deficiency might be an important cause of hyperhomocysteinemia in the general population." Supplements containing modest levels of folic acid or combinations of folic acid, B_6, and B_{12} lowered plasma levels of homocysteine (Ubbink et al. 1993).

Heart attack patients were surveyed for dietary intake of vitamins. Higher levels of folic acid were protective and this supports homocysteine as an independent risk factor for cardiovascular disease. Adequate folic acid intake from diet or supplements normalizes levels of plasma homocysteine (Verhoef et al. 1996).

Niacin

Niacin (nicotinic acid) is a B vitamin that has been used in high doses (1.0–4.5 grams per day) as a treatment for hyperlipidemia, a condition characterized by elevated blood levels of cholesterol and/or fats as triglycerides (TGs). High concentrations of TGs are associated with increased risk of CHD. Niacin reduces cholesterol and TG levels, and increases the concentration of *high-density lipoprotein* (HDL) associated with reduced risk of CHD (Crouse 1996). Niacin is usually effective at modulating blood lipids, but side effects sometimes dampen enthusiasm for therapy.

Although side effects are dose-related, few studies have determined an optimal dose of nicotinic acid that alters lipid levels with the fewest side effects. Martin-Jadraque et al. (1996) demonstrated that low-dose nicotinic acid treatment significantly lowered TGs, raised HDL concentrations by approximately 22%, and favorably altered the ratio of total cholesterol to HDL in all subjects. Improvement in blood lipid levels was observed in 75% of subjects who tolerated low-dose nicotinic acid therapy. Although the changes induced by lower doses were less than higher doses, the lower dose was better tolerated. Nicotinic acid may also be useful in combination drug therapy for prevention of CHD if higher doses cannot be tolerated. Use of a lower dose should still be beneficial in for producing a moderate rise in HDL levels. Women seem to have a greater LDL response to niacin, but experience more side effects at higher dosages. Lower doses of niacin may be more desirable for women (Goldberg 1998).

Long-term treatment with nicotinic acid (4 g/day for 6 weeks) not only corrects serum lipoprotein abnormalities, but also reduces the fibrinogen concentration in plasma and stimulates fibrinolysis (Johansson et al. 1997).

Epidemiologic evidence (Framingham Heart Study) indicates that a low level of HDL is an independent predictor of CHD. Other findings related to low HDL revealed that (1) it is an independent predictor of the number and severity of atherosclerotic coronary arteries, (2) it predicts total mortality in coronary artery disease patients when total cholesterol is in a desirable range (<200 mg/dL), and (3) it is associated with increased restenosis after angioplasty. Study conclusions were that most medications used to treat dyslipidemias will raise HDL levels modestly; however, niacin appears to have the greatest potential to do so, increasing HDL up to 30% (Kwiterovich 1998).

CAUTION Side effects associated with niacin consumption include flushing, itching, minor gastrointestinal symptoms, and the possibility of liver damage. A blood test to measure liver enzyme levels is mandatory every 3–6 months because of the potential of niacin to cause liver damage in a minority of people. Niacin cannot be used in individuals with existing liver disease (e.g., hepatitis C, cirrhosis of the liver).

It is possible that niacin raises homocysteine levels because of increased methylation of niacinamide. Niaspan, an extended-release niacin, raised homocysteine levels in a dose-dependent manner in some people, by an amount generally between 1–4 micromoles/L. Niacinamide formed from excess niacin may deplete SAMe, the body's normal agent for methylation. If niacinamide is methylated, it is likely that there would be an elevation of plasma homocysteine.

Individuals may be able to use smaller amounts of niacin if chromium accompanies the dosage. Niacin in combination with chromium lowered cholesterol levels by an average of 14% and improved total cholesterol and HDL/LDL ratio by 7%. This finding is valuable since the side effects of niacin may make it less useful in large doses (Urberg et al. 1987; Cichoke 2004; Berkeley Heart Lab). The typical daily dose of niacin (bound to chromium) is less than 2 mg (not the usual 500–4,500 mg). When niacin-bound chromium is used, mega doses of niacin are no longer needed to lower cholesterol. Niacin-bound chromium can significantly increase levels of protective HDL and decrease the LDL (Cichoke 2004).

Vitamin C

A widely publicized study showed that men who took 800 mg daily of vitamin C lived about 6 years longer than those consuming the RDA of 60 mg per day. This study evaluated 11,348 participants over 10 years and demonstrated that high vitamin C intake prolonged average life span and reduced mortality from cardiovascular disease by 42% (Enstrom et al. 1992). A study of 11,178 elderly subjects; aged 67 to 105 years compared vitamin C and vitamin E supplemented subjects to subjects using no vitamin supplements: Use of vitamin E alone reduced death from myocardial infarction (MI) by 63%, cancer mortality by 59%, and overall mortality by 34%. When the vitamin C and E were used together, overall mortality was reduced by 42% (Losonczy et al. 1996).

When vitamin C was co-administered with nitrate drugs (nitroglycerine, NTG), the adverse effects of nitrate tolerance were virtually eliminated. The most significant change was a 310% improvement in the arterial conductivity test (Bassenge et al. 1998). Nitrate drugs sometimes induce dangerous up-regulated activity of platelets that can be reversed with vitamin C supplementation. The findings demonstrated that dietary supplementation with vitamin C can eliminate vascular tolerance and up-regulation of platelet activity during long-term, non-intermittent administration of nitrate drugs (NTG) in humans.

Vitamin supplementation is effective in congestive heart failure (CHF). CHF is associated with a reduced dilation (capacity) of the endothelial lining of the arterial system (flow-dependent dilation). High-resolution ultrasound and Doppler measurements of artery diameter and blood flow following vitamin C (25 mg/min, intra-arterially) determined that vitamin C restored arterial dilatory responses and blood flow in CHF (Hornig et al. 1998). Studies have indicated that antioxidant intake is associated with decreased risk for CHD. Low plasma levels of ascorbic acid predict the presence of an unstable coronary syndrome possibly by influencing the activity surrounding an arterial wall lesion rather than the overall extent of the disease (Vita et al. 1998).

Vitamin E

Evidence demonstrates that vitamin E protects against development of atherosclerosis by retarding oxidation of LDL, inhibiting proliferation of smooth muscle cells, reducing platelet adhesion and aggregation, and altering the expression and function of adhesion molecules. Vitamin E attenuates the synthesis of leukotrienes and potentiates release of prostacyclin (which inhibits platelet aggregation and acts as a vasodilator) by up-regulating the expression of cytosolic phospholipase A2. These biological functions of vitamin E may protect against the development of atherosclerosis (Chan 1998).

Studies substantiate the involvement of free radical reactions in the early or developing stages of human disease. Improvement of diet (by increasing antioxidants) lessens degenerative diseases. Degenerative disease is lower following diets with high levels of antioxidants or diets supplemented with vitamin E. By increasing intake of vitamin E-rich foods or vitamin E supplements, it is possible to reduce the risk of many common, disabling human diseases and improve the quality of life, particularly in the elderly (Diplock 1997).

Antioxidant supplements, particularly vitamin E, reduce oxidation of lipoproteins, which promote atherosclerosis. A large study that examined the relationship between the intake of dietary carotene, vitamin C, and vitamin E and subsequent coronary mortality found an inverse association between dietary vitamin E and coronary mortality, supporting the hypothesis that antioxidant vitamins provide protection against CHD (Knekt et al. 1994). Compared to subjects receiving placebo, a significant savings in health-related costs was reported in patients receiving supplemental vitamin E. This was primarily attributed to the fact that the vitamin E-supplemented group had fewer hospital admissions and a 4.4% lower risk of acute MI than the placebo group (Davey et al. 1998).

Large epidemiological studies revealed that higher vitamin E levels in plasma result in a reduced incidence of CHD. Dose-response studies in humans have demonstrated that 400 IU per day of vitamin E increased vitamin E plasma levels twofold and delayed oxidation of LDL (Suzukawa et al. 1998). A study to determine the effects of long-term vitamin E supplementation in 17,894 people (aged 50-98) revealed that the length of time the individual used vitamin E was more important than the amount of the nutrient used. This trend was particularly apparent beyond nine years of usage. Taking 400 IU of vitamin E daily for 10 years or more strikingly reduced the occurrence of heart disease prior to 80 years of age (Passwater 1977).

The type and blend of vitamin E selected for supplementation can affect the end results. Studies show that tocopherol may offer better protection against CHD when it is combined with gamma tocopherol. Both tocopherol and gamma tocopherol can decrease platelet aggregation, inhibit blood clot formation, protect LDL against oxidation, and increase endogenous *superoxide dismutase* production (an enzyme with antioxidant activity); however, gamma tocopherol shows greater activity on each function. Unfortunately, gamma tocopherol can be obtained from food, but it is poorly retained because it is excreted in urine following liver metabolism. An a-tocopherol transfer protein, selectively transports a-tocopherol over other forms of vitamin E. Consequently, a-tocopherol is more abundant in body tissues. This does not provide for maximum protection against free radical attack. It is recommended that individuals seeking protective cardiovascular effects from vitamin E include gamma tocopherol, by complexing a-tocopherol (80%) with gamma tocopherol (20%) as an ideal blend.

Coenzyme Q_{10}

Coenzyme Q_{10} (CoQ$_{10}$; ubiquinone) is a fat-soluble *cofactor* substance. It is a naturally occurring substance that prevents cell damage due to myocardial ischemia (hypoxia) or subsequent to reestablishment of blood flow to the heart after temporary ischemia.

CoQ$_{10}$ is involved in several key enzymes in energy production within a cell, and has membrane-stabilizing activity. It functions primarily as an antioxidant. CoQ$_{10}$ has been used to treat cardiovascular disorders including angina pectoris, hypertension, CHF, and periodontal disease. The inflammatory process within the lining of atherosclerotic blood vessels parallels the chronic inflammation of periodontal disease. People with gum disease carry a greater risk for cardiovascular disease and hypertension. Research suggests that topical application of CoQ$_{10}$ improves adult periodontitis when used alone, but also in combination with traditional periodontal therapy (Greenberg et al. 1990; Hanioka et al. 1994; Genco 1997).

Numerous studies provide details of the efficacy of CoQ$_{10}$ in the prevention and treatment of heart disease, as detailed below.

Oral CoQ$_{10}$ (150 mg daily in 3 doses) was given for 4 weeks to exercising angina patients. Average levels of CoQ$_{10}$ in plasma increased after CoQ$_{10}$ treatment and were significantly related to an increase in exercise duration. Side effects were minimal. The study suggested that: "CoQ$_{10}$ is a safe and promising treatment for angina pectoris" (Kamikawa et al. 1985).

Pretreatment with intravenous CoQ$_{10}$ minimized myocardial injury caused by cardiac bypass graft (CABG) surgery and improved heart function. Patients undergoing CABG were evaluated for reduced left ventricular capacity following reperfusion. Patients received CoQ$_{10}$ (5 mg/kg, intravenously) 2 hours before cardiopulmonary bypass. Left ventricular stroke work capacity was significantly elevated at 6 and 10 hours after reperfusion following CAB. The results suggested: "pretreatment with intravenous CoQ$_{10}$ prevented left ventricular depression in early reperfusion and minimized myocardial cellular injury during CAB followed by reperfusion" (Sunamori et al. 1991).

CHF is characterized by depleted energy status and low CoQ$_{10}$ levels. Individuals experiencing heart failure (2664 individuals from 173 centers) were administered 50–150 mg of CoQ$_{10}$ daily. After 90 days of CoQ$_{10}$ treatment, patient improvement in clinical signs and symptoms was significant: cyanosis, 78.1%; edema, 78.6%; enlarged liver area, 49.3%; dyspnea, 52.7%; palpitations, 75.4%; sweating, 79.8%; subjective arrhythmia, 63.4%; insomnia, 662.8%; vertigo, 73.1%; and nocturia, 53.6%. Improvement of at least three symptoms was observed in 54% of patients, which was interpreted as improved quality of life. The incidence of side effects was low (1.5%) (Baggio et al. 1994).

Effects of oral treatment with CoQ$_{10}$ (120 mg daily) were compared after 28 days in patients with *acute myocardial infarction* (AMI). After treatment with CoQ$_{10}$, angina pectoris, total arrhythmias, poor left ventricular function, and total cardiac events were significantly reduced in the CoQ$_{10}$ group. The antioxidants (vitamins A, E, C, and beta-carotene), which were initially lower following the AMI, increased more in the coenzyme CoQ$_{10}$ group. CoQ$_{10}$ can provide rapid protective effects in patients with AMI if administered within 3 days of the onset of symptoms (Singh et al. 1998).

Many elderly individuals will soon require heart surgery as the general population ages. The outcome of surgery in the elderly, compared to younger individuals, is compromised by age-related reduction of cellular energy production in the myocardium during surgery. Elderly subjects were given CoQ$_{10}$ prior to heart surgery to improve surgical outcomes and to determine if contractile function of muscle fibers in response to ischemia (and aging) could be reversed. Fibers from subjects over age 70 showed poor recovery of force after simulated ischemia compared to younger patients. This age-associated effect was prevented by pretreatment with CoQ$_{10}$ (Rosenfeldt et al. 1999). It was hypothesized that CoQ$_{10}$ pretreatment prior to stress improved recovery of the myocardium after stress (Rosenfeldt et al. 2002). CoQ$_{10}$ improves heart function in two ways: by fighting free radical attacks during cardiac stress (angioplasty, thrombolysis, and surgery) and improving cellular energy production (Rosenfeldt et al. 1999).

Note: *Because of the popular use of "statin" drugs (Zocor®, Lipitor®, Pravachol®, Lescol®, and Mevacor®) it is important to emphasize that statins act by inhibiting HMG-CoA reductase, the rate-limiting enzyme in cholesterol biosynthesis. Drugs inhibiting HMG-CoA reductase activity decrease CoQ$_{10}$ levels (Folkers et al. 1990) because HMG-CoA reductase is required for CoQ$_{10}$ synthesis. Individuals using statins ought to increase their intake of CoQ$_{10}$ to negate the decrease in CoQ$_{10}$ biosynthesis caused by the statin drugs. Some mainstream physicians are aware of this side effect and administer CoQ$_{10}$ with statin therapy. CoQ$_{10}$ is free of toxicity and typically produces no side effects. CoQ$_{10}$ may change the insulin requirements of people with diabetes so talk to your physician if you have diabetes and plan on taking CoQ$_{10}$.*

Essential Fatty Acids

Omega-3 Oils

Omega-3 fatty acids, EPA (eicosapentaenoic acid) and DHA (docosahexaenoic acid), from fish, flax, or perilla oils, are essential for optimal health. Most Western diets contain predominantly omega-6 fatty acids, in proportions greatly exceeding the omega-3 fatty acids. The so-called "bad" saturated fatty acids and their metabolites (those fats that are solid at room temperature) compete with beneficial EPA and DHA fatty acids. Increasing dietary alpha-linolenic acid and omega-3 fatty acids, while limiting dietary polyunsaturated fat and calorie intake, have important cardiac benefits, including reduction of risk of heart attack and mortality by as much as 70% (Guize et al. 1995).

Scientific studies demonstrate that alpha-linolenic acid (from flax or perilla oil) reduced the incidence of atherosclerosis, stroke, and second heart attacks. When perilla or flax oil is consumed, it requires the enzyme *delta-6 desaturase* to convert the alpha-linolenic acid into EPA and DHA. Many individuals (particularly those over 50 years of age, who show declining activity of this enzyme) should consider using high-potency fish oil because these products directly provide EPA and DHA. Compared with no fish consumption, a lower risk of death was associated with fish consumption. High proportions of omega-3 fatty acids found in serum lipids were associated with a substantially reduced risk of death (Erkkila et al. 2003).

Thromboxane A2 promotes abnormal blood-clot formation, however, seven days of dietary perilla oil (versus soybean oil) effectively reduced inflammatory cytokine formation and thromboxane A2 production by platelets in rats (Ikeda et al. 1995). Excessive platelet-activating factor (PAF) is a major cause of arterial blood clots that can lead to heart attack and stroke. When compared with high dietary linoleic acid-containing safflower oil (an omega-6 fatty acid), high dietary alpha-linolenic acid-containing perilla oil (an omega-3 fatty acid) decreased PAF production by nearly one half in experimental animals (Oh-hashi et al. 1997). Perilla oil alleviates chronic inflammation, prevents certain types of arrhythmia, maintains cardiac cellular energy output, and preserves cell membrane structure.

Studies reflect the advantages of healthy eating (Renaud 2001). A Mediterranean-type diet has been evaluated after the first heart attack. The diet emphasizes fruits, vegetables, bread, cereals, potatoes, beans, nuts, seeds, and olive oil. Red meat and eggs are restricted. Servings of fish, poultry, and wine are restricted to low to moderate amounts. After four years, there was a 50-70% lower risk of recurrent heart disease (AHA 2004a).

Note: *Because EPA/DHA can interfere with blood clotting those who suffer from any type of hemorrhagic disease or who take anticoagulant drugs should inform their doctor they are taking these supplements. Physicians may wish to adjust the dosage of anticoagulant medication based on measures of blood coagulation.*

Herbal Supplements

One fourth of prescription drugs in the United States have at least one active ingredient derived from plant material. The World Health Organization estimates that 80% of the world population uses herbal treatments as part of their primary healthcare. Herbal extracts are among the most-studied preparations in the world. Most of modern medicine is directly or indirectly derived from folk medicine and herbal treatments.

Bromelain

Bromelain (*Ananas comusus*) is derived from the stem of the pineapple plant. Bromelain is a protein-digesting (proteolytic) enzyme capable of reducing atherosclerotic plaque. Proteolytic enzymes work directly at sites of inflammation, digesting damaged cell tissue (recall that inflammation is one of the newer risk factors recognized as a promoter of cardiac disease). Bromelain has fibrinolytic activities (the ability to break down fibrin). Fibrin forms a matrix that walls off an inflamed area, resulting in vessel blockage, inadequate tissue drainage, and edema (Felton 1980; Lotz-Winter 1990; Metzig et al. 1999; Maurer 2001). Bromelain may improve cardiac health by opposing platelet aggregation, and relieve angina attacks possibly through fibrinolytic properties. Bromelain is nontoxic up to 10 grams per kilogram. The only side effect noted has been allergic reactions in sensitive individuals (Murray 1995; Maurer 2001). Because bromelain is an anticoagulant it should be used with the advice of a physician if used with prescription anticoagulants. Individuals with cardiovascular disease who take bromelain should periodically have blood tests to measure their fibrinogen level to determine if serum fibrinogen is in a safe range.

Curcumin

Ground turmeric is used worldwide as a seasoning (as curry) and is a source for curcumin (turmeric contains approximately 4% curcumin). Turmeric is a member of the *Curcuma* botanical group, which is part of the ginger family of herbs (Zingiberaceae).

Curcumin has been used for over 3000 years in traditional Ayurvedic medicine, but more recently has showed cardiovascular-related activities (anti-platelet aggregating and anti-inflammatory activity) and antioxidant properties (Chainani-Wu 2003). Curcumin may control platelet aggregation by directly inhibiting thromboxane (a promoter of aggregation) and increasing prostacyclin activity (an inhibitor of aggregation). Some of curcumin's functions may lessen the risk of forming blood clots (Srivastava et al. 1985; Toda et al. 1985). Animal studies showed impressive cholesterol-lowering benefits. Rats fed 0.1% curcumin, on a cholesterol-containing diet, had one-half of the levels of blood cholesterol than rats without curcumin (Rao et al. 1970; Srivastava et al. 1986; Srinivasan et al. 1991).

Curcumin reduced serum levels of cholesterol and lipid peroxides in humans receiving 500 mg of curcumin daily for seven days (a short span of time to enact a change in lipid parameters). A significant decrease in the level of serum lipid peroxides (33%), an increase in HDL (29%), and a decrease in total serum cholesterol (12%) suggest that curcumin may prevent arterial diseases (Soni et al. 1992). A review of human trials determined that curcumin is without toxicity (Chainani-Wu 2003). If you are using a supplement called Super Curcumin with Bioperine in conjunction with drug therapy, your physician should be made aware of the supplementation. Piperine enhances the body's natural absorptive functions so it is possible bioperine may increase the absorption rate of drugs. The physician will schedule the dosages so that the drug and bioperine are taken at different times during the day. Because curcumin increases the excretion of cholesterol-bile acids, individuals with

biliary tract obstruction should not use curcumin. Pregnant or lactating women should not use curcumin. High doses of curcumin taken on an empty stomach might cause stomach ulcers.

Garlic

High cholesterol (hypercholesterolemia) has been recognized as a risk factor in atherosclerosis. Oxidized LDL is a key player in the initiation and progression of atherosclerosis. Short-term supplementation of garlic in humans increased resistance of LDL to oxidation, suggesting that the suppression of LDL oxidation may be one mechanism for garlic's anti-atherosclerotic action (Lau 2001; Dillon et al. 2003). Garlic may reduce other risk factors in the genesis and progression of arteriosclerosis: garlic decreases total and LDL; increases HDL; reduces serum triglyceride and fibrinogen concentrations; lowers arterial blood pressure; inhibits platelet aggregation and reduces plasma viscosity (Siegel et al. 1999).

Reduction in arteriosclerotic plaque (5–18%) in femoral and carotid arteries of subjects receiving high-dose garlic was reported after continuous, high-dose garlic intake. These results substantiated that not only a preventive, but possibly also a curative role in arteriosclerosis therapy (plaque regression) may be ascribed to garlic remedies (Koscielny et al. 1999). Studies with 280 subjects showed a 9–18% reduction and a 3% regression in plaque volume following use of standardized garlic powder (900 mg). LDL decreased 4%, HDL increased 8%, blood pressure dropped by 7%, resulting in a reduced risk for infarction and stroke of over 50% (Siegel et al. 1999).

Ginger (Zingiber officinale)

Ginger may be of benefit in the fight against atherosclerosis. Ginger inhibits abnormal platelet aggregation through two mechanisms. It acts as a potent inhibitor of thromboxane synthetase, which increases the production of thromboxane A2. Thromboxane A2 makes platelets sticky, promoting blood clotting. Formation of thromboxane A2 is blocked by aspirin (AHA 2002b), but ginger also inhibits thromboxane synthesis. Unlike aspirin, ginger also raises prostacyclin, which inhibits abnormal platelet aggregation (Backon 1986). The maximum inhibitory values of gingerol G3 and G4 (the active components of ginger) were two-fold greater than aspirin (Koo et al. 2001).

Aqueous extracts of ginger, onion, and garlic were found to inhibit aggregation in a dose-dependent manner *in vitro*. There was a good correlation between the amount of ginger extract needed to inhibit platelet aggregation and platelet thromboxane synthesis (Srivas 1984).

Ginger can increase contractile strength of the heart (a "cardiotonic" function). Ginger may increase ATP production in the heart and enhance calcium transport within heart cells. Energy derived from ATP is necessary to transport calcium ions through membranes within heart muscle cells. The cycling of calcium within the heart, sustained by ATP, is vital to the development of contractile force (UM 1997).

Ginkgo biloba

Two groups of substances possess pharmacological activity in ginkgo biloba: flavonoids, effective as oxygen-free radical scavengers, and terpenes (or ginkgolides), highly specific for their action as PAF inhibitors.

Important clinical indications for ginkgo biloba extracts are atherosclerotic disease of the peripheral arteries (intermediate severity) and cerebral insufficiency. Symptoms of cerebral insufficiency have been effectively and significantly influenced using ginkgo biloba extracts (Z'Brun 1995). Ginkgo has been used in the treatment of less severe cases of arteriosclerosis and orthostatic dysfunction (Uehleke 1994). Symptoms of orthostatic dysfunction include tachycardia, unstable blood pressure, lightheadedness, visual disturbances, and presyncope (temporarily reduction in oxygen to the brain, usually secondary to diminished blood flow).

Ischemia denotes a decreased supply of oxygenated blood to a tissue. Patients with stage II claudicating atherosclerotic arterial occlusive disease (ischemia) received 320 mg daily of ginkgo extract for 4 weeks. Subsequent tests showed that ischemic areas decreased by 38%. The rapid anti-ischemic action of ginkgo may be of value in the management of peripheral arterial occlusive disease at the stage of intermittent claudication (Mouren et al. 1994). Caution is advised when consuming more than 120 mg a day of ginkgo as excessive bleeding could result.

Green Tea Extract

Green tea is made from *Camellia sinesis*. Green tea contains polyphenols with antioxidant properties. Green tea extracts are used in Asia to lower blood pressure and reduce elevated cholesterol (ACS 2003). The ability of green tea to reduce cholesterol in rats was comparable to the drug probucol (Lorelco®, Bifenabid®), an antioxidant and hypocholesterolemic agent. Although higher amounts of polyphenol were needed to reduce total cholesterol and LDL levels (compared to probucol), green tea polyphenols effectively inhibited LDL oxidation and elevated serum anti-oxidative activity to the same degree as the drug. Green tea polyphenols increase HDL, leading to dose-dependent improvement of the atherogenic index, an effect not seen with probucol (Yokozawa et al. 2002).

The ability of green tea flavonoids to modify LDL oxidation was demonstrated in laboratory ODS rats unable to synthesize ascorbic acid (vitamin C). Rats on restricted dietary vitamin C showed deceased plasma ascorbic acid and tocopherol levels and an accelerated oxidation of LDL *in vitro*. Dietary green tea extract maintained plasma ascorbic acid and delayed LDL oxidation, suggesting flavonoids may suppress LDL oxidation by preserving levels of tocopherol in LDL or plasma levels of vitamin C (Kasaoka et al. 2002).

Antioxidants and flavonoids (in green tea) inhibit abnormal platelet aggregation associated with arterial clots preceding acute myocardial infarction or stroke. The predominant polyphenol found in green tea EGCG (epigallocatechin-3-gallate) inhibited platelet aggregation by hindering proteolysis of thrombin (Deana et al. 2003).

Side effects associated with green tea consumption are rare (aside from the occasional allergic reactions that always occur in the population). Green tea contains caffeine that acts as a stimulant, particularly in those who are sympathetic dominant. Decaffeinated green tea is an alternative choice. Pregnant or breast-feeding women should not drink green tea in large amounts (ACS 2003).

Trace Mineral Supplements

The US Department of Agriculture first suggested the importance of adequate mineral supplementation for cardiovascular disease (Anderson 1986).

"Evidence linking marginal intakes of the trace elements chromium, zinc and selenium with abnormal lipid metabolism and ultimately cardiovascular diseases is accumulating from both animal and human studies. Chromium supplementation of normal adult men as well as diabetics has been reported to increase HDL and decrease triglycerides and total cholesterol. Subjects with the highest total cholesterol and triglycerides usually respond the most to supplemental chromium. Selenium may also affect cardiovascular diseases since selenium is postulated to be involved in platelet aggregation. These data demonstrate that the trace elements chromium and selenium have beneficial effects on risk factors associated with cardiovascular diseases suggesting that a decreased risk of cardiovascular disease may be achieved by adequate intake of trace elements."

Trace elements such as selenium, zinc, and copper are essential for the activity of the antioxidant enzymes glutathione peroxidase and superoxide dismutase. Epidemiological studies suggested an increased risk of cardiovascular disease when blood concentrations of lipophilic antioxidants such as vitamin A, E, and beta-carotene are low.

Subjects with normal or elevated cholesterol who were treated by LDL-apheresis (to remove LDL from blood) were not deficient in vitamin E, beta-carotene, and copper, but did have low plasma levels of selenium, zinc, and vitamin A. The lower selenium and vitamin A levels resulted from LDL-apheresis; however, hypercholesterolemia may have caused the low levels of zinc. Supplementation of patients treated by LDL-apheresis should include selenium, zinc, and vitamin A (Delattre et al. 1998). A decrease in selenium levels parallels the increase in severity of CHD, suggesting an association of heart disease with subclinical levels of selenium. These trace elements might be used to assess the severity of CHD and adequate mineral intake might contribute to vascular disease therapy (Yegin et al. 1997).

Supplements for Healthy Coronary Arteries

Aspirin

Aspirin is used as a popular analgesic, but is also useful in maintaining cardiovascular health. Low-dose aspirin (81 mg) provides protection against abnormal blood clot formation via long-lasting effects on blood platelets. Platelets become less sticky so the risk of a heart attack and transient ischemic attacks is reduced (Diener 1998; Hart et al. 2000; Sacco et al. 2000; Califf et al. 2002).

Aspirin reduces C-reactive protein (CRP) and cardiac inflammation, which are newer risk factors in cardiovascular disease. Low-dose aspirin reduced heart attack risk by about 44% and the risk was 55% lower in men with high CRP levels. This suggests that aspirin's antagonism of platelet aggregation and its anti-inflammatory mechanisms combine to attenuate thrombosis (*Physicians Weekly* 1998).

Aspirin reduces inflammation by inhibiting the rate-limiting enzyme, cyclooxygenase that begins the inflammatory process (Newmark 2000). One molecule of aspirin will disable cyclooxygenase for 4–6 hours by acetylating the enzyme. (See *C-Reactive Protein* and the *Link between Infections and Inflammation in Heart Disease* in the protocol *Cardiovascular Disease: Comprehensive Analysis* in this book to learn how inflammatory processes contribute to cardiac disease.)

An overview of four large-scale studies substantiated that aspirin therapy reduced nonfatal myocardial infarctions (MIs or heart attacks) by 32%. The researchers concluded that aspirin therapy could prevent a third of the MIs occurring in healthy individuals. There was a small but insignificant increase in the risk of vascular disease-related death and nonfatal stroke with aspirin therapy. When strokes were subdivided by type, there was no significant effect of aspirin therapy on the risk of ischemic stroke, but, while based on small numbers, there was a statistically significant 1.7-fold increase in the risk of hemorrhagic stroke (Hebert et al. 2000).

A large study over three years determined that aspirin was beneficial for individuals with coronary disease and reduced mortality risk (Gum et al. 2001).

Aspirin's benefit is greater among diabetic patients, significantly reducing the death rate from cardiac disease in diabetic patients with CHD. Diabetic patients using aspirin had a 11% mortality risk from cardiac diseases, while diabetic patients not using aspirin had a 16% risk (Harpaz et al. 1998).

Aspirin benefits carotid endarterectomy patients. Low-dose aspirin (81–325 mg daily) reduced risk of MI, stroke, and death following surgery. Individuals receiving 650–1300 mg were not similarly protected (Taylor et al. 1999).

All individuals over 50 years of age, with one cardiac risk factor and no condition that would negate treatment (e.g., increased prothrombin time, disturbed gastric mucosa, or hypertension), should consider using aspirin therapy. *Note:* Studies demonstrate that aspirin is not sufficient to prevent MI if fibrinogen levels are excessively high. Concomitant use of ibuprofen (but not rofecoxib, acetaminophen, or diclofenac) antagonizes the platelet inhibition caused by aspirin. Treatment with ibuprofen may limit the cardiovascular benefits of aspirin (Catella-Lawson et al. 2001).

A review of 287 studies involving 135,000 patients determined that over 40,000 lives are lost worldwide yearly because aspirin is underused. Aspirin (or other anti-platelet drugs) protects most patients at risk for occlusive vascular events (acute MI, ischemic stroke, unstable or stable angina, previous MI, cerebral ischemia, peripheral arterial disease, or atrial fibrillation) (ATC 2002). A daily dosage of 75–150 mg of aspirin is an effective anti-platelet regimen. An initial loading dose of at least 150 mg might be required in acute cases. Some clinical conditions are benefited by adding a second anti-platelet drug (ATC 2002). Aspirin can reduce the amount of damage to the heart during MI. Aspirin usage following a suspected heart attack is best chewed rather than swallowed, and is most beneficial if taken within 30 minutes of the onset of symptoms. *Note:* The use of warfarin alone or in combination with aspirin was superior to aspirin in reducing the severity of an acute MI. Warfarin is associated with a higher risk of bleeding (Hurlen et al. 2002).

CAUTION Any amount of aspirin is contraindicated for individuals who are at risk for hemorrhagic stroke. If you take anticoagulants, have a blood clotting disorder, have experienced a hemorrhagic stroke, have experienced an allergic reaction to aspirin, or have a history of gastrointestinal ulcers, do not take any aspirin product without consulting your physician. Take aspirin with a meal to decrease stomach irritation. Discontinue taking aspirin two weeks before surgery. (Aspirin in low doses minimizes stomach irritation.)

Policosanol

Clinical trials using policosanol, derived from sugar cane, demonstrated similar clinical improvement in measures of cholesterol compared to commonly prescribed statin drugs such as Mevacor® (lovastatin), Zocor® (simvastatin), and Pravachol® (pravastatin) (Castano et al. 1999; Prat et al. 1999). Policosanol reduced harmful damaging LDL and increased the beneficial HDL. Policosanol (5 to 20 mg/day) decreased the risk of atheroma formation by reducing total cholesterol levels, inhibiting platelet aggregation, endothelial damage, and foam cell formation in animals (Varady et al. 2003).

Policosanol (20 mg/day) is as effective as 100 mg of aspirin per day in opposing platelet aggregation. Aspirin combined with policosanol is advantageous as each drug influences platelet activity through different mechanisms. (The combination of aspirin with other platelet inhibitors cannot be recommended without physician supervision.) Policosanol decreased systolic blood pressure providing an additional advantage for high-risk coronary patients (Arruzazabala et al. 1997; Castano et al. 2002).

Postmenopausal women receiving policosanol (5 mg/day for 8 weeks and 10 mg/day during the next 8 weeks) revealed decreased LDL levels (17% and 27%, respectively), total cholesterol levels (13% and 20%), and lower ratios of LDL to HDL (17.2% and 26.5%), and total cholesterol to HDL (16% and 21%). HDL levels were 7% higher at the end of the study. Policosanol was effective and well-tolerated in hypercholesterolemic postmenopausal women, showing additional health benefits for this subgroup (Mirkin et al. 2001).

No side effects are typically noted with policosanol therapy. Policosanol is available at less than half the cost of prescription statin medications. Side effects of nausea, headaches, dizziness, sleep disturbances, liver problems, muscle weakness, and pain reduce enthusiasm for statins by some practitioners. Policosanol does not interfere with the biosynthesis of coenzyme Q_{10} that is associated with statin usage. If you are already taking a prescription cholesterol medication, do not begin policosanol without physician consent.

TMG

TMG is used to lower homocysteine levels. Impaired homocysteine remethylation, induced by ethanol in animals, is reversed by TMG. TMG may be effective in correcting methylation defects (Barak et al. 2003). TMG lowers homocysteine, but regular dosing must continue to sustain this effect (Hoffman 1997; Fanapour et al. 1999; James et al. 2002; Baker-Racine 2002). There are no reports of side effects with TMG other than brief tension headaches when taken in large quantities without food. TMG should be taken with vitamin B_{12}, B_6, creatine, folic acid, and various sources of choline for homocysteine management.

Choline and Choline Derivatives

Any dietary supplement that contains choline or a choline derivative will lessen the need for SAMe. This is because much of the choline in the body is made by methylation reactions that require SAMe and generate homocysteine. This homocysteine must then be detoxified. Because homocysteine is linked to cardiovascular disease, supplements that reduce homocysteine production are potentially beneficial (Devlin 2002).

The biosynthesis of choline as phosphatidylcholine (lecithin) creates homocysteine in the liver for the synthesis of lipoproteins, especially HDL (Devlin 2002; Noga 2003; Lobley et al. 1996). Circulating HDL contains an enzyme that allows HDL to remove free cholesterol from arterial cell walls for metabolism by the liver as HDL-cholesterol (Lehninger et al. 1993; Devlin 2002). This is why HDL-cholesterol is called the "good cholesterol."

To lower your homocysteine, increase intake of 'pre-methylated' choline-containing products. Good sources of choline-containing products include: CDP-choline, α-GPC, lecithin and choline.

Creatine

Humans excrete 1,400 mg of creatinine in urine per day that must be replaced by the synthesis of creatine from SAMe (Devlin 2002). Supplemental creatine of 2–4 grams daily would probably cut production of homocysteine in half. Creatine supplementation reduces the formation of homocysteine and lessens the need to remethylate homocysteine back into methionine. Supplemental dietary creatine for two weeks lowered plasma levels of homocysteine by 25% (Stead et al. 2001). Doses of SAMe (1600 mg daily) increased phosphocreatine levels in human brain (Silveri et al. 2003), indicating that SAMe is important in the biosynthesis of creatine.

CONVENTIONAL MEDICAL THERAPY

This section includes examples of drugs used in the conventional treatment of CHD. The list provides examples of the various types of medications available. Surgical procedures will be briefly described. More comprehensive information may be found in *Cardiovascular Disease: Comprehensive Analysis.*

Beta-Blockers

Beta-blockers "block" the effects of adrenaline (and norepinephrine) on beta-receptors. This slows the nerve impulses that travel through the heart and the heart does not work as hard. This lessens the work output of the heart and less blood and oxygen are required for the heart to perform work. Typically, beta-blockers are prescribed to treat high blood pressure (hypertension), congestive heart failure (CHF), abnormal heart rhythms (arrhythmias), and chest pain (angina). Beta-blockers are sometimes used in heart attack patients to prevent future attacks.

Medications can alter the effects of beta-blockers. Physicians and pharmacists follow these interactions if they learn from the patient which medications are being used. While on beta-blockers, you should avoid caffeinated beverages (coffee, tea, and some soft drinks), over-the-counter cough and cold medicines, antihistamines, and antacids containing aluminum. Avoid alcohol because it decreases the efficacy of beta-blockers and inhibits methionine synthase, the most important enzyme in remethylating homocysteine to methionine. Common side effects associated with beta-blockers include drowsiness, fatigue, cold hands and feet, weakness or dizziness, and dry mouth, eyes, and skin. Less common side effects include difficulty breathing, bradycardia (slow heartbeat), and swelling of the hands and feet. Impotence, gastrointestinal disturbances, joint discomfort, and depression occur rarely (Texas Heart Institute 2003a).

According to physicians and pharmacists, even though beta-adrenergic blockers can significantly reduce mortality after a myocardial infarction, these agents are prescribed to only a minority of patients. Underutilization of beta-blockers may be attributed to fear of adverse effects, especially by the elderly, and in patients with disorders such as diabetes or heart failure. With careful dosing and monitoring, the benefits of beta-blockers after myocardial infarction far outweigh the potential risks in most patients (Howard et al. 2000). Commonly prescribed beta-adrenergic blockers drugs include: atenolol (Tenoretic®, Tenormin®), metoprolol (Lopressor®, Toprol XL®), nadolol (Corgard®), and propranolol (Inderal®).

Natural agents having beta-blocking activity include grape seed extract (procyanidins), green tea, hawthorn, magnesium, and the amino acid taurine.

Calcium Channel-Blockers

Calcium-channel blockers slow the rate at which calcium passes to the contractile fibers of heart muscle and into the vessel walls, a sequence that relaxes the vessels. Relaxed vessels allow the blood to flow more easily, thereby reducing blood pressure. In addition to treating hypertension, calcium channel blockers are used to treat chest pain (angina), and irregular heartbeats (arrhythmia).

Because various drugs (beta-blockers, ACE inhibitors, anti-arrhythmics, diuretics, some eye medications, and corticosteroids) and large doses of calcium and vitamin D may interact with calcium channel blockers, the prescribing physician should be aware of the individual's list of all drugs and supplements. Avoid smoking while taking calcium-channel blockers because it may cause rapid heartbeat (tachycardia).

Common side effects associated with calcium channel blockers are fatigue, flushing, swelling of the abdomen, ankles, or feet, and heartburn. Less common side effects are changes in heart rate, either tachycardia or bradycardia (slow heart rate), shortness of breath, difficulty swallowing, and dizziness, numbness in hands and feet, and gastrointestinal disturbances. Chest pains, jaundice, and fainting are rarely reported (Texas Heart Institute 2003b).

Calcium channel blockers are classified as short-, intermediate-, and long-acting. Most short-acting calcium channel blockers have been taken off the market, and replaced by the longer-acting ones that have not been associated with increased risk for heart disease (Estacio et al. 1998; Mirkin 2002).

Calcium channel blockers increase the risk of developing cancer (Pahor et al. 1996), perhaps through interference with apoptosis, or programmed cell death, a defense against cancer. Reports of cancer with calcium channel blocker usage are controversial (Kizer et al. 2001). The use of particular types of antihypertensive medications, including immediate-release calcium channel blockers, may modestly increase the risk of breast carcinoma among older women. Reports have demonstrated an increased risk of cancer among users of verapamil, but it is too early to conclude that calcium channel blockers are associated with cancer (Beiderbeck-Noll et al. 2003; Li et al. 2003).

Commonly prescribed calcium-channel blockers are diltiazem (Cardizem CD®, Cardizem SR®, Dilacor XR®), nifedipine (Procardia XL®), and verapamil (Calan®, Calan SR®, Isoptin®, Isoptin SR®, Verelan®).

Angelica, garlic, ginger, ginkgo biloba, grape seed, green tea (*Camellia* sinensis), hawthorn, magnesium, and olive leaf have some calcium-channel blocking activity.

Angiotensin-Converting Enzyme (ACE) Inhibitors

The juxtaglomerular cells in the kidneys stimulate renin secretion when either blood volume or serum sodium decreases. The enzyme renin participates in the conversion of angiotensinogen to angiotensin I, which is rapidly hydrolyzed to form the active compound angiotensin II. The vasoconstrictive action of angiotensin II decreases glomerular filtration rate while its action on aldosterone release (a mineralocorticoid hormone produced by the adrenal cortex) promotes sodium retention, causing fluid and sodium reabsorption. Drugs that inhibit the angiotensin-converting enzyme (ACE) decrease sodium and water retention, reduce blood pressure, improve cardiac output, and typically decrease heart size.

ACE inhibitors are used to treat congestive heart failure (CHF) and hypertension. Following a heart attack, patients are often prescribed ACE inhibitors to prevent further damage to the heart. ACE inhibitors are prescribed for kidney problems associated with diabetes.

The physician will evaluate all drug and supplement use before initiating ACE-inhibiting therapy, especially diuretics and supplements containing potassium. A common side effect is a dry cough, sometimes making speech difficult. Less common side effects include gastrointestinal disturbances, numbness or tingling in the hands and feet, joint pain, fever, lightheadedness, and fatigue. Jaundice and edema are reported rarely (Texas Heart Institute 2003c).

Some commonly prescribed ACE inhibitors are captopril (Capoten®), enalapril (Vasotec®), and lisinopril, (Prinivil®, Zestril®).

Angiotensin II Receptor Blockers

Angiotensin-converting enzyme (ACE) converts angiotensin I to angiotensin II. There are definite benefits to selective blockade of angiotensin II receptors, which mediate the very potent vasoconstricting actions of angiotensin II on arterial vasculature. Any of the drugs described in this section (or for high blood pressure) are beneficial for those with atherosclerosis because they lower blood pressure. High blood pressure in combination with atherosclerosis is common, but high blood pressure predisposes arterial plaque to rupturing, causing strokes or heart attacks. Angiotensin II is the most powerful vasoconstricting hormone affecting the arterial vasculature. Because the diseased arterial wall cells are already compromised by atherosclerosis, it is dangerous to stimulate such compromised cells with a strong vasoconstricting hormone like angiotensin II without risking the rupture of the plaque lining those cells. For this reason, angiotensin II receptor blockers are the best drug choice. These drugs specifically block the arterial vascular cells from excessive constriction mediated by angiotensin II.

Losartan was the first marketed angiotensin II receptor antagonist. It shows no risk of angioedema or cough. The AT1 subtype of angiotensin II receptors, which losartan blocks, occurs in vascular and myocardial tissue. Losartan is available alone as Cozaar®, or in combination with hydrochlorthiazide (a common diuretic) marketed as Hyzaar®. Both drugs will lower blood pressure (Oates and Brown 2001).

Years ago the Life Extension Foundation recommended angiotensin II receptor blockers for first line therapy by naming the first drugs approved in this class: Cozaar® and Hyzaar®. There is now a new member to this class called Benicar® that shows once-daily dosing (Neutel et al. 2002). Benicar® is usually given at a dose of 20 mg with a possible dose increase to 40 mg after two weeks. The Life Extension Foundation recommends that Benicar® is the best blood pressure-lowering drug product available for use in the individual that has high blood pressure that is further complicated by atherosclerosis.

Vasodilators

Vasodilating drugs act on blood vessels, opening the vessel by relaxing the muscular walls. There are four types of drugs that influence vasodilation: (1) beta-blockers, (2) direct-acting vasodilators, (3) ACE inhibitors, and (4) calcium channel blockers.

Some beta-blockers have vasodilator properties, others do not. The drugs Coreg® and pindolol block beta-1 and beta-2 receptors and are classified as direct vasodilators (enlarging arteries and increasing blood flow). Coreg® has some alpha-blocking ability as well as antioxidant potential. Labetalol (Normodyne®), blocks alpha, beta-1 and beta-2 receptors, causing greater vasodilation. Vasodilating and non-vasodilating beta-blockers reduced total hospitalizations and hospitalizations due to CHF (Bonet et al. 2000).

Hydralazine, minoxidil (Rogaine®) and nitroglycerin (NTG) are direct vasodilators (NTG is frequently used for angina) (*American Family Physician* 1998). ACE inhibitors vasodilate by inhibiting the formation of the body's most powerful constricting hormone, angiotensin II. By blocking its formation, arteries can dilate and blood pressure is typically reduced. Calcium channel blockers relax the tone of vascular smooth muscles, which promotes dilation. Certain calcium channel blockers affect the heart more than blood vessels (i.e., diltiazem and verapamil), while others (nifedipine and nicardipine) have greater effects on blood vessels than on the heart. Some vitamins, minerals, and various herbs have vasodilating potential: angelica, garlic, ginger, ginkgo biloba, hawthorn, magnesium, niacin, and olive leaf.

Cardiac Glycosides/Anti-Arrhythmics

Cardiac glycosides are obtained from digitalis purpurea and digitalis lanata, other plants that contain steroid glycosides, or their semi-synthetic derivatives. Cardiac glycosides are commonly used for CHF because they increase the force of cardiac contraction without significantly affecting other cardiovascular parameters. Cardiac glycosides are toxic at larger doses. Cardiac glycosides include Digoxin®, digitoxin, Lanoxin®, Purgoxin®, and Crystodigin®.

Bugleweed (*Lycopus virginicus*) and taurine (a non-essential amino acid synthesized during the catabolism of homocysteine) have digitalis-like activity; however, never substitute a natural substance for a prescription drug without the supervision of a physician.

Diuretics

Diuretics reduce edema and lower blood pressure by reducing sodium and water retention. The three types of diuretics (thiazides, potassium-sparing diuretics, and high-loop diuretics) all work differently, but each reduces total body salt and water, and thus, reduces blood pressure. Thiazides are the most commonly used in hypertension. If thiazides fail to lower blood pressure, an additional diuretic may be prescribed.

CAUTION Although the use of thiazide diuretics and potassium-sparing diuretics modestly increased risks of breast carcinoma and, the use of certain diuretics may increase the risk of breast carcinoma among older women (Li et al. 2003).

Angelica, bugleweed, curcumin, garlic, ginger, grape seed, green tea, hawthorn, olive leaf, taurine, vitamin B$_6$, vitamin C, and vitamin E have diuretic properties.

Cholesterol-Lowering Drugs

When cholesterol levels remain high despite adequate dietary changes, weight loss, and regular exercise, or if other risk factors for cardiovascular disease exist, cholesterol-lowering drugs are often prescribed. (See the chapter entitled *Drug Overdosing* for a detailed discussion on this topic.)

The drugs most commonly used to lower LDL are the statin drugs: lovastatin (Mevacor®), pravastatin (Pravachol®), simvastatin (Zocor®), and atorvastatin (Lipitor®). Bile acid sequestrants are another class of drugs prescribed for reducing LDL levels: cholestyramine (LoCHOLEST®, Questran®) and colestipol (Colestid®). Typically, gemfibrozil (Lopid®), clofibrate (Atromid-S®), and probucol (Lorelco®) moderately reduce LDL levels (AHA 2004b).

Policosanol, gugulipid, niacin, artichoke extract, chromium, ginger, CLA, grapefruit pectin, curcumin, proanthocyanidins, soy protein, and tocotrienols have cholesterol-lowering effects. CoQ$_{10}$ and garlic extract help to inhibit the oxidation of LDL.

Treating "Bad" Cholesterol with "Good" Cholesterol: A New Drug on the Horizon

ApoA-1 (*Apolipoprotein* A-1) is a protein component of HDL. ApoA-1 Milano is a rare genetic variant of ApoA-1 that was isolated in the blood of a family living in Italy. This genetic mutation has been found to promote an exceptionally healthy arterial system in spite of low levels of protective HDL and high levels of triglycerides. A middle-aged man with high triglyceride levels had very low levels of HDL, had no evidence of heart disease, but had the variant apolipoprotein A-1, that was subsequently named *ApoA-1 Milano*.

ApoA-1 Milano has an amino acid which has been replaced by the amino acid cysteine. Cysteine contains a *sulfhydryl* group. About 70% of ApoA-1 Milano comes in pairs, linked by the sulfhydryl groups. This restricts HDL size and growth, but allows the remaining 30% (of monomeric ApoA-1 Milano) to act as an antioxidant, protecting lipids from free radical oxidation. The monomeric form literally traps free radicals and prevents oxidization of healthy tissue and lipids lining arterial walls, preventing injury, and cholesterol deposits. Only the monomeric form protects lipids from oxidation. After over 20 years, despite unhealthy diets, ApoA-1 Milano carriers remain free of cardiovascular disease (Bieleicki et al. 2002). Less than 40 people have been identified as carriers of the Milano variant (Gualandri et al. 1985).

ETC-216 (developed by Esperion) is an investigational synthetic version of ApoA-1 Milano, which is combined with a phospholipid to form a complex that imitates the beneficial properties of HDL. ETC-216 might remove cholesterol deposits and prevent oxidation that causes cholesterol deposits (Bielicki et al. 2002). Studies demonstrated that ETC-216 rapidly removed plaque from diseased arteries. Phase II clinical trials are underway. The "ApoA-1 Milano Trial" enrolled 47 patients, 21 were given 15 mg/kg of ETC-216; 45 mg/kg of ETC-216 (15 patients); or placebo (11 patients) as weekly intravenous infusions for 5 weeks. ETC-216 was well tolerated (Nissen et al. 2003; Newton et al. 2002). Plaque volume decreased by 1.0% (3.2%) in the combined ETC-216 groups and slightly increased by 0.14% (3.1%) in the placebo group, with an absolute reduction in the combined treatment groups of 4.2% from baseline. It was concluded that five doses of intravenous ETC-216 at weekly intervals did produce significant regression of coronary atherosclerosis (Nissen et al. 2003). "We now know that it is possible to actively remove cholesterol plaques from the coronary arteries with drugs…eventually this approach will make a significant difference in the care of patients with CHD" (Nissen et al. 2003).

Combining a synthetic HDL with mechanisms similar to ApoA-1 Milano and conventional cholesterol-lowering therapies represents a new drug regimen to prevent lipid oxidation leading to cholesterol deposits and may cause regression of existing plaques (Bielicki et al. 2002).

Invasive Procedures

Coronary Artery Bypass

An estimated 200,000 Americans undergo coronary artery bypass grafting (CABG) surgery each year. Bypass surgery, once considered to be difficult or complicated, is now an almost routine surgical procedure in many medical centers. The procedure itself is relatively simple. A segment of healthy blood vessel, usually a chest artery (mammillary artery) or leg vein (saphenous vein), is grafted to bypass blocked segments of the coronary arteries. In appropriate persons, arm veins might be used because healing occurs faster in the arms than in the legs. Cedars-Sinai uses a chest artery instead of a leg vein in 95% of its cases, believing it improves long-term survival rates (Cedars-Sinai Heart Center 2003).

Usually after surgery (depending upon the individual's condition), 2–3 days are spent in an intensive care recovery unit with another few days required in the hospital. Costs also vary according to a patient's condition and geographic locale, but the average is $32,000 to $35,000. (See the *Anesthesia and Surgical Precautions* protocol to learn how to reduce surgical complications.)

Surgery is recommended for disabling angina uncontrolled by conventional therapy only in good surgical candidates. Disagreement remains for the indications for CABG. The Coronary Artery Surgery Study demonstrated that patients with healthy hearts but with one, two, or all three of the major coronary arteries blocked did surprisingly well, without surgery. Regardless of the number or severity of the blockages, each group had a low death rate of 1% a year (Anon. 1984; Graboys et al. 1987; Alderman et al. 1990; Murray 1999).

The severity of blockage does not determine blood flow in the artery. There is no correlation between blood flow and the severity of blockage. The majority of coronary arteries with a 96% blockage, had the most brisk blood flow while similar arteries, with only 40% blockage had severe flow restriction. The authors concluded that the blockages found on heart catheterization do not correlate with blood flow restriction (White et al. 1984; Winslow et al. 1988; Murray 1999).

The critical factor regarding whether a patient needs CABG or angioplasty is how well the left ventricular pump is working (not the degree of blockage or the number of arteries affected). Bypass is only helpful when the ejection fraction is less than 40%. 90% of bypass procedures are performed with ejection fractions greater than 50%, which is adequate for meeting circulatory needs. As many as 90% of all bypass procedures may be unnecessary (Murray 1999).

When CABG or angioplasty is necessary based on these accepted criteria, the procedures increase long-term survival and relieve symptoms for 85% of patients. The controversy as to when CABG is appropriate remains among the most respected of physicians.

CAUTION Although CABG greatly improves how most patients feel, it does not cure heart disease. Unless preventive steps are taken, the processes that originally caused the disease will continue. Following CABG, it is important for patients to make prudent lifestyle changes.

Angioplasty

Angioplasty is used to widen arteries in the heart that are narrowed or blocked due to plaque formation. The technique used depends on where the blockage is, its shape, and whether the blockage is hard or soft plaque. Angioplasty offers a few advantages over coronary bypass surgery: (1) although invasive, it does not require use of a heart-lung machine; (2) it is performed under local anesthesia; and (3) it is not as costly as CABG. Ordinarily, only one or two days of hospitalization are required.

Percutaneous transluminal coronary angioplasty (PTCA; or *balloon angioplasty*) involves threading a catheter with an inflatable balloon-like tip through the arteries to the blocked area. The balloon is inflated, flattening the fatty deposits and widening the arterial channel, allowing more blood to reach the heart muscle.

Laser angioplasty uses a catheter with a laser tip rather than a balloon tip. The laser-tipped catheter is guided to the blockage and the laser tip is used to destroy the plaque. Each layer is vaporized into gaseous and liquid particles (AHA 2002a; HIP 2002). Lasers have been used with both angioplasty and bypass procedures but the risks have been high and the treatment is expensive.

Angioplasty can also be used in plaque-blocked arteries in the legs and the *internal* carotid artery, the major vessel carrying blood to the brain. But, angioplasty is not appropriate for all types of CHD and it is not effective in all individuals. Patients with diabetes mellitus have better survival odds with CABG compared to PTCA (Brooks et al. 2000). Diabetic patients do much worse in heart attacks and mortality when undergoing PTCA. In treated diabetics, the 7-year survival rate was 76% in the CABG group and 56% in the PTCA group. Among non-diabetics, the survival rates were 86% in the CABG group and 87% in the PTCA group.

Women have better success rates than men because the introduction of lower-profile stents has allowed their use in small and tortuous vessels, which are more predominant in women (Presbitero et al. 2003). Success rates have been estimated as high as 90% (Choicemedia 2001).

Standard angioplasty is associated with complications because the procedure traumatizes the vessel wall. Damaged cells try to heal and regenerate, forming scar tissue that re-clogs the artery (restenosis). Six to nine months after treatment, restenosis recurs in leg arteries (50-60%) and in the heart arteries (20-30%). The procedure is often repeated or surgery is performed instead (PCI 2002). The use of stents has improved the odds of a favorable outcome, providing the procedure is done in a hospital performing a high volume of angioplasty/stent procedures.

Balloon-induced arterial wall injury is the main cause of abrupt vessel closure and subsequent problems in PTCA. The most significant injury to the diseased wall occurs when high-pressure balloon inflations are employed (University of Edinburgh http://www.cpa.ed.ac.uk/news/research/17/6.html).

Restenosis research projects are evaluating the effects of various adjuncts to improve angioplasty outcome, including radiated stents, antibiotic-covered stents, stent products that release medications into the artery to prevent closure, and a new approach referred to as cryoplasty (PCI 2002).

During cryoplasty a tiny balloon is threaded into the clogged artery and filled with nitrous oxide. As pressurized liquid nitrous oxide is delivered into the balloon, it expands and turns into a gas, causing it to cool to sub-zero temperatures. The cooling prompts apoptosis (programmed cell death, presumably in the plaque cells), a natural occurrence that is gentler and less traumatic to the tissue than the compression of plaque against the tissue wall. The low temperature produces beneficial physiological changes in the cell wall. Because the treatment is gentler than standard angioplasty, it doesn't promote a "scarring" response, frequently evidenced in standard angioplasty (AHA 2002a; *New Haven Register* 2004; Wisconsin Heart and Vascular Clinic 2004). Like CABG, angioplasty does not cure atherosclerosis. Patients need to improve their lifestyle to improve influence cardiovascular outcomes.

Stenting

A coronary stent is a tube usually made from stainless steel mesh that comes in many sizes to match the size of coronary arteries. Often a stent is placed inside a coronary artery following angioplasty so that the artery will remain expanded. Once the artery has been widened by an angioplasty procedure, a stent catheter is threaded into the artery and placed around a deflated balloon. When the balloon is exactly positioned in the artery, it is inflated to expand the stent against the artery walls. Then the balloon catheter is removed, but the stent is left in place to hold the artery open (Columbia Weill Cornell Heart Institute 2003).

Intra-Coronary Radiation

In about a third of angioplasty patients, the expanded area of the artery narrows (restenosis) within six months. Cardiologists (Columbia Weill Cornell Heart Institute) have developed a technique called *intra-coronary radiation*, which uses radiation to prevent restenosis of an opened artery. In intra-coronary radiation, a balloon containing a solution of beta radiation is inserted into the expanded heart vessel. The heart vessel is irradiated for 10 minutes and the balloon is removed. Intra-coronary radiation has shown great promise in preventing artery restenosis (Columbia Weill Cornell Heart Institute 2003).

Atherectomy

In atherectomy, specialized devices are used to remove or cut away plaque, particularly blockages that are too hardened (calcified) for balloon angioplasty. Atherectomy procedures include *extraction* (a tiny rotating blade trims away plaque on the inside of artery walls); *rotational* (a high-speed, diamond-tipped drill penetrates fatty deposits, particularly hard, calcified deposits); and *directional* (a combination of a balloon and a shaving blade hone away deposits) (HIP 2002).

Chest pain is the most common complication of atherectomy, but other complications might include injury to the blood vessel lining, restenosis, blood clots, and bleeding at the site of insertion. More serious but less frequent complications are blood vessel holes, tears, or reduced blood flow to the heart. It is estimated that atherectomy is successful about 95% of the time; plaque reforms in 20-30% of patients (De Milto 2003).

⬤ SUMMARY

Nutritional supplements are multifaceted therapeutic agents. Nutrients often participate in a variety of biochemical functions, affording them diverse mechanisms impacting multiple health conditions. In this summary, only the function specific to the heading will be illustrated. The reader is strongly advised to consult the foregoing text for a full description of the therapeutic potential of each of the nutrients. A compendium of each of the highlighted nutrients also appears in the protocol *Cardiovascular Disease: Comprehensive Analysis*.

Nutritional supplements listed in the summary contribute to the prevention of atherosclerosis and arterial blockage by:

- Lowering and inhibiting the oxidation of cholesterol and LDL
- Improving HDL levels
- Lowering serum triglycerides, fibrinogen, blood glucose, homocysteine, and iron levels
- Inhibiting abnormal blood clot formation

- Reducing inflammatory markers such as C-reactive protein

To inhibit oxidation of LDL:

1. Coenzyme Q_{10} works synergistically with vitamin E to prevent LDL oxidation. Use 30 to 400 mg daily. Superior assimilation and cardiac benefits are provided when CoQ_{10} is in a base of rice bran oil.

2. Garlic protects against the oxidation of LDL and arterial wall damage. Use 1000 to 2000 mg (aged garlic) twice daily with meals or 1800 to 7200 mg of Pure-Gar Caps daily with food.

3. Life Extension Herbal Mix: This formula contains pharmacological levels of premium-grade herbal extracts that provide protection against oxidized LDL. Among the ingredients contained in the herbal mix are green tea (which contains large amounts of catechin flavonoids to protect against the oxidation of LDL); ginkgo biloba (thought to protect LDL against oxidative stress caused by superoxide, peroxyl- and hydroxyl-radicals); grape seed-skin extract (short-term ingestion of purple grape juice reduces the susceptibility of LDL to oxidation in coronary artery disease. The prevention of LDL oxidation is a mechanism by which flavonoids in purple grape products may prevent adverse cardiovascular events, independent of alcohol use); bilberry extract (because bilberry protects cholesterol from oxidizing in test tubes, it is theorized that it protects against arteriosclerosis). The suggested dose of Life Extension Herbal Mix is 1 tablespoon mixed with water or juice, taken early in the day.

4. Life Extension Mix contains a potent spectrum of antioxidants that have been shown to inhibit the oxidation of cholesterol. The mix's trace elements zinc and selenium are essential elements required for the activity of antioxidant enzymes, thus providing physiological antioxidant protection. Use 3 tablets, 3 times per day, preferably with meals.

5. Policosanol's many biochemical properties include protecting LDL against oxidation. Some individuals need only 5 to 10 mg of policosanol while others require 20 mg a day.

To lower cholesterol levels:

1. Artichoke extract: A suggested dosage is one capsule three times per day, containing 300 mg of artichoke standardized to contain 13-18% caffeoylquinic acid.

- *L*-glutamine, a nonessential amino acid that increases the number of cells in the small intestine along with the number and height of villi on those cells

- Butyric acid, a short-chain fatty acid that enhances function and integrity in the large intestine and is an anticancer agent

- The fatty acids DHA (from fish oil) and GLA (from borage oil), which decrease inflammation and improve intestinal functioning

Appendix A of this protocol provides specific information relating to dietary and intestinal factors involved in autoimmune disease.

Reducing Stress

Stress is a major risk factor in developing disease. Even prolonged low-level stress stimulates the adrenal glands to produce cortisol, which, in excess, impairs immune function. Lack of proper rest and sleep, depression, and emotional disturbance contribute to immune dysfunction. In addition, there is a connection between the limbic system, the part of the brain that gives rise to emotion, and immune function. Therefore, to balance the immune system, one must balance the mind and emotions. Biofeedback, guided imagery, yoga, deep breathing, musical participation, positive affirmations, meditation, and prayer all help maintain balance (Hughes 1997; Long et al. 2001; Kuhn 2002; Lehrer et al. 2002; Vempati et al. 2002).

A supplemental approach to stress reduction would be obtained from *Garum armoricum* extract (Adapton), which contains a class of unique polypeptides that act as precursors to endorphins and other neurotransmitters. These polypeptides exert a regulatory effect on the nervous system enabling an individual to adapt to mentally and physically stressful conditions (Crocq et al. 1978). Another antidote to stress is an amino acid found in green tea called theanine. Although theanine creates a tranquilizing effect on the brain, it appears to increase concentration and focus thought (Juneja et al. 1999). DHEA supplementation is the most effective way of blocking the effects of excess cortisol secretion.

Improving Liver Health

The liver plays a critical role in all aspects of metabolism and health. It is important in the synthesis and secretion of albumin (a blood clotting protein), in the storage of glucose, and in the synthesis of vitamins and minerals. Because the liver has a major role in the purification and clearance of waste products, drugs, and toxins, disease states may be improved by supporting liver function. The herb milk thistle and

its components silymarin and silibinin have two therapeutic mechanisms. First, they alter the structure of the outer cell membrane of the hepatocyte to prevent penetration of liver poison into the interior of the cell. Second, they stimulate the action of nucleolar polymerase A, resulting in an increase in ribosomal protein synthesis, thus stimulating the regenerative ability of the liver and the formation of new hepatocytes (Flora et al. 1998; Luper 1998).

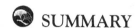 **SUMMARY**

Autoimmune diseases may be greatly improved by strengthening the immune system with nutritional supplements and by making healthy lifestyle changes in diet and stress reduction. The protocols needed may include prescription drugs as well as the following supplements.

1. Omega-3 and omega-6 fatty acids will help reduce systemic inflammation that accompanies autoimmune diseases. Life Extension recommends Super GLA/DHA, which has a balanced blend of both EFAs. EPA is also added to the formula to reduce the effects of arachidonic acid, the inflammatory agent found in meat products. Take 6 softgels daily.

2. DHEA is a steroidal hormone that can reduce the effects of inflammatory cytokines; 25–50 mg daily is recommended. DHEA is contraindicated in men with prostate cancer and in women with estrogen related cancer (*refer to the DHEA Replacement Therapy protocol for complete information*).

3. Free-radical damage is a byproduct of normal metabolic functioning and exposure to toxic substances. The following supplements have proven to be effective free radical scavengers:

- Vitamin C, 2.5–6 grams daily.

- Vitamin E, 1 softgel daily of Gamma E Tocopherol/Tocotrienols. (The most balanced form of vitamin E is Gamma E Tocopherol/Tocotrienols, which provides broad spectrum protection.)

- Green tea extract, two to four 300-mg (90% polyphenols) decaffeinated capsules daily.

- Beta-carotene, one 25,000-IU softgel daily.

- Grape seed-skin extract, two 100-mg capsules daily.

- CoQ$_{10}$, 100–200 mg daily.

- SeMSc (selenium) may be the most effective selenium derivative to fight inflammation and neutralize free radicals; 1 capsule daily between meals.

4. Alkylglycerols from Norwegian Shark Liver Oil may modulate the immune system in certain forms of autoimmune disease; one 1000-mg softgel daily.

5. Acetyl-*L*-carnitine enhances the transport of EFAs into the cell's mitochondria and may modulate the effects of damaging saturated fats. Suggested dose is two 500-mg softgels twice daily.

6. Super Carnosine will help protect against the formation of glycated proteins; two to three 500-mg capsules daily.

7. Moducare containing plant sterinols improves the immune system by balancing the Th1/Th2 response; 1 capsule 3 times daily between meals.

8. Life Flora is a probiotic that can reinoculate the gut with healthy bacteria; 1–4 capsules daily for maintenance of GI health.

9. NutraFlora is a prebiotic containing FOS, a nutrient for intestinal flora; 1–4 tsp daily for people with chronic disease states.

10. Butyric acid is a short-chain fatty acid needed for healthy functioning of the large intestine. Butyrate enemas may help reduce the intestinal inflammation that accompanies certain autoimmune conditions. Butyrate enemas must be prescribed by a physician.

11. *L*-glutamine will aid the small intestines by increasing the number and health of intestinal cells; 1–2 grams daily.

12. Adapton acts as a precursor to endorphins, which help to reduce stress. To begin dosing, take 4 softgels first thing in the morning for 15 days and then reduce amount as needed.

13. *L*-theanine, the amino acid derived from green tea, reduces stress by creating a sense of well-being; 1–4 capsules daily.

14. The liver is the most important organ in the body for detoxification. Silymarin and Silibinin Plus improve liver function. Suggested dosage is 2 capsules daily of Silibinin Plus, which provides 250 mg of silibinin and 60 mg of silymarin.

PRODUCT AVAILABILITY

Super GLA/DHA, perilla oil, flax seed oil, borage oil, evening primrose oil, cod liver oil, DHEA, vitamin C, Gamma E Tocopherol/Tocotrienols, Green Tea Extract, beta-carotene, grapeseed-skin extract, CoQ10, SeMSc (selenium), Super Carnosine, Norwegian Shark Liver Oil, acetyl-*L*-carnitine, Moducare, Life Flora, NutraFlora, *L*-glutamine, Adapton, *L*-theanine, and Silibinin Plus are available by calling (800) 544-4440 or order online at www.lef.org.

APPENDIX A

Leaky Gut Syndrome

The healthy gastrointestinal tract (gut) performs a multitude of functions. It digests foods; absorbs small food particles that are converted into energy; transports vitamins and minerals across the intestinal lining and into the bloodstream; contributes to the chemical detoxification system of the body; and contains immunoglobulins or antibodies that act as the first line of defense against infection.

Leaky gut syndrome represents a condition in which large spaces develop in the intestinal mucosa, allowing bacteria, toxins, and food to leak into the bloodstream. This hyperpermeable condition leads to inflammation and atrophic damage to the mucosal lining. Once the gut lining becomes inflamed or damaged, the functioning of the GI system is disrupted, allowing large food molecules and toxic pathogens that are foreign to our natural defense system to be absorbed into the body. The result is the production of antibodies that launch an attack on the foreign invaders, with our own healthy tissue often being damaged in the process. Food allergies often complicate leaky gut syndrome. An elimination diet should be undertaken to determine food irritants. See the section entitled Supporting the GI Tract for nutritional supplements that will aid digestion and repair a hyperpermeable condition.

Maintaining Proper pH Balance in the Gut

Diet can significantly impact complete immune function. Because 80% of immune system cells reside in the area of the small intestine, numerous potential antigens can form from the incomplete breakdown of food products. Autoimmune states can be induced by food sensitivities that cause intestinal gut permeability and complicate leaky gut syndrome (Kitts et al. 1997). A first defense against the alteration of protein structure that produces autoimmunity is in the consumption of food sources as close to natural as possible. In addition, the body should be kept in the proper acid/alkaline balance. The correct ratio by volume would be 25% acidifying to 75% alkalizing foods. The following chart provides guidelines on proper food selection. In general, it is important to eat a diet that contains both alkalizing and acidifying foods. Allergic reactions and other forms of stress tend to produce acids in the body. The presence of high acidity indicates that more of your foods should be selected from the alkalizing group.

Alkalizing Foods

Vegetables

Garlic	Celery	Mustard greens	Sea veggies
Asparagus	Chard	Nova Scotia dulse	Spirulina (algae)
Fermented veggies	Chlorella (algae)	Dandelions	Sprouts (all types)
Watercress	Collard greens	Edible flowers	Squashes
Bets	Cucumbers	Onions	Alfalfa grass
Broccoli	Eggplant*	Parsnips (high-glycemic)	Barley grass
Brussels sprouts	Kale	Peas	Wheat grass
Cabbage	Kohlrabi	Peppers*	Wild grass
Carrot	Lettuces (all types)	Pumpkins	Cauliflower
Mushrooms	Rutabaga		

Fruits

Apple	Cantaloupe	Nectarine	Tangerine
Apricot	Cherries, Currants	Orange, Lemon	Tomato*
Avocado	Dates, Figs	Peach, Pear	Tropical fruits
Banana (high-glycemic)	Grapes	Pineapple	Watermelon
Blackberry	Grapefruit, Lime	Raspberry (all berries)	Blueberry
Honeydew	Strawberry		

Protein

Free-range eggs	Organic yogurt	Flax seeds	Sunflower seeds
Whey protein powder	Almonds	Pumpkin seeds	Millet
Fat-free cottage cheese	Chestnuts	Tempeh (fermented)	Sprouted seeds, Nuts
Lean chicken breast	Tofu (fermented)	Squash seeds	

Other

Apple cider vinegar	Bee pollen	Lecithin granules	Dairy-free probiotic cultures

Beverages

GREENS+	Veggie juices	Fresh fruit juice (unsweetened)	Mineral water (non-carbonated)
Organic milk (unpasteurized)	Quality water		

Teas

Green tea	Herbal tea	Dandelion tea	Bancha tea
Ginseng	Kombucha		

Sweeteners

Stevia

Spices and Seasonings

Cinnamon	Curry	Mustard	Miso
Ginger	Chili peppers	Tamari	Salt (Sea, Celtic)
All herbs			

Oriental Vegetables

Maitake	Shiitake	Nori	Sea veggies
Daikon	Kombu	Umeboshi	Wakame
Dandelion root	Reishi		

Acidifying Foods

Fats and Oils

Avocado oil	Hemp seed oil	Lard	Sesame oil
Canola oil	Flax oil	Olive oil	Sunflower oil
Corn oil	Grape seed oil	Safflower oil	

Fruits

Cranberries

Grains

Rice cakes	Buckwheat	Rice (brown, basmati)	Wheat
Wheat cakes	Corn	Rye	Hemp seed flower
Amaranth	Barley	Oats (rolled)	Spelt
Quinoa	Kamut		

Dairy (Milk and Hard Cheeses)

Cheese, cow	Cheese, goat	Cheese, processed	Milk
Cheese, sheep	Butter		

Nuts and Butters

Cashews	Brazil nuts	Peanut butter	Tahini
Filberts	Peanuts	Pecans	Walnuts

Animal Protein

Beef	Lamb	Rabbit	Turkey
Carp	Lobster	Salmon	Venison
Clams	Mussels	Shrimp	Duck
Oysters	Scallops	Fish, white meat	Pork
Tuna			

Pasta (White)

Noodles	Macaroni	Spaghetti

Other

Distilled vinegar	Brewers yeast	Wheat germ	Potatoes*

Drugs and Chemicals

Drugs, medicinal	Drugs, psychedelic	Pesticides	Herbicides

Sweets and Sweeteners

Molasses	Maple syrup	Sugar	Fruit-flavored drinks
Candy	Saccharin	Aspartame	Soft drinks
Honey			

Alcoholic Beverages

Beer	Spirits	Hard liquor	Wine

Beans and Legumes

Black beans	Lentils	Soybeans	Almond milk
Chick peas	Lima beans	Soy milk	Green peas
Pinto beans	White beans	Kidney beans	Red beans
Rice milk			

* Nightshade family foods

Note: Use organically grown foods whenever possible.

Bacterial Infections

Bacterial infections are caused by the presence and growth of microorganisms that damage host tissue. The extent of infection is generally determined by how many organisms are present and the toxins they release. Worldwide, bacterial infections are responsible for more deaths than any other cause. Symptoms can include inflammation and swelling, pain, heat, redness, and loss of function. The most important risk factors are burns, severe trauma, low white blood cell counts, patients on immunotherapy treatment, and anyone with malnutrition or vitamin deficiency.

Bacteria are generally spread from an already infected person to the newly infected person. The most common invasion routes are inhalation of airborne bacteria, ingestion into the stomach from dirty hands or utensils, or through contaminated food or water, direct contact with an infected area of another person's body, contaminated blood, or by insect bite.

The first of the body's three primary lines of defense includes naturally occurring chemicals such as the lysozymes found in tears, gastric acid of the stomach, pancreatic enzymes of the bowel, and fatty acids in the skin. The body's immune response becomes involved only if the infective organism manages to invade the body. Nonspecific immune response—the body's second line of defense—consists primarily of inflammation, whereas specific immune response—the third line of defense—relies on the activation of lymphocytes, which send T- and B-cells to try to recognize the specific type of organism involved. T-cells marshal cytotoxic cells, which are sent to destroy the organism, and B-cells produce the antibodies—immunoglobulins—that can destroy specific types of bacteria (*for more information about preventing infections in general, please refer to the Immune Enhancement protocol*).

Acute bacterial infections require immediate conventional medical care. If FDA-approved antibiotics fail to work, European antibiotics, which are several years more advanced than American antibiotics, may be effective.

LIMITATIONS OF MODERN ANTIBIOTICS

When antibiotics were discovered in the 1940s, they were incredibly effective in the treatment of many bacterial infections. Over time many antibiotics have lost their effectiveness against certain types of bacteria because resistant strains have developed, mostly through the expression of "resistance genes." In 1998 a potentially deadly bacterium, *Staphylococcus aureus* ("staph"), which causes widespread nosocomial (infections contracted in a hospital or clinic) infections, failed to respond to the most potent antibiotic, vancomycin. The most troubling aspect was that this failure occurred in three patients in widely separated geographic areas.

There are several ways in which bacteria become resistant to antibiotic therapy. One way is that some bacteria have now developed "efflux" pumps. When the bacterium recognizes invasion by an antibiotic, the efflux pump simply pumps the antibiotic out of its cells. Resistance genes code for more than pumps, however. Some lead to the manufacture of enzymes that degrade or chemically alter (and therefore inactivate) the antibiotic. Where do these resistance genes come from? Usually, bacteria get them from other bacteria. In some cases they pick up a gene containing plasmid from a "donor" cell. Also, viruses have been shown to extract a resistance gene from one bacterium and inject it into a different one. Furthermore, some bacteria "scavenge" DNA from dead cells around them, and occasionally, scavenged genes are incorporated in a stable manner into the recipient cell's chromosome or into a plasmid and become part of the recipient bacterium. A few resistance genes develop through random mutations in the bacterium's DNA.

Research shows great promise for a novel concept: the introduction of susceptible strains of bacteria following treatment by antibiotics. The idea is for the susceptible strain to colonize the resistant strain. The resulting colony is then antibiotic sensitive.

The Last Line of Antibiotic Defense

As the problems of antibiotic resistance become ever more global, scientists see an increasing role for aminoglycosides in clinical practice. Aminoglycosides are chemical compounds that are present in a variety of antibiotics. Some are derived naturally from microorganisms, while others are synthesized. Their broad antimicrobial spectrum and ability to act synergistically with other drugs make them very useful in treating serious nosocomial (hospital-induced) infections.

Aminoglycosides are given for serious Gram-negative bacilli infections, such as *Mycobacterium avium, Mycobacterium tuberculosis, Pseudomonas aeruginosa,* and enterococcal endocarditis. Aminoglycosides exhibit a significant postantibiotic effect for up to 8 hours after antimicrobial action falls to zero, making them superior to other classes of antibiotics. Common side effects may include a loss of hearing, clumsiness, dizziness, increased or decreased urination, increased thirst, loss of appetite, and nausea or vomiting. Some of these effects may last several weeks after the last dose. The following medications compose the aminoglycoside family: streptomycin, amikacin, gentamicin, kanamycin, netilmicin, and tobramycin. Aminoglycosides are administered under physician supervision by means of inhalation solution, irrigation solution, or injection.

Enterococci are bacteria found in the feces of most humans and some animals. In healthy people, two strains of enterococci, *Enterococcus faecalis* and *Enterococcus faecium*, may cause urinary tract infections or wound infections that can be cured by tetracycline or penicillin. In severely ill patients in a hospital setting, these same two strains may cause life-threatening conditions such as bacteremia (infection of the blood stream), endocarditis (infection of the heart valves), and meningitis (infection of brain fluid).

Until the mid-1980s, all enterococcal bacteria were effectively killed by vancomycin (Vancocin), an antibiotic administered by bolus injection that was considered the last line of defense against the most life-threatening bacterial infections. However, since then, several strains of enterococci that are vancomycin-resistant have appeared in hospitals all over the world. The problem is so serious that in the United States alone over 14,000 people die each year from antibiotic-resistant bacteria picked up in the hospital.

S. aureus is another potentially lethal bacterium found in hospitals. *Staphylococcus* sp. were at one time responsive to treatment with methicillin. Now, almost all strains of *Staphylococcus* are resistant to methicillin and are becoming increasingly resistant to vancomycin as well. Hospitals are struggling to improve hygiene and take more aggressive action to contain contaminated areas, with only limited success. Both staphylococcal and enterococcal strains of bacteria resistant to the most potent antibiotics have been found in otherwise healthy people outside the hospital setting.

To combat the problem, pharmaceutical companies continue to develop new and stronger antibiotics as the last line of defense. Currently only one, Synercid, approved for use by the FDA in 1999, has proven safe, with limited effectiveness, for treatment of staphylococcal and enterococcal infections.

Synercid is administered intravenously as a drug of last resort.

NATURAL ALTERNATIVES

Lactoferrin

Lactoferrin is a subfraction of whey with well-documented antiviral, antimicrobial, anticancer, and immune modulating/enhancing effects. Whey is a complex protein made up of many smaller protein subfractions (peptides). Many of these subfractions are found only in very minute amounts in cows' milk, normally at less than 1%. For example, lactoferrin makes up only 0.5–1% or less of whey protein derived from cows' milk. Mothers' milk, on the other hand, will contain up to 15% lactoferrin.

Lactoferrin is found throughout the human body and occurs in all secretions that bathe mucous membranes, such as saliva, tears, bronchial and nasal secretions, hepatic bile, and pancreatic fluids, and is an essential factor in the immune response (Nikolaev et al. 1985). Lactoferrin is concentrated in oral cavities where it will come in direct contact with pathogens (e.g., viruses, bacteria, etc.) and kill or greatly suppress these pathogens through a variety of different mechanisms. In fact, there are specific receptors for lactoferrin found on many key immune cells, such as lymphocytes, monocytes, and macrophages (Yamada et al. 1987). Lactoferrin is known to be directly involved in the upregulation of natural killer (NK) cell activity. One study with baby pigs found that only 17% of the pigs died when fed lactoferrin and injected with a toxin—*Escherichia coli*—as opposed to 74% of the pigs that died without the lactoferrin (Lee et al. 1998).

Lactoferrin's best-known role is as an iron-binding protein. It's referred to as hololactoferrin in its iron-bound form and apolactoferrin in its iron-depleted form. Studies have found that it is the apolactoferrin form that has the most powerful effects as an antimicrobial agent (Tomita et al. 1994).

Lactoferrin is a powerful antimicrobial able to inhibit a wide range of pathogenic bacteria and other microbes. The mechanism appears to lie with lactoferrin's ability to bind iron because it is known to have an extremely high affinity for this metal. Many pathogenic bacteria need a supply of free iron to multiply and in the presence of lactoferrin are strongly inhibited or killed. One study added lactoferrin to the drinking water of mice and subjected them to the toxic microbe called *S. aureus*. The study found that in the mice getting the lactoferrin as 2% of their caloric intake, kidney infections were reduced by 40–60% and bacterial counts were reduced five- to twelvefold. Bhimani et al. (1999)

concluded, "The results suggest a potential for the use of lactoferrin as natural antibacterial proteins for preventing bacterial infections."

Another study looked at lactoferrin as a "natural antibiotic" and found that lactoferrin both *in vitro* and *in vivo* strongly inhibited the toxic bacteria *Helicobacter pylori*. Researchers stated, "It is concluded that bovine (cow's) lactoferrin has significant antimicrobial activity against *Helicobacter* species *in vitro* and *in vivo*" (Dial et al. 1998).

When fed to adult animals and human infants, lactoferrin showed a dramatic increase in good microflora—such as *Bifidobacterium bifidum* (Bifidus)—and a decrease in bad bacteria, such as *E. coli*, *Streptococcus* sp., *Clostridium* sp., and others. The result was desirable intestinal flora, which is known to be essential for optimal health, immunity, and resistance to disease. An extensive review that examined the role of lactoferrin in inflammation and the health of the intestinal tract stated, "The possibility that lactoferrin limits the autodestructive inflammatory response presents a new alternative for the future management of systemic inflammation" (Kruzel et al. 1998). Some research also suggests that lactoferrin is able to stimulate intestinal cell growth and may lead to better digestive functions, in addition to its ability to enhance the growth of "good" microflora in the intestine. There is little doubt that in addition to its immunomodulating effects, this natural peptide derived from whey has powerful probiotic properties.

Interestingly, some studies have found lactoferrin from cows to be more effective than lactoferrin from humans for antibacterial properties (Vorland et al. 1998) (although it is well established that human mother's milk confers a great deal of protection to the newborn due to many factors, including a high lactoferrin content). Studies have found lactoferrin to inhibit a wide range of Gram-positive and Gram-negative bacteria, yeasts, and even certain intestinal parasites. Cholera, *E. coli*, *Shigella flexneri*, *Staphylococcus epidermidis*, *P. aeruginosa*, *Candida albicans*, and others have all been found to be strongly or partially inhibited in the presence of lactoferrin (Percival 1997; Kuwata et al. 1998; Haversen et al. 2000). (It should be noted that not every microbe that is pathogenic to humans is suppressed by lactoferrin.)

Maybe most promising and interesting, there is research that points to lactoferrin being able to improve the efficiency of antibiotic treatments in the fight against pathogenic microbes.

Oregano Oil

Oil of oregano is a powerful antiseptic and considered one of the most potent antibacterials of all the essential oils (Marino et al. 2001). Carvacrol and thymol, the two active ingredients in oregano, are phenols—agents that kill microscopic bacteria. Oregano oil has been used for centuries in Far Eastern and Middle Eastern cultures to treat respiratory infections, chronic inflammation, urinary tract infections, dysentery, jaundice, and even to increase sexual excitability. Medicinal oregano grows wild in mountainous areas of Greece and Turkey and is rich in minerals such as calcium, magnesium, zinc, iron, potassium, copper, boron, and manganese, which adds to its therapeutic value. Oregano oil has become popular in recent years as an alternative to prescription antibiotics.

Grapefruit Seed Extract

Grapefruit seed extract is derived from the bioflavonoids found in the seed and pulp. Its antigermicide action has shown a growth-inhibiting effect on bacteria, fungi, parasites, and viruses in several *in vitro* studies. The effectiveness of grapefruit seeds was discovered accidentally by a doctor who noticed that the seeds did not decompose in his compost pile. Further examination revealed that the grapefruit seeds killed any microorganism that tried to decompose it. Laboratory studies have shown it to be effective in inhibiting bacteria such as *S. aureus*, *E. coli*, *P. aeruginosa*, and *M. tuberculosis*. Grapefruit seed extract has been formulated by a number of manufacturers for various uses, including an internal bactericide, water disinfectant, skin cleanser, and first-aid spray. Grapefruit seed extract is also a treatment for house pets and livestock that may be susceptible to bacterial infections from a variety of sources.

Sarsaparilla Root

Sarsaparilla root (*Smilax officinalis*) attacks and neutralizes microbial substances in the bloodstream through its antibiotic activity. By acting as a diuretic and diaphoretic (promotes perspiration), sarsaparilla encourages excretion of toxins and waste materials and acts as an antidote for various poisons. Heavy metallic contaminants in the blood can be extracted from the system with the judicious use of sarsaparilla. Sarsaparilla exerts strong power over fibers and tissues of the nervous system, which is an added benefit of its use.

Alkylglycerols

Alkylglycerols (AKGs) are a family of compounds that have been found to play a crucial role in the production and stimulation of white blood cells. They occur in freshwater fish and in cow, sheep, and mother's milk. AKGs help give nursing mammals, including breast-fed babies, protection against infection until their own immune systems can develop fully. Alkylglycerols are thought to act as immune boosters against infectious diseases. No side effects have been seen in patients taking 100 mg 3 times a day. Shark liver oil capsules containing a minimum of 200 mg of alkylglycerols a capsule, at a dose of 5 capsules a day, can have a direct antibiotic effect.

CAUTION Do not take shark liver oil for more than 30 days, because it may cause overproduction of blood platelets.

Enzymes

Bromelain, a proteolytic digestive enzyme, can potentiate—augment or strengthen—the effects of conventional antibiotics, making them more effective in killing bacteria (Chandler et al. 1998). (Proteolytic substances contribute to the hydrolysis of proteins or peptides and help form simpler, soluble products.) Bromelain should be taken with meals. The suggested dose is 2000 mg a day of a highly concentrated bromelain.

Amino Acids

Arginine, a crystalline basic amino acid derived from guanidine, can stimulate antibacterial components of the immune system when taken in doses ranging from 6–20 grams a day. Arginine promotes the synthesis of nitric oxide that is believed to help protect against bacterial infections. The role of nitric oxide was studied in host defense against *Klebsiella pneumoniae* infection of the lung. The results suggested that nitric oxide plays a critical role in antibacterial host defense against *K. pneumoniae*, in part by regulating macrophage phagocytic and microbicidal activity (Wang et al. 1999).

Fruit Juice

Cranberry juice has proven to be an effective non-drug therapy against urinary tract infections (Fleet 1994; Kontiokari et al. 2001). The active ingredients of the juice keep bacteria from attaching to the walls of the bladder and urinary tract. Research concludes that cranberry juice also helps to prevent the formation of dental plaque that can eventually lead to tooth decay (Weiss et al. 1998). Because the recommended daily intake of this juice is so great, a dietary supplement has been developed called Cran-Max that provides the equivalent of sixteen 8-oz glasses of cranberry juice in just 1 capsule. One capsule a day provides the equivalent of the recommended amount of cranberry juice for proven results in fighting urinary tract infections.

Honey and Bee Propolis

Before the discovery of antibiotics, honey was known to have antibacterial properties. Research has confirmed those earlier findings (Tosi et al. 1996). In addition, electron microscope studies show that bee propolis has a potent antibacterial effect by preventing cell division and inhibiting protein synthesis (Takaisi-Kikuni et al. 1994).

CAUTION Bee products should not be administered to children under the age of three.

Trace Elements

Zinc has been found to potentiate antiseptic agents (Zeelie et al. 1998). A South African study concluded that zinc is also critical in the maintenance of a healthy immune system.

Other Herbal Antimicrobials

Researchers around the world are taking another look at folk medicine, herbal remedies, and other alternatives to pharmacological drugs. Research has confirmed the antibacteriological value of herbal extracts from many parts of the world. Examples of useful herbal remedies abound. Goldenseal may be an effective natural antibiotic (Scazzocchio et al. 2001). Raw garlic has potent antibacterial effects (Kumar et al. 1998). Kyolic, an aged garlic product, does not kill bacteria directly, but does boost immune function, enabling the body to fight off some chronic bacterial infections.

Restoring Intestinal Flora

Antibiotics often destroy friendly bacteria in the intestinal tract that are needed to digest food and prohibit the growth of fungal infections and pathogenic bacteria. Fortunately, these beneficial bacteria can be restored by supplementing with a product such as Life Flora that helps to recolonize the natural floral balance that antibiotics can destroy.

Oxygenation Therapy

Hyperbaric oxygenation helps the body heal from conditions that have low oxygen in the tissues causing or complicating the outcome. Repetitive hyperbaric sessions can help many different conditions such as anemia, burns, and crush injuries. Compromised skin grafts often improve with hyperbaric oxygenation. The use of hyperbaric oxygen therapy (HBO) has become more widespread in recent years for difficult-to-heal infections, since antibiotics often fail to clear resistant strains of pathogens. Treatable infections include actinomycosis, osteomyelitis, diabetic wounds, gangrene, and other deadly soft tissue infections.

HBO consists of a monoplace chamber, in which only one patient is entirely enclosed in a pressure chamber, breathing oxygen at a pressure greater than atmospheric pressure. Each treatment lasts about 60 minutes. HBO is regarded as a therapeutic modality because significant physiological mechanisms are activated as a result. HBO delivers 10–15 times the oxygen to tissues as normal breathing. HBO is used in the formation of new capillaries around a wound area, and to treat anemia, ischemia, and some poisonings.

The flooding of the body with oxygen, as in hyperbaric therapy, tends to remove other gases, such as carbon monoxide and acute cyanide poisoning. HBO inhibits the growth of a number of anaerobic, as well as aerobic, organisms by enhancing phagocytic activity. This effect complements the improved action of host disease-fighting factors and is useful in disorders involving immunosuppression. Studies have demonstrated a prolonged postantibiotic effect when hyperbaric oxygen is combined with therapeutic dosages of antibiotics.

CONCLUSION

Ironically, the advent of the new "miracle drugs," the antibiotics developed in the 1940s and since, also set the stage for drug-resistant bacteria that do not respond to antibiotics. Avoiding or neutralizing bacterial infections requires a strong, effective immune response. Research demonstrates preventive benefits from herbal and natural alternatives. Natural and herbal remedies can provide effective treatment when FDA-approved American antibiotics fail.

🌑 SUMMARY

1. With the arrival of drug-resistant bacteria, prevention becomes more important than ever. The body's immune system can be strengthened by vitamin and trace-element supplementation. Three Life Extension Mix tablets 3 times a day (at meal times) provide the essential vitamins and trace elements for basic immune-system health.

2. Life Extension Herbal Mix incorporates 27 different herbs into a powder designed to make 1 daily drink. One tsp a day mixed in fruit juice supplies immune-enhancing nutrients.

3. Lactoferrin, a powerful antimicrobial, is able to inhibit a wide range of pathogenic bacteria and other microbes. Its mechanism of action appears to lie with its ability to bind iron. Up to 900 mg daily (3 capsules) are recommended when fighting an infection. The maintenance dose of lactoferrin is one 300-mg capsule a day.

4. Oregano oil contains potent phenols that kill microscopic bacteria. Thirty drops (1 mL) may be taken daily with water.

5. Grapefruit seed extract has been shown to inhibit bacteria, viruses, and fungi. One-fourth tsp liquid extract diluted in water or juice can be taken up to 3 times a day.

6. Sarsaparilla root (*S. officinalis*) attacks and neutralizes microbial substances in the bloodstream through its antibiotic activity. Thirty to 60 drops (1–2 mL) of tincture of sasaparilla may be taken daily.

7. Shark liver oil contains alkylglycerols, a family of compounds proven to be beneficial to the production and stimulation of white blood cells; 1000 mg a day of shark liver oil capsules can have a direct antibiotic effect.

8. Bromelain, a proteolytic digestive enzyme, augments conventional antibiotics and makes them more effective in killing bacteria. The suggested dose is 2000 mg a day with meals.

9. Arginine, an amino acid, stimulates the immune system's antibacterial components when taken at the rate of 6–20 grams a day.

10. The active ingredients of cranberry juice interfere with harmful bacteria that adhere to the walls of the urinary tract, preventing and actually helping to cure urinary tract infections. These ingredients have also been found to help prevent dental cavities. Cran-Max, a purified extract of cranberry juice, contains the equivalent of 16 glasses of juice in each capsule. The recommended dose is one 500-mg capsule a day.

11. Both honey and bee propolis are known to have antibacterial properties. They work by preventing bacterial cell division and inhibiting protein synthesis.

CAUTION Do not administer bee products to children under the age of three.

12. Zinc potentiates antiseptic agents and is critical to the maintenance of a healthy immune system. When treating a bacterial infection, 90–120 mg a day of zinc is suggested.

13. Life Flora will help to recolonize friendly intestinal flora that can be destroyed by antibiotics. Two capsules 3 times daily are recommended.

14. A hyperbaric oxygen chamber kills both anaerobic and aerobic bacteria, while improving immune function and displacing noxious gases.

 PRODUCT AVAILABILITY

Life Extension Mix, Life Extension Herbal Mix, lactoferrin, oregano oil, Kyolic garlic, Norwegian shark liver oil, bromelain, echinacea, goldenseal, Optizinc, arginine, Cran-Max (cranberry juice concentrate), Life Flora, and bee propolis can be obtained by calling (800) 544-4440 or by ordering online at www.left.org. Ask for a listing of offshore companies that sell European antibiotics.

Balding

TYPES OF HAIR LOSS

Balding is usually a result of genetic factors, aging, local skin conditions, diseases, and the taking of certain medicines. Balding is always symmetrical in both male- and female-pattern baldness. If hair loss is nonsymmetrical, for example, hair loss on only one side of the head, more than likely there is another reason for the hair loss, and a biopsy may have to be performed.

Male-Pattern Balding

Male-pattern balding, the most common type of balding in men, is controlled by a single dominant autosomal gene. This type of balding usually starts at the temples and then will gradually recede to form an "M" shape on the head. The hair on the top of the head will start to thin out. Over time, the male is left with a horseshoe-shaped pattern of hair around his head. Some males will have only a receding hairline or bald spots on the crowns of their heads. The hair that remains in the balding areas starts out as long, thick, and pigmented and changes into fine, unpigmented sprouts that grow at a slower rate. If a man begins losing his hair during his mid-teen years, there is a good chance he will become completely bald on top of his head.

Androgenic alopecia (AGA) is another factor that can cause male-pattern baldness. Androgenic alopecia is caused by three factors: advanced age, an inherited tendency to bald early, and an overabundance of dihydrotestosterone (DHT), a highly active form of testosterone within the hair follicle. DHT influences male behavior, from the sex drive to aggression. Testosterone converts to DHT by 5-alpha-reductase, an enzyme produced in the prostate, adrenal glands, and the scalp. What appears to happen is that DHT (and perhaps other androgenic hormones) causes the immune system to react to the hair follicles in the affected areas as foreign bodies. This is suggested by the presence of hair-follicle antibodies, as well as by the infiltration of immune system cells around the hair follicles of balding men (as well as women).

Female-Pattern Baldness

Female-pattern baldness is caused by aging, genetic susceptibility, and levels of endocrine hormones known as androgens. This type of balding usually begins around the age of 30 and becomes more noticeable at age 40, and can be more evident after menopause. Female-pattern baldness usually causes the hair to thin out all over the head, but it rarely progresses to total or near baldness as it does in men. This type of hair loss is permanent.

Females may also suffer hair loss because of temporary shedding, known as telogen effluvium; breaking of the hair due to styling treatments and twisting or pulling of the hair; alopecia areata, an immune disorder temporarily causing patchy areas of total hair loss; oral medications; and certain skin diseases.

Toxic Baldness

Toxic baldness occurs in males, as well as females. Hair may fall out for as long as 3–4 months before it grows back. Many cancer chemotherapy medications, as well as certain cholesterol-lowering drugs, Parkinson's medications, ulcer drugs, anticoagulants, antiarthritics, drugs derived from vitamin A, anticonvulsants for epilepsy, antidepressants, beta-blocker drugs for high blood pressure, antithyroid agents, blood thinners, and anabolic steroids, can cause baldness. When a doctor prescribes any drug, he should be asked if it causes hair loss. If he does not know, have him look it up in the *Physicians' Desk Reference*, which lists the side effects of all prescription drugs. A pharmacist can also be asked for this information.

Alopecia Areata, Universalis, and Totalis

Sudden hair loss in a certain area, such as the scalp or beard, is called alopecia areata and is sometimes caused by an autoimmune illness. Alopecia universalis is a condition in which all body hair may be lost. The total loss of all body hair, including eyebrows, eyelashes, facial and body hair, and hair on top of the head, is known as alopecia totalis. Unless hair loss is widespread, new hair may grow back within a few months, but with no color.

Trichotillomania and Scarring Alopecia

Trichotillomania, also known as hair pulling, is found primarily in children, although it can prevail throughout a person's lifetime. Children with trichotillomania have an abnormal desire to pull out their hair, chronically scratch, or brush their hair for no apparent reason.

Scarring alopecia describes skin that is scarred because of burns, x-ray therapy, skin cancer, or a severe injury that results in hair loss.

TREATMENT

A doctor may need to perform a biopsy to determine what type of baldness a person is experiencing. The biopsy will ascertain whether the follicles are normal. There are four conventional choices a person has in regard to treating hair loss: begin to take better care of the scalp, use products such as minoxidil (Rogaine) and/or Proscar, get a hair transplant or a scalp reduction, or have the hair replaced nonsurgically. More aggressive approaches to treating hair loss are discussed later in this protocol.

Successful prevention and treatment of accelerated hair loss necessitates dealing with some, if not all, of the factors involved in the process, except for the genetic component of baldness, which is still in the research phase.

Because the male hormone dihydrotestosterone (DHT) is involved in premature hair loss, scientists have experimented with a wide variety of antiandrogens in an attempt to prevent or reverse the process. Among the antiandrogens that have been used to treat hair loss are progesterone, spironolactone (Aldactone), flutamide (Eulexin), finasteride (Proscar), cimetidine (Tagamet), serenoa repens (Permixon), and cyproterone acetate (Androcur/Diane). Of these antiandrogens, the most effective has proven to be oral finasteride (Propecia and Proscar).

In the hair-loss process, it is the immune reaction caused by male hormones, such as DHT (the balding hormone), that plays, perhaps, the most significant role. Stimulated by androgens, the immune system targets hair follicles in genetically susceptible areas, causing the premature loss of hair that is characteristic of male-pattern baldness.

Among the most potent hair-growth stimulators are topical oxygen radical scavengers, such as the superoxide dismutases (SODs), enzymes that play a critical role in countering excessive free-radical activity throughout the body.

SODs not only inhibit oxygen radicals but may also inhibit the localized immune response implicated in so much hair loss and may offset some of the damage and inflammation already incurred. Unless the immunologic factors involved in the hair-loss process are dealt with effectively, the potential for significant hair regrowth may be very limited.

There are many available agents (such as Rogaine) that can stimulate some degree of hair growth in some people, but they cannot by themselves produce the kind of health and cosmetic benefits that balding people desire. What's needed is a multi-modal approach that combines antiandrogens with autoimmune protective agents, oxygen free-radical inhibitors, and other hair-growth stimulators to halt hair loss and generate hair regrowth to a degree well beyond the abilities of single compounds.

Finasteride (Propecia)

Propecia is the FDA-approved drug for treating hair loss. It comes in a 1-mg pill form and is available by prescription only for men for around $45–50 a month. Originally developed by Merck Pharmaceuticals for treating benign prostatic hyperplasia (BPH), finasteride is also sold under the name Proscar in a 5-mg pill form. At first, finasteride was thought to be useless as a treatment for androgenic alopecia because it primarily affects the Type 2 of the DHT-inducing enzyme 5-alpha-reductase. However, doses of finasteride as low as 0.2 mg a day have been shown to maximally decrease both scalp skin and serum DHT levels (Drake et al. 1999). Additional clinical trials of finasteride have confirmed its beneficial effects in AGA in males, but not in females.

Finasteride can produce visible hair growth in most men with mild to moderate alopecia, but more importantly, it can stop hair loss in a majority of patients. A 5-year study found finasteride, 1 mg per day over 5 years, was well-tolerated, led to durable improvements in scalp hair growth, and slowed the further progression of hair loss that occurred without treatment (FMPHLSG 2002). The most common side effect of finasteride is decreased sexual desire or lowered amount of ejaculate in less than 2% of men, although almost as many men who received the placebo experienced these side effects as well.

Future Treatments

Dutasteride (GG745) is a drug similar to Propecia/finasteride in that it blocks the enzyme that converts testosterone to DHT. Unlike finasteride, Dutasteride blocks both of the enzymes that create DHT instead of just one, so it may be a more potent treatment for hair loss (Bramson et al. 1997). Dutasteride was given preliminary approval for the treatment of benign prostatic hyperplasia on November 20, 2001.

Azulfidine (sulfasalazine) is an anti-inflammatory sulfa drug used to treat autoimmune disorders, such as rheumatoid arthritis and Crohn's disease. Researchers have found that it may be an effective treatment for some people with alopecia areata. Of 30 patients tested, Azulfidine led to a complete reversal of the condition in seven (23%). Others had some hair regrowth, but for the majority of test subjects (more than half), the medication had no effect (Ellis et al. 2002).

Dr. Proctor's Hair Regrowth Formulas

Dr. Peter Proctor is the only hair-treatment practitioner in the world who has developed unique, patented, multi-ingredient hair formulas that address all the known factors in the balding process. He is the author of more than 30 scientific articles and book chapters and holds several broad patents for hair-loss treatment.

Dr. Proctor offers both prescription and nonprescription hair-treatment formulas that vary both in potency and cost. However, even the least potent of Dr. Proctor's formulas has been shown to be superior to Rogaine, the only FDA-approved hair-treatment product on the market.

The least expensive of Dr. Proctor's hair growth formulas is sold under the name Dr. Proctor's Hair Regrowth Shampoo. This formula includes an abundant supply of the most potent natural hair growth stimulator available, 3-carboxylic acid pyridine-N-oxide (NANO), which is known as "natural" minoxidil.

Dr. Proctor's Hair Regrowth Shampoo has worked effectively for many people who did not respond to Rogaine. It may be all that is needed if only small to moderate hair loss is experienced or if the primary need is for a prophylactic program that will prevent hair loss in the future. Dr. Proctor's Hair Regrowth Shampoo should be used whenever the hair is washed (at least 3 times a week) and can be used just like any other shampoo.

The second formula developed by Dr. Proctor, which is sold under the name Dr. Proctor's Advanced Hair Regrowth Formula, includes a potent dose of "natural" minoxidil (NANO) combined with the following natural hair protection and hair growth agents: endothelium-derived relaxing factor (EDRF) enhancers, SODs, and various free-radical scavengers. Zinc sulfate and copper peptides are the antiandrogens that enhance the production of in the formula.

This multiagent natural formula is the most potent natural hair-growth formula available. It includes every type of natural hair treatment agent available to counter the DHT, autoimmune, and inflammatory effects that are at the root of hair loss and baldness. Dr. Proctor's Advanced Hair Regrowth Formula is a liquid that is applied to the scalp.

Dr. Proctor's Advanced Hair Regrowth Formula should be applied 8–10 drops once or twice a day to the thinning areas. Its side effects include contact dermatitis (an itchy, scaly rash at the site of application).

For serious hair-loss problems, Dr. Proctor has developed a multidrug prescription formula that contains all the known drugs that are effective when applied topically. The name of this product is Dr. Proctor's European Prescription Hair Regrowth Formula, and it contains an array of natural hair-growth protectors combined with several drugs compounded into a cream base. Natural agents in Dr. Proctor's European Prescription Hair Regrowth Formula include topical antiandrogens, which increase EDRF levels, and oxygen free-radical scavengers. These agents are combined with the following drugs: minoxidil, phenytoin (Dilantin), tretinoin (Retin-A), and spironolactone.

The protocol for using Dr. Proctor's European Prescription Hair Regrowth Formula is as follows: apply 1/10 tsp (a dab on the end of your finger) once a day for 8–12 months, and then apply every other day for maintenance.

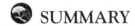 **SUMMARY**

Balding is in most cases a cosmetic problem and is usually the result of genetic influences, aging, skin conditions, or the ingesting of certain medications. The most common form of balding is male- and female-pattern baldness. At this time there is no known cure for baldness, and there are limited choices on how to cope with it. Oral prescription drugs, such as Propecia, and over-the-counter preparations, such as minoxidil, have shown benefit and are available in pharmacies.

Dr. Peter Proctor has developed unique, patented multi-ingredient hair formulas that address all the known factors in the balding process. These include Dr. Proctor's Hair Regrowth Shampoo (use like any shampoo), Dr. Proctor's Advanced Hair Regrowth Formula (8–10 drops applied once or twice a day to the thinning areas), and/or Dr. Proctor's European Prescription Hair Regrowth Formula (1/10 tsp—a dab on the end of your finger—applied once a day for 8–12 months, and then applied every other day for maintenance).

It is possible that there may be new drugs approved in the future that could be more effective than existing therapies. Most hair-growth drugs *prevent* hair from falling out better than they *regrow* hair on a balding scalp. Therefore, taking aggressive steps today to maintain healthy hair could enable one to benefit from better medications in the future.

information regarding radiation therapy, please see the *Cancer Radiation Therapy* protocol.)

ADJUVANT TREATMENT

The goal of an adjuvant treatment is to systemically eliminate any cancer cells or micrometastases that may have spread from the breast tumor to other parts of the body as well as to eliminate any microscopic cancer cells that may remain in the local breast/lymph node area. These therapies are referred to as adjuvant, meaning "in addition to," because they are used with surgery and radiation. It is called adjuvant systemic therapy because the entire system of the body is treated. Several types of adjuvant systemic treatments are used for early-stage breast cancer: chemotherapy and hormone therapy are well established conventional adjuvant therapies; nutritional supplementation and diet modification may be incorporated in any conventional adjuvant treatment plan.

Except for some women with very small tumors (less than 1 cm) and with lymph nodes that do not have cancer, adjuvant therapy is usually recommended for women with early-stage breast cancer. Which therapies, and in what combination, depends on many things, such as the woman's age, whether the tumor has estrogen receptors, and the number of positive lymph nodes.

Chemotherapy

Chemotherapy uses drugs that can be taken in oral form or injected intravenously to kill cancer cells; sometimes, a combination is used. However, intravenous drugs are usually given in a hospital or doctor's office. Depending on the drugs used, chemotherapy is administered once or twice a month for 3–6 months. Sometimes the range might be extended to 7 or 8 months. Chemotherapy usually begins 4–6 weeks after the final surgery and is administered in a combination of 2–3 drugs that have been found to be the most effective. Unfortunately, chemotherapy drugs have many side effects that can damage or destroy normal healthy tissues throughout the body.

Although the exact schedule depends on the specific drugs used, drugs may be given on day 1 of a 3-week cycle or there may be a period of a week or two on the drugs, followed by a period of about 2 weeks off the drugs. This cycling allows the body a chance to rest and recover between treatments; however, it also gives the cancer cells an opportunity to rest, recover, and possibly mutate into a type of cancer that is chemotherapy-resistant. An entire course of chemotherapy lasts about 4–6 months, depending on the drugs used. Recent studies indicate that a more efficacious approach would be to lower the dose of conventional chemotherapy agents, reschedule their application, and combine them with agents designed to interfere with cancer's ability to produce new blood vessels (anti-angiogenic agents) (Holland et al. 2000).

This lower-dose approach, known as "metronomic dosing," uses a dosing schedule as often as every day. An amount as low as 25% of the maximum tolerated dose (MTD) in combination with anti-angiogenesis agents targets the tumor endothelial cells making up the blood vessels and microvessels feeding the tumor. Tumor endothelial cells can be killed with much less chemotherapy than tumor cells, and the side effects to healthy tissue and the patient in general are dramatically reduced (Hanahan et al. 2000). While chemotherapy is an effective treatment for many women, it is associated with a number of well-known and traumatic side effects, such as hair loss, and exhausting bouts of nausea and vomiting, which many patients find difficult to tolerate. (For more information on chemotherapy, please refer to the *Cancer Chemotherapy* protocol.)

Hormone Therapy

Breast tumors often require hormones for growth, which poses a unique problem because the hormones involved in tumor growth are either estrogen, progesterone, or both. Estrogen and progesterone are naturally occurring and necessary hormones, produced mainly in the ovaries and adrenal glands in varying amounts throughout a woman's lifetime. These hormones are essential for many physiological functions, such as bone integrity, which will be discussed later in this protocol.

Hormone receptor-positive tumors can consist of cancer cells with receptor sites for estrogen, progesterone, or both. The hormones attach to receptor sites and promote cell proliferation. Hormone therapy blocks the hormones from attaching to the tumor receptor sites and may slow or stop the cancer's growth. The drug most often used in this type of endocrine therapy is tamoxifen, with a response rate from 30–60%. Other therapies are sometimes used, such as aromatase inhibitors (that inhibit the conversion of precursors to estrogens) or oophorectomy (the removal of the ovaries).

The effective role of some newer hormonal therapies in the treatment of both pre- and post-menopausal women with early breast cancer has been studied. Hormonal therapy with goserelin, either with or without tamoxifen, has been endorsed as an alternative to chemotherapy for young women with hormone-sensitive disease since it is equally effective and better tolerated. Twenty-five percent of all women diagnosed with breast cancer are premenopausal; of these women approximately 60% have hormone-sensitive tumors.

While chemotherapy kills cancer cells by destroying all rapidly dividing cells in the body, goserelin suppresses the supply of estrogen from the ovaries, which stimulates the cancer cells to grow. This is achieved by inhibiting production of another hormone called luteinizing hormone (LH), which stimulates the ovaries to make estrogen. Since many breast cancers grow more rapidly in the presence of estrogen, this can help to reduce tumor growth.

Tamoxifen prevents estrogen from stimulating cancer cell growth by blocking the estrogen receptors in the cancer cells. Cutting off the cancer's supply of estrogen provides an effective alternative method of combating the disease and avoids the distressing side effects of chemotherapy. Based upon evidence from adjuvant studies, hormonal therapy with goserelin is better-tolerated and equally effective as an alternative to chemotherapy. This gives physicians and patients a real choice in treatment following initial surgery (Goldhirsch et al. 2003).

Tamoxifen (Nolvadex)

Tamoxifen is an anti-estrogenic drug used to treat women whose tumors are estrogen or progesterone receptor-positive. This endocrine therapy blocks the female hormone estrogen from binding to the tumor cells. Tamoxifen has been the gold standard hormonal agent used for the treatment of breast cancer for more than 8 years. It is a prototype for a class of compounds called selective estrogen receptor-modulators (SERMs) of breast cancer but is also an effective primary treatment for advanced disease. Women with early-stage breast cancer who take tamoxifen have, on average, a 25% proportional increase in their chances of surviving 5 years after diagnosis.

Tamoxifen does not work equally well in all women. As the name implies, estrogen receptor-negative tumors do not have estrogen receptors, and therefore do not respond to tamoxifen. A Phase III study of 2691 high-risk cancer patients tested the effectiveness of tamoxifen with both pre- and postmenopausal subsets of receptor-negative and receptor-positive tumors. Both the 5-year disease-free and overall survival in patients with receptor-positive tumors treated with the addition of tamoxifen to chemotherapy was significantly higher than with chemotherapy alone, while no such advantage in disease-free or overall survival was found in receptor-negative patients. Further, in the receptor-positive postmenopausal group, the addition of tamoxifen showed a significant improvement in both disease-free and overall survival. However, in

the premenopausal receptor-negative patients, tamoxifen led to a worse outcome, as indicated by the significantly reduced survival rate (ONI 2000). Women with estrogen receptor-negative tumors may receive chemotherapy instead of tamoxifen.

Therefore, for the patient whose breast cancer's growth is estrogen-dependent, tamoxifen can keep estrogen from these cells, slowing or stopping their growth. Tamoxifen is a pill taken daily for 5 years. To date, studies do not show any benefit to taking tamoxifen for longer than 5 years (NCI 1998). Studies show that the use of tamoxifen as a post-surgical adjuvant therapy can reduce the chances of the cancer recurring.

Tamoxifen has a host of side effects, including hot flashes, weight gain, mood swings, abnormal secretions from the vagina, fatigue, nausea, depression, loss of libido, headache, swelling of the limbs, decreased number of platelets, vaginal bleeding, blood clots in the large veins (deep venous thrombosis), blood clots in the lungs (pulmonary emboli), cataracts (Fisher et al. 1998), and—the side effect of the greatest concern—endometrial cancer (Harris et al. 1997).

Studies have shown an increase of early-stage endometrial cancer (cancer of the lining of the uterus) among women taking tamoxifen, and the risk increases if the drug is taken for more than 5 years. Endometrial cancer is usually diagnosed at a very early stage and is usually curable by surgery. The studies have also shown an increased risk of uterine sarcoma (a rare cancer of the connective tissues of the uterus) among women taking tamoxifen. Unusual vaginal bleeding is a common symptom of both of these cancers. The treating physician should be notified immediately if vaginal bleeding occurs.

Raloxifene

Raloxifene is a drug similar to tamoxifen. It is a selective estrogen receptor-modulator (SERM) that blocks the effect of estrogen on breast tissue and breast cancer. It is currently in the testing phase to assess its effectiveness in reducing the risk of developing breast cancer. Pending testing completion, this drug is not recommended as hormonal therapy for women who have been diagnosed with breast cancer.

Toremifene (Fareston)

Toremifene (Fareston) is an anti-estrogen drug closely related to tamoxifen that may be an option for postmenopausal women with breast cancer that has metastasized. Fareston is a type of anti-estrogen medication that is used in tumors that are estrogen-receptor-positive or estrogen receptor-unknown.

Some patients treated with anti-estrogens who have bone metastasis may experience a tumor flare with pain and inflammation in the muscles and bones that will usually subside quickly. Blood calcium level should be monitored because tumor flare can cause a raised level of calcium in the blood (hypercalcemia) with symptoms of nausea, vomiting, and thirst. Often a short stay in the hospital is necessary until the calcium levels have been reduced or treatment may need to be stopped. Fareston is being studied in clinical trials for use in earlier stages of breast cancer.

Anastrozole (Arimidex), Femara (Letrozole), and Aromasin (Exemestane)

Anastrozole (Arimidex), Femara (Letrozole), and Aromasin (Exemestane) are three hormonal therapy drugs referred to as aromatase inhibitors. Aromatase is the enzyme that converts male hormones (testosterone) into female hormones (estrogens) in postmenopausal women. Premenopausal women get most of their estrogen from the ovaries. But postmenopausal women still have estrogen in their bodies, and it is this conversion to estrogen of androgens coming from adrenal glands in the body that needs to be interrupted so the breast cancer cells no longer have estrogen to stimulate their growth. Unlike tamoxifen, which slows the growth of breast cancer by preventing estrogen from activating its receptor, anastrozole blocks an enzyme needed for the production of estrogen, inhibiting the conversion of precursors to estrogens, and is effective in hormone receptor-positive breast cancers. Anastrozole is currently an option for women whose advanced breast cancer continues to grow during or after tamoxifen treatment.

Studies are ongoing to compare tamoxifen and anastrozole as adjuvant hormonal therapies. Anastrozole (Arimidex) was better than tamoxifen at preventing the recurrence of breast cancer in a study conducted in 381 centers in 21 countries, involving 9366 patients, and examining three treatment arms: tamoxifen alone, tamoxifen in combination with other therapy, and anastrozole alone. The trial results showed that women taking anastrozole experienced fewer side effects than women taking tamoxifen. However, women taking tamoxifen experienced fewer musculoskeletal disorders. The study was only conducted for a relatively short period of time, 2 years, and the long-term effects (5 years and beyond) are not yet known. Longer-term studies are needed to assess both the benefits and risks of this therapy. However, most recent studies have showed anastrozole to be slightly superior to tamoxifen (Susman 2001).

In a primary trial of 33 months, anastrozole was superior to tamoxifen in terms of disease-free survival (DFS), time to recurrence (TTR), and incidence of contra-lateral breast cancer (CLBC) in adjuvant endocrine therapy for postmenopausal patients with early-stage breast cancer. After an additional follow-up period of 47 months, anastrozole continued to show superior efficacy.

When compared with tamoxifen, anastrozole has numerous advantages in terms of tolerability. Endometrial cancer, vaginal bleeding and discharge, cerebrovascular events, venous thromboembolic events, and hot flashes all occurred less frequently in the anastrozole group. However, musculoskeletal disorders and fractures continued to occur less frequently in the tamoxifen group. The study concluded that the benefits of anastrozole are likely to be maintained in the long term and provide further support for the status of anastrozole as a valid treatment option for postmenopausal women with hormone-sensitive early-stage breast cancer (Baum 2003).

The biological basis for the superior efficacy of neo-adjuvant letrozole versus tamoxifen for postmenopausal women with estrogen receptor (ER)-positive locally advanced breast cancer was investigated. Letrozole inhibited tumor proliferation more than tamoxifen. While the molecular basis for this advantage was complex, it appeared to include a possible tamoxifen agonist effect on the cell cycle in both HER1/2+ and HER1/2- tumors. Letrozole inhibits tumor proliferation more effectively than tamoxifen independent of HER1/2 expression status (Ellis et al. 2003).

Letrozole (2.5 mg per day) and anastrozole (1 mg per day) were compared as endocrine therapy in postmenopausal women with advanced breast cancer previously treated with an anti-estrogen. Letrozole was significantly superior to anastrozole in the overall response rate (ORR) and both agents were well tolerated. Advanced breast cancer is more responsive to letrozole than anastrozole as a second-line endocrine therapy, as letrozole has the greater aromatase-inhibiting activity (Rose et al. 2003). These results support previous studies which showed that letrozole (Femara) was significantly more potent than anastrozole (Arimidex) in inhibiting aromatase activity *in vitro* and in inhibiting total body aromatization in patients with breast cancer.

A once a day oral dose of Femara lowered the risk of breast cancer recurrence by 43% in 5000 older women who had already completed 5 years of treatment with tamoxifen. After just over 2 years, 207 women had a recurrence of cancer—75 in the Femara group and 132 in the placebo group. There were 31 deaths in women receiving Femara and 42 deaths in women receiving placebo. Compared with placebo, Femara therapy after the completion of standard tamoxifen treatment significantly improved disease-free survival. This is a significant finding because in more than 50% of women treated for breast cancer, the cancer recurs 5 or more years after the original diagnosis (Goss et al. 2003).

Possible side effects of aromatase-inhibitor drugs include those associated with menopausal-like estrogen deficiency, such as hot flashes, night sweats, menstrual irregularity, depression, bone or tumor pain, pulmonary embolism (a blood clot in the lung), musculoskeletal disorders, and generalized weakness.

Megestrol Acetate

Megestrol acetate (Megace) is another drug used for hormonal treatment of advanced breast cancer, usually for women whose cancers do not respond to tamoxifen or have stopped responding to tamoxifen. Megestrol acetate is a man-made substance called progestin that is similar to the female hormone progesterone.

As with other therapies, there are reported side effects, including an increase in appetite causing weight gain, fluid retention causing ankle swelling, and nausea at the onset of therapy, which usually subsides. In rare cases, allergic reactions, jaundice, and raised blood pressure have been reported.

Trastuzumab (Herceptin Genentech)

Trastuzumab (Herceptin Genentech) is an anticancer drug therapy for women with HER2-positive metastatic breast cancer. This monoclonal antibody therapy differs from traditional treatments, such as chemotherapy and hormone-blocking therapy. Herceptin works by specifically targeting tumor cells that overexpress the HER2 protein. A monoclonal antibody blocks the receptors and prevents activation of genes that induce cell division, thereby slowing the growth of the tumor.

The reported side effects are chills, diarrhea, nausea, weakness, headache, vomiting, and possibly damage of the heart muscle, anemia, and nerve pain. Trastuzumab can be used alone or in combination with the drug paclitaxel (Taxol) and is prescribed for metastatic breast cancer.

Paclitaxel (Taxol)

Paclitaxel (Taxol) belongs to the group of medicines called antineoplastics (anticancer drugs) that interfere with the growth of cancer cells and eventually destroy them. Because the growth of normal cells may also be affected by paclitaxel, side effects can occur. Some

side effects may not occur until months or years after the medicine was used.

Side effects include neutropenia (decreased white blood cell count), anemia (decreased red blood cell count), thrombocytopenia (decreased platelet count), increased risk of infection, fatigue, bruising, hemorrhage, rash, itching, redness, hives, facial flushing, chest pain, difficulty breathing, high or low blood pressure, decreased heart rate, lightheadedness, dizziness, increased perspiration, shortness of breath, headache, numbness or tingling of the hands and/or feet, muscle aches, bone pain, mouth ulcers (sores), alopecia (loss or thinning of scalp and body hair), decreased appetite, diarrhea, nausea, vomiting, skin burns and ulcers, nail changes, hot flashes, and vaginal dryness.

Oophorectomy

Oophorectomy is surgery in which the ovaries are removed, therefore eliminating the body's main source of estrogen and progesterone in premenopausal women. Prior to the advent of anti-estrogen drugs, an oophorectomy was commonly used to treat breast cancer in premenopausal women.

Occasionally this procedure is still used in premenopausal women. However, chemotherapy drugs can alter the ovaries and reduce estrogen production. Tamoxifen may block any remaining estrogen effect on cancer cells, allowing many women to avoid surgery.

NATURAL THERAPIES

Protecting Breast Cells Against Dangerous Estrogens

The stronger form of estrogen, estradiol, can be converted into the weaker form, estriol, in the body without using drugs. Estriol is considered to be a more desirable form of estrogen. It is less active than estradiol, so when it occupies the estrogen receptor, it blocks estradiol's strong "growth" signals. Using a natural substance the conversion of estradiol to estriol increased by 50% in 12 healthy people (Michnovicz et al. 1991). Furthermore, in female mice prone to developing breast cancer the natural substance reduced the incidence of cancer and the number of tumors significantly. The natural substance was indole-3-carbinol (I3C).

I3C is a phytochemical isolated from cruciferous vegetables (broccoli, cauliflower, Brussels sprouts, turnips, kale, green cabbage, mustard seed, etc.). I3C given to 17 men and women for 2 months reduced the levels of strong estrogen, and increased the levels of weak estrogen. But more importantly, the level of an estrogen metabolite associated with breast and endometrial cancer, 16-α-hydroxyestrone, was reduced by I3C (Bradlow et al. 1991).

When I3C changes "strong" estrogen to "weak" estrogen, the growth of human cancer cells is inhibited by 54–61% (Telang et al. 1997). Moreover, I3C provoked cancer cells to self-destruct (kill themselves via apoptosis). Induction of cell death is an approach to suppress carcinogenesis and is the prime goal of cytotoxic chemotherapy. The increase in apoptosis induced by I3C before initiation of new tumor development may contribute to suppression of tumor progression. Nontoxic I3C can reliably facilitate apoptosis (12 week treatment in rats); thus, this phytonutrient may become a standard adjunct in the treatment of breast cancer (Zhang et al. 2003).

I3C inhibits human breast cancer cells (MCF7) from growing by as much as 90% in culture; growth arrest does not depend on estrogen receptors (Cover et al. 1998). Furthermore, I3C induces apoptosis in tumorigenic (cancerous) but not in nontumorigenic (noncancerous) breast epithelial cells (Rahman et al. 2003).

I3C does more than just turn strong estrogen to weak estrogen. 16-α-Hydroxyestrone (16-OHE) and 2-hydroxyestrone (2-OHE) are metabolites of estrogen in addition to estriol and estradiol. 2-OHE is biologically inactive, while 16-OHE is biologically active; that is, like estradiol, it can send "growth" signals. In breast cancer, the dangerous 16-OHE is often elevated, while the protective 2-OHE is decreased. Cancer-causing chemicals change the metabolism of estrogen so that 16-OHE is elevated. Studies show that people who take I3C have beneficial increases in the "weak" estriol form of estrogen and increases in protective 2-OHE.

African-American women who consumed I3C, 400 mg for 5 days, experienced an increase in the "good" 2-OHE and a decrease of the "bad" 16-OHE. However, it was found that the minority of women who did not demonstrate an increase in 2-OHE, had a mutation in a gene that helps metabolize estrogen to the 2-OHE version. Those women had an eight times higher risk of breast cancer (Telang et al. 1997).

I3C Stops Cancer Cells from Growing

Tamoxifen is a drug prescribed to reduce breast cancer metastases and improve survival. I3C has modes of action similar to tamoxifen. I3C inhibited the growth of estrogen-receptor-positive breast cancer cells by 90% compared to 60% for tamoxifen. The mode of action attributed to I3C's impressive effect was interfering with the cancer cell growth cycle. Adding tamoxifen to I3C gave a 5% boost (95% total inhibition) (Cover et al. 1999).

In estrogen-receptor-negative cells, I3C stopped the synthesis of DNA by about 50%, whereas tamoxifen had no significant effect. I3C also restored p21 and other proteins that act as checkpoints during the synthesis of a new cell. Tamoxifen showed no effect on p21. Restoration of these growth regulators is extremely important. For example, tumor suppressor p53 works through p21 that I3C restores. I3C also inhibits cancers caused by chemicals. If animals are fed I3C before exposure to cancer-causing chemicals, DNA damage and cancer are virtually eliminated (Cover et al. 1999).

A study on rodents shows that damaged DNA in breast cells is reduced 91% by I3C. Similar results are seen in the liver (Devanaboyina et al. 1997). Female smokers taking 400 mg of I3C significantly reduced their levels of a major lung carcinogen. Cigarette chemicals are known to adversely affect estrogen metabolism (Taioli et al. 1997).

There is no proven way to prevent breast cancer, but the best and most comprehensive scientific evidence so far supports phytochemicals such as I3C (Meng et al. 2000). The results from a placebo-controlled, double-blind dose-ranging chemoprevention study on 60 women at increased risk for breast cancer demonstrated that I3C at a minimum effective dosage of 300 mg per day is a promising chemopreventive agent for breast cancer prevention (Wong et al. 1997). The results of a single-blind phase I trial which studied the effectiveness of I3C in preventing breast cancer in nonsmoking women who are at high risk of breast cancer are awaited. The rationale for this study is that I3C, ingested twice daily, may be effective at preventing breast cancer.

I3C was found to be superior to 80 other compounds, including tamoxifen, for anticancer potential. Indoles, which down-regulate estrogen receptors, have been proposed as promising agents in the treatment and prevention of cancer and autoimmune diseases such as multiple sclerosis, arthritis, and lupus. Replacement of all the chemically altered estrogen drugs, such as tamoxifen, with a new generation of chemically altered indole drugs that fit in the aryl-hydrocarbon (Ah) receptor and regulate estrogen indirectly may prove beneficial to cancer patients (Bitonti et al. 1999). An I3C tetrameric derivative (chemically derived) is currently a novel lead inhibitor of breast cancer cell growth, considered a new, promising therapeutic agent for both ER+ and ER- breast cancer (Brandi et al. 2003).

A summary of studies shows that indole-3-carbinol (I3C) can:

- Increase the conversion of estradiol to the safer estriol by 50% in healthy people in just 1 week (Michnovicz et al. 1991)

- Prevent the formation of the estrogen metabolite, 16-α-hydroxyestrone, that prompts breast cancer cells to grow (Chen et al. 1996), in both men and women in 2 months (Michnovicz et al. 1997)

- Stop human cancer cells from growing (54–61%) and provoke the cells to self-destruct (apoptosis) (Telang et al. 1997)

- Inhibit human breast cancer cells (MCF7) from growing by as much as 90% in vitro (Ricci et al. 1999)

- Inhibit the growth of estrogen-receptor-positive breast cancer cells by 90%, compared to tamoxifen's 60%, by stopping the cell cycle (Cover et al. 1999)

- Prevent chemically induced breast cancer in rodents by 70–96%. Prevent other types of cancer, including aflatoxin-induced liver cancer, leukemia, and colon cancer (Grubbs et al. 1995)

- Inhibit free radicals, particularly those that cause the oxidation of fat (Shertzer et al. 1988)

- Stop the synthesis of DNA by about 50% in estrogen-receptor-negative cells, whereas tamoxifen had no significant effect (Cover et al. 1998)

- Restore p21 and other proteins that act as checkpoints during the synthesis of a new cancer cell. Tamoxifen has no effect on p21 (Cover et al. 1998)

- Virtually eliminate DNA damage and cancer prior to exposure to cancer-causing chemicals (in animals fed I3C) (Grubbs et al. 1995)

- Reduce DNA damage in breast cells by 91% (Devanaboyina et al. 1997)

- Reduce levels of a major nitrosamine carcinogen in female smokers (Taioli et al. 1997)

How to Use I3C

While the evidence is compelling, it is too soon to know exactly how effective I3C will be as an adjuvant breast cancer therapy (*see the Breast Cancer References for citations pertaining specifically to I3C*).

Suggested dosage: Take one 200-mg capsule of I3C twice a day, for those under 120 pounds. For those who weigh more than 120 pounds, three 200-mg capsules a day are suggested. Women who weigh over 180 pounds should take four 200-mg I3C capsules a day.

Note: *A little is good; a lot is not necessarily better. Too much I3C can have the opposite effect; therefore, do not exceed the suggested dosage.*

CAUTION Pregnant women should not take I3C because of its modulation of estrogen. I3C appears to act both at the ovarian and hypothalamic levels, whereas tamoxifen appears to act only on the hypothalamic-pituitary axis as an anti-estrogen. Both I3C and tamoxifen block ovulation by altering preovulatory concentrations of luteinizing hormone (LH) and follicle stimulating hormone (FSH) (Gao et al. 2002). The reported aversion to cruciferous vegetables by pregnant women may be associated with their ability to change estrogen metabolism. Estrogen is a necessary growth factor for the fetus.

Curcumin

Curcumin is extracted from the spice turmeric and is responsible for the orange/yellow pigment that gives the spice its unique color. Turmeric is a perennial herb of the ginger family and a major component of curry powder. Chinese and Indian people, both in herbal medicine and in food preparation, have safely used it for centuries.

Curcumin has a number of biological effects in the body. However, one of the most important functions is curcumin's ability to inhibit growth signals emitted by tumor cells that elicit angiogenesis (growth and development of new blood vessels into the tumor).

Curcumin inhibits the epidermal growth factor receptor and is up to 90% effective in a dose-dependent manner. It is important to note that while curcumin has been shown to be up to 90% effective in inhibiting the expression of the epidermal growth factor receptor on cancer cell membranes, this does not mean it will be effective in 90% of cancer patients or reduce tumor volume by 90%. However, because two-thirds of all cancers overexpress the epidermal growth factor receptor and such overexpression frequently fuels the metastatic spread of the cancer throughout the body, suppression of this receptor is desirable.

Other anticancer mechanisms of curcumin include:

- Inhibition of the induction of basic fibroblast growth factor (bFGF). bFGF is both a potent growth signal (mitogen) for many cancers and an important signaling factor in angiogenesis (Arbiser et al. 1998).

- Antioxidant activity. *In vitro* it has been shown to be stronger than vitamin E in prevention of lipid peroxidation (Sharma 1976; Toda et al. 1985).

- Inhibition of the expression of COX-2 (cyclooxygenase 2), the enzyme involved in the production of prostaglandin E2 (PGE-2), a tumor-promoting hormone-like agent (Zhang et al. 1999).

- Inhibition of a transcription factor in cancer cells known as nuclear factor-kappa B (NF-KB). Many cancers overexpress NF-KB and use this as a growth vehicle to escape regulatory control (Bierhaus et al. 1997; Plummer et al. 1999).

- Increased expression of nuclear p53 protein in human basal cell carcinomas, hepatomas, and leukemia cell lines. This increases apoptosis (cell death) (Jee et al. 1998).

- Increases production of transforming growth factor-beta (TGF-beta), a potent growth inhibitor, producing apoptosis (Park et al. 2003; Sporn et al. 1989).

- TGF-beta is known to enhance wound healing and may play an important role in the enhancement of wound healing by curcumin (Mani H et al. 2002; Sidhu et al. 1998).

- Inhibits PTK (protein tyrosine kinases) and PKC (protein kinase C). PTK and PKC both help relay chemical signals through the cell. Abnormally high levels of these substances are often required for cancer cell signal transduction messages. These include proliferation, cell migration, metastasis, angiogenesis, avoidance of apoptosis, and differentiation (Reddy et al. 1994; Davidson et al. 1996).

- Inhibits AP-1 (activator protein-1) through a non-antioxidant pathway. While curcumin is an antioxidant (Kuo et al. 1996), it appears to inhibit signal-transduction via protein phosphorylation thereby decreasing cancer-cell activity, regulation, and proliferation (Huang et al. 1991).

Based on the favorable, multiple mechanisms listed above, higher-dose curcumin would appear to be useful for cancer patients to take. However, as far as curcumin being taken at the same time as chemotherapy drugs, there are contradictions in the scientific literature. Therefore, caution is advised. Please refer to the *Cancer Chemotherapy* protocol before considering combining curcumin with chemotherapy.

Curcumin's effects are a dose dependent response, and a standardized product is essential. The recommended dose is four 900-mg capsules 3 times per day, preferably with food.

Green Tea

As a tumor grows it elicits new capillary growth (angiogenesis) from the surrounding normal tissues and diverts blood supply and nutrients away from the tissue to feed itself. Unregulated tumor angiogenesis can facilitate the growth of cancer throughout the body. Antiangiogenesis agents, including green tea, inhibit this new tumor blood vessel (capillary) growth.

Green tea contains epigallocatechin gallate EGCG, a polyphenol that helps to block the induction of vascular endothelial growth factor (VEGF). Scientists consider VEGF essential in the process of angiogenesis and tumor endothelial cell survival. It is the EGCG fraction of green tea that makes it a potentially effective adjunct therapy in the treatment of breast cancer. *In vivo* studies have shown green tea extracts to have the following actions on human cancer cells (Jung et al. 2001b; Muraoka et al. 2002):

- Inhibition of tumor growth by 58%

- Inhibition of activation of nuclear factor-kappa beta

- Inhibition of microvessel density by 30%

- Inhibition of tumor-cell proliferation *in vitro* by 27%

- Increased tumor-cell apoptosis 1.9-fold

- Increased tumor endothelial-cell apoptosis threefold

The most current research shows that green tea may have a beneficial effect in treating cancer. While drinking green tea is a well-documented method of preventing cancer, it is difficult for the cancer patient to obtain a sufficient quantity of EGCG anticancer components in that form. Standardized green tea extract is more useful then green tea itself because the dose of EGCG can be precisely monitored and greater doses can be ingested without excessive intake of liquids. A suggested dose for a person with breast cancer is 5 capsules of 350-mg lightly caffeinated green tea extract 3 times a day with each meal. Each capsule should provide at least 100 mg of EGCG. It may be desirable to take a decaffeinated version of green tea extract in the evening to ensure that the caffeine does not interfere with sleep. Those sensitive to caffeine may also use this decaffeinated form.

However, there are benefits to obtaining some caffeine. Studies show that caffeine potentiates the anticancer effects of tea polyphenols, including the critical EGCG. Caffeine will be discussed in further detail later in this protocol. Green tea extract is available in a decaffeinated form for those sensitive to caffeine or those who want to take the less-stimulating decaffeinated green tea extract capsules for their evening dose.

Conjugated Linoleic Acid (CLA)

Conjugated linoleic acid (CLA) found naturally, as a component of beef and milk, refers to isomers of octadecadienoic acid with conjugated double bonds. CLA is essential for the transport of dietary fat into cells, where it is used to build muscle and produce energy. CLA is incorporated into the neutral lipids of mammary fat (adipocyte) cells, where it serves as a local reservoir of CLA. It has been proposed that CLA may be an excellent candidate for prevention of breast cancer (Ip et al. 2003). Low levels of CLA are found in breast cancer patients but these do not influence survival. Nevertheless, it has been hypothesized that a higher intake of CLA might have a protective effect on the risk of metastasis (Chajes et al. 2003).

CLA was shown to prevent mammary cancer in rats if given before the onset of puberty. CLA ingested during the time of the "promotion" phase of cancer development conferred substantial protection from further development of breast cancer in the rats by inducing cell kill of pre-cancerous lesions (Ip et al. 1999b). It was determined that feeding CLA to female rats while they were young and still developing conferred life-long protection against breast cancer. This preventative action was achieved by adding enough CLA to equal 0.8% of the animal's total diet (Ip et al. 1999a).

CLA inhibits the proliferation of human breast cancer cells (MCF-7), induced by estradiol and insulin (but not EGF). In fact, CLA caused cell kill (cytotoxicity) when tumor cells were induced with insulin (Chujo et al. 2003). The antiproliferative effects of CLA are partly due to their ability to elicit a p53 response that leads to growth arrest (Kemp et al. 2003). CLA elicits cell killing effects in human breast tumor cells through both p53-dependent and p53-independent pathways according to the cell type (Majumder et al. 2002). Refer to *Cancer Treatment The Critical Factors*, for more information on determining the p53 status of cancer. The effects of CLA are mediated by both direct action (on the epithelium) as well as indirect action through the stroma.

The growth suppressing effect of CLA may be partly due to changes in arachidonic distribution among cellular lipids and an altered prostaglandin profile (Miller et al. 2001). Intracellular lipids may become more susceptible to oxidative stress to the point of producing a cytotoxic effect (Devery et al. 2001). CLA has the ability to suppress arachidonic acid. Since arachidonic acid can produce inflammatory compounds that can promote cancer proliferation, this may be yet another explanation for CLA's anticancer effects.

Life Extension's recommendation for CLA is a dose of 3000–4000 mg daily, which is approximately 1% of the average human diet. The suggested amount required to obtain the overall cancer-preventing effects is only 3000–4000 mg daily in divided doses.

CLA may work via a mechanism similar to that of antidiabetic drugs not only by enhancing insulin-sensitivity but also by increasing plasma adiponectin levels, alleviating hyperinsulinemia (Nagao et al. 2003) protecting against cancer. A number of human cancer cell lines express the PPAR-gamma transcription factor, and agonists for PPAR-gamma can promote apoptosis in these cell lines and impede their clonal expansion both *in vitro* and *in vivo*. CLA can activate PPAR-gamma in rat adipocytes, possibly explaining CLA's antidiabetic effects in Zucker fatty rats. A portion of CLA's broad-spectrum anticarcinogenic activity is probably mediated by PPAR-gamma activation in susceptible tumor (McCarty 2000). However, CLA's anticarcinogenic effects could not be confirmed in one epidemiologic study in humans (Voorips et al. 2002). (*Note:* The term PPAR-gamma is an acronym for peroxisome proliferator-activated-receptor-gamma. A PPAR gamma agonist such as Avandia, Actos, or CLA activates the PPAR-gamma receptor. (This class of drug is being investigated as a potential adjuvant therapy against certain types of cancer.)

Note: *A combination product called Super CLA with Guarana may be used instead of CLA alone. Guarana is an herb that contains a form of caffeine called guaranine, which is 2.5 times stronger than the caffeine found in coffee, tea, and caffeinated soft drinks. What makes guaranine a unique source of caffeine is its slower release due to the guarana seed, which is fatty (even in powder form) as opposed to water-soluble. Caffeine has an inhibitory effect on the growth of cancer and is synergistic with other natural anticancer compounds.*

Caffeine

Caffeine occurs naturally in green tea and has been shown to potentiate the anticancer effects of tea polyphenols. Caffeine is a model radio-sensitizing agent that is thought to work by abolishing the radiation-induced G2-phase checkpoint in the cell cycle. Caffeine can induce apoptosis of a human lung carcinoma cell line by itself and it can act synergistically with radiation to induce tumor cell kill and cell growth arrest. The cancer cell killing effect of caffeine is dependent on the dose (Qi et al. 2002).

Caffeine enhances the tumor cell killing effects of anticancer drugs and radiation. A preliminary report on radiochemotherapy combined with caffeine for high-grade soft tissue sarcomas in 17 patients, (treated with cisplatin, caffeine, and doxorubicin after radiation therapy) determined complete response in six patients, partial response in six and no change in five patients. The effectiveness rate of caffeine-potentiated radiochemotherapy was therefore 17%, and contributed to a satisfactory local response and the success of function-saving surgery for high-grade soft tissue sarcomas (Tsuchiya et al. 2000).

In a randomized, double blind placebo-controlled crossover study, the effects of caffeine as an adjuvant to morphine in advanced cancer patients was found to benefit the cognitive performance and reduce pain intensity (Mercadente et al. 2001).

Cancer patients should note that one study demonstrated that caffeine reduced the cytotoxic effect of paclitaxel on human lung adenocarcinoma cell lines (Kitamoto et al. 2003).

To ascertain the inhibitory effects of caffeine, mice at high risk of developing malignant and nonmalignant tumors (SKH-1), received oral caffeine as their sole source of drinking fluid for 18–23 weeks. Results revealed that caffeine inhibited the formation and decreased the size of both nonmalignant tumors and malignant tumors (Lou et al. 1999).

In cancer cells, p53 gene mutations are the most common alterations observed (50–60%) and are a factor in both carcinomas and sarcomas. Caffeine has been shown to potentiate the destruction of p53-defective cells by inhibiting p53's growth signal. The effects of this are to inhibit and override the DNA damage-checkpoint and thus kill dividing cells. Caffeine uncouples cell-cycle progression by interfering with the replication and repair of DNA (Sakurai et al. 1999; Ribeiro et al. 1999; Jiang et al. 2000; Valenzuela et al. 2000).

Caffeine inhibits the development of Ehrlich ascites carcinoma in female mice (Mukhopadhyay et al. 2001). Topical application of caffeine inhibits the occurrence of cancer and increases tumor cell death in radiation-induced skin tumors in mice (Lu et al. 2002). Caffeine inhibits solid tumor development and lung experimental metastasis induced by melanoma cells (Gude et al. 2001).

Consumption of coffee, tea, and caffeine was not associated with breast cancer incidence in a study of 59,036 Swedish women (aged 40–76 years) (Michels et al. 2002).

Melatonin

One of the most important supplements for a breast cancer patient is the hormone melatonin. Melatonin inhibits human breast cancer cell growth (Cos et al. 2000) and reduces tumor spread and invasiveness *in vitro* (Cos et al. 1998). Indeed, it has been suggested that melatonin acts as a naturally occurring anti-estrogen on tumor cells, as it down-regulates hormones responsible for the growth of hormone-dependent mammary tumors (Torres-Farfan 2003).

A high percentage of women with estrogen-receptor-positive breast cancer have low plasma melatonin levels (Brzezinski et al. 1997). There have been some studies demonstrating changes in melatonin levels in breast cancer patients; specifically, women with breast cancer were found to have lower melatonin levels than women without breast cancer (Oosthuizen et al. 1989). Normally, women undergo a seasonal variation in the production of certain hormones, such as melatonin. However, it was found that women with breast cancer did not have a seasonal variation in melatonin levels, as did the healthy women (Holdaway et al. 1997).

Low levels of melatonin have been associated with breast cancer occurrence and development. Women who work predominantly at night and are exposed to light, which inhibits melatonin production and alters the circadian rhythm, have an increased risk of breast cancer development (Schernhammer et al. 2003). In contrast, higher melatonin levels have been found in blind and visually impaired people, along with correspondingly lower incidences of cancer compared to those with normal vision, thus suggesting a role for melatonin in the reduction of cancer incidence (Feychting et al. 1998).

Light at night, regardless of duration or intensity, inhibits melatonin secretion and phase-shifts the circadian clock, possibly altering the cell growth rate that is regulated by the circadian rhythm (Travlos et al. 2001). Disruption of circadian rhythm is commonly observed among breast cancer patients (Mormont et al. 1997; Roenneberg et al. 2002) and contributes to cancer development and tumor progression. The circadian rhythm is a statistically significant predictor of survival time for breast cancer patients (Sephton et al. 2000).

Melatonin differs from the classic anti-estrogens such as tamoxifen in that it does not seem to bind to the estrogen receptor or interfere with the binding of estradiol to its receptor (Sanchez-Barcelo 2003). Melatonin does not cause side effects, such as those caused by the conventional anti-estrogen drug tamoxifen. Furthermore, when melatonin and tamoxifen are combined, synergistic benefits occur. Moreover, melatonin can increase the therapeutic efficacy of tamoxifen (Lissoni et al. 1995) and biological therapies such as IL-2 (Lissoni et al. 1994).

How melatonin interferes with estrogen signaling is unknown, though recent studies suggest that it acts through a cyclic adenosine monophosphate (cAMP)-independent signaling pathway (Torres-Farfan 2003).

It has been proposed that melatonin suppresses the epidermal growth factor receptor (EGF-R) (Blask et al. 2002) and exerts its growth inhibitory effects by inducing differentiation ("normalizing" cancer cells)(Cos et al. 1996). Melatonin directly inhibits breast cancer cell proliferation (Ram et al. 2000) and boosts the production of immune components, including natural killer cells (NK cells) that have an ability to kill metastasized cancer cells.

In tumorigenesis studies, melatonin reduced the incidence and growth rate of breast tumors and slowed breast cancer development (Subramanian et al. 1991). Furthermore, prolonged oral melatonin administration significantly reduced the development of existing mammary tumors in animals (Rao et al. 2000).

In vitro experiments carried out with the ER-positive human breast cancer cells (MCF-7 cells), demonstrated that melatonin, at a physiological concentration (1 nM) and in the presence of serum or estradiol (a) inhibits, in a reversible way, cell proliferation, (b) increases the expression of p53 and p21WAF1 proteins and modulates the length of the cell cycle, and (c) reduces the metastatic capacity of these cells and counteracts the stimulatory effect of estradiol on cell invasiveness. Further, this effect is mediated, at least in part, by a melatonin-induced increase in the expression of the cell surface adhesion proteins E-cadherin and beta (1)-integrin (Sanchez-Barcelo et al. 2003).

Melatonin can be safely taken for an indefinite period of time. The suggested dose of melatonin for breast cancer patients is 3–50 mg at bedtime. Initially, if melatonin is taken in large doses vivid dreams and morning drowsiness may occur. To avoid these minor side effects melatonin may be taken in low doses nightly and the dose slowly increased over a period of several weeks.

Se-Methylselenocysteine

Se-methylselenocysteine (SeMSC), a naturally occurring organic selenium compound found to be an effective chemopreventive agent is a new and better form of selenium. SeMSC is a selenoamino acid that is synthesized by plants such as garlic and broccoli.

Methylselenocysteine (MSC) has been shown to be effective against mammary cell growth both *in vivo* and *in vitro* (Sinha et al. 1999) and has significant anticancer activity against mammary tumor development (Sinha et al. 1997). Moreover, Se-methylselenocysteine was one of the most effective selenium chemoprevention compounds and induced apoptosis in human leukemia cells (HL-60) *in vitro* (Jung et al. 2001a). Exposure to MSC blocks expansion of cancer colonies and premalignant lesions at an early stage by simultaneously modulating pathways responsible for inhibiting cell proliferation and enhancing apoptosis (Ip et al. 2000a).

Se-methylselenocysteine has been shown to:

- Produce a 33% better reduction of cancerous lesions than selenite.
- Produce a 50% decrease in tumor development.
- Induce cell death (apoptosis) in cancer cells.
- Inhibit cancer-cell growth (proliferation).
- Reduce density and development of tumor blood vessels.
- Down-regulate VEGF (vascular endothelial growth factor).

(Ip et al. 1992; Sinha et al. 1997; Sinha et al. 1999; Ip et al. 2000a, b; Dong et al. 2001)

Unlike MSC, which is incorporated into protein in place of methionine, SeMSC is not incorporated into any protein, thereby offering a completely bioavailable compound. In animal studies, SeMSC has been shown to be 10 times less toxic than any other known form of selenium. Breast cancer patients may consider taking 400 mcg of SeSMC daily.

CoQ10

Coenzyme Q10 (CoQ10) is synthesized in humans from tyrosine through a cascade of eight aromatic precursors. These precursors require eight vitamins, which are vitamin C, B_2, B_3 (niacin) B_6, B_{12}, folic acid, pantothenic acid, and tetrahydrobiopterin as their coenzymes.

Since the 1960s, studies have shown that cancer patients often have decreased blood levels of coenzyme Q10 (Lockwood et al. 1995; Folkers 1996; Ren et al. 1997). In particular, breast cancer patients (with infiltrative ductal carcinoma) who underwent radical mastectomy were found to have significantly decreased tumor concentrations of CoQ10 compared to levels in normal surrounding tissues. Increased levels of reactive oxygen species may be involved in the consumption of CoQ10 (Portakal et al. 2000). These findings sparked interest in the compound as a potential anticancer agent (NCCAM 2002). Cellular and animal studies have found evidence that CoQ10 stimulates the immune system and can increase resistance to illness (Bliznakov et al. 1970; Hogenauer et al. 1981; NCCAM 2002).

CoQ10 may induce protective effect on breast tissue and has demonstrated promise in treating breast cancer. Although there are only a few studies, the safe nature of CoQ10 coupled with this promising research of its bioenergetic activity suggests that breast cancer patients should take 100 mg up to 3 times a day. It is important to take CoQ10 with some kind of oil, such as fish or flax, because dry powder CoQ10 is not readily absorbed.

In a clinical study, 32 patients were treated with CoQ10 (90 mg) in addition to other antioxidants and fatty acids; six of these patients showed partial tumor regression. In one of these cases the dose of CoQ10 was increased to 390 mg and within one month the tumor was no longer palpable, within two months the mammography confirmed the absence of tumor. In another case, the patient took 300 mg of CoQ10 for residual tumor (post non-radical surgery) and within 3 months there was nonresidual tumor tissue (Lockwood et al. 1994). This overt complete regression of breast tumors in the latter two cases coupled with further reports of disappearance of breast cancer metastases (liver and elsewhere) in several other cases (Lockwood et al. 1995) demonstrates the potential of CoQ10 in the adjuvant therapy of breast cancer.

There are promising results for the use of CoQ10 in protecting against heart damage related to chemotherapy. Many chemotherapy drugs can cause damage to the heart (UTH 1998; ACS 2000; NCCAM 2000; Dog et al. 2001), and initial animal studies found that CoQ10 could reduce the adverse cardiac effects of these drugs (Combs et al. 1977; Choe et al. 1979; Lubawy et al. 1980; Usui et al. 1982; Shinozawa et al. 1993; Folkers 1996).

CAUTION Some studies indicate that CoQ10 should not be taken at the same time as chemotherapy. If this were true, it would be disappointing, because CoQ10 is so effective in protecting against adriamycin-induced cardiomyopathy. Adriamycin is a chemotherapy drug sometimes used as part of a chemotherapy cocktail. Until more research is known, it is not possible to make a definitive recommendation concerning taking CoQ10 during chemotherapy. For more information please see the *Cancer Chemotherapy* protocol.

EPA and DHA

Dietary polyunsaturated fatty acids (PUFAs) of the omega-6 (n-6) class, found in corn oil and safflower oil, may be involved in the development of breast cancer, whereas long chain (LC) omega-3 (n-3) PUFAs, found in fish oil can inhibit breast cancer (Bagga et al. 2002).

A case control study examining levels of fatty acids in breast adipose tissue of breast cancer patients has shown that total omega-6 PUFAs may be contributing to the high risk of breast cancer in the United States and that omega-3 PUFAs, derived from fish oil, may have a protective effect (Bagga et al. 2002).

A higher omega-3:omega-6 ratio ((n-3)):(n-6) ratio) may reduce the risk of breast cancer, especially in premenopausal women (Goodstine et al. 2003). In a prospective study of 35,298 Singapore Chinese women aged 45–74 years, it was determined that high levels of dietary omega-3 fatty acids from marine sources (fish/shellfish) were significantly associated with reduced risk of breast cancer. Furthermore, women who consumed low levels of marine omega-3 fatty acids had a statistically significant increased risk of breast cancer (Gago-Dominguez et al. 2003)

Omega-3 fatty acids, primarily eicosapentanoic acid (EPA) and docosahexaneoic acid (DHA) found naturally in oily fish and fish oil, have been consistently shown to retard the growth of breast cancer *in vitro* and in animal experiments, inhibit tumor development and metastasis. Fish oils have antiproliferative effects at high doses, which means they can inhibit tumor cell growth, through a free radical-mediated mechanism, while at more moderate doses, omega-3 fatty acids inhibit Ras protein activity, angiogenesis, and inflammation. The production of pro-inflammatory cytokines can be modified by dietary omega-3 PUFAs (Mancuso et al. 1997).

High consumption of fatty fish is weakly associated with reduced breast cancer risk (Goodstine et al. 2003). Flaxseed, the richest source of alpha-linoleic acid inhibited the established growth and metastasis of human breast cancer implanted in mice. This effect was found to be due to its down-regulation of insulin-like growth factor I (IGF-1) and epidermal growth factor receptor (EGF-R) expression (Chen et al. 2002). The recommended dosage is to consume a fish-oil concentrate supplement that provides 3200 mg of EPA and 2400 mg of DHA a day taken in divided doses.

Vitamins A, D, and E

Vitamin A and vitamin D_3 inhibit breast cancer cell division and can induce cancer cells to differentiate into mature, noncancerous cells. Vitamin D_3 works synergistically with tamoxifen (and melatonin) to inhibit breast cancer cell proliferation. The vitamin D-3 receptor as a target for breast cancer prevention was examined. Pre-clinical studies demonstrated that vitamin D compounds could reduce breast cancer development in animals. Furthermore, human studies indicate that both vitamin D status and genetic variations in the vitamin D-3 receptor (VDR) may affect breast cancer risk. Findings from cellular, molecular and population studies suggest that the VDR is a nutritionally modulated growth-regulatory gene that may represent a molecular target for chemoprevention of breast cancer (Welsh et al. 2003).

Daily doses of vitamin A, 350,000 to 500,000 IU, were given to 100 patients with metastatic breast carcinoma treated by chemotherapy. A significant increase in the complete response was observed; however, response rates, duration of response and projected survival were only significantly increased in postmenopausal women with breast cancer (Israel et al. 1985).

Breast cancer patients may take between 4000 to 6000 IU of vitamin D_3 every day. Water-soluble vitamin A can be taken in doses of 100,000–300,000 IU every day. Monthly blood tests are needed to make sure toxicity does not occur in response to these high daily doses of vitamin A and vitamin D_3. After 4–6 months, the doses of vitamin D_3 and vitamin A can be reduced.

Vitamin E is the term used to describe eight naturally occurring essential fat-soluble nutrients: alpha-, beta-, delta-, and gamma-tocopherols plus a class of compounds related to vitamin E called alpha-, beta-, delta-, and gamma-tocotrienols. Vitamin E from dietary sources may provide women with modest protection from breast cancer.

Vitamin E succinate, a derivative of fat-soluble vitamin E, has been shown to inhibit tumor cell growth *in vitro* and *in vivo* (Turley et al. 1997; Cameron et al. 2003). In estrogen receptor-negative human breast cancer cell lines vitamin E succinate, inhibited growth and induced cell death. Since vitamin E is considered the main chain breaking lipophilic antioxidant in plasma and tissue, its role as a potential chemopreventative agent and its use in the adjuvant treatment of aggressive human breast cancers appears reasonable. Those with estrogen-receptor-negative breast cancers should consider taking 800–1200 IU of vitamin E succinate a day. Vitamin E supplementation, 800 IU daily for 4 weeks, was shown to significantly reduce hot flashes in breast cancer survivors (Barton et al. 1998).

CAUTION   Refer to the symptoms of vitamin A toxicity in *Appendix A: Avoiding Vitamin A Toxicity*. When taking doses of vitamin D3 in excess of 1400 IU a day, regular blood chemistry tests should be taken to monitor kidney function and serum calcium metabolism. Vitamin E has potential blood thinning properties, individuals taking anticoagulant drugs should inform their treating physician if supplementing with vitamin E and have their clotting factors monitored regularly.

Tocotrienols

When vitamin E was isolated from plant oils, the term tocopherols was used to name the initial four compounds that shared similar structures. Their structures have two primary parts—a complex ring and a phytyl (long-saturated) side chain—and have been designated as alpha, beta, delta, and gamma tocopherol. Tocopherols (vitamin E) are important lipid-soluble antioxidants that can protect the body against free radical damage.

However, there are four additional compounds related to tocopherols—called tocotrienols—that are less widely distributed in nature. The tocotrienol structure, three double bonds in an isoprenoid (unsaturated) side chain, differs from that of tocopherols. While tocopherols are found in corn, olive oil, and soybeans, tocotrienols are concentrated in palm, rice bran, and barley oils.

Tocotrienols elicit powerful anticancer properties, and studies have confirmed tocotrienol activity is much stronger than that of tocopherols (Schwenke et al. 2002).

Tocotrienols provide more efficient penetration into tissues such as the brain and liver. Because of the double bonds in the isoprenoid side chain, tocotrienols move freely and more efficiently within cell membranes than tocopherols, giving tocotrienols greater ability to counteract free radicals. This greater mobility also allows tocotrienols to recycle more quickly than alpha-tocopherol. Tocotrienols are better distributed in fatty cell membranes and demonstrate greater antioxidant and free-radical-scavenging effects than vitamin E (alpha-tocopherol) (Serbinova et al. 1991; Theriault et al. 1999).

Tocotrienol's antioxidant function is associated with lowering DNA damage, tumor formation, and cell damage. Animals exposed to carcinogens that were fed corn oil- or soybean oil-based diets had significantly more tumors than those fed a tocotrienol-rich palm oil diet. Tocotrienol-rich palm oil did not promote chemically induced breast cancer (Sundram et al. 1989).

Tocotrienols possess the ability to stimulate the selective killing of cancer cells through programmed cell death (apoptosis) and to reduce cancer cell proliferation while leaving normal cells unaffected (Kline et al. 2001). Tocotrienols are thought to suppress cancer through the isoprenoid side chain.

Isoprenoids are plant compounds that have been shown to suppress the initiation, growth, and progression of many types of cancer in experimental studies (Block et al. 1992). They are common in fruits and vegetables, which may explain why diets rich in these foods have consistently been shown to reduce the incidence of cancer.

Isoprenoids induce cell death (apoptosis) and arrest cell growth in human breast adenocarcinoma cells (MCF-7) (Mo et al. 1999). Isoprenoids may suppress the mevalonate pathway, through which mutated Ras proteins transform healthy cells into cancer cells. Mutated ras is the most common cellular defect found in human cancers. The mevalonate pathway escapes regulatory control in tumor tissue but remains highly sensitive to regulation by tocotrienols. Tocotrienols are at least five times more powerful than farnesol, the body's regulator of the mevalonate pathway. Interestingly, human breast cancer cells have been shown to respond very well to treatment with tocotrienols (Parker et al. 1993).

Tocotrienols cause growth inhibition of breast cancer cells in culture independent of estrogen sensitivity and have great potential in the prevention and treatment of breast cancer (Nesaretnam et al. 1998).

In vitro studies have demonstrated the effectiveness of tocotrienols as inhibitors of both estrogen-receptor-positive (estrogen-responsive) and estrogen-receptor-negative (nonestrogen-responsive) cell proliferation. The effect of palm tocotrienols on three human breast cancer cells lines, estrogen-responsive and estrogen-nonresponsive (MCF7, MDA-MB-231, and ZR-75-1), found that tocotrienols inhibited cell growth strongly in both the presence and absence of estradiol. The gamma- and delta-fractions of tocotrienols were most effective at inhibiting cell growth, while alpha-tocopherol was ineffective. Tocotrienols were found to enhance the effect of tamoxifen (Nesaretnam et al. 2000).

Delta-tocotrienol was shown to be the most potent inducer of apoptosis (programmed cell death) in both estrogen-responsive and estrogen-nonresponsive human breast cancer cells, followed by gamma- and alpha-tocotrienol (beta-tocotrienol was not tested). Interestingly, delta-tocotrienol is more plentiful in palm tocotrienols than in tocotrienols derived from rice. Of the natural tocopherols, only delta-tocopherol showed any apoptosis-inducing effect, although it was less than one tenth of the effect of palm and rice delta-tocotrienol (Yu et al. 1999).

Tocotrienols effectively arrested the cell cycle and triggered cell death of mammary cancer cells (from mice) whereas tocopherols (alpha, gamma, and delta) did not cause inhibition of tumor cell growth. Highly malignant cells were most sensitive to the antiproliferative effects of tocotrienols, whereas less aggressive precancerous cells were the least sensitive (McIntyre et al. 2000).

Tocotrienols were found to be far more effective than alpha-tocopherol in inhibiting breast cancer cell growth. Tocotrienols in combination with tamoxifen proved more effective than either compound alone in both estrogen-responsive and nonresponsive breast cancer cells. The synergism between tamoxifen and tocotrienols may reduce the risk of adverse side effect from tamoxifen (Guthrie et al. 1997).

Tocotrienols are considered important lipid-soluble antioxidants, with potent anticancer and anti-inflammatory activity. Therefore, a daily dose of 240 mg of tocotrienols should be considered as an adjuvant breast cancer therapy.

PREVENTING BREAST CANCER CELL METASTASIS

Breast cancer cells frequently metastasize to the bone, where they cause severe degradation of bone tissue. Metastatic cancer affects more than half of all women during the course of their disease. Bone metastases are a significant cause of morbidity due to pain, pathological fractures, hypercalcemia (abnormally high levels of calcium in blood plasma), and spinal cord compression. The bisphosphonates, including alendronate (Fosamax), tiludronate (Skelid), pamidronate (Aredia), etidronate (Didronel), risedronate (Actonel), ibandronate, and zoledronic acid (Zometa), are a class of drugs that protect against the degradation of bone, primarily by inhibiting osteoclast-mediated bone resorption (bone breakdown).

Bisphosphonates are analogs of a naturally occurring compound, called pyrophosphate, which serves to regulate calcium and prevent bone breakdown. Bisphosphonates are a major class of drugs used for the treatment of bone diseases as they have a marked ability to inhibit bone resorption. Bisphosphonates are considered standard care for tumor-associated hypercalcemia and have been shown to reduce bone pain, improve quality of life, and to delay and reduce skeletal events (Hortobagyi 1996; Roemer-Becuwe et al. 2003).

Bone Remodeling

The renewal of bone is responsible for bone strength throughout our life. Old bone is removed (resorption) and new bone is created (formation). This process is called bone remodeling. Healthy bone is continually being remodeled. Two main types of cells are responsible for bone renewal: the osteoblasts involved in bone formation and the osteoclasts involved in bone resorption. There are several stages involved in bone remodeling. The first is *activation*. This process involves preosteoclasts that are stimulated and differentiated under the influence of cytokine and growth factors to mature into active osteoclasts. The next step is *resorption*, in which osteoclasts digest mineral matrix (old bone). The third step is *reversal*, which ends resorption and signals for the final phase, *formation*. During this stage, osteoblasts are responsible for bone matrix synthesis (collagen production). Two other noncollagenous proteins are also formed: osteocalcin and osteonectin, together they form new bone.

Bone Metastases Affects Remodeling

In patients with bone metastases, bone resorption by the osteoclasts is increased and exceeds bone reformation. Calcium lost from the bones appears in increased amounts in the patient's blood serum and urine. This increase in bone resorption may result in pain, bone fractures, spinal cord compression, and hypercalcemia.

Normally, the activity of the osteoclasts and osteoblasts is well-balanced, with the osteoclasts cleaning out the fatigued bone and the osteoblasts rebuilding new bone. In metastatic cancer, there is increased osteoclast activity caused by factors called osteoclastic activating factors (OAFs). These OAFs are released by tumor cells and include parathyroid hormone-related peptide (PTHrP), growth factors, and cytokines.

Among inhibitors of osteoclast activity, the bisphosphonates are the most promising drugs available (by prescription) to women with breast cancer who have a high risk of advancing cancer. Bisphosphonates interrupt the "vicious cycle" of bone metastases. Bisphosphonates inhibit bone turnover directly by decreasing resorption of bone and inhibiting the recruitment and function of osteoclasts.

Bisphosphonates may stop bone metastases from occurring if they are included at the onset of cancer diagnosis and treatment (ONI 2000). Bisphosphonates may delay the occurrence of bone metastases in women with breast cancer who do not have metastases.

In patients with bone metastases, bisphosphonates are useful as an adjuvant therapy to decrease bone pain, fractures, hypercalcemia, and progression of bone metastases (Delmas 1996). Treatment with bisphosphonates can also prevent the destruction of bone by cancer metastases and reduce the progression of metastatic tumors. A new bisphosphonate, risedronate, slows the progression of bone metastases in breast cancer patients, either by inhibiting the resorption of bone, which reduces the release of tumor growth factors, or by inhibiting the adhesion of breast cancer cells to bone matrix (Delmas 1996).

In women with early and advanced breast cancer and bone metastases, the use of bisphosphonates (oral or intravenous) in addition to hormone therapy or chemotherapy reduced bone pain, the risk of developing a fracture, and increased the time to a fracture (Pavlakis et al. 2002). Monthly infusions of pamidronate in 382 women with Stage IV breast cancer and bone metastases significantly reduced the incidence and prolonged the median time of skeletal complications (Hortobagyi et al. 1996).

Bisphosphonates are now third generation and are often used in the treatment of lytic bone metastasis. They inhibit the osteoclast activity that causes elevation of the blood calcium level and osteolytic bone weakening. Osteolytic holes form as the cancer degrades the bone, making it prone to fracture (Cristfanilli et al. 1999). The bisphosphonates, zoledronate and ibandronate, manage tumor-induced hypercalcemia, Paget's disease of the bone, and multiple myeloma-associated bone resorption. These bisphosphonate drugs are three orders of magnitude more potent than the first-generation drugs: etidronate, clodronate, and tilundronate. Patients newly diagnosed with lytic bone metastasis of breast cancer are offered bisphosphonate therapy, such as intravenous zoledronate or pamidronate every 3 or 4 weeks, as long as it proves effective. Oral clodronate offers equivalent results but is less well-tolerated.

Women with primary breast cancer who receive chemotherapy, hormone therapy, aromatase therapy, or oophorectomy may experience ovarian failure or early menopause, leading to a loss of bone mineral density.

The mechanisms by which tumor cells degrade bone involve tumor-cell adhesion to bone, as well as the release of compounds from tumor cells that stimulate osteoclast-induced bone degradation. Bisphosphonates inhibit cancer-cell adhesion and inhibit osteoclast activity. By preventing tumor-cell adhesion, bisphosphonates are useful agents for the prophylactic treatment of patients with cancer that is known to preferentially metastasize to bone.

There is evidence that growth factors, such as insulin-like growth factor and transforming growth factor, are released when the bone matrix is degraded. These growth factors could stimulate tumor-cell proliferation throughout the body and may attract cancer cells to the degraded bone ripe for clonal development, which may be a reason that early use of bisphosphonates significantly improved survival and may ward off metastasis.

Based upon the mounting research, it is strongly recommended that the use of bisphosphonates be considered at onset of breast cancer treatment to potentially stop bone metastases from developing. Patients are urged to discuss the use of bisphosphonates with their physicians.

Note: *Administration of bisphosphonate therapy should be accompanied by an adequate intake of a bone supplement that supplies all the raw materials to make healthy bone. These include calcium, magnesium, boron, silica, vitamin D, and vitamin K. Do not take vitamin K with Coumadin or other anticoagulant drugs or blood thinners.*

Bone Loss and Fatty Acids

While people often use omega-3 fatty acids to reduce the inflammation associated with arthritis, these fatty acids may actually help prevent bone loss. French researchers found in a group of 105 patients that high levels of pro-inflammatory omega-6 fatty acids were strongly associated with bone loss. However, the use of omega-3 supplements—360 mg a day of eicosapentanoic acid (EPA) and 240 mg a day of docosahexaneoic acid (DHA)—appeared to decrease production of pro-inflammatory prostaglandin E2 in bone and significantly stopped bone loss (Requirand et al. 2000).

Hormone Therapy and Metastasis

In primary breast cancer the estrogen receptor (ER) status represents an important prognostic factor and therefore, has a profound impact on the type of therapy employed. Yet, there is little research into the ER expression of disseminated breast cancer cells even though these cells are the main targets in adjuvant therapy.

A small pilot study involving 17 patients evaluated the ER expression profile on disseminated epithelial cells in bone marrow, one of the preferential organs for manifestation of distant metastases in breast cancer. Eleven patients (64.7%) were found to have ER-positive primary carcinomas. Of those eleven, only two patients revealed ER-positive epithelial cells in bone marrow. Additionally, one of these two patients expressed both ER-positive and ER-negative epithelial cells in bone marrow. Although in both of these cases the ER-positive epithelial cells in bone marrow derived from ER-positive primary tumors, in this small patient cohort none of the prognostically relevant clinical and pathological factors tested (i.e., TNM-classification, grading, and ER status in primary breast cancer) correlated with the ER status in bone marrow. A striking discrepancy between ER expression in primary breast cancers and the corresponding disseminated epithelial cells in bone marrow was found. This suggests either the selective dissemination of ER-negative tumor cells into the bone marrow or a negative impact of the bone marrow microenvironment on epithelial ER expression. While further research is required before conclusions can be drawn, this phenomenon might influence therapeutic effects of anti-hormonal treatment (Ditsch et al. 2003).

Diet

Cancer has an appetite for sugar and requires sugar for survival. Sugar plays an active role in reducing the immune response and energizes cancer, as tumors are primarily obligate glucose metabolizers.

There is a relationship between lactic acid, insulin, and angiogenesis. In tumors, hypoxic conditions occur through both inflammation, which reduces blood flow, and the chaotic development of blood vessels within tumors. These hypoxic conditions alter the pathways by which immune cells and tumor cells burn fuel (glucose) for energy, creating excessive lactic acid. In an oxygen-rich (aerobic) environment, glucose is burned in an efficient process that produces a maximum amount of energy and a minimal amount of lactic acid. However, tumor cells in chronic hypoxic conditions produce excessive lactic acid and inefficient utilization of glucose. Thus, there is a vicious cycle in which the reduced energy output stimulates the tumor cells to burn more glucose, which in turn produces more lactic acid. Tumor cells consume glucose at a rate three to five times higher than normal cells, creating a highly stimulated glycolysis (glucose-burning) pathway.

This glucose consumption can waste the cancer patient's energy reserves, and the increased production of lactic acid can stimulate increased production of angiogenic factors. The macrophage-mediated angiogenesis creates a complex interplay between opposing regulators. Insulin plays an active roll in promoting angiogenesis. Insulin is a growth factor that stimulates glycolysis and the proliferation of many cancer-cell lines through tyrosine kinase growth factors (Boyd 2003). In cancer patients, elevated levels of insulin are common in cancerous tissue and blood plasma. Obesity, and early stages of Type-II noninsulin-dependent diabetes mellitus (NIDDM), has been implicated as risk factors in a variety of cancers.

Based upon cancer's sugar dependency, a sugar-deprivation diet is strongly recommended. An effective tool in eliminating sugar from the diet is through following the Glycemic Index. The index is a list that rates the speed at which foods are digested and raise blood sugar levels. The ratings are based upon the rate at which a measured amount of pure glucose affects the body's blood sugar curve. Glucose itself has a rating of 100, and the closer a food item is to a rating of 100, the more rapidly it raises blood glucose levels. Foods with a low Glycemic Index, such as vegetables, protein, and grains, are suggested (please refer to the *Obesity* protocol for specific information about low glycemic foods).

With regard to depleting sugar from the diet, the following should be considered:

- Limit or avoid all white foods, including (but not limited to) sugar, flour, rice, pasta, breads, crackers, cookies, etc.

- Read labels. Sugar has many names (brown sugar, corn syrup, honey, molasses, maple syrup, high-fructose corn syrup, dextrin, raw sugar, fructose, polyols, dextrose, hydrogenated starch, galactose, glucose, sorbitol, fruit juice concentrate, lactose, brown rice syrup, xylitol, sucrose, mannitol, sorghum, maltose, and turbinado, to mention only a few).

- Limit all fruit juices; per glass they contain the juice of many pieces of fruit and a large amount of fructose (fruit sugar) but no fiber. Instead, infrequently eat low glycemic-rated fruit in small portions.

Natural compounds have also been reported to inhibit the cancer-promoting effects of insulin. For example, vitamin C has been reported to increase oxygen consumption and reduce lactic acid production in tumor cells. In addition, some natural compounds may help reduce insulin production by reducing insulin resistance. Insulin resistance occurs when cells are no longer sensitive to insulin and thus more insulin is produced in an effort to reduce glucose levels. Insulin resistance has been implicated as a risk factor for breast cancer, and diets high in saturated fats and omega-6 fatty acids promote insulin resistance. Although the exact pathway is unknown, it is thought that the mechanism of action is via chronic activation of PKC. Some of the known natural compounds that can reduce insulin resistance include omega-3 fatty acids, curcumin, flavonoids, selenium, and vitamin E.

As discussed earlier in the protocol, estrogen is a growth factor for most breast cancers. High-fat diets and associated increases in fat tissue can increase estrogen availability in a number of ways:

- Fat tissue is a major source of estrogen production in postmenopausal women. Therefore, there is an association between high body weight and decreased survival in breast cancer patients.

- Obesity and possibly insulin resistance can decrease the levels of sex hormone binding globulin (SHBG) in both men and women and increase breast cancer risk or cancer progression. This is an important factor in estrogen-dependent breast cancer cells because it is adequate levels of SHBG that act as an anti-proliferative and provides an anti-estrogenic effect. Obesity can alter liver metabolism of estrogen, allowing the retention of high estrogen byproducts with high estrogenic activity within the body.

- High-fat diets may reduce the amount of estrogen excreted in the feces. In contrast, low-fat/high-fiber diets can reduce circulating estrogen.

Another consideration when discussing diet and breast cancer is the reduction of dietary estrogen. Several foods contain *naturally occurring hormones* (found in animal sources); *synthetic hormones* that can mimic estrogen in the human body (found in commercially packaged meat, poultry, and dairy products); or *naturally estrogenic properties* that can encourage the body's production of estrogens (natural foods such as soy). Regardless of the source, try to avoid all commercial animal products (including, but not limited to, meats, poultry, and dairy). Also avoid the use of soft plastic food-storage products that can give off large amounts of polymers (e.g., by leaching into food contents), thought by environmentalists and some researchers to be a possible cause of breast cancer.

In order to reduce estrogen, a breast cancer patient should consider increasing dietary intake of fish high in omega-3 fatty acids, whey, eggs, and nuts, occasionally including hormone-free poultry and hormone-free, low-fat dairy products.

BLOOD TESTING

Monthly blood tests should include complete blood chemistry, with tests for liver function and serum calcium levels, prolactin, parathyroid hormone, and the tumor marker CA 27.29 (or CA 15.3). Additional blood tests to consider are the CEA and GGTP tests. These tests monitor the progress of therapies used and also detect toxicity from high doses of vitamin A and vitamin D3. The patient should insist on obtaining a copy of their blood workups every month.

⬤ SUMMARY

When considering breast cancer treatment options, physicians and patients alike must sort through an overwhelming amount of information. This protocol attempts to simplify complicated scientific research and bring to the forefront the most up-to-date, multimodality approach to cancer treatment. It integrates surgery, anticancer drugs, irradiation, hormone therapy, nutritional supplementation, and diet modification in a comprehensive approach to counteract breast cancer.

As discussed in this protocol, cancer growth is based on many complicated interactions via numerous physiological pathways within the body. Despite the huge strides in scientific research, there are still many unanswered questions regarding cancer's growth and development. What we do know is that there is overwhelming research supporting an integrated approach to the treatment of cancer. Additionally, research supports using nutritional supplementation to improve the efficacy of chemotherapy drugs and radiotherapy (see the *Cancer Chemotherapy* and *Cancer Radiation* protocols for more information). In fact, combining certain supplements can create a synergism that can effectively block or impede certain cancer pathways.

Therefore, the supplementation regimen following is suggested. Please read the entire protocol before considering this regimen because there are certain cautions to consider. As always, consult your physician before beginning any nutritional supplementation regimen.

1. Indole-3-carbinol (I3C), a 200-mg capsule twice daily, if you weigh under 120 lbs or three 200-mg capsules daily in two divided doses if you weigh over 120 lbs. Take two 200-mg capsules twice daily, if you weigh over 180 lbs.

CAUTION   Pregnant women should not take indole-3-carbinol because of its modulation of estrogen.

2. Curcumin, four 900 mg capsules, 3 times daily on an empty stomach for a total of 10.8 g per day. Note the caution earlier in this protocol.

3. Lightly caffeinated green tea extract, five 350 mg capsules, 3 times daily with meals for a total of 5.25 g per day. Use decaffeinated green tea extract if you are sensitive to caffeine or want to use the less-stimulating version with the evening dosage.

4. CLA or CLA with Guarana, 3000 to 4000 mg daily of CLA and about 300 mg of guarana, early in the day.

5. Melatonin, 3 to 50 mg at bedtime.

6. PhytoFood Powder (broccoli, cabbage, and other cruciferous vegetables that provide sulphoraphane and other cancer-fighting plant extracts), 1–2 tbsp daily.

7. Se-methylselenocysteine, 200 to 400 mcg daily.

8. CoQ10, three 100 mg softgels in divided doses. Note the caution stated in this protocol.

9. Mega EPA (with DHA), 8 capsules daily, supplying 3200 mg of EPA and 2400 mg of DHA. Take with nonfiber meals.

10. Vitamin D3, 4000 to 6000 IU taken daily with monthly blood testing to monitor for toxicity. Reduce dosage at 6 months.

11. Water-soluble vitamin A, 100,000 to 300,000 IU daily with monthly blood testing to monitor for toxicity. Reduce dosage at 6 months (*refer to vitamin A precautions in Appendix A*).

12. Vitamin E succinate (tocopheryl succinate), 1200 IU daily.

13. Gamma E Tocopherol/Tocotrienol, 1 capsule daily. Take an additional 200 mg of palm-oil tocotrienols as an adjuvant therapy.

14. Vitamin C, 4000 to 12,000 mg throughout the day.

15. Gamma linolenic acid, 1200 mg a day (4 capsules of a borage oil supplement called Mega GLA will supply this amount).

16. Whey protein concentrate-isolate, 30 to 60 grams daily in divided doses.

17. Bone Assure provides calcium, magnesium, and bone-protecting nutrients. Take 6 capsules at bedtime.

18. Vitamin K, 10 mg daily.

19. Silicon, 6 mg daily. (Jarrow's Biosil is recommended.)

20. Life Extension Mix without Copper (multinutrient formula), 3 tablets 3 times daily.

Reminder: Bisphosphonate (injectable Zometa or Aredia) drug therapy is strongly encouraged for all breast cancer patients as well as aromatase-inhibitor therapy (Arimidex, Femara, or Aromasin) if appropriate.

Note: *If chemotherapy and/or radiation are being considered, refer to the Cancer Chemotherapy and Cancer Radiation protocols. Also refer to the protocols titled Cancer Treatment: The Critical Factors and Cancer Adjuvant Therapy.*

FOR MORE INFORMATION

Contact the American Cancer Society, 1 (800) ACS-2345. Sources for National Cancer Institute Information.

- Cancer Information Service, (800) 4-CANCER (1-800-422-6237); TTY (for hearing impaired callers), (800) 332-8615
- NCI Online /Internet, use http://cancer.gov to reach the NCI website.
- CancerMail Service, to obtain a contents list, send e-mail to cancermail@cips.nci.nih.gov with the word "help" in the body of the message.

 PRODUCT AVAILABILITY

Indole-3-carbinol (I3C), curcumin, green tea, CLA, CLA with guarana, melatonin, SeMsc (Se-methylselenocysteine), CoQ10, Mega EPA/ DHA, vitamin D3 caps, water-soluble vitamin A liquid, vitamin E succinate, Gamma E Tocopherol/ Tocotrienols, vitamin C, Mega GLA, enhanced whey protein, Bone Assure, Phyto Food, vitamin K, Biosil, and Life Extension Mix can be ordered by calling (800) 544-4440 or by ordering online at www.lef.org.

STAYING INFORMED

The information published in this protocol is only as current as the day the manuscript was sent to the printer. This protocol raises many issues that are subject to change as new data emerge. Furthermore, cancer is still a disease with unacceptably high mortality rates, and none of our suggested regimens can guarantee a cure. The Life Extension Foundation is constantly uncovering information to provide to cancer patients. A special website has been established for the purpose of updating patients on new findings that directly pertain to the published cancer protocols. Whenever Life Extension discovers information that may benefit cancer patients, it will be posted on the website www.lefcancer.org. Before utilizing this cancer protocol, we suggest that check www.lefcancer.org to see if any substantive changes have been made to the recommendations described herein. Based on the sheer number of newly published findings, there could be significant alterations to the information you have just read.

DISCLAIMER

This information (and any accompanying printed material) is not intended to replace the attention or advice of a physician or other health care professional. Anyone who wishes to embark on any dietary, drug, exercise, or other lifestyle change intended to prevent or treat a specific disease or condition should first consult with and seek clearance from a qualified health care professional. The information published in the protocols is only as current as the day the manuscript was sent to the printer. This protocol raises many issues that are subject to change as new data emerge. None of our suggested protocol regimens can guarantee a cure.

Cancer: Overview of Protocols

Those diagnosed with cancer today find themselves at a historical crossroad. Despite multiple therapies from which to choose, no medical facility integrates cancer therapies into a comprehensive program. The result is that cancer patients are not provided an optimal opportunity to achieve long-term survival.

Discoveries are occurring in the research setting more quickly than they are being incorporated into clinical practice.

The challenge for cancer patients is to acquire enough information to take advantage of as many treatment options as is practical. Cancer is a complex disease that requires a multimodality therapy to provide the best odds of attaining a cure. Many of the recommendations contained in the following protocols require the cooperation of a motivated oncologist.

The protocols you are about to view are complicated and will probably require several readings for most people to comprehend. One reason for the complexity is that individual variables significantly affect therapy options.

Curing cancer is not simple. Until a medical facility is developed that integrates all potential therapies into individualized treatments, patients must become self-empowered and fully educated about their disease.

The purpose of these protocols is to translate the vast amount of current knowledge into practical formats for cancer patients and their oncologists. Tens of thousands of published papers were reviewed in order to propose novel methods for overcoming the multiple survival mechanisms that cancer cells use to resist eradication by conventional therapies.

For the first time in medical history, the cancer patient can delve deep into the molecular aspects behind their disease and use this information in a practical manner. Those who believe in controlling their own destiny will appreciate how translational research is available to help them battle their disease. Here are the cancer protocol chapters that can be found in alphabetical order:

Breast Cancer

Cancer Adjuvant Therapies

Cancer Chemotherapy

Cancer: Clinics Offering Alternative Therapies

Cancer: Gene Therapies, Stem Cells, Telomeres, and Cytokines

Cancer Prevention

Cancer Radiation Therapy

Cancer: Should Patients Take Dietary Supplements?

Cancer Surgery

Cancer Treatment: The Critical Factors

Cancer Vaccines

Colorectal Cancer

Leukemia and Lymphoma (Hodgkin's and Non-Hodgkin's Disease)

Pancreatic Cancer

Prostate Cancer

STAYING INFORMED

The information published in this protocol is only as current as the day the book was printed. This cancer protocol raises many issues that are subject to change as new data emerge. Furthermore, cancer is still a disease with unacceptably high mortality rates, and none of our suggested treatment regimens can guarantee a cure.

The Life Extension Foundation is constantly uncovering information to provide the cancer patient with more ammunition to battle their disease. A special website has been established for the purpose of updating patients on new findings that directly pertain to the cancer protocols published in this book. Whenever Life Extension discovers information that points to a better way of treating cancer, it will be posted on the website www.lefcancer.org

Before utilizing the cancer protocols in this book, we suggest that you log on to www.lefcancer.org to see if any substantive changes have been made to the therapeutic recommendations described in this protocol. Based on the sheer number of newly published findings, there could be significant alterations to the information you have just read.

www.lefcancer.org

DISCLAIMER

This information (and any accompanying printed material) is not intended to replace the attention or advice of a physician or other health care professional. Anyone who wishes to embark on any dietary, drug, exercise, or other lifestyle change intended to prevent or treat a specific disease or condition should first consult with and seek clearance from a qualified health care professional. The information published in the protocols is only as current as the day the manuscript was sent to the printer. This protocol raises many issues that are subject to change as new data emerge. None of our suggested protocol regimens can guarantee a cure.

Cancer Adjuvant Therapy

The good news is that many of the 4 million people being treated for cancer in America will survive the disease and go on to live full and productive lives.

While the numbers that survive are far too low (about 44%), many of the more than 1500 daily cancer deaths occur because patients and their families are unaware of the depth of the resources currently available. Unfortunately, some die avowing they would never resort to natural medicine, while others are interested but lack the expertise to implement the program to their best advantage. Regrettably, some turn to alternative care fairly late in the course of the disease process, weakening the probability of recovery.

Mainstream medicine (relying upon surgery, chemotherapy, and radiation) may initially appear successful, but the indications of the disease process are less often addressed. Conventional cancer treatments are not for those individuals who are frail in body or spirit. For the past 30 years, cancer therapies have experienced tremendous setbacks because of an associated toxic response, resulting in significant numbers of treatment-induced deaths rather than disease-induced fatalities. Awareness regarding historic numbers of unsuccessful outcomes has forced patients to look for alternatives to bolster survival odds. Many who use alternative therapies report doing so without their oncologist's knowledge, fearful of criticism or rejection by a physician (Richardson et al. 2000).

The University of Texas M.D. Anderson Cancer Center (Houston) found that 99.3% of patients had heard of complementary medicine, and 68.7% of patients reported having used at least one unconventional therapy (Richardson et al. 2000). About 75% of the patients surveyed, however, yearned for more information concerning complementary medicine and about one-half of those participating in the survey wanted the information to come from their physician.

Until most recently, major medical schools granted only a few hours to nutritional education out of the hundreds of academic hours required to complete medical school. The exclusion began when Abraham Flexner (commissioned to correct inequities occurring in medical schools) penned the Flexner Report of 1910. His contribution, entitled *Medical Education in the United States and Canada*, closed smaller medical schools and forced those that survived to adopt a uniform curriculum that excluded nutritional courses. Thus, some physicians emerged from medical schools, scoffing at the concept of nutrition influencing health or overcoming disease.

Sir William Osler (1849–1919), chief physician at Johns Hopkins's School of Medicine, drilled into students that medical research must be validated and replicated to be good medicine. This led to controlled experiments (as randomized, controlled trials) that became the backbone of mainstream medicine. Nutritional protocols often used multiple nutrients, a difficult model to apply in clinical trials. Testing a single nutraceutical denied the patient full support of nutritional pharmacology, an injustice when treating a seriously ill patient. In addition, trials are expensive to conduct and early natural healers (by and large) did not represent an affluent subset of society.

But, ever so slowly, the medical scene is being revolutionized. According to the American College for Advancement in Medicine, physicians (in many cases) are showing eagerness to learn more about natural medicine and how to best implement it into their practice (Corbin-Winslow et al. 2002). Scientists, teaching at nutritional seminars, report attendees are often medical doctors, a vast departure from years past.

PREVENTING AND CONTROLLING CANCER

While some individuals will be reading this protocol looking for help managing a malignancy, others will be focusing upon prevention and recurrence. The alphabetical list that follows provides quick guidelines for structuring a program, highlighting major nutrients in the prevention and treatment of cancer.

These recommendations *should not* be implemented individually in aggressive cancers without careful consultation of the remainder of the material. Cancer patients (and physicians) should be deliberate about reading the entirety of this protocol in order to avoid missing information that could prove to be lifesaving. *Note:* It is important that the reader also consult the protocols entitled *Cancer Treatment: The Critical Factors* and *Cancer: Should Patients Take Dietary Supplements?*

The dosages required for treating cancer (which are considerably larger than those required for prevention) can change the effects that a nutrient has on the body. The risk is multidirectional. Overdosing or underdosing, as well as a lack of patient awareness regarding the full potential of natural pharmaceuticals, hampers recovery.

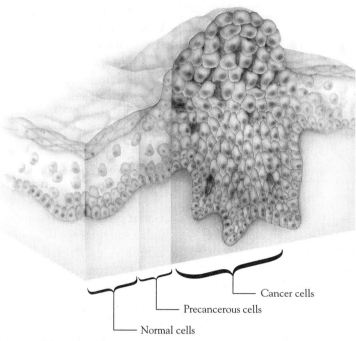

Cancer cells

Precancerous cells

Normal cells

What is cancer? Cancer is a destructive (malignant) growth of cells which invades nearby tissues and may metastisize (spread) to other areas of the body. Dividing rapidly, these cells tend to be very aggressive and out of control. In contrast, a benign tumor is simply a localized mass of slowly multiplying cells resembling its original tissue and is seldom life-threatening. (Anatomical Chart Company 2002®, Lippincott , Williams & Wilkins)

Table 1: *Type of Cancers and the Tumor Marker Used for Assessment*

Type of Cancer	Tumor Marker Blood Test
Ovarian cancer	CA 125, CK-BB
Prostate cancer	PSA, PAP, prolactin, testosterone
Breast cancer	CA 27.29, CEA, alkaline phosphatase, and prolactin (or CA 15-3 rather than the CA 27.29)
Colon, rectum, liver, stomach, and other organ cancers	CEA, CA 19-9, AFP, TPS, and GGTP
Pancreatic cancer	CA 19.9, CEA, and GGTP
Leukemia, lymphoma, and Hodgkin's disease	LDH, CBC with differential, immune cell differentiation and leukemia profile

THE CRITICAL IMPORTANCE OF SCHEDULED BLOOD TESTS

It is important to measure the successes or losses in regard to treatment-associated tumor response. Evaluating tumor markers in the blood or tumor imagery provides a basis for calculating regression of the disease. In addition, tumor markers provide direction for introducing other therapies if failures are evidenced.

It is also important to evaluate the effectiveness of immune-boosting therapies and guard against anemia and therapeutic toxicities. At a minimum, a monthly complete blood chemistry (CBC) test that includes assessment of hematocrit, hemoglobin, and liver and kidney function should be done in all cancer patients undergoing treatment.

An immune cell test should be performed bimonthly, measuring total blood count, CD4 (T-helper), CD4/CD8 (T-helper-to-T-suppressor) ratio, and NK (natural killer) cell activity. Also consider tests measuring cortisol levels (Cortisol am and pm) and HCG (human chorionic gonadotropin), a hormone that may be elevated 10–12 years prior to a diagnosis of cancer. For information regarding test availability call (800) 208-3444.

COMPLEMENTARY THERAPIES

When describing the various complementary cancer therapies, it is not possible to endorse one supplement, hormone, or drug over another. We have provided as much evidence as space allows so that patients and their physicians can evaluate what approach may be suited for the individual situation.

A great deal of effort has been made to identify therapies that are substantiated in published scientific literature or that provide a cancer patient with the opportunity to experiment with cutting-edge treatment strategies. The focus of our effort has been to identify potentially lifesaving therapies that have been overlooked by mainstream oncology. We also attempt to discuss both positive and negative studies when applicable.

The Life Extension Foundation can assume no responsibility for outcome, apart from a self-assigned duty to stay abreast of the most promising of therapies and to share the data with members. No warranties (expressed or implied) accompany the material; neither is the information intended to replace medical advice. As always, each reader is urged to consult professional help for medical problems, especially those involving cancer. All supplements, drugs, and hormones are listed alphabetically and not in order of importance.

Alpha-Lipoic Acid—is a powerful antioxidant that regulates gene expression and preserves hearing during cisplatin therapy

Lester Packer, Ph.D. (scientist and professor at the Berkeley Laboratory of the University of California), refers to lipoic acid as the most powerful of all the antioxidants; in fact, Packer says that if he were to invent an ideal antioxidant, it would closely resemble lipoic acid (Packer et al. 1999). Alpha-lipoic acid claims anticarcinogenic credits because it independently scavenges free radicals, including the hydroxyl radical (a free radical involved in all stages of the cancer process and linked to an increase in the likelihood of metastasis).

Lipoic acid increases the efficacy of other antioxidants, regenerating vitamins C and E, coenzyme Q10, and glutathione for continued service. In fact, lipoic acid boosts the levels of glutathione by 30–70%, particularly in the lungs, liver, and kidney cells of laboratory animals injected with the antioxidant. In addition, glutathione tempers the synthesis of damaging cytokines and adhesion molecules by influencing the activity of nuclear factor kappa B (NF-kB), a transcription factor (Exner et al. 2000). *Note:* A great deal of material relating to NF-kB is presented in the protocol *Cancer Treatment: The Critical Factors.*

Lipoic acid can down-regulate genes that accelerate cancer without inducing toxicity. So responsive are cancer cells that laboratory-induced cancers literally soak up lipoic acid, a saturation that increased the lifespan of rats with aggressive cancer by 25% (Karpov et al. 1977).

Alpha-lipoic acid was preferentially toxic to leukemia cells lines (Jurkat and CCRF-CEM cells). The selective toxicity of lipoic acid to Jurkat cells was credited (in part) to the antioxidant's ability to induce apoptosis. Lipoic acid activated (by nearly 100%) an enzyme (caspase) that kills leukemia cells (Pack et al. 2002). Other researchers showed that lipoic acid

acted as a potentiator, amplifying the anti-leukemic effects of vitamin D. It is speculated that lipoic acid delivers much of its advantage by inhibiting NF-kB and the appearance of damaging cytokines (Sokoloski et al. 1997; Zhang et al. 2001). Finding that lipoic acid can differentiate between normal and leukemic cells charts new courses in treatment strategies to slow or overcome the disease (Packer et al. 1999).

As with all antioxidants, the appropriateness of using lipoic acid with chemotherapy arises. Animal studies indicate that alpha-lipoic acid decreased side effects associated with cyclophosphamide and vincristine (chemotherapeutic agents) but did not hamper drug effectiveness (Berger et al. 1983). More recently, a combination of alpha-lipoic acid and doxorubicin resulted in a marginally significant increase in survival of leukemic mice (Dovinova et al. 1999). Nonetheless, the definitive answer regarding coupling antioxidants with conventional cancer therapy is complex. Factors, such as type of malignancy, as well as the nature of the cytotoxic chemical and even the time of day the agents are administered, appear to influence outcome (please consult the protocol *Cancer: Should Patients Take Dietary Supplements* to learn more about the advisability of antioxidant therapy during conventional treatments).

To its credit, lipoic acid appears able to counter the hearing loss and deafness that often accompanies cisplatin therapy. Depreciated hearing occurs as free radicals, produced as a result of treatment, plunder the inner ear; lipoic acid preserves glutathione levels and thus prevents deafness in rats (Rybak et al. 1999).

A suggested alpha-lipoic acid dosage for healthy individuals is from 250–500 mg a day. Degenerative diseases usually require larger dosages (sometimes as much as 500 mg 3 times a day). Packer et al. (1999), in their book *The Antioxidant Miracle*, recommend taking biotin supplements with alpha-lipoic acid when the daily intake exceeds 100 mg. (Alpha-lipoic acid may compete with biotin and interfere with biotin's activities in the body.) Hyper-alertness and insomnia are also associated with mega-dosages.

Arginine

Various scientists have attempted to describe the complex role of arginine in cancer biology and treatment. L-arginine is the common substrate for two enzymes, arginase and nitric oxide synthase. Arginase converts L-arginine to L-ornithine, a pathway that can increase cell proliferation. Nitric oxide synthase converts L-arginine to nitric oxide, a conversion process with uncertain effects regarding cancer.

A positive study conducted by a team of German researchers showed that arginine contributed significantly to immune function by increasing levels of white blood cells. Scottish scientists added that dietary supplementation with arginine in breast cancer patients enhanced NK cell activity and lymphokine cytotoxicity (Brittenden et al. 1994). (Lymphokines are chemical factors produced and released by T-lymphocytes that attract macrophages to a site of infection or inflammation in preparation for attack.) Various researchers have shown that increasing arginine increases neutrophils (white blood cells that remove bacteria, cellular debris, and solid particles), significantly upgrading host defense (Muhling et al. 2002).

Apart from enhancing immune function, arginine increases a number of amino acids, creating the possibility of an amino acid imbalance. Oversupplying some amino acids while undersupplying others is thought to destabilize the tumor. All cells, both healthy and diseased, have amino acid requirements; if not met, the cell is significantly disabled (Muhling et al. 2002). Amino acid manipulation has been applied in oncology for decades with varying degrees of success.

Interesting studies have emerged regarding arginine or arginine analogs in cancer treatment. For example, infusions of arginine significantly reduced the incidence of liver and lung metastasis in laboratory mice. Earlier research found that supplemental arginine altered the number of tumor-infiltrating lymphocytes in human colorectal cancer, offering important implications for new strategies in cancer treatment (Heys et al. 1997). Though many factors are involved (including appropriate dosages), Japanese researchers found that arginine induced apoptosis in pancreatic (AR4-2J) cells, inhibiting cell proliferation (Motoo et al. 2000).

The two faces of arginine, however, cloud dosing with confidence. The role of nitric oxide (NO), a molecule synthesized from arginine, remains controversial and poorly understood. While a few reports indicate that the presence of NO in tumor cells or their microenvironment is detrimental to tumor-cell survival, and subsequently their metastatic potential, a large body of data suggests that NO actually promotes tumor progression. Illustrative of its fickleness, NO was recently identified as a downstream regulator of prolactin, an inhibitor of apoptosis. However, arginine stimulated proliferation of prolactin-dependent Nb2 lymphoma cells in laboratory rats (Dodd et al. 2000). In addition, NO production (by murine mammary adenocarcinoma cells) promoted tumor cell invasiveness. Whereas, introducing NO inhibitors resulted in an antitumor, antimetastatic profile (Orucevic et al. 1999).

Ambiguity and nonconformity reduce arginine's role at the present time to adjunctive support with either traditional cancer treatment or fish oil supplementation. A heartening report regarding arginine, fish oil, and doxorubicin therapy appears in this protocol in the section devoted to Essential Fatty Acids (Ogilvie et al. 2000). Nonetheless, the diverse biological properties of L-arginine demand further careful studies, clarifying chemopreventive advantages and endangerments (Szende et al. 2000).

Carotenoids—have antioxidant activity, inhibit cellular proliferation, and offer protection against numerous types of malignancies

Carotenoids, acting as immune enhancers and free-radical scavengers, are important substances in oncology. When using carotenoids for antioxidant and cancer protection, it appears wise to use mixed carotenoids, that is, alpha-carotene, lycopene, zeaxanthin, canthaxanthin, beta-crytoxanthine, and lutein rather than emphasizing only beta-carotene.

The following are illustrative of the worth of mixed carotenoids:

Lycopene offers targeted protection against cancers arising in the prostate (Kucuk et al. 2001), pancreas (Burney et al. 1989), digestive tract (De Stefani 2000), and colon (Nair et al. 2001).

- *The American Journal of Clinical Nutrition* added that individuals seeking broad-spectrum colon protection should also include lutein-rich foods in their diet (spinach, broccoli, lettuce, tomatoes, oranges, carrots, celery, and greens) (Slattery et al. 2000).

- Canthaxanthin, a less well-known carotenoid, was shown to induce apoptosis and inhibit cell growth in both WiDR colon adenocarcinoma and SK-MEL-2 melanoma cells (Palozza et al. 1998).

- Researchers showed that the risk of breast cancer approximately doubled (2.21-fold) among subjects with blood levels of beta-carotene in the lowest quartile, compared with those in the highest quartile. The risk of breast cancer associated with low levels of other carotenoids was similar, that is, a 2.08-fold increased risk if lutein is deficient and a 1.68-fold greater risk if beta-cryptoxanthin is lacking (Toniolo et al. 2001). A Swedish study found that menopausal status has an impact on the protection delivered by carotenoids. Analysis showed that lycopene was associated with decreased breast cancer risk in postmenopausal women, but in premenopausal women, lutein offered greater protection (Hulten et al. 2001).

- Leukoplakia (an often precancerous condition marked by white thickened patches on the mucous membranes of the cheeks, gums, or tongue) is responsive to spirulina, a source of proteins, carotenoids, and other micronutrients (Sankaranarayanan et al. 1995). An inverse relationship between beta-carotene and thyroid carcinoma was observed in both papillary and follicular carcinomas (D'Avanzo et al. 1997). A high dietary intake of beta-carotene appears a protective (though modest) factor for the development of ovarian cancer (Huncharek et al. 2001).

- Lastly, Japanese researchers showed that all the carotenoids inhibited hepatic (liver) invasion, probably through antioxidant properties (Kozuki et al. 2000).

Men who consume 10 or more servings of tomato products per week reduce their risk of prostate cancer by about 35%. The American Chemical Society in August 2001 reported that 32 (largely African-American) patients diagnosed with prostate cancer and awaiting radical prostatectomy were placed on diets that included tomato sauce, providing 30 mg a day of lycopene. After 3 weeks, mean serum prostate specific antigen (PSA) concentrations fell by 17.5%, oxidative burden by 21.3%, DNA damage by 40%, while programmed cell death increased threefold in cancer cells (Holzman 2002). Part of lycopene's protection involves the ability of carotenoids to counteract the proliferation of cancer cells induced by insulin-like growth factors (Agarwal et al. 2000a).

Beta-carotene exhibited a radio-protective effect among 709 children exposed to radiation inflicted by the Chernobyl nuclear accident. For example, the Chernobyl accident showed that irradiation increases the susceptibility of lipids to oxidative damage and that natural beta-carotene may act as an *in vivo* lipophilic antioxidant or radio-protective agent (Ben-Amotz et al. 1998). Therefore, using beta-carotene following radiotherapy may reduce the tissue damage caused during treatment.

Beta-carotene, perhaps the most controversial of the family of carotenoids, has come under attack several times in the past few years. For example, smokers who received synthetic beta-carotene (as a prophylactic) in the CARET study had a higher rate of lung cancer and death than smokers not supplemented. In fact, the study was terminated by the National Cancer Institute (NCI) because of the widespread discrepancy between the two groups. The CARET study is not new, but because it still concerns beta-carotene users, we will attempt to explain the unexpected results of the study.

Dr. Packer described the subjects as "walking time bombs." Many were victims of asbestos exposure or heavy smoking. The form of beta-carotene selected for the study (synthetic versus natural) was also cited as another possible explanation for the negative outcome.

Dr. Leo Galland, M.D. (practitioner and director of the Foundation of Integrated Medicine, New York City), also explains that high-dose beta-carotene (25,000 IU a day) administered to smokers results in a particular pattern of metabolism (Galland 2000). The process is orchestrated as cytochrome p450 enzymes (Phase I detoxification system) are summoned into action by tars in cigarette smoke. As beta-carotene is acted on by cytochrome p450, oxidized end products are formed, as well as toxic derivatives.

Simultaneously, vitamins C and A, as well as glutathione, are depleted, severing antioxidant protection. This sequence can damage DNA and increase the likelihood of lung cancer, particularly in an environment with initially high oxidative stress, a profile common to smokers. Without full spectrum antioxidant support, the single dose of beta-carotene produces an oxidative environment rather than one of protection. (*Comment:* As one free radical is neutralized by an antioxidant, another oxidant may be formed. It is well established that vitamin C can serve as a pro-oxidant through the formation of ascorbyl radicals. It is also known that this radical is quenched by vitamin E to yield a tocopheryl radical, which in turn is reduced by the conversion of glutathione to glutathione disulfide. Thus, the full spectrum of antioxidants is preferable, rather than emphasizing single antioxidants.)

Beta-carotene is largely considered nontoxic even at high doses; for example, some nonconventional cancer therapies recommend large amounts of carrot juice. One large glass of carrot juice can contain 100,000–200,000 IU of provitamin A or carotene. The problem with carrot juice is that it is loaded with fructose (sugar). Cancer cells feed on sugar, and drinking carrot juice may induce an insulin spike that could potentially fuel cancer cell propagation.

Cancer patients should consider natural beta-carotene supplements in lieu of carrot juice. Suggested phytonutrient dosages are from 9–20 mg of sulphoraphane, 10–30 mg a day of lycopene, and 15–40 mg of lutein, along with a mixed carotenoid blend that includes alpha- and beta-carotene. A product called PhytoFood Powder provides potent amounts of sulphoraphane, while carotenoid extracts are available in a variety of encapsulated preparations. *Note: What Should the Cancer Patient Eat*, appearing later in this protocol, contains a discussion regarding the value of sulphoraphanes in the diet.

cer (http://clinicaltrials.gov/ct/search.?term=soy). When the findings of these studies are published, perhaps more definitive recommendations can be made about soy supplements. Based on the information available to us as of this writing, those concerned about cancer may consider these guidelines: a suggested dosage is five 700-mg capsules 4 times a day of a soy extract providing a minimum of 40% isoflavones. For prevention purposes, as little as 135 mg of a 40% soy isoflavone extract once a day may be adequate.

Theanine—increases efficacy of chemotherapeutic drugs

Researchers speculate that drinking 1 cup of green tea favors a positive mental attitude and increases the efficacy of chemotherapy. However, components of green tea have been identified (caffeine, epigallocatechin gallate (EGCG), flavonoids, and theanine) that better explain the chemotherapeutic advantage beyond its soul-soothing effects (Sadzuka et al. 2000a).

Japanese researchers focused specifically on theanine and its influence on the anti-tumor activity of Adriamycin (doxorubicin). In vitro, theanine inhibited the outflow of Adriamycin (ADR) from cancerous cells, increasing concentrations within the cell by almost three-fold. An increase in ADR concentrations was not observed in normal tissues, suggesting theanine protects healthy organs, such as the heart and liver (Sadzuka et al. 1996). Illustrative of the enhancing qualities of theanine, injecting ADR into ovarian sarcoma-bearing (M5076) mice did not inhibit tumor growth, whereas a combination of theanine and ADR reduced tumor weight 62% (Sugiyama et al. 1998).

When theanine was added to pirarubicin, intracellular concentrations of pirarubicin increased 1.3-fold and the overall therapeutic efficacy of the drug increased 1.7-fold (Sugiyama et al. 1999). Satisfying results were also found when theanine was used with Idarubicin (IDA), which is highly toxic to bone marrow and an anti-leukemia agent similar to doxorubicin. Risk factors permitted only about one-fourth of the standard IDA dose to be used in combination with theanine. However, theanine reduced toxicities and increased IDA anti-tumor activity, rendering the chemotherapeutic agent a possibility for the treatment of leukemia (Sadzuka et al. 2000b).

Part of theanine's anticancer effects can be attributed to mimicking glutamate, an amino acid that potentiates glutathione. Glutathione detoxifies chemotherapeutic agents, barricading chemicals from cells, and inhibiting tumor cell kill. Theanine is structurally similar to glutathione and crowds out glutamate transport into tumor cells. Cancer cells (in confusion) erringly take in theanine and theanine induces glutathione production. Glutathione (derived from theanine) does not detoxify like natural glutathione, and instead blocks the ability of cancer cells to neutralize cancer-killing agents. Deprived of glutathione, cancer cells cannot remove chemotherapeutic agents, and the tumor cell dies as a result of chemical poisoning (Sadzuka et al. 2001).

Administered with doxorubicin, the suggested dose of theanine is 500–1000 mg a day, although no human studies have been conducted with chemotherapy and theanine.

Thymus Extract—improves T-cell response and regulates the activity of cytokines

The thymus gland was at one time removed as an unnecessary appendage. It is an essential organ of the immune system, increasing stamina, energy, well-being, and the ability to ward off infections and cancer. Since 1965, when Burnet was awarded the Nobel Prize for demonstrating the endocrine function of the thymus gland, medical interest has focused on the thymus. It is now largely accepted that the thymus gland plays a central role in the mammalian immune system.

The immune system is made up of B-cells that protect against bacterial and viral infections and T-cells that guard against viral and fungal infections, as well as cancer. This powerful body of cells normally treats a developing cancer as foreign tissue, destroying aberrant cells before rapid multiplication occurs.

The effectiveness of T-cell mediated immunity depends upon the activity of T-lymphocytes (T-cells), which are programmed by proteins from the thymus gland. Immature (naïve) T-4 cells do not function properly until programmed by thymic proteins. As new T-lymphocytes migrate from the bone marrow to the thymus, they are programmed to distinguish between self-tissue (the host) and nonself tissue (an invading pathogen).

The thymus gland, a lymphoid organ situated in the anterior superior mediastinum, reaches its maximum weight near puberty and then undergoes involution, or degenerative change, shrinking to about one-sixth of its original size. By the age of 40, the thymus gland is scarcely functional in many individuals; therefore, the essential thymus-provided protein is no longer available to program T-4 cells. More than 20 years ago, thymic protein A was isolated and purified from bovine thymus cells (by Dr. Terry Beardsley, an immunologist). Dr. Beardsley patented a technology to grow thymus cells in the laboratory and then purify a specific thymus protein (Thymic Protein A) that helps T-cells to mature with immune competency.

The active ingredient in Thymic Protein A is the precise thymus protein that programs the T-4 lymphocytes to locate abnormal cells and then directs T-8 killer cells to destroy them.

Three types of cells emerge from the thymus: T-4 helper cells (master regulators), T-8 cytotoxic killer cells (guided by T-4 helper cells to attack and destroy invading cells), and T-8 suppressor cells. T-4 helper cells regulate many key functions, including the activity of IL-2 and interferon.

High dose thymosin, a humoral factor secreted by the thymus, in conjunction with intensive chemotherapy was administered to 21 patients with advanced lung cancer. Ordinarily, patients with late stage lung cancer live about 240 days; the median survival rate more than doubled (500 days) among patients receiving thymosin. Some of the thymosin-treated group were alive and disease-free 2 years after treatment (Chretien et al. 1979).

Blood tests to measure the immune response are extremely valuable when detailing either a preventive or a therapeutic program to fight cancer. While determining T-lymphocyte numbers is important, assessing their activity is even more crucial. It is possible for a person with a total count of 1000 T-4 cells to have only 50% of these cells activated by the thymus. It is important that the patient know the degree of immune impairment in order to structure a corrective program. Tests to evaluate the activity of the immune system are performed at the Immuno-Science Laboratory (Los Angeles), (310) 657-1077.

Suggested dosage: For healthy individuals 1 packet of BioPro Thymic Protein A daily or every other day. Cancer patients may wish to increase this amount. For example, HIV patients use 3 doses a day until blood tests remain normal for 3–6 months. For maintenance, reduce to 1 dose a day. Use the thymic protein under the tongue, retaining for 3 minutes to allow for maximum absorption. Typically, patients undergoing chemotherapy maintain acceptable white blood cell counts if Thymic Protein A accompanies treatment.

Vitamin A—offers protection against radiation induced tissue damage, down-regulates telomerase activity, and is involved at almost every juncture of cancer control

Retinoids induce cell differentiation, control cancer growth and angiogenesis, repair precancerous lesions, prevent secondary carcinogenesis and metastasis, and act as an immunostimulant. After FAR therapy (5-fluorouracil-retino palmitate with radiation and surgery), the disease-specific, 5-year survival was nearly 50% in various head and neck cancers (Yamamoto 2001). Retinoids, at pharmacological levels, assist in preventing the appearance of secondary tumors following curative therapy for epithelial malignancies.

It is well-established that a vitamin A deficiency (in laboratory animals) correlates with a higher incidence of cancer and an increased susceptibility to chemical carcinogens. This is in agreement with epidemiological studies, which indicate that individuals with a lower dietary vitamin A intake are at a higher risk of developing cancer (Sun et al. 2002). The chemotherapeutic possibilities surrounding vitamin A are plentiful.

Two vitamin A analogs currently in large chemoprevention, intervention trials, or epidemiological studies are all-trans-retinoic acid (ATRA) and 13-cis-retinoic acid (13-cis-RA).

Note: *Retinoic acid is biologically active in two forms: all-trans-retinoic acid and 9-cis-retinoic acid. Vitamin A and 13-cis-RA are converted to these biologically active forms.*

Thirty-two women with previously untreated cervical carcinoma (ages 14–60) were treated for at least 2 months using oral 13-cis-RA (1 mg per kg body weight a day) and alpha-interferon subcutaneously (6 million units daily): 16 of the women (50%) had major reactions, including four complete clinical responses. Remission occurred in 15 of the patients within 2 months and in one patient within 1 month; toxicity to treatment was described as manageable (Espinoza et al. 1994). The positive results were replicated in other studies using a similar model (Hansgen et al. 1998, 1999).

The role of 13-cis-RA on a human prostate cancer cell line (LNCaP) was studied. It was found that 13-cis-RA significantly inhibited PSA secretion and the ability to form new tumors. It was also noted that tumors that appeared (having escaped 13-cis-RA inhibition) were smaller compared to tumors in nontreated animals (Dahiya et al. 1994). During the course of 13-cis-RA therapy, prostate cancer cells became more differentiated, that is, they resembled (microscopically) normal prostate cells.

A combination of phenylbutyrate and 13-cis-RA as a differentiation and anti-angiogenesis strategy against prostate cancer was evaluated. Phenylbutyrate, considered nontoxic, is used to arrest tumor growth and induce differentiation of premalignant and malignant cells. Tissue examination of tumors showed decreased cell proliferation and increased apoptosis, as well as reduced microvessel density in animals treated with 13-cis-RA and phenylbutyrate; tumor growth was inhibited by 82–92%. In contrast, researchers reported 13-cis-RA and phenylbutyrate, when used singularly, were suboptimal in terms of clinical benefit (Pili et al. 2001).

A pilot study conducted at M.D. Anderson Cancer Center found ATRA alone ineffective as a long-term treatment for chronic myelogenous leukemia (CML). Only four of 13 subjects showed a transient, nonsustaining indication of an anti-leukemic effect (Cortes et al. 1997). However, combinations of therapeutic agents that included ATRA were promising in the treatment of CML. The combination included alpha-interferon plus ATRA, which reduced proliferation 50–60% (Marley et al. 2002).

Cisplatin (a popular chemotherapeutic agent) shares a similar chemotherapeutic profile with ATRA (the ability to induce cytotoxicity through apoptosis). A combination of ATRA and cisplatin induced apoptosis in significantly more cancer cells, particularly in ovarian and head and neck carcinomas, than either drug alone (Aebi et al. 1997). A combination of ATRA and IL-2 showed therapeutic value in treating resistant metastatic osteosarcoma, a malignant tumor of the bone (Todesco et al. 2000).

For decades, researchers have searched for ways to minimize the damage to the heart during Adriamycin therapy. Adriamycin, though relatively effective, damages the heart muscle. Several animal studies indicated that supplemental vitamin A reduced Adriamycin-induced inflammation and preserved heart tissue. Vitamin A appears not only to counter Adriamycin damage, but also to increase survival in animals (Tesoriere et al. 1994). Vitamin A extends similar protection to patients using cisplatin, a drug often used for bladder and ovarian cancer, as well as small cell carcinoma.

Radiation-induced lung injury frequently limits the total dose of thoracic radiotherapy that can be delivered to a patient undergoing treatment, restricting its effectiveness. Animal studies suggest that supplemental vitamin A may reduce lung inflammation after thoracic radiation and modify radiotherapy damage to the lungs (Redlich et al. 1998).

Vitamin A (in dosages of 25,000 IU a day) offers significant protection against radiation-induced tissue damage. Various cancer patients use more than 100,000 IU of a water-soluble vitamin A liquid a day, a dosage that must be supervised by a physician. Do not supplement with vitamin A if the cancer involves the thyroid gland or if the liver is damaged. Both professionals and patients should consult Appendix A to read about avoiding vitamin A toxicity.

Good food sources of vitamin A include liver and fish liver oils, green and yellow fruits and vegetables such as apricots, asparagus, broccoli, cantaloupe, carrots, collards, papayas, peaches, pumpkins, spinach, and sweet potatoes. High-potency water-soluble vitamin A is available as a dietary supplement.

Vitamin C (ascorbic acid)—has a chemotherapeutic effect on many cancers, promotes collagen production, sequestering the tumor, and reduces the toxicity of conventional therapies

Linus Pauling, winner of the Nobel Prize for chemistry in 1954 and the Nobel Prize for Peace in 1963, believed strongly that vitamin C could play an important role in cancer treatment. Dr. Pauling suggested 10 grams of vitamin C a day for patients with advanced cancer for whom conventional treatments had ceased to be of benefit (Cameron et al. 1993). Over an 8-year period, 500 patients with varying stages and types of cancer were treated with vitamin C therapy. Those receiving 10 grams of vitamin C a day improved their state of well-being, as measured by increased appetite and mental alertness, as well as a decreased need for pain-killing drugs. A retrospective analysis showed that those using vitamin C lived considerably longer than those not supplemented.

Various clinics are using intravenous vitamin C and with positive results. Dr. Hugh Riordan, recognized as a world authority on this procedure, practices from Wichita, KS, at the Center for the Improvement of Human Functioning International. Dr. Riordan's vitamin C story began in 1984 when he treated his first cancer patient; a 70-year-old renal cell carcinoma patient with metastasis to the lung and liver, using injectable vitamin C. Renal cell carcinoma has only a 5% response rate.

The initial treatment began with 15 grams of vitamin C administered intravenously 2 times a week; showing excellent tolerance, the vitamin C dosage was increased to 30 grams twice weekly. Within 6 weeks, the patient showed a favorable response to treatment and at the 12-week interval was pronounced tumor-free. The patient lived 14 additional years and died of congestive heart failure with no evidence of tumors.

In light of the favorable initial response to intravenous (IV) vitamin C, ascorbic acid was investigated. Vitamin C is preferentially toxic to tumor cells, that is, it kills tumor cells but not normal cells.

In low doses, vitamin C assumes the nature of an antioxidant; in high dosages, vitamin C changes roles and becomes a prooxidant, inducing peroxide production. Tumor cells have a relative catalase deficiency, an enzyme necessary to detoxify hydrogen peroxide to water and oxygen. A 10- to 100-fold difference in catalase concentrations exists between tumor cells and normal cells. Without the protection of catalase, peroxide accumulates in cancerous cells, along with aldehydes (toxic byproducts of the reaction), causing death to malignant cells. On the other hand, normal, healthy tissues have the protection of the detoxification enzyme and are spared destruction by peroxide and aldehyde. Vitamin C, a virtually nontoxic nutrient (Bowie et al. 2000), could cause a transient diarrhea if not absorbed properly.

Vitamin C is safe compared to standard chemotherapeutics and has an ability to preserve immune function. Many patients succumb, not because of cancer, but rather from a post-chemotherapeutic toxicity, resulting from a damaged immune system. Vitamin C protects the immune system. Vitamin C is preferentially toxic to many types of cancer cells, including 20 different melanoma cell lines. Ovarian cell lines are more susceptible to vitamin C-induced toxicity than pancreatic cells. Breast cancer appears to be one of the most responsive cancers to IV vitamin C.

Much higher concentrations of vitamin C are required to kill cancer cells than originally thought, about 600 mg/dL. Also, as the density of the cells increases, the efficacy of vitamin C decreases. It is extremely difficult to reach vitamin C concentrations greater than 200 mg/dL even when administered intravenously (Riordan et al. 2000). To increase the sensitivity of tumor cells to vitamin C, other approaches need to be employed.

Alpha-lipoic acid, a water- and lipid-soluble antioxidant that recycles vitamin, enhances the toxic effect of ascorbic acid. Lipoic acid decreases the dose of vitamin C required to kill tumor cells from 700 to 120 mg/dL (Riordan et al. 2000). Vitamin C toxicity is further enhanced by 1000 mcg of vitamin B12, which forms cobalt ascorbate, a benign but cancer-cell toxic agent. Vitamin K, selenium, quercetin, niacinamide, biotin, and grape seed extract are also regarded as potentiation factors.

The goal is to achieve and maintain 400 mg/dL of vitamin C in the plasma. At this concentration, every cancer cell line so far tested has been found to be sensitive to vitamin C. After reaching an ascorbic acid peak, as occurs during infusion, the level returns to near baseline levels 24 hours after the IV infusion.

Vitamin C has an ability to increase collagen production. Vitamin C is required for the hydroxylation of proline, which in turn is required for collagen production. Vitamin C has the ability to inhibit enzymes that degrade or break down the extracellular matrix. Vitamin C dramatically increased the collagen within tumor cells, an act that tended to immobilize the cells.

Vitamin C (supported by lipoic acid) has been used as a cancer therapy. It is strongly advised that patients contact a physician trained in administering infusions and monitoring progress. By giving vitamin C intravenously, doctors can achieve a blood saturation that far exceeds that attained by administering vitamin C orally (200% versus 2%). A high dose of vitamin C is critical to achieve tumor cell kill.

A Hickman line allows large doses of vitamin C to be self-administered at home on a daily to weekly basis over a period of months, modulating down or up in frequency according to response. Otherwise the treatment can be administered as an outpatient. Contraindications to vitamin C therapy are few but include individuals with kidney failure and on dialysis, as well as those with hemochromatosis. Also, physicians should screen patients for a red blood cell glucose-6 phosphate dehydrogenase deficiency, a rare condition whose presence can lead to a hemolytic crisis involving red blood cell breakdown.

Large doses of vitamin C should be reached gradually to establish tolerance. For example, 15 grams for one or two sessions and then 50 grams to 100 grams if necessary. The exact dose is determined by the individual's plasma saturation immediately after an infusion. The therapy should not be stopped abruptly because a rebound effect could result in scurvy. Patients should allow weeks or even months to wean off the treatment, with oral vitamin C therapy used on the days between infusions.

A 10-year research project using high dose IV vitamin C has been completed. While a number of orthomolecular physicians are using IV vitamin C therapy, it is recommended that Dr. Riordan's protocol become the backbone of the therapy. Instructions are available to physicians upon request from the center (Riordan et al. 2003).

Center for the Improvement of Human Functioning
3100 North Hillside Avenue
Wichita, KS 67219
(316) 682-3100

Other chemotherapeutic credits awarded to vitamin C:

- Vitamin C prolongs the lives of animals undergoing conventional cancer treatment by protecting normal cells against chemotherapy-induced toxicity; in tandem, vitamin C increases the cytotoxicity targeted at the cancer (Antunes et al. 1998; Giri et al. 1998). When 5-FU was administered together with vitamin C, the tumor cell kill rate was boosted from 38% to 95.5%. X-ray therapy decreased cancer growth 72%, but adding vitamin C to the regime decreased cancer growth by 98.2%. Full spectrum antioxidants rather than isolated nutrients are suggested (Prasad et al. 1999; Moss 2000).

- Infection: *Heliobacter pylori* increases the risk of developing stomach cancer (Uemura et al. 2001), as well as pancreatic cancer (Stolzenberg-Solomon et al. 2001). High doses of vitamin C inhibit the growth of *H. pylori*, both *in vitro* and *in vivo* (Zhang et al. 1997). A study showed vitamin C levels to be consistently low in individuals with the *H. pylori* infection (The Analyst 2002).

- Frequent intake of vitamin C from food and supplement sources was associated with a protective effect against multiple myeloma, particularly among Caucasians. African Americans benefited less from ascorbic acid intake (Brown et al. 2001).

- NF-kB is a central mediator of altered gene expression during inflammation and is implicated in cancer. Vitamin C inhibited the activation of NF-kB by multiple stimuli, including IL-1 and TNF-alpha (Bowie et al. 2000).

It should be re-emphasized that oral vitamin C does not bestow equal benefits compared to intravenous vitamin C. If a patient with a solid tumor elects to use oral vitamin C, ascorbic acid buffered with sodium may produce better results. If the cancer is bloodborne (leukemia, lymphoma, or myeloma), ascorbic acid crystals buffered with calcium appears to offer greater efficacy. The majority of the patients use 6–12 grams a day. Food sources of vitamin C are berries, citrus fruits, papayas, and pineapple, as well as tomatoes, broccoli, Brussels sprouts, dandelion and mustard greens, peas, red peppers, and spinach.

Vitamin D—promotes differentiation, inhibits angiogenesis, regulates cell division

Current recommendations to avoid natural sunrays to thwart the possibility of deadly melanoma may be allowing other endangerments. For more than 50 years, medical literature has affirmed that regular sun exposure is associated with a substantial decrease in death rates from certain types of cancers. It is estimated that moderate sun exposure without sunscreen—enough to stimulate vitamin D production but not enough to damage the skin—could prevent 30,000 cancer deaths in the United States each year (Ainsleigh 1993). The most damaging of the sun's rays occur between the hours of 10 a.m. and 3 p.m. and are thus the hours demanding the greatest watchfulness.

Evidence points to a prostate, breast, and colon cancer belt in the United States, which lies in northern latitudes under more cloud cover than other regions (Studzinski et al. 1995). Certain regions in the United States, such as the San Joaquin Valley cities and Tucson, AZ; Phoenix, AZ; Albuquerque, NM; El Paso, TX; Miami, FL; Jacksonville, FL; Tampa, FL; and Orlando, FL; have a lower incidence of breast and bowel cancers. Conversely, New York; Chicago; Boston; Philadelphia; New Haven, CT; Pittsburgh; and Cleveland, OH; have the highest rates of breast and intestinal cancer of the 29 major cites in the United States. The greater hours of year-round sunlight correlate to a lower rate of breast and intestinal cancer in the U.S.A.

Vitamin D is formed in the skin of animals and humans by the action of shortwave UV light, the so-called fast-tanning sunrays. Precursors of vitamin D in the skin are converted into cholecalciferol, a weak form of vitamin D3, which is then transported to the liver and kidneys where enzymes convert it to 1,25-dihydroxycholecalciferol, the more potent form of vitamin D3 (Sardi 2000). Although vitamin D exists in two molecular forms, vitamin D3 (cholecalciferol) found in animal skin and vitamin D2 (ergocalciferol) found in yeast, vitamin D3 is believed to exhibit more potent cancer-inhibiting properties and is therefore the preferred form.

Dark-skinned people require more sun exposure to produce vitamin D because the thickness of the skin layer (the stratum corneum) affects the absorption of UV radiation. Black human skin is thicker than white skin and thus transmits only about 40% of the UV rays needed for vitamin D production. Darkly pigmented individuals who live in sunny equatorial climates experience a higher mortality rate from breast and prostate cancer when they move to geographic areas that are deprived of sunlight exposure in winter months (Angwafo 1998; Sardi 2000).

Women with polymorphisms (genetic variations) of the vitamin D receptor gene may be less able to benefit from the nutrient. There is some evidence that vitamin D receptor gene polymorphisms play a role in the breast cancer (Bretherton-Watt et al. 2001); however, recent studies do not support this evidence (Buyru et al. 2003). Identifying the at-risk groups, through the assessment of genetic variations in the vitamin D receptor, appears to be a forthcoming tool for planning intervention strategies.

Human leukemia cells cultured in the presence of vitamin D exhibited a reduced rate of tumor growth when injected into mice. Cells grown in vitamin D3 failed to form detectable tumors in 11 of 12 inoculated mice (Wang et al. 1997). The anticarcinogenic properties of vitamin D, confronts multiple stages of cancer development, including apoptosis, differentiation, angiogenesis, and metastasis, as well as regulating the cell growth cycle (van den Bemd et al. 2002).

Since vitamin D can cause calcium to be released from bones (a condition referred to as hypercalcemia), large doses of vitamin D cannot be used in patients whose medical history or genetics puts them at increased risk. Using a combination of Vitamin D3 and vanadium (a metallic element) enables vitamin D to retain its anticancer activity and vanadium addresses the problem of hypercalcemia (Basak et al. 2000).

Rats were supplemented with vanadium or vitamin D3 or both vanadium and D3 four weeks prior to induced liver cancer and continued thereafter until the 20th week. After 20 weeks of supplementation, the vitamin D3-vanadium combination had significantly reduced the number and size of abnormal hepatic nodules. The combination also showed an additive effect, reducing the number and size of hyperplastic nodes from 83.3% to 37.5%. In addition, vanadium effectively blocked the entry of calcium into cells.

A modified form of vitamin D (referred to as a deltanoid) delays the onset and reduces the number of skin cancers in laboratory mice. The microscopically altered structure of vitamin D produced a potentially effective cancer therapeutic. The vitamin D analog retains its anticancer profile but diminishes the threat of hypercalcemia. The most effective of four analogs tested was a doubly modified hybrid compound containing fluorine (Posner 2000).

During one study, mice painted with a chemical substance, inducing cancerous tumors were concurrently the animals were given the deltanoid. After 20 weeks, the fluorine-containing analog had reduced the incidence of tumors more than 28%, while the actual number fell 63% (Kensler et al. 2000). Deltanoids are in the early stages of development and, unfortunately, it may take 10 years before they become available (Guyton et al. 2003). It is possible that deltanoids could lessen the need for hormone treatments or aggressive chemotherapy. Patients could theoretically stay on the treatment for the remainder of their life to keep the cancer from advancing.

Studies indicate that moderate or severe hypovitaminosis D was present in 66% of patients taking daily vitamin D in amounts less than the recommended dosage for their age. Adults may need a minimum of 5 times the 200-IU RDA, (or 1000 IU daily), to protect against cancer (Vieth 1999). Therapeutic dosages of vitamin D typically range from 800–4000 IU a day. Monthly kidney function blood tests (creatine, BUN, etc.) should be performed if daily vitamin D intake exceeds 1400 IU. These tests are included in most standard blood chemistry tests that cancer patients regularly perform to guard against anemia and overt immunosuppression.

Food sources of vitamin D include egg yolks, organ meats, fortified dairy products, butter, cod liver oil, and cold-water fish, such as salmon, herring, and mackerel. Vitamin D enhancers are vitamins A and C, calcium, magnesium, phosphorus, and choline. Antagonists are mineral oil, phenobarbital, and laxatives.

Vitamin E—is an antioxidant that can protect smokers, reduces radiation damage, potentiates chemotherapy, and inhibits many types of cancers

The inhibitory role of vitamin E in the growth of a number of human tumor cells, as well as its defensive functions in overcoming treatment-induced toxicity have been examined. The impact of vitamin E (perhaps acting through its antioxidant strengths) is significant, as evidenced by the following studies:

- After examining 29,000 male smokers in Finland, researchers found that high blood levels of alpha-tocopherol reduced the incidence of lung cancer by approximately 19%. The relationship appears stronger among younger persons and among those with less cumulative smoke exposure. These findings suggest that high levels of alpha-tocopherol, if present during the early critical stages of tumorigenesis, may inhibit lung cancer development (Woodson et al. 1999).

- A combination of vitamin E and pentoxifylline (PTX), a drug that inhibits abnormal platelet aggregation, allowing more blood to reach irradiated areas, resulted in a 50% regression of superficial radiation-induced fibrosis (the proliferation of fibrous connective tissue) in half of the patients studied (Gottlober et al. 1996; Delanian 1998). A suggested dosage is 800 mg a day of PTX and 1000 IU per day of vitamin E.

- An anti-melanoma effect obtained from vitamin E succinate *in vivo* has been reported (Malafa et al. 2002).

- Gamma-tocopherol inhibits COX-2 activity, demonstrating anti-inflammatory properties (Jiang et al. 2001; *Life Extension Magazine* 2002).

- The use of vitamin E, in combination with vitamins A and C, led to a four-fold reduction in p53 mutations (Brotzman et al. 1999). This is an extremely important finding because p53 mutations indicate a more malignant, aggressive form of cancer.

- Men with a high intake of vitamin E are 65% less likely to develop colorectal adenomas (precursors to colon cancer) compared to men with low vitamin E intake (Tseng et al. 1996).

- Lower morbidity and mortality from prostate cancer in men taking 50 mg of synthetic alpha-tocopherol daily. Subsequent testing determined gamma-tocopherol to be superior, however, to alpha-tocopherol in terms of tumor cell inhibition (Moyad et al. 1999). Men in the highest fifth of the distribution for gamma-tocopherol had a five-fold reduction in the risk of developing prostate cancer compared to those in the lowest fifth. In addition, statistically significant protection from high levels of selenium and alpha-tocopherol occurred only when gamma-tocopherol concentrations were also high (Helzlsourer et al. 2000).

- Vitamin E's mode of efficacy in regard to prostate protection: Vitamin E interferes with two proteins (the receptor for testosterone and prostate-specific antigen [PSA]). The fewer androgen receptors there are on a prostate cancer cell, the less capable the remaining receptors are of turning on genes that stimulate prostate cancer growth and progression. PSA serves as a good marker molecule for androgen receptor activity (Mercola 2002b).

- Tocotrienols, quite similar to a tocopherol (but for the addition of an unsaturated tail in its chemical structure), accumulate in adipose tissues, including mammary glands. If a cell becomes diseased, the tocotrienol is prepared for action, ready to inhibit growth and regulate aberrant cellular activity at onset. Curiously, the more cancerous the cell, the more susceptible it is to tocotrienols. Scientists apparently have been focusing upon the wrong form of vitamin E (the tocopherols), which show little protection against breast cancer. Tocotrienols appear to inhibit proliferation of human breast cancer cells by as much as 50% (Nesaretnam et al. 1998). Results suggest that tocotrienols are effective inhibitors of both estrogen receptor-negative and estrogen receptor-positive cells and that combination with tamoxifen should be considered as a possible improvement in breast cancer therapy. This strategy could significantly reduce the amount of tamoxifen required to affect the cancer (Guthrie et al. 1997).

- Cortisol (associated with poorer survival) and IL-6 (a negative marker for various cancers) were significantly lower in laboratory animals that received alpha-tocopherol before a cortisol-IL-6 challenge (Webel et al. 1998).

Vitamin E	Chemotherapeutic Agent	Combination with Vitamin E
47% growth inhibition	Bleomycin, 46% tumor reduction	71% reduction
	5-FU, 37% tumor reduction	85% reduction
	Adriamycin, 58% tumor reduction	88% reduction
	Cisplatin, 57% tumor reduction	82% reduction

A suggested vitamin E dosage is from 400–1200 IU a day of alpha-tocopherol together with gamma E tocopherol. For optimal results, use 80% alpha-tocopherol and 20% gamma-tocopherol. A tocotrienol dosage is 240 mg each day. Good food sources of vitamin E are cold-pressed vegetable oils, wheat germ, eggs, dark green vegetables, nuts, brown rice, and butter.

Vitamin K—is a growth regulator, promotes apoptosis, and decreases pro-inflammatory cytokines

A novel form of vitamin K that appears extremely promising in the treatment of primary liver cancer, a type notoriously resistant to chemotherapy has been discovered by scientists at the University of Pittsburgh Cancer Institute (UPCI). The research published in the *Journal of Biological Chemistry* described an innovative approach to treat, and possibly prevent, cancer by triggering apoptosis (Ni et al. 1998).

The UPCI team found that a vitamin K analog, Compound 5 (CPD5), causes an imbalance in the normal activity of enzymes that controls the addition or removal of small molecules (phosphate groups) from proteins inside cells. Specifically, CPD5 blocks the activity of enzymes (protein-tyrosine phosphatases) that normally remove phosphate groups from selected proteins inside liver cancer cells. CPD5, however, does not interfere with another group of enzymes called protein tyrosine-kinases, which add phosphate groups to the same proteins. The result is an excess of tyrosine-phosphorylated proteins, which triggers a variety of activities within cells, including the shutting down and subsequent death of the cell.

It may be possible to remove some individuals from liver transplant waiting lists if CPD5 is as effective in humans as it is experimentally. However, the vitamin K compound is not limited to killing liver cancer; in tissue culture the compound was also effective against melanoma and breast cancers. Although the new vitamin K is not in clinical testing at this time, clients and physicians may contact the UPCI's Cancer Information and Referral Service at (800) 237-4PCI (4724) or (412) 624-1115 for periodic updates regarding the treatment. Inquirers can also visit the university's website at http://www.upci.upmc.edu.

Vitamin K compounds inhibited IL-6 production by lipopolysaccharide-stimulated fibroblasts, which are recognized as rich sources of cytokines (Reddi et al. 1995). This finding has significant anticancer implications because over-expression of IL-6 is intricately involved in the inflammatory process, bone resorption, the activation of telomerase, and cancer proliferation. A suggested vitamin K dosage is 10 mg a day. Interesting research relating to the use of vitamin K concurrent with anticoagulant therapy (not usually a recommended practice) appears in the protocol *Cardiovascular Disease: Comprehensive Analysis* in the section dedicated to vitamin K.

OTHER FACTORS AFFECTING PATIENT OUTCOME

What Should Cancer Patients Eat?

For a cancer patient who appreciates the importance of a properly planned diet, the task is daunting. The diversity of the population minimizes the likelihood of a universal diet; nonetheless, most diets are hyped as being nutritionally correct for everyone. This section explores dietary variables, conceding that many generalities exist, that is, eat organic when available and eat on schedule to avoid blood glucose swings. Select foods characterized by color and texture. Avoid synthetic and refined foods: white flour products and sugar as well as trans fats (those fats altered by overheating, hydrogenation, and refining). Avoiding well-done meats and exposure to heterocyclic amines (formed during high temperature cooking) eliminates another significant cancer source (Zheng et al. 1998).

Tumors are primarily obligate glucose metabolizers, meaning they require sugar for survival. Even though the brain normally uses high amounts of glucose, hepatomas (a tumor of the liver) and fibrosarcomas (a sarcoma that contains fibrous connective tissue) consume roughly as much glucose as the brain. Some Americans continuously satisfy cancer's appetite, ingesting as much as 295 pounds of sugar a year.

Nobel laureate Otto Warburg, Ph.D., discovered in 1955 that cancer cells use glucose for fuel. But glucose accomplishes another strategic maneuver that strongly favors the cancer: it immobilizes internal defenses, the actions of the immune system. A study involving 10 healthy human volunteers assessed fasting blood glucose levels and the phagocytic index of neutrophils, a type of white blood cell. Glucose, fructose, sucrose, honey, and orange juice all significantly decreased the capacity of neutrophils to engulf bacteria. A diet structured away from sugars deprives cancer of its energy and increases the reliability of the immune response.

Dr. Jeff Bland advises selecting foodstuffs low on the glycemic index to avoid gratifying the tumor's appetite. The glycemic index lists the relative speed at which different foods are digested and raise blood sugar levels. Each food is compared to the effect of the same amount of pure glucose on the body's blood sugar curve. Glucose itself has a glycemic index rating of 100. Foods that are broken down and raise blood glucose levels quickly have higher ratings. The closer to 100, the more the food resembles glucose. The lower the rating, the more gradually that food affects blood sugar levels.

Common foods have the following glycemic ratings: baked potatoes, 95; white bread, 95; mashed potatoes, 90; chocolate candy bar, 70; corn, 70; boiled potatoes, 70; bananas, 60; white pasta, 55; peas, 50; unsweetened fruit juice, 40; rye bread, 40; lentils, 30; soy, 15; green vegetables; and tomatoes, < 15.

Note: *The glycemic index should not be relied upon without factoring in the glycemic load, which is the glycemic index of a food times its carbohydrate content in grams, a concept developed at Harvard School of Public Health in 1997. Carrots, for instance, have a high glycemic index, but a very low glycemic load. This means that carrots consumed in moderation usually do not present a problem. Refer to the Obesity protocol for complete information about the glycemic index load.*

An admonition, based more on folk medicine than scientific certainty, to avoid the white foods (all sugar-containing foods, as well as rice, and white flour and flour-based products) appears to have validity when applied to the glycemic index. A diet structured principally around carbohydrates that promotes hyperglycemia (high blood sugar level) and hyperinsulinemia (high blood insulin level) provides an environment that feeds the fire of cancer. High blood insulin levels drive protein tyrosine kinase (leading to cell division) and high blood glucose metabolically feeds cancer cells. On the other hand, a diet centered on fiber-, vitamin-, and mineral-rich foods that cause no blood glucose rise or insulin rush is an excellent target for healthy eating.

The diseases such as obesity and diabetes mellitus (often characterized by hyperinsulinemia) are associated with an increased risk of endometrial, colorectal, and breast cancers. The mechanisms underlying insulin-mediated neoplasias appear to include enhanced DNA synthesis (with the resultant tumor cell growth), inhibited apoptosis, and an altered sex hormone milieu. The reduced insulin levels seen with physical activity, weight loss, and a high fiber diet may in fact account for the decreased cancer incidence observed in individuals who maintain normal glucose and insulin levels (Gupta et al. 2002). *Comment:* Reducing blood insulin levels may result in remarkable improvements in men with prostate disease, with a concurrent drop in PSA levels (Hsing et al. 2001).

Unfortunately, glucose modulation is an underutilized component of cancer treatment. Some aspects of traditional treatments actually contribute to higher blood levels of glucose. For example, consider hospital meals, often favoring sugar-based foodstuffs. In addition, if the patient is on an IV solution, the infusion is largely dextrose-based, feeding the cancer and perpetuating its growth.

The American Cancer Society believes that 30% of all cancer is due to inadequate consumption of vegetables and fruits. About 91% of Americans fail to achieve target recommendations, that is, 5 vegetable servings a day or 2–3 pounds a week. Asians who consume from 15–20 servings of fruits and vegetables a day have a much lower incidence of some cancers.

Vegetables of the cruciferous family isolate the anticarcinogenic constituents of *Brassica* plants. Glucosinolates (appearing in cruciferous vegetables) can inhibit, retard, or even reverse experimental multistage carcinogenesis (Fimognari et al. 2002). As enzymatic processes hydrolyze glucosinolates, isothiocyanates are released, including sulphoraphane. Sulphoraphane wields a strong arm against cancer, promoting apoptosis, inducing Phase II detoxification enzymes, increasing p53 and participating in the regulatory mechanisms of the cell's growth cycle. Necrosis (localized death of diseased tissues) is typically observed after prolonged exposure to elevated doses of sulphoraphane.

For the past several years, researchers at Johns Hopkins University have urged the inclusion of broccoli sprouts in the diet. According to Dr. Paul Talalay, broccoli sprouts have 20–50 times more anticancer sulphoraphanes than grown vegetables (Fahey et al.

1997). Eating a few tablespoons of sprouts daily can supply the same amount of chemoprotection as 1–2 pounds of broccoli eaten weekly (Talalay 1997).

Broccoli sprouts contain a chemical that kills *H. pylori,* even in antibiotic-resistant conditions. The release of anticarcinogenic chemicals from *Brassica* vegetables is a sequential process that occurs as the plant tissue is broken down. Indole-3-carbinol (I3C), a product of cruciferous metabolism, is referred to as a secondary metabolite, meaning it is not found in a preformed state in the vegetables. Rather, I3C is formed after myrosinase (an enzyme inherent to the plant) is exposed to a phytochemical in the vegetable (glucobrassicin), a glucosinolate that subsequently delivers indole-3-carbinol. This occurs only when vegetable cells are crushed or eaten, a process known as enzymatic hydrolysis. I3C, thus formed, is then broken down in the presence of stomach acid to various byproducts including diindolylmethane (DIM), another powerful defense against cancer (Lukaczer 2001). It appears highly possible that the breakdown products of I3C may be delivering as much protection as I3C itself (Katchamart et al. 2001; Lukaczer 2001; Lord et al. 2002).

An undesirable effect is the conversion of estrone to a carcinogenic material called 16-alpha hydroxyestrone that damages DNA and inhibits apoptosis. The ratio of 2-hydroxyestrone to 16-hydroxyestrone indicates a woman's risk for developing breast and ovarian cancer. Levels of 2-hydroxyestrone are typically higher in women who do not get cancer; 16-hydroxyestrone is higher in women with cancer. When breast cancer cells are treated with I3C (*in vitro*) 90% of cells undergo growth inhibition, whether the cells are estrogen positive or negative (Galland 2000).

Broccoli (500 grams for 12 days) increased the average 2-alpha-hydroxyestrone: 16-alpha-hydroxyestrone ratio (Kall et al. 1997). Hence, consuming vegetables rich in indole-3-carbinol gives hope that as 2-hydroxyestrone increases, cancers will be decreased in both men and women. The ability of I3C to neutralize estrogen metabolites as well as to block aflatoxin (a mycotoxin that promotes prostate cancer) makes cruciferous vegetables equally important to men.

By inhibiting protein kinases and other growth factors, restoring p21 activity, and encouraging apoptosis, I3C appears an effective chemopreventive/therapeutic agent against many types of malignancies (Chinni et al. 2001; Roman-Gomez et al. 2002). Evidencing its benefits, I3C reduced the incidence of cervical cancer from 76 to 8% in laboratory mice (Jin et al. 1999), and administered together with tamoxifen, I3C inhibited the growth of estrogen-dependent human MCF-7 breast cancer more effectively than either agent used alone (Cover et al. 1999).

If vegetables providing I3C are in short supply in the diet, indole-3-carbinol capsules are available. For those under 120 pounds, one 200-mg capsule taken 2 times a day is suggested; those between 120–180 pounds could take 200 mg 3 times a day, while those over 180 pounds could take four 200 mg a day. If the diet generally lacks adequate amounts of vegetables, powdered vegetable extracts are available, an example is PhytoFood; a suggested dosage for cancer patients is 1–2 tbsp daily (with food).

Cholesterol (Can It Be Too Low?)

Hypocholesterolemia (abnormally low levels of cholesterol) has been shown in several epidemiological studies to be related to increased mortality from human cancer. Cholesterol and triglyceride levels in 135 patients with squamous cell and small cell lung carcinoma were evaluated. All lung cancer patients had higher rates of hypocholesterolemia as well as lower triglyceride levels compared to a healthy control group. Total cholesterol concentrations were lower in both histological types, but triglyceride levels were lower only in patients with squamous cell lung cancer (Siemianowicz et al. 2000).

An article in *Hematology and Oncology* reported that 90% of 83 patients with acute myeloid leukemia were hypocholesterolemic (Zyada et al. 1990). Additionally, another article in the *European Journal of Haemtology* reported that remission in acute myelogenous leukemia was associated with a significant increase in cholesterol levels in those patients with low cholesterol concentrations or high leukocyte counts at diagnosis (Reverter et al. 1988).

Various reports have emerged showing that low cholesterol levels are associated with higher death rates (particularly among elderly people), from cancer and infection (Weverling-Rijnsburger et al. 1997; Schatz et al. 2001). These findings raise concerns regarding hypocholesterolemic drug therapy and diet manipulation to drastically lower cholesterol levels in a subset of the population.

STRESS AND CANCER

Few events are as stressful as a diagnosis of cancer. As the stress level increases, the outpouring of the adrenal cortex hormone (cortisol) also increases. Women with breast cancer who had abnormal cortisol rhythms survived an average of 3.2 years, while those with normal rhythms survived an average of 4.5 years (more than a year longer). The difference in survival times began to emerge about 1 year after the cortisol testing and continued for at least 6 additional years (Richter 2000).

Animal studies, mostly involving rats, demonstrated stress as a causal factor in cancer. The onset of cancer appears similarly allied in humans, with the immune system highly responsive to emotional pitfalls. It is well established that when the individual is emotionally challenged, cancer has a significant advantage (Levy et al. 1987).

Psychobiologist Shamgar Ben-Eliyahu, Ph.D., has been working for the past decade on stress, tumor development, and the activity of NK cells (Ben-Eliyahu et al. 2000). Considering all immune system cells, NK cells show the strongest activity in preventing metastasis and the strongest response to stress. Even short-term stress decreases NK cell activity in laboratory animals, significantly increasing the risk of certain types of cancer and metastasis. Gender plays a significant role in the NK cell response to stress, with men more adversely affected than women (Irwin 2000). The stress of abdominal surgery promotes the growth of cancerous tumors in rats, a sequence thought orchestrated by NK cell suppression (Ben-Eliyahu et al. 1999).

High levels of neuropeptide-gamma are observed in the bloodstream of depressed individuals, an elevation synonymous with immune suppression (Ader et al. 1981; Scanlan et al. 2001). Macrophages (pathogen scavengers) have receptor sites that attract endorphins (mood enhancers with analgesic traits). With the right emotional programming, white blood cells swim through the bloodstream with determination; conversely, under stress, immune competence falters, and the immune attack becomes lethargic.

Breast cancer patients with the most anxiety had a weaker immune response and were less equipped to fight the disease. The following stress-associated situations and personality types are associated with breast cancer: (1) the use of denial or repression as a coping strategy, (2) an experience of separation or loss, (3) a history of stressful life experiences, (4) a tendency toward melancholy and hopelessness (this trait has, since antiquity, been associated with uterine and breast cancers), and (5) a personality type characterized by conflict avoidance. It is theorized that the genes that cause one to avoid conflict are the same genes that increase susceptibility to cancer (Goodkin et al. 1986; Darmon 1993).

Also, psychological stress induces the production of pro-inflammatory cytokines, such as TNF-alpha, IL-6, and IL-10 (Maes et al. 2000). Please turn to the protocol *Cancer: Gene Therapies, Stem Cells, Telomeres, and Cytokines* for a full discussion regarding pro-inflammatory cytokine's role in malignancies.

The effect of chronic stress on the immune system of 116 recently treated breast cancer patients found (reproducibly) that stress levels significantly predicted (1) lower NK cell activity, (2) diminished response of NK cells to interferon-gamma, and (3) decreased proliferation of lymphocytes, white blood cells considered the army of the immune system (Andersen et al. 1998). Oncologists often suggest stress management, such as meditation, yoga and breathing exercises, guided imagery, or spirituality, to help bring about calm.

Because the cells responsible for cancer surveillance work best in an environment favoring confidence and calm, it is important that the message springing from our thoughts and transmitted to cells is commensurate with healing. Fright, pessimism, and melancholy send uncertain instructions and the cells respond with a feeble effort. The enduring message (fear or assurance, despair or hopefulness, laughter or tears) reflects our hour-to-hour psyche and sets the tone for health victories or failures. Expect little more from your body than the quality of your thoughts at this very moment: "As a man thinks in his heart, so is he" (Proverbs 23:7).

⚫ SUMMARY

The drugs, hormones, and nutrients discussed in this protocol have documented mechanisms of action that may benefit the cancer patient. The objective of implementing an adjuvant regimen consisting of multiple agents is to increase the odds of achieving a long remission. Once a remission is achieved, preventing recurrence and secondary cancers becomes a lifetime commitment.

Few oncologists aggressively seek to prevent recurrence once the primary disease appears to have been eradicated. However, the regrettable facts are that colonies of cancer cells can remain dormant in the body for years or decades before reappearing as full-blown disease that is highly resistant to treatment. This has been documented in autopsy studies of people who died of diseases other than cancer but nonetheless showed significant residual metastatic tumors in their bodies.

In too many cases, a breast, melanoma, or other cancer reemerges that was supposed to have been cured. Scientists speculate that the body has natural anticancer control mechanisms that may diminish with age and exposure to physical and emotional stress factors. It is thus important for cancer patients to be vigilant in maintaining an inhospitable environment for cancer cells to propagate and protecting against age-associated immune dysfunction.

We have prepared the following chart to summarize recommendations on the basic dietary supplements and suggested doses for cancer prevention and adjuvant treatment. In addition to the agents listed here, a number of other potential adjuvant approaches are discussed in this protocol. For long-term control of cancer, some cancer patients attempt to incorporate as many of these adjuvant approaches as are tolerable and affordable. Others pick and choose which drugs, hormones, and supplements they want to consume over the long term.

Patients should read the other cancer protocols in this book, with special attention given to *Cancer: Should Patients Take Dietary Supplements?* and *Cancer Treatment: The Critical Factors*. If surgery, radiation, or chemotherapy is being considered, please refer to these specific protocols: *Cancer Surgery, Cancer Radiation,* and *Cancer Chemotherapy*.

Note: *While it would be wholly inappropriate for the Life Extension Foundation to steer individuals in decisions of omission or commission regarding therapies, it would be equally improper to shun responsibility. Because we are challenged by a professional and moral commitment to assist in overcoming appalling statistics, we have discussed some controversial issues in this protocol. We look forward to new findings to better substantiate optimal therapeutic approaches.*

Nutrient	Preventive Dose	Cancer Adjuvant Dose
Super Alpha-Lipoic Acid w/Biotin	250–500 mg/day	500–1000 mg/day
Coenzyme Q10	30–300 mg/day	Up to 400 mg/day
EPA-DHA fatty acids	1400 mg/day	2000–4000 mg/day
Garlic (PureGar Caps) or	900 mg/day	Up to 7200 mg/day
Kyolic Aged Garlic (1000 mg)	1 caplet daily	3 caplets daily
Green Tea (350 mg)	1–2 caps/day	5 capsules 3 times/day
Life Extension Mix*	1 tbsp of powder, 9 tabs, or 14 capsules daily	or 14 capsules daily 1 tbsp of powder, 9 tabs, or 14 capsules daily
Liquid Emulsified Vitamin A	Up to 35,000 IU/day**	Up to 100,000 IU/day**
Vitamin C (included in LE Mix)	6–12 grams/day	
Vitamin D3	Up to 1400 IU/day	800–4000 IU/day**
Gamma Tocopherol/Tocotrienol Formula	1 capsule/day	2–4 capsules/day
Grape Seed Extract	100 mg/day	300 mg/day
Phyto-Food (cruciferous vegetable concentrate)	1 tbsp/day	1–4 tbsp/day
Melatonin	300 mcg–6 mg/day	3–50 mg/day
Selenium (included in LE Mix)	200–400 mcg/day	200–400 mcg/day
Silibinin	260 mg/day	Up to 2000 mg/day
Curcumin	900 mg/day	2700 mg 3 times/day
GLA (gamma-linolenic acid)	900 mg/day	900 mg/day

*Those individuals using the Life Extension Mix (powder, tablets, or capsules) are receiving a storehouse of nutrients targeted at maintaining good health. Very few of the cornerstone nutrients are not contained in the Life Extension Mix Formula, but exceptions are alpha-lipoic acid, coenzyme Q10, essential fatty acids, garlic, and melatonin. If indicated, the reader may wish to emphasize these nutrients for maximum support. Some people bolster their nutritional program by incorporating the Life Extension Booster (complete with gamma E tocopherol) together with the Life Extension Mix. These formulas are popular from both financial and convenience perspectives. While individuals with cancer will benefit from these suggestions, a more comprehensive program is recommended, such as supplements with precise anticancer mechanisms, targeted at specific cancer cell lines or established weaknesses.

**Refer to safety precautions that appear in this protocol when taking high doses of vitamins A and D.

PRODUCT AVAILABILITY

Alpha-lipoic acid, alpha-tocopherol succinate, L-arginine, buffered ascorbic acid, Bio Pro Thymic Protein A, biotin, calcium, Cell Forte with IP-6, Chloroplex, coenzyme Q10, conjugated linoleic acid (CLA), flaxseed oil, Gamma-E-Tocopherol/Tocotrienols, glutathione, goldenseal, grape seed-skin extract, green tea bags (organic), Kyolic Garlic, indole-3-carbinol, lactoferrin, L-glutamine, Life Extension Mix (caps, powder, or tablets), Mega EPA, Mega GLA, melatonin, N-acetyl-cysteine, Pecta-Sol, perilla oil, Phyto-Food, Pure-Gar Caps, Super Curcumin, Super Max EPA, Super GLA/DHA, selenium, Silibinin Plus, Ultra Soy Extract, Super Green Tea Extract, theanine, tocotrienols, vitamin A, vitamin B12, vitamin D, and vitamin E are available by calling (800) 544-4440 or by ordering online.

STAYING INFORMED

The information published in this protocol is only as current as the day the book was sent to the printer. This cancer protocol raises many issues that are subject to change as new data emerge. Furthermore, cancer is still a disease with unacceptably high mortality rates, and none of our suggested treatment regimens can guarantee a cure. The Life Extension Foundation is constantly uncovering information to provide the cancer patient with more ammunition to battle their disease. A special website has been established for the purpose of updating patients on new findings that directly pertain to the cancer protocols published in this book. Whenever Life Extension discovers information that points to a better way of treating cancer, it will be posted on the website

www.lefcancer.org.

Before utilizing the cancer protocols in this book, we suggest that you log on to www.lefcancer.org to see if any substantive changes have been made to the recommendations described in this protocol. Based on the sheer number of newly published findings, there could be significant alterations to the information you have just read.

Alternatively, call 1-800-226-2370 and ask a Health Advisor if your topic of interest has been updated on the website

www.lefcancer.org

DISCLAIMER

This information (and any accompanying printed material) is not intended to replace the attention or advice of a physician or other health care professional. Anyone who wishes to embark on any dietary, drug, exercise, or other lifestyle change intended to prevent or treat a specific disease or condition should first consult with and seek clearance from a qualified health care professional.

The information published in the protocols is only as current as the day the book was sent to the printer. This protocol raises many issues that are subject to change as new data emerge. None of our suggested treatment regimens can guarantee a cure for these diseases.

Cancer Chemotherapy

Cancer cells are everything we would like healthy cells to be: They quickly adapt to toxic environments, they readily alter themselves to assure their continued survival, and they utilize biologic mechanisms to promote cellular immortality. All of these factors make cancer an extremely difficult disease to treat.

Chemotherapy drugs have a high rate of failure because they usually kill only specific types of cancer cells within a tumor or the cancer cells mutate and become resistant to the chemotherapy. Cancer chemotherapy could save more lives if the latest scientific findings were incorporated into clinical medicine.

What concerns us is that respected cancer journals are publishing articles that identify safer and more effective treatment regimens, yet few oncologists are incorporating these synergistic methods into their clinical practice. Cancer patients often suffer through chemotherapy sessions that do not integrate the latest scientific findings. Our objective is to provide the patient with more options to discuss with their oncologist and to bring about multi-modality approaches to improve the probability of a successful outcome.

It is impossible to design a single chemotherapy protocol that is effective against all types of cancer. The oncologist might need to administer several chemotherapy drugs at varying doses because tumor cells express survival factors with a wide degree of individual cell variability. This protocol conveys the findings from published scientific studies so that a cancer patient will have a logical basis to augment the effects of chemotherapy and also reduce the potential for side effects.

HOW DOES CHEMOTHERAPY WORK?

According to the National Cancer Institute, almost all normal cells grow and die in a controlled way through a process called *apoptosis*. Cancer cells, on the other hand, keep dividing and forming more cells without a control mechanism to induce normal apoptosis.

Anticancer drugs destroy cancer cells by stopping them from growing or dividing at one or more points in their growth cycle. Chemotherapy may consist of one or several cytotoxic drugs that kill cells by one or more mechanisms. The chemotherapy regimen chosen by most conventional oncologists is based on the type of cancer being treated. As you will read later in this protocol, there are factors other than the type of cancer that can be used to determine the ideal chemotherapy drugs that should be used to treat an individual patient.

The goal of chemotherapy is to shrink primary tumors, slow the tumor growth, and kill cancer cells that may have spread (metastasized) to other parts of the body from the original, primary tumor. However, chemotherapy kills both cancer cells and healthy normal cells. Oncologists try to minimize damage to normal cells and to enhance the cell killing (cytotoxic) effect on cancer cells. Too often, unfortunately, this delicate balance is not achieved.

Clinical studies show that for certain types of cancer chemotherapy prolongs survival and increases the percentage of patients achieving a remission. A *partial remission* is defined as 50% or greater reduction in the measurable parameters of tumor growth as may be found on physical examination, radiologic study, or by biomarker levels from a blood or urine test. A *complete remission* is defined as complete disappearance of all such manifestations of disease. The goal of all oncologists is to strive for a complete remission that lasts a long time—a durable complete remission, or *CR*. Unfortunately, the vast majority of remissions that are achieved are partial remissions. Too often, these are measured in weeks to months and not in years. Some types of cancer do not show any meaningful response to chemotherapy.

CHOOSING THE BEST CHEMOTHERAPY DRUGS TO KILL YOUR TUMOR

It is highly desirable to know what drugs are effective against your particular cancer cells before these toxic agents are systemically administered to your body. A company called Rational Therapeutics, Inc., performs chemosensitivity tests on living specimens of your cancer cells to determine the optimal combination of chemotherapy drugs.

Dr. Robert Nagourney, a prominent hematologist/ oncologist, founded Rational Therapeutics, Inc., in 1993. Rational Therapeutics pioneers cancer therapies that are specifically tailored for each individual patient. They are a leader in individualized cancer strategies. With no economic ties to outside healthcare organizations, recommendations are made without financial or scientific prejudice.

Rational Therapeutics develops and provides cancer therapy recommendations that have been designed scientifically for each patient. Following the collection of living cancer cells obtained at the time of biopsy or surgery, Rational Therapeutics performs an Ex-Vivo Apoptotic (EVA) assay on your tumor sample to measure drug activity (sensitivity and resistance). This will determine exactly which drug(s) will be most effective for you. They then make a treatment recommendation. The treatment program developed through this approach is known as *assay-directed therapy*.

At present, medical oncologists, according to fixed schedules, prescribe chemotherapy. These schedules are standardized drug regimens that correspond to specific cancers by type or diagnosis. These schedules, developed over many years of clinical trials, assign patients to the drugs for which they have the greatest statistical probability of response.

Patients with cancers that exhibit multidrug resistance will likely receive treatments that are wrong for them. A failed attempt at chemotherapy is detrimental to the physical and emotional well being of patients, is financially burdensome, and may preclude further effective therapies.

Rational Therapeutics' EVA assay uses your living tumor cells to determine which drug or drug combination induces apoptosis in the laboratory. Each patient is highly individualized with regard to sensitivity to chemotherapy drugs. A patient's responsiveness to chemotherapy is as unique as their fingerprints.

Rational Therapeutics, leading the way in custom-tailored, assay-directed therapy, provides personal cancer strategies based on the tumor response in the laboratory. This eliminates much of the guesswork prior to the patient undergoing the potentially toxic side effects of chemotherapy regimens that could prove to be of little value against their cancer. Rational Therapeutics may be contacted at:

Rational Therapeutics, Inc.

750 East 29th Street

Long Beach, CA 90806

Telephone: (562) 989-6455; Fax: (562) 989-8160

Web site: www.rationaltherapeutics.com

In addition to the EVA chemosensitivity testing, we advocate immunohistochemistry testing of your tumor to provide additional data that will assist in making treatment decisions. The importance of the immunohistochemistry test is described in the *Cancer Treatment: The Critical Factors* protocol. The immunohistochemistry test can be done if your physician sends a specimen of your tumor to a specialty laboratory called Impath (www.impath.com). Impath can be reached by calling (800) 447-5816. Impath also performs chemosensitivity testing of living tumors (fresh specimens). Because many chemotherapy patients' primary tumors were previously removed or irradiated, Impath can perform the immunohistochemistry test with a frozen or paraffin-preserved tissue sample that is accessible through the pathology laboratory that examined your previous tumor(s).

Protecting Against Anemia

The importance of maintaining or enhancing the oxygen-carrying capacity of blood cannot be overemphasized. Blood oxygen-carrying capacity may be the single most important factor in determining whether chemotherapy is successful.

In response to a low-oxygen environment, cancer cells send out growth signals that result in increased angiogenesis (blood vessel growth into the tumor). Oxygen deprivation not only induces angiogenesis, but also causes cancer cells to express additional survival factors that make them highly resistant to the toxic effects of chemotherapy.

It is an established fact that a low-oxygen environment (hypoxia) promotes tumor growth. If nothing else in this protocol is followed, correcting a hypoxic state could vastly enhance the odds of long-term survival.

The first step in correcting hypoxia is to guard against anemia. Anemia is common in cancer patients, and the result is that less oxygen is delivered to the tumor, that is, hypoxia occurs. The importance of avoiding anemia is well established in scientific literature. A study was conducted to systematically review and obtain an estimate of the effect of anemia on the survival of cancer patients. This study found that the increased risk of mortality in cancer patients who were anemic was an astounding 65% (Caro et al. 2001)!

Chemotherapy often induces anemia that then exacerbates hypoxia in the tumor. The best way of evaluating blood oxygen-carrying capacity is to measure *hematocrit* and *hemoglobin* levels. These are standard components of the complete blood count (CBC) test that should be routinely performed in all cancer patients.

Since cancer cells thrive in a hypoxic environment, the cancer patient's hematocrit and hemoglobin should be maintained in the upper one-third of normal range prior to the initiation of chemotherapy. Table 1 describes the optimal ranges of hematocrit and hemoglobin for cancer patients.

Table 1: *Optimal Ranges of Cancer Patients' Hematocrit and Hemoglobin Levels*

Based on findings from survival studies, cancer patients should fall within the optimal ranges of the following two blood tests that measure the oxygen-carrying capacity of blood:

Blood measure		Normal laboratory reference range	Optimal range for cancer patients
Hemoglobin	(men)	12.5–17 grams/dL	15.5–17 grams/dL
	(women)	11.5–15 grams/dL	13.83–15 grams/dL
Hematocrit	(men)	36–50%	45–50%
	(women)	34–44%	41–44%

Source: Normal reference ranges based on Labcorp's standards as of May 14, 2002.

Hypoxia (low oxygen) promotes tumor growth by inducing angiogenesis and causing cancer cells to express survival factors that interfere with the ability of chemotherapy to kill them. Chemotherapy drugs are supposed to promote apoptosis. In a hypoxic environment, however, cancer cells develop survival mechanisms that protect them against apoptosis.

There are nutrients that help improve anemic states, but any cancer patient who does not have his or her hematocrit and hemoglobin in the upper one-third of the normal range (as described in Table 1) should consider the drug Procrit (or Epogen) to achieve such levels. Procrit is a natural erythropoietin that stimulates the production of red blood cells. There is also a new long-acting erythropoietin agent approved by the FDA called Aranesp, which allows dosing every 2 weeks instead of weekly injections.

If an oncologist fails to address anemia, the patients should assume the role of advocate, demanding that attention be paid to the quality of his blood counts.

A problem that cancer patients will encounter is that oncologists normally view low blood counts as normal in cancer patients and are reluctant to prescribe Procrit unless anemia is demonstrated. Because Procrit is an expensive drug, most insurance companies refuse to pay for it unless a cancer patient is severely anemic (<10 g/dL). Remember, anemia means hematocrit and hemoglobin are *below* the *low-normal* laboratory reference ranges. A cancer patient, on the other hand, should aim to have levels in the high upper-third range of normal for hematocrit and hemoglobin. Some insurance companies will not pay for Procrit until hematocrit levels are at least 20% *below* the lowest normal range. Is it any wonder that chemotherapy fails for so many cancer patients?

Since most insurance companies will not pay for Procrit for the purpose of boosting hematocrit and hemoglobin to the upper ranges of normal, patients may have to pay for this drug as an out-of-pocket expense. The first hurdle is convincing the oncologist to prescribe Procrit. The good news is that most cancer patients may only need Procrit for a few months, so the high cost does not have to be borne indefinitely.

The Life Extension Foundation has located pharmacies that will sell Procrit at lower prices. If your insurance company will not reimburse for this costly drug, call (800) 544-4440 for referrals to pharmacies that may charge less than conventional retail prices.

Inhibiting the COX-2 Enzyme

Some progressive oncologists are prescribing cyclooxygenase-2 (COX-2) inhibitor drugs along with chemotherapy to improve the odds of successful treatment. COX-2 is an enzyme that many types of cancers use in order to propagate. COX-2 and its byproducts such as prostaglandin E2 (PGE2) have been shown to help fuel the growth of cancers such as colon, pancreas, estrogen-negative breast, prostate, bladder, and lung cancer.

Drugs that inhibit the cyclooxygenase enzyme are known as *COX-2 inhibitors*. Celebrex and Vioxx are two popular COX-2 inhibitors. Both Celebrex and Vioxx are nonsteroidal anti-inflammatory drugs (NSAIDs) that are usually prescribed to treat the symptoms of rheumatoid arthritis and osteoarthritis. There appears to be more research on Celebrex in the treatment of cancer than Vioxx.

Since chemotherapy can cause gastrointestinal bleeding, careful physician monitoring is needed when using a COX-2 inhibiting drug such as Celebrex. Caution is urged for those with known kidney disease, poor heart-lung function, liver disease, or susceptibility to stress-induced ulcers. The protocol entitled *Cancer Treatment: The Critical Factors* has a detailed description of the connection between COX-2 and cancer and why inhibiting the COX-2 enzyme is so important in treating many cancers.

In 1996, Life Extension recommended that most cancer patients take a COX-2 inhibiting drug because of solid evidence that cancer cells use the COX-2 enzyme to sustain their rapid division. In 1996, Americans had to import a COX-2 inhibitor named nimesulid from other countries because this class of drug was not widely available in the United States.

Experiments in laboratory animals suggest that drugs such as Celebrex could help cure cancer, especially if combined with chemotherapy or radiation (Hsueh et al. 1999; Pyo et al. 2001; Swamy et al. 2002). There are 100 separate cancer studies involving COX-2 inhibitors going on worldwide at this time.

Doctors are predicting that COX-2 inhibiting drugs may become standard therapy in 5–10 years. There was adequate evidence in 1996, however, to recommend COX-2 inhibiting drugs available to cancer patients. There are three potent COX-2 inhibiting drugs on the American marketplace. You may ask your physician to prescribe one of the following COX-2 inhibitors:

Lodine XL, 1000 mg once a day or

Celebrex, 200–400 mg every 12 hours or

Vioxx, 12.5–25 mg once a day

Controlling Cancer Cell Growth

A family of proteins known as ras oncogenes often governs the regulation of cancer cell growth. The ras family is responsible for modulating the regulatory signals that direct the cancer cell cycle and rate of proliferation. Mutations in genes encoding ras proteins have been intimately associated with unregulated cell proliferation, that is, cancer.

There is a class of cholesterol-lowering drugs known as *statins* that has been shown to inhibit the activity of ras oncogenes. Some of these cholesterol-lowering drugs are lovastatin, simvastatin, and pravastatin (Ura et al. 1994; Narisawa et al. 1996; Tatsuta et al. 1998; Wang et al. 2000; Furst et al. 2002; van de Donk et al. 2002).

In advanced primary liver cancer (hepatoma or hepatocellular carcinoma), patients who received 40 mg of pravastatin survived twice as long compared to those who did not receive this statin drug (Kawata et al. 2001). Interestingly, statins are also associated with the preservation of bone structure and improvement in bone density (Edwards et al. 2000; 2001; Pasco et al. 2002).

Some types of cancer (breast and prostate) have a proclivity to metastasize to the bone (Waltregny et al. 2000; Pavlakis et al. 2002). This results in bone pain that also may be associated with weakening of the bone and an increased risk of fractures (Papapoulos et al. 2000; Plunkett et al. 2000). Patients with prostate cancer, for example, are found to have a very high incidence of osteoporosis even before the use of therapies that lower the male hormone testosterone (Berruti et al. 2001; Smith et al. 2001).

In prostate cancer, when excessive bone loss is occurring, there is a release of bone-derived growth factors, for example, TGF-b1 (transforming growth factor-beta 1), that stimulate the prostate cancer cells to grow further (Reyes-Moreno et al. 1998; Shariat et al. 2001). In turn, prostate cancer cells elaborate substances such as interleukin-6 (IL-6) that facilitates the further breakdown of bone (Paule 2001; Garcia-Moreno et al. 2002).

Thus, a vicious cycle results: bone breakdown-stimulation of prostate cancer cell growth that results in production of IL-6 and other cell products, which leads to further bone breakdown. When there is a breakdown of bone, the growth factors released can fuel cancer cell growth. (All cancer patients should refer to the *Osteoporosis protocol* in order to optimally maintain bone integrity and prevent the release of these cancer cell growth factors. The *Prostate Cancer protocol* has an extensive discussion about the importance of maintaining bone integrity.)

As far as statin drug dosing, higher amounts than are required to lower cholesterol are suggested for a period of several months. Cancer patients, for instance, have used 80 mg a day of lovastatin (Mevacor). This should be considered during chemotherapy in some cases. A monthly SMAC/CBC blood test is also recommended while taking a statin drug to monitor liver function. A rare potential side effect that can occur with the use of statin drugs is a condition known as *rhabdomyolysis* in which muscle cells are destroyed and released into the bloodstream. If muscle weakness should occur, alert your doctor so you can have a creatine kinase (CK) test to determine if muscle damage has occurred.

Combining a COX-2 Inhibitor with a Statin Drug and Chemotherapy

Depending on the type of cancer, a logical approach would be to combine a statin (such as Mevacor) with a COX-2 inhibitor and the appropriate dosing of chemotherapy.

Mevacor augmented up to five-fold the cancer-killing effect of the COX-2 inhibitor Sulindac (Agarwal et al. 1999). In this study, three different colon cancer cell lines were induced to undergo apoptosis by depriving them of COX-2. When Mevacor was added to the COX-2 inhibitor, the kill rate increased five-fold.

Physician involvement is essential to mitigate potential side effects of these drugs. Those who are concerned about potential toxicity should take into account the fact that the types of cancers that these drugs might be effective against have extremely high mortality rates. Please note that the use of statin drugs and COX-2 inhibitors for cancer is considered an off-label use of these drugs. You may ask your doctor to prescribe one of the following statin drugs to inhibit the activity of ras oncogenes:

Mevacor (lovastatin), 40 mg twice a day or

Zocor (simvastatin), 40 mg twice a day or

Pravachol (pravastatin), 40 mg once a day

medicine. Surgeons, for instance, strongly endorse surgical removal of the tumor(s), although radiologists often recommend various forms of radiotherapy to kill cancer cells. Medical oncologists, on the other hand, are proponents of chemotherapy, immune-augmentative, and hormone modulation therapies. In many cases, a particular type of cancer may warrant utilization of all conventional therapies, that is, surgery, radiation, and chemotherapy.

When it comes to alternative approaches, there are a wide variety of choices that can be accessed on the Internet. The challenge is separating the hype from credible science. The difficulty in achieving control over many forms of cancer has enabled inexperienced practitioners to flourish.

Conventional oncology has long criticized the efficacy of alternative methods. The irony is that the treatments offered at mainstream cancer centers provide little hope for those afflicted with the most deadly cancers. Until a cure is found, there will be a constant political and scientific struggle to capture the attention and gain financially from the 1.3 million Americans who are diagnosed with cancer each year.

The purpose of this protocol is to provide options that would not normally be offered by practicing oncologists. These various alternative therapies raise many issues that are subject to change as new data emerges. Patients are encouraged to check www.lefcancer.org for updated information about reported successes or failures of treatments offered by alternative cancer clinics.

It is important that cancer patients also read the protocols in this book titled *Cancer Adjuvant Therapies* and *Cancer Treatment: The Critical Factors* to learn about other potential treatment strategies.

STAYING INFORMED

The information published in this protocol is only as current as the day the manuscript was sent to the printer. This protocol raises many issues that are subject to change as new data emerge. Furthermore, cancer is still a disease with unacceptably high mortality rates, and none of our suggested regimens can guarantee a cure.

The Life Extension Foundation is constantly uncovering information to provide to cancer patients. A special website has been established for the purpose of updating patients on new findings that directly pertain to the published cancer protocols. Whenever Life Extension discovers information that may benefit cancer patients, it will be posted on the website www.lefcancer.org.

Before utilizing this cancer protocol, we suggest that you log on to www.lefcancer.org to see if any substantive changes have been made to the recommendations described herein. Based on the sheer number of newly published findings, there could be significant alterations to the information you have just read.

DISCLAIMER

This information (and any accompanying printed material) is not intended to replace the attention or advice of a physician or other health care professional. Anyone who wishes to embark on any dietary, drug, exercise, or other lifestyle change intended to prevent or treat a specific disease or condition should first consult with and seek clearance from a qualified health care professional.

The information published in the protocols is only as current as the day the manuscript was sent to the printer. This protocol raises many issues that are subject to change as new data emerge. None of our suggested protocol regimens can guarantee a cure.

Cancer: Gene Therapies, Stem Cells, Telomeres, and Cytokines

The media reports on many medical breakthroughs but usually issues a disclaimer stating that it will take many years before the discovery becomes part of standard practice. Interestingly, there are steps a cancer patient can take right now to gain access to this state-of-the-art knowledge. In some instances, a patient will have to travel to a research facility. In other cases, these therapies can be incorporated into a cancer treatment program utilizing existing therapeutic approaches.

We describe some of these exciting advances in this protocol and reveal how cancer patients may take advantage of them today. It is important to caution that the information provided in this chapter is highly technical and some lay readers may have difficulty fully understanding it.

HOW GENES CONTROL CANCER CELLS

One of the main categories of genes responsible for cancer includes those that (when working properly) suppress the development of malignancies. Various cancers result from the loss or malfunction of the key regulatory proteins that tumor suppressor genes encode, primarily p53 and pRB proteins. (pRB is named from retinoblastoma, the type of tumor in which its gene, RB, was first identified.) In its active form, pRB serves as a brake on DNA replication, blocking the activity of another protein (E2F) which promotes the synthesis of DNA. Loss of pRB protein therefore leads to uncontrolled E2F action and rampant cell division. Research indicates the RB gene is mutated in about 40% of human cancers, rendering its protein inactive (Oliff et al. 1996).

Another infinitely important regulatory molecule is the p53 protein. Often called the guardian of the genome, p53 prevents replication of damaged DNA in normal cells and promotes suicide or apoptosis of cells with abnormal DNA (Oliff et al. 1996). Faulty

p53 molecules allow cells (carrying damaged DNA) to survive when they would normally die and to replicate when they would normally stop. Cell cycle constraints are when pass, repair, and apoptotic mechanisms falter and disturbed cells pass mutations down to offspring. Thus, a lack of p53 regulation promotes the spontaneous emergence of mutant cells, a cellular distortion that is an invitation to cancer (Greenblatt et al. 1994).

Researchers compared the expression of more than 7000 genes and found that about 30 genes are activated by p53; the 14 most often stimulated by p53 are involved in cell regulation. The inactivation of the p53 gene is observed in about 50% of all solid tumors, affording prognostic and therapeutic implications. For example, researchers from the Mayo Clinic announced that analyzing p53 gene mutations identifies a subset of breast cancer patients who, despite lack of conventional indications of poor prognosis, are at high risk of early disease recurrence and death (Blaszyk et al. 2000).

Therapeutically, studies demonstrate that injecting wild type p53 into a malignant cell has positive effects when the p53 gene is either absent or mutated. In a 3-month study, nine men with advanced lung cancer (displaying a mutation in the tumor suppressor gene p53) were injected with healthy copies (genetically engineered) once a day for 5 days. The lung tumors treated with the p53 solution stopped growing in three patients; regression occurred in another three. Although all of the subjects eventually failed treatment, the major finding from the study, that is, "proof of principle," suggests that gene therapy can be an effective way to halt tumor cell growth (Modica et al. 1996). This therapeutic approach may have a potential application in at least 50% of all human tumors.

The highest frequency of p53 mutations reported in human cancers are lung, 56%; colon, 50%; esophagus, 45%; ovary, pancreas, and skin, 44%; stomach, 41%; head and neck, 37%; bladder, 34%; prostate, 30%; and breast, endometrial, and mesothelioma, 22% (Greenblatt et al. 1994). Nearly 20% of women treated for ovarian cancer develop other tumors beyond the abdomen. A mutation in the p53 tumor suppressor gene appears to predispose some women with ovarian cancer to distant and rapid tumor spread, according to data from the University of Iowa Health Care Study.

A mutant p53 gene seems able to escape destruction even when confronted with normally lethal concentrations of cytotoxic drugs and ionizing radiation (Buttitta et al. 1997). Furthermore, a dysfunctional p53 gene affects the outcome of traditional therapies because toxic treatments depend upon DNA damage and p53-induced cell death. The p53 gene induces cells to kill themselves by producing free radicals (charged molecules) causing cellular oxidation. Oxidation damages protein as well as the membranes and eventually the cell dies (Choisy-Rossi et al. 1998).

The character and therapeutic value of p53 is illustrated in the following studies:

- The tumors of 30 patients were directly injected with the p53 gene. Among 17 patients with non-resectable tumors, five stabilized and two exhibited partial regression (defined as at least a 50% reduction in the size of the mass). Among the 13 patients with resectable tumors, three died of their cancer, and five (38%) remained free of disease for 6 months post-injection (Kigawa et al. 2000).

- Progesterone induces apoptosis and markedly up-regulates p53 expression in ovarian cell lines. It is, thus, suspected that p53 plays a significant role in progesterone-induced apoptosis (Bu et al. 1997).

- Australian researchers found that interactions between telomerase and p53 indicate the activity of telomerase may be regulated by p53; down-regulation of p53 would (in turn) favor up-regulation of telomerase activity in cancer cell development (Li et al. 1999). Please consult the Telomere/Telomerase Connection appearing later in this protocol for additional information.

- Vitamin E, in combination with vitamins A and C, led to a four-fold reduction in p53 mutations (Brotzman et al. 1999).

Part of the body's natural defense against cancer may have a downside. Mice with high activity of the tumor-suppressing p53 gene had low rates of cancer, but aged prematurely. The surprise finding suggests that aging might occur, in part, because of the body's innate vigilance against cancer. Mutant mice with "revved up" p53 were more resistant to cancer than normal mice, but despite this protection, the mutant mice had (roughly) a 20% shorter lifespan. Instead of cancer, the animals experienced bone thinning, organ breakdown, vulnerability to physical stress, and the equivalent of sagging skin and balding in humans. Researchers speculate that hyperactivity in the p53 gene may disable the body's reserve of stem cells sooner than normal. This would keep primitive cells from replenishing certain body tissues and lead to premature tissue degeneration (Ferbeyre et al. 2002).

Protein Kinase Inhibitors

According to the Laboratory of Molecular Biophysics, of the hundreds of protein kinases in the human genome, only about 27 protein kinase structures have been solved to date. Yet, so important are the family of kinases, oncogenes that encode (program) protein kinases are under ongoing study for their participation in cancer (Johnson 2002). In normal cells, protein kinases are involved in signals sent between the cell membrane and the nucleus, regulating progression through the cell cycle. Protein kinases control these processes by activating other proteins in response to stimuli. Mutated kinase genes have been found in a number of malignancies, including chronic myelogenous leukemia and breast and bladder cancers.

Kinases can lead to cancer though various pathways including overproduction, an event caused by mutations in the control regions of their genes. Compared to normal cells, tumor cells often overproduce kinases, encouraging the cell to divide. A commonly overproduced kinase in cancerous tissue is the receptor for epidermal growth factor (EGF), an up-regulation strongly favoring cancer.

Kinases can also contribute to cancer if their structure is abnormal. Many tumor cells possess protein kinases that (because of a structural defect) are permanently turned on, goading the cell into division. Examples of kinases that behave abnormally in certain human cancers are the Abl, Src, and cyclin-dependent kinases (Oliff et al. 1996).

Obviously, an inhibitor of dysfunctional kinases is a worthy cancer therapy research objective. The challenge is finding a substance that can distinguish one kinase from another. Many of the protein kinases in mammalian cells have similar structures, particularly in biochemically active regions. Hence, an inhibitor of any single protein kinase might disrupt the activity of others, that is, an unrelated kinase crucial to normal cell function.

Despite limitations, pharmaceutical researchers have synthesized and tested a number of kinase inhibitors. Most target the kinases themselves, but others attack at the genetic level (preventing the kinases from being formed). Remarkably, kinase inhibitors can be quite selective. In the test tube, some find their intended target 1000 times more frequently than they do unrelated kinases. More important are findings that several of these compounds inhibit the growth of cancer cells possessing mutated kinase genes.

Various natural agents appear able to inhibit protein kinase activity:

- Flavonoid analogues inhibit protein-tyrosine kinase. The most active substance used in this study was compound 17c, which is approximately one order greater in potency than quercetin. After a series of reduction mechanisms, 3-(alkoxycarbonyl)-2-arylflavones is produced and then converted to a variety of flavonoids, including 17c (Cushman et al. 1991).

- Genistein and daidzein, isoflavones found in soy, are specific inhibitors of protein tyrosine kinase (PTK). By modulating pathways involved in signal transduction, isoflavones acting upon PTK put the brakes on rapidly dividing cells (Bland 2001).

- Oxidants selectively react with the regulatory center of protein kinase C (PKC), signaling tumor promotion and cell growth. In contrast, antioxidants (selenium and polyphenolic agents, such as curcumin, and vitamin E analogues) inhibit cellular PKC activity and thus interfere with the action of tumor promoters (Gopalakrishna et al. 2000). Other polyphenolic phytochemicals, that is, the constituents of green tea and resveratrol, respond similarly, displaying significant PKC inhibition (Stoner et al. 1995; Atten et al. 2001).

- As protein kinase C (PKC) is stimulated, tumor activity in the colon increases. Retinol, retinoic acid, and beta-carotene (in nanomolar concentrations) block stimulation of PKC. At higher doses, retinol and retinoic acid can stimulate kinase activity; beta-carotene does not have this effect and could thus be useful in the prevention and treatment of colorectal cancer (Kahl-Rainer et al. 1994).

This growing body of knowledge about the effect of kinases on cell regulatory genes helps explain why soy extracts (genistein and daidzein), curcumin, beta-carotene, and certain types of vitamin E have anticancer effects. The problem is that we don't have precise data to predict how a particular dose of a *protein kinase C* inhibiting agent will affect gene expression on cancer cells. There are findings, however, from related studies indicating that the following doses of nutrients might be beneficial in suppressing *protein kinase C* that is involved in controlling cancer cell propagation:

- Curcumin, 3600 mg a day
- Genistein, 2700 mg a day
- Tocopheryl succinate, 800 mg a day
- Beta-carotene, 25,000 IU a day
- Retinal palmitate, 25,000 IU a day

THE TELOMERE/TELOMERASE CONNECTION

One of the crucial features that distinguish a cancer cell from a normal cell is its ability to divide indefinitely. Telomerase, an enzyme in the cell nucleus, is intricately involved in the cancer process through interactions with telomeres, the protective structures at the ends of chromosomes. In most normal human cells, the action of telomerase is repressed and subsequently telomeres shorten progressively with each cell division. In contrast, most human tumors utilize telomerase, resulting in stabilized telomere length. For tumor cells to proliferate, they must maintain the telomeres. Thus, cancer cells turn on genes responsible for telomerase production which in humans normally ceases after birth. Suppressing telomerase is an obvious target for the development of anticancer therapies (Hahn et al. 1999).

Telomerase is composed of at least two units: hTR and hTRT, genes whose activity correlate with the malignancy and metastatic potential of the tumor. The combination of hTR and hTRT activates telomerase, lengthening telomeres and extending the cell's replicative lifespan. hTR and hTRT were detected in 85% and 82% of primary tumors, respectively; in surrounding, healthier tissue, the positive incidence of hTR/hTRT was only ~3% (Bodnar et al. 1998; Yuan et al. 2000).

Because telomerase activity is increased in the vast majority of human tumors (about 90%), its gene product appears to be the first molecule common to all tumors (Cairns et al. 2000; Minev et al. 2000). In analyzing human cancers, the positive frequency of hTR and hTRT was overwhelmingly displayed in cancers of the breast, colon, gallbladder, lung, stomach, and esophagus. Telomere length and telomerase activity are also evidenced in chronic lymphocytic leukemia, often proving predictive of survival (Bechter et al. 1998). In addition, multiple myeloma patients with high levels of telomerase activity were also found to have a significantly shorter survival time. Telomerase, thus, is proving a reliable marker for the proliferating capacity and tumor mass of cancer patients (Shiratsuchi et al. 2002).

Retinoids employ two different pathways to impact telomerase activity; the second means (down-regulating hTRT) results in a suppression of telomerase that develops slowly during 2 weeks of retinoic acid therapy, terminating in telomere shortening, growth arrest, and cell death. Telomerase expression is an efficient and selective target of retinoids in the therapy of tumors (Pendino et al. 2001).

Retinoids are not alone in their capacity to inhibit telomerase.

- Epigallocatechin gallate (EGCG), a green tea catechin, strongly and directly inhibited telomerase (Naasani et al. 1998).

- Antioxidants reduce telomerase activity (Liu et al. 2002)

- Administering NSAIDs (indomethacin and ibuprofen) resulted in a dose-dependent reduction in telomerase activity (Thurnher et al. 2001).

- Scientists from USCD School of Medicine and Cancer Center in corroboration with the Institute Pasteur in Paris are successfully using telomerase in a prototype vaccine to activate cytotoxic T-lymphocytes. By immunizing lymphocytes against telomerase, killer cells targeting telomerase are generated. The vaccine specifically targets the hTRT peptide, and the proliferative patterns common to immortal cells are destroyed (Zanetti et al. 2000). Researchers (University of California) suggest that hTRT has the potential to serve as a universal cancer vaccine (Minev et al. 2000).

- Two pharmaceutical groups (Geron Corporation and Ribozyme Pharmaceuticals) have joined forces to elaborate GRN163, a short, modified oligonucleotide designed as a telomerase antagonist. A Geron Corporation spokesperson said that inhibiting telomerase represents a novel mechanism for the treatment of cancer with potentially broader utility and greater selectivity against cancer cells than currently available agents. The companies are also exploring a ribozyme-based telomerase inhibitor with apoptotic activity, as well as the ability to shorten telomeres (BW 2001). Isolating anticancer drugs targeted at telomerase inhibition is a global effort, one considered crucial to understanding and subsequently overcoming cancer.

Telomerase inhibitors are exciting potential therapies against cancer (Cairns et al. 2002; Mokbel 2003). Several human clinical trials are expected in the year 2004. A Phase II clinical trial for individuals fighting metastatic cancer using a vaccine that contains a telomerase peptide (piece of a telomerase protein) is currently underway at the National Cancer Institute:

http://clinicaltrials.gov/ct/show/NCT00016640?order=1

Although much of this work is still in the research phase, there is evidence that high-dose green tea extract and retinoid compounds may inhibit the telomerase enzyme that allows cancer cells to proliferate out of control (L'Allemain 1999; Pendino et al. 2003). You may consider one or both of the following potential telomerase-inhibiting therapies available right now:

- Vesanoid (all-trans retinoic acid) is a drug already approved to treat certain cancers (Ozpolat et al. 2001). Based on its potential telomerase-inhibiting property, you may want to ask your oncologist to prescribe an individualized dose for you.

- High-potency green tea extracts are available as dietary supplements. A dose used by some cancer patients is five 350-mg capsules of green tea (95%) extract with each meal (3 meals per day). Each capsule should be standardized to provide a minimum of 100 mg of epigallocatechin gallate (EGCG). It is the EGCG fraction of green tea that has shown the most active anticancer effects. These high-potency green tea extract capsules are available in decaffeinated form for those who are sensitive to caffeine or who want to take the less stimulating decaffeinated green tea extract capsules in their evening dose. The brand name of the 95% green tea extract is Super Green Tea Extract Caps.

For information regarding telomerase-inhibiting drug clinical trials, call the National Cancer Institute (NCI) at (800) 422-7237 or visit the NCI's clinical trials Web site. One company that may start clinical trials in 2004 is Geron Corporation.

STEM CELL TRANSPLANTS

Many of the most respected cancer centers in the United States are using stem cells rather than bone marrow for transplants. According to the Fred Hutchinson Cancer Research Center (Seattle, WA), stem cell transplants are substantially more effective for certain high-risk patients, particularly patients with blood borne tumors who are beyond first remission or who have experienced refractory relapse.

In a multicenter trial, 168 patients between the ages of 12–55 with various blood malignancies (leukemia, lymphoma, and myelodysplasia) were randomized to receive either bone marrow or peripheral blood stem cell transplants from HLA-identical sibling donors (Stephenson 2000). The trial was stopped prematurely because a safety monitoring committee determined there was a statistically significant difference in outcome between the two groups. An analysis of 138 of the patients showed that engraftment of platelets and neutrophils was more rapid by about a week in patients who received stem cells. (Engraftment refers to the interval when the donor's marrow cells "attach" to the transplant patient's site and begin to produce healthy cells.) This is momentous because infection looms as a major threat to survival among transplant patients; thus, hastily restoring blood cell production and the efficiency of the immune system is paramount.

Even more impressive were the differences in survival; the 2-year survival rate was 45% among patients with bone marrow transplants compared to 70% among patients with stem cell transplants. The survival advantage was most apparent in patients with more advanced disease. Data were insufficient to determine whether stem cells offer similar advantage over bone marrow for patients with less advanced cancers.

A stem cell transplant involves replacing the diseased marrow with healthy stem cells that match the recipient's. The transplanted stem cells travel through the recipient's blood to the marrow spaces where they begin to grow, producing healthy new blood cells. This occurs after massive amounts of cytotoxic agents have been administered in a courageous attempt to kill the cancer. Unfortunately, the agents that kill cancer cells also kill bone marrow, a spongy tissue in the cavities of large bones that produces blood cells. Without bone marrow, stem cell activity ceases and subsequently so does production of platelets (cells necessary for blood coagulation), white blood cells (cells essential to fight infections and cancer), and red blood cells (cells required for oxygen transport). Without a healthy supply of these vital cells, life expectancy is extremely short.

Not all recipients survive the intensive pretransplant chemotherapy or radiation treatment, which (until recently) were considered the only curative phases of the procedure. Other complications (apart from infections and nonengraftment) include graft-versus-host disease (white blood cells in the marrow fight the patient's body) and relapse (recurrence of the original disease). To find out if you are eligible for this stem cell therapy, contact the Fred Hutchinson Cancer Research Center (Seattle) at (800) 804-8824.

PERIPHERAL BLOOD STEM CELL TRANSPLANT PROGRAM

The Peripheral Blood Stem Cell Transplant Program allows patients to restore their own supply of blood cells degraded during chemotherapy. Apheresis, a process that withdraws blood and circulates it through a machine, removes the stem cells. Remaining components of the blood are then returned to the patient. The harvested stem cells are stored at a very low temperature, and (after high-dose chemotherapy or radiation

therapy) the cells are thawed and returned to the patient through a central venous catheter. Once the stem cells are reinfused into the bloodstream, they return to the bone marrow and begin producing mature red blood cells, white cells, and platelets.

Allogeneic stem cells (donated by another person) are more likely to muster an immune attack against the cancer than autologous stem cells (those harvested from the patient). According to Richard E. Champlin, M.D., chairman of the Department of Blood and Marrow Transplantation at the University of Texas M.D. Anderson Cancer Center, physicians found that allogeneic transplantation harbored unexpected benefits, that is, immunoreactivity against the cancer. In some cases, the graft versus malignancy effect proved curative.

In the past, the threat of graft versus host disease limited the number of patients who were able to undergo allogeneic transplantation but advances in immunosuppressive therapies and cell manipulation techniques have steadily increased the numbers (Wright 2000). Treatment-related mortality rate is about 20% for allogeneic transplants, with the hospital stay about 4 months; autologous transplants have less than a 5% treatment-related mortality and require hospitalization of about 1 month. Transplantation studies are currently being expanded to include ovarian, breast, lung, and renal cell cancers.

For aged and very ill patients, reliance upon high-dose chemotherapy has changed to emphasis upon immune modulation generated by the donor cells. The process, referred to as a mini-transplant, allows for a graft versus malignancy effect with the chemotherapeutic drug limited to a low-dose application. A minitransplant can now be performed in senior patients with comorbid conditions, such as hepatitis or cardiac and lung abnormalities. Myeloablative regimens (bone marrow removal) are still used for younger patients and nonablative regimes are used for older or badly compromised patients.

The success rate of transplants varies, but M.D. Anderson Cancer Center reported the results of 13 patients with low-grade lymphoma who underwent a mini-transplant: All 13 survived and are in remission. Survival variables include the specific disease, the stage of the disease, and the age and condition of the patient. Typically, the survival rate (measured at 2–3 years) is in the range of 40–60%. The Peripheral Blood Stem Cell Transplant Program is ongoing. Contact the M.D. Anderson Cancer Center information line at (800) 392-1611.

UMBILICAL CORD BLOOD TRANSPLANTS

Umbilical cord blood, a source of cells for transplant, has been life-saving to children who are without an acceptable donor. In about a 4-year time frame, M.D. Anderson Cancer Center has performed 25 umbilical cord blood transplants, all from mismatched donors, on pediatric patients (most with advanced acute leukemia). After a median follow-up of 22 months, 14 of the young patients were alive, and 12 were in remission. (Chalaire 2000). Fatal complications in umbilical cord blood transplants exceed 30% in the first 100 days.

Umbilical cord blood transplants, unlike bone marrow transplants, can tolerate mismatches in HLA (as many as 2–6 antigens), but unfortunately (if the mismatch is large) it increases the time of engraftment (the point when the donor's marrow cells have "attached" to the transplant patient's site and start to produce healthy cells). In addition, umbilical cord blood contains about 10 times fewer cells than bone marrow. The period of engraftment is thus extended to 40–60 days, as compared to 10–20 in bone marrow transplants. During this period of pancytopenia (a marked reduction in the numbers of the formed blood cells), life-threatening infections are a significant threat. Thus, recipients (until recently) have been restricted to children and low-weight adults (Chalaire 2000). A new protocol, that is, combining umbilical cord blood from two or three donors, appears to amend blood cell shortages, making future transplants available to more individuals in diverse age groups.

According to Dr. Champlin, "The important message is that the whole field of blood and marrow transplantation is probably the most dynamic area in all of medicine, where advances in chemotherapy, immunosuppressive agents, genetic therapy, and cellular therapy are all coming together." For more information regarding transplants, contact Dr. Richard E. Champlin at (713) 792-3618 or Dr. Ka Wah Chan at M.D. Anderson Cancer Center (713) 792-7751.

SUPPRESSING PRO-INFLAMMATORY CYTOKINES

There is a growing body of evidence showing that the net biological response of pro- and anti-inflammatory cytokines affects the outcome of several degenerative diseases, including cancer (Dinarello 1997). Cytokines are one of a large group of proteins secreted by various cell types. These relatively small peptides are involved in cell-to-cell communication, coordinating antibody/ T-cell immune interactions, and amplifying immune reactivity. The broad family of cytokines includes colony stimulating factors (as G-CSF and GM-CSF), interferons, interleukins, tumor necrosis factor, and macrophage activating and inhibiting factors.

Some cytokines were named for the cellular modulating property with which they were initially associated. For example, tumor necrosis factor has anticancer properties, causing death (necrosis) to certain tumors. But, in inflammatory diseases TNF-alpha (like IL-1) can increase cellular responsiveness to growth factors, inducing signaling pathways that lead to proliferation. In addition, by acting synergistically with epidermal growth factors, TNF-alpha can induce expression of a number of oncogenes, as well as several potentially damaging interleukins (ISU 2001).

Illustrative of TNF-alpha's capriciousness, short-term culture with tumor necrosis factor increases apoptosis (programmed cell death), but extended culture with TNF-alpha suppresses it, probably through induction of IL-8 (Dunican et al. 2000). *In vitro*, TNF acts as an antiangiogenic; *in vivo* it assumes the nature of an angiogenic, unless redirected by interferon-gamma, another cytokine (Frater-Schroder et al. 1987).

Tumor necrosis factor (TNF) is secreted by macrophages, monocytes, neutrophils, T-cells, and natural killer cells (following stimulation by bacterial lipopolysaccharides). (Lipopolysaccharide is a major component of the cell wall of Gram-negative bacteria.) Production of TNF (also induced by oxidative stress) can activate nuclear factor-kappa-B (NF-kB), a transcription factor. NF-kB, so named because of its cellular location, is normally maintained in an inactive state due to inhibitory molecules. Once activated, NF-kB becomes a potent stimulus to cytokine production. Agents that act at various levels, including antioxidants to repress the production of free radicals, as well as suppressants of TNF and/or NF-kB production, can assist in regulating cytokine production (Martin 2002; *Pathfinder Encyclopaedia* 2002).

Interleukins (one arm of the cytokine family) are not created equally. Although some show promise in cancer control, that is, IL-2, IL-7, IL-12, IL-15, IL-18, interferon alpha, interferon gamma, GM-CSF, IP-10, and Flt-3 ligand, others can have a deleterious effect. For example, IL-6 attacks the skeletal system and induces telomerase (an enzyme delivering immortality to cancer cells) (Sotiriou et al. 2001); IL-8 inhibits apoptosis and is one of the strongest promoters of inflammation (Harada 1994); IL-10 suppresses NK cell and macrophage function (Ho et al. 1994); IL-13 suppresses T-cell mediated immunity and may be involved in the progression of Hodgkin's disease (de Waal Malefyt et al. 1995; Skinnider et al. 2001); IL-4 activates B-cells (promoting their proliferation) while inhibiting the positive effects of IL-2 (Kay et al. 2003); IL-9 can increase IL-6 levels (Cavaillon 1990).

It is important to note that the production of pro-inflammatory cytokines occurs rapidly following trauma or invasion of the body by disease-causing organisms. But, inflammation is not an efficient means of tumor surveillance. Inflammation, in fact, significantly works against the cancer patient by contributing to weight loss, inhibiting beneficial interleukins, suppressing cell-mediated immunity, and promoting angiogenesis (CIC 2000).

Once an infection or injury stimulates production of IL-1 or TNF-alpha, these two pro-inflammatory compounds can further stimulate each other, as well as IL-6. In addition, IL-1 and TNF-alpha trigger the production of free radicals, which encourage the production of more pro-inflammatory cytokines. According to Jack Challem (reporting in *Let's Live* Magazine), the pro-inflammatory reaction essentially feeds on itself, setting the stage for chronic inflammation. Although a cytokine response is (at times) essential, excessive production of pro-inflammatory cytokines or the production of cytokines in the wrong biological context is regarded as poor indicators of stability and even survival among individuals with degenerative disease (Grimble et al. 1998).

Researchers at the University of Colorado Health Sciences Center explain that the cytokine system is self-regulating through the action of anti-inflammatory cytokines, opposing cytokines, and cytokine receptor antagonists. If cytokine regulation becomes deranged (with cytokine numbers favoring those considered inflammatory), the risks of morbidity and mortality markedly increase. Imbalance of pro-inflammatory and anti-inflammatory cytokines (deregulation) is strongly linked with cardiovascular disease and arthritis and, as the following list indicates, with cancer as well (Arend 2001; Kurzrock 2001).

IL-6 is elevated in the following cancers:

- Brain Tumor: IL-6 appears involved in tumor progression in some glioblastomas, that is, tumors of the cerebrum (the largest and uppermost section of the brain) or spinal cord (Sasaki et al. 2001).

- Breast Cancer: IL-6 levels are nearly 10 times higher in patients with metastatic breast cancer. Elevated IL-6 levels are the most distinguishing factor separating healthy controls from women with breast cancer (Benoy et al. 2002).

- Chronic Lymphocytic Leukemia: Elevations in IL-6 and IL-10 correlate with adverse disease features and short survival in leukemia patients (Fayad et al. 2001).

- Colorectal Cancer: IL-6 is reported to be responsible for loss of lean body mass during cancer cachexia in colon-26 adenocarcinoma (C-26)-bearing mice (Fujita et al. 1996). Data also suggest that carcino-embryonic-secreting tumors (such as colon cancers) induce the production of IL-6 and that IL-6 stimulates tumor cell growth at metastatic sites (Belluco et al. 2000).

- Gynecological Cancers: Higher IL-6 levels are found in women with gynecological cancers, making them less responsive to chemotherapy (Scambia et al. 1996). Consistent elevations in IL-8 and IL-6 are observed in ovarian cancer, the latter proving a negative prognosticator regarding outcome (Penson et al. 2000).

- Lung Cancer: Increased levels of serum IL-6 are found in patients with lung cancer and appear part of a systemic inflammatory response syndrome (Dowlati et al. 1999).

- Lymphoma: Vascular endothelial growth factor (VEGF), an angiogenesis promoter, and IL-6 levels are often higher in patients with aggressive lymphoma. Disease-free survival rates for patients displaying high levels of VEGF or IL-6 are poor, but the prognosis becomes worse if VEGF/IL-6 elevations coexist (Niitsu et al. 2002).

- Multiple Myeloma: IL-6 is an important cytokine in myeloma cell growth and proliferation. Close cell-to-cell contact between myeloma cells and the bone marrow stromal cells triggers a large amount of IL-6 production, which supports the growth of malignant cells, as well as protecting them from apoptosis. Elevations in IL-6 are deemed (by some) highly predictive of survival (Blade et al. 2002; Hussein et al. 2002).

- Obstructive Jaundice: Elevations in TNF-alpha and IL-6 are observed in patients with malignant obstructive jaundice, especially those with a poor immediate prognosis (Puntis et al. 1996).

- Pancreatic Cancer: IL-6 and IL-8 play a role in several pancreatic diseases, including pancreatic cancer (Blanchard et al. 2001).

- Prostate Cancer: Prostate cancer cells produce factors that increase IL-6, a known activator of bone resorption (Garcia-Moreno et al. 2002).

- Renal Cell Carcinoma: IL-6 is implicated in osteoclastic bone resorption and hypercalcemia, factors associated with metastatic renal cell cancer (Paule 2001).

Important information was released in 2002 regarding the impact of too little sleep upon IL-6 production. Researchers found that getting adequate sleep lessened IL-6 production and exposure of tissues to its potentially detrimental actions. Sleep deprivation caused a 40–50% average increase in IL-6 (in both men and women) and a 20–30% increase in tumor necrosis factor in men. Dr. Alexandros Vgontzas (professor of psychiatry at Pennsylvania State University) stated at the annual meeting of the Endocrine Society (June 22, 2002) that 8 hours of sleep is not a nice bonus but a necessity if one is concerned with good health. Considering the risks imposed by over-expression of pro-inflammatory cytokines, every precaution should be implemented to preserve equilibrium between pro- and anti-inflammatory cytokines. Thus, if insomnia is a problem, please consult the *Insomnia protocol* for assistance in overcoming this disorder (Vgontzas et al. 1999; 2001).

Therapies that influence the tumor and its microenvironment are being aggressively pursued with the goal of converting active malignancies to chronic disease states, with the patient maintaining a normal lifestyle (Hussein et al. 2002). Much of current research, thus, focuses upon modulation of the family of pro-inflammatory cytokines with anti-inflammatory drugs, cytokine receptor antagonists, and nutrients (Di Girolamo et al. 1997; Grimble et al. 1998).

There are natural agents and prescription drugs that suppress pro-inflammatory cytokines. Many nutrients are broad-spectrum cytokine inhibitors, meaning they are capable of inhibiting several pro-inflammatory cytokines. Although relying upon a single nutrient (as a cytokine inhibitor) is not recommended, it is not necessary to incorporate the full list of inhibitors into a therapeutic program.

The following list comprises dietary supplements that suppress inflammatory cytokines:

1. DHEA inhibits TNF-alpha by 98% and IL-6 by 95% (Kipper-Galperin et al. 1999).

2. Alpha Tocopherol (Vitamin E) significantly lowered levels of C-reactive protein and IL-6 at a dosage of 1200 IU a day (Devaraj et al. 2000).

3. DHA and EPA may reign supreme as an inhibitor of dangerous cytokines. IL-6 is potentiated when endothelial cells are stimulated. Omega-3 fatty acids restrain stimulating factors, such as TNF-alpha, IL-4, or lipopolysaccharides. Void of stimulation, endothelial cells are inhibited in their production of IL-6 (Khalfoun et al. 1997). Fish oil inhibited IL-1 and TNF-alpha by approximately 90% (James et al. 2000). It should also be noted that psychological stress induces the production of pro-inflammatory cytokines, such as TNF-alpha, IL-6, and IL-10. Increasing omega-3 PUFAs lessened the pro-inflammatory response to psychological stress (Maes et al. 2000). DHA and EPA can be obtained directly from fish oil concentrates or indirectly from perilla or flax oils.

4. N-Acetylcysteine (NAC) inhibited the production of IL-6 and IL-8 induced by TNF-alpha or lipopolysaccharides (Munoz et al. 1996; Gosset et al. 1999).

5. Vitamin K inhibited IL-6 production by lipopolysaccharide-stimulated human fibroblasts. Fibroblasts are recognized as rich sources of cytokines (Reddi et al. 1995).

The transcription factor (NF-kappa-B) is implicated in several types of malignancies. Once activated, NF-kB is responsible for an onslaught of pro-inflammatory cytokines. Generally, suppression of NF-kB correlates well with inhibition of various damaging cytokines, including IL-6 and IL-8. NF-kB can be inhibited by:

1. Alpha-Lipoic Acid, antioxidants that eliminate reactive oxygen species, also blocks NF-kB. Lipoic acid is particularly effective, completely inhibiting NF-kB at a fifth of the dosage required by N-acetyl-cysteine (Suzuki et al. 1992).

2. Alpha Tocopherol Succinate (Vitamin E) prevents monocytic cell adhesion to cytokine-stimulated endothelial cells by inhibiting the activation of NF-kappa B (Erl et al. 1997).

3. Curcumin blocks NF-kB activation and a generation of pro-inflammatory cytokines (Jobin et al. 1999).

4. Feverfew contains a lactone or chemical compound called parthenolide according to Newmark et al. (2000).

5. Researchers at Children's Hospital Medical Center (Cincinnati, OH) determined that parthenolide inhibits nuclear factor-kB activity (Sheehan et al. 2002).

6. Genistein, an isoflavone in soy, inhibits both basic and inducible NF-kB activation (Tabary et al. 1999).

7. Green Tea, the EGCG fraction, displays a potent inhibitory effect on NF-kB expression in hypoxic cells (Yang et al. 1998; Muraoka et al. 2002).

8. Quercetin has the ability to inhibit NF-kB and inflammatory mediators produced by it (Ishikawa et al. 1999).

9. Silymarin, a bioflavonoid, potently suppresses NF-kB, a key in inflammatory and immune reactions (Saliou et al. 1998).

10. Stinging Nettle (standardized plant extracts from the leaves of stinging nettle, IDS23) reliably inhibits NF-kB (Riehemann et al. 1999).

11. Vitamin C inhibits the activation of NF-kB by multiple stimuli, including IL-1 and TNF-alpha (Bowie et al. 2000).

Note: *For specific information about the nutrients detailed in the list, refer to the* Cancer Adjuvant Therapy *protocol.*

Comments On These Findings

The fact that many antioxidants are strong inhibitors of NF-kB activation appears to explain another of the pathways antioxidants utilize to defend against cancer. Various chemotherapeutic agents increase expression of both good and bad cytokines. Thus, questions regarding safe usage of natural agents that elicit production of both pro- and anti-inflammatory cytokines arise.

Most of our knowledge regarding pro-inflammatory cytokines (such as IL-1 or TNF-alpha) is derived from experiments in which humans or animals have been injected with either a single or a combination of inflammatory cytokines (Dinarello 1997). However, in models of inflammation where several cytokines are produced, specific blockade of either IL-1 or TNF-alpha (or both) results in a reduction in the severity of inflammation. This may explain the success when using agents that lift expression of many of the family of cytokines, both pro- and anti-inflammatory in nature.

It is possible to test one's blood level of pro-inflammatory cytokines such as TNF-alpha, interkeukin-6 (IL-6), interleukin-8 (IL-8), and interleukin-1(b). For information regarding cytokine blood testing, call (800) 208-3444.

Although there are many supplements that can suppress pro-inflammatory cytokines and inhibit the expression of NF-kB, the following are the ones most commonly used by cancer patients:

1. Fish oil: 1300 mg DHA and 500 mg EPA a day to suppress inflammatory cytokines. (*Note:* This potency of DHA and EPA can be obtained by taking 8 capsules a day of a product called Super GLA/DHA.)

2. DHEA: 15–75 mg a day to suppress inflammatory cytokines. Refer to *DHEA Replacement Therapy protocol* for precautions.

3. Curcumin (with Bioperine): 3600 mg a day to mitigate NF-kB activation and to inhibit protein kinase C. (*Note:* This potency can be obtained by taking four capsules of Super Curcumin with Bioperine once a day with a heavy meal containing fat.)

4. Green Tea Extract (95%): 1500 mg 3 times a day to mitigate NF-kB activation and to inhibit the telomerase enzyme. (*Note:* This potency can be obtained by taking 5 Super Green Tea Extract capsules 3 times a day.)

5. Genistein: 2700 mg a day to inhibit protein kinase C and to mitigate NF-kB activation. (*Note:* This potency can be obtained by taking 5 Ultra Soy Extract capsules 4 times a day.)

6. Tocopheryl Succinate (dry vitamin E): 400–1200 IU a day to mitigate NF-kB activation and to inhibit protein kinase C.

SUMMARY

The cancer patient has a wide range of treatment choices to inhibit molecular mechanisms that cancer cells utilize for survival and propagation. It is interesting to note that nutrients such as green tea extract, curcumin, and tocopheryl succinate function in several different ways to inhibit tumor cell proliferation.

For a more thorough description of how certain dietary supplements may be of benefit to the cancer patient, refer to the *Cancer Adjuvant Therapy protocol.*

Note: *Data were collected (in part) from the work of Dr. Frank McCormick, chief scientific officer at Onyx Pharmaceuticals, and Dr. Allen Oliff, executive director for cancer research, and Dr. Jackson Gibbs, senior director of cancer results, both at Merck Research Laboratories.*

 ## PRODUCT AVAILABILITY

Super GLA/DHA, Mega EPA, tocopheryl succinate capsules (vitamin E), vitamin C, alpha-lipoic acid, quercetin, DHEA, Ultra Soy, Super Curcumin w/Bioperine, Super Green Tea Extract, silymarin, and Silibinin Plus can be ordered by calling (800) 544-4440 or by ordering online at www.lef.org.

STAYING INFORMED

The information published in this protocol is only as current as the day the manuscript was sent to the printer. This protocol raises many issues that are subject to change as new data emerge. Furthermore, cancer is still a disease with unacceptably high mortality rates, and none of our suggested regimens can guarantee a cure.

The Life Extension Foundation is constantly uncovering information to provide to cancer patients. A special website has been established for the purpose of updating patients on new findings that directly pertain to the published cancer protocols. Whenever Life Extension discovers information that may benefit cancer patients it will be posted on the website www.lefcancer.org.

Before utilizing the cancer protocols in this book, we suggest that you check www.lefcancer.org to see if any substantive changes have been made to the recommendations described in this protocol. Based on the sheer number of newly published findings, there could be significant alterations to the information you have just read.

Alternatively, call 1-800-226-2370 and ask a Health Advisor if your topic of interest has been updated on the website – www.lefcancer.org

DISCLAIMER

This information (and any accompanying printed material) is not intended to replace the attention or advice of a physician or other health care professional. Anyone who wishes to embark on any dietary, drug, exercise, or other lifestyle change intended to prevent or treat a specific disease or condition should first consult with and seek clearance from a qualified health care professional.

The information published in the protocols is only as current as the day the manuscript was sent to the printer. This protocol raises many issues that are subject to change as new data emerge. None of our suggested protocol regimens can guarantee a cure.

Cancer Prevention

Just a few years ago, the federal government released an optimistic report stating that the rate of cancer was leveling off or declining. In late 2002, the National Cancer Institute disclosed that the data used to prepare this report was seriously flawed. According to the National Cancer Institute, the incidences of some of the most deadly cancers are actually sharply increasing.

The American Cancer Association responded to these startling statistics by urging that more research be devoted to ascertain why prevention programs are failing. It has become strikingly apparent that the most respected cancer institutions have no explanation for why more Americans than ever before are contracting this devastating disease.

Regrettably, most cancer cases occur needlessly. Thousands of published scientific findings provide a clear road map as to what one can do to reduce their risk of developing cancer. The problem is that people are overwhelmed by the volume of cancer prevention data and have largely failed to take the necessary steps to reduce their personal risk.

In this protocol, we will reveal the fundamental factor that causes all cancers. We will then suggest relatively simple lifestyle changes that can help keep normal cells from transforming into malignant cells.

GENE MUTATION AND CANCER

Causes

Cancer is a disease caused by genetic mutation. Most people have a difficult time grasping the molecular complexities of genes and their relationship to cancer. To bring this down to the simplest level, the following definition from the *New England Journal of Medicine* (Haber 2000) should enable lay persons to understand how genes are intimately involved in cancer processes: "Cancer results from the accumulation of mutations in genes that regulate cellular proliferation."

This one sentence description enlightens us to the critical importance of maintaining gene integrity if we are to prevent cancer from developing in our bodies.

Cells operate under the direction of genes located in the DNA. Our existence is dependent on the precise genetic regulation of all cellular events. Healthy young cells have nearly perfect genes. Aging and environmental factors cause genes to mutate, resulting in cellular metabolic disorder. Gene mutations can turn healthy cells into malignant cells. As gene mutations accumulate, the risk of cancer sharply increases.

What Causes Genes to Mutate

Human studies show that about 70% of gene mutations are environmental and, thus, relatively controllable based on what we eat, whether we smoke, or exposure to genotoxins or radiation (Ljungquist et al. 1995; Herskind et al. 1996; Finch et al. 1997). Antioxidant supplements have become popular because they reduce gene damage inflicted by free radicals. However, it takes more than antioxidants to adequately protect genes against environmental mutation.

The most prevalent cause of environmental genetic mutation is the food we eat every day. While certain foods are particularly genotoxic, even healthy foods result in the body being exposed to small amounts of carcinogens. A consistent finding in epidemiological studies is that people who consume the most calories have significantly higher incidences of cancer (Kuska 2000; Winick 1991). There are several mechanisms that explain why overeating causes cancer, but one reason is that more gene mutations occur in response to higher food intake.

It is well known that foods cooked at high temperatures inflict massive damage to the genes. Women who eat very well cooked hamburgers have a 50% greater risk of breast cancer than women who eat rare or medium hamburgers. A nested, case-control study among 41,836 cohort members of the Iowa Women's Health Study found that women who consistently consumed well cooked beef steak, hamburgers, and bacon had a 4.62-fold increased risk of breast cancer (Zheng et al. 1998). Cooking foods at high temperatures causes the formation of gene-mutating heterocyclic amines. This is one reason why eating deep-fried foods is dangerous. Heterocyclic amines have been linked to prostate, breast, colorectal, esophageal, lung, liver, and other cancers. While health-conscious people try to avoid foods that are known carcinogens, even grilled salmon contains a potent dose of gene-mutating heterocyclic amines (Madrigal-Bujaidar et al. 1997).

While one can reduce his exposure to cancer-causing heterocylic amines, it may be impossible to prevent them from forming in the body. This is because enzymatic activities that naturally occur in the liver can inadvertently manufacture heterocyclic amines from otherwise harmless organic compounds (Guengerich et al. 1991). The carcinogenic dangers of heterocyclic amines have been thoroughly discussed in the scientific literature, yet the public is largely unaware of these dangers and continues to consume foods that inflict massive numbers of gene mutations.

Studies indicate that heterocyclic amines cause more cases of cancer than previously indicated (Terry et al. 2003; Turesky 2002). However, heterocyclic amines are not the only dietary culprit involved in gene mutation. Other mutagenic agents found in food are nitrosamine preservatives, aflatoxin molds, and pesticide/herbicide residues.

The bottom line is that we need to eat a certain number of calories, and this inevitably exposes us to agents that mutate our genes. Because avoiding all dietary carcinogens is impossible, identifying methods to protect genes against mutation becomes a critical part of a life extension program.

How Cancer Cells Form

As quoted earlier in this text, "Cancer results from the accumulation of mutations in genes that regulate cellular proliferation" (Haber 2000). A common pathway toward cancer occurs when dietary mutagenic agents cause adducts to be formed on DNA genes. Adducts (gene alterations) are formed when a carcinogen binds to DNA. When a high enough percentage of DNA adducts form along critical gene segments, normal cells can be transformed into cancer cells (Strauss et al. 1991). Roughly 90% of DNA adducts are removed within a 24-hour period by DNA repair enzymes and other natural gene protective mechanisms (Hart et al. 1974). Humans possess the most efficient DNA repair mechanisms in the entire animal kingdom. Mice and other small mammals, on the other hand, have a 0–13% repair rate over 24 hours (which correlates with the mouse average lifespan of only 3.4 years) (Hart et al. 1974). DNA adducts represent genetic mutation. If the adducts are not repaired, this can lead to tumor formation. Preventing these adducts from forming in the first place would dramatically lower cancer risk.

PREVENTING GENE MUTATION

The first line of defense against the many carcinogens in the human diet are agents that prevent gene mutation. Many antimutagenic agents have been identified in fruits and vegetables, the most potent being the indole-3-carbinols, the chlorophylls, and chlorophyllin (Negishi et al. 1997). The traditional dietary antioxidants should be considered only as a secondary line of defense against cancer because it is more important to inactivate or neutralize carcinogens in the first place than to try to protect the cells and proteins downstream from their effects. Chlorophyllin is the modified, water-

soluble form of chlorophyll that has been tested as an antimutagenic agent for more than 20 years. In one of the great ironies of natural product science, we now have a very large body of data concerning the anticancer, antimutagenic, antioxidant, and potentially life-extending benefits of chlorophyllin but much less information on the effects of natural chlorophyll itself (Negishi et al. 1997; Tsunoda et al. 1998).

For example, chlorophyllin can cross cell membranes, organelle membranes, and the blood-brain barrier while chlorophyll cannot. Chlorophyllin even enters into the mitochondria, the energy-producing organelles of the cell where 91% of oxygen reduction occurs and where the majority of free radicals are produced (Boloor et al. 2000; Kamat et al. 2000). Chlorophyllin quenches all major reactive oxygen species, such as the superoxide radical, hydrogen peroxide, singlet oxygen, and even the most dangerously reactive hydroxyl radical at very low doses (Kamat et al. 2000). Chlorophyllin has been shown to be a potent mitochondrial antioxidant that not only protects mitochondria from their own auto-oxidation (considered to be one of the major causes of aging), but also protects mitochondria from a variety of external chemical, biological, and radiation insults (Boloor et al. 2000; Kamat et al. 2000; Wei et al. 2001).

History of Chlorophyllin

The Life Extension Foundation introduced its members to the antimutagenic effects of chlorophyllin in 1989. Life Extension based its recommendation to supplement with chlorophyllin on a study in the journal *Mutation Research*, showing that this plant extract was more effective than all other known anticancer vitamins at that time (Ong et al. 1989). An earlier study also in *Mutation Research* reported that chlorophyllin suppressed the mutagenic activity of carcinogens such as fried beef and pork, red wine, chewing tobacco and snuff, cigarette smoke, diesel emissions, and coal dust by more than 90% (Ong et al. 1986)! No other supplement came close to the ability of chlorophyllin to inhibit deadly gene mutations. In 1989, the cost of chlorophyllin was exorbitant, and only relatively low amounts could be used in dietary supplements. The good news is that the price of chlorophyllin has plummeted, enabling consumers to obtain high potencies at affordable prices.

Detoxifying Dietary Mutagens

The great majority of studies about chlorophyllin's health benefits concern its antimutagenic and anticarcinogenic properties. Unlike other antioxidants, which merely quench free radicals, chlorophyllin traps heterocyclic hydrocarbon carcinogens by reacting with their backbone, making it impossible for them to form adducts with DNA (Dashwood et al. 1996; Hernaez et al. 1997). There are more than 50 cancer-causing agents known to occur in the human diet that chlorophyllin has been shown to protect against, including benzopyrene, dimethylbenzanthracene (DMBA), dibenzopyrene, TRP-P2, aflatoxin B-1 and aflatoxin B-2, 2-aminoanthracene, 2-nitrofluorene, 1-nitropyrene, 1-methyl-6-phenylimidazo [4,5-pyridine] (PHIP), and 2-amino-3-methylimidazo [4,5-f] quinoline (IQ). Tea epigallocatechins have no effect on the degradation rate of N-hydroxy IQ, but chlorophyllin rapidly degrades it by combining with it (Hernaez et al. 1997; Madrigal-Bujaidar et al. 1997; Negishi et al. 1997; Tang et al. 1997; Breinholt et al. 1999; Cabera et al. 2000; Chung et al. 2000; Kamat et al. 2000; Egner et al. 2001).

Many of these carcinogens are found in ordinary broiled, boiled, baked, and otherwise high-temperature cooked foods (Guengerich et al. 1991). For instance, PHIP is considered the most abundant heterocyclic amine in fried ground beef. It causes colon cancers in F344 rats and is considered a leading cancer suspect agent in humans (Guengerich et al. 1991; Guo 1995). Chlorophyllin 0.1% in the drinking water of rats reduced aberrant crypt foci 50% in the colon when exposed to PHIP (Guo 1995). In another study with F344 rats, a diet with 2000-ppm chlorophyllin significantly protected them from diethylnitrosamine-induced liver neoplasms (Sugie 1996). Diethylnitrosamine is commonly found in many types of distilled spirits and beers (Guengerich et al. 1991).

The most notorious of all human dietary carcinogens is aflatoxin B-1. Aflatoxins occur all over the world in fungus-infected rice, wheat, rye, and other staple grains. They have also been found in a variety of U.S. crops. Aflatoxin-infected crops are more of a problem in developing countries such as China where, in certain provinces, the farmers experience the highest liver cancer rates in the world (Egner et al. 2001). In a landmark study entitled "Chlorophyllin Intervention Reduces Aflatoxin-DNA Adducts in Individuals at High Risk for Cancer," researchers demonstrated a 55% reduction in aflatoxin urinary bio-markers compared to controls by giving the farmers 100 mg of chlorophyllin 3 times a day with their meals (Egner et al. 2001).

The scientists estimated that the induction period needed for this type of cancer to develop was extended from 20–40 years by supplementing with chlorophyllin. Chlorophyllin tablets were found to be the least expensive and most cost effective means of preventing these types of cancers (Egner et al. 2000; 2001). Several studies have noted that there is a powerful relationship between dietary aflatoxin reduction, DNA adducts, and lowering of cancer rates in both humans and animals (Dashwood et al. 1998; Kensler et al. 1998; Breinholt et al. 1999; Egner et al. 2001).

The effective dose of chlorophyllin as an antimutagenic agent is far lower than teas and other antioxidants, usually in the range of 0.5–4 mg per kilogram of body weight, making chlorophyllin the most potent antimutagen available on a weight basis. The best results in animals at suppressing carcinogenesis are in the 2–4 mg per kilogram range (Madrigal-Bujaidar et al. 1997), the same as the dosage used in the human intervention trials (Egner et al. 2000, 2001). At this dose range, it protected mouse bone marrow from benzopyrene toxicity 80.9% and 77.5%, respectively.

The anticancer properties of green tea, black tea, and chlorophyllin were compared, and it was found that chlorophyllin is a far more potent antimutagenic agent, protecting against a wider range of carcinogens than tea (Hernaez et al. 1997). In one study, teas did not degrade the mutagen IQ found in cooked meat, while chlorophyllin rapidly degraded IQ.

In human breast cell studies, chlorophyllin was one of the most effective compounds protecting against DNA adduct formation. Chlorophyllin inhibited adduct formation 65% at 30 micromolar concentrations, and it was also a very effective inhibitor at 15 micromoles/L, a level obtainable in vivo in the tissues of humans (Smith et al. 2001).

In vitro studies with chlorophyllin show it to be an inhibitor of the cytochrome P-450 liver enzymes (Tachino et al. 1994). All in vivo [whole animal] studies where cytochrome P-450 enzyme activity is reduced resulted in lower cancer rates and longer life span (Guengerich et al. 1991). In Stage II liver detoxification, enzymes called glutathione transferases cause glutathione to react with the carcinogens formed from cytochrome P-450 activity to produce harmless byproducts, but this process is not very efficient (Finch et al. 1997). Chlorophyllin, however, makes this conversion more efficient by lowering cytochrome P-450 enzyme activity in the first place and by reacting with carcinogens to produce harmless complexes in a similar manner to the glutathione transferases. Thus, chlorophyllin is not an inducer of glutathione transferases but mimics glutathione transferase activity.

When to Take Chlorophyllin

The primary purpose of taking chlorophyllin supplements is to neutralize dietary carcinogens before they can mutate our DNA genes. People are exposed to more carcinogens in their diet than from cigarette smoke. It has been established that overcooked meat, fried meat, meat containing nitrosamine, and aflatoxin-contaminated plants contain known carcinogens. There are, however, mutagenic agents in virtually all foods. The benefit of eating fresh fruits and vegetables is that they often provide more antimutagenic phytochemicals (such as chlorophyll) than harmful ones.

There is a considerable amount of animal research, and some human data to recommend that a 100-mg capsule of chlorophyllin should be taken with each meal or at least with meals that are known to contain a lot of carcinogens. While some people may not be able to take chlorophyllin with every meal, there would appear to be considerable benefit in taking at least a 100-mg chlorophyllin capsule with the most dangerous meal of the day, that is, the meal that contains the most carcinogens. If your dinner consists of grilled fish or barbecued steak, it might be wise to take 200–300 mg of chlorophyllin to help neutralize the heterocyclic amines and many other carcinogens formed in the cooking process. Because the main benefit of supplementing with chlorophyllin is to detoxify dietary mutagens, it should be taken with food and not wasted on an empty stomach.

Chlorophyllin Side Effects/Contraindications

The only reported side effects with chlorophyllin after 40 years of experience are occasional reports of diarrhea (transient), a green color imparted to the stool, and a pale green color conferred to serum (Egner et al. 2000, 2001). When this coloring of sera was first noticed, the authors of the study noted it to be a good sign. In other words, chlorophyllin is probably acting as an antioxidant and antimutagenic agent in the bloodstream, having been shown to be an inhibitor of ascorbate-iron induced lipid peroxidation (Kamat et al. 2000). Chlorophyllin is sold as an expensive prescription drug to reduce fecal odors in nursing home patients. Some institutions mandate that the chlorophyllin drug be given to every patient to suppress unpleasant odors. When taken by healthy people, chlorophyllin has been reported to reduce fecal aroma and possibly halitosis (Ui et al. 1991; Hideshi et al. 1996).

Persons who have Wilson's disease should avoid chlorophyllin supplements. Wilson's disease is a genetic defect that causes toxic amounts of copper to accumulate in the blood because the body lacks the ability to metabolize copper. Persons with Wilson's disease should avoid any copper supplement because

of the excess copper already in their bodies. Those with active cancer may also want to avoid chlorophyllin based on a current theory that copper may promote angiogenesis. Physicians who subscribe to this theory often attempt to reduce copper to extremely low levels to better enable the patient to gain control over their active cancer. Healthy people do not have this concern because most of the copper in chlorophyllin is in the bound form and is not bioavailable to the body. Additional information about free versus bound copper appears in the next section.

Choosing a Chlorophyllin Product

There are many chlorophyllin products sold on the supplement market. They can all be expected to provide benefits in reducing fecal odor and possibly halitosis (Ui et al. 1991; Hideshi et al. 1996). In order to derive the maximum antimutagenic effects of chlorophyllin, a supplement should contain standardized potencies of these specific constituents.

A 100-mg capsule of chlorophyllin should contain very little or no free copper. The copper that is naturally part of the chlorophyllin should be tightly sequestered (bound) in the chlorophyllin molecule (Meydani et al. 2002) so that it is not freely available to the body. Consumers should insist on a standardized chlorophyllin supplement that provides optimal percentages of active chlorophyll constituents and verifies that the free copper is very low. To reduce the absorption of any free copper that may be in the product, 10 mg of zinc could be taken with chlorophyllin or be included in the supplement itself.

🌑 SUMMARY

The evidence presented here clearly shows that avoiding substances known to inflict gene mutations can reduce one's risk of developing cancer. Epidemiological studies document that people who expose themselves to gene-mutating toxins develop cancer far more frequently than those who follow a healthier lifestyle.

Each human cell sustains about 10,000 DNA gene mutations every day (Seo et al. 2002). If it were not for DNA repair enzymes, these mutations would quickly lead to cancer or functional cell failure. There is a limit to the cell's ability to repair these multiple DNA alterations. That is why protecting genes against mutation is so important.

Most gene mutations occur from environmental factors, the most prevalent being the food we eat (Guengerich et al. 1991; Herskind et al. 1996; Finch et al. 1997). While a healthy diet helps protect our genes, it has been established that gene mutations occur as a part of normal metabolic processes. If we live long enough, the accumulation of gene mutations can result in cancer, neurological disorders, and other degenerative diseases.

While it is possible to reduce exposure to substances that mutate genes, it is impossible to avoid them altogether. Even if one consumed the perfect diet and minimized environmental mutagen exposure, the aging process itself results in gene mutations that can lead to cancer. It, thus, becomes imperative to both detoxify dietary mutagens as well as protect one's genes against mutagenic transformation into cancer cells.

Antioxidants help to protect genes against mutation. This is one reason why humans who consume higher levels of antioxidants and other plant extracts often have lower incidences of cancer. A number of published studies show that chlorophyllin may be the most effective antimutagenic agent ever discovered.

Because the accumulation of gene mutations is the underlying cause of cancer and a host of other diseases, it appears logical to add chlorophyllin to one's supplement program. Chlorophyllin is an antioxidant that quenches a wide variety of reactive oxygen species and exhibits a multitude of anticancer effects at very low doses.

While cholorophyllin is an important nutrient to prevent excess gene mutations, there are other supplements that protect against cancer via different mechanisms. A number of these anticancer supplements are discussed in the *Prevention* protocol in this book.

 ## PRODUCT AVAILABILITY

Standardized chlorophyllin (100-mg) capsules and Life Extension Super Booster (multinutrient formula that includes 100 mg of standardized chlorophyllin), and Zinc are available by telephoning (800) 544-4440 or by ordering online at www.lef.org.

STAYING INFORMED

The information published in this protocol is only as current as the day the manuscript was sent to the printer. This protocol raises many issues that are subject to change as new data emerge. Furthermore, cancer is still a disease with unacceptably high mortality rates, and none of our suggested regimens can guarantee a cure.

The Life Extension Foundation is constantly uncovering information to provide to cancer patients. A special website has been established for the purpose of updating patients on new findings that directly pertain to the published cancer protocols. Whenever Life Extension discovers information that may benefit cancer patients, it will be posted on the website www.lefcancer.org.

Before utilizing this cancer protocol, we suggest that you check www.lefcancer.org to see if any substantive changes have been made to the recommendations described herein. Based on the sheer number of newly published findings, there could be significant alterations to the information you have just read.

DISCLAIMER

This information (and any accompanying printed material) is not intended to replace the attention or advice of a physician or other health care professional. Anyone who wishes to embark on any dietary, drug, exercise, or other lifestyle change intended to prevent or treat a specific disease or condition should first consult with and seek clearance from a qualified health care professional.

The information published in the protocols is only as current as the day the manuscript was sent to the printer. This protocol raises many issues that are subject to change as new data emerge. None of our suggested protocol regimens can guarantee a cure.

Cancer Radiation

Therapy Radiation therapy is given to about 60% of all cancer patients, but it can inflict significant damage on healthy normal tissues. Radiotherapy can also cause secondary cancers after the primary cancer has been treated, which typically occur several years later. Other secondary diseases such as pneumonitis and radiation fibrosis may also occur. Radiation therapy is associated with both acute and delayed disturbances in nutritional status.

Radiation therapy relies on the free radical disruption of cellular DNA. The rationale behind damaging cancer cell DNA is that it may preclude successful division into more cancer cells or trigger cancer cell *apoptosis* (also known as programmed cell death). Radiation therapy can be delivered from both external or internal sources, may be high or low dose, and is often delivered with computer-assisted accuracy to the site of the tumor. Brachytherapy (or interstitial radiation therapy) places the source of radiation directly into the tumor as temporarily implanted ribbons and seeds or as permanently implanted seeds.

Newer radiotherapy technologies, such as stereotactic radiosurgery, which uses tightly focused x-rays or gamma rays to target tumors without widespread irradiation of surrounding tissues, may improve radiotherapy results. However, these approaches are limited to certain types of cancers.

REVERSING HYPOXIA

Cancer often outgrows the ability of the host to supply blood vessels and oxygen. Cancer cells are therefore often found in a low-oxygen (hypoxic) environment. Hypoxic cancer cells are *radio-resistant*, an effect that contributes significantly to the inability of radiotherapy to control large cancers. Therapies that provide more oxygen to cancer cells help radiation work more effectively by enabling more free-radical formation. *Remember:* Radiation kills cancer cells by concentrating massive amounts of free radicals directly into tumors. L-arginine is a promising natural agent for enhancing oxygenation of tumor cells due to its ability to increase the serum nitric oxide level, which enhances blood flow by expanding arterial elasticity. Enhanced blood flow provides more oxygen to tumors

that in turn enables radiation therapy to generate more cell-killing free radicals.

Consuming 20–30 grams of arginine 30–60 minutes prior to each radiation session could significantly increase the number of cancer cells killed in persons undergoing radiation therapy. Many people find it difficult to consume 20–30 grams of arginine orally. As an alternative, a physician could administer the arginine via an IV (intravenous) infusion 30 minutes before each radiation session. Arginine is available to doctors in IV dosing packs for the purpose of testing pituitary growth hormone response. However, conventional physicians are reluctant to try innovative approaches. Patients seeking to use high dose arginine prior to each radiation session have the following options:

1. Swallowing 23–33 arginine (900 mg per capsule) capsules

2. Mixing 2.5–3.5 tablespoons of unpleasant-tasting arginine powder and drinking the mixture

3. Taking 4–6 tablespoons of an arginine-based drink called sugar-free PowerMaker II. (This makes normally unpalatable arginine acceptable to taste.)

4. Finding a physician in your area who will have trained a medical technician to administer the 20–30 grams of arginine by IV therapy prior to each radiation session. (To find an innovative physician who might accommodate this IV arginine request, call (800) 544-4440.)

To further saturate the tumor with more oxygen, some patients breathe pure oxygen during the radiation therapy (Kaanders et al. 2002; Zajusz et al. 1995; Evans et al. 1975)

Guarding Against Blood's Oxygen-Carrying Deficiencies

Arginine will not be of much benefit if there is a deficiency in the ability of blood to carry oxygen (anemia). Anemia is common in cancer patients. Conventional cancer therapies, such as surgery, chemotherapy, radiation, and testosterone blockade, often induce anemia. Elevated levels of certain cytokines such as tumor necrosis factor-alpha (TNF-alpha), commonly seen in cancer patients, also suppress red blood cell formation.

The adverse effect of anemia in cancer patients is well established in scientific literature. A study conducted to systematically review the effect of anemia on survival in cancer patients found that the increased risk of mortality associated with anemia in

example, IMPATH can determine whether certain types of lymphomas have recurred before they can be detected by any other method. The earlier tumor recurrence is detected, the greater the likelihood of therapeutic success.

IMPATH not only offers a full range of diagnostic and prognostic cancer analyses, but also emphasizes client service. Typically within 48 hours after receiving a specimen, IMPATH returns the stained slides along with a thorough and detailed case report to a physician. If your oncologist wants to consult with a member of the IMPATH staff, telephone lines are open. In *Appendix A* at the end of this protocol are examples of typical IMPATH laboratory reports that your oncologist receives.

Contact information for IMPATH is as follows:

New York
521 West 57th Street, Sixth Floor
New York, NY 10019

Los Angeles
5300 McConnell Avenue
Los Angeles, CA 90066

Phoenix
810 East Hammond Lane
Phoenix, AZ 85034

Telephone: (800) 447-5816
Website: www.impath.com

HOW TO IMPLEMENT STEP ONE

Make certain your surgeon sends a specimen of your tumor to IMPATH for immunohistochemistry testing, using the contact information just provided. You may have to pay out of pocket for this test because not all insurance plans reimburse for it. Please note that this test may not be of benefit to all cancer patients. While it provides a basis for improved treatment, not all cancers are effectively treatable with today's technologies.

STEP TWO: ANALYZING THE PATIENT'S LIVING TUMOR CELLS TO DETERMINE SENSITIVITY OR RESISTANCE TO CHEMOTHERAPY

If chemotherapy is being considered, it is desirable to know which of the chemotherapy drugs will have a high probability of being effective against your particular cancer before any toxic agents are administered into your body. It is equally as important, if not more important, to know if your particular cancer cells

exhibit extreme drug resistance (EDR) to specific chemotherapy drugs. EDR implies a probability of 95% that the chemotherapy drugs exhibiting EDR will be *ineffective* in killing the cancer cells. A company called Rational Therapeutics, Inc. performs chemosensitivity tests on the living specimens of your cancer cells to determine the optimal combination of chemotherapy drugs, as well as determining EDR.

Rational Therapeutics, Inc., was founded in 1993 by Dr. Robert Nagourney, a prominent hematologist and oncologist. Rational Therapeutics pioneers cancer therapies that are specifically tailored for each individual patient and is a leader in individualized cancer strategies. With no financial ties to outside healthcare organizations, recommendations are made without financial or scientific prejudice.

Rational Therapeutics develops and provides cancer therapy recommendations which have been designed scientifically for each patient. Following the collection of living cancer cells obtained at the time of biopsy or surgery, Rational Therapeutics performs an *Ex-Vivo* Apoptotic (EVA) assay on your tumor sample to measure drug activity (sensitivity and resistance). *Ex-vivo apoptotic* means that your tumor cells are grown outside of your body for the purpose of determining which drug or drug combination most effectively induces cell death (apoptosis) in the laboratory. Each patient is highly individualized with regard to his or her sensitivity to chemotherapy drugs. Your responsiveness to chemotherapy is as unique as your fingerprints. Therefore, this test will help to exactly determine which drug(s) will be most effective for *you*. Dr. Nagourney will then make a treatment recommendation based on these findings.

The treatment program developed through this approach is known as *assay-directed therapy*. In 1999, there were more than 1.2 million newly diagnosed cases of cancer in the United States, with 563,000 deaths attributed to this disease. Unfortunately, 50% of newly diagnosed cancer patients have advanced disease that is beyond the hope of a surgical or radiation cure. Patients with advanced disease and those with recurrent disease are candidates for systemic therapy, which is administered usually in the form of chemotherapy. Despite the enormity of the cancer problem, in the last 45 years, there has been virtually no major change in the outcome for the common advanced solid tumors such as those of the lung, prostate, colon, and breast. While there have been improvements in treating lymphomas, certain types of leukemia, and some earlier-stage cancers, the grim facts indicate more aggressive tumor diagnostic tests are needed to provide the medical oncologist with better prognostic information about your individual tumor.

At present, cancer chemotherapies are prescribed by medical oncologists, according to fixed schedules. These schedules are standardized drug regimens that correspond to specific cancers by type or diagnosis. These schedules, developed over years of clinical trials, assign patients to the drugs for which they have the greatest statistical probability of response.

Patients with cancers that exhibit multidrug resistance are on the wrong side of the probability curve, that is, they will likely receive treatments that are wrong for them. A failed attempt at chemotherapy is detrimental to the physical and emotional well-being of patients, is financially burdensome, and may preclude further effective therapies.

Rational Therapeutics provides custom-tailored, assay-directed therapy based on your tumor response in the laboratory. This eliminates much of the guess work prior to your undergoing the potentially toxic side effects of chemotherapy regimens that could prove to be of little value against your cancer. In *Appendix B* at the end of this protocol are typical laboratory reports your oncologist receives from Rational Therapeutics.

Here is the contact information for Rational Therapeutics:

Rational Therapeutics, Inc.

750 East 29th Street

Long Beach, CA 90806

Telephone: (562) 989-6455; Fax: (562) 989-8160

Email: www.rationaltherapeutics.com

HOW TO IMPLEMENT STEP TWO

Get in touch with Rational Therapeutics using the contact information provided so that your surgeon can follow the precise instructions required to send a living specimen of your tumor for chemosensitivity testing. It is important that your surgeon carefully coordinate with Rational Therapeutics in order to ensure your cells arrive in a viable condition. You may have to pay for this test yourself because your insurance may not reimburse for it. Please note that this test may not be of benefit to all cancer patients. While it provides a basis for improved treatment, not all cancers are effectively treatable with today's technologies.

STEP THREE: PROTECTING AGAINST ANEMIA

Anemia diminishes the chances that a cancer patient will survive. Since red blood cells carry oxygen, fewer numbers of red blood cells result in less oxygen transport. When normal cells are oxygen deprived, they lack the vigor to overcome cancer. Cancer cells, on the other hand, thrive in a low oxygen environment. The journal *Cancer* reported that anemia increased the risk of mortality in cancer patients by about 65% (Caro et al. 2001).

Anemia is defined functionally as lack of sufficient red blood cells to maintain tissue oxygenation. Anemia develops when the demand for new red blood cells exceeds the capacity of the bone marrow to produce them. This may be due to inadequate red blood cell production, as occurs when cancer or cancer therapies inhibit the production of erythropoietin, a glycoprotein hormone secreted by the kidney, which acts on stem cells of the bone marrow to stimulate red blood cell production (Spivak 1994).

Cancer-related anemia also results from activation of the immune and inflammatory systems (responses orchestrated by the tumor), leading to an increased release of *tumor necrosis factor-alpha* (TNF-alpha) and *interleukin-1* (IL-1). Such cytokines circumvent the ability of the bone marrow to respond to available circulating erythropoietin, resulting in lesser numbers of oxygen-carrying red blood cells being produced (Cazzola 2000). In addition, the lifespan of red blood cells (normally 120 days in men and about 110 days in women) is shortened in cancer-related anemia; thus, production cannot compensate sufficiently for the shorter survival time. The energy-depleting cycle of abnormal metabolism (leading to malnutrition and wasting disease) also is a contributing factor to the progression of anemia.

Anemia appears to contribute to angiogenesis—the vascular network supplying life to the tumor. Vascular endothelial growth factor (VEGF) is an endothelial cell specific mitogen, an agent that induces cell division. The expression of VEGF appears to be an indicator of the angiogenic potential and correlates with the biological aggressiveness of a tumor. The serum levels of VEGF, as well as hemoglobin levels (which ranged from 8.9–15.6 g/dL), were determined in a total of 54 cancer patients. An association between low hemoglobin levels and increased serum VEGF was seen in 26 patients whose hemoglobin was less than 13 g/dL as compared to 28 patients with hemoglobin levels greater than 13 g/dL. A correlation was also established between anemia and intratumoral hypoxia (reduced oxygen supply within the tumor). The increased serum-VEGF levels in patients with low hemoglobin may be explained via hypoxia-induced VEGF secretion. This suggests that anemia may stimulate angiogenesis through intratumoral hypoxia (Dunst et al. 1999).

Weakness, fatigue or faintness, shortness of breath and increased heart rate, headaches, confusion, dementia, depression, cold extremities, dizziness, pallor, and sore mouth are complaints of anemia that complicate recovery. Severe anemia may also result in heart failure.

Where Cancer Patients' Hematocrit and Hemoglobin Levels Should Be

Based on findings from survival studies, cancer patients should fall within the optimal ranges of the following two blood tests that measure the oxygen-carrying capacity of blood:

Normal Laboratory Reference Range	Optimal Range for Cancer Patients
Hemoglobin	
Men: 12.5–17 (g/dL)	15.5–17 (g/dL)
Women: 11.5–15 (g/dL)	13.83–15 (g/dL)
Hematocrit	
Men: 36–50%	45–50%
Women: 34–44%	41–44%

Note: Normal references ranges based on Labcorp's standards as of October 2002.

If the oncologist fails to address anemia, the patient should assume the role of advocate, demanding attention be paid to the quality of the blood. Please note that it will be difficult to convince most oncologists that cancer patients should be in the optimal ranges indicated on this chart. One reason is that even healthy people are often below the optimal ranges for cancer patients. The problem is that insurance companies will not reimburse for a drug such as Procrit for the purposes of elevating hematocrit and hemoglobin to the high optimal ranges for cancer patients. Most insurance companies, in fact, will not pay for Procrit unless severe anemia is demonstrated.

Procrit, a synthetic erythropoietin that stimulates the production of red blood cells, is often prescribed for the treatment of cancer-related anemia.

HOW TO IMPLEMENT STEP THREE

1. If your hemoglobin or hematocrit levels are not in the optimal ranges described on the chart in this section, ask your physician to prescribe an individualized dose of Procrit.

2. In order for Procrit to effectively boost red blood cell production, it is essential that your body have adequate iron stores. Even if you have adequate iron stores prior to Procrit therapy, the rapid production of red blood cells induced by Procrit may eventually deplete total body iron stores. Therefore, it is important to obtain baseline studies to exclude the presence of iron deficiency.

Note: *Iron deficiency is best diagnosed by checking the serum ferritin to see if the values are low. Many physicians obtain a serum iron and serum iron binding capacity and divide the former by the latter to obtain the transferrin saturation. If this result is < 10%, there is a probability of iron deficiency anemia (IDA). A more modern approach to a diagnosis of iron deficiency anemia, however, is to check the serum ferritin; if it is greater than 220, IDA is essentially ruled out. However, if the serum ferritin level is lower than 220, a blood test called the soluble transferrin receptor (sTfR) assay should be obtained. This measures the receptors for transferrin— receptors that bind to the available iron. If this value is 28 or higher, there is a significant chance of IDA. Regular blood tests to assess ferritin and, when indicated, sTfR will assist your doctor in determining whether or not you need iron supplementation.*

3. Dietary supplements that can help protect against anemia include folic acid (800 mcg/day), vitamin B_{12} (500 mcg/day), and melatonin (3–10 mg/day, taken at night) (Vaziri et al. 1996; Herrera et al. 2001).

STEP FOUR: INHIBITING THE CYCLOOXYGENASE-2 (COX-2) ENZYME

Our diet, the amount of saturated and polyunsaturated fat we eat, and the unfavorable fats that we create in our bodies play a crucial role in the development and progression of malignancy. A critical pathway that represents a "Rosetta Stone" to all aspects of our health is that involving the metabolism of omega-6 fatty acids leading to either di-homo gamma-linolenic acid (DGLA) or to arachidonic acid (*see Figure 1*).

These "roads" are called the *eicosanoid pathways*. The metabolism of DGLA leads to the production of fats that are actually beneficial to our health, that is, good eicosanoids. Unfortunately, in today's world, this is the "road less traveled" for most people. The metabolism of arachidonic acid, the bad eicosanoid pathway, leads to most of the health maladies currently faced by our society. A key enzyme in the bad eicosanoid pathway is cyclo-oxygenase (cyclooxygenase or COX). It is the COX-2 enzyme that results in the production of prostaglandin E_2 or PGE_2 (*see Figure 1*).

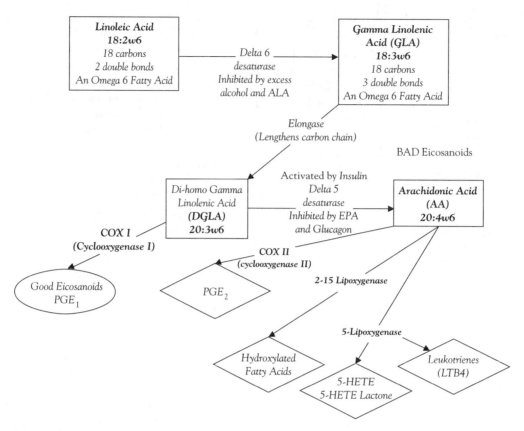

Figure 1. The Eicosanoid Pathways

Initially, scientists believed COX-2 was merely an inducible response to inflammation. It is now speculated that COX-2 performs biological functions in the body, particularly in the brain and kidneys as well as the immune system. COX-2 becomes troublesome when up-regulated (sometimes 10- to 80-fold) by pro-inflammatory stimuli (interleukin-1, growth factors, tumor necrosis factor, and endotoxin). When over-expressed, COX-2 participates in various pathways that could promote cancer, that is, angiogenesis, cell proliferation, and the production of inflammatory prostaglandins (Sears 1995; Newmark et al. 2000).

A number of researchers have established the COX-2 cancer connection:

• The *Wall Street Journal* (September 7, 1999) reported the results of a trial involving a group of rats given a potent carcinogen along with a COX-2 inhibitor. Rats treated with the COX-2 inhibitor experienced a 90% reduction in cancer compared to a group of rats not given a COX-2 inhibitor. Also, the tumors that appeared were 80% smaller and less numerous than in the control group.

• An article in the journal *Cancer Research* showed that COX-2 levels in pancreatic cancer cells are 60 times greater than in adjacent normal tissue (Tucker et al. 1999).

• Solid tumors contain oxygen-deficient or hypoxic areas, that is, a reduction of oxygen supply to a tissue below physiological levels. Cells low in oxygen cloud prognosis, promoting up-regulation of COX-2 and angiogenesis, as well as establishing a resistance to ionizing radiation (Gately 2000).

• Greater microvessel density was observed in cancers over-expressing COX-2, compared to those with less COX-2 activity (Uefuji et al. 2000).

Within the nonsteroidal anti-inflammatory drug (NSAIDs) class is a subclass referred to as COX-2 inhibitors (cyclooxygenase inhibitors). COX-2 inhibitors are popularly prescribed to relieve pain but now have found a place in oncology. It began when scientists recognized that people who regularly take NSAIDs lowered their risk of colon cancer by as much as 50% (Reddy et al. 2000).

COX-2 inhibitors also significantly reduced colon polyps (considered precursors to cancer) in individuals with a propensity to polyp formation. Laboratory animals showed a similar benefit, that is, about 52% fewer polyps among mice treated with COX-2 inhibitors (Nakatsugi et al. 1997; Moran 2002). JAMA reported that a 9.4-year epidemiological study showed that COX-2 upregulation was related to more advanced tumor stage, tumor size, and lymph node metastasis as well as diminished survival rates among colorectal cancer patients (Sheehan et al. 1999). With more regular use of aspirin (a COX-2 inhibitor), the risk of dying from the disease decreased (Brody 1991; Knorr 2000). The journal *Gastroenterology* reported additional encouragement, showing that three different colon cell lines underwent apoptosis (cell death) when deprived of COX-2; when lovastatin was added to the COX-2 inhibitor, the kill rate increased another fivefold (Agarwal et al. 1999). The benefits, however, observed with COX-2 inhibitors extend beyond colon protection (Tsujii et al. 1998).

The COX-2 enzyme is increased in neoplastic epithelium in a number of other types of cancers (breast, bladder, lung, prostate, and head and neck cancers) as well as the blood vessel network surrounding the cancerous mass. Tumors expressing COX-2 are considered more treacherous than tumors that lack COX-2 (in part) because of the angiogenic (blood vessel-promoting) nature of cyclooxygenase. It appears cancer cells use COX-2 as a biological mechanism to fuel rapid cell division, growing larger tumor cells than those that lack COX-2 stimulation (Tsujii et al. 1998).

The Life Extension Foundation predicts that COX-2 inhibitors will eventually be approved to treat cancer. Progressive oncologists already have COX-2 inhibitors in their anticancer war chest, but the numbers are few. Unfortunately, the risks associated with traditional NSAIDs include gastrointestinal perforation, ulceration and bleeding, and less frequently, renal and liver disease. Vioxx and Celebrex, the most popular prescription COX-2 inhibitors, are often under fire due to potential kidney damage.

The *Archives of Internal Medicine* reported that seven cases of aseptic meningitis appear suspiciously linked with Vioxx (Bonnel et al. 2002). JAMA published a report raising a cautionary flag concerning the risk of cardiovascular events among users of COX-2 inhibitors (Mukherjee et al. 2001). Blood tests to assess liver and kidney function are essential, along with serum tumor markers and imagery testing to determine gains or losses during COX-2 inhibiting therapy.

While there are potential side effects to COX-2 inhibiting drugs, some cancer patients accept this small risk in exchange for the anticancer benefit. Since the COX-2 enzyme appears an excellent target for pharmacological intervention, a number of natural COX-2 inhibitors, safe and with diverse anticancer properties, are detailed in the protocol entitled *Cancer Adjuvant Therapy*.

HOW TO IMPLEMENT STEP FOUR

Ask your physician to prescribe one of the following COX-2 inhibiting drugs:

Lodine XL, 1000 mg once daily, or
Celebrex, 100–200 mg every 12 hours, or
Vioxx, 12.5–25 mg once daily

STEP FIVE: SUPPRESSING ras ONCOGENE EXPRESSION

The family of proteins known as ras plays a central role in the regulation of cell growth. It fulfills this fundamental role by integrating the regulatory signals that govern the cell cycle and proliferation (*see Figure 2*).

Defects in the ras-Raf pathway can result in cancerous growth. Mutant ras genes were among the first oncogenes identified for their ability to transform cells to a cancerous phenotype, that is, a cell observably altered because of distorted gene expression. Mutations in one of three genes (H, N, or K-ras) encoding ras proteins are associated with upregulated cell proliferation and are found in an estimated 30–40% of all human cancers. The highest incidences of ras mutations are found in cancers of the pancreas (80%), colon (50%), thyroid (50%), lung (40%), liver (30%), melanoma (30%), and myeloid leukemia (30%) (Bartram 1988; Bos 1989; Minamoto et al. 2000).

According to information in *Scientific American*, the differences between oncogenes and normal genes are slight. The mutant protein that an oncogene ultimately

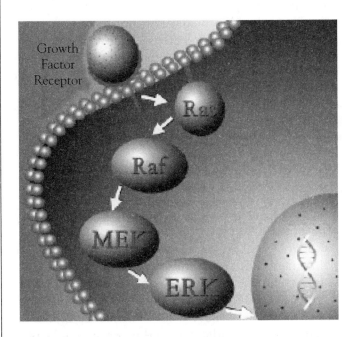

Figure 2. The ras-Raf Pathway. The ras-Raf pathway is used by human cells to transmit signals from the cell surface to the nucleus. Such signals direct cells to divide, differentiate, or even undergo programmed cell death (apoptosis). (With permission from Onyx Pharmaceuticals.)

creates may differ from the healthy version by only a single amino acid, but this subtle variation can radically alter the protein's functionality.

A ras gene usually behaves as a relay switch within the signal pathway that tells the cell to divide. In response to stimuli transmitted to the cell from outside, cell-signaling pathways are activated; in the absence of stimulus, the Ras protein remains in the "off" position. A *mutated ras* gene behaves like a switch stuck on the "on" position, continuously misinforming the cell, instructing it to divide when the cycle should be turned off (Gibbs et al. 1996; Oliff et al. 1996). Researchers have known for some time that injecting anti-ras antibodies, specific for amino acid 12, cause a reversal of excessive proliferation and a transient alteration of the mutated cell to one of a normal phenotype (Feramisco et al. 1985).

To establish new methods for diagnosing pancreatic cancer, K-ras mutations were examined in the pancreatic juice of pancreatic cancer patients. Pancreatic juice was positive for K-ras in 87.8% (36/41) of patients. When combined with p53 mutations in the stool and CA 19-9 (a blood marker for pancreatic cancer), it may be possible to identify the disease in its earliest stage. Thus, a program can be implemented that includes addressing mutant K-ras and p53 to achieve a more favorable outcome (Lu et al. 2001).

Greater understanding regarding the activity of mutant ras genes opens exciting avenues of treatment. Researchers found that newly formed ras molecules are functionally immature. Precursor ras genes must undergo several biochemical modifications to become mature, active versions. After such maturation, the ras proteins attach to the inner surface of the cells outer membrane where they can interact with other cellular proteins and stimulate cell growth.

The events resulting in mature ras genes take place in three steps, the most critical being the first, referred to as the farnesylation step. A specific enzyme, farnesyl-protein transferase (FPTase), speeds up the reaction. One strategy for blocking ras protein activity has been to inhibit FPTase. Inhibitors of this enzyme block the maturation of ras protein and reverse the cancerous transformation induced by mutant ras genes (Oliff et al. 1996).

A number of natural substances impact the activity of ras oncogenes. For example, a historic body of literature indicates individuals consuming large quantities of citrus products have a lower incidence of cancer. One of the essential oils within citrus products is limonene, a monoterpene that has been shown to act as a farnesyl transferase inhibitor. Administering high doses of limonene to cancer-bearing animals blocks the farnesylation of ras, thus inhibiting cell replication (Bland 2001; Asamoto et al. 2002). A study conducted at Mercy Hospital of Pittsburgh also showed that diallyl disulfide, a naturally occurring organosulfide from garlic, inhibits p21 H-ras oncogenes, displaying a significant restraining effect on tumor growth (Singh et al. 2000).

Researchers at Rutgers University investigated the ability of different green and black tea polyphenols to inhibit H-ras oncogenes. The Rutgers team found that all the major polyphenols contained in green and black tea except epicatechin showed strong inhibition of cell growth (Chung et al. 1999). Texas A&M University also found that fish oil decreased colonic ras membrane localization and reduced tumor formation in rats. In view of the central role of oncogenic ras in the development of colon cancer, the finding that omega-3 fatty acids modulate ras activation likely explains why dietary fish oil protects against colon cancer (Collett et al. 2001).

Statins are a class of popular cholesterol-lowering drugs. Mevacor (lovastatin), Zocor (simvastatin), and Pravachol (pravastatin) are statin drugs shown to inhibit the activity of ras oncogenes (Wang et al. 2000). Statin drugs block the hydroxymethylglutaryl-coenzyme A (HMG-COA) reductase enzyme, which depletes cells of farnesyl pyrophosphate. Levels of total ras do not decrease but rather shifts when Ras protein occurs, that is, farnesylated Ras decreases and unmodified, nonfarnesylated ras increases (Hohl et al. 1995).

Illustrative of the potential of statin therapy, patients with primary liver cancer were treated with either the chemotherapeutic drug 5-FU or a combination of 5-FU and 40 mg/day of pravastatin. Median survival increased from 9 months, among patients treated with only 5-FU, to 18 months when using 5-FU combined with the statin drug pravastatin (Pravachol®). Increased survival was attributed to decreased cellular proliferation and incidence of metastasis (Wang et al. 2000).

If a statin drug is co-administered with chemotherapy, some patients are medicated cyclically, that is, 3 weeks of a statin drug such as lovastatin (80 mg/day) followed by a 2-week break before restarting the statin. Other regimens involve using the statin drug for 6 continuous months or until signs of toxicity develop.

Note: *Some cancer patients may benefit from coenzyme Q_{10} supplementation when taking statin therapy. For a detailed explanation, please consult the Coenzyme Q_{10} section in the Cancer Adjuvant Therapy protocol.*

Individuals with cancer should consider an immunohistochemistry test of their cancer tissue for mutated ras genes at IMPATH Laboratories (*see the beginning of this protocol*), a recommendation the Life Extension Foundation first made in 1997. The Life Extension Foundation strongly believes all cancer patients should undergo immunohistochemical testing to determine p53 and ras status. As mentioned previously, the following laboratory can perform the test:

IMPATH Laboratories (www.impath.com),
Telephone: (800) 447-5816

HOW TO IMPLEMENT STEP FIVE

Ask your physician to prescribe one of the following statin drugs to inhibit the activity of ras oncogenes:

Mevacor (lovastatin), 40 mg twice each day, or
Zocor (simvastatin), 40 mg twice each day, or
Pravachol (pravastatin), 40 mg once a day

Note: *These statin drugs can produce toxic effects in patients. Physician oversight and careful surveillance with monthly blood tests (at least initially) to evaluate liver function, muscle enzymes, and lipid levels are suggested.*

In addition to statin drug therapy, consider supplementing with the following nutrients to further suppress the expression of ras oncogenes:

Fish Oil Capsules: 2400 mg of EPA and 1800 mg of DHA day (6 Mega EPA fish oil capsules provide this potency)
Green Tea Extract: 1500 mg of tea polyphenols a day (5 Super Green Tea Extract Caps provide this potency)
Aged Garlic Extract: 1200 mg a day (1 Kyolic One Per Day caplet provides this potency)

STEP SIX: CORRECTING COAGULATION ABNORMALITIES

Both experimental and clinical data have shown that coagulation disorders are common in patients with cancer, although clinical symptoms occur less often. Many cancer patients reportedly have a hypercoagulable state, with recurrent thrombosis due to the impact of cancer cells and chemotherapy on the coagulation cascade (Samuels et al. 1975). Pulmonary embolism is a particular problem for patients with pancreatic and gastric cancer, cancer of the large bowel, and women with ovarian cancer (Cafagna et al. 1997). Thus, momentum is building for anticoagulant therapy through reports, the vast majority of which are derived from secondary analyses of clinical trials on the treatment of thromboembolism.

Research on low-molecular-weight heparin (LMWH), an anticoagulant, shows promise in regard to increasing cancer survival rates. Data comparing unfractionated heparin to LMWH indicate that LMWH is equally beneficial if not more beneficial to cancer patients in terms of survival. The improved life expectancy gathered from anticoagulant therapy is not solely a result of the reduced complications from thromboembolism, but also from enzyme interactions, cellular growth modifications, and anti-angiogenic factors (Cosgrove et al. 2002). It appears heparin inhibits the formation of cancer's vascular network by binding to angiogenic promoters, that is, basic fibroblast growth factor and VEGF (Mousa 2002).

Another important aspect of anticoagulant therapy involves breaking down fibrin, a coagulation protein found in blood. Fibrin has various strategies it employs to accommodate the tumor. For example, fibrin covers maverick cells with a protective coat, hindering recognition by the immune system. In addition, fibrin relays a signal to the cancer cell to start angiogenesis, the growth of new blood vessels. As fibrin encourages a healthy vascular network and tumor growth increases, it sets the stage for metastasis.

German scientists evaluated whether cancer fatalities in women with previously untreated breast cancer were reduced using LMWH therapy. The study showed that breast cancer patients receiving LMWH, compared to women receiving unfractionated heparin, had a lower rate of mortality during the first 650 days following surgery. The survival advantage was evidenced after even a short course of therapy (von Tempelhoff et al. 2000). In another study of 300 breast cancer patients, none of the trial participants developed metastasis while receiving anticoagulant therapy although 37 (12.3%) died from the disease (Wellness Directory of Minnesota 2002).

Similar advantages were evidenced among small cell lung cancer patients undergoing anticoagulant therapy in union with conventional treatments. When anticoagulants were a part of the program, subjects enjoyed a better prognosis, that is, greater numbers of complete responses, longer median survival, as well as better survival rates at 1, 2, and 3 years compared to patients denied treatment (Lebeau et al. 1994; however, see also Zacharski et al. 1984, 1987; Chahinian et al. 1989).

HOW TO IMPLEMENT STEP SIX

1. Ascertain if you are in a hypercoagulable state by having your blood tested for prothrombin time (PT), partial thromboplastin time (PTT), and D-dimers. A hypercoagulable state is suggested if the shortening of the PT and PTT are seen in conjunction with elevation of D-dimers (*see table on laboratory tests for hypercoagulability*).

2. If there is any evidence of a hypercoagulable (prethrombotic) state, ask your physician to prescribe the appropriate individualized dose of low-molecular-weight heparin (LMWH). Repeat the prothrombin blood test every 2 weeks to guard against overcoagulation. If you cannot afford LMWH, ask that lower-cost Coumadin be prescribed instead.

Lab Tests for Hypercoagulability

Tests routinely available	Results if hypercoagulable	Tests requiring dedicated coagulation laboratory	Results if hypercoagulable
Protime (PT)	Less than normal	Alpha-1 antitrypsin (A1AT)	Elevated
Partial thromboplastin time (PTT)	Less than normal	Euglobulin clot lysis time (ECLT)	Prolonged
Platelet count (part of CBC)	Elevated	Factor VIII levels	Elevated
Fibrin split products (FSP)	Elevated	D-dimers (DD)	Elevated
Fibrinogen	Elevated		

STEP SEVEN: MAINTAINING BONE INTEGRITY

Some types of cancer (breast and prostate) have a proclivity to metastasize to the bone (Hohl et al. 1995; Wang et al. 2000). The result may be bone pain, which also may be associated with weakening of the bone and an increased risk of fractures (Spivak 1994; Caro et al. 2001).

Patients with prostate cancer have been found to have a very high incidence of osteoporosis or osteopenia even before the use of therapies that lower the male hormone testosterone (Cazzola 2000). In settings such as prostate cancer, when excessive bone loss is occurring, there is a release of bone-derived growth factors, such as TGF-beta-1, which stimulate the prostate cancer cells to grow further (Samuels et al. 1975; Dunst et al. 1999). In turn, prostate cancer cells elaborate substances such as interleukin-6 (IL-6), which has as one of its main effects the further breakdown of bone (Cafagna et al. 1997; Mousa 2002). Thus, a vicious cycle results: bone breakdown, the stimulation of prostate cancer cell growth, and the production of IL-6 and other cell products, which leads to further bone breakdown (*see Figure* 3).

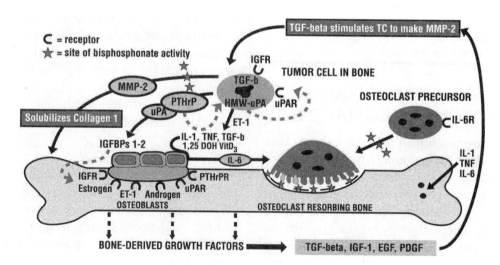

Figure 3. The vicious cycle of bone loss and release of bone-derived growth factors appears to be operative in prostate cancer. Growth factors such as IGF-1, EGF, and TGF-B1 appear to correlate with more aggressive and extensive PC. The use of bisphosphonate compounds to shut off bone resorption also reduces PSA. (Courtesy of Dr. Stephen Strum, *A Primer on Prostate Cancer* 2002.)

The intravenous (IV) or oral administration of any of the drugs called bisphosphonates, such as Aredia (IV), Zometa (IV), and Fosamax or Actonel (oral), can be used to stop this vicious cycle. Such agents stop excessive bone breakdown (resorption) and favor bone formation (Zacharski et al. 1984; Zacharski 1987; Chahinian et al. 1989; von Templehoff et al. 2000). Administration of bisphosphonates should be accompanied by an adequate intake of a bone supplement that supplies all raw materials to make healthy bone. These include calcium, magnesium, boron, silica, and vitamin D.

The problem that prostate and breast cancer patients face is that bisphosphonate therapy is approved for treatment only after cancer cells have metastasized to the bone and become clinically apparent by a nuclear medicine bone scan. If bisphosphonates were administered monthly to those with certain types of cancers, the risk of bone metastasis could be significantly reduced (Zurborn et al. 1982; Kohli et al. 2002). The Life Extension recommended bisphosphonate drugs (similar to those mentioned above) for certain types of cancer patients more than a decade ago. For many cancer patients, it would be ideal to continue bisphosphonate drug therapy a year or longer. Insurance companies, however, do not pay for bisphosphonates until after the cancer has metastasized to the bone.

Maintaining bone integrity may inhibit the growth of a wide range of cancers. Even when bone is broken down as a result of normal aging, the release of growth factors, such as IL-6 and transforming growth factor, can fuel tumor cell propagation.

Bisphosphonate class drugs, along with the appropriate mineral supplements and exercise to stimulate bone formation, can help to maintain bone integrity and, thus, save the lives of cancer patients.

The Life Extension Foundation strongly advises that the status of bone integrity should be evaluated periodically by means of a quantitative computerized tomography bone mineral density study called QCT. At the very least, this should be done annually. We prefer to use the QCT scan over the DXA since the QCT is not falsely affected by arthritis or calcifications in blood vessels that are commonly seen in men and women in their 50s and over. It is fairly common to see patients with a normal DXA scan and yet the QCT will be blatantly abnormal.

QCT sites possibly near you can be found via Mindways, Inc. at (877) 646-3929 (www.qct.com) or Image Analysis at (800) 548-4849 (www.image-analysis.com).

Tests that assess bone breakdown are inexpensive and involve a random urine collection obtained in the morning at the time of the second voided specimen.

One such highly accurate test of bone resorption is called DPD (deoxypyridinoline). This test provides information on excessive bone breakdown (resorption).

The deoxypyridinoline (DPD) cross links urine text can be ordered through the Life Extension Foundation by calling 1-800-208-3444.

HOW TO IMPLEMENT STEP SEVEN

1. If you have a type of cancer with a proclivity to metastasize to the bone (breast or prostate), ask your physician for a bisphosphonate drug before evidence of bone metastasis occurs. An oral bisphosphonate drug to consider is Actonel in the high dose of 30 mg twice a week. Alternatively, Fosamax can be used at a dose of 70 mg once a week. These agents should be taken on an empty stomach at least 1 hour and optimally 2 hours before breakfast. Some people experience gastroesophageal side effects from oral bisphosphonate drug therapy and prefer administration directly into the vein. An IV-administered bisphosphonate drug such as Aredia may be administered monthly beginning at 30 mg the first month, 60 mg the second month, and working up to 90 mg for subsequent months. Alternatively, Zometa can be given at a dose of 4 mg intravenously over 15 minutes every 3–4 weeks. When taking a bisphosphonate drug, it is important to take a wide array of bone-protecting supplements such as calcium, magnesium, zinc, manganese, and vitamin D_3. Six capsules a day of a product called Bone Assure provides optimal potencies of bone-protecting nutrients.

2. Because excessive bone breakdown releases growth factors into the bloodstream that can fuel cancer cell growth, the DPD urine test should be done every 60–90 days to detect bone loss. A QCT bone density scan should be done annually. If either of these tests reveals bone loss, ask your physician to initiate bisphosphonate drug therapy. Every cancer patient should take a bone-protecting supplement such as Bone Assure to protect against excess bone deterioration.

STEP EIGHT: INHIBITING ANGIOGENESIS

Angiogenesis, the growth of new vessels from pre-existing blood vessels, is critical during fetal development but occurs minimally in healthy adults. Exceptions occur during wound healing, in inflammation, following a myocardial infarction, in female reproductive organs, and in pathologic conditions such as cancer (Shammas et al. 1993; Suh 2000).

Angiogenesis is a strictly controlled process in the healthy, adult human body, a process regulated by endogenous angiogenic promoters and inhibitors. Dr. Judah Folkman, the father of the angiogenesis theory of cancer, explains: "Blood vessel growth is controlled by a balancing of opposing factors. A tilt in favor of stimulators over inhibitors might be what trips the lever and begins the process of tumor angiogenesis."

According to the National Cancer Institute, solid tumors cannot grow beyond the size of a pinhead, that is, 1–2 cubic mm, without inducing the formation of new blood vessels to supply the nutritional needs of the tumor. Since rapid vascularization and tumor growth appear to occur concurrently, interrupting the vascular growth cycle is paramount to overcoming the malignancy.

Tumor angiogenesis results from a cascade of molecular and cellular events, usually initiated by the release of angiogenic growth factors. At a critical phase in the growth of a tumor, the tumor sends out signals to nearby endothelial cells to activate new blood vessel growth. The pro-angiogenic growth factors diffuse in the direction of preexisting blood vessels, encouraging development (Folkman 1992; Folkman et al. 1992).

Various agents are known to activate endothelial cell growth, including angiogenin, estrogen, interleukin-8, fibroblast growth factors (both acidic and basic), prostaglandin E2, tumor necrosis factor, granulocyte colony-stimulating factor, and VEGF. VEGF and basic fibroblast growth factors are expressed by many tumors and appear particularly important to tumor development and angiogenesis (NIH/NCI 1998).

A number of substances from orthodox and natural pharmacology (angiostatin, endostatin, interferons, interleukin-2, curcumin, green tea, lactoferrin, N-acetyl-cysteine (NAC), resveratrol, grape seed-skin extract, retinoic acid (vitamin A), and vitamin D) are antiangiogenic in nature (*to read more about natural products with an anti-angiogenesis profile, please turn to the Cancer Adjuvant Therapy protocol*). Endostatin, a fragment of collagen XVIII, and angiostatin, a fragment of plasminogen involved in the coagulation process, have produced remarkable results in animal models.

While endostatain and angiostatin are still in clinical trials, the anti-angiogenesis drug Avastatin® has been approved by the FDA to treat colon cancer and is being studied to treat other cancers as well.

HOW TO IMPLEMENT STEP EIGHT

1. There are a number of clinical trials using anti-angiogenesis agents such as angiostatin and endostatain. Call (800) 422-6237 or log on to www.cancer.gov/clinicaltrials to find out if you are eligible to participate.

2. In the *Cancer Adjuvant Therapy* protocol of this book, there are nutrients that have demonstrated potential ant-iangiogenesis effects such as green tea extract and curcumin. Refer to the *Cancer Adjuvant Therapy* protocol for information and dosing recommendations.

3. Ask your doctor to consider prescribing Avastatin®, as it is the only currently available approved drug.

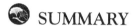 **SUMMARY**

This protocol has described therapies that a leading-edge oncologist can prescribe to improve the odds of long-term survival and possible cure.

The fundamental message is to have your oncologist thoroughly assess the individual characteristics of your tumor, your blood system, and available treatments. Based on this evaluation, patients can interact with their oncologists to determine what therapies may work synergistically with standard conventional treatments.

The objective of this multimodality approach is to attack tumor cells where they are most vulnerable. The primary determining factor in choosing the specific drugs is finding the various tumor cell and blood tests recommended in this protocol, along with historical statistical data that can help ascertain how your tumor will respond to specific therapies.

The following summary is a succinct reiteration of the eight approaches discussed in this protocol:

Step One: Evaluating the Molecular Biology of the Tumor Cell Population

How to implement: Make certain your surgeon sends a specimen of your tumor to IMPATH (Telephone: (800) 447-5816, website: www.impath.com) for immunohistochemistry testing, using the contact information provided. You may have to pay out-of-pocket for this test.

Step Two: Analyzing the Patient's Living Tumor Cells to Determine Sensitivity or Resistance to Chemotherapy

How to implement: Get in touch with Rational Therapeutics (Telephone: (562) 989-6455, website: www.rationaltherapeutics.com) using the contact information provided so that your surgeon can follow the precise instructions required to send a living specimen of your tumor for chemosensitivity testing. It is important that your surgeon carefully coordinate with Rational Therapeutics in order to ensure your cells arrive in a viable condition. You may have to pay for this test yourself because insurance may not reimburse you for it.

Step Three: Protecting Against Anemia

How to implement: If your hemoglobin or hematocrit levels are not in the optimal ranges described on the following chart, ask your physician to prescribe an individualized dose of Procrit.

Normal Laboratory Reference Range	Optimal Range for Cancer Patients
Hemoglobin	
Men: 12.5–17 (g/dL)	15.5–17 (g/dL)
Women: 11.5–15.0 (g/dL)	13.83–15 (g/dL)
Hematocrit	
Men: 36–50%	45–50%
Women: 34–44%	41–44%

Step Four: Inhibiting the COX-2 Enzyme

How to implement: Ask your physician to prescribe one of the following COX-2 inhibiting drugs:

Lodine XL, 1000 mg once daily, or

Celebrex, 100–200 mg every 12 hours, or

Vioxx, 12.5–25 mg once daily

Step Five: Suppressing ras Oncogene Expression

How to implement: Ask your physician to prescribe one of the following statin drugs to inhibit the activity of ras oncogenes:

Lovastatin, 40 mg twice daily, or

Zocor, 40 mg twice daily, or

Pravachol, 40 mg once daily

Note: *These statin drugs can produce toxic effects in a minority of patients. Physician oversight and monthly blood tests to evaluate liver function are suggested.*

In addition to statin drug therapy, consider supplementing with the following nutrients to further suppress the expression of ras oncogenes:

Fish Oil Capsules: 2400 mg of EPA and 1800 mg of DHA a day (6 Mega EPA fish oil capsules provide this potency)

Green Tea Extract: 1500 mg of tea polyphenols a day (5 Super Green Tea Extract Caps provide this potency)

Aged Garlic Extract: 2000 mg a day (2 Kyolic One Per Day caplets provide this potency)

Step Six: Correcting Coagulation Abnormalities

How to implement: Ascertain if you are in a hypercoagulable (prethrombotic) state by having your blood tested for prothrombin (PT), partial thromboplastin time (PTT), and D-dimers. A prethrombotic state is indicated by a shortening of PT and/or PTT and an increase in D-dimers.

If there is any evidence of a prethrombotic state, ask your physician to prescribe the appropriate individualized dose of LMWH. If you cannot afford LMWH, ask that lower-cost Coumadin be prescribed instead. Anticoagulation requires significant patient education and monitoring of laboratory tests to minimize the risks of hemorrhage due to overanticoagulation. As in all biological systems, a balance must be established if health is to be restored.

Step Seven: Maintaining Bone Integrity

How to implement: If you have a type of cancer with a proclivity to metastasize to the bone (breast or prostate), ask your physician for a bisphosphonate drug before evidence of boney metastasis occurs. An oral bisphosphonate drug to consider is Actonel at a dose of 30 mg twice a week or Fosamax at a dose of 70 mg once a week. Either drug must be taken at least 1 hour before breakfast and with water only. Some people experience gastroesophageal side effects from oral bisphosphonate drug therapy and prefer administration directly into the vein. An IV-administered bisphosphonate drug such as Aredia may be administered monthly beginning at 30 mg the first month, 60 mg the second month, and working up to 90 mg for subsequent months.

A newer, more potent IV bisphosphonate, Zometa, can be used at a starting dose of 1–2 mg for the first dose and then 4 mg every 3–4 weeks thereafter. Zometa is routinely given as a 15-minute infusion. When taking a bisphosphonate drug, it is important to take a wide array of bone-protecting supplements such as calcium, magnesium, zinc, manganese, and vitamin D_3. Six capsules a day of a product called Bone Assure provide optimal potencies of bone protecting nutrients. Some physicians also prescribe a synthetic vitamin D such as Calcitriol (Rocaltrol) or Hectorol.

Since excessive bone breakdown releases growth factors into the bloodstream that can fuel cancer cell growth, the Pyrilinks-D urine test should be done every 60–90 days to detect bone loss. A QCT bone density scan should be done annually. If either of these tests reveals bone loss, ask your physician to initiate bisphosphonate drug therapy. Every cancer patient should take a bone-protecting supplement like Bone Assure to protect against excess bone deterioration.

Step Eight: Inhibiting Angiogenesis

How to implement: There are a number of clinical trials using anti-angiogenesis agents such as angiostatin. Call (800) 422-6237 or log on to www.cancer.gov/clinicaltrials to find out if you are eligible to participate. In the *Cancer Adjuvant Therapy* protocol of this book, there are nutrients that have demonstrated potential anti-angiogenesis effects such as green tea extract and curcumin. Refer to the *Cancer Adjuvant Therapy* protocol for information and dosing recommendations. The drug Avastatin® is now approved, and may be considered as an anti-angiogenesis therapy against a variety of cancers.

Implementing the Eight Steps

As can be seen from the eight-step list, a patient might be prescribed several treatments in addition to standard therapy for the purposes of inhibiting the COX-2 enzyme, suppressing the ras oncogene, protecting against anemia/hypercoagulation, inhibiting blood vessel growth in the tumor (angiogenesis), maintaining bone integrity, and so forth.

While these therapies are substantiated in the published scientific literature and most are part of mainstream medicine, few cancer patients are benefiting from this knowledge.

If you are determined to wage modern medicine against your tumor, some or all of these therapies should be considered, depending on your individual situation. The reader is advised to refer to the *Cancer Adjuvant Therapy* protocol for additional guidance. If standard therapies such as radiation or chemotherapy are being contemplated, please refer to the *Cancer Surgery*, *Cancer Radiation* and/or *Cancer Chemotherapy* protocols.

PRODUCT AVAILABILITY

Mega EPA, green tea extract, Kyolic® Aged Garlic Extract and high-allicin PureGar® garlic extract, melatonin, folic acid, vitamin B12, and Bone Assure are available by telephoning (800) 544-4440 or by ordering online at www.lef.org.

STAYING INFORMED

The information published in this protocol is only as current as the day the manuscript was sent to the printer. This protocol raises many issues that are subject to change as new data emerge. Furthermore, cancer is still a disease with unacceptably high mortality rates, and none of our suggested regimens can guarantee a cure.

The Life Extension Foundation is constantly uncovering information to provide to cancer patients. A special website has been established for the purpose of updating patients on new findings that directly pertain to the published cancer protocols. Whenever Life Extension discovers information that may benefit cancer patients it will be posted on the website www.lefcancer.org.

Before utilizing the cancer protocols in this book, we suggest that you check www.lefcancer.org to see if any substantive changes have been made to the recommendations described in this protocol. Based on the sheer number of newly published findings, there could be significant alterations to the information you have just read.

Alternatively, call 1-800-226-2370 and ask a Health Advisor if your topic of interest has been updated on the website – www.lefcancer.org.

DISCLAIMER

This information (and any accompanying printed material) is not intended to replace the attention or advice of a physician or other health care professional. Anyone who wishes to embark on any dietary, drug, exercise, or other lifestyle change intended to prevent or treat a specific disease or condition should first consult with and seek clearance from a qualified health care professional.

The information published in the protocols is only as current as the day the manuscript was sent to the printer. This protocol raises many issues that are subject to change as new data emerge. None of our suggested protocol regimens can guarantee a cure.

APPENDIX A

The following pages show examples of IMPATH laboratory reports that provide your oncologist with immunohistochemistry and chemosensitivity testing of your tumor cells. Refer to Step One (Evaluating the Molecular Biology of the Tumor Cell Population) for information about these particular tests.

IMPATH's mission is to develop and offer innovative products and services that lead to more accurate diagnosis and more effective treatments for cancer patients. IMPATH helps to improve outcomes for cancer patients as a leading source of cancer information and analyses. IMPATH Physician Services uses sophisticated technologies to provide patient-specific cancer diagnostic and prognostic information to more than 8,300 pathologists and oncologists in over 2,000 hospitals and 570 oncology practices.

An accurate diagnosis is the vital first step in the successful management of cancer. Thereafter, identifying key prognostic indicators such as hormone receptor status, oncogene expression, and tumor aggressiveness provide treatment-defining information to help maximize the patient outcome. IMPATH currently performs more specialized analyses to identify complex tumors and provide prognostic information than any other institution—anywhere.

IMPATH's unique combination of resources includes a growing network from which well-characterized cancer tissue specimens and corresponding serology are procured with informed patient consent. IMPATH's GeneBank™ initiative provides the infrastructure to support collection and extraction of key biological materials and the subsequent tracking of longitudinal (treatment and outcomes) data on donors. Further, utilizing extensive databases and physicians networks, IMPATH Clinical Trials Network (ICTN) can identify appropriate patients for clinical trials, which is essential for optimizing clinical outcome while accelerating the development process and mitigating costs incurred by unnecessary over-recruitment.

Telephone: (800) 447-5816	Website: www.impath.com	
New York	**Los Angeles**	**Phoenix**
521 West 57th Street, Sixth floor	5300 McConnell Avenue	810 East Hammond Lane
New York, NY 10019	Los Angeles, CA 90066	Phoenix, AZ 85034

IMPATH DRA™

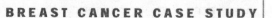

BREAST CANCER CASE STUDY

Excluding what isn't, to find what is"

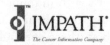

New York | Los Angeles | Phoenix

PATIENT - 48 yr. old female

- 4.5 cm tumor and axillary lymph nodes removed
- ER +
- 3 nodes positive for microscopic tumor
- No distant metastases

IMPATH DRA™

- 1 gm tissue forwarded to IMPATH
- Extreme resistance to doxorubicin (Adriamycin)
- Low resistance to cyclophosphamide and fluorouracil

TREATMENT DECISION

- Patient at high risk of recurrence
- Effective chemotherapy would include CMF, CA, or CAF
- Due to extreme resistance to doxorubicin, patient treated with CMF, followed by Tamoxifen

Cost Effectiveness

Conventional Therapy   = $5,818
DRA Directed Therapy   = $3,112

IMPATH DRA™

Cost Savings   = $2,706

OUTCOME

Patient is clinically disease-free six years post-surgery

IMPATH DRA™ RESULTS

Drug Tested	Percentile Rank	Degree of Resistance	Probability of Response	
			Untreated	Prior Chemotherapy
Doxorubicin	86	Extreme	3	3
Doxil	81	Extreme	3	3
Gemcitabine	74	Intermediate	12	6
Vinorelbine	51	Intermediate	32	16
Docetaxel	39	Low	56	28
Paclitaxel	35	Low	58	29
Fluorouracil	25	Low	59	30
Cyclophosphamide	14	Low	60	30

Percentile Rank:

Percentile Rank is a measure of the relative resistance of the patient's cancer cells to each drug tested. The Percentile Rank can range from 100 (complete resistance) to 0 (no resistance).

Reference Ranges:	Percentile Rank	Degree of Resistance
	80-100	Extreme
	51-79	Intermediate
	0-50	Low

Degree of Resistance:

Extreme - Extreme resistance indicates the drug was inactive against the tumor and the patient is, therefore, highly unlikely to respond to the drug. The IMPATH DRA™ is highly accurate at predicting clinically inactive drugs. In one landmark study, patients whose cancer cells had extreme resistance to an anticancer agent had <1% response rate to that agent. The IMPATH DRA™ can be used to avoid exposing patients to the toxicity of drugs that are unlikely to be effective.

Low - Low resistance indicates that little or no resistance to the drug was detected and the drug was active against this tumor. The patient is much more likely to respond to anticancer drugs that are active *in vitro* than to inactive drugs. Clinical data suggest a therapeutic advantage in the activity of agents to which a tumor is highly responsive *in vitro*. Treatment based on drugs that are active *in vitro* may improve response rates and survival if second choice drugs exist that are active on tumors resistant to first-line agents.

Intermediate - A moderate degree of drug resistance was detected and the patient has a finite but less than average likelihood of responding to the drug.

Probability of Response:

As the degree of drug resistance *in vitro* increases, the probability that the patient will respond to an anticancer drug decreases. The probability of response is an estimate of the likelihood that the patient will respond to a particular drug. IMPATH's probability of response was derived from the percentile rank of the drug and the expected response for the patient's cancer type.

---

(800) 447-5816   (212) 698-0300 international   www.impath.com   DRA CS01/0101

Cancer Vaccines

Billions of dollars are being invested in cutting-edge research to find solutions to cancer. Vaccines are among the most promising pursuits, representing the next generation in cancer treatment. Vaccines have come to the attention of many because they appear more effective and less toxic than commonly used conventional therapies. According to Elizabeth M. Jaffee (Johns Hopkins University), the goal is to make the host immune system responsive to antigens characteristic of cancer cells, just as a classic vaccine makes the system responsive to a viral or bacterial pathogen. A subsequent exposure to the antigen will evoke a response that ultimately eliminates or destroys the invader, in this case, cancer.

> **Note:** *An antigen is a substance capable of stimulating a specific immune response. Antigens may be soluble substances, such as toxins and foreign proteins, or particulates, such as bacteria and cells.*

Unlike chemotherapeutic drugs that directly attack a tumor, cancer vaccines attempt to prompt the body's own immune system to destroy cancer cells. This has been a difficult task because cancer cells have proven to be adept at fooling the body into treating tumors as natural parts of the body. A few years ago, it was believed cancer occurred because of a breakdown in immune surveillance; it is now thought that cancers may develop (in part) because the normal, healthy host immune system fails to fully realize a malignancy is present.

Lest vaccines sound new as a cancer treatment, they are not. In 1880, William B. Coley pioneered one of the earliest efforts to produce an effective vaccine against cancer. Coley, a general surgeon, observed that occasional patients who developed an infection in the vicinity of the cancer experienced a reduction in tumor size. He took the bold step of injecting live bacterial organisms into growing soft tissue tumors. To Coley's delight, some of the tumors shrank after developing a brisk inflammatory response. It was theorized that the immune system was activated by the bacterial inoculation and, in its heightened state, also destroyed the tumor. Other bacterial agents that have been examined by investigators include bacillus Calmette-Guerin (BCG), a tuberculosis immunization, and Corynebacterium parvum, a microbial species (Milas et al.1976). Unfortunately, several clinical trials evaluating nonspecific antigens or their products largely proved to be disappointing (Decroix et al. 1984).

According to Alfred Chang, M.D., chief, division of surgical oncology, University of Michigan Comprehensive Cancer Center, bacterial agents are now being combined with tumor-associated antigens (TAAs) in an effort to induce specific immunity to the tumor. TAAs are proteins, enzymes, or carbohydrates that are present on tumor cells and relatively absent or diminished on normal cells. Examples include carcinoembryonic antigen (CEA) produced by colon cancers and other adenocarcinomas such as breast, gastric, lung, and pancreatic cancers; prostate specific antigen (PSA) produced by prostate cancers; and alpha-fetoprotein (AFP) produced by liver cancers. By virtue of being fairly unique to the tumor cell, TAAs provide targets for the immune system to recognize and attack. Clinical trials are underway in which patients are vaccinated against the appropriate secreting protein in an attempt to destroy the tumor. For additional information relating to vaccine therapies, call (800) 4-CANCER or visit http://www.cancer.gov/clinicaltrials.

RESAN: A VACCINE WITH A PREVENTIVE PROFILE

RESAN, an antitumor vaccine introduced in 1992, is regarded not only as a vaccine against cancer, but also as a therapeutic agent (RESAN 2002). According to a spokesperson at Providence Pacific Hospital (Mexico), RESAN has shown results in producing cancer prophylaxis, as well as in therapeutic results. According to physicians at the hospital, the chances of complete tumor destruction depends upon (1) the size of the tumor and its mitotic potential, (2) the type of tumor-histological structures, antigen structures, and the number of HLA class molecules on tumor cells, and (3) the initial state of the immune system.

RESAN, purported to be effective against most cancers, is regarded as an anti-metastatic drug. If the cancer is at Stage III or Stage IV, the vaccine is used in combination with surgical procedures, interleukin-2, and gamma-interferon (cytokines).

RESAN is not toxic to normal cells, has no mutagenic or teratogenic potential, and does not contain any cells or tissues of the tumor. The main components of the vaccine are glycoproteins, which "imitate particular fragments of tumor antigens." RESAN gains pharmacological value as glycoproteins (conjugated proteins in which the nonprotein substance is a carbohydrate) stimulate the production of specific antitumor, immune-competent cells. The vaccine targets the following population groups:

- Individuals at high risk for cancer because of family history

- Patients showing no visible sign of a tumor, but displaying tumor markers higher than normal

- Individuals who, after radical surgery, need protection against relapse

- Individuals preparing for surgical removal of a tumor

- Patients with benign conditions, such as benign prostatic hypertrophy (BPH) and fibroid conditions, are often able to avoid surgical procedures with RESAN vaccines

Absolute contraindications are few, but the vaccine is not recommended during pregnancy or for 3–4 weeks following an infection. Providence Pacific Hospital, (619) 972-3831, is actively involved in administering RESAN vaccines. Individuals wanting more information concerning RESAN may also consult resan@anticancer.net. *Note:* A spokesman for RESAN is quick to add that the vaccine has no backing or endorsement among orthodoxy. Submitting documentation of RESAN's mode of operation (successes and limitations) for mainstream evaluation was unsuccessful. Yet, the hospital continues to administer RESAN and, in their estimation, with positive results.

DENDRITIC CELL VACCINE

Perhaps the most promising area of active research in cancer vaccines is with a unique cell known as a *dendritic* cell. A dendritic cell captures antigens and then travels to lymph nodes and the spleen where it presents the processed antigen to T-cells. Dendritic cells (spiked with cancer proteins from the patient's own tumor) can generate an immune response that may result in stabilization or regression of metastatic disease. *Note:* Dendritic cells are aptly named: the name infers tree-like or branching. Dendritic cells (with the antigen attached to the cell's long branches) present the alien material to the immune system for recognition and destruction.

Experimental studies show that cancer-bearing animals given an infusion of dendritic cells (trained to deliver tumor antigens) resulted in cure rates of 40% in MBT-2 bladder tumors. Immunization with dendritic cells was also remarkably effective in the B16 melanoma lung metastasis model (Nair et al. 1997). Illustrative of the enthusiasm surrounding dendritic cells, in 1998 the University of Pittsburgh was granted a 5-year, $7.7-million award from the National Cancer Institute for research.

In a study involving end-stage pediatric cancer patients, dendritic cells (considered pacemakers of the immune system) were isolated from the patient's blood and enticed to replicate. The process begins as cancerous cells undergo freezing and thawing, allowing the antigen to be extracted from the ruptured cells. A tumor cell *lysate* results. The lysates from the tumor are then mixed with a protein and added to the dendritic cells, a process that activates the cells.

After being injected back into the body, dendritic cells find a cancerous cell and sound the alarm to the remainder of the immune system by displaying pieces of the digested tumor proteins (antigens) on their long projections. Dendritic cells present the antigen to white blood cells until a match is found, that is, lymphocytes with receptors that fit the antigen. Once a match is found, T-lymphocytes (equipped with the exact receptor needed to attack and destroy one specific type of tumor cell) attack the cancer cells. Among the 13 children participating in the study (neuroblastoma, sarcoma, osteosarcoma, and fibrosarcoma patients), a 16-year-old girl with metastatic cancer to the lungs and spine displayed a significant regression of tumors following treatment; five other children experienced a stabilization of their condition (Geiger 2001; UniSci 2001b).

Cancer cells can hide from lymphocytes by becoming almost invisible. Instead of displaying all of their proteins on their surfaces, cancer cells keep most of their proteins inside where the T-lymphocytes cannot find them. Dendritic cells can super-sensitize T-lymphocytes to recognize the few proteins that remain on the cancer cell surface, triggering an intense immune reaction. Early results suggest that dendritic cells may have the most potential of all cancer vaccines.

Some of the Many Cancer Centers Involved in Dendritic Cell Vaccines and Research:

- University of Michigan Comprehensive Cancer Center, Ann Arbor, MI, (800) 865-1125.

- University of Pittsburgh Cancer Institute, (800) 237-4724.

- Neurosurgical Institute, a subsidiary of Cedars-Sinai Medical Center, Los Angeles, CA, (310) 423-7900.

- Duke Comprehensive Cancer Center, Durham, NC, (919) 684-3377 for general vaccine information; Dr. Douglas S. Tyler: dendritic cell vaccines for pancreatic and gastric cancers, as well as melanoma; call (919) 684-2137 for appointments.

- Pacific Northwest Cancer Center Hospital, Seattle, WA, (206) 633-4636 or (888) 694-7333.

- University of Minnesota Department of Neurosurgery (brain tumors), Minneapolis, MN, (612) 273-1913.
- M.D. Anderson Cancer Center, Houston, TX, (713) 792-2830; Dr. Robert J. Amato (renal cell carcinoma).

Note: *Make certain that your type of malignancy is one that the center either focuses on or can give statistical data relating to patient outcome.*

FAVORABLE RESULTS OF CLINICAL TRIALS INVOLVING VARIOUS VACCINES

Colon Cancer Scientists at Intracel, a Rockville, MD, biotech firm, reported that a Phase III clinical trial (based at the Vrije Universiteit in Amsterdam using the company's OncoVAX product) showed the vaccine reduced the recurrence of Stage II colon cancer by 61% (Hanna et al. 2001; Vermorken et al. 1999). Stage II colon cancer, sometimes referred to as Dukes B, means the cancer has spread outside the colon to nearby tissue but has not invaded the lymphatic system.

Another large-scale study (1400 patients) is underway to evaluate the effectiveness of a vaccine (CEA-targeted) to prevent new tumors from occurring following surgery for colon cancer. Trials employing a similar model have been encouraging. For example, a woman whose colon cancer had spread to 22 lymph nodes has lived cancer-free for 7 years following surgery and vaccine therapy. If proven effective as a follow-up treatment, the vaccine might be considered for preventive use for high-risk colon cancer patients, much like the Tamoxifen trials for breast cancer (Bonfield 2000).

CEA-Secreting Tumors

The human carcinoembryonic antigen (CEA) that is expressed in several cancer types (colorectal, breast, esophageal, cervical, gastric, and pancreatic cancers) induces a strong T-cell response when inserted into a vaccine (Tsang et al. 1995). Researchers at Georgetown University's Lombardi Cancer Center found that vaccinia-CEA (V) and ALVAC-CEA (A) that was developed by Therion Biologics prompted an immune response in five out of nine late-stage metastatic cancer patients. The vaccines are pox virus-based that specifically target the carcinoembryonic antigen, a protein found on the surface of CEA secreting tumors. These vaccines, referred to as a *prime-boost protocol*, are able to sustain a powerful anticancer immune response over a period of time. Responders were still alive at 2 years (receiving vaccinia-CEA followed by three vaccinations with ALVAC-CEA) compared to zero long-term survivors in other treatment groups (UniSci 2001c).

Breast Cancer

Biomira Inc. is currently involved in the largest metastatic breast cancer trial ever, with 1000 evaluable patients in the Phase III study. Theratope, a synthetic, carbohydrate-based vaccine, is the focus of the trial. In an earlier study, Theratope-treated patients with metastatic breast cancer had a median survival of 26.6 months compared with 9.2 months in the placebo group. Interim results from a study conducted at the Fred Hutchinson Cancer Research Center in Seattle, WA (using a newer Biomira formulation) showed 27 of 28 patients injected with the Theratope vaccine developed an antibody response to the vaccine after only two vaccinations. Of the 21 patients who received three vaccinations, 29% achieved a higher response than the maximum seen using the previous formulation at the same point. Theratope is not limited to breast cancer therapy. It also lengthened survival rates of colorectal cancer patients (Biomira 1999; Holmberg et al. 2001).

Note: *Biomira Inc., a pharmaceutical company, does not treat patients at its facility. Instead, Biomira provides the vaccines to physicians at various cancer clinics in North America and Europe where government-approved clinical trials are ongoing. The vaccines are provided only to physicians who are currently involved in vaccine exploration and who have extensive experience with these agents. To speak to Biomira's Medical Information Assistant, call(609) 655-5300.*

Prostate Cancer

A Phase II trial conducted at Pacific Northwest Cancer Foundation in Seattle, WA, (888) 694-7333, demonstrated the efficacy of a dendritic cell-based vaccine in patients with advanced prostate cancer. Subjects in the metastatic group (Group A-2) were followed for an average of 291 days; the local recurrence group (Group B) was observed for 557 days. The average duration of response was 149 days for Group A-2 and 187 days for Group B. A majority of responders (11 of 19; 58%) were still responsive at the end of the follow-up. This study suggests that dendritic cell-based cancer vaccines may provide an additional therapy for advanced prostate cancer (Tjoa et al. 1999). Memorial Sloan-Kettering (MSK) reported similar results, suggesting vaccines as an alternative treatment for cancer patients who have rising PSA levels following primary prostate therapies.

404

MSK used a carbohydrate-glycoprotein conjugate vaccine in their trials (Slovin et al. 1999).

Lymphoma

Researchers at UCLA's Jonsson Cancer Center are seeking volunteers for a final-phase clinical trial that will test the safety and effectiveness of individually tailored vaccines to fight follicular lymphoma, a disease that is most often incurable. The vaccine, manufactured from samples obtained through needle biopsy, targets proteins unique to each patient's lymphoma. Volunteers will undergo 8 rounds of chemotherapy and then receive 5 weekly injections of the vaccine.

The UCLA study is structured similarly to highly successful trials conducted at Stanford University (UCLA 2001). In 1997, Stanford researchers reported in the journal *Blood* that in a similar model, B-cell lymphoma patients (showing an immune response following chemotherapy and vaccines) experienced 7.9 years of freedom from disease progression compared to 1.3 years in patients classed as nonresponders (Hsu et al. 1997). For more information on the UCLA study or to volunteer for the vaccine therapy, call (310) 825-2516 or (310) 794-4376.

Lung Cancer

A vaccine (in Phase I and II trials) demonstrated a major response rate in 18% of 22 individuals (four patients) with advanced nonsmall cell lung cancer who had failed chemotherapy and/or radiation therapy. Three patients showed a complete disappearance of metastatic tumors following treatment with Cell Genesys' GVAX lung cancer vaccine. Another patient experienced a greater than 50% reduction in tumor volume, while four other patients were deemed stable (showing nonprogressive disease status) following treatment (UniSci 2001a). *Note:* Apart from lung cancer, Cell Genesys, (650) 425-4400, is also conducting clinical trials using GVAX vaccines in myeloma, prostate, and pancreatic cancers.

Ovarian Cancer

Metastasis to the abdominal cavity is the primary cause of morbidity and mortality in patients with ovarian cancer. Recently designed tumor vaccines (coupled with cytokine therapy, i.e., interleukin-2 and interleukin-12) afford a higher level of immune sophistication and (it is hoped) a better outcome in women with ovarian cancer (Butts 1999). Currently there are eight clinical trials utilizing vaccine therapy in ovarian cancer patients ongoing at the National Cancer Institute, for further information call 1(800) 4-CANCER or check the NCI clinical trials website:

http://clinicaltrials.gov/ct/search?term=ovarian+AND+vaccine

Melanoma

National Cancer Institute researchers reported that a vaccine plus IL-2 prompted tumor regression in 13 of 31 melanoma patients (42%). At least half of the cancers disappeared, and in some cases there was a complete response (Rosenberg et al. 1998). David Berd and colleagues at Jefferson Medical College of Thomas Jefferson University (Philadelphia, PA), (215) 955-6000, had previously shown that an autologous vaccine (from the patient's own cancer cells) was effective in treating patients with malignant melanoma.

Before injecting the cells into patients, the cells are inactivated and then treated with dinitrophenyl (DNP), a chemical that modifies the cells. The altered cells appear foreign to the immune system for it to react against them. Dr. Berd gave the vaccine to 37 postoperative patients with advanced Stage IV melanoma that had spread beyond the lymph nodes. Dr. Berd found that giving the DNP vaccine to patients following surgery resulted in an estimated 59% of patients living 3 years. Only 10–20% of patients typically live more than 5 years with surgery alone. In an expanded trial, 47% of 214 melanoma patients with disease spread to one or two lymph node areas lived 5 years. Those with cancer spread to only one lymph node area did even better, experiencing a 50% 5-year survival (TJUH 2001).

Brain Tumors

Dendritic cell immunotherapy, using a vaccine derived from a patient's own cells to fight the malignancy, is being used to treat brain tumors at Cedars-Sinai Medical Center (Los Angeles, CA). According to principal investigator Keith Black, M.D., foreign proteins are taken from a tumor after surgical removal. These proteins are introduced to antigen-presenting dendritic cells taken from the patient's blood and grown in a petri dish. The new dendritic cells, when reinjected into the patient, are intended to work like a vaccine, recognizing and destroying lingering malignant tumor cells.

Several such injections are typically scheduled over a 6-week interval. Cedars-Sinai profiled a brain tumor patient having undergone surgery, radiation, and vaccine therapy. She was described about 1 year later as "feeling fine," returning to the Neurosurgical Institute only for follow-up laboratory work and MRIs (CSMC 1999). *Note:* Researchers from Cryoma Labs, (877) 604-4111, stress that if you are having brain cancer surgery or a biopsy, it is critical that brain tissue be stored for a future personalized cancer vaccine.

Cervical Cancer

Cervical cancer develops from the cells lining the cervix, i.e., the canal that connects the uterus to the vagina. There are approximately 500,000 new cases of cervical cancer worldwide per year and 300,000 deaths according to the World Health Organization. About 5000 cervical cancer deaths occur annually in the United States (SLU 1998; BBC News 1999). Illustrative of the potential of vaccines to prevent and control cancer, an article that appeared in the *New England Journal of Medicine* announced that vaccines appear to be "the beginning of the end for cervical cancer" (Crum 2002).

Although the majority of the human papillomavirus (HPV) infections will not lead to cancer, researchers at Saint Louis University (SLU) published that a percentage of women who are infected with a specific type of HPV (Type 16) ultimately increase their risk of cervical cancer. SLU researchers state that persistent HPV infection increases a woman's risk of cervical cancer 40-fold. It is estimated that up to 40 million Americans have one of the ten HPV strains; persons infected worldwide number untold millions (SLU 1998).

Researchers from Brown University announced that oncogenic proteins E6 and E7 of HPV-16 and HPV-18 are the primary focus of the most current clinical trials for cervical cancer patients (Steller 2002). Studies indicate that the E6 and E7 gene products interfere with p53 and pRB functions, respectively, and deregulate the cell cycle. The HPV DNA is integrated into the host's chromosomes along with disruption of the E2 gene. This disruption promotes the expression of E6 and E7, leading to the accumulation of DNA damage and the development of cervical cancer (Furumoto et al. 2002). (To read more about p53 and pRB please consult the protocol *Cancer: Gene Therapies, Stem Cells, Telomeres, and Cytokines*.)

The scientific advance in 1991 that led to the successful HPV-16 vaccine trial was the creation of papillomavirus-like particles in the laboratory (Zhou et al. 1991). Virus-like particles are devoid of DNA and are therefore noninfectious. However, they mimic the natural structure of the complete viral particle, generating a potent immune response. It was determined that vaccines derived from species-specific, virus-like particles protected animals from wart viruses. Immunologists questioned whether such vaccines could protect the highly vulnerable cervical epithelium from the cancer-causing papillomavirus infection.

Laura Koutsky and colleagues, University of Washington (Seattle, WA) appear to have favorably answered the question by randomly assigning 2392 young women (16–23 years of age) to receive either 3 doses of a placebo or the HPV-16 virus-like particle vaccine. The women were followed for a median of 17.4 months after completing the vaccination regimen. The incidence of persistent HPV-16 infection was 3.8 per 100 woman-years at risk in the placebo group and 0 per 100 woman-years at risk in the vaccine group (100% efficacy). The vaccine not only prevents the disease from developing, it also prevents its causative agent from residing in the genital tract where it can infect new sexual partners (Crum 2002; Koutsky et al. 2002).

Several hundred young women have been vaccinated without adverse side effects (Muderspach et al. 2000). The most common complaint is soreness at the site of the injection (Koutsky et al. 2002). Although the duration of protection, as well as the vaccine's adeptness at treating cervical neoplasia once it has developed is uncertain, the Cancer Research Campaign (University of Wales) says that (with continued preventive successes) vaccines will most likely be used on women with less advanced cervical cancer (van Driel et al. 1999). A papillomavirus vaccine that prevents HPV infection, on the one hand, and acts against established disease on the other could have a profound impact on one of the major cancers affecting women globally (Davidson et al. 2002).

Comment: The Koutsky team evaluated a monovalent HPV-16 vaccine; from a public health perspective, a vaccine that prevents infection with a broad spectrum of types of HPV would be more advantageous. Five HPVs-types: 16, 18, 31, 33, and 45 are responsible for most cervical cancers, but the more pernicious cancers most often appear with HPV-16 and HPV-18. If young women were vaccinated against these types of HPV before they become sexually active, there should be a reduction of at least 85% in the risk of cancer and a decline of 44% to 70% in the frequency of abnormal Papanicolaou smears attributable to HPV. It is estimated that the level of protection from death due to cervical cancer could exceed 95% (Walboomers et al. 1999; Koutsky 2002; Crum 2002). According to French researchers, more than 20 different types of prophylactic and therapeutic vaccines against HPV are currently being evaluated in clinical or preclinical studies worldwide (Franceschi 2002).

A Negative Opinion on the Efficacy of Testing

In the midst of jubilation regarding an effective cervical cancer vaccine, various reporters and scientists are challenging the breakthrough. Dr. Howard Urnovitz, a scientist dealing in molecular issues and a regular contributor to *redflagsweekly.com*, noted that initially

2392 women were enrolled in the Koutsky study; from those numbers, 36% were disqualified because of detectable HPV markers. Urnovitz states that women selected for the study showed robust natural immunity that kept them from expressing HPV markers.

In addition, the Papanicolaou's (Pap) test was used as a means of cancer detection in the study. Those who doubted the recent study contend that Pap smears (a test currently used in the United States to screen women for signs of cervical cancer) are known to be inaccurate. Some estimate the rate of false negative tests results to be from 1–93%. (A false negative result means that women who have cervical cancer or precancerous tissues are not being identified when they have a Pap smear.) So displeased with the mode of testing used in the cervical cancer vaccine study, cynics assert the rest of the study is rendered highly suspect.

At present, the gold standard for diagnosis of HPV is detection of HPV DNA by polymerase chain reaction (PCR). According to Dr. E. Mordechai (Medical Diagnostics Laboratories), PCR can provide an extremely accurate diagnosis of HPV subtypes, thereby determining the risk for cervical cancer (Mordechai 1999). Laura Koutsky and her colleagues employed the PCR-based method in their study. A positive result was defined as any signal that exceeded the background level associated with an HPV-negative sample of human DNA (Koutsky et al. 2002).

Dissenters challenge that this is a risky protocol because PCR tests are plagued with false positive reactions. Dr. Urnovitz contends that since no data or reference to data on a secondary test confirms the gene sequence of a positive signal, researchers cannot conclude that they are measuring HPV.

According to Dr. Urnovitz, "The proper conclusion of this study should be: administration of the HPV-16 vaccine reduced the incidence of an uncharacterized PCR signal from a poorly defined cohort which was strongly biased toward a natural immunity (Mercola 2002).

Good science considers both sides of controversial issues. Reporting positive and negative positions provides Life Extension members with the most current of research that might affect health and longevity.

ONGOING TRIALS

These few studies represent only a glimpse of the immunotherapy vaccine trials ongoing in the United States sponsored by the National Cancer Institute, academic medical centers, and several pharmaceutical companies. If the numbers of survivors appear disappointingly low, recall that (for the most part) subjects were classed as "late-stage:" those patients for whom all other therapeutic doors had (largely) closed. If you have an advanced cancer which has failed standard treatments, you may be eligible for a research vaccine trial. You are strongly urged to pursue vaccine therapy, a procedure that has (in many cases) reversed a grim prognosis. We must caution however, that the FDA can make it extremely difficult for early-stage cancer patients to participate in these vaccine therapy trials.

A source of information is the National Cancer Institute Trials Database which lists and describes many clinical trials occurring at different locations across the country. This is referred to as the PDQ listing and can be accessed via the Internet at http://cancertrials.nci.nih.gov/ or by calling Cancer Information Service, (800) 4-CANCER. Other sources of information are NCI-designated cancer centers, of which there are approximately 30. These centers are reviewed and certified by the NCI for quality of research. For information, visit

http://www3.cancer.gov/cancercenters/centerslist.html.

STAYING INFORMED

This published information is only as current as the day the protocol was sent to the printer. This cancer protocol raises many issues that are subject to change as new data emerges. Furthermore, cancer is still a disease with unacceptably high mortality rates, and none of our suggested regimens can guarantee a cure.

The Life Extension Foundation is constantly uncovering information to provide the cancer patient with more ammunition to battle their disease. A special website has been established for the purpose of updating patients on new findings that directly pertain to the cancer protocols published. Whenever Life Extension discovers information that points to a better way of treating cancer, it will be posted on the website, www.lefcancer.org.

Before utilizing Life Extension cancer protocols, we suggest that you check www.lefcancer.org to see if any substantive changes have been made to the recommendations described in this protocol. Based on the sheer number of newly published findings, there could be significant alterations to the information you have just read.

DISCLAIMER

This information (and any accompanying printed material) is not intended to replace the attention or advice of a physician or other health care professional. Anyone who wishes to embark on any dietary, drug, exercise, or other lifestyle change intended to prevent or treat a specific disease or condition should first consult with and seek clearance from a qualified health care professional.

The information published in the protocols is only as current as the day the book was sent to the printer. This protocol raises many issues that are subject to change as new data emerge. None of our suggested treatment regimens can guarantee a cure for these diseases.

Candida

Candidiasis is an infection caused by various species of the *Candida* yeast, the most common being *Candida albicans*. *Candida* are normally present in the digestive tract and the vagina. During certain favorable conditions, such as warm, humid weather or when an individual's immune system is impaired, the yeast can infect the skin. Mucous membranes in the mouth and vagina are commonly infected. In rare instances, *Candida* can invade blood and deeper tissues, causing a life-threatening infection.

People may sometimes develop a *Candida* infection after taking antibiotics (Still et al. 1995; Witsell et al. 1995). The antibiotics kill the bacteria that normally keep the *Candida* under control, allowing the *Candida* organism to grow unchecked. Pregnant women, diabetics, and obese people are also prone to *Candida* infections. Corticosteroids given after organ transplantation can also promote growth of *Candida*.

COMMONLY INFECTED AREAS

- *Skin folds*, including the navel and anus. Symptoms include a red rash with patchy areas oozing whitish fluid. Pus may also appear. The area will itch or burn. Perlèche is a *Candida* infection at the corners of the mouth that creates cracks and tiny cuts. It is often caused by ill-fitting dentures.

- *Vagina* (vulvovaginitis), occurring most often in pregnant women, those taking antibiotics, or those with diabetes. Symptoms include a white or yellow discharge, with burning, itching, and redness on the walls and the external areas of the vagina.

- *Penis*, occurring mostly in men having diabetes or whose sexual partner has a vaginal *Candida* infection. A red, scaly, often painful rash appears on the underside of the penis. However, a fungal infection of the penis (or vagina) will not always cause discernible symptoms.

- *Mouth* (thrush), (caused by a candida infection in the mouth) where creamy white patches will appear on the tongue or sides of the mouth. Thrush can appear in a healthy child; however, in an adult it may be a symptom of a more serious disorder, such as diabetes or AIDS. The use of antibiotics can also cause thrush.

- *Nails* (paronychia), (caused by a candida infection in the nail bed) resulting in a painful swelling and secretion of pus from the nail beds. Infected nails may turn white or yellow and separate from the surrounding skin.

CANDIDIASIS AND THE YEAST SYNDROME

Most conventional physicians restrict a diagnosis of candidial infection to the previously mentioned conditions. When there is doubt, cultures may be obtained to prove the diagnosis and to check for susceptibility to antifungal agents. Conventional physicians may also encounter the particularly vexing problem of women who have multiple vaginal yeast infections that are difficult to control. Many of these women are treated with repeated courses of potent antifungal drugs, often without relief.

Another more controversial perspective was popularized by Dr. W. G. Crook (1986, 1999). Dr. Crook used the term "candidiasis" or "yeast syndrome" to refer to a syndrome in which the predominant features are fatigue, a generalized malaise, gastrointestinal complaints, recurrent chronic infections, allergies, skin problems, decreased concentration, depression, irritability, and craving for sweets or carbohydrates. The underlying cause is purported to be an overabundance of yeast in the bowel and perhaps elsewhere. While this theory has not been investigated and subjected to the rigorous scrutiny of peer review, there is certainly substantial clinical and anecdotal evidence that this syndrome exists and appears to be connected with the overuse of antibiotics. Many patients who have been diagnosed with yeast syndrome do get better when they follow a diet essentially devoid of sugar, yeast-containing substances, and wheat.

If you utilize the questionnaire following this protocol, which comes from Dr. Crook, you may better understand the problem. Physicians experienced with this condition can also look for *Candida* antibody levels in the blood and do an ELISA-ACT test for T-cell mediated allergy. (*See the Allergies protocol for a discussion of this very useful test.*) It is also useful to check the acidity of the stomach and the alkalinity of the first part of the duodenum with a Heidelburg test. This is a noninvasive test utilizing a small capsule, containing a sensitive pH probe and radio transmitter, that is swallowed by the patient. A radio receiver picks up the signals and measures the perspective values. The capsule passes harmlessly into the test probe afterlife. Abnormalities of stomach and pancreatic secretions can be corrected with the proper supplements.

TREATMENT

Treatment of Candida depends upon the location of the infection. Infection of the skin is easily treated with medicated creams and lotions, often containing nystatin. Suppositories may be used for vaginal and anal infection. Thrush medications may be taken as a liquid swished around the mouth or as a slowly dissolving lozenge. Along with an antifungal cream, hydrocortisone for skin infection may be used to relieve pain and itching. Keeping the skin dry will help to clear up the infection and prevent its return.

Most people have a bout with a candidial infection at one time or another in their lives. This discussion is directed to the patients that either have recurrent infections or suffer from yeast syndrome. It is very important to screen for the more obvious and common predisposing factors like diabetes or chronic steroid use. The challenge is to look for more subtle problems that impair immunity. One must realize that there is a vicious cycle, especially in yeast syndrome. A person may become predisposed to a yeast infection because of antibiotic overuse. Then when the syndrome takes hold, immune function is further impaired, making it all the more difficult to treat. Therefore, based on the clinical experience of many physicians, it is fair to say that anyone suffering from either recurrent yeast infections or the yeast syndrome should adhere to most of the suggestions that follow, especially with respect to dietary changes.

Removal of Sugar

The importance of the removal of sugar from the diet cannot be overemphasized. For reasons that are not entirely clear, many patients suffering from this problem have serious sugar and carbohydrate cravings that are of an addictive nature. There is no magic bullet. Failure to change the diet will result in failure to recover from the problem. Anyone who tells you that you can merely take an antifungal drug to cure the problem is mistaken! If ELISA-ACT testing reveals food allergies, those foods need to be avoided during the recovery period.

Some authorities suggest that decreasing honey and fruit juice during the period of recovery is sufficient. Many physicians feel that people may need to eliminate these foods entirely during the recovery period and reintroduce them slowly following recovery. The same may be said for dairy products. Yeast-containing products are a definite no. The reader is referred to Dr. Crook (1986, 1999) for an exhaustive description of the proper diet. In addition, as mentioned, consideration should be given to supplemental hydrochloric acid and pancreatic enzymes if indicated.

Many readers are probably thinking "how long must I stay on this diet?" The truth is that as far as sugar is concerned, one should never resume its use. The other foods may often be reintroduced slowly. Again, it is wise to work with a physician experienced with recurrent yeast infections. It may also be said that as a person gets more attuned to their body's health a certain sensitivity develops letting one know that eating certain things leaves one feeling "not right." This question is the same as when a patient asks how long they should avoid using an injured limb. The answer, of course, is "when it no longer hurts!" Your body knows what is right and wrong for it. It always knew. One just has to relearn by self-observation.

Often a person will report that after following this diet for 2 to 4 weeks they begin to feel worse. This is most probably a result of the yeast dying off and releasing toxins. It is for this reason that the diet should include plenty of fiber to ensure proper elimination. Additionally, 2–4 weeks of a proper diet should be undertaken before initiating treatment with antifungal agents, natural or otherwise.

Probiotics

Natural agents are frequently neglected for the treatment and prevention of selected intestinal and vaginal infections. Placebo-controlled studies demonstrated that natural agents have been used successfully to prevent antibiotic-associated bacterial infections and *Candida* vaginitis (Collins 1980). Few adverse effects have been reported. There is now significant evidence that administration of selected microorganisms is beneficial in the prevention and treatment of certain intestinal infections, and possibly in the treatment of vaginal infections (Jack et al. 1990; Elmer et al. 1996). These are called probiotics and are particularly useful in treating yeast syndrome.

The intake of *bifido* bacteria concentrate capsules every day can dramatically increase the quantity of beneficial bacteria in the gut to help fight *Candida* infections. *Acidophilus* bacteria also can help to fight *Candida* in the upper intestinal tract. *Bifido* bacteria (a beneficial bacteria located in the lower intestines) feed on a special sugar called fructo-oligosaccharides found in a product called NutraFlora. One teaspoon (4 grams) a day of fructo-oligosaccharide promotes the proliferation of friendly *bifido* bacteria in the gut (Howard et al. 1995; Oyarzabal et al. 1995; Buddington et al. 1996).

Studies have shown that the daily ingestion of 150 mL of yogurt enriched with live *Lactobacillus acidophilus* is associated with an increased colonization of friendly bacteria in the rectum and vagina (Shalev et al. 1996). This results in reduced episodes of bacterial vaginitis. Yogurt is often used by women with chronic vaginal *Candida* infections (Hilton 1992). This should not be used for treating yeast syndrome or for those with known milk sensitivity.

Natural Yeast Fighters

Garlic, biotin, and caprylic acid have a direct yeast-killing effect in the intestine (Dausch 1990). Fiber in the diet also can help remove yeast and fungus from the intestines. A product called Yeast Fighters, made by Twin Lab, contains an odorless garlic concentrate, caprylic acid, biotin, *Acidophilus* sp, and a fiber blend to control *Candida* overgrowth in the intestine before it spreads to other parts of the body.

Other supplements to consider are goldenseal (*Hydrastis canadensis*) and volatile oil from oregano (Hammer et al. 1999). Both have antifungal properties. Goldenseal is probably best taken as an infusion such as in a tea bag or about 4 grams, 3 times a day in capsule form. Oregano oil comes in an enteric-coated capsule to protect you from a bad bout of dyspepsia (heartburn.) Take 1 capsule on an empty stomach 3 times a day.

A possibility for treating a yeast infection is a sub-fraction of whey protein called lactoferrin. Several studies have found lactoferrin to inhibit a wide range of gram positive and gram negative bacteria, yeasts, and even certain intestinal parasites. *C albicans*, in particular, has been proven to be inhibited by lactoferrin (Percival, 1997; Kuwata et al., 1998). One to two capsules of lactoferrin should be taken daily, with or without meals.

Although research has not yet proven orthomolecular therapies to be useful for this, some physicians who practice complementary therapies administer nutritional intravenous vitamins, particularly vitamin C, during the recovery period (Wu et al. 1998). Clinically, patients seem to feel stronger more quickly when this is done.

Studies have demonstrated the antifungal properties of tea tree oil (*Melaleuca alternifolia*) against a wide range of fungal isolates including species of *Candida* (Hammer et al. 1997; Rushton et al. 1997). Studies indicate that controlled doses of tea tree oil may be used as an effective topical treatment for dermatologic *Candida* infection and paronychia.

Shark liver oil has demonstrated an antifungal effect in laboratory studies. Shark liver oil capsules containing 200 mg of alkyl glycerol can be taken in doses of 5 capsules a day for up to 30 days. After 30 days, reduce the dose to 2 capsules a day or stop altogether. Shark liver oil promotes the healthy production of blood cells, particularly platelets.

Note: *If you have been diagnosed with thrombocytosis (too many platelets), then do not take shark liver oil supplements.*

Antifungal Drugs

When diet and "natural" therapies fail, a number of antifungal drugs can be considered. One is nystatin, which works only in the bowel and is not absorbed systemically. The dosage is variable and is usually given mixed in water. Infection of the skin is easily treated with medicated creams and lotions containing nystatin. Suppositories may be used for vaginal and anal infection. Thrush medications may be taken as a liquid swished around the mouth or as a slowly dissolving lozenge.

The other drug, Diflucan, is the most potent FDA-approved antifungal drug available. One month's treatment with Diflucan can temporarily eradicate a systemic *Candida* infection (Dmitrieva et al. 1993) so that anti-*Candida* nutritional supplements like Yeast Fighters, Life Flora (*bifido* bacteria), and NutraFlora (fructo-oligosaccharides) can prevent a new *Candida* infection from occurring.

Along with an antifungal cream, hydrocortisone for skin infection may be used to relieve pain and itching. Keeping the skin dry will help to clear up the infection and prevent its return.

🌑 SUMMARY

1. Investigate carefully for underlying health problems.

2. For one-time infection, use traditional local treatment with a topical antifungal or systemic treatment with Diflucan to eradicate the primary yeast infestation.

3. Follow the yeast syndrome diet for 2–4 weeks prior to initiating antifungal therapy, but probiotics (see #4) may be initiated during this time.

4. Take probiotics with *Lactobacillus acidophilus* and *Lactobacillus bifidum*, such as Life Flora (1 tsp a day up to 3 times a day) or Primal Defense (1 capsule 3 times daily).

5. Consider ELISA-ACT allergy testing.

6. Consider Heidelberg testing for gastrointestinal secretions.

7. Use HCl and/or pancreatic enzymes if indicated.

8. Consider Yeast Fighters containing garlic, biotin, and caprylic acid, 5 capsules daily.

9. Consider goldenseal infusion, or about 4 grams in capsule form, taken 3 times a day.

10. Consider oregano oil, enterically coated. One 400-mg softgel twice daily with a small amount of warm water between meals is recommended.

11. Consider shark oil, up to 5 capsules a day for no more than 30 consecutive days. After 30 days, reduce the dose to 2 capsules a day or stop altogether. Each capsule should contain 200 mg of alkyl glycerol. Shark liver oil promotes the healthy production of blood cells, particularly platelets. *Note:* if you have been diagnosed with thrombocytosis (too many platelets), then do not take shark liver oil supplements.

12. Consider lactoferrin, 300–600 mg a day with or without food.

13. Consider orthomolecular therapy with intravenous vitamins, in particular vitamin C, 50 grams IV, 1–3 times a week.

Please note that studies have not been done to ascertain exact dosing. It is also unclear whether to combine the antifungals or use them one at a time. It is probably best to begin with single agents and add others if necessary.

14. Refer to the *Obesity* protocol for information about cutting carbohydrate (sugar) craving.

 FOR MORE INFORMATION

Contact the National Women's Health Network, (202) 628–7814. A staffer will answer questions on vaginitis and yeast infections. An information packet costs $6 for members and $8 for nonmembers. Also refer to Crook (1986, 1999).

 PRODUCT AVAILABILITY

Yeast Fighters capsules (combination anti-fungal nutrients), Life Flora, Primal Defense (both containing *bifido* bacteria), Kyolic Garlic Formulas, Pure-Gar Formulas, standardized shark liver oil capsules, lactoferrin, goldenseal, oregano oil (Gaia Herbs), pancreatic enzymes, and Nutraflora can be ordered by calling (800) 544–4440, or order online at www.lef.org. Diflucan is an expensive prescription drug that needs to be prescribed by your physician.

Candida Questionnaire

History	Point	Score
1. Have you taken tetracycline or other antibiotics for acne for 1 month or longer?	25	_____
2. Have you at any time in your life taken other "broad-spectrum" antibiotics for respiratory, urinary, or other infections for 2 months or longer, or in short courses 4 or more times in a 1-year period?	20	_____
3. Have you ever taken a broad-spectrum antibiotic (even a single course)?	6	_____
4. Have you at any time in your life been bothered by persistent prostatitis, vaginitis, or other problems affecting your reproductive organs?	25	_____
5. Have you been pregnant?		_____
One time?	3	_____
Two or more times?	5	_____
6. Have you taken birth-control pills?		
For 6 months to 2 years?	8	_____
For more than 2 years?	15	_____
7. Have you taken prednisone or other cortisone-type drugs?		
For 2 weeks or less?	6	_____
For more than 2 weeks?	15	_____
8. Does exposure to perfumes, insecticides, fabric shop odors, and other chemicals provoke:		_____
Mild symptoms?	5	_____
Moderate to severe symptoms?	20	_____
9. Are your symptoms worse on damp, muggy days or in moldy places?	20	_____
10. Have you had athlete's foot, ringworm, "jock itch," or other chronic infections of the skin or nails?		_____
Mild to moderate	10	_____
Severe or persistent	20	_____

Candida Questionnaire

11. Do you crave sugar?	10	_____
12. Do you crave breads?	10	_____
13. Do you crave alcoholic beverages?	10	_____
14. Does tobacco smoke really bother you?	10	_____
Total Score for This Section		_____

Major Symptoms

For each of your symptoms, enter the appropriate figure in the Point Score column

If a symptom is occasional or mild	score 3 points
If a symptom is frequent and/or moderately severe	score 6 points
If a symptom is severe and/or disabling	score 9 points

1. Fatigue or lethargy _____
2. Feeling of being "drained" _____
3. Poor memory _____
4. Feeling "spacey" or "unreal" _____
5. Depression _____
6. Numbness, burning, or tingling _____
7. Muscle aches _____
8. Muscle weakness or paralysis _____
9. Pain and/or swelling in joints _____
10. Abdominal pain _____
11. Constipation _____
12. Diarrhea _____
13. Bloating _____
14. Persistent vaginal itch _____
15. Persistent vaginal burning _____
16. Prostatitis _____
17. Impotence _____
18. Loss of sexual desire _____
19. Endometriosis _____
20. Cramps and/or other menstrual irregularities _____
21. Premenstrual tension _____
22. Spots in front of eyes _____
23. Erratic vision _____
     Total Score for This Section _____

Other Symptoms

For each of your symptoms, enter the appropriate figure in the Point Score column

If a symptom is occasional or mild	score 3 points
If a symptom is frequent and/or moderately severe	score 6 points
If a symptom is severe and/or disabling	score 9 points

1. Drowsiness _____
2. Irritability _____
3. Lack of coordination _____
4. Inability to concentrate _____
5. Frequent mood swings _____
6. Headache _____
7. Dizziness/loss of balance _____
8. Pressure above ears, feeling of head swelling and tingling _____
9. Itching _____
10. Other rashes _____
11. Heartburn _____
12. Indigestion _____

Candida Questionnaire

13. Belching and intestinal gas ⎯⎯⎯
14. Mucus in stools ⎯⎯⎯
15. Hemorrhoids ⎯⎯⎯
16. Dry mouth ⎯⎯⎯
17. Rash or blisters in mouth ⎯⎯⎯
18. Bad breath ⎯⎯⎯
19. Joint swelling or arthritis ⎯⎯⎯
20. Nasal congestion or discharge ⎯⎯⎯
21. Postnasal drip ⎯⎯⎯
22. Nasal itching ⎯⎯⎯
23. Sore or dry throat ⎯⎯⎯
24. Cough ⎯⎯⎯
25. Pain or tightness in chest ⎯⎯⎯
26. Wheezing or shortness of breath ⎯⎯⎯
27. Urinary urgency or frequency ⎯⎯⎯
28. Burning on urination ⎯⎯⎯
29. Failing vision ⎯⎯⎯
30. Burning or tearing of eyes ⎯⎯⎯
31. Recurrent infections or fluid in ears ⎯⎯⎯
32. Ear pain or deafness ⎯⎯⎯
　　Total Score for This Section ⎯⎯⎯

Interpretation

	Women	Men
Yeast-connected health problems are almost certainly present	> 180	> 140
Yeast-connected health problems are probably present	120–180	90–140
Yeast-connected health problems are possibly present	60–119	40–89
Yeast-connected health problems are less likely to be present	< 60	< 40

Source: (Taken from W. G. Crook, The Yeast Connection 1986.)

Cardiovascular Disease: Overview

A staggering number of people are destined to experience a cardiovascular-related disorder sometime in their lives. Almost 1 million Americans die each year as a result of cardiovascular disease, whereas 556,000 die each year from cancer. Despite these facts, people are often more afraid of cancer than they are of vascular disease.

Americans have become complacent about the dangers of arterial disease. One reason is that the percentage of young people dying from acute heart attack has plummeted over the past 50 years. Explanations for these reductions include lifestyle changes, greater use of dietary supplements/preventive medications, and improved cardiac medical care.

The question is why are so many Americans continuing to die from heart attack and stroke? The fundamental answer is that people are living longer. What has happened is that much of the human population has succeeded in delaying the development of arterial disease. So instead of suddenly dying from a heart attack at age 50, the vascular symptoms do not manifest until the 60s or 80s are reached. At this point, systemic arteriosclerosis has damaged the major organ systems, and multiple degenerative diseases result in diminished quality and quantity of life.

Many of the underlying causes of arterial disease have been identified in the scientific literature. Regrettably, cardiologists have only addressed a limited number of these factors, such as prescribing cholesterol-lowering drugs, controlling hypertension, etc. By ignoring the other proven causes for the epidemic of vascular-related diseases, a significant number of Americans are experiencing needless suffering and are dying prematurely.

This overview presents some of the more important missing pieces of the puzzle about why cardiovascular disease remains the nation's leading crippler and killer. It provides solid information about what can be done to significantly reduce cardiovascular risk today.

For those who want to learn about every identified risk factor, the protocol that follows entitled *Cardiovascular Disease: Comprehensive Analysis* provides meticulous data that is especially important for anyone who already has a heart or vascular-related disorder.

INFLAMMATION AND HEART DISEASE

A growing consensus among scientists is that common disorders such as heart attack, stroke, and other vascular-related diseases are all caused in part by a *chronic inflammatory syndrome*. Numerous published articles demonstrate that the presence of blood indicators of inflammation are strong predictive factors for determining who will develop coronary artery disease and have cardiac-related death (Lindahl et al. 2000; Packard et al. 2000; Rader 2000).

The good news is lifestyle changes and certain dietary supplements can suppress these dangerous inflammatory components of blood.

One of the dangerous inflammatory markers that has been identified is a coagulation protein called *fibrinogen*. High fibrinogen levels can induce a heart attack via several mechanisms, including increased platelet aggregation, hypercoagulation, and excessive blood thickening. The findings of published scientific studies show that persons with high levels of fibrinogen are more than twice as likely to die of a heart attack.

Another inflammatory marker is *C-reactive protein*. This marker indicates an increased risk for destabilized atherosclerotic plaque and abnormal arterial clotting. When arterial plaque becomes destabilized, it can burst open and block the flow of blood through a coronary artery, resulting in an acute heart attack. Some studies show that people with high levels of C-reactive protein are almost three times as likely to die from a heart attack.

Why Cardiologists Are So Slow to React

In 1996 the Life Extension Foundation published an article showing that high levels of fibrinogen represented a significant risk factor for heart attack and ischemic stroke (Ridker et al. 2000). The article was based on studies dating back to the 1980s showing that people with elevated fibrinogen levels were more likely to die from a cardiovascular-related disease.

Despite numerous studies linking elevated fibrinogen to increased heart attack risk, few physicians bother to check their patient's blood levels of fibrinogen or other correctable risk factors such as homocysteine and C-reactive protein.

Many cardiologists are still demanding a higher standard of proof before they routinely test their patients' blood for what they consider to be "newly identified" cardiac risk factors. Even when a physician is aware of the importance of testing a patient's blood for the presence of inflammatory risk factors, a common problem is that managed care organizations (HMOs and PPOs) refuse to pay for them.

The sad fact is that the majority of practicing physicians are not yet aware of how to properly correct for elevated inflammatory risk factors (such as C-reactive protein and fibrinogen).

As a result of physician ignorance or insurance company stinginess, many Americans experience progressive debilitating congestive heart failure or cerebral circulatory impairment, when the underlying causes could have been corrected if the physician ordered and then properly interpreted these blood tests.

Correcting Inflammatory Risk Factors

Cardiovascular risk factors such as fibrinogen and C-reactive protein are produced in the liver by pro-inflammatory cytokines called interleukin-1B, interleukin-6, and tumor necrosis factor alpha (TNF-a) (Ridker et al. 2000). Supplements such as highly concentrated DHA fish oil and DHEA suppress excess production of some of these dangerous cytokines.

Another study showed that interleukin-6 by itself increased the risk of heart attack, even after adjustment for the elevation in C-reactive protein induced by interleukin-6 (Rader 2000). Both vitamin K and DHEA suppress interleukin-6, which helps explain why these supplements have been shown to protect against such a wide range of age-related diseases (Reddi et al. 1995; Kipper-Galperin et al. 1999; Haden et al. 2000).

Concerning the suppression of the dangerous tumor necrosis factor alpha and interleukin-1B cytokines, nettle leaf extract appears to be the most effective dietary supplement (Obertreis et al. 1996; Teucher et al. 1996).

Protection Against Fibrinogen-Induced Heart Attacks

Agents that *inhibit* platelet aggregation reduce the risk that fibrinogen will cause an abnormal arterial blood clot. Platelet aggregation inhibitors include aspirin, green tea, ginkgo, garlic, and vitamin E (Bossavy et al. 1998; Kang et al. 1999; Logani et al. 2000; Rahman et al. 2000). For optimal protection against heart attack, it also makes sense to utilize therapies that directly *lower* elevated fibrinogen levels.

High serum vitamin A and beta-carotene levels have been associated with reduced fibrinogen levels in humans. Animals fed a vitamin A-deficient diet have an impaired ability to break down fibrinogen. When animals are injected with vitamin A, they produce tissue plasminogen activator (tPA), which breaks down fibrinogen (Lagente et al. 1993; Back et al. 1995; Ceriello et al. 1997).

Excessive homocysteine blocks the natural breakdown of fibrinogen by inhibiting the production of tissue plasminogen activator (tPA) (Midorikawa et al. 2000). Folic acid, TMG, vitamin B_{12}, and vitamin B_6 reduce elevated homocysteine levels. High doses of fish or olive oil have also been shown to lower fibrinogen in humans with elevated fibrinogen levels (Flaten et al. 1990; Oosthuizen et al. 1994).

Vitamin C, in pharmacological doses, has been shown to break down excess fibrinogen. In one study, heart disease patients were given either 1000 or 2000 mg a day of vitamin C to measure the fibrinogen breakdown effect. At 1000 mg a day, there was no detectable change in fibrinolytic activity or cholesterol. At 2000 mg a day of vitamin C, there was a 27% decrease in the platelet aggregation index, a 12% reduction in total cholesterol, and a 45% increase in fibrinolysis (fibrinogen breakdown) activity (Bordia 1980).

A Lethal Misconception Among Vitamin Supplement Users

The medical establishment woke up to the dangers of homocysteine when *The New England Journal of Medicine* (Welch et al. 1998) and the *Journal of the American Medical Association* (Tucker et al. 1996) published articles suggesting that vitamin supplements be used to lower homocysteine levels. (Many years earlier, this same message appeared in the November 1981 issue of a Life Extension Foundation publication entitled *Anti-Aging News*, pp. 85–86.)

Conventional medical journals have published hundreds of new studies in recent years that unequivocally link elevated homocysteine to greater risk of heart attack and stroke. As a result of these findings, some cardiologists suggest that coronary artery disease patients take a multivitamin supplement to lower their homocysteine levels. Patients who follow this advice but fail to have their blood tested for homocysteine could be making a fatal mistake.

The Life Extension Foundation uncovered a flaw in the theory that a person can blindly take vitamin supplements to adequately reduce homocysteine levels. While folic acid, vitamin B_{12}, vitamin B_6, and trimethylglycine (TMG) all lower homocysteine levels, it is impossible for any individual to know if they are taking the proper amount of nutrients unless they have a homocysteine blood test.

The clear message from new scientific findings is that there is no safe "normal range" for homocysteine. While commercial laboratories state that normal homocysteine can range from 5–15 micromoles per liter (umol/L) of blood, epidemiological data reported in the American Heart Association's journal *Circulation* reveal that blood levels of homocysteine levels above 6.3 cause a steep progressive risk of heart attack (Robinson et al. 1995). Another study reported in *The American Journal of Epidemiology* found that each 3-unit increase in homocysteine equals a 35% increase in myocardial infarction (heart attack) risk (Verhoef et al. 1996).

People taking vitamin supplements think they are being protected from the lethal effects of homocysteine when, in reality, even supplement users can have homocysteine levels far above the *safe* level of 6.3.

The Life Extension Foundation has identified several cases of people with coronary artery disease who had lethal levels of homocysteine despite taking the recommended dose (and higher) of vitamin supplements. One case involved a 60-year-old man who had previous bypass surgery, but was again experiencing angina pain with significant restenosis (reclogging of the coronary arteries) verified by angiography. This man knew about the dangers of homocysteine and had been taking more than 15,000 mcg daily of folic acid, along with other homocysteine-lowering vitamins. Because of the angina pain and re-stenosis, The Foundation recommended a homocysteine blood test. The results showed this man had the shockingly high homocysteine reading of 18. (Homocysteine levels over 15 have been shown to be extremely dangerous.) The Foundation immediately suggested that this man take 6 grams of TMG (trimethylglycine) daily. Within 1 month, his homocysteine level had dropped to 4. This case was a wake-up call that one or more homocysteine-lowering factors are not always the solution to keeping homocysteine levels in the safest range (below 7 micromoles per liter of blood).

How to Detoxify Homocysteine

Elevated homocysteine can be reduced (or detoxified) in two ways: via the remethylation process and via the trans-sulfuration pathway.

The most common way to reduce homocysteine is via the remethylation process in which "methyl groups" are donated to homocysteine to transform it into methionine and S-adenosylmethionine (SAMe). TMG (tri-methyl-glycine) is a potent remethylation agent. The "tri" means there are three "methyl" groups on each "glycine" molecule that can be transferred to homocysteine to transform (remethylate) it into methionine and SAMe. The remethylation (or detoxification) of homocysteine requires adequate levels of folic acid and vitamin B_{12} in addition to TMG.

The other pathway by which elevated homocysteine is reduced is via its conversion to cysteine and eventually to

glutathione via the "trans-sulfuration" pathway. This pathway is dependent on vitamin B_6. The amount of vitamin B_6 required to lower homocysteine has considerable individual variability. Methionine is the only amino acid that creates homocysteine. People who eat foods that are high in methionine such as red meat and chicken may need more vitamin B_6. Elevated homocysteine can occur when there are insufficient vitamin co-factors (such as folate and vitamin B_6) to detoxify the amount of methionine being ingested in the diet.

Elevated homocysteine can also be caused by a genetic defect that blocks the trans-sulfuration pathway by inducing a deficiency of the B_6-dependent enzyme cystathionine-B-synthase. In this case, high doses of vitamin B_6 are required to suppress excessive homocysteine accumulation. Since one would not want to take excessive doses of vitamin B_6 (greater than 300–500 mg daily for a long time period), a homocysteine blood test can help determine whether you are taking enough B_6 to keep homocysteine levels in a safe range. There are some people who lack an enzyme to convert vitamin B_6 into its biologically active form *pyridoxal-5-phosphate*. In this case, if low-cost vitamin B_6 supplements do not sufficiently lower homocysteine levels, then a high-cost pyridoxal-5-phosphate supplement may be required.

For many people, the daily intake of 500 mg of TMG, 800 mcg of folic acid, 1000 mcg of vitamin B_{12}, 250 mg of choline, 250 mg of inositol, 30 mg of zinc, and 100 mg of vitamin B_6 will keep homocysteine levels in a safe range. But the only way to really know is to have your blood tested to make certain your homocysteine levels are under 7.

If homocysteine levels are too high, then up to 6000 mg of TMG may be needed along with higher amounts of other remethylation cofactors. Some people with cystathione-B synthase deficiencies will require 500 mg daily or more of vitamin B_6 to reduce homocysteine to a safe level. For the prevention of cardiovascular disease, you would also want your homocysteine blood level to be under 7 micromol per liter of blood.

THE SILENT STROKE EPIDEMIC

Stroke is a common threat to aging humans. Most people believe a stroke can either kill suddenly or induce a state of paralysis requiring institutional care. However, newer studies reveal that most strokes cause no obvious symptoms, but over time these "silent" strokes lead to memory loss, neurologic disorders, and more strokes. According to one study, 11 million Americans have "silent" strokes annually, and by the time people reach their 70s, 1 in 3 experiences a silent stroke every year (Leary et al. 2000).

Health-conscious people should be comforted in knowing that following the proper lifestyle and consuming specific dietary supplements may dramatically reduce the risk of ever having a stroke. For example, a meta-analysis of 15 published studies showed that mild-to-moderate elevations in homocysteine were independently associated with an astounding 86%

increase in the risk of stroke (Kelly et al. 2000). The use of extra vitamin B$_6$, vitamin B$_{12}$, and folic acid is one way of lowering homocysteine levels.

What Is a STROKE?

Stroke is the third leading cause of death in developed countries. About 25% die as a result of a stroke or its complications, and almost 50% have moderate-to-severe health impairments and long-term disabilities. Only 26% recover most or all normal health and function.

The majority of strokes occur when a blood clot blocks the flow of oxygenated blood to a portion of the brain. This type of stroke, caused by a blood clot blocking a blood vessel, is called "ischemic stroke." An ischemic stroke can result from a blood clot that forms inside the artery of the brain (thrombotic stroke) or by a clot formed somewhere else in the body that travels to the brain (embolic stroke).

In the case of ischemic stroke, abnormal blood clotting blocks large or small arteries in the brain, cutting off blood flow. Ischemic strokes account for 83% of all strokes and occur as either an embolic or thrombotic stroke. The other 17% of strokes are called "hemorrhagic stroke" and these occur when a blood vessel in the brain ruptures.

Thrombotic stroke represents 52% of all ischemic strokes. Thrombotic stroke is caused as the result of unhealthy blood vessels becoming clogged with a buildup of fatty deposits, calcium, or blood clotting factors such as fibrinogen, homocysteine, and LDL-cholesterol. We generally refer to this as *atherosclerosis disease*. More recent information indicates that a chronic inflammatory process is also a cause of the arterial damage that leads to stroke. Elevated C-reactive protein is an indicator of underlying inflammatory disease (Fichtlscherer et al. 2000; Ijem et al. 2000; Pasceri et al. 2000).

Elevated fibrinogen is also a significant risk factor for developing the most common form of stroke (Audebert et al. 2000; Bai et al. 2000; Chen et al. 2000; Trouillas et al. 2000). Some of the nutrients that can lower fibrinogen include at least 2000 mg a day of vitamin C, 2400 mg of flush-free niacin, 2800 mg of EPA/DHA from fish oil, and 2000 mg a day of bromelain. To protect against fibrinogen inducing an arterial blood clot that can cause an ischemic stroke, we suggest low-dose aspirin, vitamin E, and garlic, along with ginkgo and green tea extracts.

One of the best-documented ways of determining who will have a stroke is to measure levels of C-reactive protein in the blood. One study showed that elevated C-reactive protein posed a two-to-three times greater risk of stroke (Kelly et al. 2000). Another study showed that in those who have a major stroke, persons who had higher levels of C-reactive protein had a much greater likelihood of having another vascular event (such as a heart attack or stroke) or dying within the following year. In this study, stroke patients with the highest C-reactive protein levels had nearly a 2.4 times greater chance of experiencing death or a vascular event within the next year compared to patients with the lowest levels (Di Napoli et al. 2001).

High levels of C-reactive protein also indicate a potentially destructive inflammatory autoimmune condition that could predispose a person to a host of degenerative diseases. C-reactive protein can be suppressed by ibuprofen, aspirin, or vitamin E (McMillan et al. 1995; Ikonomidis et al. 1999; Devaraj et al. 2000). Some of the pro-inflammatory immune cytokines that cause elevated C-reactive protein include interleukin-6, interleukin 1(b), and TNF-a. Supplements such as DHEA, vitamin K, nettle leaf extract, and high levels of DHA fish oil can help suppress these dangerous inflammatory cytokines that can cause C-reactive protein elevation (Reddi et al. 1995; Teucher et al. 1996; Kipper-Galperin et al. 1999).

One of the strengths of C-reactive protein testing is its ability to detect at-risk patients with normal cholesterol levels. The Physician's Health Study found that apparently healthy men with the highest C-reactive protein levels had twice the risk of future stroke, three times the risk of future heart attack, and four times the risk of future peripheral vascular disease (Ridker et al. 1997). The Women's Health Study reported that C-reactive protein was the single strongest predictor of future vascular risk (Ridker et al. 1998).

Taking Steps to Reduce Your Stroke Risk Profile

For the last 50 years, physicians have concentrated on controlling blood pressure as the primary method of preventing stroke. While guarding against even borderline hypertension is critical in reducing stroke risk, there are factors that can be tested in the blood to further determine stroke risk. Everyone over age 40 should have their blood tested to be certain their homocysteine, fibrinogen, C-reactive protein, LDL-cholesterol, etc. levels are in the safe range.

If any of these risk factors for stroke are elevated, they can be safely lowered with therapies that are proven to work. Since these same risk factors also predispose one to heart attack and other diseases, anyone concerned with living a long and healthy life should keep them in the optimal ranges. (See the table on the next page for list of recommended blood tests.)

Blood Test	What the "Standard Reference Range" Allows	The "Optimal" Level: Where YOU Want to Be
Fibrinogen	Up to 460 mg/dL	Under 300 mg/dL
C-reactive protein	Up to 4.9 mg/L	Under 2 mg/L [Some studies indicate C-reactive protein levels should be below 1.3 mg/L (Kaneko et al. 1999; Sandrick 2000)]
Homocysteine	Up to 15 micromol/L	Under 7 micromol/L
Glucose	Up to 109 mg/dL	Under 100 mg/dL
Iron	Up to 180 mg/dL	Under 100 mcg/dL
Cholesterol	Up to 199 mg/dL	Between 180–220 mg/dL
LDL cholesterol	Up to 129 mg/dL	Under 100 mg/dL
HDL cholesterol	No lower than 35 mg/dL	Over 50 mg/dL
Triglycerides	Up to 199 mg/dL	Under 100 mg/dL
DHEA	Males: no lower than 80 mcg/dL Females: no lower than 35 mcg/dL	Between 400–560 mcg/dL Between 350–430 mcg/dL
Fasting Insulin	6–27 uIU/mL	0–5 uIU/mL

If your physician will not prescribe these blood tests, or if your insurance company will not pay for them because the cost is too expensive, call (800) 208-3444 to inquire about obtaining these tests via mail order.

All of this new research points to the fact that the common forms of mental impairment, disability, and death in the aging population (vascular dementia, stroke, and heart attack) are potentially avoidable. While conventional physicians focus solely on blood pressure control, they are failing to recommend important blood tests, drugs, and supplements to reduce the stroke epidemic that continues to plague the aging human population. HMOs and insurance companies often refuse to pay for these important blood tests even though overall medical costs could be significantly reduced if common diseases like stroke were prevented.

TESTING YOUR BLOOD TO AVOID CARDIOVASCULAR DISEASE

Do not let complacent physicians put you at risk for heart disease and stroke. The following table provides the most common blood tests that can help reveal underlying cardiovascular disease risk factors.

As can be seen from the table, blood test results that conventional physicians accept as being "normal" can be lethal for you. In other words, what the "Standard Reference Range" allows is not always a practical indicator for where your "optimal" level should be.

In many cases, a "standard reference range" reflects what is expected in the average population. Since cardiovascular disease remains the number one killer of Americans, you do not want to ever be part of the "average" range when it comes to cardiovascular disease risk factors.

By keeping your blood levels in the "Optimal Range," rather than the average "Standard Reference Range," you take advantage of the increasing volume of evidence showing that most heart attacks and strokes are preventable.

In the table, you can also see that the "Standard Reference Range" differs (often dangerously) from what the published research indicates is protective against cardiovascular disease.

HOW EXCESS INSULIN CAUSES HEART ATTACKS

According to the Centers for Disease Control (CDC), results of the National Health and Nutrition Examination Survey (NHANES) indicate that 35% of U.S. adults aged 20–74 were overweight and almost 20% of adults in the same population were obese (CDC 2002a,b). A Harris Poll of a smaller population of 1011 people indicated that an even higher level (79%) were overweight, based on their body mass index (CNN 2002). Despite aggressive use of existing weight-loss therapies, far more Americans have excess body fat today than at any prior time. Weight gain has most often been associated with cardiovascular disease and diabetes, but new studies reveal that other age-related disorders such as cancer (endometrial, breast, prostate, and colon) occur at sharply higher rates in overweight individuals (CDC 2002c). The government is now encouraging people to lose weight to protect their health. In 2002, U.S. Surgeon General David Satcher stated that obesity may soon become a greater health hazard than cigarette smoking and issued a *Call to Action* urging the nation to find solutions to the problem of obesity and overweight (Surgeon General 2002).

As people age, they accumulate unwanted body fat even though they may be consuming fewer calories than when they were young. The overlooked culprit responsible for unwanted body fat and bulging waistlines is the hormone insulin. We are not talking about normal insulin secretion. Instead, it is the *overproduction* of insulin that causes so many people to uncontrollably gain weight. Because insulin is required to sustain life, the public mistakenly "sees" this hormone in a favorable light. As you will learn, too much insulin not only causes weight gain, but it is also a prime factor contributing to a multitude of diseases associated with obesity.

There are serious misconceptions about why people accumulate so much body fat as they age. One overlooked factor is that overweight people have startlingly high levels of insulin in their blood. When the blood is saturated with insulin, the body will not release significant fat stores, even when a person restricts calorie intake and exercises.

Additionally, persons who are overweight face a significant risk for developing Type II diabetes (Jallut et al. 1990; Kadowaki et al. 1994; McCance et al. 1994). The treatment of obesity and Type II diabetes is interrelated. By effectively treating either one of these diseases, one can mitigate or control the other.

Having diabetes also sharply increases the risk of heart attack and stroke. It is critical that persons concerned about preventing cardiovascular disease reverse the diabetic process. Losing excess body fat is a mandate for most persons seeking to control a Type II diabetic condition.

Hyperinsulinemia is the medical term used to describe a condition in which too much insulin is produced. One way that excess insulin makes people gain weight is that it causes them to be chronically hungry. This happens because high insulin levels rapidly deplete glucose from the blood. This causes a state known as "reactive hypoglycemia," meaning the blood becomes deficient in glucose because there is too much insulin in the blood.

The May 8, 2002, issue of the *Journal of the American Medical Association* (JAMA) featured an article that described the effects of consuming high-glycemic index foods and the subsequent hyperinsulinemia,

hunger, and weight gain that occurred (Ludwig 2002). The author of this JAMA article summarized his position by stating: "It is possible that the hunger incident to hyperinsulinemia may be a cause of overeating and therefore the obesity that so often precedes diabetes."

A surprising number of studies show that excess serum insulin (hyperinsulinemia) is a major health problem (Despres et al. 1996; Chu et al. 2001; Thakur et al. 2001). For people trying to reduce body fat, excess insulin suppresses the release of growth hormone in addition to preventing fat from being released from cells. High serum insulin is associated with the development of abdominal obesity and the number of health problems this induces, including atherosclerosis and impotence (Aversa et al. 1998; Jeremy et al. 1998; Despres et al. 2000).

Perhaps the simplest method of evaluating the toxic effects of excess insulin is to look at its effects on human mortality. One study showed that over a 10-year period, the risk of dying was almost twice as great for those with the highest levels of insulin, compared to those with the lowest. The scientists who authored this study stated that hyperinsulinemia is associated with increased all-cause and cardiovascular mortality independent of other risk factors (Pyorala et al. 2000).

Another study showed that the risk of developing coronary artery disease increased by 60% for each single-digit increase in fasting insulin level among men aged 45–76 years (after other risk factors were controlled) (Despres et al. 1996). In optimal health, fasting insulin levels should be in the range of 0–5 (uIU/mL). As people age, their fasting insulin levels normally increase by several single digits. Fasting insulin levels in the obese often exceed 20.

Having too much insulin in the blood has become so commonplace that laboratory reference ranges now indicate that fasting insulin levels of 6–27 are "normal." While it is normal for aging individuals to have high fasting insulin, it is by no means desirable. Unfortunately, aging people experience a wide range of vascular diseases, such as kidney failure, heart attack, stroke, etc., that are directly attributable to elevated insulin.

Standard laboratory reference ranges can sometimes be misleading. For instance, it was once considered normal to have a cholesterol reading of up to 300 (mg/dL). While it is true that a cholesterol count of 300 was normal at that time in history, so was an epidemic of heart attacks. Once the danger of high cholesterol became known, laboratories reduced the high normal reference range to 200.

As more research substantiates the dangers of excess insulin, we believe that laboratory reference ranges will show that fasting insulin levels of 0–3 are desirable and that levels in excess of 5 put an individual at increased risk for developing a host of age-related ailments.

However, suppressing excess serum insulin is not as easy as lowering cholesterol or homocysteine. To access an in-depth protocol dealing with proven methods to lower excess insulin, refer to the *Obesity protocol* in this book.

TESTOSTERONE AND THE HEART

Normal aging results in gradual weakening of the heart, even in the absence of significant coronary artery disease. If nothing else kills an elderly male, his heart will just stop beating at some point.

Testosterone is a muscle-building hormone, and there are many testosterone-receptor sites in the heart (Bricout et al. 1994). Weakening of the heart muscle can sometimes be attributed to testosterone deficiency (Sewdarsen et al. 1990; Phillips et al. 1994). Testosterone is not only responsible for maintaining heart muscle protein synthesis, but it is also a promoter of coronary artery dilation (Rosano et al. 1999; Webb et al. 1999) and helps to maintain healthy cholesterol levels (Zgliczynski et al. 1996; Gelfand et al. 1997).

There is an ever-increasing number of studies indicating an association between high testosterone and low cardiovascular disease rates in men (Gelfand et al. 1997). In the majority of patients, symptoms and EKG measurements improve when low testosterone levels are corrected. One study showed that blood flow to the heart improved 68.8% in elderly male coronary heart disease patients who received testosterone therapy (Wu et al. 1993b). In China, physicians successfully treat angina with testosterone therapy (Wu et al. 1993a, b, c).

The effects of low testosterone on cardiovascular disease are given in the following list:

- Cholesterol, fibrinogen, triglycerides, and insulin levels increase (Glueck et al. 1993; Winkler 1996; De Pergola et al. 1997).

- Coronary artery elasticity diminishes.

- Blood pressure rises.

- Human growth hormone (HGH) declines (weakening heart muscle).

- Abdominal fat increases (increasing the risk of heart attack).

Persons with cardiovascular disease should have their blood tested for free testosterone and estrogen. Some men (who have the full cooperation of their physicians) may be able to stop taking expensive drugs to stimulate cardiac output, to lower cholesterol, and to keep blood pressure under control if a testosterone deficit or a testosterone-estrogen imbalance is corrected. A compelling study of 1100 men showed that men with serum DHEA-S in the lowest quarter (<1.6 mcg/mL) were significantly more likely to incur symptoms of heart disease (Feldman et al. 2001). In a review of several studies, other authors have confirmed this association (Porsova-Dutoit et al. 2000). *Note:* DHEA is produced by the adrenal gland and is a precursor hormone for the manufacturing of testosterone.

Despite numerous studies substantiating the beneficial effects of testosterone therapy in treating heart disease, conventional cardiologists continue to overlook the important role this hormone plays in keeping their cardiac patients alive (Tripathi et al. 1998; Webb et al. 1999; Rosano et al. 1999).

Testosterone replacement therapy is normally indicated in aging men who do not have prostate cancer. It should be done in cooperation with a knowledgeable physician. To learn the facts about safely restoring testosterone levels, refer to the *Male Hormone Modulation protocol* in this book.

SUMMARY

This cardiovascular disease overview has addressed the following five significant cardiovascular risk factors that conventional physicians often overlook to the detriment of their patients:

1. Elevated C-reactive protein
2. Elevated fibrinogen
3. Elevated homocysteine
4. Excess insulin
5. Too little free testosterone (men)

Persons concerned about arterial system health should have their blood tested for all of the potential indicators of a pending cardiovascular event. A table has been provided in this protocol so that the reader will know what blood tests to ask for and what the optimal ranges should be.

If any of the indicators are out of the optimal range, appropriate corrective actions should be taken. A number of suggested methods to restore blood indicators to optimal ranges have also been discussed. A review of the approaches that may be considered to specifically correct the five cardiovascular disease risk factors outlined in this protocol will now be provided:

1. Elevated C-Reactive Protein

To reduce C-reactive protein to below 1.3 mg/L of blood, first try the following natural supplements that reduce pro-inflammatory cytokine production and oxidative stress:

- Vitamin E (alpha tocopherol), 1200 IU daily along with 400 mg of gamma tocopherol.
- DHEA, 15–75 mg a day. (Refer to *DHEA Replacement protocol* for precautions.)
- Essential fatty acids, a supplement that provides at least 1000 mg of DHA and 400 mg of EPA from fish oil along with 900 mg of gamma-linolenic acid (GLA) from borage oil.
- Vitamin K, 10 mg a day.
- Nettle leaf extract, 1000 mg a day.

If the natural supplements do not work, consider trying:

- Ibuprofen, 200–800 mg a day, or aspirin, 81–325 mg a day.
- A statin drug such as Pravacol, 40 mg a day (as long as total cholesterol levels do not drop substantially below 180 mg/dL).

Persons taking ibuprofen or doses of aspirin in excess of 81 mg a day should take 900–1800 mg a day of polyenylphosphatidylcholine (PPC) to protect against damage to the stomach lining. (Statin drugs are available only by prescription.)

2. Elevated Fibrinogen

To reduce fibrinogen to below 300 mg/dL of blood, try:

- Flush-free niacin (inositol hexanicotinate), 2400–3000 mg a day.
- Vitamin C, 4000 mg a day.
- Bromelain, 2000 mg a day.
- Fish oil, a supplement that supplies 2400 mg of EPA and 1800 mg of DHA a day.
- Vitamin A 25,000 IU a day. (Refer to Vitamin A Precautions in *Appendix A*.)

Note: *When taking high doses of niacin or flush-free niacin, have a blood liver enzyme test done within 60 days, at which time the blood should also be tested to ascertain if adequate fibrinogen reduction has occurred.*

If the natural fibrinogen-lowering supplements do not work, consider trying:

- Pentoxiphylline (Trental), 400 mg two times a day. (Trental is a prescription drug.)

3. Elevated Homocysteine

If homocysteine levels are above 6.3 micromol/L of blood, try:

- Folic acid, 800–2400 mg a day.
- Vitamin B_{12}, 300–1000 mcg a day.
- Vitamin B_6, 100–250 mg a day.
- Trimethylglycine (TMG), 500–2000 mg a day.

If the homocysteine-lowering supplements do not work, consider:

- Reducing dietary sources of methionine (the precusor to homocysteine). This means cutting back on red meat, chicken, and dairy proteins.
- Increasing vitamin B_6 to 500–750 mg a day. Note that long-term use of vitamin B_6 in excess of 250 mg has been associated with peripheral neuropathy that normally goes away upon cessation of the high B_6 intake. Taking other B-complex vitamins and magnesium has been reported to reduce neu-ropathy risk.
- Increasing TMG to 3000–9000 mg a day.

4. Excess Insulin

Attempt to reduce fasting insulin levels to below 5 uIU/mL of blood:

- Consume a low-glycemic diet. (Refer to the *Obesity protocol* for specifics.)
- Take 200 mg of *d*-mannoheptulose (avocado sugar extract) 1 hour after the evening meal.

If these natural approaches to reducing fasting insulin do not work, consider taking:

- A standardized avocado extract after dinner and possibly before bedtime. For specific dosage instructions, refer to the *Obesity protocol* in this book.
- 500–1000 mg a day of Metformin (a prescription drug).
- Refer to the *Diabetes protocol* in this book.

5. Low Testosterone (Men Only)

If blood tests reveal free testosterone in lower ranges of normal, consider asking your physician for a prescription for a testosterone patch, gel, or cream, usually in a dose of 5 mg a day. If estrogen levels are significantly above 30 pg/mL, ask your physician for a prescription for an aromatase-inhibiting drug such as Arimidex (0.5 mg twice a week). Super MiraForte, a dietary supplement, inhibits the aromatase enzyme, which boosts free testosterone and lowers estrogen in some men. Testerone replacement therapy cannot be used by men with prostate cancer. Refer to the *Male Hormone Modulation protocol* for complete information.

Because cardiovascular disease remains the number one killer in Western societies, there is more published scientific information about prevention and treatment than exists for other diseases. Based on the sheer volume of information available, we only discussed five commonly overlooked factors in this chapter. We urge persons who want to be fully informed about proven methods to reduce arterial disease risk to review the entire *Cardiovascular Disease: Comprehensive Analysis protocol* that follows.

 PRODUCT AVAILABILITY

Trimethylglycine (TMG), avocado sugar extract, vitamin K, flush-free niacin, folic acid/B_{12} caps, vitamin C capsules and powders, fish/borage oil capsules, alpha and gamma tocopherol caps, bromelain, nettle leaf extract, vitamin B_6 caps, and vitamin A emulsified liquid are available by calling (800) 544-4440 or by logging on to www.lef.org. Metformin, Pravachol, and pentoxiphylline are prescription drugs, while ibuprofen and aspirin are over-the-counter drugs. If your physician will not cooperate by ordering the blood tests recommended in this protocol or if your insurance company refuses to pay for them, call (800) 208-3444 to inquire about low-cost blood testing, which is available by mail order.

benign materials, such as vitamin C, are available to protect the vessel from injury and to participate in vascular repair, the need for Lp(a) is moot. Without adequate amounts of vitamin C, Lp(a) becomes indispensable (Rath 1993).

There is a vast difference between the materials used to repair vascular injuries. For example, vitamin C repairs the wound, leaving the vessel wall smooth, but stronger; Lp(a) repairs the injury, leaving residual trappings, a sticky compress, capable of continued growth. Although Lp(a) has an important function in the body, Matthias Rath, M.D., considers Lp(a) 10 times more dangerous than LDL cholesterol.

The risk of a major cardiovascular event nearly tripled among middle-aged men (participating in a Lp(a)/heart study) whose Lp(a) levels fell within the highest 20% of the study group compared to those with lower levels (von Echardstein et al. 2001). The risks escalate even higher if Lp(a) coexists with high LDL cholesterol, low HDL cholesterol, and hypertension.

Elevated Lp(a), above 30 mg/dL, has been noted in 20% of all thromboembolism patients compared to 7% of healthy controls (von Depka et al. 2000). Lp(a) may prove to be one of the most predictive of the risk factors for strokes, re-stenosis (recurrent narrowing of a vessel), or heart attack following either coronary bypass surgery or angioplasty. Recent studies also incriminated Lp(a) in angina pectoris, citing accumulations of Lp(a) in the plaque of unstable angina patients. *Comment:* According to the American Heart Association, the lesions on artery walls contain substances that may interact with Lp(a), leading to the buildup of fatty deposits (American Heart Association 2002).

Aortic stenosis, the narrowing of the valve separating the left ventricle from the aorta, is often described as a calcification process. Lp(a) appears to play a role in this process; as Lp(a) is deposited on the aortic valve, it creates a binding site for calcium (Shavelle et al. 2002). Researchers at the University of Washington (Seattle) hypothesized that HMG CoA reductase inhibitors (statins) might slow aortic calcification: 28 patients receiving statin therapy for approximately 2.6 years had a 62–63% lower rate of aortic valve calcium accumulation; 44–49% fewer statin patients experienced definite progression of the disease process (Shavelle 2002) (*please consult the section devoted to valvular disease for an in-depth discussion regarding aortic stenosis*).

The reference interval for Lp(a) is 0–30 mg/dL. Reference ranges are valuable only as generic markers. Depending upon the test, risk may be significantly increased as values reach upper or lower limits of normal.

Various reputable cardiologists strive for an Lp(a) less than 10 mg/dL among patients (Sinatra 2002). Read about essential fatty acids, *L*-lysine, *L*-proline, niacin, vitamin A, and vitamin C (nutrients that assist in maintaining healthy Lp(a) levels) in the *Therapeutic section* of this material.

Introduction to Homocysteine

For a discussion relating to detoxification mechanisms and nutrients to reduce homocysteine levels, *consult the Homocysteine Lowering Nutrients and Elimination Pathways subsections in the Therapeutic Section of this protocol.*

Although the dangers imposed by hyperhomocysteinemia are not a new discovery, most of the medical community has until recently ignored homocysteine as a cardiovascular risk. Decades ago, Kilmer McCully, M.D., pioneered the homocysteine/cardiovascular hypothesis; the Life Extension Foundation focused upon the dangers of homocysteine and outlined a vitamin protocol to reduce hyperhomocysteinemia in an article released in November 1981 (*Anti-Aging News* pp. 85–86). Eric Braverman, M.D., joined the crusade, describing homocysteine as a substance that is worse than cholesterol (Braverman 1987).

Homocysteine is regarded as more dangerous than cholesterol because homocysteine damages the artery and then oxidizes cholesterol before cholesterol infiltrates the vessel. Craig Cooney, Ph.D., says that homocysteine is now widely recognized by scientists as the single greatest biochemical risk factor for heart disease, estimating that homocysteine may be a participant in 90% of cardiovascular problems.

Although homocysteine's role in atherosclerosis and atherothrombosis is confirmed, it should be noted that most naturally occurring substances have purpose in physiology. The American Academy of Family Physicians explains that homocysteine is typically changed into other amino acids for use in the body's normal functions (American Family Physician 1997). For example, homocysteine is an intermediate product of methionine metabolism. Two pathways detoxify homocysteine, the remethylation pathway (which regenerates methionine) and the transsulfuration pathway (which degrades homocysteine into cysteine and then to taurine). The amino acids cysteine and taurine are important nutrients for cardiac health, hepatic detoxification, cholesterol excretion, bile salt formation, and glutathione production. Because homocysteine is located at a critical metabolic crossroad, it either directly or indirectly impacts the metabolism of all methyl and sulfur groups occurring in the body (Miller et al. 1997).

In addition, a select group of researchers contend that the residuals (metabolites) of homocysteine appear to support adrenal gland function and contribute to neurotransmitter synthesis and the regeneration of bones and cartilage. If their undocumented speculations prove valid, it should be strongly emphasized that homocysteine must be detoxified in order for its byproducts to offer any biological advantage. If disposal systems (remethylation and transsulfuration) are nonfunctional, allowing homocysteine to accumulate, the results can be deadly. Remethylation and transsulfuration are discussed in detail in the *Therapeutic section* of this protocol, under the subsections *Homocysteine Lowering Nutrients* and *Elimination Pathways*.

The Hazards of Hyperhomocysteinemia

Experiments show that if homocysteine accumulates in the cell, all methylation reactions are inhibited. Because methylation is used for so many body processes (apart from homocysteine metabolism), if this system becomes dysfunctional, essential pathways are foiled. For example, methylation is fundamental to maintaining healthy DNA, lessening the possibility of mutations and strand breaks. Since DNA strand breaks have been detected in the biopsies of diseased cardiac tissue, it is suspected that strand breaks fuel the progression of heart disease. In addition, DNA strand breaks are associated with accelerated aging and a greater cancer risk (Domagala et al. 1998; Seki et al. 1998).

If homocysteine is not detoxified and begins to accumulate, plaque builds up in the endothelial cells lining the arteries through various mechanisms. For example, homocysteine speeds the oxidation of cholesterol, which then becomes bound to small, dense LDL particles. Macrophages then take up the particles to become foam cells in plaque. The earliest detectable lesion of atherosclerosis is the fatty streak (consisting of lipid-laden foam cells that are macrophages that have migrated as monocytes from the circulation into the subendothelial layer of the intima) that later become fibrous plaque (Naruszewicz et al. 1994; Cranton et al. 2001). Dr. Kilmer McCully, a crusader for the homocysteine theory of heart disease, says that homocysteine plays a key role in every pathophysiological process that leads to arteriosclerotic plaque (McCully 1996).

A heart attack or stroke is more likely to occur as homocysteine promotes coagulation factors, favoring clot formation (Magott 1998). The *European Journal of Clinical Investigation* reported that 40% of all stroke victims have elevated homocysteine levels compared to only 6% of controls (Brattstrom et al. 1992). Other studies chronicled similar findings: the elevations in homocysteine in 16 of 38 patients with cerebrovascular disease (42%), seven of 25 with peripheral vascular disease (28%), and 18 of 60 with coronary vascular disease (30%) but in none of the 27 normal subjects (Clarke et al. 1991).

In addition to causing cardiovascular disease by increasing the incidence of blood clots, hyperhomocysteinemia triggers atherosclerosis by encouraging smooth muscle cell proliferation, intimal-medial wall thickness, thromboxane A2 activity, lipid abnormalities, and the binding of Lp(a) to fibrin (Magott 1998; Sandrick 2000).

Vascular integrity is compromised as homocysteine blocks production of nitric oxide in the cells of blood vessel walls, causing vessels to become less pliable and even more susceptible to plaque buildup (Boger et al. 2000; Holton 2001). Scientists explain that vessels lose their expansion capacities as homocysteine reduces nitric oxide's availability (Tawakol et al. 2002). Homocysteine significantly hampers coronary microvascular circulation by impairing dilation functions.

Drs. Allen Miller and Gregory Kelly explain that homocysteine facilitates the generation of hydrogen peroxide. By creating oxidative damage to LDL cholesterol and endothelial cell membranes, hydrogen peroxide can then promote injury to vascular endothelium (Starkebaum et al. 1986; Stamler et al. 1993; Miller et al. 1997). Nitric oxide (also known as endothelium-derived relaxing factor) normally protects endothelial cells from damage by reacting with homocysteine, forming S-nitrosohomocysteine, which inhibits hydrogen peroxide formation. However, as homocysteine levels increase, this protective mechanism can become overloaded, allowing damage to the endothelial cells to occur (Stamler et al. 1992, 1993, 1996).

Genes are also involved in homocysteine attack. This has a significant impact upon the cardiovascular system, as homocysteine activates genes in blood vessels, encouraging the coagulation process and the proliferation of smooth muscles (Outinen et al. 1999).

Since homocysteine wields such a powerful cardiovascular blow from so many different directions, it is estimated that a 3-unit increase in homocysteine equates to a 35% increase in heart attack risk (Verhoef et al. 1996). The risk becomes even greater if hyperhomocysteinemia occurs with other risk factors. For example, a hypertensive woman with elevated homocysteine levels has a 25-fold increased risk of vascular disease.

Other homocysteine/disease associations are:

- High concentrations of homocysteine and low levels of folate and vitamin B_6 are associated with an increased risk of extracranial carotid-artery stenosis, particularly in the elderly (Selhub et al. 1995).

- Higher levels of homocysteine predispose deep venous thrombosis (den Heijer et al. 1996).

- The link between hyperhomocysteinemia-hypercholesterolemia and hypothyroidism is clearly drawn in the section devoted to *Thyroid Disease* appearing in this protocol.

- Plasma homocysteine levels predictably increase with elevations in creatinine. As chronic renal failure occurs, hyperhomocysteinemia is frequently observed (Wilcken et al. 1979; Chauveau et al. 1993).

- Homocysteine metabolism is impaired in patients with Type II diabetes. Intramuscular injections of 1000 mcg of methylcobalamin (a homocysteine-lowering nutrient) once a day for 3 weeks reduced elevations of plasma homocysteine in diabetic test subjects (Araki et al. 1993).

- While the focus of this protocol is upon cardiovascular disease, it should be noted that individuals suffering with Alzheimer's disease, depression, eye problems, liver damage, Crohn's disease, ulcerative colitis, irritable bowel disease, pernicious anemia, and Parkinson's disease often present with elevated homocysteine levels (Refsum et al. 1991; Savage et al. 1994; Mayer et al. 1996; Cattaneo et al. 1998; Clarke et al. 1998; Romagnuolo et al. 2001; Duan et al. 2002).

- A large-scale prospective study of 4700 Norwegian men and women (65–67 years of age) showed that for each 5-millimol/L increase in plasma homocysteine levels, the number of deaths from all causes jumped 49%. This included a 50% increase in cardiovascular deaths, a 26% increase in cancer mortality, and a 104% increase in noncancer and noncardiovascular fatalities (Vollset et al. 2001).

Chronically high levels of homocysteine normally affect 30–40% of healthy elderly people. But in older individuals with severe illnesses, the prevalence of hyperhomocysteinemia may almost double. Based on a random testing of 600 hospitalized elderly patients (ages 65–102 years), researchers found evidence of hyperhomocysteinemia in over 60% of those with serious chronic conditions): 70% presented with vascular disease and 63% presented with cognitive impairment (Ventura et al. 2001). Impaired kidney function, the use of drugs (particularly diuretics), and malnutrition were suspected as causes of age-related hyperhomocysteinemia. Of the senior population in the United States, 67% have one or more vitamin levels within 15% of the lower recommended range, suggesting the need for review of reference values in elderly people.

While cholesterol does not normally pose a cardiac risk until levels exceed 240 mg/dL, some researchers consider homocysteine so capricious that even so-called normal levels may contribute to heart disease. Homocysteine levels should be kept as low as possible, below 7 micromol/L of blood plasma. Laboratories usually regard levels up to 15 micromol/L as normal, but epidemiological data reveal that homocysteine levels above 6.3 reflect a steep, progressive increase in the risk of a heart attack (Robinson et al. 1995). Although the incidence of hypertension, thrombotic stroke, peripheral vascular disease (gangrene), blood vessel toxicity, and the risk of heart attack escalate as homocysteine levels increase, homocysteine levels are not routinely evaluated in a cardiovascular work-up.

The *Therapeutic section* and the sections *Homocysteine Lowering Nutrients* and *Elimination Pathways* detail a program to assist in managing hyperhomocysteinemia. *Note:* Because of homocysteine's role in the metabolism of sulfur and methyl groups, elevated levels of homocysteine would be expected to negatively impact the biosynthesis of SAMe, carnitine, chondroitin sulfate, coenzyme Q_{10}, creatine, cysteine, dimethylglycine, glucosamine sulfate, glutathione, melatonin, pantethine, phosphatidylcholine, and taurine. Many of these substances are profiled in the *Therapeutic section* for their cardioprotection and restorative qualities. The short supply of these agents could severely disable cardiac performance (Miller 1997).

Syndrome X

For the past 20 years, eclectic physicians have judged Syndrome X to be a powerful indicator of an eventual heart attack. For clarity, let it be understood that a syndrome represents clusters of symptoms. In Syndrome X, the symptoms are an inability to fully metabolize carbohydrates; hypertriglyceridemia; reduced HDL levels; smaller, denser LDL particles; increased blood pressure; visceral adiposity; disrupted coagulation factors; insulin resistance; hyperinsulinemia; and, often, increased levels of uric acid. *Note:* For years, high uric acid levels have been associated with cardiovascular disease, but the relationship was poorly understood. Dr. Gerald Reaven unraveled the link when he determined that elevations in uric acid are often prompted by Syndrome X, a forerunner to heart disease (Fang et al. 2000).

Until hyperinsulinemia is diagnosed and a therapeutic course is charted, the arteries are under severe attack and the risk of a blood clot increases. Lesions, or wounds and injuries, damage the arteries; the attempts at vascular repair corrode the vasculature with atheromatous material, blockading and closing off vital circulatory routes. The population of sticky platelets increases along with the production of free radicals. Lipogenesis (the production and accumulation of fat in arterial tissue) encourages smooth muscles in the vasculature to proliferate. Along with excessive amounts of fibrinogen (a plasma protein that encourages the clotting of blood), PAI-1 is induced, further increasing the likelihood of a blood clot. HMG-CoA reductase, the rate-limiting enzyme involved in hepatic cholesterol production, appears to be simulated in both diabetic and nondiabetic animal studies amidst high levels of insulin (Dietschy et al. 1974).

Syndrome X interferes with glucose delivery, a consequence initiated by insulin's nonresponsiveness at the receptor site on the cell. Normally, ordinary levels of insulin will escort glucose into the cell, leaving a bloodstream favoring neither hyper- or hypoglycemia. In Syndrome X, the receptor turns a cold shoulder to the hormone, and insulin is no longer able to deposit its cargo; as a result, glucose loads up in the bloodstream. The pancreas is aware of the problem and attempts to resolve it by discharging more and more insulin. The logic appears to be that since normal levels of insulin cannot get the job done, perhaps greater and greater amounts of circulating insulin will be able to drive glucose, the principal metabolic fuel, into our 100 trillion cells.

In most cases of Type II diabetes, the problem is insulin resistance and inadequate compensatory insulin; in Syndrome X, insulin resistance and excessive amounts of insulin are the hallmarks. The vast difference between the two conditions is that in Syndrome X, the pancreas does not falter in its effort to pump out insulin (Reaven 2000). It sounds as if the host has won, but the following reasons discredit this logic.

1. The pancreas can tire in its endless effort to supply compensatory insulin, and insulin-dependent diabetes will result.

2. Hormones are powerful substances with an equally meaningful purpose. When insulin is not used for its intended functions, insulin builds up in the bloodstream, and from various perspectives, the risk of heart disease increases.

For example, the Quebec Cardiovascular Study found that individuals with elevated levels of triglycerides and LDL cholesterol, plus low HDL cholesterol, had 4.4 times the risk of heart disease compared to men with none of the risk factors. But the risk soars to 20-fold for men with a triad of elevated fasting insulin, apolipoprotein B, and small, dense LDL particles. According to Dr. Benoit Lamarche (Laval University),

hyperinsulinemia should not be overlooked as an independent risk factor for ischemic heart disease. His case-controlled study of 91 patients and 105 controls found fasting insulin levels 18% higher in cases than controls. For each 30% increase in insulin concentration, there was a 70% increase in the risk of ischemic heart disease over 5 years (Despres et al. 1996; *Physician's Weekly* 1998b).

Insulin growth factor-1 (IGF-1), a hormone that increases the body's sensitivity to insulin and promotes clearance of glucose and toxic metabolites, appears critical to surviving the crisis and aftermath of a heart attack (Conti et al. 2001). Lower levels of IGF-1 during the early phase of a myocardial infarction are associated with poorer clinical outcomes, arrhythmias, ischemia, and death.

Italian researchers measured IGF-1 levels in the blood of patients within 24 hours of the onset of heart attack symptoms. IGF-1 (a hormone that enhances the elasticity of blood vessels, strengthens heartbeat, and increases blood flow) was about 5 times lower compared to healthy controls (47 ng/mL versus 189 ng/mL). The transient reduction of IGF-1 during the early phase of infarction appears to cause an acute worsening of insulin resistance.

A decline in IGF-1 is also linked to poorer prognosis following a heart attack. Of the 23 patients evaluated regarding IGF-1 levels (postinfarction), 12 experienced adverse clinical events in the 90-day follow-up period. The two individuals with the lowest IGF-1 levels died from the heart attack or its complications. Negative end results were attributed to reduced insulin sensitivity, glucose clearance, fat metabolism, and cardiac function. Interestingly, infusing IGF-1 into rats (programmed to develop metabolic syndrome) alleviated hyperphagia (overeating), obesity, hyperinsulinemia, hyperleptinemia (excesses of a hormone frequently found in the bloodstream of overweight, cardiac-prone individuals), and hypertension (Vickers et al. 2001).

The IGF-1 system is regulated by various stimuli, including hormones, growth factors, and nutritional status (Fu et al. 2001). For example, IGF-1 increased when protein foods were emphasized in the diet, in combination with adequate levels of vitamin D and calcium (Rizzoli et al. 2001).

Unfortunately, many physicians fail to consider insulin resistance as a forerunner to Type II diabetes and cardiovascular disease. A fasting blood glucose level above 115 mg/dL, triglycerides above 160 mg/dL, low HDL cholesterol, blood pressure persistently over 140/90 mmHg, total cholesterol above 240 mg/dL, and 10–15 pounds of extra weight are important evaluations regarding the likelihood of insulin resistance (Challem et al. 2000). A normal 2-hour postprandial glucose is generally between 70–139 mg/dL. If fasting or 2-hour postprandial insulin levels are measured, a normal range is 6–35 mcIU/mL. The Life Extension Foundation believes that fasting insulin levels over 5 mcIU/mL may be a cause for concern, and respected physicians and scientists are aligning with this projection.

Even if these tests are run, physicians often err in properly assessing the cumulative values of multiple irregularities. The signs are all there, but a failure to connect the dots can lead to a treatment that never addresses the source of the ill health. Syndrome X is largely a nutritional disease that is manageable with dietary corrections, reducing carbohydrates such as sweets, pastas, and breads and instating good fats in carbohydrates' place (*consult the section entitled Essential Fatty Acids in this protocol for a discussion regarding good and bad fats*).

The Harvard University School of Public Health announced that women between the ages of 38–63 increased their risk of heart attack by about 40% if their diet contained quantities of carbohydrates, particularly refined carbohydrates (Liu et al. 2000). It has been determined that the type of food selected and the quantity consumed determine how much insulin must be supplied.

Dr. Gerald Reaven believes an appropriate breakdown of the food groups should be about 45% of calories from carbohydrates, 40% from fat, and 15% from protein. Substituting appropriate fats for carbohydrates quiets an insulin release from the pancreas, and a primary step in Syndrome X has been averted. Dr. Reaven cautions that current dietary recommendations, that is, replacing fats with carbohydrates, may be fine for some individuals, but it is a grievous, even fatal, suggestion for those who are insulin resistant (Reaven et al. 2000). *Note:* Nutritionists reviewing the concept of macronutrient fractions stress the importance of selecting healthy foods to supply requirements. Eating ad libitum from unwise food choices, but within acceptable percentages, could still render the diet unhealthy from many perspectives.

To read more about Syndrome X, consult the sections entitled *Hypertension, Obesity, Sedentary Lifestyle, Fibrinolytic Activity*, and *Beta-Blockers*. Also, the *Therapeutic section* has supplemental recommendations to assist in controlling Syndrome X, including alpha-lipoic acid, conjugated linoleic acid, DHEA, essential fatty acids, magnesium, vitamin A, and vitamin C.

C-Reactive Protein (CRP)

CRP is a marker for systemic inflammation that rises several hundredfold in response to acute tissue injury but stays relatively stable in the absence of inflammation. CRP appears in the serum before the erythrocyte sedimentation rate begins to rise, often within 24–48 hours of the onset of inflammation. Elevated CRP levels can indicate the presence of chronic low-grade inflammation, with linkage to blood vessel damage and vascular disease (Pasceri et al. 2000). High levels of CRP appear to mark inflammatory processes that have the potential to disrupt fatty plaque buildup inside blood vessels, causing a critical rupture; the end result is a blood clot.

When CRP levels are factored in as a cardiovascular risk, along with hypertension, diabetes, elevated cholesterol, family history, and BMI, there is significant improvement in predicting cardiac health compared with models that exclude CRP testing. Ten prospective studies (six in the United States and four in Europe) have consistently shown that hs-CRP is a powerful predictor of a future first coronary event in apparently healthy men and women. ("hs" refers to high sensitivity testing, the only method able to discriminate the subtle differences in CRP in a range that accurately predicts coronary risk.)

As new as CRP is to many as a risk factor in coronary artery disease, Rudolf Virchow, a German pathologist (1821–1902), hypothesized that inflammation was the causative factor in the atherogenic process. Decades later, scientists confirmed that increased monocytes (white blood cells critical in early plaque development) and macrophages (mononuclear phagocytic cells capable of scavenging and ingesting dead tissue and degenerated cells) are present, particularly at points of plaque rupture. It appears that CRP and several other inflammatory markers may be elevated many years prior to a coronary event.

However, data from the University of Texas Health Sciences Center indicate that CRP is more than a measurable antecedent preceding a cardiac problem. CRP, along with the cooperative efforts of an unidentified serum factor, acts directly upon the blood vessels to activate adhesion molecules in endothelial cells: the intercellular adhesion molecule (ICAM-1) and the vascular cell adhesion molecule (VCAM-1). VCAM-1 appears to be an early molecular marker of lesion-prone areas as a response to experimental hypercholesterolemia. In humans, ICAM-1 and VCAM-I expression is increased in the endothelium of atherosclerotic plaque. Researchers concluded that CRP appears intricately involved in the inflammatory process, thus proving to be a potential target for the treatment of atherosclerosis (Pasceri et al. 2000; Biomedical Science 2001; Alvaro et al. 2002).

The journal *Circulation* reports that CRP appears able to affect the activity of LDL cholesterol (increasing atherogenesis). The cycle begins as stranded LDL is taken up by macrophages; macrophages, gorged with fats contained in blood, become bloated and develop into foam cells. When foam cells have reached their maximum load, they explode, discharging their fatty contents into the blood vessel wall at the site of injury. The presence of added fat signals the need for more macrophages to clean up the mess. They stuff themselves, explode, and the cycle starts anew. Since native LDL does not induce foam cell formation, CRP appears to ready LDL for uptake by the macrophages, initiating the sequence (Braley 1985; Zwaka et al. 2001).

In the Physicians' Health Study, middle-aged men deemed healthy at baseline were evaluated over an 8-year period in regard to CRP levels and a cardiovascular event. This study showed that those in the highest quartile of hs-CRP had a twofold higher risk of (future) stroke, a threefold higher risk of (future) heart attack, and a fourfold higher risk of (future) peripheral vascular disease (Rifai et al. 2001a, 2001b). Stroke patients with the highest CRP levels were nearly 2.4 times more likely to die within the next year compared to patients with the lowest levels (DiNapoli et al. 2001). Another of hs-CRP's strengths is its ability to detect at-risk patients with normal cholesterol levels.

The risk of stroke, according to data reported in the *New England Journal of Medicine*, decreased among those using statin drugs (White et al. 2000). The Cholesterol and Recurrent Events Trial concluded that pravastatin (administered long term) appears to be doing more than reducing cholesterol, perhaps acting as an anti-inflammatory. Another study (also published in the *New England Journal of Medicine*) reported that pravastatin reduced CRP levels after both 12- and 24-weeks' administration, independent of LDL cholesterol levels. It appears statin therapy may prevent coronary events among individuals with relatively low lipid levels but with elevated levels of CRP (Ridker et al. 2001). Conversely, some drugs, including hormone replacement therapy, actually increase CRP levels and the inflammatory response.

Researchers hypothesized in the *Journal of the American College of Cardiology* that the cytomegalovirus (CMV) (herpes-type viruses) may stimulate an inflammatory response, reflected by elevated CRP levels. The journal *Circulation* reported that older people who have IgG antibodies to the herpes simplex-I virus experienced a twofold increase in the risk of a myocardial infarction or coronary heart disease death. Since the relationship between CMV and coronary heart disease is not observed in all people, researchers consider the ability of individuals to control CMV inflammatory activities, the variable in the progression to a myocardial infarction (Zhu et al. 1999; Siscovick et al. 2000).

The infectious process in heart disease is chronicled in numerous studies, but the microorganisms involved remain of interest. Subsequently, a group of researchers from Johannes Gutenberg University (in Mainz, Germany) evaluated 572 heart patients. They tested for antibodies in the bloodstream that would show that the immune system had at some stage been exposed to a variety of different viruses and bacteria. These included herpes simplex-1 and -2, which cause cold sores and genital herpes; Epstein-Barr virus, which causes mononucleosis, chlamydia, and flu virus; and *Helicobacteria pylori*, which causes stomach ulcers. Then they looked at the patients again 3 years later to see how many had survived. The death rate was 3.1% in patients who tested positive for only a few of the viruses or bacteria, 9.8% for those with four or five, and 15% in those positive for six to eight. Among those who had the most advanced artery hardening, 20% of those exposed to between six and eight infections had died, compared to 7% of those with three or fewer (BBC 2002b).

Japanese researchers concentrated upon finding a method to distinguish between bacterial and viral infection by measuring inflammatory markers, among them C-reactive protein (CRP). They found that during the acute stage of bacterial infections, CRP levels were moderately or highly increased, whereas in viral infections, CRP levels were normal or slightly increased. The researchers propose that the measurement of CRP (among various inflammatory markers) during the acute phase of illness, that is, within 5 days of onset, is of value to determine whether the infection is caused by a bacteria or virus (Sasaki et al. 2002). For an opposing view regarding the association between viruses and CRP levels, please consult the section entitled *Link Between Infections and Inflammation in Heart Disease* in this protocol.

Figure 4 shows the risk factors associated with CRP (data extracted from publications authored by Dr. Paul Ridker). It is important to note that risk factors vary according to individual publications and may change with future publications.

Current research indicates that persistent CRP elevation, lasting longer than 96 hours following a

MEN CRP (mg/L)	RELATIVE RISK FOR:[1]	
	Future MI (heart attack)	Future Stroke
>2.11	2.9	1.9
1.15-2.10	2.6	1.9
0.56-1.14	1.7	1.7
<0.55	1.0	1.0
WOMEN CRP (mg/L)	RELATIVE RISK FOR:	
	Future MI (heart attack)	Future Stroke
>7.3	5.5	5.5
3.8-7.3	3.5	3.5
1.5-3.7	2.7	2.7
<1.5	1.0	1.0

[1]Relative risk is the ratio of the chance of a disease developing among members of a population exposed to a factor compared to a similar population not exposed to the factor.

Source: Ridker et. al. (1998); Ridker et. al. (1997).

Figure 4   Risk Factors Associated with CRP

successful coronary stent implantation, is predictive of prolonged inflammation leading to re-stenosis (Gottsauner-Wolf et al. 2000). Patients who developed re-stenosis within the first 6 months had increases in CRP levels for up to 96 hours following the procedure, although their baseline CRP had been normal. Patients without re-stenosis displayed an increased CRP level that was sustained for no longer than 48 hours and subsequently decreased. Higher CRP levels appear predictive of less satisfactory end results, following angioplasty and stent procedures.

Although many of the newer risk factors are not yet standardized, some laboratories are using a CRP reference range of 0.24–1.69 mg/L. Recent medical events resulting in tissue injury, infections, or inflammation may increase CRP levels and, if not factored into clinical interpretations, can distort results.

To read more about factors affecting CRP levels, consult the sections referring to *Smoking, Obesity, Sedentary Lifestyle, Gender, Gum Disease,* and *The Link Between Infections and Inflammation in Heart Disease.* Improved glycemic control and normalizing blood pressure may also assist in reducing inflammation and (subsequently) CRP levels.

CRP appears responsive to aspirin, DHEA, fish oil, pravastatin, vitamin C, vitamin E, and vitamin K supplementation (*consult the* Therapeutic Section *to learn more about natural products*). As research continues, it may be found that many other nutrients and herbs known for their anti-inflammatory properties are equally valuable in maintaining healthy CRP levels. *Note:* CRP appears to reduce levels of vitamins A, C,

and E, as well as carotenoids, zinc, and selenium. Individuals with elevations in CRP may wish to emphasize these nutrients for their contribution to cardiac health.

THE LINK BETWEEN INFECTIONS AND INFLAMMATION IN HEART DISEASE

Infections are of particular interest because of the increasing attention paid to the role of inflammation in heart disease, according to David S. Siscovick, M.D., professor of medicine and epidemiology at the University of Washington. The data incriminate the infectious process in various phases known to contribute to heart disease. For example, current research suggests that infection may be an important determinant of fibrinogen levels, offering one possible explanation for the association between chronic or acute infection and vascular events (Woodhouse et al. 1997). Many researchers class inflammation as worse than cholesterol at triggering heart attacks. *Note:* Men with hypercholesterolemia and inflammation have a significantly higher risk of cardiovascular death (2.4) compared to those with only high cholesterol levels (1.4) (Engstrom et al. 2002).

Dr. Paul Ridker (Boston's Brigham and Women's Hospital) recently explained that everyone reaching middle age has some degree of fat buildup, that is, plaque in the vasculature. New evidence suggests the plaque becomes threatening if weakened by inflammation, which makes the buildup squishy and fragile. Even a small lump can burst, promoting the formation of a clot that in turn chokes off blood flow and causes a heart attack. Thus, reducing the inflammatory process is of equal importance to lipid monitoring in controlling the dangers of plaque (Associated Press 2002).

Researchers observed that mortality from ischemic heart disease markedly increases during the flu season, particularly among the elderly. One reason for this appears to be that patients with influenza A, a flu virus, tend to have much higher levels of CRP. Researchers at Rochester General Hospital and Rochester School of Medicine and Dentistry showed that CRP increased 370% during infection and that old age magnified the increase (Falsey et al. 2001; Horan et al. 2001).

A higher white blood cell count, common when the body is fighting off infection, is associated with an increased coronary risk by diminishing blood flow to the heart muscle and encouraging blood clot formation. The higher the white blood cell count, the greater the patient's risk of death from a heart attack or of developing congestive heart failure (Barron et al. 2000).

In fact, angina pectoris appears less a prognosticator of a forthcoming heart attack than a febrile (flu-like, feverish) infection prior to the attack. Peter Ammann, M.D. (Switzerland), stated that he has observed significantly higher numbers of myocardial infarctions among patients with febrile conditions, mainly of the upper airways, within 2 weeks prior to infarction (Ammann et al. 2000; Healthlink 2000).

Bacteria appear to gain entry into the heart via immune cells, most likely activated in the process of clearing infections from the respiratory passages. The bacteria most suspected of initiating coronary problems are *Chlamydia pneumoniae, Pasteurella aerogenes, Enterococcus endocarditis, Staphylococcus aureus, Enterococcus faecalis, Candida albicans,* and *Viridan streptococcus.* (Some researchers add *H. pylori,* a bacteria associated with duodenal ulcers, peptic ulcers, and chronic gastritis, to the list.)

Tissue specimens from patients who had undergone a carotid endarterectomy showed high levels of *C. pneumoniae* in 11 of 17 cases (64%). The American Heart Association also reported that *C. pneumoniae* was found in the infected arteries of autopsied cardiac patients. Dr. Tatu Juvonen (Oulu University Hospital in Finland) explains that *C. pneumoniae* is a specific microbial antigen that causes inflammation and atherosclerotic cells to proliferate (Mosorin et al. 2000; Vink et al. 2001).

An alternative to this dismal situation may be antibiotic therapy, controlling the inflammatory process attacking the vessel wall. An American study of more than 16,000 British patients showed that people treated with two types of antibiotics had a significantly reduced risk of heart attack. Those treated with tetracyclines were at 30% less risk than patients not given antibiotics, while those who took quinolones (antimicrobials) had a 55% reduced risk. It appears antibiotics may act in the same fashion as anti-inflammatory drugs, reducing inflammation in the arteries (BBC News 1999, 2002a).

Inflammation appears to be an independent risk factor that may explain cardiovascular disease in the presence of normal cholesterol, blood pressure, and coronary arteries. MINC patients, individuals experiencing a myocardial infarction with normal coronary arteries, should be at lower risk for a cardiac event because they most often have normal electrocardiograms, higher HDL levels, and no significant impairment in LDL cholesterol. Dr. Ammann believes the trigger may be systemic inflammation or specific infective agents, advancing a benign complaint to a life-threatening condition. Interestingly, migraine headaches have also been observed as forerunners to a heart attack in otherwise healthy individuals (Ammann et al. 2000; HealthLink 2000).

IS ATRIAL FIBRILLATION PREDICTIVE OF CARDIAC MORTALITY?

Atrial fibrillation, a condition shared by over 2 million Americans, occurs when the atria, the upper chambers of the heart, beat faster than the lower two chambers, the ventricles. Many problems can cause atrial fibrillation, including a leaky heart valve, hypertension, obesity, stimulants (including caffeine and alcohol), medications (such as sumatriptan, a headache drug), and thyroid disorders. Dr. Robert Atkins, M.D., adds that patients should be evaluated for heavy metal intoxication and mycoplasmal infections, factors also capable of provoking atrial fibrillation.

Although not immediately life-threatening, atrial fibrillation may cause up to a 30% reduction in cardiac output, resulting in shortness of breath, fatigue, and reduced exercise capacity. In fact, the American Heart Association no longer regards atrial fibrillation as a benign disorder. About 75,000 strokes related to atrial fibrillation occur each year in the United States. Up to 23% of such patients die, and 44% experience significant neurologic deficits. (The mortality rate from other causes of stroke is about 8%.) Nonetheless, Dr. H.J. Crijns (University Hospital Gröningen, the Netherlands), declares that even patients with heart failure should not be in greater danger because of atrial fibrillation *if the condition is well managed* (Kennedy 1999; Alpert 2000; Crijns et al. 2000).

Blood thinners are often prescribed for atrial fibrillation, but a program based in natural medicine is also helpful. While full correction of the chaotic rhythm associated with atrial fibrillation is often difficult to achieve, nutritional supplements can lessen the risk of a blood clot. Dr. William Campbell Douglass, M.D., states that vitamin E (800 IU daily), cod liver oil capsules (4 daily), olive oil (1 tbsp daily), and bromelain (about 750 mg 3 times a day on an empty stomach) have similar action to Coumadin and aspirin, thinning the blood and reducing the risk of a thrombotic event (Douglass 1996). Other heart nutrients such as CoQ_{10}, hawthorn, carnitine, taurine, magnesium, and ginkgo biloba are also important. To read more about the supplements recommended for atrial fibrillation, please consult the *Therapeutic section* of this protocol. Also refer to the *Thrombosis Prevention protocol* in this book.

ARRHYTHMIA

An estimated 4 million Americans have recurring cardiac arrhythmias. Arrhythmia is any change in the normal sequence of electrical impulses in the heart that results in an abnormal rhythm. The heart might skip a beat, beat irregularly, beat very slowly, or beat very fast. The symptoms of a more serious arrhythmia and benign palpitations are very similar. An arrhythmia might be brief and harmless or it might be associated with cardiac disease. Therefore, arrhythmia should always be addressed by a qualified physician because the end result can be quite dissimilar (although not representative of the norm, some types of arrhythmias can be extremely dangerous or even fatal). The major types of cardiac arrhythmias are:

- *Tachycardia* (a heart rate in excess of 100 beats per minute). A reduction in parasympathetic tone or an increase in sympathetic stimulation will increase the frequency of heartbeats. An elevation in body temperature or a toxic condition can also result in tachycardia. The abnormally fast heart rhythm of tachycardia can prove dangerous because the racing rhythm interferes with the heart's ability to contract properly (Seeley et al. 1991; Ozdemir et al. 2003).

- *Bradycardia* (the ventricles beat at a rate less than 60 beats per minute). Bradycardia, even as low as 50 beats per minute, can be normal in athletes and in individuals who lead a physically active lifestyle (AHA 2002; NASPE 2002). In these people, regular exercise maximizes the ability of the heart to pump blood efficiently, so fewer heart contractions are required to supply the body's needs. In other cases, bradycardia can be caused by excessive vagus nerve stimulation (vagus stimulation is principally responsible for parasympathetic control over the heart) (Merck Manuals 2003a). In addition, a dysfunctional sinoatrial node (SA; specialized heart tissue that controls heartbeat), as well as hypothyroidism, severe liver disase, hypothermia, and typhoid fever can result in bradycardia. Medications including propranolol (Inderal), atenolol (Tenormin), metoprolol (Toprol-XL), sotalol (Betapace), verapamil (Calan, Isoptin, Verelan), and diltiazem (Cardizem, Dilacor-XR) can slow the heart rate to bradycardia status (IH/HMS 2002; Stein 2003). In some instances, the weak pace may indicate the heart is not beating well enough to ensure adequate blood flow.

Note: *When the parasympathetic nervous system is active, the heart rate tends to be slower; conversely, the heart rate is accelerated when the sympathetic nervous system is active.*

- *Sinus Arrhythmia* (a normal increase in heart rate that occurs during inspiration, the act of drawing air into the lungs). On inspiration, there is a decrease in vagal tone (parsympathetic stimulation) and an increase in sympathetic tone. This produces an increase in heart rate. Conversely, on expiration there is an increase in vagal tone and a decrease in sympathetic tone, resulting in a decrease in sinus rate. Sinus arrhythmia (occurring most often in young healthy people) does not result in symptoms and is generally classified as benign (Michaels 1995; MHI 1999).

- *Paroxysmal Atrial Tachycardia* (a sudden increase in heart rate to 160–200 beats per minute that can last for only a few seconds or for several hours). Paroxysmal atrial tachycardia starts with a premature P wave that is superimposed on the T wave. The series of early beats in the atria is responsible for the accelerated heart rate. Paroxysmal atrial tachycardia (the most common form of arrhythmia is children) is not regarded as a disease and is seldom life-threatening. The episodes are usually more unpleasant than they are dangerous and the prognosis is generally good.

Note: *The P wave results from depolarization of the atrial myocardium and precedes the onset of atrial contractions (atrial contraction begins at about the middle of the P wave); the T wave represents repolariztion of the ventricles (Seeley et al. 1991).*

- *Atrial Flutter* (the atria beat more often than the ventricles). This means that the atria have a shorter time to push all of their blood into the ventricles and the ventricles may not fill with sufficient blood. Depending upon how fast the atria are beating, the body may not receive enough oxygen-rich blood. The faster the atria beat, the more difficult it is for the body to receive ample oxygen. Atrial flutter is subdivided into two types: typical and atypical. Typical atrial flutter has a very characteristic electrocardiogram (ECG) pattern and is caused by localized reentry with impulse pathways occupying large portions of the right atrial wall. Because the circuit is fixed and accessible, typical atrial flutter can often be treated by destroying a portion of the circuit during a procedure known as ablation. Conversely, atypical atrial flutter exhibits a more variable ECG pattern and more than one circuit may be responsible. Atypical atrial flutter behaves much more like atrial fibrillation (pounding heart rate or pulse, shortness of breath, or dizziness) than does typical atrial flutter. Thyroid disorders, heart valve disease, coronary artery disease, and heart failure as well as a swelling or irritation near the heart are possibilities that can provoke atrial flutter. If a fast atrial flutter goes untreated, the body could become oxygen deprived. As a result, a heart attack or fluid accumulation in the lungs are possible consequences. The sooner treatment is begun, the better the chances are of avoiding serious cardiac or respiratory endangerments (Seeley et al. 1991; PDR 1997).

- *Atrial Fibrillation* (the two small upper chambers of the heart, the atria, quiver instead of beating effectively). Because blood is not completely pumped out of the atria, blood may pool and clot. If a piece of a blood clot in the atria leaves the heart and becomes lodged in an artery in the brain, a stroke results. It is estimated that about 15% of strokes occur in individuals experiencing atrial fibrillation. An individual with atrial fibrillation does not always have blockages in the arteries (coronary arteries) that serve the heart muscle or other serious heart problems, but the odds favor a cardiac association. Chronic hypertension (high blood pressure); abnormalities of the heart valves (thin tissue flaps that keep blood flowing in one direction through the heart); and abnormalities of the heart's pumping function are causes of atrial fibrillation. About one third of individuals with atrial fibrillation have no structural heart disease and no identifiable cause for their heart rhythm problem. In these instances, atrial fibrillation may be due to (1) microscopic abnormalities of the muscle of the atria; (2) abnormalities within individual heart cells; (3) abnormal electrical properties of groups of heart cells; and (4) exposure to heart stimulants such as alcohol, caffeine, or too much thyroid hormone (Seeley et al. 1991; MC 2003).

- *Ventricular Tachycardia* (a rapid heart beat initiated within the ventricles and characterized by three or more consecutive premature ventricular beats known as ectopic beats). Ventricular tachycardia (occurring in approximately 2 out of 10,000 individuals) is a potentially lethal arrhythmia that can cause the heart to become unable to pump adequate amounts of blood throughout the body. The heart rate might be between 160–240 beats per minute. Ventricular tachycardia can occur spontaneously or

it can develop as a complication of a heart attack, cardiomyopathy, mitral valve prolapse, and myocarditis or after heart surgery. It may also be a result of scar tissue formed following an earlier heart attack or an undesired effect of anti-arrhythmic drugs. Disrupted blood chemistries (a low potassium level), pH (acid/base) changes, or insufficient oxygenation can trigger ventricular tachycardia. Reentry (re-stimulation of the electrical conductive pathway from a single initial stimulus) may also be a mechanism in ventricular tachycardia. Sustained ventricular tachycardia is dangerous because it can worsen until it becomes ventricular fibrillation, a form of cardiac arrest (Seeley et al.1991; *Illustrated Health Encyclopedia* 2002; Merck Manual 2003b).

- *Ventricular Fibrillation* (a pulseless arrhythmia with irregular and chaotic electrical activity and ventricular contractions in which the heart immediately loses its ability to function as a pump). Sudden loss of cardiac output with subsequent tissue hypoperfusion (a process that intensifies anaerobic metabolism and instigates the formation of lactic acid which further deteriorates the systolic performance of the myocardium) creates global tissue ischemia. The brain and myocardium (the middle layer of the heart, consisting of cardiac muscle) are most susceptible to injury. Without immediate emergency treatment (an electric shock to restore normal rhythm), an individual loses consciousness within seconds and dies within minutes. Ventricular fibrillation is the primary cause of sudden cardiac death (Seeley et al. 1991; Kazzi et al. 2001).

Symptoms of more serious arrhythmias and symptoms of benign palpitations can be very similar. Palpitations are often described as a sensation in the chest and throat that the heart is flopping or pounding, seeming to beat harder and faster than usual, or beating irregularly. Some individuals experiencing palpitations report feeling faint, dizzy, or out of breath. When no medical or cardiac cause can be found, lifestyle events such as exercise, stress, or fear or using tobacco, caffeine, alcohol, cough and cold remedies, or diet pills might be determined to be the cause of the arrhythmia. Palpitations that recur, become sustained or uncomfortable, or are associated with other symptoms require further investigation (Hendrickson 2001; DeRoin 2003; NHLBI 2003).

However, most individuals who experience heart palpitations have some type of cardiac arrhythmia. Virtually any arrhythmia can cause palpitations. The most common cardiac causes of palpitations are premature atrial complexes, premature ventricular complexes, episodes of atrial fibrillation, and episodes of supraventricular tachycardia. In some cases, palpitations are caused by a more dangerous arrhythmia such as ventricular tachycardia. Because life-threatening arrhythmias are usually seen in individuals with underlying heart disease, it is especially important to identify the cause of palpitations in individuals who have fundamental heart disease. The same recommendation applies to palpitations in individuals who have significant risk factors for heart disease: family history, tobacco habits, high cholesterol, excess weight, or sedentary lifestyle (Fogoros 2003).

The Cardiac Cycle

Dysfunction in the heart's electrical conduction system can make the heart beat too fast, too slow, or at an uneven rate. The cardiac cycle (the period from the beginning of one heartbeat to the beginning of the next) is the sequence of events that occurs when the heart beats. This cycle is regulated by specialized cardiac muscle cells in the wall of the heart that form the conduction system of the heart. The heart beats normally when an electrical impulse from the SA node (sinoatrial node) moves uninterrupted in a set pattern throughout the heart. The normal flow of an electrical impulse is:

SA node ® right atrium ® AV node (atrioventricular node) ® atrioventricular bundles ® bundle branches ® special conducting fibers (His-Purkinje system) ® ventricles

The SA node, which functions as the pacemaker of the heart, is located in the upper wall of the right atrium and initiates contractions of the heart. Action potentials originate in the SA node and spread over the right and left atria causing them to contract. A second area of the heart called the atrioventricular node (AV node) is located in the lower portion of the right atrium. When action potentials reach the AV node, they spread slowly through the AV node and into a bundle of specialized cardiac muscle called the bundle of His or atrioventricular bundle. The slow rate of action potential conduction in the AV node allows the atria to complete their contraction before action potentenials are delivered to the ventricles.

After the action potentials pass through the AV node, they are transmitted rapidly through the atrioventricular bundle, which projects through the connective tissue separating the atria from the ventricles, to two branches of conduction tissue called the left and right bundle branches. At the tips of the left and right bundle branches, the conducting tissue branches further to many small bundles of Purkinje fibers. The Purkinje fibers rapidly deliver action potentials to all the cardiac muscle of the ventricles. As long as this exact route is followed, the heart pumps and beats regularly (a normal heart rate, or number of contractions, is about 70–80 beats per minute) (Seeley et al. 1991; AHA 2002; NHLBI 2003).

Arrhythmia may also result from an abnormal impulse rate in the SA node or when a condition called "heart block" exists. In heart block, electrical signals are delayed, partially conducted, or completely interrupted (NHLBI 2003).

Another common cause of arrhythmia is damage to the heart's "wiring" resulting from decreased blood flow from clogged coronary arteries or from heart muscle that died as a result of a heart attack (myocardial infarction). Other factors affecting heart rhythm are ingested toxins, congenital heart arrhythmia, anemia, thyroid conditions, hypoglycemia, mitral valve prolapse, and high blood pressure (DeRoin 2003; THI 2003). These underlying factors must also be treated to correct the arrhythmia.

Diagnostic tools used in arrhythmia are an electrocardiogram (ECG); intracardiac electrophysiology study (EPS, a study that involves placing wire electrodes within the heart to determine the characteristics of heart arrhythmias); and tilt table examinations (tilt table study is mainly used in diagnosing vasovagal syncope, a classic fainting episode). Once serious arrhythmia is diagnosed, it might be treated with drugs; an implantable device that sends electrical shocks or impulses to restore normal heart rhythm, i.e., an implantable cardioverter defibrillator (ICD) or pacemaker; or surgery that can remove misfiring heart tissue (radiofrequency and surgical ablation) or create a new electrical pathway (maze surgery) (ACC 2002; DeRoin 2003; NHLBI 2003).

Frequently used anti-arrhythmic drugs are anticoagulants (warfarin); sodium channel blockers (class I); beta-blockers (class II); potassium channel blockers (class III); calcium channel blockers (class IV); and digitalis (Chaudhry et al. 2000; ACC 2002). Almost all medications have side effects including the antiarrhythmic drugs. One side effect is a potentially life-threatening *pro-arrhythmia* (meaning the drug itself causes arrhythmia). Because studies show that antiarrhythmics have no mortality benefit and can even increase mortality, patient benefit vs. risk must be considered before using anti-arrhythmics (Brendorp et al. 2002; Sanguinetti et al. 2003; Yamreudeewong et al. 2003). Overall there is still no ideal anti-arrhythmic agent and drug selection remains highly individualized (Tsikouris et al. 2001).

Arrhythmia and Myocardial Infarction

Patients are monitored very closely in a coronary intensive care unit immediately following a myocardial infarction (MI) because this is a time period when life-threatening dysrhythmias can develop. Life-saving thrombolytic treatment that is used to open a clogged coronary artery ("clot busters") can also cause an increased risk of dysrhythmia. Successfully opening an artery results in a sudden influx of blood (reperfusion) into the blood-starved area of the heart. Reperfusion has the potential to cause a fatal arrhythmia. In part, the culprit is thought to be a free-radical reaction. Therefore, reducing the free-radical burden on the heart offers potentially helpful benefits. In a post-MI setting, studies have demonstrated the importance of cardio-protective treatment.

Natural Approaches

Compared to placebo, when coenzyme Q10 (120 mg daily) was given to patients with acute MI, there was significant reduction in total arrhythmias and symptoms of angina pectoris. There was also better left ventricular function. Total cardiac events, including cardiac deaths and nonfatal infarction, were also significantly reduced in the CoQ10 group compared to the placebo group (15.0% vs. 30.9%) (Singh et al. 1998). Subsequent studies demonstrated that CoQ10 significantly reduced serum lipoprotein(a) and decreased oxidative stress overall. After 1 year of follow-up, even subjects receiving optimal lipid-lowering therapy (lovastatin) had a significant reduction in total and low-density lipoprotein (LDL) cholesterol compared to baseline levels. Fatigue was found to be more common in the placebo group which did not receive CoQ10 (Singh et al. 1999, 2003).

Omega-3 fatty acids (fish oil) given within 18 hours to patients with acute MI also demonstrated protective benefits, and after 1 year of follow-up, total cardiac events were significantly reduced (including nonfatal infarctions, cardiac deaths, total cardiac arrhythmias, left ventricular enlargement, and angina pectoris) (Singh et al. 1997). Other benefits provided by omega-3 fatty acids were reduced rates of heart attacks; reduced susceptibility to sudden death from ventricular arrhythmia; and reduced inflammation and lowered serum triglycerides (O'Keefe et al. 2000; De Caterina et al. 2003; Lee et al. 2003). Lee et al. (2003) concluded that "the use of omega-3 fatty acids should be considered as part of a comprehensive secondary prevention strategy post-myocardial infarction." Flaxseed, perilla, and fish oils are sources of omega-3 fatty acids. Perilla oil works well (Ezaki et al. 1999); does not have an unpleasant taste; and does not cause the gastrointestinal side effects which limit the use of fish oil for some.

Note: *Because EPA/DHA can interfere with blood clotting, individuals with any type of hemorrhagic disease related to excessive bleeding should consult their physician before supplementing with fatty acids. In addition, individuals taking anticoagulant drugs such as Coumadin should inform their physician that they are taking EPA/DHA supplements. The dose of anticoagulant medication they are taking might require adjustment based on template bleeding time tests.*

Ensuring that the heart gets enough blood and protecting it from free radical reactions are essential. Natural medicine offers tremendous possibilities for individuals with arrhythmia, but it is important to remember that no treatment should be undertaken without the guidance of a cardiologist or physician trained in natural medicine as well as the approval of your personal cardiologist or physician. In particular, close professional medical supervision is essential with larger doses. Pregnant women should never take any supplement without consulting their personal physician. Additionally, persons with cardiac arrhythmias should avoid caffeine, heavy alcohol intake, and saturated fats. Chelation therapy might also be an option.

The *Therapeutic Section* of this protocol includes discussions of numerous supplements that offer protective and supportive benefits for individuals with arrhythmias: acetyl-L-carnitine, alpha lipoic acid, angelica, bugleweed, coenzyme Q10, fish oil, garlic, Ginkgo biloba, hawthorn, magnesium, olive leaf extract, perilla and flaxseed oil, potassium, selenium, taurine, thiamine, and vitamin E.

WARNING Some supplements are regarded as pro-arrhythmic in susceptible individuals (e.g., Ma Huang and excessive dosages of supplemental choline). Additionally, before supplementing with the nicotinic acid form of vitamin B_3, cardiac patients with arrhythmias should consult with a physician (NASPE 2003; NTC website).

CONGESTIVE HEART FAILURE

Congestive heart failure (CHF) reflects the heart's inability to pump sufficient amounts of oxygenated blood to supply the body's needs. It does not mean the heart has ceased to work, but rather that the heart's pumping mechanism is performing inadequately. Conditions that damage the heart, such as a heart attack, ischemic heart disease (a lack of oxygen in tissue cells), cardiomyopathy (fibrous tissue partially replaces heart muscle and blood no longer moves efficiently), alcohol abuse, rheumatic fever, arrhythmias, pericarditis (inflammation of the thin sac covering the heart), or drug toxicity can result in CHF. Symptoms of CHF are fluid retention, fatigue, weakness, and unjustified dyspnea (shortness of breath after slight exertion). In some cases, liver and kidney function are also disrupted.

CHF occurs when the heart fails to adequately pump blood through the largest organ of the human body, 65,000 miles of blood vessels (the vascular system). This breakdown causes increased pressure in the circulatory system, allowing fluid to escape from the bloodstream and accumulate in tissues and organs. More than 100 years ago, CHF would have been diagnosed as dropsy, an abnormal accumulation of a clear watery fluid in a body tissue or cavity. Dropsy was the most common of all forms of heart problems until the current epidemic of coronary diseases.

The heart is a two-sided instrument, having a right and left atrium and a right and left ventricle. The atria of the heart receive blood from veins and function as reservoirs before the blood enters the ventricles. The ventricles are the major pumping chambers of the heart, ejecting blood into the arteries and forcing it throughout the vascular system.

Just as there are two sides to the heart, there are two types of heart failure (right-sided and left-sided). The right side of the heart has the job of moving the blood through the pulmonary blood supply to the lungs, where it picks up oxygen. If the failure occurs on the right side of the heart, it means the right side is not keeping pace with the left side and the blood accumulates in the vessels leading to the heart. Excess fluid (as peripheral edema) occurs in the lower legs, ankles, and feet (Atkins 1988).

In left-sided failure, the ventricle that normally pumps blood from the lungs through the aorta to the body lags in its effort compared to the right ventricle. Blood accumulates in the veins leading from the lungs, and the lungs become congested. Terms such as *pulmonary edema* or fluid in the lungs usually mean the left side of the heart is failing, allowing the congestion. The patient may experience shortness of breath (most evidenced upon exertion) or paroxysmal nocturnal dyspnea (shortness of breath occurring after several hours of sleep). Often, left-sided and right-sided failures coexist, meaning the patient may experience both at the same time. Acute pulmonary edema can be fatal.

Traditional medicine treats CHF with diuretics and inotropic drugs that increase the contractility of the heart. If overweight, a weight-loss program will probably be recommended, as well as an individualized exercise regime. Abstinence from tobacco, either direct or secondhand, is essential. Experimental studies have shown that nonsteroidal anti-inflammatory drugs (NSAIDs) can lead to the development of congestive heart failure when given to susceptible individuals. Researchers feel that there have been few epidemiological investigations equal to the importance of this finding (Page et al. 2000).

The *Archives of Internal Medicine* clarified the risks, reporting that NSAIDs appear to cause fluid retention and an increase in blood pressure in patients with prevalent heart failure. Patients who have had congestive heart failure, angina, heart attacks, bypass surgery, or angioplasty with stent placement should seriously consider safer alternatives. This warning is not restricted to prescription NSAIDs but to over-the-counter anti-inflammatory drugs as well (Feenstra et al. 2002).

Dispersed throughout the *Therapeutic section* of this protocol are numerous supplemental suggestions to benefit the patient with CHF. (Read about alpha-lipoic acid, *L*-arginine, *L*-carnitine, coenzyme Q_{10}, hawthorn, vitamin B_6, selenium, taurine, and thiamine.) Diet also plays an important role. For example, carbohydrate restriction exerts a diuretic effect, prompting an immediate loss of salt and water. Removing water accumulations from saturated tissue is of great advantage to individuals with high blood pressure and congestive heart failure.

VALVULAR DISEASE

The purpose of heart valves is uncomplicated. Valves simply route the blood in a forward direction, preventing its backward flow. Functioning properly, valves are control devices, opening and closing with each beat of the heart, warranting a healthy lap around the circulatory system. But valves can be damaged by rheumatic fever, infections, injuries, tumors, and calcification, hampering their ability to direct the blood supply.

Some valves, once injured, pose more serious health hazards than others. Those include the mitral, aortic, and the tricuspid valves and are the focus of this section of the protocol. *Note:* This material was collected in part from the ACC/AHA Guidelines for the Management of Patients with Valvular Heart Disease (Bonow et al. 1998).

Mitral Valve

The mitral valve, or bicuspid valve, is located between the left atrium and the left ventricle. (The mitral valve is the only valve with two rather than three cusps.) The mitral valve allows oxygenated blood to flow from the left atrium into the left ventricle but prevents blood from flowing back into the atrium. As blood is forced against the valve, it closes the two cusps, allowing a smooth trajectory from the ventricle to the aorta.

Mitral Valve Prolapse

Mitral valve prolapse (MVP), or floppy valve syndrome, is a slight deformity in the valve separating the left atrium from the left ventricle, a condition that affects 5–10% of the population. During MVP, one or both of the cusps protrude back into the left atrium, causing the floppy valve appearance.

Mitral valve prolapse is fairly benign in most patients, but about 1–10% of MVP patients have serious problems such as chest pain, arrhythmias, and leakage of the valve, leading to congestive heart disease. Coenzyme Q_{10} and magnesium (detailed in the *Therapeutic section* of this protocol) are of significant advantage to individuals with MVP.

Mitral Valve Regurgitation

Mitral regurgitation, the backflow of blood from the left ventricle into the left atrium, occurs because the valve is too leaky. The mitral valve can become regurgitant for many reasons, including the aging process, rheumatic valvular disease, endocarditis, chest trauma, or a previous heart attack. Mild but chronic regurgitation does little to alter the overall cardiac health of the patient, but if the condition is moderate to severe, the left ventricle and left atrium can enlarge because of the increased volume of blood. The enlargement of the left atrium can cause symptoms of fatigue, pulmonary edema, atrial fibrillation, and atrial thrombi. The enlargement of the left ventricle can lead to congestive heart failure.

The leakage can be repaired by surgery and/or insertion of a metal ring around the valve to assist in holding the valve in shape. If surgical replacement is elected, the diseased valve is cut out and replaced with a prosthetic heart valve.

Knowing when to perform the surgery is critical. The consequences of waiting too long may negate any surgical advantage because of enlargement and damage to the left ventricle. Leakiness occurring in a damaged valve can actually make the job of the left ventricle easier. The effort expended by the left ventricle when the valve is leaking is less than when the valve is repaired. The weakened left ventricle may not be strong enough to keep pace with the efficiency of the repaired or artificial valve. Therefore, the first sign of left ventricular impairment may be the best clue that it is time to consider surgery.

Mitral Valve Stenosis

Mitral stenosis occurs when the mitral valve is too tight, and the blood cannot flow easily from the left atrium to the left ventricle. To compensate, the left atrium will enlarge to develop the extra pressure to push the blood into the ventricle. As pressure in the left atrium increases, blood pools in pulmonary vessels. The excess blood then seeps out into the air spaces of the lungs and shortness of breath results.

If the condition is mild, there is a minimal effect on the overall health of the person. However, some patients experience significant symptoms such as fatigue, dyspnea, orthopnea (requires sitting or standing to breathe comfortably), and cyanosis (a bluish discoloration of the skin and mucous membranes). Mitral valve stenosis can lead to atrial fibrillation, which if not well managed increases the risk of stroke. People who have the combination of atrial fibrillation and mitral stenosis have a high rate of stroke, on the order of 5% per year.

Therapeutic options include balloon valvuloplasty (a procedure in which one or more balloons are placed across a narrowed valve and inflated to decrease the severity of stenosis), mitral commissurotomy (a procedure to increase the size of the opening by separating adherent, thickened leaflets), or replacement with a prosthetic valve. The two methods of repair are not permanent; the valve will become stenotic in about 5–15 years. A mechanical prosthetic valve requires chronic anticoagulation therapy.

Tricuspid Valve

The tricuspid valve has three main cusps and is situated between the right atrium and the right ventricle of the heart. The right atrium receives blood returning from the body and pushes the blood into the right ventricle. As the right and left ventricles relax (during the diastolic phase of the heartbeat), the tricuspid valve opens, allowing blood to enter the ventricle. During the systolic phase of the heartbeat, both blood-filled ventricles contract, pumping out their contents while the tricuspid and mitral valves close to prevent any backflow.

Tricuspid Regurgitation

Tricuspid regurgitation is a condition in which the tricuspid valve becomes leaky, allowing blood to flow backward from the right ventricle into the right atrium. It can occur by itself or in combination with a disease process that elevates right ventricular pressure.

When tricuspid regurgitation occurs by itself, perhaps due to subacute bacterial endocarditis, regurgitation does not pose much of a problem. But when tricuspid regurgitation occurs in union with mitral stenosis or lung disease, fatigue, abdominal discomfort, nausea, and swelling of the legs and feet result. If surgery is scheduled to correct another cardiac problem, the tricuspid valve should be evaluated for surgical repair at that time. Otherwise, medical treatment includes a low-salt diet, diuretics, and digoxin.

Tricuspid Stenosis

Tricuspid stenosis is a condition in which the tricuspid valve is too tight. Symptoms of tricuspid stenosis closely parallel those of tricuspid regurgitation, that is, nausea, fatigue, abdominal discomfort, and swelling of the legs and feet. Patients are frequently advised to follow a low-sodium diet and to use diuretics; if atrial fibrillation develops, digitalis may be prescribed. Balloon valvuloplasty or valve replacement is usually recommended if medical treatment proves ineffective. Because the risk of thrombus on the valve is higher in the tricuspid position than in the mitral position, bioprosthetic valves are better than mechanical valves, despite their limitations.

Aortic Valve

The aortic valve, composed of three semilunar cusps, is located between the left ventricle and the aorta. The aortic valve prevents blood from flowing back into the left ventricle from the aorta.

Aortic Stenosis

Aortic stenosis is a condition in which the aortic valve is too tight. This means that the opening through which blood must flow is too small; consequently, the left ventricle must generate higher pressure to maintain normal blood flow. It usually takes decades for the condition to fully develop. Not until the aortic valve area has narrowed to about one-fourth of its normal size do circulatory problems become significant.

The most common cause of aortic stenosis in adults is a degenerative calcification process that immobilizes the aortic valve cusps. The calcification process can either decrease worthiness of the valve or result in total fusion. Studies implicate a chronic inflammatory process in calcium buildup, leading to aortic valvular stenosis. Therefore, long-term anti-inflammatory therapy may be beneficial.

The degree of closure does not always correlate to symptoms. Thus, aortic valve replacement is usually reserved for patients experiencing symptoms, rather than those with narrowing who are asymptomatic. Eventually, angina, syncope (fainting), and heart failure may develop. After the onset of symptoms, the average survival is usually less than 2–3 years.

Fifty-one asymptomatic patients with severe aortic stenosis were followed for an average of 17 months. During this period, two patients died (with cardiac symptoms preceding their deaths). Other studies have shown similar survival trends among asymptomatic patients. (Sudden death occasionally occurs in the absence of symptoms, but the numbers are small, less than 1% per year.)

Once symptoms have become apparent, surgery becomes the patient's best option. Not all experts agree on when to do valve replacement surgery in asymptomatic patients with aortic stenosis. The *rationale* for early surgery is that the first symptom of aortic stenosis can be sudden death.

In theory, the aortic valve can be replaced in almost all patients, even octogenarians, who are otherwise in good health. Insertion of a prosthetic aortic valve is associated with low perioperative morbidity and mortality; complications arise at the rate of at least 2–3% a year, with death due directly to the prosthesis at about 1% a year. Symptomatic but inoperable patients are usually prescribed digitalis, diuretics, and an ACE (angiotensin converting enzyme) inhibitor.

Aortic Regurgitation

Aortic regurgitation occurs when the blood flows from the aorta back into the left ventricle. Some of the blood that should be flowing to the body from the heart flows back into the left ventricle. As a result, the left ventricle has to pump harder to move the blood though the circulatory route and back to the heart. A few of the factors provoking aortic regurgitation include congenital deformities, calcification, rheumatic fever, infective endocarditis, systemic hypertension, and anorexic drugs.

Acute aortic regurgitation is a medical emergency. During acute, severe aortic regurgitation, the left ventricle does not have time to make the necessary adjustments to accommodate the backflow and, as a result, forward stroke volume decreases. Tachycardia (a heartbeat over 100 beats a minute) occurs as a compensatory mechanism, but the effort is usually not equal to the task. Pulmonary edema and/or cardiogenic shock, a condition of critically low cardiac output, can result. (About 80% of events involving cardiogenic shock are fatal.)

Conversely, in chronic aortic regurgitation, a number of compensatory adjustments occur, rendering aortic regurgitation less dangerous. In fact, the majority of patients remain asymptomatic through this compensated phase, which may last for decades.

With time, the left ventricle progressively enlarges and depressed myocardial contractility increases. This can progress to the extent that the full benefits of surgical correction, that is, recovery of left ventricular function and improved survival, are no longer possible.

The results of several studies, involving 490 asymptomatic patients with chronic aortic regurgitation who were followed for an average of 6.4 years, give a brief history regarding the developmental patterns of the condition.

- The rate of progression to symptoms and/or left ventricle dysfunction averaged 4.3% a year. (As the left ventricle goes, so goes the heart.)

- Sudden death occurred in six of the 490 patients (an average mortality rate of < 0.2% a year).

Are Artificial Valves as Good as Natural Valves?

The replacement of diseased natural heart valves with artificial valve can be life-saving, but the replacement valves are never considered as good as healthy natural ones. There are two general types of valves: mechanical and bioprosthetic (usually taken from pigs). The mechanical valves last longer but require the patient to take anticoagulants. The bioprosthetic valves do not require long-term anticoagulation therapy, but they frequently must be replaced after about 10 years in adults. Their replacement comes quicker in children and persons on kidney dialysis. The major risk of prosthetic heart valves is stroke. Those taking anticoagulants reduce the incidence of stroke, but the risk is not totally eliminated.

The following natural products may be of value to patients with valvular disease. The herbs profiled have one or more chemicals that convey the biological property delineated and are subsequently not equal in therapeutic strengths (Duke Database). Researchers state that carnitine may provide independent benefit in ischemia when used as monotherapy, or additional benefit when used in combination with conventional beta-blockers or calcium antagonists (Jackson 2001). To learn more about the following supplements, please consult the *Therapeutic section*.

- *Vasodilators.* Angelica, garlic, ginger, ginkgo biloba, hawthorn, magnesium, niacin, and olive leaf

- *ACE inhibitors.* Angelica, garlic, ginger, ginkgo biloba, grape seed, green tea, hawthorn, olive leaf, procyanidins, and taurine

- *Calcium blocking properties.* Angelica, garlic, ginger, ginkgo biloba, grape seed, green tea, hawthorne, magnesium, and olive leaf

- *Digitalis-like activity.* Bugleweed and taurine

- *Diuretic activity.* Angelica, bugleweed, curcumin, garlic, ginger, grape seed, green tea, hawthorn, olive leaf, taurine, vitamin B_6, vitamin C, and vitamin E

- *Anti-inflammatories.* Angelica, bromelain, bugleweed, chondroitin, curcumin, DHEA, EFAs, garlic, ginger, ginkgo biloba, grape seed, green tea, hawthorn, olive leaf, and vitamin C

- *Beta-blocking activity.* Grape seed, green tea, hawthorn, magnesium, and taurine

THERAPEUTIC SECTION

The following therapeutics are arranged alphabetically and not by order of importance, providing greater accessibility to readers.

Alpha-Lipoic Acid (a.k.a. Thiotic Acid)— beneficial in preventing and treating Syndrome X, has antioxidant and antidiabetic activity, protects LDL cholesterol against oxidation, lowers total cholesterol, is beneficial in congestive heart failure and strokes, inhibits protein glycation, and stabilizes arrhythmias

Some researchers credit alpha-lipoic acid with being the principal supplement for preventing and reversing Syndrome X. Lipoic acid earned this reputation by increasing the burning of glucose. The mitochondria (the powerhouse of the cell) are one of the benefactors of enhanced glucose utilization, via the Krebs's cycle, a process that utilizes glucose, amino acids, and fatty acids to yield high energy. Many of the B vitamins assist in maximizing production from the Krebs's cycle, but perhaps none is as efficient as lipoic acid (Challem et al. 2000).

Note: *Free radicals are produced as a byproduct of the energy generated during the Krebs's cycle. Alpha-lipoic acid appears to quench free radicals that are not contained during the reactions.*

As glucose is provided to fuel the Krebs's cycle, blood glucose and insulin levels decrease and simultaneously another perk occurs: insulin sensitivity increases. Lipoic acid resulted in a 50% increase in insulin-stimulated glucose disposal and a significant improvement in insulin sensitivity compared to a nonsupplemented placebo group. Blood glucose levels often drop 23–45% in lipoic acid-treated diabetic animals. The journal *Hypertension* also reported alpha-lipoic acid, a thiol compound known to increase tissue cysteine and glutathione levels, reduced systolic blood pressure in spontaneously hypertensive rats (Jacob 1995, 1996, 1997; Vasdev et al. 2000).

Lipoic acid is of value in treating diabetic and non-diabetic subjects with congestive heart failure. Researchers from Beijing University added that lipoic acid, because of its free-radical scavenging effects, is able to protect the myocardium from free-radical damage and subsequently decrease the incidence of malignant arrhythmias (Gao et al. 1991). Antioxidants are extremely important in cardiac health, for the heart is one of the most susceptible of all organs to free-radical damage. (There are three times more free radicals produced in aging hearts compared to young hearts.)

Alpha-lipoic acid is, in fact, regarded as the universal antioxidant because it enhances the activity of other antioxidants. It acts like a big brother in regard to vitamin E, coenzyme Q_{10}, and vitamin C, assisting in recycling these important antioxidants for continued service. Lipoic acid's antioxidant qualities appear greater than vitamin E's because vitamin E works only in the fatty parts of cells, whereas lipoic acid works in both watery and fatty portions (Challem et al. 2000).

Stroke deaths dropped from 78% to 26% in lipoic acid animal studies conducted by Lester Packer. The journal *Stroke* confirmed that alpha-lipoic acid reduced stroke infarct volume and free-radical activity, inhibited platelet-leukocyte activation and adhesion, and increased cerebral blood flow (Clark et al. 2001).

Lipoic acid reduced the formation of glycosylated end products (AGEs) (Jain et al. 1998). Glycation occurs when proteins react with sugar to form AGEs. This process increases the risk of cardiovascular disease by oxidizing LDL cholesterol and rendering blood vessels tough and inflexible. This gradually affects the left ventricle, reducing its ability to pump oxygen-rich blood into the circulation. Stiffness occurring in the myocardium increases diastolic pressure, and arterial rigidity increases systolic pressure. Also, glycosylated cholesterol-carrying proteins are no longer capable of binding to receptors on liver cells to signal the cessation of cholesterol manufacturing. A healthy cholesterol-carrying protein halts the copious supply of cholesterol. Without this binding process, cholesterol continues to be pumped out. Lipoic acid interrupts all of these processes at the starting point, by inhibiting glycation.

Note: Although a normal byproduct of oxidative metabolism, free radicals in excess are considered germane to the onset of vascular disease. When out of control, these highly unstable electrons can cause extensive damage to lipid membranes, organelles, and DNA itself. But most all of nature is two-pronged, having a good side as well as a bad. For example, free radicals participate in many positive reactions, including mitochondrial respiration, prostaglandin synthesis, platelet activation, and leukocyte-phagocytosis, (the engulfing and destruction of microorganisms and cellular debris). It is thus extremely important to supply sufficient nutrient cofactors to support endogenous antioxidant enzyme systems (such as superoxide dismutase, catalase, and glutathione peroxidase) but to retain enough free-radical oxidative activity to carry on essential life processes (Sinatra 2001).

Some researchers believe 50–250 mg a day (in concert with other antioxidants) may be sufficient to protect against Syndrome X. Most Life Extension members have been taking between 250–500 mg a day of alpha-lipoic acid. If the patient has unstable blood glucose levels, higher doses of lipoic acid will be required. German practitioners frequently use 600 mg daily as adjunctive therapy in coronary artery disease and 600–1800 mg of alpha-lipoic acid to improve insulin sensitivity and diabetic conditions. Higher doses should be administered with the help of a qualified physician who can adjust insulin requirements as indicated. *Note:* Dr. Lester Packer, in *The Antioxidant Miracle*, recommends taking biotin supplements with alpha-lipoic acid when the daily intake exceeds 100 mg. Alpha-lipoic acid may compete with biotin and interfere with biotin's activities in the body.

Reader's guide to lipoic acid food sources. Liver, yeast, spinach, broccoli, potatoes, and red meat.

Angelica (*Angelica archangelica*)—an anti-anginal, anti-inflammatory calcium antagonist, ACE inhibitor, and diuretic

Angelica, a member of the carrot family, contains 15 compounds considered to be calcium channel blockers. One of the calcium antagonists in angelica is, in fact, more potent than verapamil (Calan, Isoptin), a popular calcium channel blocker prescribed for angina, atrial fibrillation, and spasms occurring in the blood vessels (Duke 1997).

James Duke, Ph.D. (botanist), comments that it is well known that vegetarians have a low incidence of heart disease. Usually their low-fat diet gets the credit, but Dr. Duke speculates that it may be because they eat lots of plants from the carrot family, such as carrots, celery, fennel, parsley, and parsnips, which (like angelica) contain compounds with calcium channel blocking activity. Calcium channel blockers (whether natural or pharmaceutical) are powerful anti-anginals.

Angelica bestows its cardiac advantage through various pathways. For example, angelica not only reduces the incidence of angina attacks, but also regulates an erratic heartbeat. It has diuretic properties, making it of value in the treatment of congestive heart failure and hypertension. Chemicals contained in angelica exhibit another mechanism to reduce blood pressure, that is, the inhibition of ACE, the angiotensin-converting enzyme (Duke Database 1992).

Inflammation, one of the newer risk factors for heart disease, is also reduced by angelica (*read about the inflammation-heart disease connection in the sections dedicated to Newer Risk Factors*). A suggested angelica dosage is 15–30 drops 1–3 times a day.

Comments: How many milligrams (mg) of herb are in a drop of extract? According to Herb Pharm, a respected name in the herbal industry, the milligrams represented by 1 milliliter of extract (about 30-40 drops) from a dried herb are given by the herb-to-menstruum ratio (menstruum is a solvent—a liquid that dissolves a solid). This number varies for extracts made from fresh herbs due to the increased yield of these extracts. Liquid extracts are more assimilable than powdered herbs so the weights are not comparable. If trying to follow a recommendation, the form of the recommendation (powdered herb, liquid extract, etc.) needs to be considered. Quality and quantity are separate issues and even liquid extracts cannot be accurately compared on a mg-to-mg basis. Many factors determine the quality of an herbal extract, including the makeup of the menstruum, extraction technique, and raw herb quality. The following is only an approximate calculation, but it may be helpful:

1 mL is equal to about 33 drops of many extracts
1 mL of a 1:4 ratio contains extractives from ¼ gram of herb (0.25 gram = 250 mg)

The strength ratio does not directly address quality. Quality is dependent on other factors such as the quality of the herb, the plant part used, special handling, the extraction process and technique, as well as storage. Always follow dosage instructions (and caveats) appearing on the label.

L-Arginine—dilates blood vessels, reduces blood pressure, replicates the activity of nitroglycerine, and is needed to produce nitric oxide

L-arginine, along with a properly planned exercise program, assists in amending abnormalities occurring in blood vessels. Individuals with congestive heart failure often have blood vessels that fail to dilate in response to certain drugs, a sign that the inner blood vessel wall, or endothelium, is compromised.

A study reported in the *American College of Cardiology* concluded that treatment with *L*-arginine produced a fourfold increase in blood vessel dilation from 2.2–8.8% (Hambrecht et al. 2000). Regular forearm exercises increased the dilation response by the same amount, but the combination of *L*-arginine and exercise training resulted in an improvement from 2.9–12%. Doses of 5.6–12.6 grams of arginine increased blood flow to the extremities 29%; the distance walked on a treadmill in 6 minutes increased 8% (Rector et al. 1996).

Much of *L*-arginine's effectiveness comes by way of increasing nitric oxide, a blood vessel dilator and clot buster produced in endothelial cells by the enzyme nitric oxide synthase (Brunini et al. 2002). Nitric oxide counteracts the vasoconstriction and platelet-aggregating effects of the stress hormone adrenaline (epinephrine) and assists in maintaining vascular elasticity. Nitric oxide (the endothelial relaxing factor) is needed for expansion and contraction of the arterial system (Rohdewald 1999). *L*-arginine *increases* nitric oxide, but hypertension, hyperhomocysteinemia, diabetes, and smoking *decrease* it.

Because of arginine's vasodilating properties, it is frequently used as a treatment for angina pain and hypertension. Researchers at the University of Southern California (Los Angeles) speculate that a defect in nitric oxide production may be a possible mechanism of hypertensive disease (Campese et al. 1997). Some cardiologists, in fact, recommend *L*-arginine over nitroglycerine, since the two substances appear to replicate a similar vascular function: the ability to relax smooth muscles and dilate blood vessels.

In their current book, *The Arginine Solution*, Drs. Robert Fried and Woodson C. Merrell note that as people age and develop disorders such as hypertension, hypercholesterolemia, and atherosclerosis, their ability to make sufficient amounts of nitric oxide from arginine is impaired, contributing to a decline in their cardiovascular health. Drs. Fried and Merrell contend that increasing arginine intake addresses various cardiovascular risks associated with decreased nitric oxide synthesis, often improving symptomatic and clinical evaluations (Fried et al. 1999). A suggested dosage is 2 grams before bedtime. *Arginine caveat:* Individuals who have frequent herpes outbreaks may find arginine-rich foodstuffs or supplementation contraindicated.

Reader's guide to arginine food sources. Most protein foods and carob, chocolate, nuts, seeds, beans, oats, peanuts, and wheat and wheat germ.

Artichoke Extract—reduces cholesterol and triglycerides

Artichoke (*Cynara scolymus*), a delicious table vegetable, has a reputation that extends beyond culinary enhancement. It has long been used to improve digestive and liver complaints, but more recently artichoke has become popular as a hypolipidemic. Studies have shown that the more lipid correction needed, the greater artichoke's cholesterol-lowering effects. Caffeoylquinic acids and flavonoids, constituents of artichoke, appear to deliver much of the plant's positive effects.

In a multicenter, placebo-controlled, randomized trial, 143 patients with initial cholesterol levels greater than 280 mg/dL took either a placebo or 450 mg of artichoke dry extract 4 times a day. After 6 weeks, those taking the artichoke extract showed an 18.5% reduction in cholesterol compared to a 5.6% reduction in the placebo group. LDL-cholesterol decreased 22.9% among those taking the artichoke extract and 6.3% in the placebo group. The LDL/HDL ratio showed a decrease of 20.2% among the artichoke users (Englisch et al. 2000). Another short-term study (6 weeks) showed that artichoke reduced triglycerides from 214.97 mg/dL to 188.07 mg/dL (Fintelmann 1996a, 1996b). There were no drug related adverse events during the course of these studies, indicating an excellent tolerability.

Artichoke reduces cholesterol by decreasing the synthesis of cholesterol in the liver and increasing the conversion of cholesterol to bile acids. (Cholesterol is a building block for bile acids.) According to Michael Murray, N.D., cholesterol levels are sometimes high because of the impaired conversion of cholesterol to bile acids. Thus, low bile acid levels send a powerful signal to the liver to provide more cholesterol. Artichoke extract intercepts this signal, and the liver complies with less cholesterol production (Murray 1998b).

The flavonoid luteolin appears to be pivotal in the hypocholesterolemic effects of artichoke. Statin drugs reduce cholesterol by competitively inhibiting the binding of HMG-CoA reductase. Tocotrienols also degrade this enzyme. Artichoke research has found no direct inhibition of HMG-CoA reductase. Other enzymatic steps occurring later in the biosynthesis of cholesterol appear unaffected. It seems luteolin inhibits cholesterol below the level of HMG-CoA reductase and therefore spares coenzyme Q_{10} synthesis. Recall that the cholesterol cascade begins with acetyl-CoA being converted to HMG-CoA. HMG-CoA reductase reduces HMG-CoA to mevalonic acid. Mevalonic acid participates in several steps that reduce it to squalene. Squalene is then converted to cholesterol (Murray 1998b; Sardesai 1998).

A suggested dosage is 1 capsule 3 times a day, containing 300 mg of artichoke standardized to contain 13–18% caffeoylquinic acid. *Note:* The *American Journal of Clinical Nutrition* recently reported that chlorogenic acid, a component of black tea and coffee, could increase homocysteine levels (Olthof et al. 2001). Chlorogenic acid also appears in artichoke and would therefore be contraindicated in refractory hyperhomocysteinemia. Lastly, individuals with gallstones or biliary tract obstruction should not use artichoke.

Aspirin—reduces C-reactive protein (CRP), platelet aggregation, and cardiac inflammation

Aspirin has been used for over a century to relieve pain; research suggests that it may play an equally important role in heart health. A study involving 51,085 participants showed a total of 2284 cardiovascular endpoints occurring during an aspirin trial. The risk of a first nonfatal heart attack was reduced 32% among aspirin users compared to nonusers. The researchers concluded that aspirin therapy could prevent a third of myocardial infarctions occurring in apparently healthy individuals (Hebert et al. 2000). *JAMA* also reported that aspirin usage was associated with reduced all-cause mortality, particularly among older subjects with known coronary artery disease and impaired exercise capacity (Gum et al. 2001).

Three studies looked at the incidence of stroke subtypes among aspirin users. A 1.69-fold increase in the risk of hemorrhagic stroke occurred among aspirin users, but no increase in ischemic strokes was noted. Secondary prevention trials, evaluated by Drs. Patricia R. Hebert (Yale University) and Charles Hennekens (University of Miami) indicated that aspirin therapy administered to 10,000 persons would prevent about 67 myocardial infarctions and cause approximately 11 hemorrhagic strokes. In November 2001, the *New England Journal of Medicine* published that over a 2-year period, no difference was found between aspirin and warfarin in the prevention of recurrent ischemic stroke or death or in the rate of major hemorrhage (Hebert et al. 2000; Mohr et al. 2001).

The drug disposition of aspirin is persuasive when applied to a cardiovascular model. For example, low-dose aspirin (81 mg) appears to provide partial protection against abnormal blood clot formation, having a 2-day lasting effect on blood platelets. Platelets become less sticky and the risk of a heart attack and transient ischemic attacks (TIAs) is subsequently reduced.

Aspirin exerts some of its cardioprotection by inhibiting the enzyme cyclooxygenase, a trigger in the inflammatory process (Newmark et al. 2000). One molecule of aspirin will destroy the cyclooxygenase enzyme for 4–6 hours (*read the sections devoted to C-Reactive Protein and The Link Between Infections and Inflammation in Heart Disease to learn how the inflammatory process advances cardiac disease*).

Aspirin appears to lower C-reactive protein (CRP). In the Physician's Health Study, participants were randomly assigned at baseline to receive 323 mg of aspirin on alternate days and were then followed through first myocardial infarction. The study showed that low dose aspirin reduced heart attack risk by about 44% compared to the control group; the risk was 55% lower than that of placebo-treated men with high CRP levels. The results of this study suggest that in addition to aspirin's antagonism toward platelet clumping, it may also attenuate thrombosis through anti-inflammatory mechanisms (*Physicians Weekly* 1998a).

Aspirin significantly cut the death rate from cardiac disease among 2368 noninsulin-dependent diabetic patients with coronary artery disease. (The aspirin benefit was greater among diabetic patients than nondiabetics.) Diabetic patients using aspirin had a 10.9% mortality risk from cardiac diseases, while diabetics not using aspirin had a 15.9% risk (Harpaz et al. 1998).

The aspirin advantage extended to include carotid endarterectomy patients. Individuals using low-dose aspirin (81–325 mg a day) reduced the risk of myocardial infarction, stroke, and death for a 30-day to 3-month interval following surgery. Individuals taking 650–1300 mg were not similarly protected, illustrating that the dose can alter the end response (Taylor et al. 1999).

Current information indicates that aspirin can also reduce the level of heart damage during a heart attack. When taking aspirin because one believes they are experiencing an acute heart attack, the aspirin should be chewed rather than swallowed and is best taken within 30 minutes of the onset of symptoms.

In conclusion, the Antithrombotic Trialists' Collaboration (representing a review of 287 studies involving 135,000 patients) announced that over 40,000 lives are lost worldwide every year because aspirin is underused. According to the report, aspirin (or other antiplatelet drugs) is protective in most patients at increased risk of occlusive vascular events, including those with acute myocardial infarction or ischemic stroke, unstable or stable angina, previous myocardial infarction, cerebral ischemia, peripheral arterial disease, or atrial fibrillation (Antithrombotic Trialists' Collaboration 2002).

Aspirin (75–150 mg a day) appears to be an effective antiplatelet regimen for long-term usage, but in acute settings, an initial loading dose of at least 150 mg may be required. Adding a second antiplatelet drug to aspirin may produce additional benefits in some clinical circumstances (Antithrombotic Trialists' Collaboration 2002). *Note:* The *New England Journal of Medicine* recently published that warfarin, in combination with aspirin or given alone, was superior to aspirin alone in reducing the incidence of composite events following an acute myocardial infarction. Warfarin was, however, associated with a higher risk of bleeding (Hurlen et al. 2002).

The American College of Chest Physicians suggests that all people over 50 years of age, with one cardiac risk factor and no condition that would negate treatment, consider aspirin therapy. The cautionary includes those individuals who have increased prothrombin time, disturbed gastric mucosa, or hypertension. As acclaimed as low-dose aspirin is, studies have shown that aspirin does not appear comprehensive enough to prevent a heart attack if fibrinogen levels are excessively high. It should also be noted that a concomitant administration of ibuprofen (but not rofecoxib, acetaminophen, or diclofenac) antagonizes the platelet inhibition activity induced by aspirin. Thus, treatment with ibuprofen in patients with increased cardiovascular risk may limit the cardioprotective effects of aspirin (Catella-Lawson et al. 2001).

Bromelain—is an anti-inflammatory, reduces fibrinogen, lessens risk of blood clots, is beneficial in atrial fibrillation, is hypotensive, relieves angina, and is basic to smokers

Bromelain, derived from pineapple (*Ananas comusus*), is regarded as a natural anti-inflammatory, acting as a protein-digesting enzyme. Since the revelation that inflammation may be causal to cardiovascular disease, bromelain has attained new stature. Proteolytic enzymes work directly on the

• Niacin can also increase blood glucose levels. In nondiabetic patients, 1500 mg a day of Niaspan (an extended-release niacin) increased fasting blood glucose levels 2.5–11% following a 2-hour glucose load. Using 3000 mg a day of immediate-release niacin, fasting blood glucose increased 4.1% and 11.6% following a 2-hour glucose load. The niacin effect in Type II diabetic patients is currently under investigation (Berkeley Heart Lab). However, it is speculated that individuals predisposed to Type II diabetes may have a poorer response to niacin (in regard to glucose management) compared to individuals without a diabetic inclination.

Considering these negatives, large-dose niacin may be too great a price to pay for the benefits. If a decision is made to use high-dose niacin, some practitioners report that an aspirin taken 30 minutes before the dose markedly reduces some of the lesser side effects, for example, the allergic-like symptoms.

Reader's guide to vitamin B₃ sources, enhancers, and antagonists. Good sources of niacin are lean meats, whole grains, brewer's yeast, peanuts, eggs, poultry, fish, and green, leafy vegetables. Milk; some cheeses, for example, cheddar cheese; bananas; and turkey are good sources of tryptophan (a precursor to niacin) (Braly 1985).

Vitamin B_3 enhancers (in regard to absorption) are the B-complex (especially vitamins B_1, B_2, and B_6), vitamin C, magnesium, zinc, protein, and essential fatty acids. Antagonists to niacin absorption are alcohol, coffee, excess sugar, antibiotics, and steroids.

Olive Leaf Extract—according to botanist James Duke, the cardiac properties found in olive leaf extract include antioxidants, anti-aggregates, anti-arrhythmics, anti-inflammatories, cyclooxygenase inhibitors, diuretics, hypotensives, vasodilators, antispasmodics, antidiabetics, platelet activating factor inhibitors, weight modulators, antiperiodontics, antihyperlipidemics, and plaque fighters

Olive leaf extract (*Olea europaea*), although historically regarded as a medicinal for fever and malaria, is also valuable in the treatment of cardiovascular disease. Olive leaf extract has been shown in both laboratory and clinical settings to have antidiabetic,

hypotensive, and vasodilating properties (Petkov et al. 1972; Gonzalez et al. 1992; Fehri et al. 1994). Researchers documented that an aqueous extract of olive leaves inhibits ACE, the enzyme that converts angiotensin I to angiotensin II (Duke 1992). The vasoconstricting nature of angiotensin II terminates in an increase in blood pressure, a sequence that olive leaf extract disrupts.

According to Dr. Duke, chemicals contained in *O. europaea* are regarded as calcium antagonists, diuretics, and anti-inflammatories. In addition, olive leaf protects LDL cholesterol against oxidation and inhibits the production of thromboxane A2 and platelet-activating factor (PAF). These functions discourage vasoconstriction and platelet clumping (Duke 1992; Petroni et al. 1995; Mindell 1998).

Chelation therapy, in conjunction with an aggressive supplemental program that relied heavily upon olive leaf extract, has proved remedial among select senior subjects who have suffered multiple heart attacks and arrhythmias. A suggested dosage is one to two 500-mg olive leaf extract capsules, administered 3 times daily with meals.

Pantethine—reduces cholesterol, discourages platelet clumping, and has antioxidant activity

Pantethine, a biologically active, intermediate form of pantothenic acid (vitamin B_5) and a precursor to coenzyme A, is a powerful natural pharmaceutical that reduces cholesterol, increases heart muscle contractility, slows the heart rate, and has antioxidant activity.

Pantethine (300 mg 3 times daily) reduced serum triglycerides 32%, total cholesterol 19%, and LDL cholesterol 21%; HDL cholesterol levels increased 23% (Arsenio et al. 1986, Murray 1996b). Pantethine further reduces cardiovascular risk by inhibiting platelet clumping and the production of the inflammation-producing chemical, thromboxane A2 (CVR, http://www.thewayup.com/products/0012.htm). A dosage suggestion is 300 mg 3 times a day.

Policosanol—is a hypocholesterolemic, protects LDL cholesterol against oxidation, inhibits thromboxane and the proliferation of vascular cells, discourages blood clot formation, inhibits platelet aggregation, and increases exercise tolerance

Policosanol, derived from sugar cane, is a new face on the cholesterol scene in the United States but is a popular hypocholesterolemic in other countries (Mas et al. 1999). The main ingredient in sugar cane is octacosanol, a long-chain fatty alcohol found in the waxy film that covers the leaves and fruit of plants.

Policosanol represents an effective alternative to lowering cholesterol for many people. For example, 10 mg a day of policosanol (over a 6- to 12-week period) lowered LDL cholesterol 20%, reduced total cholesterol 15%, and raised the beneficial HDL cholesterol 7–28%. Doubling the dose (20 mg a day) resulted in the following lipid improvements: LDL cholesterol reduced about 28%, total cholesterol about 20%, and HDL increased by 7–10%. Triglycerides were unaffected. During the course of the trial, participants continued on a low cholesterol diet.

The hypolipidemic effects of policosanol are comparable to many cholesterol-lowering drugs (Prat et al. 1999). The results of a head-to-head study classing popular hypocholesterolemic drugs against policosanol follow in Figure 6.

Policosanol also outclassed the drugs in regard to increasing levels of the beneficial HDL cholesterol. Yet, a combination of policosanol and gemfibrozil (Lopid) was more hypocholesterolemic than either used singularly. In fact, policosanol even upgraded the efficiency of bezafibrate, a once touted fibrinogen-lowering drug that yielded disappointing results in the Bezafibrate Infarction Prevention Study (Castano et al. 1998; Behar 1999). Bezafibrate in union with policosanol dramatically reduced LDL and total cholesterol. In addition, policosanol appears to replicate another of the objectives of statin drugs, reducing the proliferation of cells. A telltale sign of a diseased vessel is that the smooth lining of the vessel becomes thickened and overgrown with cells.

When comparing the value of a drug to a natural alternative, the safety factors must be considered. Usually, the ramifications of a nutrient, in contrast to a drug, are not side *effects* but side *benefits*. For example, the oxidation of LDL cholesterol (a particularly destructive form of cholesterol that creates chronic inflammation) is inhibited by policosanol. As less inflammation and blood vessel destruction occur, fewer foam cells appear (Noa et al. 1996). Conversely, if the oxidation of LDL is not inhibited, metalloproteinase enzymes are aroused, further damaging the vasculature by interfering with the protective nature of HDL cholesterol.

Policosanol combines well with aspirin to inhibit the formation of clots, with each influencing the activity of different platelets (Arruzazabala et al. 1997; Carbajal et al. 1998). The synergistic approach provides more comprehensive protection against platelet aggregation. Another factor in blood clot formation, thromboxane, is repressed after a couple of weeks of policosanol therapy.

Policosanol users can expect an improvement in exercise tolerance. When patients with heart disease were given 10 mg a day of policosanol, exercise capacity and oxygen uptake increased, but ischemia decreased. The improvement in treadmill-ECG tests confirmed that policosanol benefits heart patients, but healthy, physically active individuals also reported increases in exercise tolerance and strength (Stusser et al. 1998). Policosanol not only improved cardiovascular capacity, but also protected against atherosclerotic lesions (thickened fatty streaks in the vasculature).

Policosanol does not appear to interfere with other heart medications. However, it may potentiate the effects of propranolol, a beta-blocker used to treat hypertension. The 10-mg dose has had more than 2 years of clinical testing with no significant ill effects noted, except some patients reported an unexpected weight loss. Blood tests (after about 2 months of policosanol therapy) will allow the individual to adjust the dose commensurate with need. Some individuals will need only 5–10 mg of policosanol to maintain healthy cholesterol levels; others will require 20 mg a day. *Note:* Policosanol has undergone as many clinical trials as most drugs.

Polyenylphosphatidylcholine (PPC)—is a hypolipidemic, improves exercise tolerance and apoB/apoA-1 ratio, lessens angina attacks, and increases levels of HDL2b

Phosphatidylcholine, the main component of lecithin (a soy product), has a long history as a preventive in arteriosclerosis, cardiovascular disease, and brain derangements. PPC, a newer, polyunsaturated soy derivative, has shown extraordinary promise in managing hypercholesterolemia. It appears that PPC delivers its value by traversing into cholesterol, where direct modulation of the substance occurs. In a study involving 100 participants, PPC lowered total LDL cholesterol by about 15%, reduced triglycerides 32%, and raised HDL levels by about 10% (Klimov et al. 1995; Jordon 2000).

PPC significantly increased apolipoprotein A-1 and only slightly increased apolipoprotein B, while decreasing postprandial triglycerides, VLDL, and IDL (Klimov et al. 1995; Zeman et al. 1995). ApoB is a cholesterol particle that is believed to promote heart disease by affecting how cholesterol is transported in arteries and other tissues. It is found not only in LDL cholesterol, but also in VLDL and IDL, other potentially bad cholesterols. On the other hand, apoA-1 is a protective, anti-atherogenic particle found in the highly beneficial HDL cholesterol. Researchers concluded that PPC appeared to be an appropriate supplement for patients with decreased concentrations of HDL cholesterol and plasma apoA-1.

CHOLESTEROL-LOWERING AGENT	DOSAGE	LIPOPROTEIN EVALUATED	AMOUNT REDUCED
Lovastatin (Mevacor)	20 mg	LDL Cholesterol	22%
Simvastatin (Zocor)	10 mg	LDL Cholesterol	15%
Policosanol	10 mg	LDL Cholesterol	24%

Figure 6   Comparison of Policosanol to Classic Drug Therapy

The Lancet recently reported the results of a 5 1/2-year trial (the AMORIS, Apoliprotein-Related Mortality Risk Study) evaluating the cardiovascular health of 175,553 men and women. Although all conventional markers were assessed (triglycerides, total cholesterol, and LDL–HDL cholesterol ratio), persons with the greatest absolute risk of dying from a heart attack tended to have the highest ratios of apoB to apoA-1 (Srinivasan et al. 2001; Walldius et al. 2001; GSDL 2001).

Over the course of the study, 864 men and 359 women died from acute myocardial infarctions. When researchers compared their blood results, the apoB:apoA-1 ratio was the strongest predictor of fatal heart attacks. Men with the highest apoB and lowest apoA-1 levels were nearly 4 times as likely to experience a deadly heart attack compared to those with a favorable apo ratio. (In women the relative risk was threefold greater.) apoB proved to be a stronger predictor of risk than LDL cholesterol in both sexes.

The study also showed that the apo ratio remained a strong marker in all age groups, including those patients over age 70, a group in which total cholesterol levels are not considered to be accurate risk indicators for heart attack. Assessing apoB:apoA-1 ratio appears to identify high-risk individuals who have normal-to-low LDL cholesterol, as well as those with diabetes and insulin resistance. Recall that PPC's credits include increasing the desirable apoA-1.

PPC has a positive effect upon HDL levels, particularly the most protective of the HDL family, HDL$_{2b}$. Individuals attaining longevity often display HDL differentials favoring HDL$_{2b}$, suggesting that this sub-fraction renders, among other health benefits, greater cardio-protection. Another of the restorative capacities of PPC is its ability to increase exercise tolerance (Klimov et al. 1995).

Alcohol in moderation appears to prevent atherosclerosis. Heavy drinking has the opposite effect, in part by promoting oxidation of LDL cholesterol. Administering PPC at 2.8 grams/1000 kcal to baboons made alcoholic for experimentation lessened the expected ethanol-induced increase in LDL oxidation (Navder et al. 1999).

Russian researchers compare PPC to niacin in the treatment of angina and hyperlipidemia. While nicotinic acid is a reliable hypocholesterolemic, the clusters of annoying symptoms (flushing and itching) and less benign side effects (liver disruption and GI disturbance) discredit megadose usage in some individuals. Conversely, PPC therapy has no contraindications, side effects, or drug interactions. A suggested dosage is two 900-mg capsules daily.

Potassium—reduces blood pressure, maintains fluid balance, encourages parasympathetic nervous system, and increases insulin sensitivity

Potassium, considered by some to be the major electrolyte, is found almost exclusively in the intracellular fluids of the cell. Sodium is found in the extracellular fluid, but it is equilibrium between potassium and sodium that determines fluid balance and blood pressure regulation. A high potassium–low sodium intake reduces the blood vessel constricting effects of adrenaline, a hormone associated with sympathetic nervous system arousal; the result is lower blood pressure.

Adults (37 in number) with diastolic blood pressure less than 110 participated in a crossover trial of 32 weeks duration to determine the hypotensive nature of minerals. Sixty mmol/day of potassium (about 2.5 grams) reduced systolic pressure by an average of 12 mmHg and decreased diastolic pressure 16 mmHg (Patki et al. 1990; Murray 1996). *Comment:* Results of the DASH study illustrate the necessity for providing adequate amounts of potassium, magnesium, and calcium to control blood pressure. To read more about the study, please turn to the subsection entitled, *Does Sodium Restriction Lower Blood Pressure?* in this protocol (Bland 2000b).

Hypertensive individuals over 65 years of age may find particular value in potassium, since medications are not always as effective among senior subjects. Administering 2.5 grams a day of potassium for 4 weeks to 18 untreated elderly hypertensive patients resulted in a systolic drop of 12 mmHg and a diastolic reduction of 7 mmHG. All entered the study with systolic blood pressure greater than 160 mmHg and diastolic pressure greater than 95 mmHg

(Fotherby 1992; Murray 1996). The results were impressive considering the brevity of the study and the fact that potassium's value is cumulative, meaning a greater response is generally seen with longer supplementation.

Researchers at the Johns Hopkins University School of Medicine advocate increasing potassium to treat and prevent hypertension. A group of seven medical researchers reviewed 33 randomized, controlled trials involving over 2600 participants. The researchers concluded that increased potassium intake is effective in lowering both systolic and diastolic blood pressure (systolic blood pressure dropped an average of 3.11 mmHg and diastolic was reduced 1.97 mmHg) (Whelton et al. 1997).

The hypotensive nature of potassium benefited a group of rats made stroke-prone for experimentation. The rats were divided into two groups. Only 2% of the potassium-supplemented group experienced a fatal stroke, compared to 83% of the untreated group (Alternative Medical News Staff). Cardiologists report using 400 mg of magnesium, 500–1000 mg of calcium, and 500–1000 mg of potassium to treat patients with arrhythmias (Sinatra 1997).

Several factors influence potassium levels. For example, insulin therapy appears to cause a potassium deficiency. Conversely, a diabetic supplementing with potassium may observe increased insulin secretions and responsiveness, reducing insulin requirements. Physical exertion (producing heavy perspiration) or diarrhea and vomiting (resulting in loss of body fluids) can cause a mineral depletion. Always replace minerals, for if not replaced, heart function can quickly depreciate. Symptoms of potassium deficiency are weakness, fatigue, mental confusion, and heart disturbances (Murray 1996).

While the results of potassium studies are impressive, it must be noted that though self-poisoning is uncommon, the consequences are often fatal (Colledge 1988). Potassium supplementation in the form of oral potassium tablets is generally not needed if you are on a good anti-aging diet that includes several servings of fruits and vegetables per day (The estimated safe and adequate daily dietary intake of potassium, as set by the Committee on Recommended Daily Allowances, is 1.9 grams to 5.6 grams per day.)

Most individuals can tolerate excesses of potassium, but individuals taking digitalis, potassium-sparing diuretics, and ACE inhibitors, or individuals with diagnosed kidney disease, should never supplement unless physician prescribed. This cautionary is valid for anyone considering therapeutic dosages of potassium. Due to the potential side effects of potassium on cardiac function, the FDA limits the amount of potassium permitted in nutritional supplements to 99 mg per serving.

Recall that many foods offer reliable potassium stores; subsequently, eating from foods delineated in the potassium food source section should be especially important to individuals with hypertension and cardiac irregularities. It becomes increasingly difficult, however, to provide adequate levels of potassium if taking a diuretic. Patients are commonly told to replace potassium by consuming potassium-rich foodstuffs. Yet, if every milligram of potassium in a banana were retained, it would require eating an entire stock of bananas every day to offset the potassium lost during diuretic therapy (Cuneo et al. 1985; Alternative Medical News Staff).

Reader's guide to potassium food sources, enhancers, and antagonists: Potassium is abundant in most food selections, e.g., 1 banana has 440 mg, 1 medium orange (263 mg), 1 medium peach (308 mg), ¼ cup of apricots (318 mg), ½ avocado (680 mg), ¼ cantaloupe (341 mg), ½ cup cooked lima beans (581 mg), 1 medium potato (782 mg), 1 medium raw tomato (444 mg), 1 stalk of celery (130 mg), 3 ounces of light chicken (350 mg), 3 ounces of cod (345 mg), 3 ounces of flounder (498 mg), and 3 ounces of salmon (378 mg). Asparagus, carrots, spinach, apples, plums, strawberries, watermelon, roast beef, pork, haddock, and tuna are other reliable sources.

Potassium enhancers (regarding absorption) are vitamin B_6, calcium, magnesium, and essential fatty acids. Antagonists to potassium include excesses of sodium, sugar, stress, alcohol, and coffee, plus steroids, diuretics, and laxatives.

Proanthocyanidins—are antioxidants, ACE inhibitors, and beneficial to smokers; reduce platelet aggregation, protect endothelium against white blood cell adherence, increase exercise tolerance

Many names aptly describe the flavonoids found in pine bark, grape seed, citrus peel, lemon tree bark, peanuts, and cranberries. The scientific community once referred to this entire family as pycnogenols, a term now considered outdated. Today pycnogenols are recognized by terms such as proanthocyanidins, oligomeric proanthocyanidin complexes (OPCs), or procyanidolic oligomers (PCOs). In the United States, Pycnogenol is a registered trademark for Horphag Ltd. of Switzerland, identifying a PCO derived from French maritime pine trees.

Much discussion as to whether pine bark or grape seed extract delivers the most medicinal advantage still leaves the question unresolved. Dr. Michael Murray states that while both are excellent sources of proanthocyanidins, grape seed extracts are available that contain from 92–95% PCO content; pine bark extracts vary from 80–85%. An overwhelming majority of the published clinical and experimental trials over the past 20 years have been performed using the grape seed extract, not the extract of pine bark (Murray 1995b).

Peter Rohdewald, Ph.D., reported that nitric oxide (NO) became the molecule of the year in 1993 when, among other functions, it was determined that NO was a powerful vasodilator (Rohdewald 1999). NO is produced in the endothelial cells from arginine, a process controlled by the enzyme, endothelial nitric oxide synthase. Scientists became additionally excited when it was determined that PCOs stimulate endothelial nitric oxide synthase, producing more NO. This action counteracts the vasoconstricting effects of the stress hormone adrenaline and also diminishes the threat of platelets clumping.

Studies indicate that PCOs may be an alternative to aspirin. Among 180 post-stroke patients receiving 500 mg a day of aspirin for 2 years, 21% were forced to stop medication because of side effects; more than 41% experienced an increase in bleeding time. John D. Folts (University of Wisconsin) reported that flavonoids benefited laboratory monkeys, reducing the incidence of platelet aggregation and blocked arteries with efficiency equal to or greater than aspirin. Adrenaline can completely wipe out the positive effects of aspirin, but it has no degrading effect on flavonoids. PCOs offer neither GI toxicity nor an effect on coagulation, suggesting a better risk–benefit ratio compared to aspirin (Folts 1997; Watson 1999; Duke 2000b).

Research cited in *The Lancet* showed an inverse relationship between flavonoid intake and the risk of heart attack, that is, the more flavonoids ingested, the less the incidence of heart disease (Hertog et al. 1993). PCOs provide some of the most beneficial classes of plant flavonoids available.

Consider the multiple pathways PCOs employ to protect against heart disease:

- Inhibits ACE (the angiotensin-converting enzyme) (Duke 2000b). This means that the production of angiotensin II (a vasoconstricting compound) is blocked and sodium and water retention decreases. These actions decrease blood pressure and improve cardiac output; a decrease in heart size usually follows.

- Protects the endothelium from leukocyte adherence, a process that lessens the threat of occlusion (Cooke et al. 1997; Rohdewald 1999).

- Increases intracellular vitamin C levels, a function that strengthens capillary and blood vessel walls (Schwitters et al. 1993; Murray 1995b).

- Appears to offer about 50 times more antioxidant protection than vitamin C or vitamin E, an action that assists in shielding LDL cholesterol from the cardiac damaging oxidation process (Murray 1995b).

- Lowers blood cholesterol levels, even shrinking the size of cholesterol deposits appearing in the arteries of laboratory animals (Wegrowski et al. 1984).

- Increases treadmill endurance (improvement confirmed by electrocardiograms and stress tests) and reduces myocardial ischemia and cardiovascular deterioration (Petry et al. 2001).

- Regarded as beta-adrenergic receptor blockers, reducing sympathetic nervous system activity and the "fight or flight syndrome" (Duke Database 1992).

- Reports from the Institute of Pharmaceutical Chemistry (Germany) indicate that PCOs lower platelet aggregation in heavy smokers without increasing the risk of bleeding (Rohdewald 1999). Tests confirm that the platelet aggregation index was reduced to levels closely challenging those found in nonsmokers, in part by inhibiting the synthesis of thromboxane, a compound derived from inflammatory prostaglandins that increases platelet aggregation (Putter et al. 1999).

For most individuals, 100 mg daily of PCO (grape seed-skin extract) appears adequate. Therapeutic doses are 150–300 mg a day.

Note: *While proanthocyanidins do not prolong bleeding time when used independently, if used with anticoagulant drugs, caution is advised.*

Selenium—prevents ventricular tachycardia, is a hypolipidemic, and improves diabetic symptoms, congestive heart failure, and cardiomyopathy

Cardiomyopathy is defined as any disease that affects the structure and function of the heart. For example, the heart may become disabled as fibrous tissue partially replaces the heart muscle; the fibrous tissue degrades the heart's performance, and the blood no longer moves efficiently. The World Health Organization recognizes cardiomyopathy as a selenium deficiency. In addition, French researchers showed that chronic heart failure (associated with oxidative stress) appears to be relieved by selenium supplementation. Selenium may play a role in the clinical severity of the disease, rather than in the degree of left ventricular dysfunction (de Lorgeril 2001).

Selenium limited the incidence of ventricular tachycardia—that is, at least three consecutive ventricle complexes with the heart rate more than 100 beats a minute—from 91% in the control group to 36% in the selenium-treated group; irreversible ventricular fibrillation was reduced from 45% in the control group to 0% in the selenium group (Tanguy et al. 1998). Luoma et al. (1984) noted that 97 mcg of selenium a day increased the ratio of HDL:LDL cholesterol, while inhibiting platelet aggregation. It is reported that a 1% increase in HDL reduces the risk of a heart attack or stroke 4%.

Korpela et al. (1989), in a 6-month double-blind trial involving 81 heart attack patients, found that 100 mcg of selenium reduced the number of cardiovascular events to one nonfatal heart attack, while the group not receiving the selenium suffered four fatal heart attacks and two nonfatal heart attacks. Among men free of stroke at the outset, low serum selenium was associated significantly with stroke mortality, an adjusted relative risk of 3.7 (Virtamo et al. 1985).

Selenium brought blood glucose levels, malondialdehyde (a breakdown product of peroxidized polyunsaturated lipids), and glutathione concentrations to near control levels in almost all diabetic patients. A suggested dosage is 200–300 mcg daily.

Reader's guide to selenium food sources, enhancers, and antagonists. Quantities found in foods are dependent upon the selenium content of the soil, but typically whole grains, wheat germ, broccoli, onions, tomatoes, Brazil nuts, brewer's yeast, garlic, eggs, and seafood are classed as selenium sources.

Selenium enhancers include most antioxidants and essential fatty acids. Antagonists to selenium absorption are heavy metals (mercury and cadmium), excesses of iron, saturated and *trans* fats, unresolved stress, and indulgences in alcohol and tobacco.

Taurine—has hypotensive and diuretic activity, tempers the sympathetic nervous system, is beneficial in CHF and arrhythmias, and has digitalis-like mentality

Taurine is the most important and abundant of the amino acids in the heart, surpassing the combined quantity of all the others. Under high stress conditions—hypertension and many forms of heart disease—the need for taurine increases to compensate for either an accompanying impairment of taurine metabolism or increased requirements. Dr. H. Kohaski and colleagues

(Japan) suggest that entry-level taurine may have been low and, as the stress of hypertension progresses, taurine levels drop even lower (Kahashi 1983; Braverman et al.1987).

Taurine has a diuretic action that benefits hypertensive individuals, as well as patients with congestive heart failure. Taurine elicits much of its diuretic action by preserving potassium and magnesium and by promoting sodium excretion (Atkins 1996b).

Taurine also reduces blood pressure by acting as an antagonist to the blood pressure-increasing effect of angiotensin, a circulating protein that is activated by renin, a hormone secreted by the juxtaglomerular cells in the kidneys in response to a drop in blood pressure (Braverman et al. 1987). When both blood and urine taurine levels decrease, renin is activated and angiotensin is formed. As a result blood vessels vasoconstrict, water and salt are retained, and blood pressure increases. Taurine suppresses renin and breaks the renin-angiotensin feedback loop. Dr. Robert Atkins, a complementary physician with a creditable cardiology background, amplifies the positive results of scientific literature, stating that taurine would be his choice were he selecting a single nutrient to treat hypertension.

Dr. Y. Yamori (a Japanese researcher who established an amino acid–stroke association) studied a strain of rats, genetically susceptible to strokes. Yamori found the rats had a much lower incidence of stroke, dropping from 90% to 20%, if their diet was supplemented with methionine, taurine, and lysine (Yamori et al. 1983; Braverman et al. 1987).

Japanese researchers found that 3 grams of taurine, administered daily to patients with congestive heart failure, was more effective than 30 mg of CoQ_{10} (Azuma et al. 1992). The Japanese, who use taurine widely in the treatment of various forms of heart disease, found that 4 grams of taurine, given for 4 weeks, brought relief to 19 of 24 patients with congestive heart failure. Taurine appears to act much like the drug digitalis, increasing the contractility of cardiac muscle and the force of the pumping action.

Taurine appears to impact cardiac arrhythmias through various pathways. For example, some forms of cardiac irregularities are helped by taurine because it regulates membrane excitability and scavenges free radicals. In addition, taurine protects potassium levels inside heart cells, which, when imbalanced, can cause electrical instability and cardiac arrhythmias (Braverman 1987; Chahine et al. 1998).

Some types of premature ventricular contractions and arrhythmias respond to taurine because the amino acid tends to dampen activity in the sympathetic nervous system (SNS) and the outpouring of epinephrine.

As the SNS is quieted, the heart tends to beat less aggressively and the blood pressure is lowered. Lastly, Lebanese researchers showed that the incidence of ventricular fibrillation and ventricular tachycardia were significantly reduced when taurine therapy was utilized (Braverman 1987; Chahine et al. 1998). A suggested dosage is 1500–4000 mg daily.

Testosterone—modulates cholesterol levels, dilates blood vessels, improves circulation, lessens angina attacks, and reduces blood pressure

Testosterone, a muscle-building hormone, appears to do far more than promote the development of male secondary sexual characteristics. There are, in fact, many testosterone-receptor sites in the heart that play a role in maintaining heart muscle protein synthesis and strength (Bricout et al. 1994).

If testosterone levels are normal, cholesterol is more easily managed, and blood has an easier route as it flows through dilated vessels. One study showed that circulation to the heart improved 68.8% in patients receiving testosterone therapy (Wu et al. 1993). A testosterone delivery patch applied to men with low testosterone levels increased exercise time on a treadmill and (according to trial participants) increased quality of life. Improved emotional health (important to the heart) and a decrease in the incidence of angina attacks reflect some of the benefits of upgrading testosterone levels (English et al. 2000).

Typically, fibrinogen, triglycerides, and insulin levels are higher if testosterone levels are low (Marin 1995; Kryger 2002). In addition, the elasticity of the coronary arteries diminishes, contributing to the development of arteriosclerosis. Blood pressure increases, but the growth hormone decreases, further weakening the heart muscle. Abdominal fat, the most dangerous form of obesity, increases.

Physicians who check for testosterone deficiencies or testosterone–estrogen imbalances have in some cases been able to discontinue cardiac and hypertension medications. Improved EKGs confirm subjective reports of improvement. Since testosterone testing is noninvasive, the risk–benefit ratio swings heavily in favor of testing. For information about safely increasing testosterone levels, refer to the *Male Hormone* or *Female Hormone Modulation* protocols.

Thiamine (Vitamin B₁)— is beneficial in some forms of cardiac arrhythmias, palpitations, enlarged heart, elevated venous pressure, and congestive heart disease

Cardiac arrhythmia refers to a deviation from the normal pattern of the heartbeat. Arrhythmias can be caused by a variety of underlying medical conditions that should be addressed by a qualified cardiologist. Arrhythmias are not always clinically significant because rather benign events can spur healthy hearts to enter irregular patterns of beating. Yet, arrhythmias should be taken seriously, and a diagnosis made as to the causative factors provoking the disturbed beat. Stress, electrolyte imbalance, ischemia, hypoxia, ventricular enlargement, occlusions, an insulin rush, or derangement in the autonomic nervous system can drive a heart into irregular rhythms.

Since thiamine has proved correctional for some types of arrhythmias, there appears to be linkage between irregular heartbeats and beriberi, a disease caused by a deficiency of or an inability to assimilate thiamine. Cultures that depended upon rice, a high carbohydrate food, as a dietary mainstay found the milling process, that is, the removal of the brown coat rich in thiamine, to be their undoing. Beriberi swept through the population with epidemic force.

Cardiac arrhythmias may manifest among heavy drinkers as thiamine deficiencies occur, and symptoms of beriberi appear. But, heavy imbibers are not the only individuals susceptible to thiamine deficiency. Infirm individuals, as well as those who are elderly and malnourished, are at particular risk. Long-term diuretic usage can also contribute to a thiamine deficiency through urinary loss. It is not uncommon for heart palpitations, deranged heart rhythms, and elevated venous pressure to occur as patients become thiamine deficient (Whiting 1989). Additional cardiovascular manifestations of wet beriberi are myocardial lesions, sodium and water retention, and biventricular myocardial failure. Typically, clinical improvement occurs quickly following vitamin B₁ therapy (Blanc et al. 2000).

In 1995, 30 patients with severe heart failure and taking furosemide (Lasix, a diuretic) were enrolled in a heart study. Although furosemide was unsuccessful in improving their cardiac condition, 200 mg of thiamine (a day) dramatically improved heart function (Shimon et al. 1995). Some patients may experience improvement from 200–250 mg a day; other individuals may require 500–1000 mg daily. (A full spectrum vitamin B supplement should always accompany single B vitamin supplementation.)

Reader's guide to vitamin B₁ food sources, enhancers, and antagonists. Lean pork, wheat germ, and whole grains (particularly brown rice) are considered to be excellent sources of thiamine. Meat, poultry, egg yolk, fish, legumes, peas, sunflower seeds, nuts, and brewer's yeast represent other good thiamine choices.

Vitamin B_1 enhancers are all others of the B complex, vitamin C, vitamin E, and manganese. Alcohol, coffee, antacids, and excesses of sugar and refined carbohydrates decrease thiamine absorption.

Tocotrienols—are antioxidants, decrease platelet aggregation, and act like statin drugs

Tocotrienols have been until recently the lesser known half of vitamin E. A major functional difference between tocotrienols and tocopherols appears to be the ability of tocotrienols to more aptly decrease cholesterol synthesis in the liver. Both tocotrienols and tocopherols appear to be potent antioxidants, with some research demonstrating greater antioxidant protection and less oxidative damage when supplementing with tocotrienols (Serbinova et al. 1991).

Cholesterol lowering statin drugs—Lipitor, Lescol, Mevacor, Pravachol, and Zocor—operate at the level of 3-hydroxy-3 methylglutaral coenzyme A (HMG-CoA) reductase. HMG-CoA reductase is a rate-limiting enzyme that participates in cholesterol synthesis. The cholesterol cascade occurs as follows: (1) acetyl-CoA is converted to HMG-CoA, (2) HMG-CoA is reduced to mevalonic acid by the enzyme HMG-CoA reductase, and (3) several steps convert mevalonic acid to squalene and then to cholesterol.

Tocotrienols, particularly gamma and delta, accelerate the degradation of HMG-CoA reductase, altering the functionality of the enzyme responsible for cholesterol synthesis (Parker et al. 1993). The statin drugs, though acting at the level of HMG-CoA reductase, approach the enzyme differently. Statin drugs do not degrade the enzyme but competitively inhibit its binding. The inhibition of the binding mechanism leads to a higher production of HMG-CoA reductase, which may explain the side effects, such as liver toxicity, associated with statin usage.

Studies indicate that roughly 75% of hypercholesterolemic individuals respond favorably to tocotrienol supplementation. The most impressive cholesterol reductions occur when tocotrienol supplements are combined with dietary changes (a high fiber/low fat diet). In a 12-week double-blind trial, those who responded to tocotrienol therapy saw a reduction of approximately 23% in total cholesterol and a 32% reduction in LDL cholesterol using dietary modification plus tocotrienol supplements. Tocotrienols alone yielded a 16% decrease in total cholesterol and a 21% decrease in LDL cholesterol (Quereshi et al. 1993; ACCM 1998). HDL levels do not appear to respond to tocotrienol supplementation, but apo-B, a protein component found in LDL, VLDL, and IDL cholesterol, is lowered. Thromboxanes are also considered tocotrienol responsive (Qureshi et al. 1997).

The Kenneth Jordan Heart Research Foundation (New Jersey) reported the results of 50 patients with narrowing of the carotid artery that were treated with either a placebo or tocotrienols: 25 patients (some with carotid stenosis greater than 49%) received 650 mg of tocotrienols plus tocopherols; a control group of 25 patients, with comparable closure, received a placebo. Each group was evaluated every 6 months for the first year and every year thereafter with ultrasonography. In the placebo group, 15 patients showed worsening of the stenosis, eight remained stable, and two showed some level of improvement. In the tocotrienol plus tocopherol group, three patients showed minor worsening, 12 remained stable, but 10 patients showed regression of stenosis. Participants experienced a simultaneous drop in triglycerides and LDL cholesterol (Papas undated; Tomeo et al. 1995; Watkins et al.1998).

The late Karl Folkers, a pioneer in CoQ_{10} research, observed that drugs inhibiting HMG-CoA reductase activity cause a simultaneous decrease in CoQ_{10} levels (Folkers et al. 1990). The reason for this is that the HMG-CoA enzyme also plays a role in CoQ_{10} synthesis. Individuals using either statin drugs or tocotrienols may wish to increase their intake of CoQ_{10}; a decrease in CoQ_{10} could negate any benefit garnered from a hypocholesterolemic drug.

According to Andreas M. Papas, Ph.D., appropriate tocotrienol dosages are as follows: 100 IU of mixed tocopherols and 100 IU of tocotrienols if young and healthy and without a family history of heart disease; 200 IU of mixed tocopherols and 200 IU of tocotrienols for young adults with some cardiac risk factors or healthy people up to 50 years of age without risk factors; 400 IU of mixed tocopherols and 400 IU of tocotrienols for people who have a personal or family history of chronic heart disease. The latter dosage includes senior subjects and those under severe stress and eating a poor diet.

Vitamin A and Beta-Carotene—lower fibrinogen levels and heart disease risks and increase insulin sensitivity

Dexter Morris, M.D. (University of North Carolina), says that phytochemicals keep your heart healthy. "The 60–80 age group has a much greater risk of heart disease than younger people do. If your diet is rich in fruits and vegetables, you can reduce risk," according to Morris. In a study begun in 1973, researchers kept track of 1883 men ages 35–59 that had high cholesterol levels. Over the next 20 years, the men who had the highest levels of carotenoids in their blood had 60% fewer heart attacks and deaths (Morris 2001).

Dr. J.E. Manson of the Women's Hospital in Boston reported that those taking 25,000 IU of beta-carotene daily had 22% fewer heart problems and strokes than those taking less than 10,000 IU daily (Friend 1991; Passwater undated). Dr. Monika Eichholzer (scientist at the University of Bern, Switzerland) reported similar findings after tracking 2974 people for 12 years. The relative risk of ischemic heart disease was increased (1.53%) among those lowest in plasma carotene concentrations (Eichholzer et al. 1992).

High vitamin A and beta-carotene serum levels have been reported to reduce fibrinogen levels in humans and animals (Green 1997). Animals fed a vitamin A-deficient diet have an impaired ability to break down fibrinogen, but when injected with vitamin A, they produce tissue plasminogen activators that break down fibrinogen, reducing the risk of clot formation.

Vitamin A is beneficial to individuals with Syndrome X and diabetes. A study involving 52 patients indicated that vitamin A enhanced insulin-mediated glucose disposal (Facchini et al. 1996a). Since beta-carotene must be converted in the body to vitamin A, an adaptation some individuals lack, diabetics may do better using vitamin A rather than beta-carotene.

It should be noted that the protection of beta-carotene is not absolute. In fact, if the individual is consuming greater amounts of alcohol, beta-carotene may actually increase the risk of intracerebral hemorrhage (Leppala et al. 2000). A blend of phytoextracts (alpha-carotene, beta-carotene, lutein, and lycopene) appears to offer more comprehensive cardiac protection than using beta-carotene alone.

For example, individuals participating in the Toulouse study who had higher blood levels of lutein also had a lower incidence of coronary artery disease (Howard et al. 1996). The Los Angeles Atherosclerosis study uncovered a relationship between thickenings in the carotid arteries (an indicator of systemic atherosclerosis) and blood levels of lutein (Dwyer et al. 2001). Participants with the highest blood levels of lutein showed virtually no artery wall thickening, while those with the lowest lutein levels showed increased arterial thickness. In addition, lutein reduces the oxidation of LDL cholesterol, a declaration the Life Extension Foundation first made to members in 1985.

A current Finnish study evaluated 725 middle-aged men free of coronary heart disease and stroke at the study baseline. Men in the lowest quartile of serum levels of lycopene had a 3.3-fold risk of an acute coronary event or stroke compared with other trial participants with higher lycopene levels. In a second study, the same researchers assessed the association between plasma concentrations of lycopene and intima-media thickness (IMT) of the common carotid artery wall in 520 asymptomatic men and women. After adjusting for common cardiovascular risk factors, low plasma levels of lycopene were associated with an 18% increase in IMT in men as compared with men in whom plasma levels were higher than median. In women, the difference did not remain significant after the adjustments (Rissenen et al. 2002).

German researchers reported that plasma levels of alpha-carotene may represent a marker of atherosclerosis in humans. Measuring alpha-carotene levels (among other antioxidants) may be of clinical importance as a practical approach to assess atherogenesis and/or its risk (Kontush et al. 1996).

Some individuals are susceptible to vitamin A toxicity even when the dosage is low. This occurs because of a challenged liver and fewer detoxification mechanisms. Beta-carotene, on the other hand, is generally regarded as nontoxic (*to read more about vitamin A toxicity, consult Appendix A*). Appropriate dosages for most individuals are 5000 IU of beta-carotene and/or 10,000 IU of vitamin A daily. Several supplements are available that provide the carotenoids alpha-carotene, beta-carotene, lutein, and lycopene.

Reader's guide to vitamin A food sources, enhancers, and agonists. The richest sources of vitamin A are foods of animal origin, i.e., liver, fish liver oil, milk and milk products, butter, and eggs. Yellow fruits and green and yellow vegetables will also help meet vitamin A requirements.

Enhancers to vitamin A absorption are vitamin C, calcium, magnesium, vitamin E, B complex, choline, and essential fatty acids. Vitamin A antagonists are laxatives and some cholesterol-lowering drugs (Questran). Coffee, alcohol, excess iron supplementation, sugar, tobacco, and mineral oil can also interfere with vitamin A absorption. Food sources of lutein are kale, brussels sprouts, corn, collards, spinach, and egg yolks. Egg yolks have tiny amounts of lutein—about 0.2 mg per yolk—because chickens eat corn (Carper 2002). Lycopene is present in tomatoes and several other red fruits.

Vitamin C—lessens risk of stroke and heart attack; strengthens blood vessels; reduces blood pressure, fibrinogen levels, Lp(a), inflammation, and C-reactive protein (CRP); promotes gingival healing; is a reliable antioxidant and diuretic; and is highly beneficial to smokers and those exposed to secondhand smoke

Linus Pauling, a Nobel Prize winner, showed that the body often forms atherosclerotic plaque to repair a wound inflicted upon an artery. When adequate amounts of vitamin C are available, an injured artery is repaired without involving atheromatous materials. In the absence of adequate levels of vitamin C, Lp(a), acting as a surrogate for vitamin C, must participate in the repair. Lp(a) does what it must, but the health of the artery is compromised as plaque is added to the vessel. If ascorbate levels had been adequate, Lp(a) would not have been necessary; without adequate vitamin C, the need for Lp(a) is enormous.

Vitamin C Lowers Lp(a)

Kathie M. Dalessandri, M.S., M.D., was inspired by a report appearing in the *Archives of Internal Medicine* relating to the ability of vitamin C to lower Lp(a). Dr. Dalessandri, a general surgeon in Point Reyes Station, CA, was displeased with her own Lp(a) levels. She was well aware of the dangers associated with Lp(a), particularly when linked with other risk factors as a family history of heart disease. Dr. Dalessandri (53 years old at the time) was taking hormone replacement therapy and niacin, but the niacin became problematic and had to be discontinued. After reviewing the literature, she decided upon 3 grams a day of both ascorbic acid and *L*-lysine monohydrochloride as a natural regime against the elevated Lp(a). Dr. Dalessandri reports that her Lp(a) dropped 14 mg/dL, a reduction of 48% after 6 months. She was also pleased that she was able to take vitamin C and lysine without side effects (Dalessandri 2001).

Matthias Rath, M.D., in *Eradicating Heart Disease*, says that animals do not have heart attacks and strokes because their bodies manufacture vitamin C, a genetic adaptation humans lack. Most mammals produce impressive amounts of vitamin C, the human equivalency of 2000–13,000 mg daily. Under periods of stress the same animal's needs for vitamin C may skyrocket, but the body complies by producing prodigious amounts. Man cannot adapt to stress with the same efficiency as lower animals because of a lack of *L*-gulonolactone oxidase, an enzyme needed to produce vitamin C from glucose. Dr. Rath states that because of this genetic flaw and inadequate dietary

vitamin C, cardiovascular disease can emerge as a form of early scurvy (Rath 1993).

An ascorbic acid deficit contributes to the development of vascular lesions (wounds or injuries) by altering collagen metabolism (Rath 1993). Vitamin C produces many collagen molecules, supporting a strong and elastic blood vessel wall. Over time, arterial collagen must be replenished. If vitamin C is not present in large enough quantities, collagen is not produced, and blood vessels become thin and weak.

Vitamin C levels are lower in patients who have had heart attacks, both fatal and nonfatal events. Randomly selected Finnish men (1605 individuals who were 42–60 years old) entered a study evidencing no signs of preexisting heart disease. Among men with a vitamin C deficiency, 13.2% had a heart attack compared to 3.8% who were not vitamin C deficient. After adjusting for other confounding factors, men who were deficient in vitamin C had 3.5 times more heart attacks than men who were not vitamin C deficient (Nyyssonen et al. 1997).

The most significant report emanated from UCLA, where it was announced that men who took 300–400 mg of vitamin C a day lived 6 years longer than those who received less than 50 mg daily. The study (which evaluated 11,348 participants over a 10-year period) showed that long-term, high vitamin C intake extended average lifespan and reduced mortality from cardiovascular disease 45% (Enstrom et al. 1992; Hansen 2000).

Researchers from the Boston University School of Medicine reported that vitamin C appears effective in lowering mild cases of hypertension. The patients lowered systolic and diastolic blood pressure by about 9% with a daily dose of 500 mg of ascorbic acid (Stauth 2001). The value of vitamin C as a hypotensive nutrient may come by way of its antioxidant activity, possibly by protecting the body's supply of NO, a vasodilator. (Free radicals appear to lower NO levels.) Depriving test animals of antioxidants, such as vitamin C, glutathione, and vitamin E, resulted in oxidative stress and higher blood pressure.

The heart is one of the most vulnerable of all organs to free-radical oxidative stress. Vitamin C can respond to this risk by exerting its antioxidant properties, acting independently, or by prompting the production of other antioxidants. For example, 3 grams of vitamin C increased white blood cell glutathione levels fourfold and plasma glutathione levels eightfold (Jain et al. 1994; Murray 1996b).

Vitamin C is beneficial in reducing fibrinogen levels. In a report published in the journal *Atherosclerosis*, heart disease patients were given either 1000 or 2000 mg a day of vitamin C to assess its effect on the break-down of fibrinogen. At 1000 mg a day, there was no significant change in fibrinolytic activity. At 2000 mg of vitamin C a day, fibrinolytic activity increased 62.5% (Bordia 1980).

Inflammation, a newer risk factor for heart disease, is reduced by vitamin C. Each winter (in most countries) there is a 15–30% increase in deaths from cardiovascular and respiratory disease. Researchers in the United Kingdom followed 96 men and women for 1 year to assess the impact of winter stress upon the heart and circulatory system. It appears some of the increase in winter cardiovascular mortality may be related not only to a rise in fibrinogen, but also to an increase in other inflammatory markers, such as C-reactive protein. This cycle may be spurred as winter infections increase and vitamin C intake (because of less availability of fruits and vegetables) decreases. The conclusion of the study was that vitamin C might be able to influence cardiovascular risk and the resulting thrombotic tendency by modulating the inflammatory response to infection (Woodhouse et al. 1997).

Vitamin C appears to lessen the negative effects of many other risk factors, including stress, diseased gums, unhealthy diet, and smoking. Smoking severely depletes the body of vitamin C; vitamin C, on the other hand, destroys free radicals produced in smoke and protects against endothelial dysfunction. Even secondhand smoke breaks down blood antioxidant defenses and accelerates lipid peroxidation, which leads to an accumulation of LDL cholesterol (Tribble et al. 1993). Vitamin C should be a part of an individual's nutritional fortress against the ravages of both firsthand and passive smoke.

A dosage suggestion is 6 grams daily in divided dosages. (A loose stool may result from higher doses of vitamin C. Should this occur simply reduce the dose to a level that is not problematic to the bowel.) Under periods of stress, a great deal more vitamin C can be taken without bowel derangement.

Reader's guide to vitamin C food sources, enhancers, and antagonists. Vegetables and fresh, uncooked fruits (especially citrus) are vitamin C-rich sources. Raw foods represent excellent choices, having escaped the rigors of processing and preparation.

All vitamins and minerals work synergistically to enhance vitamin C absorption, particularly the bioflavonoids. Alcohol, coffee, sulfa drugs, antibiotics, analgesics, antidepressants, anticoagulants, oral contraceptives, and steroids can drain vitamin C from the body. Smoking seriously depletes vitamin C levels.

Vitamin D—reduces heart disease risk in women

It was reported at the 42nd annual conference on Cardiovascular Disease and Epidemiology Prevention (in Honolulu, HI, on April 23, 2002) that women who take vitamin D supplements lowered their risk of death from heart disease by one-third. The finding was an unexpected dividend extracted from an osteoporosis trial to determine the incidence of bone fracture in nearly 10,000 older women. From the trial participants, 4200 women reported taking vitamin D supplements at the onset of the study; another 733 reported a prior history of supplementation. After tracking the women for an average of nearly 11 years, researchers found that the risk of heart disease death was 31% lower in those taking vitamin D at the time of the study (Mercola 2002b).

Recent studies indicate that moderate or severe hypovitaminosis D was present in 66% of patients taking daily vitamin D in amounts less than the recommended dosage for their age; 37% of the patients taking daily vitamin D in excess of the recommended amount for their age were nonetheless still deficient. Thus, experts recommend at least 400 IU of vitamin D a day; if the individual is elderly and not participating in outdoor activities (and sunlight exposure), 800 IU a day is recommended (Thomas et al. 2000).

Vitamin E—prevents plaque formation, protects LDL from oxidation, strengthens blood vessels, reduces blood viscosity and platelet aggregation, is helpful in atrial and ventricular fibrillation, is an antioxidant and antidiabetic nutrient, improves insulin sensitivity, is protective to smokers, reduces C-reactive protein, has diuretic activity, and is beneficial to those with hemochromatosis

Dr. Richard Passwater commented in June 2001 that good research is timeless. The following is an example of an excellent study that should not be lost in the archives. In 1974, Dr. Passwater enrolled 17,894 persons (ages 50–98) in a study to determine the effects of long-term vitamin E supplementation. He found the length of time the individual used vitamin E was more important than the amount of the nutrient used. The trend was especially apparent beyond 9 years of usage. Taking 400 IU of vitamin E daily for 10 years or more strikingly reduced the occurrence of heart disease prior to 80 years of age (Passwater 1977).

An ongoing study involving 87,245 nurses (ages 34–59) and 39,910 male health professionals (ages 40–75) showed a significant relationship between the use of vitamin E supplements and a reduced risk of heart disease (Rimm et al.1993; Stampfer et al. 1993). A study reported in *The Lancet* may have eclipsed all others, showing that 2002 individuals with documented heart disease (supplemented with 400–800 IU of vitamin E daily) reduced their risk of nonfatal heart attacks 77% (Stephens 1996; Challem 2001).

These dramatic results occur in part because vitamin E prevents white blood cells from adhering to arterial walls. Researchers from the University of Texas Southwestern Medical Center explain that when monocytes are suppressed from bonding to the artery, a primary step in arterial closure has been averted (Devaraj et al. 2000a).

According to researchers at Georgetown University Medical School, vitamin E also renders the blood less sticky and platelets less prone to clump. In animal models of endothelial dysfunction, vitamin E improved the activity of endothelium-derived nitric oxide; this effect was not dependent upon the antioxidant protection of LDL cholesterol. Instead, it appears vitamin E inhibits platelet aggregation through a mechanism that involves protein kinase C inhibition, not its antioxidant activity as previously suspected (Freedman et al. 2001).

French scientists found that alpha-tocopherol supplementation prevented lethal ventricular arrhythmias associated with ischemia and reperfusion. In addition, animals with coronary arteries occluded for experimentation experienced a significant decrease in the ventricular fibrillation threshold; animals similarly occluded, but vitamin E supplemented, realized no decrease in the threshold (Dzhaparidze et al. 1986; Fuenmayor et al. 1989; Sebbag et al. 1994). *Comment:* Ventricular tachycardia represents at least three consecutive ventricular complexes with a heart rate of more than 100 beats a minute. Ventricular fibrillation is a cardiac arrhythmia marked by rapid, disorganized depolarizations of the ventricular myocardium. Blood pressure falls to zero, resulting in unconsciousness; without defibrillation and resuscitation, death can promptly ensue.

According to Ron Kennedy, M.D., atrial fibrillation is a condition in which the regular pumping function of the atria is replaced by a disorganized, ineffective quivering caused by the chaotic conduction of electrical signals through the upper chambers of the heart. The patient has various corrective options, including anti-arrhythmic drugs, anticoagulants, radio-frequency ablation, a pacemaker, and, according to Dr. Kennedy, high-dose (2000 IU a day) vitamin E. Recall that vitamin E reduces blood viscosity and platelet aggregation. If the patient is receiving anticoagulant therapy and wishes to add vitamin E,

close monitoring by a physician is essential to avoid compromising the clotting mechanism (Kennedy 1999).

Researchers from the University of Naples reported encouraging data regarding pharmacological doses (about 900 mg a day) of vitamin E administered to elderly patients with coronary heart disease and insulin resistance. Lower fasting and 2-hour blood glucose levels, reduced plasma insulin and triglyceride concentrations, and an improved HDL:LDL ratio indicate vitamin E is useful in stabilizing insulin-resistant patients with coronary heart disease (Paolisso et al. 1995).

According to Drs. Ishwarlal Jialal and Sridevi Deveraj (University of Texas Southwestern Medical Center at Dallas), diabetics have increased inflammation and are more prone to cardiovascular disease (Deveraj et al. 2000). Vitamin E, by decreasing inflammation, may contribute to a reduction in cardiovascular disease in both diabetic and nondiabetic subjects. Vitamin E lowered levels of IL-6 50% and 1200 IU of vitamin E reduced C-reactive protein (CRP) 30% (Devaraj et al. 2000b; O'Brien 2001). CRP levels remained constant 2 months postsupplementation. For an in-depth review of CRP, consult the CRP subsection under the sections *Newer Risk Factors* and *The Link Between Infections and Inflammation in Heart Disease*, in this protocol.

Vitamin E appears to be decreased in patients with hereditary hemochromatosis or iron overload. Iron loading, in experimental studies, significantly decreases hepatic and plasma vitamin E, a shortage amenable with supplementation. Free-radical index markers increase three- to fivefold in an iron-loaded liver, but supplementation with vitamin E has been shown to reduce levels by about 50% (Brown et al. 1996).

Free radicals activate a gene that encourages overgrowth of smooth muscles in the blood vessel walls, a process that can contribute to closure (Gonzalez-Flecha 2002). Vitamin E, a reliable antioxidant, has the opposite effect, that is, it turns off the gene responsible for smooth muscle proliferation. Vitamin E's antioxidant powers extend to protect the cells and organs (particularly the lungs) from damage caused by smoking.

Vitamin E has been credited (for decades) with diuretic activity, stimulating urine excretion (Davis 1965). This action is of a significant advantage to patients with edematous tissues and elevated blood pressure.

The type and blend of vitamin E used affects the end results. Studies have shown that alpha-tocopherol may not protect as aggressively against coronary heart disease unless it is combined with the gamma-tocopherol form. Both alpha-tocopherol and gamma-tocopherol can decrease platelet aggregation, inhibit blood clot formation, protect LDL cholesterol against oxidation, and increase endogenous SOD production (an enzyme with antioxidant activity); gamma-tocopherol, however, shows greater activity on each function.

Unfortunately, gamma-tocopherol has a couple of factors working against its utilization. For example, gamma-tocopherol can be obtained from foodstuffs, but it is poorly retained, and much of it is excreted in urine after being metabolized by the liver. Furthermore, a protein, referred to as alpha-tocopherol transfer protein, identifies and selectively chooses alpha-tocopherol over other forms of vitamin E. As a result, alpha-tocopherol is found more abundantly in lipids, blood, and body tissues. This scenario does not allow for maximum protection against free-radical attack.

It is strongly recommended that individuals relying upon the cardioprotective effects of vitamin E include (as part of their intake) the gamma-tocopherol form, but the complexing process determines the benefit. A union of alpha-tocopherol (80%) with gamma-tocopherol (20%) appears ideal; too much alpha-tocopherol may oppose the antioxidant qualities of gamma-tocopherol.

In addition, the hypolipidemic value of tocotrienols, the lesser known half of vitamin E, should not be overlooked. The most dramatic cholesterol reduction is seen when tocotrienol supplements are combined with dietary changes (a high-fiber, low-fat diet). In a 12-week, double-blind trial, those who responded to tocotrienol therapy saw a reduction of approximately 23% in total cholesterol and 32% in LDL cholesterol using dietary modification plus tocotrienol supplements. Tocotrienols alone yielded a 16% decrease in total cholesterol and a 21% decrease in LDL cholesterol (Quereshi et al. 1993; ACCM 1998). apo-B, a protein component found in LDL, VLDL, and IDL cholesterol also appears to be tocotrienol responsive (Qureshi et al. 1997).

Tocotrienols degrade the enzyme 3-hydroxy-3-methylgulutaryl coenzyme A reductase, the rate-limiting enzyme that participates in cholesterol synthesis. Researchers credited this function as being the mechanism delivering tocotrienol's hypolipidemic edge (Qureshi et al. 2001). A team of researchers from Switzerland reported greater hypolipidemic value when using gamma-tocotrienol rather than a mixture of tocotrienols (Raederstorff et al. 2002). To read more about tocotrienols and dosing recommendations, please consult the *Tocotrienols* subsection appearing earlier in this section.

A suggested dosage of vitamin E is 400–1200 IU a day. *Comment:* Initially, blood pressure rose in approximately one-third of hypertensive individuals treated with vitamin E (Shute 1976). Therefore, individuals who are hypertensive should use 100 IU a day for 1 month and add 100 IU each month until 400 IU a day is reached (Balch et al. 1997). Because of the reductions in blood glucose levels, diabetic individuals wishing to use vitamin E should begin with low dosages. Gradually increase the dosage, allowing for appropriate insulin or drug adjustments. Lastly, Pracon, Inc., a hospital outcomes analysis firm in Reston, VA, estimated that healthcare expenses could be reduced $7.7 billion annually if the public regularly took vitamin E supplements.

Reader's guide to vitamin E food sources, enhancers, and antagonists. Vitamin E is found in wheat germ, whole grains (brown rice, cornmeal, oatmeal, and wheat), vegetable oils (soybean, corn, and cottonseed), egg yolk, butter, milk fat, meat (especially liver), dark green leafy vegetables, legumes, nuts, and seeds.

Vitamin E enhancers are vitamin A, B complex vitamins, vitamin C, magnesium, manganese, selenium, inositol, and essential fatty acids. For optimal vitamin E absorption, excessive fat intake should be avoided, as well as birth control pills and the chronic use of mineral oil.

Vitamin K—modulates calcium levels; reduces inflammation, C-reactive protein (CRP), IL-6, the risk of thrombosis, and the progression to valvular stenosis; and has a role in glucose management

As important as calcium is as a hypotensive and antiarrhythmic mineral, it has a detrimental side if it seeps into arteries. Arterial calcification, common to the aging process, is a risk factor leading to the development of heart disease, atherosclerosis, and mitral and aortic valve stenosis. Researchers recently reported the results of a comprehensive study evaluating 2213 individuals over a 10.4-year period in regard to coronary calcium levels. Those with a calcium score in the fourth quartile were 3.7 times more likely to die over the 10 years than were individuals in the first quartile (Buenano et al. 2000).

Harvard Medical School announced that about 25% of adults over 65 years of age have arterial calcification, increasing their risk of severe heart disease 50% (Harvard Heart Letter 1999). However, the Framingham Heart Study determined that the risks imposed by thoracic aortic calcification are not restricted to senior subjects; 35-year-old men with aortic calcification had 7 times the risk of dying of a sudden heart attack (Witteman et al. 1990).

The cumulative results of 8 years of research determined that women with severe kyphosis (increased convexity in the curvature of the thoracic spine) increased their risk of pulmonary death (likely a blood clot) by 2.6 times. Compared with women who were fracture-free, those with one or more vertebral fractures had a 1.23 times greater mortality rate. Mortality increased as the number of fractures increased (Kado et al. 1999).

It was also noted that women with atherosclerotic calcification had 7% less bone mass. Dutch researchers connected the dots and determined that postmenopausal women with calcification in bone tissue and atherosclerotic vessels had diminished vitamin K levels. It was concluded that vitamin K status affects the mineralization process in both bone and atherosclerotic plaque (Jie et al. 1996).

Vitamin K, an underutilized fat-soluble vitamin, overcomes the pathological effects of a calcium imbalance by promoting the deposition of calcium in its primary site (bone) and out of arterial walls.

Note: *Because of the number of individuals using anticoagulants, it is important to note that warfarin (Coumadin) caused extensive arterial calcification in laboratory animals (Howe et al. 2000). Humans on long-term warfarin therapy may be at an increased risk for developing arterial calcification due to a drug-induced vitamin K deficiency.*

So interrelated is bone loss to cardiovascular disease that measuring bone density has become a predictive factor for cardiovascular health. If bone density deviates one standard from the norm, the risk of stroke increases 3 times (Mitchell 2000). Vitamin K thus emerges as a star player in cardiovascular health, keeping calcium in bones and out of arteries and valves. *Note:* Be aware that the risks imposed by low bone density have no gender preference. Low bone density is a strong and independent predictor of all-cause and cardiovascular mortality in both men and women (Trivedi et al. 2001).

A group of animals with induced atherosclerosis were given vitamin K (100 mg/kg of body weight), vitamin E (40mg/kg), or a placebo to assess reversal of the atherosclerotic process. At the conclusion of the study, the control group showed aortic calcium of 17.5 microns/mg; those receiving vitamin K had approximately 1 micron/mg of calcium, and vitamin E reduced it even further (Seyama et al. 1999) (*for more*

information relating to valvular calcification, consult the section devoted to Valvular Disease in this protocol).

With age, the levels of IL-6 increase. This creates an imbalance between anti-inflammatory and pro-inflammatory cytokines (Ferrucci et al. 1999). Disproportionate numbers of good and bad cytokines increase inflammation, as well as bone degradation.

IL-6 is germane to this untoward sequence, promoting not only the inflammatory process, but also bone resorption, that is, the loss of substance from the skeletal system (Paule 2001). Vitamin K reduces the levels of IL-6; subsequently, the assault targeted at bone, as well as inflammation (a risk factor for both cardiovascular disease and cancer) is reduced (Reddi et al. 1995). Since C-reactive protein (CRP) is synthesized in response to IL-6, it appears vitamin K may be valuable in reducing elevations in CRP, as well.

Japanese researchers also found that a vitamin K deficiency can mimic the symptoms of diabetes. (The pancreas, which produces insulin, has the second highest levels of vitamin K in the body.) Low levels of vitamin K appear to induce a tendency toward a poor early insulin response and late hyperinsulinemia, following a glucose load in laboratory animals (Sakamoto et al. 1999). Lastly, vitamin K's antioxidant powers are rated (by some) as superior to either vitamin E or coenzyme Q_{10}, other highly respected free-radical fighters (Mukai et al. 1993).

Typically, vitamin K would not be indicated if a patient is on anticoagulant therapy. However, *The Lancet* reported that asymptomatic patients on warfarin should consider low-dose vitamin K if blood-clotting time, as measured by the international normalized ratio (INR), is 4.5–10.0 (Crowther et al. 2000). Follow-up studies to determine the success of vitamin K therapy (1 mg per day) showed that 4% of the patients who received vitamin K therapy had bleeding episodes, compared with 17% of those in the placebo group. The conclusion of the study was that low-dose vitamin K, an inexpensive intervention without known toxicity, might prevent a hemorrhage in patients on warfarin therapy.

A suggested vitamin K dosage for patients not on anticoagulant therapy is 10 mg a day.

Reader's guide to vitamin K food sources and antagonists. Friendly bacteria in the intestines synthesize the majority of vitamin K. However, persistent low-grade levels of intestinal bacteria in the small intestine could hamper vitamin K synthesis. *Acidophilus* cultures in the form of yogurt or kefir serve not only as a good food source, but also ensure that sufficient friendly intestinal flora are present for vitamin K production.

Green leafy vegetables are vitamin K-rich; other sources include alfalfa, egg yolks, blackstrap molasses, asparagus, Brussels sprouts, cauliflower, oatmeal, and rye. Antibiotics increase the need for vitamin K, and vitamin E (doses greater than 600 IU) antagonizes vitamin K activity.

The calcium paradox. It is important to look at the ways calcium can become an atheromatous material. Most body stores of calcium are found in the bones and teeth, and 1% is found in the bloodstream. This 1% performs so many vital functions, including cardiac health, that the body vigorously defends this minute percentage. If inadequate calcium is available, vitamin D is mobilized in the kidney and rushes to the intestinal wall to pull more calcium into the bloodstream. If inadequate amounts of vitamin D are available, the parathyroid gland delivers a message to bones to release calcium. Because the calcium mass in the bone is so great, it is easy for too much of the mineral to be extracted, overwhelming the amount needed in the blood. After compensating for deficiencies, the excess calcium binds soft tissues, the lining of arteries, and brain tissue.

Poor calcium regulation also affects arterial plaque, causing it to become harder but more brittle (*Harvard Heart Letter* 1999). This occurs as calcium deposits in the blood attach to cholesterol deposits on the walls of arteries, making an almost impenetrable union (Shappell 2000). This process further narrows the artery, causing symptoms ranging from fainting spells to sudden death due to abrupt changes in blood pressure (Doss 2001).

It is important to grasp that excesses of calcium (potentiating arterial disease) come essentially from the bone. Furthermore, the results of a test indicating adequate blood calcium levels can be totally misleading, for the supply may have been extracted from the skeletal system. Because secondary pathways, important in maintaining homeostasis, are not well-regulated, it is imperative to maintain adequate calcium levels without summoning the parathyroid gland into service.

Zinc—is important in weight and blood pressure management, regulates glucose and insulin levels, and increases testosterone

Zinc, the second most abundant trace mineral in the body, is important in glucose and insulin management, as well as weight control. Individuals with the lowest dietary intake of zinc showed the greatest prevalence of coronary artery disease, diabetes, and obesity; conversely, as patients made corrections to include more zinc in their dietary program, blood pressure, blood glucose, triglycerides, and central abdominal obesity decreased (Challem et al. 2000).

Zinc is a vital component of insulin, but its worth extends to the cellular receptors, where zinc increases insulin sensitivity. When zinc levels are too low, the pancreas cannot supply enough insulin to control blood glucose levels, and the amount that is produced is less functional (Challem 2000).

However, the emphasis is upon correcting a zinc deficiency, not dosing at will. The journal *Diabetes* reported that administering large doses of zinc sulfate (220 mg 3 times a day, 90 mg of actual zinc) increased fasting blood glucose levels in Type II diabetic patients from an average of 177 mg/dL to 207 mg/dL (Raz et al. 1989). Glycosylated hemoglobin levels also increased among a group of Type I diabetics receiving 50 mg of zinc a day (Cunningham et al. 1994). Considering these poor statistics, if prediabetic or diabetic, use no more than 35 mg of zinc a day without close blood glucose monitoring.

Zinc assists in controlling weight through various mechanisms. According to Jack Challem (the nutrition reporter), zinc is a copper antagonist (meaning it competes with copper for intestinal absorption). Challem states that this is significant because in test tube and animal experiments, excess copper increases fat (or triglyceride) synthesis from sugar. Zinc supplementation lowers copper levels, so it may decrease the synthesis of triglycerides, which show up as either triglycerides in the bloodstream or fat on the body (Challem 2000).

Lower androgen levels have an adverse effect on lipid metabolism, coagulative function, and insulin sensitivity. For the cardiovascular patient with low testosterone levels, a healthier heart profile may emerge with either testosterone therapy or supplementation to increase androgen levels (Xu et al. 2001). The benefits of zinc as an androgen potentiator were exemplified when 22 men with chronically low testosterone levels were given 50 mg of zinc sulfate daily for 45–50 days to promote fertility. (The 22 had experienced infertility longer than 5 years.) All 22 experienced a significant increase in testosterone levels during zinc therapy. In fact, nine of the 22 wives became pregnant during the study (Netter et al. 1981).

It appears that zinc therapy, although beneficial to most, is not risk-free. Occasionally, emphasizing zinc without copper can lead to copper-deficiency anemia, lower levels of HDL, and higher levels of LDL cholesterol; for some, the lack of balance between the two trace minerals can result in an irregular heartbeat (Klevay 1975). Copper is not risk-free either: it can potentiate free-radical activity.

Epidemiologic and metabolic data are convincing concerning the theory that a zinc–copper imbalance is a major factor in the etiology of coronary heart disease. For this reason, if consuming over 50 mg of zinc daily, 2 mg of copper is recommended several times a week. Since copper is widely distributed in selected foods, such as poultry, organ meats, shellfish, oysters, chocolate, nuts, dried legumes, and cereals, 2 mg per day can usually be obtained by favoring dietary selections from this list.

Reader's guide to zinc food sources, enhancers, and antagonists. Zinc content is highest in flesh foods, such as meats, poultry, liver, and oysters. Legumes and whole grain products are also sources of zinc, but larger quantities must be consumed to deliver significant amounts. Other good sources of zinc per kilocalorie (Whitney et al. 1998) are spinach, broccoli, green peas, green beans, tomato juice, plain yogurt, Swiss cheese, tofu, shrimp, and crab.

Vitamins A, B_3, B_6, and C, as well as calcium, copper, magnesium, essential fatty acids, and essential amino acids enhance zinc absorption. Alcohol, oral contraceptives, excesses of copper and calcium, saturated and *trans* fats, steroids, obesity, and smoking interfere with zinc utilization. Diarrhea, kidney disease, cirrhosis of the liver, and diabetes can also contribute to a zinc deficiency.

AUXILIARY FACTORS THAT AFFECT CARDIOVASCULAR HEALTH

Anemia—a predictor of death from acute heart attack

Anemia reflects a reduction below normal in the number of red blood cells, hemoglobin level, or hematocrit (a measure of the packed cell volume of red cells in blood). Hematocrit has emerged as an extremely important assessment in targeting individuals at high risk of succumbing to a heart attack (Wu et al. 2001).

Note: *A normal hematocrit is between 36–50%; below 36% indicates anemia.*

A study reported in the *New England Journal of Medicine* evaluated 78,974 patients, ages 65 and older, who were hospitalized with acute myocardial infarction. Patients were categorized according to hematocrit upon admission. Researchers considered the prognostic value of hematocrit percentages as well as the impact of blood transfusions on 30-day mortality. Their findings follow:

Hematocrit Percentages as Predictor of Cardiac Survival

Hematocrit 5.0%–24.0% = 78% chance of patient dying within 30 days
Hematocrit 24.1%–27.0% = 52% chance of patient dying within 30 days
Hematocrit 30.1%–33.0% = 31% chance of patient dying within 30 days
Hematocrit >33.1% = No increased risk

Reduction in Cardiac Mortality Following Transfusion

Note: Transfusion benefits with increased severity of anemia.
Patients with hematocrit < 24% reduced mortality 64% with transfusion.
Patients with hematocrit 24.1–27% reduced mortality 31%.
Patients with hematocrit 27.1–30% reduced mortality 25%.

It should be emphasized that transfusion therapy is only effective in reducing cardiac mortality among anemic patients; mortality actually increased when transfusions were given to nonanemic patients.

Does Sodium Restriction Lower Blood Pressure?

An evaluation of a hypertensive patient should include measuring plasma renin activity (PRA) to determine if renin is a factor in the pathogenesis of elevated blood pressure. In order to stimulate renin release, the individual is told to follow a diet very low in sodium for 3 days prior to the test. Normal values of adult plasma renin, measured in an upright position and sodium-depleted, are 2.9–10.8 ng/mL an hour.

Renin is an enzyme secreted by the juxtaglomerular apparatus of the kidney in response to many cardiovascular factors, such as a fall in blood pressure, reduced plasma volume, and/or sodium depletion. In an attempt to maintain homeostasis, renin is released, increasing the conversion of angiotensinogen to angiotensin I. Angiotensin I is then converted to angiotensin II, which in turn causes an increase in aldosterone secretion, a sequence that increases peripheral vascular resistance and blood pressure.

Patients with low renin levels respond best to sodium restriction and diuretic therapy. Those with high baseline renin levels will not respond to sodium restriction. According to Jeff Bland, Ph.D., most individuals who have essential hypertension are not salt sensitive. Putting those individuals on a rigorous salt-restricted diet has little impact on their hypertension. Conversely, if an individual is salt sensitive, sodium restriction will have a profound effect upon modulating blood pressure. This is an example of matching an appropriate dietary program with the right genotype (Bland 2000b).

Acknowledging that dietary salt accounts for a significant but only a minor segment of increased blood pressure in hypertensive people, it has been proposed that the larger segment of essential hypertension is caused by enhanced renal sodium retention prompted by hyperinsulinemia. Insulin resistance may also play a role by altering internal sodium and potassium distribution in a direction associated with increased peripheral vascular resistance (Zavaroni et al. 1992; Lukaczer 2000). Researchers were able to demonstrate that blood pressure increased or decreased when lesser or greater amounts of insulin were administered to obese, hypertensive patients (Tedde et al. 1989; Randeree et al. 1992).

The most effective dietary treatment for hypertension appears to be weight loss and a dietary intervention to increase calcium, magnesium, and potassium intake. Results of the Dietary Approaches to Stop Hypertension (DASH) study showed that a diet rich in fruits, vegetables, and low-fat dairy products significantly lowered blood pressure. These foods are excellent sources of potassium, magnesium, and calcium, accounting for the success of the diet. In the study, blood pressure was reduced by 5.6 mmHg and 2.8 mmHg (systolic and diastolic pressures), making dietary intervention comparable to first generation antihypertensives. Weight loss and dietary manipulation appears to control hypertension in nearly one-half of individuals with high blood pressure (Bland 2000a).

Can What You Drink Make a Difference?

Alcohol. Endorsing alcohol consumption is difficult considering the number of health risks imposed by drinking. But when considering the health of the heart and vascular system, statistics appear to flip in favor of moderate alcohol consumption. Studies involving atherosclerosis (disease authenticated by cardiac catheterization or autopsy) show less arterial closure among persons who consume moderate amounts of alcohol. A moderate drinker, in fact, decreases the possibility of heart disease by 30–50% (Gaziano 1993; Pearson 1996). This is true for both men and women, particularly imbibers middle-aged or older.

As encouraging as this information is, the line is extremely narrow in regard to the amount of alcohol one can consume and still reap benefits. For example, teetotalers or occasional drinkers lose the alcohol advantage because of inconsistent consumption. Conversely, persons consuming 3 or more drinks a day experience a rapid rise in total morbidity, that is, cardiomyopathy, hypertension, and hyperhomocysteinemia, as well as mortality. The bottom line indicates that nondrinkers, as well as individuals who aggressively imbibe, have a higher risk of succumbing from heart disease than an individual consuming 1–2 drinks a day (Rimm et al. 1996).

It is speculated that about 50% of the protective nature of alcohol is due to alcohol's ability to increase HDL cholesterol (Gordon et al. 1981). An additional edge comes by reducing blood glucose and insulin levels (Facchini et al. 1994). It appears that no advantage is gained from alcohol in regard to lowering either blood pressure or LDL cholesterol levels, but the blood clotting mechanism is altered by alcohol consumption (Renaud et al. 1992; Ridker et al. 1994). It is debatable how alcohol accomplishes this. Perhaps it is by influencing coagulation factors, such as PAI-1, t-PA, and the activity of platelets.

Reports appearing in *The Lancet* added to the benefits obtained from alcohol, citing the antioxidants found in red wine and dark beer (Maxwell et al. 1994). Antioxidants, regardless of their source, always play heroic roles in heart health. Interestingly, alcohol is still able to convey a cardiovascular advantage, even in light of a poor diet or cigarette smoking.

Is alcohol the utopia we are all searching for? Probably not, considering the dangers imposed by excessive consumption. Persons with a personal or family history of alcoholism and those with hypertriglyceridemia, pancreatitis, liver disease, certain blood disorders, or hypertension, as well as pregnant women, are not candidates for either beginning or continuing to drink alcohol. Those on diets should not forget that alcohol is a significant source of calories as well as carbohydrates. It is also important to recall that drug and alcohol interactions can be fatal. Yet, after acknowledging the negatives, if current consumers of alcohol all abstained from drinking, about 80,000 additional heart deaths would occur annually (Pearson et al. 1994). Although the research is compelling, alcohol should never be considered to be a treatment for either Syndrome X or heart disease.

Green Tea. The pleasure of a cup of green tea is well accepted, but it appears to accomplish far more than satisfy the palate. Published literature confirms the hypolipidemic nature of green tea, reporting decreases in triglycerides and LDL cholesterol, while increasing the beneficial HDL cholesterol. In addition, green tea suppressed the oxidation of LDL cholesterol, further deterring the atherosclerotic process (Chan et al. 1999).

Some researchers liken green tea to aspirin because of similar therapeutic qualities. Information published in *Beyond Aspirin* (Newmark et al. 2000), states that green tea contains salicylic acid, a naturally occurring COX-2 inhibitor. Green tea, like aspirin, inhibits thromboxane A2; the inhibition of thromboxane A2 lessens the risks of blood clot formation and the dangers imposed by arterial constriction.

Heart attacks and strokes are less likely to occur if neither fibrinogen levels nor the activity of platelet-activating factor (PAF) become excessive. Green tea lowers fibrinogen levels and is a PAF inhibitor. A 4-year study involving 5910 Japanese women (ages 40 and older) showed twice as many strokes among trial participants who used less green tea (less than 5 cups a day) than in those who used more (greater than or equal to 5 cups daily) (Sato et al. 1989).

A cup of green tea appears to be beneficial to hypertensives through various mechanisms. The loss of arterial elasticity (arteriosclerosis) is one cause of high blood pressure. Youthful arteries expand and contract in compliance with the heartbeat to move blood to peripheral sites. Damaged vessels are unable to participate in this ritual. Green tea (by inhibiting thromboxane) reduces arterial constriction and consequently blood pressure is reduced. Also many antihypertensive drugs are ACE inhibitors, meaning angiotensin pathways are disrupted. Without interruption of this feedback loop, blood vessels vasoconstrict, water is retained, and blood pressure increases. Green tea breaks this sequence, acting as a natural (although mild) ACE inhibitor (Duke Database 1992; Faloon 2000).

The 1st International Symposium on Green Tea (September 22, 1989) reported that green tea reduces blood glucose levels. During the ensuing years, the Life Extension Foundation has frequently informed members that green tea reduces the expected glucose and insulin rise after a carbohydrate load. It should also be noted that green tea contains chemicals regarded as beta-adrenergic receptor blockers, anti-inflammatories, diuretics, and calcium antagonists, proving beneficial in arrhythmias and hypertension (Duke Database 1992).

Green tea, an antioxidant, helps remove excess iron from the liver (Carper 2001). Individuals with hemochromatosis should drink several cups or use two to four 300-mg capsules a day. (Each capsule should provide 95% active polyphenols.) *Note:* Research suggests that decaffeinated green tea has a different therapeutic disposition than that containing caffeine and may be more effective in reducing iron overload. Caffeine drinks are not appropriate for sympathetic dominant individuals and those taking beta-adrenergic drugs.

As similar as green tea and aspirin are in their defensive mechanisms, it would not be wise for an individual, relying on aspirin as a cardio-protective, to depend only on green tea to the exclusion of aspirin.

Nuts: A Heart Food

According to a report published in the *American Journal of Clinical Nutrition*, one of the most unexpected and novel findings in nutritional epidemiology in the past 5 years has been that nut consumption protects against ischemic heart disease (IHD) (Sabate 1999). Phytonutrients in nuts, such as luteolin (a flavonoid), tocotrienols, fiber, fatty acids, amino acids, and vitamins and minerals, appear to work synergistically to provide heart protection, lower blood pressure, reduce the risk of stroke, and increase longevity. The protective effect of nuts applies to men and women (both black and Caucasian), all age groups, smokers, and sedentary individuals.

Of the tree nuts, walnuts are unique because they are a rich source of linolenic acid. Almonds are a good source of vitamin E and calcium; peanuts provide folate (important in controlling homocysteine) and resveratrol (inhibits blood clots and the inflammatory process). Nuts are also good sources of arginine and fiber (Kris-Etherton 1999).

The *Adventist's Health Study* reported that individuals who ate nuts 1–4 times a week reduced their risk of acute myocardial infarction 22% (Fraser et al. 1992). Eating nuts more than 5 times a week resulted in a 51% lower cardiac risk compared to individuals who consumed nuts less than 1 time a week. Persons consuming nuts more than 5 times a week reduced their lifetime IHD risk 12%, and men who developed the disease did so 5.6 years later than men who consumed nuts infrequently.

In 1993, the *New England Journal of Medicine* published results of a walnut study conducted at Loma Linda University. All trial participants conformed to the *National Cholesterol Education Program Step 1 Diet*, except that 20% of the calories of one diet were derived from walnuts, offset by lesser amounts of fatty foods. Both diets contained identical foods and macronutrients, except for the addition of walnuts in the test diet.

At the conclusion of the study, participants eating the walnut diet had total cholesterol levels 22.4 mg/dL (12.4%) lower and LDL cholesterol levels 18.2 mg/dL (16.3%) lower than those consuming the control diet. Blood pressure was unaffected on either diet. Researchers noted that subjects on the walnut diet, despite increased energy intake, did not gain weight (Sabate et al. 1993). *Comment:* Nuts, in general, are healthy foods, but select those not roasted at high temperatures in oils of uncertain quality.

The *Journal of the American Medical Association* recently expanded the potential benefits of higher nut and peanut butter consumption, showing a significantly reduced risk for Type II diabetes among women who regularly include nuts in their diet (Jiang et al. 2002).

Autonomic Balancing: Right Messages, Good Results

The autonomic nervous system, consisting of the parasympathetic (PNS) and the sympathetic divisions (SNS), play major roles in heart function. For example, when the PNS is active, heartbeat, blood pressure, and respiration rate tend to be decreased, as well as the activity of the adrenal glands. Conversely, when the SNS is dominant, the brain alerts the adrenal glands (small organs located on top of the kidneys) to supply adrenaline, the stress hormone. Adrenaline rushes through the bloodstream to all tissues, organs, and glands, heightening their responsiveness. Subsequently, blood pressure, heart rate, blood glucose levels, respiration, and perspiration increase. It is referred to as the "fight or flight" division because a general state of excitement and preparedness is evidenced.

If the individual is healthy, an adrenaline surge is inconsequential. But, if the heart is diseased or damaged, the sympathetic stimuli can be dangerous, even deadly. Type A individuals often live with chronic stimulation of the SNS, a burdening handicap to long-term survival. *Note:* Interesting data released from the Stanford University School of Medicine showed that insulin-resistant individuals, with compensatory hyperinsulinemia, have a higher nocturnal heart rate, a finding consistent with the possibility that increased heart rates are secondary to insulin-induced sympathetic activity (Facchini et al. 1996b).

Although each of us is born with a propensity toward a sympathetic, parasympathetic, or balanced response from the autonomic nervous system (ANS), Dr. Nicholas Gonzalez (an authority on autonomic balancing) is finding that chemical pollutants and life-style abuses can shift balance and disrupt the natural tendency of the individual. If either division becomes abrasively dominant, the risks imposed upon the heart can be meaningful. For example, if the PNS becomes overly dominant, the risks are as genuine as if the SNS were over-expressed. A heart receiving its instructions from the PNS may become a bit passive, and cardiac output lethargic. Unable to cope with a one-sided response from the ANS, the heart can make fatal errors.

The SNS and PNS are a two-neuron system, meaning that two sets of nerves interconnect in the ganglion. Minerals play an extremely important role in the message sent to organs and glands from the ANS. For example, Dr. Gonzalez explains that magnesium blocks transmission between the two nerves and the ganglion and is regarded as the very best turn-off for sympathetic arousal. On the other hand, calcium arouses activity in the SNS. Potassium, although not a sympathetic toner, acts directly upon the PNS, encouraging increased responsiveness. Exercise quiets the SNS, burning off sympathetic hormones and making stronger parasympathetic expression.

The pH of a parasympathetic dominant tends to be alkaline; the pH of a sympathetic dominant migrates toward acidity. This principle may best explain the benefit some cardiac patients gain when eating a predominantly fruit and vegetable diet, with protein sources limited to smaller amounts of fish and chicken. The alkalinity of a plant-based diet makes the response from the PNS stronger and the activity in the SNS more subdued. Conversely, red meat turns on the SNS and is beneficial to an individual with an overactive parasympathetic response. In fact, Dr. Gonzalez feels a cholesterol level between 210–220 mg/dL is fitting for a parasympathetic because the cholesterol then assumes the nature of a powerful antioxidant.

A cardiac patient should seek counsel with a physician who can determine metabolic type. A physician who can make this determination will also make cohesive choices regarding supplements, diet, and exercise, eliminating conflicting messages being delivered to the heart. *Note:* Tapes of Dr. Gonzalez's lectures, addressing the ANS in-depth, may be purchased from Conference Recording Service Inc., (800) 647-1110 or at www.conferencerecording.com. Although the lectures focus on treating cancer, the tapes are extremely interesting and informative.

Beta-Blockers

Since over-expression of the adrenergic system (increasing sympathetic activity) can provoke an irregular heartbeat, scientists have searched for drugs that could block its activity. Propranolol became the granddaddy of the family of beta-blockers and is one of the most prescribed drugs in America for arrhythmias, hypertension, and angina pectoris.

Beta-blockers bind to specific receptors on nerve endings in an effort to control blood pressure, anxiety, and arrhythmias occurring before or after a heart attack. The binding process blocks the effects of impulses transmitted by the adrenergic postganglionic fibers of the SNS. As beta-blockers compete with epinephrine (also known as adrenaline) for receptor sites, the excitatory nature of epinephrine is curtailed. Beta-adrenergic receptors are located mainly in the heart, lungs, kidneys, and blood vessels (PDR 1999).

Conventional cardiologists conducting propranolol studies reported satisfaction with beta-blockers, citing fewer second heart attacks among users and a 26% reduction in heart mortality. Many patients were less pleased with beta-blockers, describing clinical depression, erectile dysfunction, and fatigue as compromising factors. Also, beta-blockers have been associated with an increased risk of developing diabetes by impairing insulin sensitivity. Newer beta-blocking drugs such as Toprol are now considered superior to propranolol.

Calcium Channel Blockers

The heart is controlled by tiny electrical impulses that regulate the heart, not unlike a pacemaker. Calcium plays a key role in regulating the heart's response to these electrical signals. It flows between the heart cells and surrounding fluid through a sort of chemical turnstile, or calcium channel. The more calcium that gets through the turnstile before the electrical signal is received, the more strongly the heart contracts, an effort that increases the heart's workload. Calcium channel blockers do not totally block movement through the turnstile, but they significantly slow it down. For some, this process lessens the labor required of a damaged heart, signaling it to slow down and take it easy. Because calcium channel blockers dilate the arteries and reduce resistance to blood flow, they are also widely used to control hypertension. The FDA first approved calcium channel blockers in 1982 for the purpose of treating arrhythmias.

While most of the literature (cautiously) supports calcium channel blockers, a few clinicians adamantly oppose their usage. According to Gabe Mirkin, M.D., calcium channel blockers are classified as short-, intermediate-, and long-acting. Older studies showed that short- and intermediate-acting calcium channel blockers might increase the risk of heart attacks; a more recent study showed that longer-acting calcium channel blockers might as well (Estacio et al. 1998). Patients were followed for 67 months, at which time the Drug and Safety Monitoring Committee detected a significant difference in the rate of heart attacks among patients treated with nisoldipine (a long-acting calcium channel blocker) compared with those treated with enalapril (an ACE inhibitor). The termination of nisoldipine treatment was recommended, and patients receiving nisoldipine were switched to enalapril.

Professor Bruce Psaty (University of Washington) reported that the risk of a heart attack increased up to 60% among 2655 hypertensive patients taking calcium channel blockers (Psaty et al. 1995). In addition, *The Lancet* reported that calcium channel blockers, often hailed as an ace in cardiac pharmacology, appear to increase the risk of developing cancer (Pahor et al. 1996). Among 5000 men and women enrolled in a verapamil, diltiazem, and nifedipine study, the risk of cancer increased by about 72% (Atkins 1996c).

Other side effects associated with both calcium channel blockers and beta-blockers are congestive heart failure, lightheadedness, fatigue, low blood pressure, shortness of breath, and bradycardia (heartbeat less than 60 beats a minute). Although not enough studies exist to prove that calcium channel blockers cause heart attacks or increase the risk of cancer, the research is strong enough for doctors to use calcium channel blockers with the utmost caution (Mirkin 2002b).

Dispersed throughout the *Therapeutic section* are a few of the herbs (containing one or more chemicals) considered beta-adrenergic receptor blockers or calcium antagonists. The literature also supports magnesium as a SNS inhibitor as well as a calcium antagonist (Whitaker 1995b; Duke 2000; Gonzalez 2000). Researchers state that carnitine may provide independent benefit in ischemia when used as monotherapy or additional benefit when used in combination with conventional beta-blockers or calcium antagonists (Jackson 2001). *Never* should drug therapy be stopped and a nutraceutical started without counsel with a qualified physician.

Calcium blocking activity. Angelica, garlic, ginger, ginkgo biloba, grape seed, green tea (*Camellia sinensis*), hawthorn, magnesium, and olive leaf

Beta-blocking activity. Grape seed, green tea, hawthorn, and magnesium

RISK FACTORS ASSOCIATED WITH PRESCRIPTION DRUGS

Many people are unaware that there may be risks associated with taking commonly prescribed prescription medications. In addition, once-daily dosing of certain drugs such as anti-hypertensive agents may not provide 24-hour protection against arterial damage. Individuals who are currently taking any of the medications described in this section are urged to discuss alternative treatment options with their physician.

Nitroglycerin Drugs and Angina

Angina is a sudden intense pain in the chest that is often accompanied by a feeling of suffocation. Angina is caused by a momentary lack of adequate blood supply to the heart muscle. Individuals who have occluded coronary arteries often experience periodic bouts of angina.

Nitroglycerin temporarily dilates blood vessels and reduces workload on the heart. As early as 1879, nitroglycerin was administered to an angina patient (Kipple 1993). Nitroglycerin worked so well that nitroglycerin and other "nitrate" drugs have been used as standard angina therapy ever since. Unfortunately, while these nitrate drugs do provide temporary relief from angina, regular use of nitrate drugs may increase the risk of a future heart attack.

A startling new finding came from a Japanese study that involved 518 patients with suspected coronary artery disease (Murakami et al. 2002). The patients were categorized into groups based on their degree of *endothelial dysfunction* (a measurement of inner arterial wall damage) and the use of nitrate drugs.

These 518 patients were followed for 45 months to ascertain which patients were more likely to experience major cardiovascular events. As expected, patients with severe endothelial dysfunction had significantly more heart attacks, strokes, bypass surgeries, congestive heart failure, etc. However, the surprising finding was that those who regularly used nitrate drugs were 2.42 times more likely to experience major cardiovascular events. The researchers concluded that the effects of nitrate drugs accelerated atherogenic processes and endothelial dysfunction and that use of nitrate drugs caused future cardiovascular events (Murakami et al. 2002).

Millions of Americans with coronary artery disease have been prescribed nitrate drugs. However, there is now evidence that nitrate drugs actually accelerate arterial wall damage (endothelial dysfunction) and thus contribute to progression of coronary artery disease—the very disorder that the nitrate drugs have been prescribed to alleviate.

Angina patients who rely on nitrate drugs should bring this new information to the attention of their physician. It is important to note that *occasional* use of a nitrate drug to relieve angina symptoms was not shown to be dangerous in the most recent study. It was the *regular* use of a nitrate or nitroglycerin drug that increased the risk of heart attack by 2.42 times within a 45-month period (Murakami et al. 2002).

Commonly Prescribed Nitrate Drugs

A 2002 study indicating danger from nitrate drugs referred to *regular* use rather than *occasional* use (Murakami et al. 2002). It is highly unlikely that occasional use of a nitrate drug to relieve angina symptoms would cause a problem. However, regular use of a nitrate or nitroglycerin drug more than doubled the risk of heart attack or other pathological vascular event. Commonly prescribed nitrate and nitroglycerin drugs are:

Isosorbide	Nitro-Dur Transdermal Infusion
Isosorbide Dinitrate	Nitrolingual Pump Spray
Isosorbide Mononitrate	Nitrostat tablets
Nitroglycerin patches	Minitran Transdermal Delivery System

For information about an FDA-approved technique that has been shown to safely reduce angina symptoms, refer to "A Non-Invasive Alternative to Coronary Bypass Surgery" in the May 2003 issue of *Life Extension Magazine* (pp. 54–60). This article may also be accessed at www.lef.org.

Dietary supplements that have been shown to help protect against endothelial dysfunction include:

- Folic acid (Title et al. 2000a; Woo et al. 2002)
- Vitamin C (Richartz et al. 2001; Pullin et al. 2002)
- Vitamin E (Title et al. 2000b; Raghuveer et al. 2001)
- Arginine (Maxwell et al. 2000; Kawano et al. 2002; Lekakis et al. 2002)
- Taurine (Wang et al. 1996; Fennessy et al. 2003)
- Fish oil (Chin et al. 1994; Morita et al. 2001; Goodfellow et al. 2000)

It should be pointed out that if left untreated, endothelial dysfunction may become so severe that it will not be possible to reverse it with currently available therapies.

The term *endothelial dysfunction* is increasingly being described in scientific journals as a significant underlying cause of most forms of cardiovascular disease, including hypertension, atherosclerosis, and congestive heart failure.

Class I Anti-Arrhythmic Drugs Kill Thousands

In the June 1995 issue of *Life Extension* Magazine, an article exposed the dangers of a class of anti-arrhythmic drugs the FDA had approved to prevent lethal heart arrhythmias (LEF 1995). In this 1995 article, evidence was introduced that the FDA knew of the risks these drugs posed, but had approved them anyway. When the FDA was confronted with accusations that these drugs had been improperly approved, the reply was that the FDA had a *theory* that these drugs would save the lives of more people by preventing abnormal heartbeats than the drugs would kill by *causing* abnormal heartbeats. The problem was that the FDA had no evidence that these drugs would save even a single life.

Even after a large study conducted by the *National Heart, Lung and Blood Institute* showed that anti-arrhythmic drugs had killed large numbers of Americans, the FDA's response was not to remove the drugs, but to merely suggest changes in the labeling of the drugs (CAST 1989; NHLBI. 2002).

True to its word, the FDA did mandate a change in the labeling of at least one of these anti-arrhythmic drugs (Tambocor®). On page 1889 of the year 2003 *Physician's Desk Reference*, a large warning box appears containing the following statement:

> "An excessive mortality or non-fatal cardiac arrest was seen in patients treated with Tambocor compared with that seen in patients assigned to a carefully matched placebo-treated group. This rate was 16/315 (5.1%) for Tambocor and 7/309 (2.3%) for the matched placebo."

What this warning means is that if you take Tambocor (flecainide), your risk of dying or experiencing a heart attack is more than double compared to taking a placebo.

The sordid history of the FDA's approval of Tambocor and other lethal Class I anti-arrhythmic drugs is chronicled in the book *Deadly Medicine* by Thomas J. Moore (1995).

Are You Taking the Proper Anti-Hypertensive Medication?

The Life Extension Foundation has repeatedly warned persons with high blood pressure (hypertension) to not depend on one-a-day dosing of anti-hypertensive drugs because many of these drugs do not provide complete 24-hour protection. When an anti-hypertensive drug wears off, the patient is vulnerable to having a stroke. One solution to this problem is to take a lower dose of the anti-hypertensive drug twice a day, even though the FDA claims that one-a-day dosing is adequate.

Failure to keep blood pressure at optimal low levels (below 120/85) dramatically increases mortality risk. The United States government states that blood pressure readings as high as 140/90 are acceptable (CDC 2002), but published results of human studies clearly show that maintaining levels below 120/85 confer longevity and protection against heart attack and stroke (Stamler et al. 1993; Stamler 1999).

The best-selling anti-hypertensive drugs in the United States are not necessarily the most effective. Advertising by drug companies and physician "force-of-habit" prescribing often result in hypertensive individuals taking drugs that do not provide optimal blood pressure-lowering effects.

Life Extension long ago recommended a class of anti-hypertension drugs known as *angiotensin II receptor blockers*. Some of the first drugs approved in this class were Cozaar® and Hyzaar® and Life Extension has suggested them as first line therapy. The only drawback to these drugs was that they did not provide consistent one-a-day protection.

A new drug in this class is called Benicar®. A recent study indicated that Benicar may be the first drug to provide true 24-hour blood pressure reduction (Neutel et al. 2002). A typical starting dose of Benicar is 20 mg a day. For patients requiring further reduction in blood pressure, the dose can be increased to 40 mg a day after 2 weeks.

Optimal control of hypertension requires blood pressure checks throughout the day. This is the only way to be certain an anti-hypertensive drug is not wearing off, endangering the arterial system. Even if you take Benicar, it is still critical to verify that it is actually keeping your blood pressure suppressed during an entire 24-hour period.

INVASIVE VERSUS NONINVASIVE TESTING AND HEART PROCEDURES

Facts to Consider Before a Final Decision Is Made

Invasive heart treatment ranks ninth among the top 10 causes of death. Because of the obvious seriousness of any procedure involving the heart, consenting to invasive testing and surgery should be made rationally rather than emotionally. The intent of this protocol is not to steer the patient in regard to cardiac testing and treatment but rather to enlighten the reader concerning both options and risks. Fortunately, researchers have removed many of the uncertainties from the dilemma.

The detection of a heart problem can be made by several noninvasive tests, medical history, physical examination, electrocardiogram, stress tests, blood tests, and an echocardiogram. An echocardiogram provides a graphic outline of the movements of the heart structures, showing the valves and the action of blood flowing through them, the ability of the left ventricle to pump blood, the thickness of the walls of the heart, and an assessment of the membrane around the heart (the pericardium). It does not show the coronary arteries well enough to determine blood circulation directly to the heart. For this evaluation, the echocardiogram should be combined with a cardiac stress test. This combination will show the workings of the various parts of the heart during stress compared to rest.

The blood tests are valuable because they confirm or refute uncertainties arising from early-stage diagnosis of a heart attack. Creatine kinase (CK), an isozyme (CK-MB), and troponins are heart damage markers or cardiac enzymes measurable in the blood. CK-MB shows an increase above normal about 6 hours after the onset of a heart attack. It typically reaches its peak level within 9–30 hours and usually returns to normal within 48–72 hours (Cardiac Biomarkers 2000).

Blood tests to measure troponins, specifically troponin T (cTnT) and troponin I (cTnI)—cardiac muscle proteins—have been developed. These proteins control the interaction between actin and myosin, muscle proteins that contract or squeeze the heart muscle. Identifying troponins specific to heart muscle allowed for the development of blood assays that can detect heart muscle injury with great sensitivity and specificity. The normally low level of cTnT and cTnI increases substantially within 4–6 hours of heart muscle damage. Peak levels occur at 14–20 hours, usually returning to normal 5–7 days later (American Heart Association 2000; Cardiac Biomarkers 2000; Sobki et al. 2000).

It is now considered possible to use troponin testing to identify individuals at either low or high risk for a coronary event. Even modestly elevated troponin levels are associated with larger numbers of tiny coronary artery blood clots, complex arterial lesions, and impaired blood flow through the vasculature.

Compared to patients with the lowest levels of troponin T, those with the highest troponin T levels are almost 13 times more likely to die over a 37-month period (Lindahl et al. 2000). The type of troponin blood test used by most clinical laboratories is troponin I. If levels exceed 0.4 ng/mL, antiplatelet and antithrombotic therapy should be considered. Nutrients with an antiplatelet and antithrombotic therapeutic profile are highlighted in the *Therapeutic section* of this protocol.

Researchers at University of Texas Southwestern Medical Center (Dallas) have discovered another impressive cardiac marker, brain natriuretic peptide (BNP), showing remarkable accuracy in regard to predicting cardiac morbidity and mortality. BNP is a neurohormone synthesized in the muscular wall of the left ventricle of the heart that is released into the circulation in response to ventricular dilation and pressure overload. BNP, a counter-regulatory hormone, promotes excretion of salt by the kidneys and dilates blood vessels.

To determine the predictive value of BNP, 2525 patients were enrolled in a study (half having experienced a heart attack and the other half displaying unstable angina or chest pains). After a 30-day analysis, the researchers found that levels of BNP were higher among patients who died. Also, it was observed that patients with higher BNP were more likely to have a new or recurrent heart attack, develop heart failure, or experience progression of the disease process. Even in patients who had no detectable heart damage from a previous attack, elevated BNP levels identified individuals at high risk of dying or developing life-threatening cardiac complications (de Lemos et al. 2001).

Angiograms

An angiogram, referred to as cardiac catheterization, is a mechanism in which coronary arteries are luminated by injections of dye, a process that aids in diagnosing blocked arteries. A catheter is introduced through an incision into a large vein, usually of an arm or a leg, and threaded through the circulatory system to the heart. As the dye wends its way through the vasculature, blockages are detected by changes in flow rate at points of occlusion. An angiogram is a popular diagnostic tool, but it is not without risks. It is possible that the catheter will damage the artery or loosen a piece of plaque lining the artery wall. The dislodged plaque can block the flow of blood, causing a stroke. Thrombophlebitis, local infection, and cardiac arrhythmias are other valid concerns.

Data reported in the JAMA debated the relevancy of widespread angiogram usage (Graboys et al. 1987, 1992). A study chronicled 168 patients who were advised to have an angiogram to determine the need for either angioplasty or cardiac surgery: 80%, or 134, of the 168 patients who were evaluated noninvasively were determined not to need catheterization. From the 168 patients, an annual fatal heart attack of 1.1% was observed over a 5-year period compared to a 5–10% mortality rate from coronary bypass surgery and a 1–2% mortality rate from angioplasty. The conclusion of the published report was that noninvasive testing to access the heart's performance is a better and safer determinant of a suitable therapeutic program than searching for blocked arteries. If the patient fails some of the noninvasive tests, an angiogram is warranted to determine the need for surgery (Murray 1999).

Magnetic Resonance Imaging

Up to 70% of heart attacks occur in blood vessels that appear normal on an angiogram. The journal *Circulation* reported that plaque without any calcium deposits is not detectable by angiograms or CT scans, but it is the most common cause of sudden death from a heart attack. While calcification may lead to a more extensive form of heart disease, it is less likely to lead to a heart attack (Fayad et al. 2000, LEF 2000).

Fatty buildup on arterial walls, although not detectable by an angiogram, can result in a small fraction of plaque breaking free. The circulating particle ultimately increases the risk of a heart attack or stroke.

A special type of MRI, with a sensitive screening technique, is promising in regard to detecting even a slight buildup in coronary arteries, including plaque without calcium deposits. This is especially praiseworthy since coronary arteries are very small and the constant movement of the heart makes a clear image difficult. The newer technique, black blood imaging, blacks out the blood and produces an image of just the artery. Besides being of much greater advantage in diagnosing early-stage heart disease, this process is noninvasive. It is hoped that this newer, more responsible means of assessing the health of coronary arteries will become part of a routine check-up (Fayad et al. 2000).

Coronary Bypass Surgery

Blocked arteries are not always prognosticators of an impending heart attack. The Coronary Artery Surgery Study (CASS) demonstrated that heart patients with healthy hearts, but with one, two, or three of the heart vessels blocked, did amazingly well without heart surgery. The number of blockages did not alter the 1% a year death rate observed in the study groups (Hueb 1989; Alderman et al. 1990).

A study conducted by researchers in Iowa and published in the *New England Journal of Medicine* evaluated the efficiency of arteries that were 96% blocked (diagnosis made by angiogram) (White et al. 1984; CASS Principle Investigators, 1983, 1984). The researchers found that arteries blocked 96% had a greater thrust of blood than similar arteries only 40% blocked. The conclusion of the report was that the degree of closure did not correlate to the briskness of blood flow. Michael Murray, N.D., states that the most critical assessment regarding the heart's performance is how well the left ventricular pump is working, not necessarily the degree of closure (Murray 1999).

It seems that aggressive procedures to open the vessels do not influence the course of the disease, except in the most advanced stages of atherosclerosis. Bypass appears most helpful when the ejection fraction is less than 40%. Many bypass procedures are performed when the ejection fraction is greater than 50%, a percentage that appears adequate for meeting the demands of circulation. (White et al. 1984; Winslow et al.1988; Murray 1999).

A study by Harvard Medical School's Department of Public Health revealed that 84% of patients who obtained a second opinion after being scheduled to undergo a heart bypass procedure were told that they did not need it. During the study's 2-year follow-up, there were no deaths in the group who canceled their surgeries based upon the second opinion (Perlmutter 2002). Often individuals undergoing the surgery live no longer and with no more quality than a matched group of patients treated without surgery. Conversely, if coronary bypass surgery or angioplasty is appropriately advised, the procedures definitely increase long-term survival and give symptomatic relief to about 85% of patients (Murray 1999).

Although coronary bypass surgery can bring relief to many patients, the procedure is weighted with danger and chance. Infections, problems with blood coagulation, nerve damage, and the possibility of a heart attack or stroke are risks that must be factored into the patient's final decision. According to Harvard researchers, up to 30% of patients have their heart arteries reclog badly in just a year. Few patients survive 10 years without needing retreatment, and high risk patients—such as those who already have undergone repeat surgery—reclog at even greater rates. It should be noted that morbidity and mortality rates vary considerably between hospitals. If considering any heart procedure, ask for an analysis of patient outcome.

Steven Whiting, Ph.D., states that although the odds of surviving bypass surgery have improved since the operation was first introduced, the risk of experiencing a decline in mental function following surgery has remained consistent since the 1980s. Signals of this type of decline may include difficulty following directions, mood swings, and short tempers. Many doctors have downplayed the importance of alterations in intellectual abilities that occur in about 50–80% of patients following bypass surgery, believing the decline to be temporary. It now appears a transient display of incompetency may predict an increased risk of intellectual instability several years later.

Researchers (reporting in the *New England Journal of Medicine*) followed 261 bypass patients for 5 years. Enrollees in the study underwent intellectual testing before and after surgery, as well as at the 6-week, 6-month, and 5-year interval. Intellectual function declined by 20–53% considering presurgical and postsurgical mental status. The decline was 36% at 6 weeks and 24% at 6 months. In 5 years after surgery, 41% of the patients had experienced neurocognitive impairment. The researchers concluded that an intellectual decline in patients following heart surgery was significantly associated with diminished mental abilities 5 years postsurgery (Newman 2001).

Angioplasty

In 1977, Dr. Andreas Gruentzig introduced the procedure known as balloon angioplasty, and by 1980 balloon angioplasty had become a popular cardiac option. Angioplasty is used 3–10 times more often in the United States than in other developed nations.

Balloon angioplasty widens coronary arteries by inserting a specially designed catheter (a long, thin, bendable tube) with a balloon on its tip into a blocked coronary artery. After centering the tip of the catheter in the blocked area, the balloon is inflated, stretching the artery and compressing the plaque. The arteries do not fully constrict, which leaves a larger opening than before. Unfortunately, any procedure using an arterial catheter may cause plaque to be dislodged (resulting in a cardiovascular event) or the wall of an artery to be torn. Other concerns associated with angioplasty are arterial spasms and blood clots, fluid accumulation in the lungs, and impaired kidney function.

From the University of Giessen (Germany) comes a detailed analysis of 300 patients who underwent primary angioplasty for an acute myocardial infarction. At 1 year, 34% had experienced a cardiac event, 23% required repeat angioplasty, and 6% had died from cardiac disease (Peterson et al. 1994; Noninvasive Heart Center, http://www.heartprotect.com/mortality-stats.shtml; Waldecker et al. 1995).

Dr. Eric Peterson at Duke University Medical Center reported the following survival statistics among various age groups undergoing angioplasty:

Ages	30 Day	1 Year
	%	%
65–69	2.1	5.2
70–74	3.0	7.3
75–79	4.6	10.9
> 80	7.8	17.3

Chart extracted from material provided by *The Noninvasive Heart Center*, 2550 Fifth Avenue, Suite 706, San Diego, California 92103 hhwayne@heartprotect.com (619) 544-0200.

Figure 7   Mortality After Angioplasty in 225,915 Patients

After collaborating with several universities, Ian Gilchrist, M.D., cardiologist at the Penn State Milton S. Hershey Medical Center (Philadelphia, PA), announced that 178 angioplasty patients (from a total of 2064) experienced a heart attack, required additional surgery, or died, and 82% of those patients experienced the trauma within 18 hours of the procedure. Gilchrist said that despite efforts to minimize risk, angioplasty complications are nonetheless common (Gilchrist et al. 2000).

The original focus of the trial was to establish the worthiness and dosage of eptifibatide, an IV platelet inhibitor. Dr. James Tcheng (Associate Professor of Medicine at Duke University Medical Center, Durham, NC) reported that eptifibatide, a cost-effective drug, reduced the risk of major complications during angioplasty 40% in the first 48 hours following the procedure. While evaluating the worth of eptifibatide (a landmark study in itself) researchers were able to target the period requiring greatest watchfulness among angioplasty patients.

Angioplasty vs. Thrombolytic Therapy For Acute Heart Attack

An interesting study with far-reaching implications compared primary angioplasty to intravenous thrombolytic therapy for acute myocardial infarctions (heart attacks). An example of a thrombolytic is streptokinase (Streptase), which enhances the conversion of plasminogen to the fibrinolytic enzyme plasmin. Plasmin has a high specificity for fibrin and the particular ability to dissolve formed fibrin clots. Other drugs used to open clogged arteries during and after a heart attack are t-PA (Activase) and anistreplase (Eminase). Angioplasty is fully described in the preceding section.

Most cases of acute myocardial infarctions are caused by thrombotic occlusion of a ruptured plaque, diminishing blood circulation. Earlier research suggested there might be a time frame in human beings during which restoration of blood flow in the infarct-related artery might limit infarct size (Reimer et al. 1977). Research verified the concept, showing that timely reperfusion (a procedure in which blocked arteries are opened to reestablish forward flow of blood) resulted in less heart muscle damage and enhanced survival (Davies et al. 1985). The period from symptom onset to thrombolytic administration was related to reduced infarct size and mortality, with the greatest benefits within the first several hours following early symptoms. From these observations arose the premise that "time is muscle," establishing the need for swift treatment in progressive cardiac care (FTTCG 1994).

Based on its widespread availability, intravenous thrombolytic therapy has been the standard care for patients with acute myocardial infarction. Despite its popularity, thrombolytic therapy has limitations. Of those patients deemed candidates for anticoagulants, 10 to 15% had persistent occlusion or re-occlusion of the infarct-related artery. Consequently, primary percutaneous transluminal coronary angioplasty (primary PTCA) has been advocated as a better treatment for patients with acute myocardial infarction.

Proponents cited higher rates of opened vessels and improved blood flow to the heart among users of PTCA. In addition, avoiding thrombolytic administration virtually eliminates the approximate 1% risk of intracranial hemorrhage inherent with systemic clot-reducing procedures (Stone et al. 2001a). Naysayers point out negatives associated with primary angioplasty, citing excessive delays to treatment compared with thrombolytic therapy, unproven results in large clinical trials, and a lack of widespread availability of treatment centers.

Yet, 22 trials (involving 6889 patients) demonstrated that for every 1000 patients treated with primary angioplasty (rather than thrombolytic therapy) an additional 20 lives were saved, 43 re-infarctions were prevented, 10 less strokes occurred, and 13 intracranial hemorrhages were avoided (meta-analysis by Ellen C. Keeley, University of Texas Southwestern, and Cindy L. Grines, William Beaumont Hospital in Detroit). The angioplasty advantage was still observed even if the patient had to be transported (by 3 hour ambulance trip) to a center equipped to perform the procedure. (It typically takes about 2 hours to mobilize the medical team to perform the angiography and angioplasty in the United States compared to 60 to 90 minutes in European hospitals) (Cannon et al. 2000; Weaver et al. 2000).

Despite the inherent delays apparent with angioplasty, the evidence that primary PTCA offers advantage compared to thrombolytic therapy appears convincing. Optimizing angioplasty with coronary stents and drug regimens has significantly improved the early safety profile and long-term results of percutaneous intervention in acute myocardial infarctions (Stone et al. 2002).

In conclusion, *The Lancet* recently described the CAPTIM trial (a current appraisal of the worth of angioplasty compared to thrombolytic therapy). In CAPTIM, 840 patients (within 6 hours of the onset of a heart attack) were randomized to fibrinolysis with accelerated doses of tissue plasminogen activators or to primary PTCA. Because of funding woes and slow enrollment, the trial ended before the planned recruitment of 1200 patients was reached (the number needed to demonstrate a 40% relative reduction in 30-day composite endpoints). Even so, the results demonstrated a trend toward a 24% reduction in the occurrence of adverse events (Bonnefoy et al. 2002).

Survival trends were similar between patients undergoing angioplasty and those receiving thrombolytic therapy, but the lower-risk population initially enrolled in the study appeared to explain the similarity in mortality statistics. (The survival benefit of primary angioplasty is mostly seen in high-risk patients, such as the elderly, and those with anterior myocardial infarction, or in shock [Stone et al. 2001b; Zahn et al. 2001]). The lack of a survival benefit in low-risk patients does not diminish the clinical relevance of fewer strokes, re-infarctions, a reduction in urgent revascularization procedures, and shorter hospital stays with primary PTCA, compared to fibrinolytic therapies.

Some advocate facilitated primary PTCA trials, i.e., combining thrombolysis with primary PTCA. However, the additional costs and bleeding complications that will certainly accrue by adding thrombolytic therapy before primary angioplasty cannot be dismissed without evidence of overriding benefit. To date, four modest-sized randomized trials have found facilitated PTCA either inferior to or no better than primary PTCA alone.

PTCA enthusiasts avow that (currently) the best therapy for most patients with developing acute heart attack should no longer be debated: administer antiplatelet therapy (aspirin, a thienopyridine, and possibly abciximab), and transfer the patient for primary PTCA to an experienced center, regardless of whether the nearest catheterization suite is three floors or three hours away. To do less, they caution, can no longer be considered standard care (Stone 2002). *Comment*: According to Dr. Philip O'Dowd, the thienopyridines (clopidogrel and ticlopidine) are slightly more effective than aspirin in preventing morbid vascular events in certain patients (O'Dowd http://www.brown.edu/Departments/ Clinical_Neurosciences/articles/po401.html).

Angioplasty Among Diabetics

Although about 700,000 angioplasties are performed annually in the United States, the procedure is not a worthy consideration for everyone. Patients with diabetes mellitus, who are in need of revascularization, have better survival odds with coronary artery bypass grafting (CABG) compared to angioplasty, according to study findings published in the *Journal of the American College of Cardiology* (Bari Investigators 2000).

to cell death—and increases the mortality of animals subjected to bacterial stress (Becker et al. 2000).

A clinical human study involving bone-marrow transplant patients demonstrated, after supplementation with glutamine, a decrease in the incidence of infections and a shortening of hospital stay. In critically ill patients, parenteral glutamine reduced nitrogen loss and caused a reduction of the mortality rate (Roth et al. 1996). In surgical patients, glutamine invoked an improvement of several immunological parameters (Slotwinski et al. 2000). Moreover, glutamine exerted a nutritional (tropic) effect on the intestinal mucosa, decreased the intestinal permeability, and thus may prevent the translocation of bacteria.

In conclusion, glutamine is an important metabolic substrate of rapidly proliferating cells. It influences the cellular hydration (molecular water content) state and has multiple effects on the immune system, intestinal function, and protein metabolism (Sacks 1999). In several disease states, glutamine may become an indispensable nutrient supplement. Catabolic wasting patients should consider supplementing with 2000 mg of glutamine a day.

WHEY PROTEIN

Scientists have examined the impact of whey protein concentrate on preventing or treating catabolic wasting, immune dysfunction, and cancer. A study involving HIV-positive men fed whey protein concentrate found dramatic increases in glutathione levels, with most men reaching their ideal body weight (Bounous et al. 1993). In another study, when different groups of rats were given a powerful carcinogen, those fed whey protein concentrate showed fewer tumors and reduced tumor masses (McIntosh et al. 1995). Whey appears to inhibit the growth of breast cancer cells at low concentrations. In one clinical study, when cancer patients were fed whey protein concentrate at 30 grams a day, some patients' tumors showed a regression (Kennedy et al. 1995).

The research using whey protein concentrate has led researchers to a discovery regarding the relationships between cancerous cells, whey protein concentrate, and glutathione. Glutathione is an antioxidant that protects the body against harmful compounds. It was found that whey protein concentrate selectively depletes cancer cells of their glutathione, thus making them more susceptible to cancer treatments, such as radiation and chemotherapy (Kennedy et al. 1995; Baruchel et al. 1996). It has been found that cancer cells and normal cells will respond differently to nutrients and drugs that affect glutathione status.

The concentration of glutathione in tumor cells is higher than that in the normal cells that surround the tumor. This difference in glutathione status between normal cells and cancer cells is believed to be an important factor in the resistance of cancer cells to chemotherapy. Research has shown that cancer cells subjected to whey proteins were depleted of their glutathione and their growth was inhibited, although normal cells had an increase in glutathione and increased cellular growth. These effects were not seen with other proteins.

Not surprisingly, these researchers concluded, "Selective depletion of tumor glutathione may, in fact, render cancer cells more vulnerable to the action of chemotherapy and eventually protect normal tissue against the deleterious effects of chemotherapy."

Whey protein also appears to play a direct role in bone growth. Researchers found that rats fed whey protein concentrate showed increases in bone strength, as well as bone protein, such as collagen. Whey protein was found to stimulate total protein synthesis, DNA content, and increased hydroxyproline content of bone cells in a dose-dependent manner.

It should be noted that not all whey protein concentrates are created equal. Processing whey protein to remove the lactose and fats, but without losing its biological activity, takes special care by the manufacturer. The protein must be processed under low-temperature and low-acid conditions so as not to denature it. Maintaining the natural state of the protein is essential to its biological activity.

Whey protein has the highest biological value rating of any protein. When the biological value is high, that means protein is absorbed, used, and retained better in the body. High biological values also are associated with tissue sparing. Thus, whey protein concentrate can be beneficial for people with wasting catabolic diseases.

OTHER NUTRITIONAL SUPPLEMENTATION

Conjugated linoleic acid (CLA), a fatty acid, has anticatabolic properties. This has been demonstrated in laboratory mice injected with endotoxin to produce catabolic response. By 72 hours after feeding with linoleic acid, the mice presented body weights similar to controls. The researchers concluded that conjugated linoleic acid prevented anorexia in endotoxin-injected test subjects (Miller et al. 1994). The suggested dose of CLA for a person in a catabolic state is 2 1000-mg capsules taken 2 times a day.

The amino acid arginine can help to generate anabolic cell replacement throughout the body and can suppress excess levels of ammonia in the body, a common problem associated with catabolic breakdown (Vanaja et al. 2001; Kosenko et al. 1995; Kennedy et al. 1994; De Bandt et al. 1998). The suggested dose for arginine to counteract catabolism is 5–20 grams a day. Additional amino acid supplementation should include 2400 mg of *L*-carnitine and 4 capsules a day of a branched-chain amino acid complex which includes at least 1200 mg of leucine, isoleucine, and valine.

WARNING Some nutritionists are concerned about the use of high doses of glutamine or arginine in cancer patients. Glutamine and arginine promote cellular growth, and the concern is that these amino acids could cause cancer cells to grow faster. Scientific studies, however, show that glutamine and arginine provide beneficial effects to cancer patients. Only one study on breast cancer patients hinted at a risk for arginine supplementation.

RESISTANCE TRAINING

Resistance or strength training is defined by resisting, lifting, and lowering weights. Resistance exercise training for a period of 8–12 weeks results in significant increases in muscle mass, muscle strength, and muscle function. Even in cases where dietary intake of protein falls below recommended daily allowances, the anabolic effect of resistance training appears to improve energy intake and protein use, allowing nitrogen retention (Castaneda et al. 1998). The benefits of resistance training have been shown to improve muscle strength and functioning in people with disease-causing muscle wasting and in healthy but frail elderly people (Fielding 1995). Resistance exercise training should be considered as an adjunct treatment modality that is cost-effective, noninvasive, and a means to improve the quality of life.

APPETITE STIMULANTS

Appetite stimulants have been used in both HIV and cancer patients who have wasting syndrome.

Marinol (dronabinol) is a synthetic version of the active ingredient in marijuana, 9-tetrahydro-cannibol (THC). Marinol can be prescribed by a physician and taken orally. Results have been mixed as a treatment for nausea and vomiting due to chemotherapy. However as an appetite stimulant, results are more encouraging. In a study of 139 people with HIV, Marinol significantly improved appetite, body weight, and mood and decreased nausea and vomiting compared to those on placebo (Beal et al. 1995). Side effects from Marinol may include heightened awareness, a sense of well-being, and elation. Dizziness, drowsiness, muddled thinking, and anxiety are also possible side effects.

Megace is a synthetic progesterone used to stimulate appetite in people with wasting syndrome caused by HIV or advanced stages of cancer. It is also used as a therapy in women with breast cancer by interfering with the action of estrogen on cancer cell receptor sites. Although an increase or stabilization of weight may be seen after 6 weeks at the therapeutic dose of 800 mg a day, most of the gain will be in fat. A lower therapeutic dose along with resistance training will help to promote more muscle mass. Megace has a low incidence of adverse side effects when taken as directed.

TESTOSTERONE

Testosterone is a natural anabolic steroid and can help place patients in a positive nitrogen balance. Dosages of 100–200 mg a week can be given to most men and women. Consideration can be given to DHEA (*see the DHEA Replacement Therapy protocol*) and pregnenolone as well. The intravenous administration of vitamins—in particular, vitamin C, 25–50 grams, 2–3 times a week—may be helpful.

Testosterone supplementation in male HIV patients with wasting syndrome has been shown to increase lean body mass at doses of 200 mg daily administered intramuscularly. The most significant results were seen in combination with resistance weight training. In a study conducted at Massachusetts General Hospital, 54 men were given testosterone or placebo and placed on a 12-week exercise training program or no training at all. Lean body mass and muscle increased in those undergoing training and testosterone therapy. Levels of beneficial HDL cholesterol increased in those training, but fell in those supplementing with testosterone. Viral load fell in those taking the hormone (Fairfield et al. 2001).

Consideration should be given to "adrenal support." Patients with catabolic wasting should be assumed to have some degree of adrenal fatigue from the stress of chronic disease (*see the Adrenal Disease protocol*).

WARNING The possibilities discussed above have not been thoroughly studied with respect to potentially worsening cancer (if cancer is the source of the cachectic state). It is suggested that you discuss any potential treatment with a physician practicing complementary medicine prior to initiating therapy.

SUMMARY

Catabolic wasting can be counteracted by proper nutrient supplementation. A daily dose of 2000 mg of glutamine is suggested to prevent glutamine depletion in the tissues and the ensuing catabolic effect. Fish and borage oil supplementation, in the dose of 1300 mg of DHA, 500 mg of EPA, and 1200 mg of GLA a day, should be considered to suppress inflammatory cytokines and prostaglandins that can destroy tissue. Two 1000-mg CLA capsules should be taken 2 times a day to facilitate the transport of glucose into muscle cells. The intake of 30 grams a day of biologically active whey protein concentrate, 10–20 grams of arginine, 2400 mg of *L*-carnitine, and a branched-chain amino acid complex may produce a dramatic anticatabolic tissue-sparing effect and regulate immune system cytokines that are thought to cause cachexia.

The multinutrient Life Extension Mix formula should be given to all people with catabolic breakdown to provide the basic building blocks the body needs to start rebuilding.

A person at risk for developing catabolic wasting syndrome or who is already suffering from cachexia (tissue wasting) should consider the following supplements:

1. Glutamine, 2000 mg a day, available in capsule or powder form.

2. Super GLA/DHA oil, 8 capsules a day (provides optimal potencies of GLA from borage oil and DHA/EPA from fish oil concentrate).

3. Conjugated linoleic acid (CLA), (76%) 2000 mg 2 times a day.

4. Biologically active whey protein concentrate, 30–60 grams a day.

5. Arginine, 10–20 grams a day in divided doses.

6. *L*-carnitine, 2400 mg a day in divided doses.

7. Life Extension Mix, 9 tablets, 14 capsules, or 1 tbsp of powder daily in divided doses.

8. Consider growth hormone, DHEA, and/or testosterone replacement therapy.

9. Branched Chain Amino Acid Formula, 1200–2400 mg a day.

PRODUCT AVAILABILITY

Glutamine, enhanced whey protein, arginine, Life Extension Mix, Super GLA/DHA, CLA, Mega EPA, *L*-carnitine, DHEA, and the Branched Chain Amino Acid Formula can be ordered by calling (800) 544-4440 or by ordering online at www.lef.org. Growth hormone and testosterone are prescription drugs.

Cataracts

Cataract: from the Latin word *cataracta* meaning waterfall

Few people know that poor vision from cataracts affects 80% of people 75 years of age and older. Cataract surgery costs Medicare more money than any other medical procedure, with 60% of those who initially qualify for Medicare already having cataracts. For most people, the question is not whether you ever will suffer from cataracts, but when? We may all suffer from cataracts at some time in our lives, so taking steps to prevent the disease early in life may mean you are one of those 20% of people who enjoy good eye health and never suffer from cataracts.

A cataract is the clouding of the lens of the eye, which reduces the amount of incoming light and results in deteriorating vision. The condition is often described as similar to looking through a waterfall or a piece of waxed paper. Daily functions, such as reading or driving a car, may become difficult or impossible. Sufferers may need to change eyeglass prescriptions frequently. It is estimated that 200 million people worldwide suffer from cataracts. More than 350,000 cataract operations are performed in the United States yearly.

Many people are born with minor lens opacities that never progress, while others progress to the point of blindness or surgery. Many factors influence vision and cataract development such as age, nutrition, heredity, medications, toxins, health habits, sunlight exposure, and head trauma. Cataracts can also be caused by high blood pressure, kidney disease, diabetes, or direct trauma to the eye.

The good news is that a lot of published research exists showing that the cataract progression can be slowed or prevented by the use of natural therapies and minor lifestyle changes.

THE STAGES OF CATARACT DEVELOPMENT

The first stage of cataract development occurs when there is a separation of laminated lens (cartilage-like) protein fibers, appearing as water and/or debris in eye vacuoles (spaces) in the eye.

The second or middle stage of the disease presents with an increase in the size of the vacuole (space) area within the eye. This is when people can noticeably see a halo around lights at night, or may have an increase in visual glare, increase in nearsightedness, and decrease in farsightedness.

In the third, or maturing stage, there is a large increase in vacuole space located in the lens, taking in water and distending protein fibers. These factors in turn cause a decrease in water in the aqueous humor, increasing disintegration of the cortex and calcification of the lens capsule and the lens. The release of lens proteins into the aqueous and vitreous humor may cause inflammation leading to the development of glaucoma. The lens is drying out at this stage.

In the last stage, the disintegration causes byproducts to escape the lens capsule, leaving a shrunken, dried, yellow, or brown lens.

TYPES OF CATARACTS

There are three main types of cataracts. The first, most common type, is a *nuclear cataract* that occurs when the proteins of the nucleus (center) degenerate and darken, causing light to scatter. The second most common type of cataract occurs in the cortex (periphery) of the lens and is termed a *cortical cataract*. This forms when the regular order of fibers in the cortex is disturbed and the gaps in fibers fill with water and debris, thus altering light by scattering and/or absorbing it.

The third and least common type affects the back of the lens, called a *posterior subcapsular cataract* (behind the lens). Women taking the drug tamoxifen to prevent or treat breast cancer have a higher risk of developing this particular type of cataract (9.2% in the tamoxifen group compared with 2.5% in the control group), although their overall risk of developing cataracts is the same as women who are not taking tamoxifen. Women with preexisting cataracts may also have a slightly higher risk of needing eye surgery after starting treatment with tamoxifen. It is recommended that women taking tamoxifen receive eye examinations from an ophthalmologist at least every 2 years.

COMMON SYMPTOMS OF A CATARACT

Here are some signs of a cataract:

- Cloudy, fuzzy, foggy, or filmy vision
- Changes in the way you see colors
- Problems driving at night because headlights seem too bright

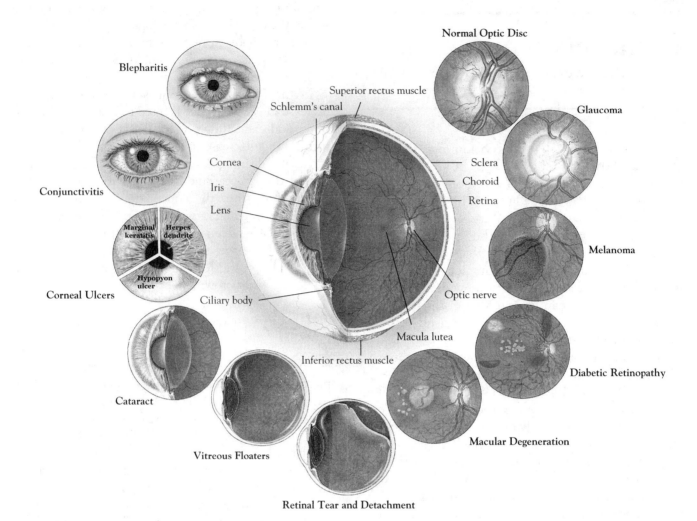

Three basic processes are required for healthy vision. (1) An image must form on the retina (refraction). (2) Photoreceptors located in the retina detect dim and bright light, different colors, and create nervous signals. (3) The optic nerve transmits the nervous signals to the visual cortex of the occipital lobe where they are interpreted as "sight." (Anatomical Chart Company 2002®, Lippincott Williams & Wilkins)

- Problems with a glare from lamps or the sun

- Frequent changes in your eyeglass prescription

- Double vision

- Better near vision for a while only in farsighted people

Note: *These symptoms also can be signs of other eye problems.*

DIAGNOSIS OF CATARACTS

A regular eye exam is all that is needed to find a cataract. Your eye physician will ask you to read a letter chart to see how sharp your sight is. You probably will get eye drops to enlarge your pupils (the round black centers of your eyes). This helps the doctor to see inside of your eyes. The doctor will use a bright light to see whether your lenses are clear and to check for other problems in the back of your eyes.

Other eye tests may also be used occasionally to show how poorly you see with a cataract or how well you might see after surgery. Only a few people need these tests:

- Glare tests

- Contrast sensitivity tests

- Potential vision tests

- Specular photographic microscopy

Source: American Society of Cataract Refractory Surgery, 1999.

CONVENTIONAL MEDICAL TREATMENT

A change in your glasses, stronger bifocals, or the use of magnifying lenses may help improve your vision and be treatment enough. The way to surgically treat a cataract is to remove all or part of the lens and replace it with an artificial lens.

Just because you have a cataract does not mean it must be removed immediately. Cataract surgery can almost always be put off until you are unhappy with the way you see.

Your eye physician will tell you whether you are one of a small number of people who must have surgery. For example, your doctor may need to see or treat an eye problem that is behind the cataract. Or surgery may be required because a cataract is so large that it could cause blindness.

Ninety-eight percent of cataract problems can be improved by surgery, and cataracts will not grow back once they are surgically removed.

Free-Radical Damage to the Aging Eye

Researchers at Brigham and Women's Hospital, Harvard Medical School (Christen 1999), stated in a scientific research report that

> Basic research studies suggest that oxidative mechanisms may play an important role in the pathogenesis of cataract and age-related macular degeneration, the two most important causes of visual impairment in older adults.

The researchers recommended that additional research be conducted in the promising area of preventive therapy and treatment.

The aging lens suffers metabolic changes that may predispose it to cataract development. Some of this occurs due to low supply of oxygen and nutrients, which leaves the eye open for free-radical damage. According to Garner et al. (1983), cataracts are initiated by free-radical hydrogen peroxide found in the aqueous humor. Free radicals, such as hydrogen peroxide, oxidize glutathione and destroy the energy-producing system of the eye and allow leakage of sodium into the lens. Water follows the sodium, and the edema phase of the cataract begins. Then, body heat in the lens of the eye oxidizes (cooks) lens protein, and it becomes opaque and insoluble (similar to egg protein).

Free radicals reside in the aqueous fluid and bathe the lens of the eye, destroying enzymes that produce energy and maintain cellular metabolism. Free radicals also break down fatty molecules in membranes and lens fibers, generating more free radicals and creating a cross-linking (denaturing or breakdown) of the laminated-like structural proteins inside the lens capsule. The lens capsule has the ability to swell or dehydrate. In doing so, the increase and/or decrease in pressure can cause breaks in the lens fiber membranes, resulting in microscopic spaces in the eye in which water and debris can reside (KaLuzny et al. 1997).

INTEGRATED AND ALTERNATIVE MEDICAL THERAPIES

Protecting Against Free Radicals

Prevention and treatment of cataracts are probably the more scientifically documented and beneficial uses of dietary supplements. Free-radical action has been directly linked to and accepted as one of the major causes of cataracts and damage to the healthy eye. Numerous well-conceived, scientific studies have been conducted to test and document the possible effect of supplements due to their capability to reduce free-radical damage, and in some cases allow the body to reverse the damage done by free radicals.

Although it is difficult to treat cataracts with oral antioxidants since there is only minimal blood circulation within the eye compared to other parts of the body, nutritional supplements have been shown to reduce the risks of cataracts as well as slow or reverse their progression (Bantseev 1997).

Maintaining Healthy Glutathione Levels

The eye consists of 65% water and 35% protein (the highest protein content in the body). The eye also contains the highest percentage of potassium in the body, along with a high percentage of vitamin C and glutathione.

If glutathione levels are abnormal, they can affect the health of the eye in a major way (Bunin et al. 1992). Glutathione helps maintain the water balance in the lens. It also is synthesized within the lens and is made of three amino acids: glycine, cysteine, and glutamic acid. Glutathione can affect the function of the lens and is essential to its normal metabolism in the following ways:

1. Preserving the physicochemical balance of proteins within the lens

2. Maintaining the action of the sodium-potassium transport pump and the molecular integrity of lens fiber (protein) membranes

3. Maintaining molecular integrity of lens fiber membranes and acting as a free-radical scavenger to protect membranes and enzymes from oxidation (cooking)

4. Maintaining an effect on proper energy production (glutathione indirectly preserves the glycolysis pathway for energy production within the lens)

Higher levels of glutathione are present in the cortex (edge) of the lens, preventing free radical-induced photochemical generation of harmful by-products. Oxyradicals (free radicals) generate cataracts, and experiments demonstrate that glutathione reactivates oxidized vitamin C, which in turn improves antioxidant potential within the lens. Vitamin C, selenium, and N-acetylcysteine (NAC) fight free-radical damage and help increase vital levels of glutathione.

Bioflavonoids

Bioflavonoids are powerful inhibitors of the enzyme, aldose reductase. Accordingly, if aldose reductase is decreased, then sorbitol will not form, reducing the danger of water accumulating in the lens. The bioflavonoids quercetin, myrcetin, and kaempferol (found in limes) are specifically noted in inhibiting diabetic cataracts (Head 2001). Ginkgo is a widely used flavonoid in maintaining microcirculation to the eye and inhibiting free radicals (Allard 1986).

Carotenoids

Carotenoids are fat-soluble yellowish pigments found in some plants, algae, and photosynthetic bacteria. Carotenoids serve as light-gathering pigments and offer protection from the toxic effects of UV radiation and oxygen (Schalch 1992). Two carotenoids of importance are lutein and zeaxanthin, found in high concentrations in the macula, retina, and crystalline lens of the eye (Sommerburg et al. 1998; Ciulla et al. 2001). There is evidence that both lutein and zeaxanthin play a role in protecting the eye from age related macular degeneration and cataract formation (Brown et al. 1999). Lutein is derived from dark green leafy vegetables such as spinach, broccoli, kale, and collard greens. Zeaxanthin is found in fruits and vegetables with a yellow hue such as corn, peaches, and mangoes.

Vitamin C

Vitamin C is crucial for normal ocular metabolism. Vitamin C occurs in the lens concentration and is 30–50 times higher than that found in circulating blood. This concentration is second only to the nervous system and the adrenal cortex. Vitamin C is found in high concentrations in the eyes of animals that are active during the daylight hours and in low concentrations in the eyes of animals that are nocturnal. Vitamin C acts to

1. Protect delicate lens-protein sulfa-hydroxyl groups from oxidation in the eyes of nocturnal animals

2. Ensure proper formation of collagen and many other structures

3. Stimulate the immune system

4. Play a major role in protecting the lens from photochemical oxidation

5. Feed the delicate membranes that regulate the transport of nutrients and ions (minerals/electrolytes) into the lens

Because the pupillary part of the eye is transparent (where the iris cannot shield and protect it), UV radiation and light can more easily generate the superoxide radical O_2, which is known to be extremely destructive in every cell of the body, including the lens. The superoxide radical can self-mutate into hydrogen peroxide and hydroxide radicals. Just prior to cataract formation, researchers have reported a significant drop of vitamin C concentrations in the eye.

B Vitamins

Vitamin B_2 (riboflavin) is necessary for the production of glutathione reductase. This enzyme is utilized within the lens to activate glutathione and glutathione-selenium peroxidase. These two glutathione forms are crucial in the protective mechanism for operation of the glutathione system.

Light, especially ultraviolet light, destroys B_2. Most B vitamins are not stored, so they must be replaced on a daily basis. Riboflavin deficiency is the prime cause of photosensitivity, making eyes more sensitive to damage; 50–150 mg a day of riboflavin can help reduce photosensitivity.

Vitamin B_6 (pyridoxine) is essential for protein metabolism, for absorption of vitamin B_{12}, and for proper synthesis of antiaging nucleic acids. Its coenzyme is necessary for many protein reactions and metabolic functions. Vitamin B_6 is suggested for nutritional support for cataract patients.

N-Acetylcysteine and Garlic

A 1998 study, Zhao et al., tested the treatment effects of diallyl disulfide (DADS) and N-acetylcysteine (NAC) using acetaminophen (the active ingredient in Tylenol) to induce rapid cataract formation. Acetaminophen is a potent generator of free radicals. Injection of acetaminophen (350 mg/kg body weight) produced acute cataract and other ocular tissue damage. However, treatment with DADS (200 mg/kg body weight), one of the major organosulfides in garlic oil, prevented cataract development and prolonged survival time. N-acetylcysteine also prolonged survival time but was only weakly effective in preventing cataract formation. The remarkable finding was that a combination of DADS and NAC completely prevented cataractogenesis, and that all of the treated animals survived the acetaminophen toxicity.

Melatonin

Melatonin is a potent antioxidant that may be especially effective in preventing and treating cataracts. A compelling study by Abe et al. (1994) showed a potent inhibitory effect of melatonin on cataract formation in newborn rats. By administering a drug that inhibited glutathione synthesis, scientists were able to induce cataracts in rats. The glutathione-depleted rats all developed cataracts, but only 6.2% of the rats given melatonin acquired them. When glutathione levels in the eye lens were measured, the melatonin group had more glutathione than the group not receiving melatonin. The scientists concluded that the inhibitory effects of melatonin on cataract formation could be due to melatonin's free-radical scavenging activity or due to its stimulatory effect on glutathione production.

Melatonin production slows down in people over the age of 40, and by age 60 there is virtually no melatonin being naturally produced. It is over the age of 60 when most cataracts develop. The suggested dosage is 500 mcg–3 mg of melatonin at bedtime.

Other Supplements for Healthy Eyes

Potassium and Magnesium

Eye lenses afflicted with cataracts have decreased concentrations of potassium and magnesium. Supplementation with 400 mg of elemental potassium and 800 mg of elemental magnesium would theoretically increase the availability of these minerals to the eye lens. Potassium and magnesium are often deficient in aging humans, and supplementation with these low-cost minerals helps protect the arterial system.

Selenium and Vitamin E

Selenium and vitamin E may work synergistically in protecting against cataracts, and these two nutrients have been shown to reduce the risk of cancer and cardiovascular disease. Therefore, 400–800 IU a day of vitamin E and 200–400 mcg a day of selenium would appear to be prudent methods of protecting against cataract formation and maintaining good overall health. A low plasma vitamin E level was shown to increase the risk of lens opacities (Rouhiainen 1996). Selenium works with alpha-lipoic acid to increase cellular

concentrations of glutathione. As previously discussed, glutathione is a critical antioxidant in protecting against free radicals in the eye lens.

Ginkgo and Bilberry

Ginkgo biloba extract has shown efficacy in treating dementia, certain arterial diseases, and disorders related to equilibrium. Bilberry, from the genus Vaccinium Myrtillus Fructus, is a proanthocyanidin that has historically been used in various eye conditions, including glaucoma, cataracts, macular degeneration, diabetic retinopathy, and retinitis pigmentosa. Both nutrients may help to restore microcapillary circulation to the eye. After taking ginkgo and bilberry for a month, add 400 mcg of the mineral selenium, 500 mg of the amino acid glutathione, and 500 mg of alpha-lipoic acid every day.

Inositol

Inositol nicotinate is a member of the B vitamin family. Research has shown that it has anticholesterol properties and may help in the management of certain peripheral vascular diseases. Inositol occurs in high concentrations within the ocular lens. It is indispensable for intercellular transport of amino acids in the lens, aiding metabolism, and accelerating the production of ATP which pumps inositol into the lens itself. Inositol performs best when taken in combination with the B-complex vitamins.

Taurine

Taurine is also recommended for the prevention of cataracts. It is the most abundant amino acid in the retina. In the 1970s, scientists discovered that taurine deficiency in cats leads to several biological abnormalities including central retinal degeneration (Hayes et al. 1975). In human studies it was found that children receiving total parenteral nutrition without taurine had low plasma taurine levels and abnormal electroretinograms (Geggel et al. 1985). Infants fed formulas lacking taurine had lower plasma levels of the amino acid than did infants fed human milk (Chesney 1985; 1988). Supplemental taurine has been added to most human infant formulas since these findings were made known. Taurine may also protect cells in the retina from harmful UV light (Gaby et al. 1993).

Inhibiting Glycation

Glycation (glycosylation) of proteins has been shown to play a prominent role in the development of diabetic cataract formation and retinopathy. Glycation occurs when proteins react with sugars and form advanced glycation end products (aptly called AGEs). AGEs physically alter proteins, DNA, and lipids, changing their chemical properties.

Acetyl-L-Carnitine

L-carnitine is an amino acid that helps to maintain healthy cellular metabolism. During aging, mitochondria, the energy-producing sites within the membrane, begin to deteriorate, resulting in the accumulation of cellular debris and the eventual death of the cell. Acetyl-L-carnitine is the more chemically stable form of L-carnitine. Acetyl-L-carnitine is absorbed more efficiently into the bloodstream and is utilized more efficiently in the mitochondria.

Acetyl-L-carnitine was shown to be effective in reducing glycation protein damage leading to cataract formation. Swamy-Mruthinti et al. (1999) stated: "This *in vitro* study shows, for the first time, that acetyl-L-carnitine could acetylate potential glycation sites of lens crystallins and protect them from glycation-mediated protein damage."

Carnosine

Carnosine not only inhibits the formation of AGEs, it can also protect normal proteins from the toxic effects of AGEs that have already formed. An elegant experiment carried out at King's College, University of London, made this point (Brownson et al. 2000; Hipkiss et al. 2000). The scientists employed a glycating agent called methylglyoxal (MG) that reacts with lysine and arginine residues in body proteins.

The scientists used MG to glycate ovalbumin (egg white protein). This produced a brown colored solution typical of the "browning" effect of glycation. They then incubated the glycated albumin with a normal protein, α-crystallin, from the lens of the eye. The glycated albumin formed crosslinks with the crystallin, but this was inhibited by carnosine.

N-acetyl-L-carnosine eye drops have been shown to delay vision senescence in humans, being effective in 100% of cases of primary senile cataract and 80% of cases of mature senile cataract (Wang et al. 2000). N-acetyl-L-carnosine eye drops are able to enter both the aqueous and lipid parts of the eye, and they have been shown to prevent and repair light-induced DNA strand breaks in the eye. In Russia, N-acetyl-L-carnosine eye drops are approved in humans for the treatment of many eye diseases. Brite Eyes II is an advanced eye formula that contains 1% N-acetyl-L-carnosine in a soothing eye drop.

Aminoguanidine

Aminoguanidine is another AGE inhibitor. In one study (Swamy-Mruthinti et al. 1996), aminoguanidine was shown to inhibit cataracts in moderately diabetic rats. Aminoguanidine functioned as an inhibitor of advanced glycation on the development of cataracts in diabetic rats. The scientists showed that aminoguanidine treatment inhibited the formation of damaging advanced glycated end-products by about 56–75% in moderately diabetic rats and by 19–52% in severely diabetic rats. The formation of cataracts, however, was observed only in the moderately diabetic rats, showing that a diabetic must maintain some degree of control over blood sugar levels if they can expect antiglycating agents like aminoguanidine to be effective in protecting against cataracts.

The recommended safe dose of aminoguanidine is 300 mg a day. Aminoguanidine is especially important for diabetics, who suffer from greatly accelerated glycosylation throughout their body. Since aminoguanidine is only available in Europe, most Americans take 1000 mg a day of carnosine based on its potent anti-glycating properties.

Alpha-Lipoic Acid

In animal studies, supplementation with alpha-lipoic acid has prevented cataract formation caused by inhibition of glutathione synthesis. These studies showed that alpha-lipoic acid reduced cataract formation by 40% by protecting the lens of the eye from the loss of vitamins C and E and glutathione, which occurred in unsupplemented control animals.

Avoid Arginine for Now

Arginine facilitates the natural synthesis of nitric oxide, and this has been shown to enhance arterial elasticity in the diabetic patient. Nitric oxide enables arteries to easily expand and contract with each heartbeat. While most people benefit from increased nitric oxide production, a study in rats suggests that nitric oxide might contribute to cataracts. Until this issue is resolved, those with cataracts might want to avoid taking large amounts of arginine since arginine promotes nitric oxide synthesis. It has long been known that nitric oxide is damaging if other antioxidants are not present. Most people who take supplemental arginine also take large amounts of antioxidant supplements like selenium and vitamin E and are probably protected against any oxidizing effects that could occur in response to elevated synthesis of nitric oxide.

PROTECTION FROM ULTRAVIOLET (UV) SUNLIGHT

It is crucial for cataract patients to wear protective eyeglasses to shield against free-radical damage induced by UV sunlight. If UV-blocking sunglasses were to be worn throughout life, the risk of cataract would be reduced greatly. Exposure to sunlight is a major risk factor in the development and progression of cataract disease. Low-cost, wrap-around sunglasses called Sun-Shields are available;

they fit over regular glasses to provide almost 100% protection against UV penetration to the eye.

CONCLUSION

Metabolic changes in the aging lens may predispose it to cataract formation. Free-radical damage due to oxygen and nutrient deficiencies in the eye can create a denaturing effect causing damage to the lens membranes. Supplements, as a preventive approach or as an adjunctive therapy, have been well-documented in the scientific literature (Gerster 1989; Seddon et al. 1994a,b; KaLuzny 1996).

 SUMMARY

Cataract surgery costs Medicare more money than any other medical procedure. Cataract is epidemic among the aged, and its incidence is often linked to controllable lifestyle factors such as cigarette smoking, unprotected sun exposure, and poor dietary practices (Jacques et al. 1991; Seddon 1994a; 1994b; Taylor et al. 1995; Tavani et al. 1996). Women taking tamoxifen should regularly have their eyes checked. The following integrated therapy may be beneficial to the prevention and/or treatment of cataracts.

1. Alpha-lipoic acid, 250 mg twice daily (to boost glutathione production)
2. Melatonin, 300 mcg–3 mg each night
3. Carnosine, 1000 mg per day
4. Glutathione, 500 mg per day
5. Super Zeaxanthin with Lutein for protection against UV radiation and oxidation, 1 capsule daily
6. *N*-acetylcysteine (NAC), 600 mg per day (to boost glutathione levels)
7. Life Extension Mix, 3 tablets 3 times a day to obtain NAC, selenium, inositol, vitamins B_2, B_6, C, and E, bioflavonoids, and many other antioxidants and anti-glycating nutrients
8. Acetyl-*L*-carnitine, two to four 500-mg capsules daily
9. Potassium, 400 mg per day
10. Ginkgo extract, 120 mg per day
11. Bilberry extract, 100 mg per day
12. High-allicin garlic powder, 1800 mg a day; or garlic oil extract, 10 mg per day; or Kyolic Garlic One Per Day Formula, one 1000-mg caplet daily
13. Taurine, 1–3 grams daily
14. Brite Eyes II Formula with *N*-acetyl-*L*-carnosine to protect against glycation, and antioxidant vitamins A and E, 1–2 drops in each eye daily

 FOR MORE INFORMATION

Contact the National Eye Health Education Program of the National Institutes of Health, (301) 496-5248, or the American Society of Cataract Surgery, (703) 591-2220.

 PRODUCT AVAILABILITY

Brite Eyes II, taurine, Super Carnosine, Sun-Shields, Super Zeaxanthin with Lutein, glutathione, vitamin C, Life Extension Mix, ginkgo biloba extract, bilberry extracts, alpha-lipoic acid, potassium, melatonin, garlic formulas, NAC, taurine, acetyl-*L*-carnitine, and selenium can be ordered by calling (800) 544-4440 or by ordering online at www.lef.org.

Cerebral Vascular Disease

Thrombotic (Ischemic) Stroke,
Hemorrhagic Stroke, and Cerebral Aneurysm

A cerebral vascular event (stroke) is defined as a sudden neurological deficit in the brain caused by either ischemia (a lack of blood supply to the brain) or a hemorrhage: 80% of all strokes occur due to arterial blockage (ischemia), and 20% occur due to bleeding (hemorrhage). Hemorrhagic strokes are classified as either occurring within the brain tissue (intracerebral or intraparenchymal) or around the brain tissue (subarachnoid).

Incidence and Epidemiology

Stroke is the leading cause of disability in the United States and the third leading cause of death. While it was originally estimated that annual stroke incidents were approximately 550,000 cases, a study in 1998, through more rigorous counting in all racial and ethnic groups, increased the yearly estimate to 731,000 cases (Broderick et al. 1998). This study showed that African Americans have a higher stroke incidence and stroke mortality than other racial groups.

Women have lower stroke rates than men at all age ranges except 75 years and older, when stroke rates are at their highest. It is of concern that the overall declining rate of stroke-related deaths slowed over the past several decades and leveled off in the 1990s (Gillum 1999).

Individual approaches for the management of ischemic and hemorrhagic stroke are discussed under Thrombotic Stroke and Hemorrhagic Stroke in this protocol. Also, the terms *thrombotic* and *ischemic* stroke will be used interchangeably.

Prognosis and Recovery

In spite of conventional advancement in acute stroke care, the majority of stroke survivors remain permanently partially disabled with neurological symptoms and limitations. While most patients develop some improvement, it is rarely complete. The more severe the initial stroke, the greater the chance of long-term disability. Recovery also varies depending on the size and location of the infarction or hemorrhage. Small infarctions, especially multiple small stroke sites, may result in little disability, whereas large infarctions may cause severe permanent disability.

It is interesting that other related conditions such as high blood pressure do not appear to affect recovery. However, younger patients have a better prognosis than older patients. Overall there is marked variability in recovery, making early disability predictions difficult. In general, recovery is greatest in the first 3 months and rarely occurs beyond 1 year after the stroke. This makes it essential that speech therapy, physical therapy, and occupational therapy be instituted as soon as possible after the stroke occurs and continued three to five times weekly throughout the first year of recovery. All too often, rehabilitative therapy is too infrequent and is stopped prematurely preventing optimal recovery.

Recovery from strokes is relatively poorly understood. While infarcted brain tissue is not able to repair itself, recovery has been theorized to occur by recruiting neighboring neurons (nerve cells) to serve new or additional functions. It is fascinating that electrical brain mapping in monkeys has demonstrated that the cerebral cortex can be functionally reorganized during recovery after an infarction (Nudo et al. 1996). In fact, MRIs in humans have shown increased activity in both hemispheres as patients improve after a stroke. This suggests recruitment of neighboring neurons as well as the corresponding larger regions of the cortex (Cramer et al. 1997).

If you or someone with you is possibly having a stroke, respond immediately! The time it takes to receive treatment is as important to stroke victims as it is for those who are having a heart attack. Not recognizing the symptoms of a stroke, or believing that stroke is untreatable, causes many people to fail to respond to the warning symptoms of stroke and to not seek immediate medical attention.

Regardless of whether the stroke is thrombotic (caused by a clot) or hemorrhagic, management at the onset is considered an acute medical emergency. Stroke patients receiving medical care within 6 hours of the onset of symptoms have a 32% greater chance for a reduced hospital stay (13 days versus 19 days) than those treated after this period (Davalos et al. 1995). Amazingly, 42% of stroke patients wait as long as 24 hours before presenting for medical treatment. That is 21 hours too late! The delay in presenting at the emergency room results in a missed opportunity to effectively treat, and possibly reverse, the damage caused by thrombotic stroke. According to one study, "patients with milder symptoms, for whom treatment might be more effective, were less likely to arrive in time for therapy" (Alberts et al. 1990).

From a preventive medicine and patient education perspective, it is therefore crucial that healthcare providers educate at-risk patients and their families about stroke-related symptoms and encourage them to call 911 if stroke symptoms occur. It is equally crucial that optimal emergency room intervention and treatment occur as soon as the patient arrives in the hospital emergency room.

From the time the patient arrives at the emergency room (ER) triage desk, a computerized tomography (CT) scan should be authorized as soon as possible (within 5 minutes). Multiple timely interventions are crucial in the acute emergency room. These vary based on a range of findings including the patient's temperature, oxygen saturation, blood pressure, glucose levels, complete blood count, electrocardiogram, airway and pulse, medical history, and hydration status. Inclusion and exclusion criteria are reviewed for the consideration of intravenous (IV) thrombolytic therapy if a thrombotic CT scan pattern is identified. The CT scan is further reviewed distinguishing a thrombotic stroke from an intracranial or a subarachnoid hemorrhage. A neurosurgeon will be consulted if an aneurysm or blood pooling is present due to an intracranial hemorrhage. Surgery may be necessary for the evacuation of a hematoma (blood pooling from a hemorrhage). In the intensive care department, blood perfusion (hemodynamics) is continually monitored and assessed. Secondary stroke prevention is initiated based on National Institutes of Health (NIH) guidelines. The treatment of stroke patients in dedicated stroke units has been shown to reduce morbidity, mortality, and disability as well as other post stroke complications (Indredavik et al. 1999).

Stroke-Related Symptoms

The sudden onset of neurological signs and symptoms developing over a few minutes or few hours are indicative of a stroke event. Most of these strokes will be ischemic, involving a thrombus (clot), rather than hemorrhagic. However, any of the following symptoms can result from a clot or bleed, depending upon the arteries in the brain involved in the stroke and their location.

According to the National Stroke Association (1999), strokes more often occur abruptly, with the following symptoms which often develop suddenly:

- Difficulty standing or walking, dizziness, loss of balance, loss of coordination
- Numbness in the face, arm or leg weakness, particularly on one side of the body
- Confusion, difficulty speaking or understanding
- Vision difficulty in one or both eyes
- Severe headaches that have no known cause

Other important, but less common stroke symptoms include:

- Nausea, fever, and vomiting that is different from a viral illness in the speed of onset (begins in minutes or hours instead of over several days)

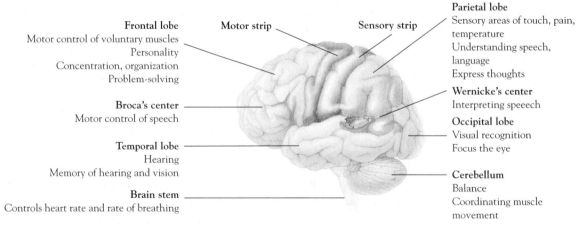

Normal Functional Areas of Brain

The brain has two sides: a right hemisphere that controls the left side of the body and a left hemisphere that controls the right side of the body. Each hemisphere has four lobes and a cerebellum that control our daily functions. Depending on what part of the brain has been affected, stroke victims experience a variety of neurological deficits. Rehabilitation is crucial to the stroke patient's recovery. Physical therapists and speech therapists help patients "relearn" their lost functions and devise ways to cope with the loss of those they cannot regain. (Anatomical Chart Company 2002®, Lippincott Williams & Wilkins)

- A brief loss of consciousness or a period when there is a reduced level of consciousness (sudden fainting, increased confusion, convulsion, or coma)

WARNING Any of these signs may be only temporary and may last only a few minutes.

Hemorrhagic Stroke Symptoms

When a bleed occurs, causing a stroke, the symptoms are less abrupt over one or several hours. The most commonly associated symptoms include headaches, vomiting, and altered states of consciousness.

Cerebral Embolism Symptoms

Symptoms vary further depending upon the nature of the developing stroke. If the stroke is caused by a thrombus (clot) suddenly passing into arteries in the brain (cerebral embolism), the symptoms are of rapid onset, often intensifying over a few seconds, causing headaches on the affected side, seizures, or both. There is often a preexisting heart disease, such as mitral stenosis or atrial fibrillation, endocarditis (an inflamed heart), or a mitral valve prolapse, in which stagnant blood has had the chance to clot and then pass from the heart suddenly into arteries of the brain, blocking blood flow to the brain.

Cerebral Thrombotic Stroke Symptoms

When a cerebral artery becomes blocked from the progressive worsening of a localized clot or a hardened artery in the brain, the symptoms develop over minutes or hours and sometimes over days or weeks. Common causes include gradual hardening and narrowing of cerebral arteries (atherosclerosis) often associated with hypertension, diabetes, coronary artery disease, peripheral vascular disease, or head trauma.

Transient Ischemic Attacks

Often patients can experience temporary symptoms that are associated with a lack of adequate blood supply to the brain. These episodes are known as *transient ischemic attacks* (TIAs). When TIA-related symptoms occur, they occur suddenly and last from 5 minutes to several hours and then resolve completely. These symptoms are often due to reduced circulation and blood supply from the two main arteries leading into the brain—the carotid arteries located in the neck supply the brain from the front, and the vertebrobasilar arteries supply the brain from the back, passing through holes in the vertebrae of the cervical spine.

The peak age of onset for TIAs is 60–70 years of age. It is interesting that a third of the time, TIAs will lead to a subsequent stroke; a third of the TIAs continue and do not lead to a stroke; and a third of the time TIAs spontaneously remit and no longer occur.

It is commonly agreed that TIAs are due to micro-embolization (small clots moving into the brain), excessive platelet aggregation, or from ulcerations in the walls of atheromatous hardened arteries. Other causes include transient episodes of low blood pressure due to dehydration or adrenal insufficiency, mechanical kinking of arteries in the head and neck during head rotation, cervical spine bone spurs compressing the vertebrobasilar artery, or heart arrhythmias.

TIA symptoms are artery-location dependent. Here is a list of the arteries and brain regions that may be temporarily restricted in blood supply and the associated symptoms that develop.

Location	Related Symptoms
Carotid artery	Effects retina, cerebral hemisphere, or both.
Retinal	Transient blackouts; the sense of a shade pulled over the eyes.
Cerebral	Contralateral (opposite sided) paralysis of a single body part; paralysis of one side of the body; localized tingling, numbness; hemianopic visual loss; aphasia (loss of speech); rare loss of consciousness.
Vertebrobasilar	Bilateral visual disturbance including dim, gray, or blurred vision or temporary total blindness; diplopia (double vision).
Labyrinth/medulla	Vertigo; unsteadiness; nausea; vomiting.
Brainstem	Slurring dysarthria (tongue weakness causing impaired speech); dysphagia (difficulty swallowing); numbness, weakness; all four limb paresthesia; drop attacks from sudden loss of postural tone are basilar in origin; a vertebrobasilar artery occlusion episode causes symptoms to be induced by abrupt position changes.
Subclavian Steal syndrome	Symptoms of claudication (lameness or limping) of an exercised arm with symptoms of vertebrobasilar insufficiency described above.

THROMBOTIC STROKE

Ischemic, Thrombotic, Embolic, and Transient Ischemic Attack

In this section, we will discuss methods of preventing primary and secondary thrombotic (ischemic) strokes, along with approaches to restoring function to brain cells that are damaged by a thrombotic stroke (i.e., inducing or accelerating rehabilitation, or both). Because some people may refer to this protocol if they have symptoms of an acute stroke, we will begin with the initial steps involved in diagnosis and immediate treatment.

Aggressive Stroke Therapy

Healthcare providers still do not treat stroke as aggressively as they do heart attack. Many therapies that are proven to work are not made available to the acute stroke patient presenting in the emergency room.

Further contributing to stroke deaths is the belief by many healthcare providers that stroke is untreatable, leading to an attitude of "watchful waiting" with an onset of a stroke instead of being focused on treating the stroke as a medical emergency. The National Stroke Association has described this opinion as being an outdated attitude that serves as the largest obstacle to effective prevention and emergency treatment of strokes.

The use of CT and Doppler ultrasonography has made radical changes in early diagnosis of ischemic and hemorrhagic strokes (Wintermark et al. 2002). These advances have resulted in declines in stroke mortality. In the 1980s, the development of magnetic resonance imaging (MRI) further improved evaluation of persons with cerebrovascular disease (Hesselink 1986; Welch et al. 2000).

Tissue Plasminogen Activator

The FDA approved the use of a tissue plasminogen activator (t-PA) in June 1996 to treat strokes. t-PA had already been approved to dissolve clots that occur in the coronary arteries (which cause an acute heart attack), but the FDA has delayed approving t-PA to treat ischemic stroke for many years. Millions of cases of death and permanent paralysis occurred because of the FDA's delay in approving t-PA in treating stroke caused by abnormal blood clotting in the brain's arteries. Physicians affiliated with the Life Extension Foundation were using t-PA in emergency rooms to treat ischemic stroke years before the FDA gave its official seal of approval.

t-PA (sold under the brand name Activase) should be administered immediately (or within 3 hours) after a stroke to dissolve the clot that is preventing blood from reaching a portion of the brain. t-PA is a natural clot-dissolving substance produced by the body and can literally "blow open" the blood clot in the brain that is causing the acute ischemic brain damage characteristic of a stroke. However, it is crucial that the attending physician review all of the inclusion and exclusion criteria associated with the use of t-PA in advance of its administration. Examples of exclusion criteria making t-PA absolutely contraindicated include an intracranial mass or hemorrhage; very low or high glucose; a previous stroke or head trauma within the last 3 months; current use of anticoagulant drugs; a seizure at the onset of the stroke; major surgery within the last 2 weeks; low platelets; gastrointestinal hemorrhage within the last 3 weeks; blood pressure greater than 185/110; or a previously known cerebral aneurysm (Adams et al. 1996).

One study has shown that 30% more stroke victims were able to regain full use of their faculties after receiving t-PA. In this study 45% of the stroke victims had a good result, defined as "complete regression or slight neurological sequelae." The subgroups with poor prognosis outcomes in three parameters showed a good outcome in 30% of those patients with each of these characteristics (Trouillas et al. 1998). Even today, patients may encounter extreme resistance from emergency room physicians who are reluctant to administer it (Alberts 1998), even if a patient's life is at stake. In some cases, surgery may be required to remove any blockage of blood vessels going to the brain because it is important to get the blood circulating to the brain.

While t-PA can dissolve the blood clot that causes a blood vessel blockage, there are other complications that occur during ischemic stroke that have to be addressed if permanent brain damage is to be prevented. Any interruption in blood flow causes an oxygen imbalance that results in massive free-radical damage. It is critically important to have antioxidants in your bloodstream when t-PA is administered to reduce the free-radical damage that will occur when blood flow is restored (Ozmen et al. 1999).

Heparin

Heparin is a natural polysaccharide normally found in mast cells. Heparin increases the activity of antithrombin III, preventing the conversion of fibrinogen to fibrin. Heparin must be administered parenterally (by IV) because it is not absorbed in the GI tract. Because of this, heparin may be used in acute care situations, but not usually in stroke prevention.

Silent Strokes

Debilitating strokes depicted on television shows or in movies have severe symptoms. Most strokes, however, are not as dramatic. Often the symptoms are minor and transient and may be ignored or dismissed as unimportant. Over time these silent strokes lead to memory loss and other neurological problems. According to one study, by the time people reach their 70s, one in three has a silent stroke every year (Leary 2001).

Of particular concern to stroke victims is that silent strokes occur frequently, causing neurological damage days or weeks after the initial crisis. A 2001 study found that one fourth of stroke survivors had at least one silent stroke during the 2 years following their initial stroke (Corea et al. 2001).

The Underlying Causes

We usually consider a heart attack a life-or-death health event. Strokes have been given less attention, but the realization that stroke is an acute event has now led to stroke being referred to as a *brain attack*. Thrombotic strokes are a major cause of brain attacks and are caused in part by atherosclerosis, hypertension, and procedures that cause abnormal arterial blood clot formation (thrombosis), such as atrial fibrillation and heart valve replacement.

As with almost all cardiovascular disease, strokes are generally the result of several underlying diseases which result in stopping or reducing the flow of blood to the brain.

The majority of strokes occur when a blood clot blocks the flow of oxygenated blood to a portion of the brain. This type of stroke, caused by a blood clot blocking or "plugging" a blood vessel, is called *ischemic* stroke. An ischemic stroke can be caused by a blood clot that forms inside the artery of the brain (a *thrombotic* stroke) or by a clot that forms somewhere else in the body and travels to the brain (an *embolic* stroke). In healthy individuals, blood clotting is beneficial. When you are bleeding from a wound, blood clots work to stop the bleeding. In the case of ischemic stroke, abnormal blood clotting blocks large as well as small arteries in the brain, cutting off blood flow and resulting in a clinical diagnosis of ischemic, thrombotic, or embolic stroke.

Ischemic strokes account for 80% of all strokes and occur as either an embolic or thrombotic stroke. Thrombotic strokes represent 52% of all ischemic strokes.

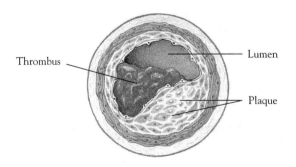

Ischemic Stroke. This type of stroke results from a blockage or reduction of blood flow to an area of the brain. This blockage may result from atherosclerosis and blood clot formation. **Atherosclerosis** is the deposit of cholesterol and plaque within the walls of arteries. These deposits may become large enough to narrow the lumen and reduce the flow of blood while also causing the artery to lose its ability to stretch. A **thrombus**, or blood clot, forms on the roughened surface of atherosclerosis plaques that develop in the wall of the artery. The thrombus can enlarge and eventually block the lumen of the artery. Part of a thrombus may break off and become an embolus. An embolus travels through the bloodstream and may block smaller arteries. (Anatomical Chart Company 2002®, Lippincott Williams & Wilkins)

Thrombotic strokes are caused by unhealthy blood vessels becoming clogged with a buildup of fatty deposits, calcium, and blood-clotting factors such as fibrinogen and cholesterol. We generally refer to this as atherosclerotic disease. Simplistically, what happens with a thrombotic stroke is that our bodies regard these buildups as multiple, infinitesimal, repeated injuries to the blood vessel wall. Our own bodies react to these injuries, just as they would if we were bleeding from a small wound, and they respond by forming blood clots. Unfortunately, in the case of thrombotic strokes, these blood clots get caught on the plaque on the vessel walls and reduce or stop blood flow to the brain. That is when we experience a brain attack.

Two types of thrombosis can cause a stroke: large vessel thrombosis and small vessel disease. Thrombotic stroke occurs most often in the large arteries, magnifying the impact and devastation of disease. Most large vessel thrombosis is caused by a combination of long-term atherosclerosis followed by rapid blood clot formation. Many thrombotic stroke patients have coronary artery disease, and heart attacks are a frequent cause of death in patients who have suffered this type of brain attack.

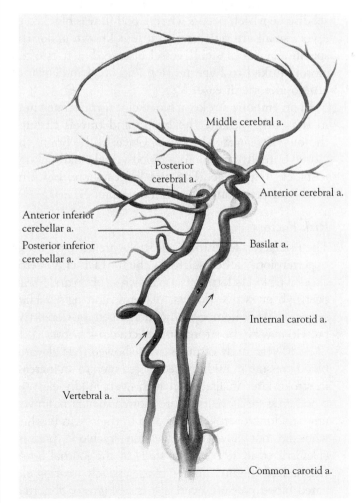

Cerebral arterial system. Shaded circles show common sites of plaque formation. (Anatomical Chart Company 2002®, Lippincott Williams & Wilkins)

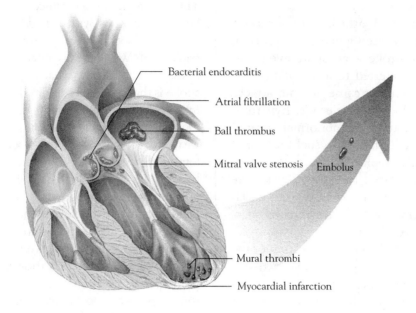

Emboli commonly come from the heart, where different diseases can cause thrombus formation.
(Anatomical Chart Company 2002®, Lippincott Williams & Wilkins)

The second type of thrombotic stroke is small vessel disease which occurs when blood flow is blocked to a very small arterial vessel. Little is known about the specific causes of small vessel disease, but it is often closely linked to hypertension and is an indicator of atherosclerotic disease.

In an embolic stroke, a blood clot forms somewhere in the body (usually the heart) and travels through the bloodstream to the brain. Once in the brain, the clot eventually travels to a blood vessel small enough to block its passage. The clot lodges there, blocking the blood vessel and causing a stroke.

Risk Factors

The risk factors for thrombotic stroke are the presence of hypertension, atherosclerosis, high LDL-cholesterol, excessive blood-clotting factors (such as fibrin and fibrinogen), heart valve defects, diabetes, and aging. High serum levels of homocysteine, fibrinogen, or C-reactive protein may be the strongest predictive risk factors.

A 30-year study of male twins showed that elevated blood pressure in midlife predisposed men to an increase in stroke later in life. Men with even mildly elevated blood pressure 25 years before showed smaller brain volumes and more strokes compared to their twin brothers who did not have the elevation in blood pressure (DeCarli et al. 1999). This study in the journal *Stroke* emphasized the importance of aggressively treating elevated blood pressure even if it is not grossly abnormal (*refer to the Cardiovascular Disease protocol for information about blood pressure control therapies and diets*).

Uncontrollable Risk Factors.

Increasing age. The chance of having a stroke more than doubles for each decade of life after age 55. While strokes are common among the elderly, substantial numbers of people less than 65 also have strokes.

Gender. Overall, men have about a 19% greater chance of a stroke than women. Among people under age 65, the risk for men is even greater when compared to that of women.

Family history. The chance of a stroke is greater in people who have a family history of strokes.

Race. African Americans have a much higher risk of death and disability from a stroke than Caucasians, in part because African Americans have a greater incidence of high blood pressure.

Diabetes mellitus. Diabetes is an independent risk factor for stroke and is strongly correlated with high blood pressure. While diabetes is treatable, having it still increases a person's risk of a stroke. People with diabetes often also have high cholesterol and are overweight, increasing their risk even more.

Controllable Risk Factors.

High blood pressure. High blood pressure is the most prominent risk factor for stroke. In fact, stroke risk varies directly with blood pressure. More widespread treatment of high blood pressure is a key reason for the decline in the death rates for strokes.

hypoxia (oxygen deficiency), and reduces abnormal coagulation of the blood.

An article in the *European Journal of Neurology* described a study of 30 patients diagnosed with acute ischemic stroke. The National Institute of Health Stroke Scale was marginally (but significantly) better in the group treated with vinpocetine at 3 months. No significant adverse effects were seen. The authors concluded that a full-scale trial of vinpocetine was feasible and warranted (Fegin et al. 2001).

Vinpocetine, derived from *Vinca minor* (lesser periwinkle), has been used as a prescription medication in Europe and Asia for over 20 years. Vinpocetine selectively increases blood flow to the brain and reduces neuronal excitotoxicity, resulting in improved stroke recovery and stroke preventive benefit. Vinpocetine has been shown to increase memory and cognition, improve intellectual performance, and enhance coordination. It has been shown to improve vision, hearing, and tinnitus (ringing in the ears) as well (Subhan et al. 1985; Balestreri et al. 1987; Hindmarch et al. 1991).

Theanine

Theanine is an amino acid found in green tea that has a tranquilizing effect on the brain. Theanine increases GABA (gamma-amino butyric acid), an inhibitory neurotransmitter, while caffeine decreases it. Theanine creates a sense of well-being and relaxation without drowsiness.

An article in *Neuroscience Letters* described a study in which theanine was given to gerbils 30 minutes before an ischemic stroke was induced by bilateral occlusion of the carotid artery. The number of intact neurons in the hippocampus was assessed 7 days after the ischemic event. Pretreatment with theanine was found to prevent neuronal death in a dose-dependant manner (Kakuda et al. 2000).

Fruits and Vegetables

An article in *JAMA* evaluated the relationship between fruit and vegetable intake and cardiovascular disease in two prospective cohort studies: the Nurses' Health Study and the Health Professionals' Follow-up Study. After controlling for standard cardiovascular risk factors, those with diets containing over five servings of fruit and vegetables per day had 31% risk reduction compared with the group that consumed the least amount. An increment of one serving per day of fruits or vegetables was associated with a 6% lower risk of ischemic stroke. Cruciferous vegetables, green leafy vegetables, citrus fruit including juice, and citrus fruit juice contributed most to the apparent protective effect of total fruits and vegetables. The authors concluded that these data support a protective relationship between consumption of fruit and vegetables (particularly cruciferous and green leafy vegetables and citrus fruit and juice) and ischemic stroke risk (Joshipura et al. 1999; Suter 1999).

Resveratrol (3,4',5-trihydroxystilbene) is a phytoestrogen (plant-based estrogen) found in the skins of most grapes. Its neuroprotective effects are attributed to its antioxidant, vasodilating, and antiplatelet aggregating actions. An article in *Life Sciences* described a study of resveratrol and infarct size. A middle cerebral artery occlusion was induced in rats 15 minutes after pre-treatment with resveratrol. Resveratrol significantly reduced the total infarction volume (Huang et al. 2001b). Supplemental grape seed-skin extract is a good source of resveratrol.

Consulting Your Physician

When over-the-counter supplements such as aspirin, vitamins, herbs, and oils are used as the primary antithrombotic therapy, the risk of undesirable side effects is reduced significantly. Although over-the-counter medications such as aspirin and natural therapies come with a lower risk of hemorrhaging, they should not be substituted for prescription medication if you are at a high risk for thrombosis.

In all circumstances requiring anticoagulation therapy or antithrombotic therapy, your physician should be consulted if you desire to substitute your medication because the risk can be life-threatening and the appropriate therapeutic dosing is crucial. Since medications such as Coumadin and heparin have a very narrow therapeutic range, anyone on these medications should have his or her blood tested frequently for one or more of the following: PT, PTT, INR. Once the effective dose is achieved, blood testing is recommended every 2–4 weeks to monitor the medication blood levels and avoid overdosing which could lead to hemorrhaging. The template bleeding time test should be conducted if over-the-counter drugs or natural supplements that affect the clotting cascade are added to the regimen. Some of these supplements include vitamins C and E, CoQ_{10}, bromelain, ginseng, garlic, ginkgo biloba, curcumin, St. John's wort, green tea, policosanol, vinpocetine (periwinkle), and fish oils. If you are taking any of these supplements, do not vary your dose of Coumadin without rechecking your PTT (and INR) and template bleeding time.

Diagnosis, Treatment, and Prevention Overview

Many people are familiar with the dramatic portrayal of strokes in movies. While strokes are clearly a medical emergency, most strokes are far less dramatic. In fact, the symptoms of most strokes are so mild that they are often dismissed as unimportant. The critical time for strokes is immediately after they occur.

- The symptoms of thrombotic strokes include nausea and dizziness; sudden, severe headaches; weakness, numbness; paralysis, particularly to one side of the body; partial or total loss of sight in one eye.

- Diagnostic procedures for thrombotic strokes include ultrasound, CT scan, and MRI.

- Treatment of thrombotic strokes consists of medication, natural supplements, and surgical interventions, based on the underlying cause. Controlling hypertension is essential prevention in the occurrence of ischemic strokes.

- Silent strokes commonly occur after thrombotic strokes and may cause damage weeks or months after the initial stroke.

Ischemic stroke is a medical emergency. Time to treatment of this brain attack is important, concerning what is done once in the emergency room.

- *Tissue plasminogen activator* is of great importance immediately after a stroke has occurred to help dissolve blood clots before they thrombose.

- *Heparin* is sometimes used in critical care settings and should be requested by stroke victims.

- *Warfarin* is the drug of choice to prevent strokes. Unfortunately, warfarin has a large number of contraindications and drug interactions with many commonly used medications.

- *Low-dose aspirin* is widely recommended to help thin the blood and prevent strokes. One 81-mg tablet of aspirin a day with a heavy meal is recommended for its anticlotting and anti-inflammatory effects.

- *Ticlopidine* may be recommended as a substitute for aspirin.

- *Mevacor*, a statin drug (HMG-reductase inhibitor), is being investigated for use in reducing the risk of stroke, primarily because of its effect on cholesterol.

The following drug strategies should be considered in stroke prevention, treatment, and rehabilitation.

- *Hydergine*, an antioxidant medication that protects brain cells, may be given in an acute situation. The recommended dosage is 10 mg given sublingually and 10 mg administered orally. Because the FDA has not approved Hydergine for this purpose, the patient or patient's advocate should request that the medication be given.

- *Piracetam*, a nootropic medication, may be useful in the prevention of thrombotic strokes because it appears to protect brain cells from injury during the stroke event. The recommended dosage for piracetam is 4800 mg a day, administered orally.

- *Nimodipine* is a prescription medication that dramatically increases cerebral blood flow by acting as a calcium channel blocker. Nimodipine may be of clinical benefit in acute stroke. The recommended dose is 30 mg 3 times a day, although up to 60 mg 4 times a day have been used in studies.

- *Aminoguanidine*, a medication that prevents glycosylation of proteins and helps prevent mental decline in the elderly, may be useful in preventing thrombotic strokes. The recommended dose is 300 mg once a day with food. This dose should not be exceeded.

An aggressive program for stroke prevention begins by addressing the known risk factors for stroke. The risk factors for ischemic strokes are hypertension, arteriosclerosis, and blood that has a propensity to clot abnormally inside vessels. Blood components that increase the risk of abnormal arterial clotting include elevated levels of LDL cholesterol, homocysteine, C-reactive protein, and/or fibrinogen. Drug and alcohol abuse, age, gender, and race are also factors.

Conventional medicine often recommends several drugs to cover some of these risk factors, including antihypertensives, cholesterol-lowering drugs (statins), and anticoagulants, such as Coumadin and aspirin. Each of these drugs has side effects and may interact with each other, particularly with Coumadin. Bleeding is of primary concern with anticoagulant therapy as it dramatically increases the risk of hemorrhagic stroke.

⬤ SUMMARY

Natural supplements can be used as an adjunct to conventional drugs. Proper testing is required to monitor the effectiveness of both drug and nutritional supplement programs. Recommended blood tests include total cholesterol, HDL, LDL, triglycerides, glucose, prothrombin time, homocysteine, C-reactive protein, fibrinogen, and template bleeding time. Further, the Life Extension Foundation highly recommends using optimal levels, instead of the standard reference ranges, for these laboratory tests. The primary objective of using the following nutrients is to help restore function to injured brain cells.

1. CDP-Choline has been shown to be effective and is currently in clinical trials in the United States for treating strokes. CDP-Choline Caps

contain 250 mg of pharmaceutical grade cytidine-5'-diphosphocholine. One capsule a day is recommended for healthy people over the age of 40. Those with neurological impairment should take two capsules daily under the care of a physician.

2. Ginkgo biloba has been shown to be very effective as an antioxidant and in treating cerebral vascular deficiency, including stroke. Super Ginkgo Extract contains 120 mg of standardized ginkgo leaf powder. One capsule daily is recommended. Use ginkgo with caution when taking anticoagulants.

3. Essential fatty acids, including alpha-linolenic acid (ALA) and docosahexaenoic acid (DHA) from fish oils are recommended. Essential fatty acids are necessary to control inflammation leading to elevated levels of C-reactive protein and to lower fibrinogen levels. Super GLA/DHA provides high potency anti-inflammatory fatty acids. Six 1000-mg capsules a day are recommended. Perilla oil provides high potencies of precursors to EPA and DHA. Six 1000-mg capsules a day are recommended.

4. Vitamin C is recommended as a daily supplement for healthy people and may also be of benefit in stroke; 1000–4000 mg of high-quality vitamin C may be taken daily. Vitamin C should be taken with lysine for maximum benefit.

5. Vitamin E is an antioxidant and blood-thinner. The recommended dose for most people is 400–500 IU of alpha tocopherol, 200 mg of gamma tocopherol, and at least 50 mg of the tocotrienols. Vitamin E should be used with caution with warfarin because it thins the blood.

6. Alpha-lipoic acid may also be considered. Super Alpha Lipoic Acid with Biotin contains 250 mg of pharmaceutical-grade alpha-lipoic acid and 3000 mcg of biotin. One to two capsules daily are suggested for healthy people. Up to 4 capsules can be taken for therapeutic effect. Alpha-lipoic acid should be taken with vitamin B_{12} because it may cause a worsening of symptoms in those with a vitamin B_{12} deficiency.

7. Minerals, including calcium, magnesium, potassium, and selenium should be considered based on the results of serum electrolytes (although serum levels may not represent mineral stores in the body). Thiazide and loop diuretics deplete potassium and coffee increases excretion. Magnesium is needed for the absorption of potassium.

- The Mineral Formula for Men contains four different forms of magnesium, two forms of calcium, potassium, and manganese. One to four capsules daily are recommended as a booster to the minerals contained in the Life Extension Mix.

- The Mineral Formula for Women contains more calcium, which reflects the greater need by women. One to four capsules daily are recommended as a booster to the minerals contained in the Life Extension Mix.

- Calcium and magnesium are available separately in several forms, including calcium citrate with vitamin D_3, calcium carbonate powder, calcium/magnesium powder, magnesium, magnesium citrate, and magnesium oxide powder.

- Super Selenium Complex contains three different forms of selenium in capsule form. One capsule per day is recommended. Selenium drops are also available. One to five drops are suggested daily. Lower doses of selenium are recommended when taking Life Extension Mix.

8. Vitamin B_6, vitamin B_{12}, folic acid, and trimethylglycine should be considered if homocysteine levels are elevated (*see the Cardiovascular Disease protocol for more information*).

- TMG tablets contain 500 mg of trimethylglycine. One to five tablets are recommended daily for healthy people. Up to 12 tablets can be taken daily if high levels of homocysteine persist.

- Vitamin B_6 may be taken at doses up to 800 mg daily to reduce homocysteine levels though high doses of 100–250 mg daily are usually adequate.

- Vitamin B_{12}, 300–1500 mcg daily.

- Folic acid, 800 mcg daily.

9. Elevated fibrinogen leads to the formation of blood clots. Many of the recommended supplements to control homocysteine and lower cholesterol levels will work synergistically in keeping fibrinogen levels in the normal range. The following supplements may also be considered:

- Green tea extract, 350 mg daily.

- Vitamin A, 20,000 IU in a liquid base.

- Beta carotene, one 25,000-IU softgel daily.

- Bromelain, one 500-mg tablet at the beginning of each meal.

- Niacin, 1500–3000 mg daily. Niacin should be monitored to avoid liver toxicity at doses above

1000 mg daily. Flush-free niacin may be taken to avoid the red face and flushing sensation of regular niacin.

10. SAMe may be considered, particularly if there is related depression. SAMe tablets contain 200 or 400 mg of pharmaceutical-grade *S*-adenosyl-methionine. The recommended total daily dose is 400–1600 mg. SAMe is best taken without food, unless GI upset occurs.

11. Policosanol has been shown to have a dramatic effect on lowering cholesterol, reducing platelet aggregation and decreasing the size of experimentally induced thrombus. Policosanol tabs contain 10 mg of policosanol. The ideal cholesterol range is between 180–200 mg/dL. The average person uses 10 mg a day to achieve optimal cholesterol levels. Some people may only need 5 mg a day, while others may require 20 mg a day. Cholesterol levels should be monitored regularly because levels below 150 may be dangerous.

12. Garlic extract, 1000–6000 mg daily, may help lower cholesterol levels. (See the *Cardiovascular Disease* protocol for more information.) Garlic is available in two effective forms. One is the aged garlic extract under the Kyolic brand name. Use the formula that provides 1000 mg of Kyolic odorless garlic in each caplet. Pure-Gar Caps provide a high-allicin garlic that is not odor-free (900 mg garlic powder), and Pure-Gar with EDTA (a chelating agent).

13. Melatonin readily crosses the blood-brain barrier and may help protect against further free radical-induced brain cell injury. Melatonin is to be taken before bed as a sleep-enhancer, 300 mcg–10 mg nightly is recommended.

14. Hormones play a clear role in neuronal functioning and repair. Blood testing is recommended for all people over 40 to determine hormonal deficiencies.

- Pregnenolone is synthesized from cholesterol. It acts as a memory enhancer and converts to progesterone and DHEA. One 50-mg capsule, 1–4 times daily.

- DHEA improves brain cell activity and suppresses overproduction of the adrenal hormone, cortisol. The usual dose for men is 50 mg daily. For women the usual dose is 15–25 mg early in the day. See the *DHEA Replacement protocol* for additional information and warnings.

- Testosterone and estrogen replacement are determined by blood testing. These hormones must be prescribed by a physician.

15. Arginine, vitamin B_2, vitamin B_3, and folic acid may be considered as a way to naturally increase nitric oxide synthesis. *L*-Arginine caps contain 900 mg of pure *L*-Arginine HCl. Arginine should be used with caution in diabetics and those with psychosis.

16. Carnosine may be useful in protecting the brain from neurological damage. Super Carnosine contains 500 mg of pure carnosine. One capsule 2–3 times a day is recommended.

17. Vinpocetine has been shown to have a positive effect on brain metabolism and to protect against excitotoxicity and may be of benefit in stroke recovery. Take 10 mg 3 times daily. For additional protection against excitotoxicity, consider a sublingual vitamin B_{12} lozenge called methylcobalamin in the dose of 5–40 mg a day.

18. Theanine, an amino acid found in green tea, produces a tranquilizing effect on the brain by increasing production of GABA, an inhibitory neurotransmitter. Theanine may also prevent ischemic damage to neurons. Up to four 100-mg capsules can be taken daily.

19. Dietary measures to lower stroke risk include high amounts of fresh fruits and vegetables every day and several servings of fish a week.

To learn about therapies that may protect arteries prior to a thrombotic stroke, or to reduce the risk of further disease or stroke attacks, refer to the protocols on *Cardiovascular Disease* and *Thrombosis Prevention*. To learn more about therapies that may restore neurological function following thrombotic stroke, refer to the protocol for *Age-Associated Mental Impairment*.

HEMORRHAGIC STROKE

For those who have experienced a hemorrhagic stroke or who have a cerebral vascular disease, such as cerebral aneurysm, it is suggested that nutrients that help build collagen and elastin be taken to help rebuild the endothelial lining of the cardiovascular arterial system. Nutrient supplements have also been reported to help reduce the risk of or damage caused by aneurysm or hemorrhage.

Of all patients diagnosed with an aneurysm or cerebral hemorrhage, 50% have hypertension. Cerebral atherosclerosis is also an underlying risk factor for cerebral vascular disease.

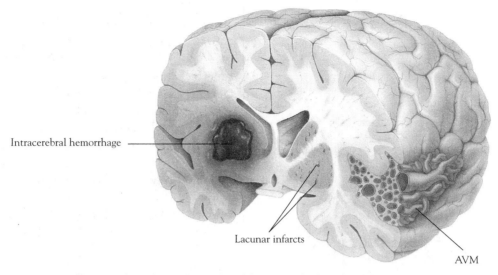

Intracerebral hemorrhage

Lacunar infarcts

AVM

An arteriovenous malformation (AVM) is an abnormality of the brain's blood vessels in which arteries lead directly into veins without first going through a capillary bed. The pressure of the blood coming through the arteries is too high for the veins, causing them to dilate in order to transport the higher volume of blood. This dilation can cause them to rupture. (Anatomical Chart Company 2002®, Lippincott Williams & Wilkins)

Although hemorrhagic strokes account for only 15% of all strokes, hemorrhagic strokes have a much higher mortality rate. There are two subcategories of hemorrhagic stroke: intracerebral hemorrhage (ICH) and subarachnoid hemorrhage (SAH). Although ICH and SAH are very similar, they generally result from different causes.

Intracerebral Hemorrhage (ICH)

ICH is defined as the rupturing of cranial blood vessels, resulting in the leakage of blood into brain tissues. Symptoms of ICH include:

- Partial or total loss of consciousness
- Vomiting or severe nausea
- Weakness, numbness, or paralysis, especially on one side of the body
- Sudden, severe headache
- Severe vertigo (unable to walk or stand)

If these symptoms occur, it is essential to receive immediate medical attention.

ICH rarely occurs in people under the age of 45; however, the risk for developing ICH doubles every 10 years thereafter. ICH accounts for 11% of stroke deaths. ICH occurs more frequently in men, and African-Americans are more likely to be affected than are Caucasians.

Risk Factors

Risk factors for intracranial hemorrhage include:

- Untreated hypertension, 50%

- Amyloid angiopathy, 17%
- Anticoagulation treatment (Warfarin), 10%
- Brain tumors, 5–10%
- Smoking, 5%
- Drug abuse, especially crack cocaine and amphetamines, 5%. (This is the most common cause of ICH for people in their 20s and 30s.)

The most common risk factor for ICH is chronic hypertension. Hypertension causes arteries and arterioles to become weakened, resulting in leakage. A Chinese study noted that there was considerable increased risk for ICH in hypertensive patients who did not regularly take their medications (Hsiang et al. 1996).

Anticoagulants, such as Coumadin or Heparin, are prescribed for a variety of conditions, including ischemic stroke, myocardial infarction, and deep vein thrombosis. Proper monitoring of these medications is essential because they increase the risk of ICH.

Aspirin has also been shown to increase the risk of ICH in elderly patients (Wong et al. 2000). An article in the journal *Stroke* identified epistaxis (nosebleed) as a risk factor for ICH in middle-aged and elderly people, both independently and combined with the use of aspirin. The authors proposed that nosebleeds may be a warning sign for increased risk of ICH in people using aspirin (Saloheimo et al. 2001).

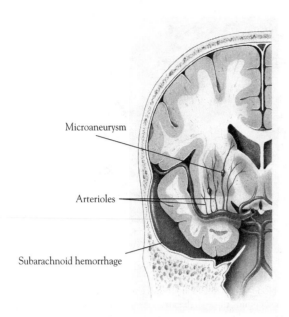

Microaneurysm

Arterioles

Subarachnoid hemorrhage

Hemorrhagic Stroke. This type of stroke is caused by bleeding within and around the brain. Bleeding that fills the spaces between the brain and the skull is called a subarachnoid hemorrhage. It is caused by ruptured aneurysms, arteriovenous malformations, and head trauma. Bleeding within the brain tissue itself is known as intracerebral hemorrhage and is primarily caused by hypertension. (Anatomical Chart Company, 2002®, Lippincott, Williams & Wilkins.)

Hepatitis C virus infection has been identified as a risk factor for ICH. ICH patients with hepatitis C infections were also found to have lower cholesterol levels, lower platelet counts, and longer prothrombin times than ICH patients without hepatitis C, although most of the values were within normal range (Karibe et al. 2001).

Subarachnoid Hemorrhage (SAH)

A SAH occurs when blood leaks into the membranes that surround the brain. The underlying causes for SAH include ruptured aneurysm (a ballooning of the arterial wall) and vascular malformations. Symptoms of SAH include:

• Sudden onset of severe headache

• Nausea or vomiting

• Stiff neck

• Light intolerance

• Total or partial loss of consciousness

After an aneurysm ruptures, a blood clot forms over the affected area. If the clot is disturbed, rebleeding occurs. Rebleeding is the leading cause of death among SAH patients. It is critical that patients with the symptoms of SAH seek immediate medical attention.

Risk Factors

Risk factors for SAH include hypertension, cigarette smoking, and family history of a primary relative with a SAH (4% risk). Other risk factors include age, gender, race, and alcohol use. The risk of rupture depends on the size of the aneurysm.

The incidence of SAH increases throughout middle age and peaks between the ages of 40 and 60. SAH affects women in 60% of all cases. African Americans have nearly twice the risk as Caucasians. Cigarettes and alcohol abuse have been shown to increase aneurysm rupture. People with a family history of aneurysm-induced SAH are at higher risk because certain types of aneurysms appear to run in families.

Diagnosis

The most common diagnostic procedures for determining the cause of hemorrhagic stroke are CT scan, MRI, and cerebral angiogram. These procedures are used to determine the type of stroke and the specific area of the brain that has been affected. Treatment of the stroke is based on the findings of these procedures.

Additional Risk Factors

Can Cholesterol Levels Be Too Low? Cholesterol has obtained such a bad reputation, that some people may be inadvertently harming themselves by intentionally keeping their serum cholesterol too low.

At the American Heart Association's Annual Stroke Conference (February 1999), a report was presented showing that people with cholesterol levels under 180 doubled their risk of hemorrhagic stroke compared to those with cholesterol levels of 230. Hemorrhagic stroke occurs when a blood vessel in the brain breaks open and is different from the more common thrombotic stroke caused by an abnormal blood clot. This study also showed that the risk of thrombotic stroke was twice as likely in those with cholesterol levels over 280 compared to those at 230. The report concluded that the optimal cholesterol level for overall stroke prevention was around 200.

An article in the journal *Neuroepidemiology* found that the proportion of intracerebral hemorrhage (ICH) cases with low cholesterol was significantly greater than in controls. The authors concluded that an increased risk for primary ICH was associated with low cholesterol, a relationship that may apply specifically to hemorrhages from hypertensive vasculopathy (Segal et al. 1999).

Some Foundation members have pushed their cholesterol levels far below 180. In the few reports of hemorrhagic stroke experienced by Foundation members, their cholesterol levels have all been far below 180 mg/dL. The Life Extension Foundation recommends that cholesterol levels be monitored regularly and medication or supplement doses regulated to maintain a range of between 180–200 mg/dL.

Drugs that May Increase Bleeding Risk.

Phenylpropanolamine (PPA). PPA is a popular ingredient in dozens of over-the-counter and prescription diet aids and cough and cold remedies. A case-control study found that the use of PPA significantly *increased* the risk of hemorrhagic stroke in women. The FDA has requested that drug companies stop marketing products containing PPA (Kernan et al. 2000; Mersfelder 2001).

Coumadin. Intracranial hemorrhage is one of the known side effects of Coumadin (warfarin). Coumadin is the drug of choice for thrombosis prophylaxis (prevention). Its uses include prophylaxis for myocardial infarction, stroke, arterial thromboembolism, and deep venous thrombosis. Coumadin is used in patients with prosthetic (artificial) heart valves and is sometimes used in combination with aspirin to thin the blood.

Coumadin interferes with the synthesis of vitamin K which forms several essential coagulation factors. It prolongs prothrombin time (PT) and thromboplastin time (APTT). Prothrombin time is the time measured in seconds for a fibrin clot to form. Thromboplastin time measures in seconds the ability of blood to clot normally. Both tests are closely related and are often ordered together. The universal standard coagulation blood test for Coumadin patients is called the INR or International Normalization Ratio.

Bleeding is the primary side effect of Coumadin therapy. Minor bleeding often occurs in the mucous membranes, particularly around the eyes and nose (causing nosebleeds). Of particular concern is easy bruising and ecchymoses (purple patches on the skin). Another side effect is "purple toe syndrome," referring to drastically reduced blood flow to the feet.

Coumadin (warfarin) has an extremely long list of contraindications and drug interactions (see page 559). Of particular concern is its use in elderly patients because they are more susceptible to the effects of anticoagulants and have an increased possibility of hemorrhage.

Those currently on anticoagulant therapy with Coumadin and aspirin should closely monitor their PT and INR and take the clinical symptoms of hemorrhage seriously. Particular attention should be given to nosebleeds. Even minor symptoms of bleeding should be cause for alarm, particularly in the elderly and those on multiple medications.

There are several natural blood-thinners that may be used in conjunction with Coumadin and aspirin. See the *Thrombosis Prevention* and *Thrombotic Stroke* protocols for more information.

Conventional Treatments

Treatment of hemorrhagic stroke is based on the underlying cause of the hemorrhage and the extent of damage to the brain: treatment includes medication and surgical intervention. In patients with hypertension-induced ICH, initial treatment involves the use of antihypertensive agents. However, lowering blood pressure in ICH remains controversial. Studies have shown that one third of ICHs expand in the first 24 hours (Brott et al. 1997). Some physicians have therefore concluded that a need to lower blood pressure exists in managing acute ICH. No trial has demonstrated the effectiveness of lowering blood pressure. Furthermore, there is significant concern about reducing cerebral blood perfusion pressures in patients with elevated intracranial pressure.

The American Heart Association guidelines recommend that mean arterial blood pressure be kept lower than 130 mmHg in patients with a history of hypertension (Broderick et al. 1997). If the hemorrhage results from the use of anticoagulants, such as Coumadin or Heparin, these medications are discontinued immediately. Protamine and vitamin K may be given to reduce bleeding in patients with anticoagulant-induced bleeding.

In patients with ruptured aneurysms, surgical intervention is the method of treatment and includes placing a clip across the aneurysm or embolization if the damaged area is difficult to approach. During embolization, a wire-packed catheter is threaded through the blood vessels until it reaches the damaged area; the wires are then detached so that they form coils that attract blood cells to promote clot formation. Patients with ICH may benefit from a surgical evacuation of the hematoma. Surgical intervention is contraindicated in patients who are 75 years old or older, who have significant pre-existing disease, or who arrive at the hospital in very poor condition.

Innovative Drug Strategies
Hydergine
Hydergine, an antioxidant medication that helps to protect brain cells, may be beneficial for the treatment

of hemorrhagic shock. In Europe, Hydergine is administered on an acute-care basis for the prevention of brain damage following stroke. The recommended dosage of Hydergine in an acute situation is 10 mg administered sublingually and 10 mg given orally. Because the FDA has not approved Hydergine for use in the treatment of stroke, emergency room physicians may not be willing to administer this medication. Patients or their surrogates can, however, request that this medication be used. Hydergine has been approved in the treatment of other diseases, so it is available through the hospital pharmacy.

Piracetam

Piracetam, a nootropic medication similar to pyroglutamate (an amino acid), may be useful in the treatment of hemorrhagic stroke. Piracetam appears to protect brain cells from injury and death during stroke, thereby lessening the potential for permanent neurological damage. The recommended dosage for piracetam is 4800 mg a day taken orally. A Belgian study indicated that piracetam may be very beneficial if administered within 7 hours after the onset of stroke (De Deyn et al. 1997). Piracetam is not currently available in the United States.

Any disruption of blood flow to the brain causes massive free radical damage that induces much of the reperfusion injury to brain cells characteristic of stroke. When blood flow is interrupted and subsequently restored (reperfused), tissues release iron that provides a catalyst for the formation of free radicals that often permanently damage brain cells. The Life Extension Foundation has spent millions of dollars conducting research that involves developing methods of protecting the brain cells from injury caused by blood flow disruption. The use of antioxidant nutrients, drugs, and hormones, along with specific calcium-channel blockers and cell membrane-stabilizing agents, provide enormous protection to brain cells.

To learn more about therapies that may restore neurological function following hemorrhagic stroke, refer to the Foundation's protocol for *Age-Associated Mental Impairment*.

Supplements

CDP-Choline

CDP-choline is a unique form of choline that readily passes through the blood-brain barrier directly into the brain. Choline is essential for proper brain and neuron function. It is used to make acetylcholine, one of the major neurotransmitters. Choline also aids the movement of fats in and out of cells. Brain tissue is composed almost entirely of fats.

An article in the journal *Stroke* described a study of citicholine sodium (cytidine-5'-diphosphocholine) in an experimental model of ICH using Swiss albino mice. Treatment with CDP-choline significantly improved neurological functional outcome and reduced the volume of ischemic injury surrounding the hematoma (Clark et al. 1998).

CDP-Choline has been approved in Europe and Japan to treat stroke, head injuries, and other neurological impairments. Its effectiveness in treating stroke has not been substantiated in more recent clinical trials, so CDP should be considered an adjuvant therapy at best.

Vitamin C

Vitamin C is well known for its health benefits. Humans, unfortunately, are not able to produce ascorbic acid. We therefore rely upon dietary sources. Pauling earned his second Nobel Prize by proposing that vitamin C deficiency was a major cause of atherosclerosis and cardiovascular disease.

A study in the journal *Stroke* measured the levels of vitamin C in 13 patients with intracranial hemorrhage and 15 patients with head trauma. Compared with 40 healthy controls, ascorbic acid (vitamin C) levels were significantly lower and inversely correlated with the severity of neurologic impairment (Polidori et al. 2001).

An article in the journal *Stroke* described a 20-year study in Japan that examined vitamin C levels and the risk of stroke (Yokoyama et al. 2000). High concentrations of vitamin C strongly predicted lower risks of cerebral infarction and hemorrhagic stroke. Those who had a dietary intake of vegetables 6–7 times per week had half the sex- and age-adjusted risks of all stroke and cerebral infarction than those consuming vegetables 0–2 times a week. The authors noted that the effects of vitamin C on stroke could not be explained by the antioxidant theory alone because an inverse association of serum vitamin C concentration was observed not only with cerebral infarction, but also with hemorrhagic stroke. The authors proposed several mechanisms by which vitamin C may protect against stroke:

- Vitamin C levels are inversely correlated with blood pressure. High blood pressure is a well known risk factor for stroke.

- Ascorbic acid promotes endothelial prostacyclin which decreases vascular tone and inhibits platelet aggregation (Srivastava 1985; Toivanen 1987; Lefer 1990).

- Oxidized LDL-induced increases in leukocyte-platelet aggregation may be prevented by ascorbic acid (Lehr et al. 1995).

Those at risk of a stroke or victims recovering from stroke may have increased demands for vitamin C. High amounts of vitamin C should not be acutely administered during the period when one is actually having a stroke. This recommendation is based on Life Extension Foundation-sponsored research indicating that during an acute ischemic event to the brain, too much vitamin C may promote iron-induced oxidative stress. This type of oxidative stress does not occur during periods of normal blood flow when other antioxidants (such as tocopherols) are available to balance the catalyzing effects of vitamin C, and iron is not being abnormally released from the tissues due to re-perfusion injury.

Whenever vitamin C supplements are used, it is important to consume antioxidants such as alpha-lipoic acid, the tocopherols-tocotrienols, and *N*-acetyl-*L*-cysteine to protect the vitamin C itself from turning into an oxidizing agent.

Strengthening Cerebral Vasculature

The skin of thick-skinned berries such as cherries and grapes, the seeds of grapes, and the skin, leaf, and flower of the Hawthorne tree are all naturally rich sources of a potent antioxidant called oligomeric proanthocyanidins (OPC). These naturally occurring antioxidant flavonoids are tissue specific for strengthening the walls of arteries and thereby reducing the risk of recurring aneurysms and hemorrhagic strokes. In addition to antioxidant protection, OPCs also support collagen and help maintain elastin throughout the entire body. These two critical proteins are major components of all our connective tissues and organs. They are responsible for maintaining structural integrity as well as the elasticity of all the tissues throughout your body. This includes joints, blood vessels, skin, ligaments, tendons, muscles, and even the heart.

By maintaining healthy levels of structural collagen and elastin, our bodies are able to continue to function more efficiently and maintain their youthful strength and flexibility longer. OPCs attach to "reactive sites" on collagen molecules and protect them from free radical attack. This is one of the reasons they are so protective and so valuable for the circulatory system (Laperra et al. 1977; Thebaut et al. 1985; Blazso et al. 1997; Rohdewald 1998; Packer et al. 1999). As noted earlier, oligomeric proanthocyanidins are found in grape seeds, Hawthorne tree skin, leaf, and flowers, thick-skinned berries, and the inner rind of citrus fruit.

Conclusion

Hemorrhagic stroke is a medical emergency. The two types of hemorrhages involved are ICH and SAH.

- The primary risk factor for ICH is hypertension, because chronic hypertension weakens blood vessels. Other risk factors include drug and alcohol abuse, anticoagulant medications, age, gender, and race.

- The underlying cause for SAH is cerebral aneurysm (an abnormal dilation of a blood vessel in the brain). Risk factors for SAH include family history of aneurysm, age, gender, and race.

Symptoms for both types of hemorrhagic stroke are similar and include sudden onset of severe headache, loss of consciousness, nausea and vomiting, and partial or total paralysis. Diagnosis of the underlying cause of hemorrhagic stroke is by CT scan, MRI, and angiography. Surgical evacuation of the hematoma may be necessary. For SAH, treatment includes clipping or embolization of the aneurysm.

The medications Hydergine and piracetam may be beneficial to patients with hemorrhagic shock. The FDA has not approved Hydergine for the treatment of stroke, but it should be available through the hospital pharmacy, and patients or their surrogates should request its use. Piracetam may be beneficial in preventing permanent neurological damage following stroke. Piracetam is not currently available in the United States.

There is little research on natural supplements for hemorrhagic stroke. CDP-Choline and vitamin C may be of some benefit in facilitating recovery and preventing future strokes. Supplements like vinpocetine and phosphatidylserine that enhance neuronal energy metabolism could also help in the rehabilitation process. See the section on *Cerebral Aneurysm* for recommendations on maintaining healthy blood vessels.

⬤ SUMMARY

1. The symptoms of intracerebral hemorrhage (ICH) include nausea and vomiting; sudden, severe headache; weakness; numbness; paralysis, particularly to one side of the body; and partial or total loss of consciousness. The symptoms of subarachnoid hemorrhage (SAH) include sudden, severe headache; nausea and vomiting; stiff neck; light intolerance; and partial or total loss of consciousness.

2. Diagnostic procedures for hemorrhagic stroke include CT scan, MRI, and cerebral angiogram. Treatment of hemorrhagic stroke consists of medication and surgical interventions, based on the underlying cause of the hemorrhage:

- For intracranial hemorrhage resulting from uncontrolled hypertension, the initial treatment is blood pressure control (*see the Cardiovascular Disease protocol for more information about natural blood-pressure lowering supplements and the Hypertension protocol*).

- Persons taking anticoagulants (Coumadin and aspirin) should exercise extreme care to prevent ICH. If signs of major hemorrhage are present, these medications should be immediately discontinued. For more information about Coumadin and natural blood-thinners, see the *Thrombosis Prevention protocol* and the *Thrombotic Stroke* section.

- Smoking should be discontinued for those at risk of ICH. The detrimental effects of smoking on the cardiovascular system are well known.

- Amyloidosis can be due to several diseases, including multiple myeloma (amyloid light chains) and Alzheimer's disease (beta-amyloid). The *Alzheimer's Disease protocol* contains information on several natural supplements that reduce beta-amyloid deposition.

3. Hydergine, an antioxidant medication that protects brain cells, may be given in an acute situation. The recommended dosage is 10 mg given sublingually and 10 mg administered orally. Because the FDA has not approved Hydergine for this purpose, the patient or patient's advocate should request that the medication be given.

4. Piracetam, a nootropic medication, may be useful in the prevention of hemorrhagic stroke because it appears to protect brain cells from injury during the stroke event. The recommended dosage for piracetam is 4800 mg a day, administered orally.

5. CDP-choline may be useful in both preventing and reducing the neurological damage following hemorrhagic stroke. CDP-Choline Caps contain 250 mg of pharmaceutical grade cytidine-5'-diphosphocholine. One capsule a day is recommended for healthy people over the age of 40. Those with neurological impairment should take 2 capsules daily.

6. Vitamin C has been shown to both lower the risk of hemorrhagic stroke and reduce the neurological damage following hemorrhagic stroke. An appropriate dosage of vitamin C depends on the dietary intake. A prophylactic dose of 2.5–6 grams daily is recommended. Up to 15 grams a day may be taken therapeutically. Large doses should be consumed with meals. Do not take high doses of vitamin C during an acute stroke.

7. For further protection from free-radical induced brain injury, consider taking 300 mcg–10 mg of melatonin (at night) and 100–200 mg of palm-oil derived tocotrienols (vitamin E) a day.

CEREBRAL ANEURYSM

Cerebral artery aneurysm, one of the cerebral vascular diseases, can be fatal. An aneurysm is a weakened portion of the heart or a blood vessel, usually an artery, that fills up with blood under pressure, causing it to balloon outward. Aneurysm can be caused by a hereditary weakness in the vessel wall, high blood pressure, atherosclerosis, direct injury, infection, and other diseases.

Approximately 30,000 people a year in the United States experience an aneurysm rupture, causing cerebral hemorrhage. It has been estimated that if five people were to experience a cerebral hemorrhage today, in 1 year: *only one of those people would be alive and well; one would be disabled; and the other three would be dead.*

Cerebral vascular hemorrhage may also produce delayed problems such as hydrocephalus ("fluid on the brain") and narrowing of the blood vessels because of the irritation of the blood on the blood vessels (known as vasospasm). Rebleeding, hydrocephalus, and vasospasm can happen days to weeks after the initial bleed. Aneurysms can and do grow. If they reach a certain size, usually more than 25 mm (1 inch), they may start applying pressure on the surrounding brain tissue and cause additional problems.

Cerebral aneurysm is very uncommon in patients under 20 years of age and is increasingly common in older patients. In people over 65, cerebral aneurysm may be found in as high as 5% of the population. It appears cerebral aneurysm is related to an absence of a muscular layer that makes up part of the blood vessels; over time, it stretches and thins and creates the aneurysm. Smoking appears to markedly increase the chance that one will develop a cerebral aneurysm.

Indications of the presence of an aneurysm depend on the location of the aneurysm. Aneurysm generally exhibits few symptoms and is discovered by accident on x-ray films or imaging scans performed for some other reason.

The rupture or hemorrhage of an aneurysm usually produces severe pain. The location of the aneurysm usually determines the amount of bleeding, shock, loss of consciousness, or if death will occur. In some cases, the aneurysm may leak blood, causing warning pain

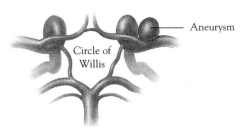

An aneurysm is a weakening of the arterial wall that causes it to stretch and balloon. It usually occurs where the artery branches. (Anatomical Chart Company 2002®, Lippincott Williams & Wilkins)

without the rapid deterioration and damage characteristic of a rupture. The threat of aneurysm goes beyond the immediate site damage it can cause. Blood clots often form in an aneurysm, creating danger of embolisms and clotting in distant organs or vessels.

Cerebral hemorrhagic problems occur when an aneurysm ruptures, causing internal bleeding. For example, aneurysm affecting the arteries supplying the brain can occur at any age, but occurs most often in people 60 years of age with a history of hypertension. The aneurysm may rupture, causing hemorrhage and blood leakage into the membrane surrounding the brain. A cerebral artery aneurysm is particularly important because it can lead to fatal subarachnoid hemorrhage which occurs underneath one of the layers of tissue lining the brain. This aneurysm frequently occurs from inherited vascular defects at the branch points of cerebral arteries.

If your physician suspects an aneurysm or the possibility of hemorrhage, he or she will probably recommend ultrasound testing, computed tomography scanning (CT scan), magnetic resonance imaging (MRI), or angiography of the area to determine the size and severity and to predict the possibility of rupture and subsequent hemorrhage.

Conventional Treatment

If an aneurysm is large and the risk of rupture is significant, surgery may be necessary.

When an aneurysm ruptures, emergency surgery is necessary to stop the bleeding. Surgical intervention into cerebral aneurysm or hemorrhage may be difficult or impossible because of the constraints of access to the damaged or threatened areas of the brain.

Hypertensive drugs may also be prescribed in an attempt to lower blood pressure and reduce the chances of additional aneurysm or cerebral hemorrhage (*see the Cardiovascular Disease protocol for more information on natural ways to reduce blood pressure*).

Integrated or Alternative Therapies

Researchers speculated in a 1998 issue of *Life Sciences Journal* that "an acute systemic oxidative stress condition might influence the rupture of intracranial aneurysm." Vitamin E was specifically identified by investigators to act as an antioxidant by scavenging free radicals and thus reducing the conditions that precipitate these cerebral vascular ruptures (Marzatico et al. 1998). We recommend taking 400–800 IU of vitamin E daily to reduce the risk of aneurysm ruptures. Vitamin C at 2000–5000 mg a day is suggested, along with 300 mg a day of the flavonoid proanthocyanidin (from grape seed or pine bark) for further protection against underlying factors that cause cerebral vascular disease.

Magnesium is crucial for arterial structure, and it is suggested that 1500 mg a day of elemental magnesium be taken along with 1000 mg a day of calcium and 500 mg a day of potassium.

Mechanisms that regulate cerebral circulation have been intensively investigated in recent years, and this research is increasingly focused on the effects of nitric oxide. Nitric oxide is an important regulator of cerebral vascular tone. Nitric oxide maintains the cerebral vasculature in a dilated state. Arginine, a natural supplement, specifically enhances nitric oxide synthesis. Persons with cerebral vascular disease may consider taking 4–5 grams of arginine 3 times a day to better maintain the health of vessels.

Activation of potassium channels appears to be a major mechanism for *dilatation* of cerebral arteries. Agents that increase the intracellular concentration of cyclic adenosine monophosphate (cAMP) produce vasodilatation. Supplementation with 500 mg a day of potassium and 5–20 mg a day of Hydergine may enhance vasodilatation in cerebral vascular disease, helping to restore vessels to a healthier state.

Additionally, alcohol consumption poses a risk for development of hypertension (high blood pressure), strokes, and sudden death through the depletion of magnesium from the body. The dietary intake of magnesium modulates the hypertensive actions of alcohol (Altura et al. 1999). Experiments indicate that chronic ethanol ingestion results in the contraction of the cerebral arteries and capillaries, a contraction that causes increased cerebral vascular resistance. Chronic ethanol ingestion increases the reactivity of intact microvessels to vasoconstrictors and results in decreased reactivity to vasodilators. However, pretreatment of animals with magnesium prevents ethanol from inducing a stroke and prevents the adverse cerebral vascular changes from taking place. Magnesium influences the response of cerebral arteries to several other natural or synthetic stimulators (agonists) and has been shown to decrease cerebral vascular resistance. Contractility of cerebral arteries is dependent upon the actions and interactions of calcium and magnesium (Altura et al. 1994).

It is clear from published studies that magnesium can induce healthy vascular tone in all types of vascular smooth muscle. Magnesium appears to act on voltage-, receptor-, and leak-operated membrane channels in vascular smooth muscle. Standard channel blocker drugs do not have this uniform capability. Calcium channel-blocking drugs, however, can block calcium infiltration into brain cells, lower cerebral vascular resistance, relieve cerebral vasospasm, and lower arterial blood pressure.

Magnesium can also cause significant vasodilatation of intact cerebral arteries. Although magnesium is three to five orders of magnitude less potent than the standard calcium channel-blocking drugs, it possesses unique and potentially useful effects in maintaining healthy cerebral vascular circulation. Those with cerebral vascular disease, and especially those who consume alcohol, should take 1500 mg a day of elemental magnesium.

Nimotop (nimodipine) is an FDA-approved calcium channel-blocking drug specific to cerebral circulation and brain-cell activity. It has been shown to work better in the restoration of cerebral circulation than any other calcium channel-blocking drug yet tested. The normal dose is 30 mg of Nimotop taken 3 times a day.

Medical Device Advances the Treatment of an Aneurysm

By using the device known as the Guglielmi coil, physicians can now correct an aneurysm that is not approachable surgically, either because of its position in the brain or because of other factors that present a high risk.

The coil is an extremely fine wire made from platinum—one of the softest metals—at the end of a longer stainless steel wire. Several coils, depending on the size of the aneurysm, are inserted inside the bubble-like aneurysm through a catheter (a long, narrow tube) threaded through the patient's blood vessels. When the coil is in the correct position—verified by a blood vessel X-ray called an angiogram—it is given a positive electrical charge. The charge causes the steel wire to dissolve at the point of a junction with the platinum coil and the positively charged coil attracts blood cells to form a clot within the aneurysm.

The coils and resulting blood clot fill up the aneurysm, essentially sealing it off. Eventually, the lining of the blood vessel grows over the "neck" of the aneurysm and the aneurysm is essentially healed.

Conclusion

Cerebral vascular disease can be life-threatening. Aneurysm and the subsequent rupture-causing hemorrhage are caused by inherited vascular defects and may be unavoidable. Aneurysm is often precipitated by atherosclerosis and hypertension. High blood pressure increases the risk of aneurysm. Reduction of high blood pressure is imperative in reducing the risk of cerebral vascular disease. Natural supplements combined with lowered blood pressure can reduce the risk and/or damage caused by cerebral vascular disease.

Refer to the *Age-Associated Mental Impairment* protocol for additional suggestions about restoring cerebral circulation. See the *Cardiovascular Disease* protocol and the *Hypertension* protocol for more information on hypertension, cholesterol reduction, and atherosclerosis.

⬤ SUMMARY

The following nutrients and drugs should be considered:

1. To maintain cerebral vasculature, thus lowering the risk of a cerebral aneurysm or hemorrhagic stroke, the following supplements should be considered:

   • Magnesium, 1500 mg daily.

   • Arginine, 4–5 grams daily.

   • Calcium, 1000 mg daily.

   • Grape-seed skin extract, two 200-mg capsules daily.

2. To enhance vasodilation and improve the health of vessels, consider the following:

   • Potassium, 500 mg daily.

   • Hydergine, 5–20 mg daily. (Hydergine may be obtained by prescription or from offshore pharmacies.)

3. Antioxidants scavenge free radicals and protect against underlying factors that lead to cerebral vascular disease:

   • Vitamin E containing tocopherols and tocotrienols provide the most broad spectrum protection, 1–2 softgels daily of Gamma E Tocopherol/Tocotrienols. (Provides 210 mg of gamma-tocopherol and full spectrum tocotrienols.)

   • Vitamin C, 2000–5000 mg daily.

FOR MORE INFORMATION

Contact the National Institute of Neurological Disorders and Stroke, (800) 352-9424.

 ## PRODUCT AVAILABILITY

Vinpocetine, low-dose aspirin, CDP-Choline Caps, Policosanol Tabs, Super Ginkgo Extract, vitamin E succinate, Gamma E Tocopherol/Tocotrienols, Super GLA/DHA, Mega EPA, alpha lipoic acid, selenium, green tea extract, liquid emulsified vitamin A, beta carotene, No Flush Niacin, policosanol, pregnenolone, DHEA, Super Carnosine, *L*-theanine, Mineral Formula for Men, Mineral Formula for Women, magnesium, calcium, arginine, potassium, vitamin C, grape seed-skin extract, TMG, vitamin B_6, Methylcobalamin (B_{12} sublingual tablets), vitamin B_{12} powder, folic acid + B_{12}, melatonin, Kyolic Garlic, and Pure-Gar Caps can be ordered by calling (800) 544-4440 or by ordering online at www.lef.org. You may also ask for a list of offshore suppliers of Hydergine, Piracetam, and Aminoguanidine. Coumadin is a prescription medication.

Cervical Dysplasia

Cervical dysplasia is an abnormal benign or premalignant (or precancerous) change that occurs in the cells of the female cervix. Cervical dysplasia or cervical intraepithelial neoplasia (CIN) is asymptomatic (Goodman 2002). Left undiagnosed or untreated, cervical dysplasia can progress to cervical cancer (Clayman 1989). Worldwide, cervical cancer is still the second leading cause of cancer death in women (WHO 1997). In the United States in 2001, there were 12,900 new cases of cervical cancer, resulting in 4400 deaths (ACS 2001; Greenlee, 2001).

Women have the ability to prevent the progression of cervical dysplasia to cervical cancer through regular Pap screening tests. However, according to the National Institute of Cancer, in developing countries, very few women receive Pap tests and invasive cervical cancer affects an estimated 350,000 women each year, resulting in death for 200,000. Even in the United States, with the known success of Pap tests for cervical cancer screening, each year about 15,000 women will learn that they have cervical cancer (NCI 2001). Some women decide to not have screening because they think they are not at risk. Other women have weakened immune systems, particularly women who are positive for the human immunodeficiency virus (HIV) and the human papillomavirus (HPV). HPV has been implicated as the primary cause of 90% of cervical cancers (NCI 2001). Many other women are at higher risk as a result of their lifestyle choices: smoking, use of oral contraceptives, multiple sex partners, nutritional vitamin and mineral deficiencies, stress, and poor dietary habits (Slattery et al. 1990; Liu et al. 1995; ACS 2001; Moore et al. 2001).

All of these reasons have prompted researchers to direct work toward discovering more effective, less invasive, and less costly preventive, diagnostic, and treatment methods for cervical cancer. The results are particularly encouraging for women who have suspicious cervical dysplasia. A refined, simplified system to classify early lesions (the Bethesda System) has been established to guide medical treatment. Vaccines to spur the immune system to attack existing HPV are also in development (NCI 2001).

DETECTION OF CERVICAL DYSPLASIA

There are three types of cervical dysplasia (also cervical intraepithelial neoplasia): mild (CINI), moderate (CINII), and severe (CINIII). Mild dysplasia is by far the most common. Mild dysplasia is not considered to be a true premalignant disease by many experts. However, mild dysplasia can represent a tissue response to the HPV virus.

Up to 70% of women who have mild dysplasia will have their abnormal cervical cells return to normal cells over time without any specific medical intervention. However, even mild dysplasia can progress to a more serious condition if it remains undetected. Moderate and severe dysplasias should be treated as soon as they are discovered. Left untreated, these types of dysplasia can lead to cervical cancer.

As noted earlier, routine screening with a regular Pap test can detect cervical dysplasia. Early diagnosis and treatment can prevent it from progressing to moderate or severe dysplasias. Therefore, do not skip your regular Pap test screen because you consider yourself to be at low risk. Even though certain lifestyle choices are often unavoidable (high stress levels, use of oral contraceptives, or just too busy to eat properly), they increase a woman's susceptibility to develop cervical dysplasia (Slattery et al. 1990; Liu et al. 1995).

A weakened immune system, whether from a medical condition or dietary deficiencies, is a factor in cervical dysplasia. Because HPV has been implicated as the primary cause of cervical dysplasia and cervical cancer (NCI 2001), if you suspect that you have been exposed to HPV, also request a test for the presence of HPV at the same time you have a Pap test. If HPV is detected, it is important to determine the specific type of HPV virus. This will ensure that the best information possible regarding HPV is available to assist you and your physician in determining the best course of treatment for your particular condition.

Exposure to Human Papilloma Virus

Some experts estimate that as high as 70% of women have had HPV or are currently infected by HPV. HPV is also the most frequent cause of cervical dysplasia (Schiffman et al. 1993; Holly 1996). HPV is commonly called the "wart virus." A papilloma is a noncancerous tumor with a branch or stalk (Glanze 1996). More than 70 types of HPV have been identified (ACS 2001). Usually, types 1, 3, and 5 can cause warts on the hands and feet of children. Types 6 and 11 can cause warts on the genital areas of males and females (genital warts). Other types, such as 16, 18, 31, 33, and 35, may not cause warts, but they can cause changes in the cells of the vagina or cervix, such as dysplasia (Hildesheim et al. 1991). Some data also provide evidence of an association between HPV activity, smoking, and subsequent dysplasia and cancer. Research is being directed to determining if the connection with HPV, dysplasia, and cancer and smoking is from direct carcinogenic effects and/or from local immunosuppression (Moore et al. 2001)

Many women do not know that they have been in contact with HPV or that they have it. A Pap smear often detects abnormal cervical cells that are caused by HPV (symptoms such as warts, are exhibited in only one person in 100 with HPV). Even if HPV is not noted on the Pap smear, there is an 80–90% chance that you have the HPV virus if you have ever been diagnosed with any type of cervical dysplasia.

Because routine testing for the presence of HPV varies across the United States, the Foundation strongly recommends that women request HPV testing with their routine Pap smear to aid in early HPV detection and to facilitate treatment by determining the type of HPV.

Protecting women from HPV is difficult. Generally, the virus is acquired through sexual contact. Condoms can prevent the spread of many diseases, but *not* HPV. Because HPV is found on *all* genital tissues, a condom on the penis will usually not prevent transmission of HPV. HPV can lie dormant on the cervix for 20 years before it causes any changes to the cells or causes warts (ACS 2001). Therefore, if a physician has just discovered that you have an abnormal Pap smear, you may not have recently acquired the virus.

Unprotected sex and even protected sex with a male who has genital warts carries high risks. Warts are lower grades of HPV that sometimes mutate to cancer-causing HPVs. Research has revealed that the earlier the age an individual first contracts genital warts, the more likely they are to develop cervical neoplasia later on in life (Kjaer 1998).

Cigarette Smoking

Cigarette smoking has also been implicated as a cause of dysplasia. More than 53% of women with cervical dysplasia are/were smokers. The bodies of women who smoke concentrate the chemicals ingested by smoking (nicotine and cotinine) in the cervix (ACS 2001). These chemicals have been shown to damage cervical cells.

Interestingly, men who smoke also concentrate these chemicals into their genital secretions and can bathe the cervix with these chemicals during intercourse. Partners who smoke may want to consider the use of condoms as a preventive approach to reduce the risk or progression of the cervical dysplasia.

There are a number of studies that link smoking directly to cervical dysplasia and neoplasia (Moore et al. 2001). Several studies also indicate that smoking at a younger age increases risk factors for cervical intraepithelial neoplasia (CIN) and squamous cell intraepithelial lesions (Lyon et al. 1983; Trevathan et al. 1983).

Smoking has also been shown to lower plasma vitamin C and beta-carotene levels. Lower plasma vitamin C and beta-carotine levels adversely affect pathology and increase the risk of contracting cervical intraepithelial neoplasia.

Smoking can cause low-grade squamous cell intraepithelial lesions (SIL) to develop into high-grade lesions and possibly progress to cancer. One study observed changes in smokers and compared smokers to nonsmokers. The authors concluded that the mutagenic effect of cigarette smoking on cervical cells has an effect on chromosomal damage of the tissue, meaning that smoking increases the risk of progression of dysplasia toward cancer (Cerqueira et al. 1998).

Additionally, the vitamin C status in cervical tissue and leukocytes in the blood has been examined to compare smokers to nonsmokers. The findings show that nonsmokers have four times as much vitamin C as leukocytes, and smokers have lower levels of vitamin C and higher levels of leukocytes in their cervical tissue. This reversal of normal levels of vitamin C and leukocytes further illustrates the ongoing damage of smoking. The study further discusses the free radical-induced cellular damage due to smoking and the possible benefits of antioxidants (Basu et al. 1990).

Use of Oral Contraceptives

The use of oral contraceptives and the duration of their use appear to increase the risk and subsequent development of cervical dysplasia and neoplasia (Ebeling et al. 1987; Brinton et al. 1990). Studies indicate that low levels of folic acid in the blood of women using oral contraceptives have a positive correlation with development of cervical dysplasia and neoplasia. Researchers have demonstrated that oral contraceptives can cause an imbalance in the nutrient status of folic acid, B_6, zinc, and vitamin A, thereby leaving the tissues void of the nutrients that would otherwise protect them.

Other studies have reported that women with mild to moderate cervical dysplasia who were using oral contraceptives experienced improvement when they received folic acid supplementation.

Another group of investigators studied the long-term effects of oral contraceptives by following 195 women for more than 12 years. They found those women were twice as likely to have adenocarcinoma of the cervix (Ursin et al. 1994).

Another study screened 726 subjects for possible factors leading to dysplasia. The researchers identified 294 cases of dysplasia (with 170 controls) as defined by coexistent cytologic and colposcopic evidence. Their results indicated that the key risk factors leading to dysplasia and cancer were the use of oral contraceptives, the number of sexual partners, and the presence of HPV-16 infection. The presence of all or one of these factors increased the risk of cervical dysplasia (Butterworth et al. 1992a; 1992b).

CAUTION Both vitamins E and B_6 should be supplemented in women who are taking oral contraceptives. However, those supplements need to be taken at different times because B_6 can nullify the effects of vitamin E on blood hematocrit.

Multiple Sex Partners

Studies indicate that the number of sexual partners is a risk factor for cervical dysplasia (Parazzini et al. 1992; de Vet et al. 1993). Often this number is taken into consideration along with other factors, such as the lack of condom use; smoking; low levels of vitamin C, beta-carotene, vitamin A, or folic acid; and oral contraceptive use. These factors seem to play a very large role in development of cervical dysplasia. Risk has been reported to be as much as 72% greater if all of these risk factors are present (de Vet et al. 1994).

Poor Dietary Choices

For women at high risk for dysplasia, or those who already have dysplasia, diets with high levels of fruits and vegetables, as well as foods which are high in carotenoids may be beneficial. A healthy diet would also include raw nuts, complex carbohydrates, and foods high in essential fatty acids, but low in animal fat.

A high-quality, easily digestible protein is also beneficial. Protein is extremely important for a strong immune system and tissue repair. Many women are "on the go" and have a low protein intake. These women are advised to consume protein. One easy approach used by many wise women is to make a protein shake in the blender each morning. Because a protein shake is convenient, fast, and easy, it can make an ideal breakfast. Whey or soy proteins would be excellent choices as ingredients in a breakfast shake, along with some frozen fruit, a banana, Udo's Multi-Blend Oil, vitamin B_{12}, and folic acid mixed at the same time in a blender.

There are also studies indicating that a diet high in fruits and vegetables, especially those higher in beta-carotene and vitamin C, has a direct protective effect against the development of cervical dysplasia into the more dangerous cervical neoplasia (Herrero et al. 1991; Goodman et al. 1998). Several studies show a positive correlation between risk factors for cervical dysplasia and consumption of fruits and vegetables, yet the risk factors for squamous cell carcinoma of the cervix were not positive in this area. It would seem that diet might be better as a preventive mechanism for cervical dysplasia. Once cervical dysplasia continues and develops into a neoplasia, diet alone will not likely be a significant factor in stopping the progression, but a good diet should be maintained to support recovery and future prevention.

In addition to a healthy diet, there is also a relationship between other supplements and nutrients and the severity of cervical dysplasia. As early as 1984, a study by Wylie-Rosett et al. (1984) revealed that there is approximately a threefold greater risk for severe dysplasia in women who had lowered vitamin A or beta-carotene intake. Therefore, adding supplements and nutrients (e.g., vitamins, minerals, folic acid, indole-3-carbinol) as a daily part of healthy diet should be carefully considered (*see the section on Integrated Natural Therapy for Cervical Dysplasia for a discussion of beneficial supplements*).

Stress

Stress and a feeling of hopelessness have been implicated as having an adverse effect on immunity. Clinical researchers reported that stress contributed to the promotion of CIN and squamous cell cervical cancer (Goodkin et al. 1987). If you have been diagnosed with cervical dysplasia, take steps to reduce your daily stress as part of an integrated therapeutic approach for the disease.

Other

Other risk factors are intercourse before the age of 18, having an immune deficiency disorder, and giving birth before the age of 22.

TRADITIONAL MEDICAL TREATMENT FOR CERVICAL DYSPLASIA

Getting rid of the HPV is difficult. Even if the entire cervix is burned using Loop Electrosurgical Excisional Procedure (LEEP) or frozen (cryosurgery), generally the virus will still remain. According to the American Academy of Dermatology (AADA 1995), the major goal of treatment is not to eliminate the virus but to assist the body's immune system in controlling the virus by:

- Increasing the patient's disease-free intervals.
- Decreasing the amount of clinically diseased tissue, both to assist the immune system in handling the virus more effectively and in reducing the spread of HPV to adjacent or distant body areas or to other persons.
- Providing a routine, life-long follow-up plan for continued early detection and treatment of further cervical dysplasia.
- Determining an appropriate treatment plan that will be the least aggressive but most effective (possibly avoiding surgical procedures that may result in scarring but still does not cure the patient).

Surgical treatment of cervical dysplasia can be accomplished by several means including techniques such as LEEP, conization, or cryosurgery (freezing). The purpose of LEEP and cryosurgery is to remove or kill abnormal cells on or around the cervix before they can develop into cancer. These surgical procedures are aimed at destroying the unhealthy tissue that has been affected by HPV. Your physician will discuss these procedures with you if they are needed.

Generally, women who have normal immune system function can limit the progression or be cured of mild to moderate cervical dysplasia without surgery (*see the Integrated Natural Therapies section*).

INTEGRATED NATURAL THERAPY FOR CERVICAL DYSPLASIA

Supplements, taken orally as well as delivered topically, have been shown to be an effective part of an integrated treatment approach for cervical dysplasia. Several vitamins and supplements have been the subject of scientific studies that demonstrated the benefits and the supportive role of supplements in a positive outcome for cervical dysplasia, including vitamins A, B_6, C, and E, beta-carotene, topical vitamin A, indole-3-carbinol, folic acid, lycopene, alpha-carotene, selenium, and zinc.

Vitamin A

In a study in which 34 women were biopsied (Volz et al. 1995), researchers concluded that supplementation with vitamin A may help prevent cervical neoplasia. Another case-control study of 87 cases and 82 controls demonstrated that with all factors considered, about a threefold greater risk for severe dysplasia or carcinoma was found in women who had lowered

vitamin A or beta-carotene intake and nutritional status (Wylie-Rosett et al. 1984). Liu et al. (1995) also found that high plasma levels of vitamin A (retinol) were related to regression of cervical dysplasia, especially in HPV-16-positive women. Nagata et al. (1999a) conducted a follow-up study in 134 women who had been histologically diagnosed with cervical dysplasia (from October 1987 to September 1988). Follow-up with the women was continued until February 1995. Every 3 months, the women were examined with cervical smears and colposcopy (a visual examination of the cervix and vagina using a lighted instrument). During follow-up, 8 women (5.9%) developed cancer *in situ* or invasive cervical cancer and 106 (79.1%) reverted to normal. The rate of progression of cancer *in situ* or cervical cancer was 4.5 times higher in women with the lower serum retinol levels than in women with higher serum retinol levels. Nagata et al. (1999a) concluded that "the results suggest an association of low serum retinol level with development of cervical cancer."

CAUTION Vitamin A is obtained from animal sources (e.g., egg yolks or liver), synthesized in our own livers, or obtained from supplements. Before supplementing with high doses of vitamin A, please refer to *Appendix A*.

Topical Vitamin A as a Therapeutic Approach to Cervical Dysplasia

Because retinoids are regulators of epithelial differentiation and are necessary for maintenance, they have been the basis for study of their potential chemopreventive effects on cervical tissues. In particular, treatment with topical vitamin A in the form of various retinoids (all-*trans*-retinoic acid or RA) has been studied, resulting in positive results for both cervical dysplasia and cervical cancers (Graham et al. 1986; Weiner et al. 1986; Meyskens et al. 1994; Ruidi et al. 1997).

Some of the research was conducted using treatment with topical vitamin A via vaginal inserts. Studies were completed using topical vitamin A applied directly to the cervical tissue using a cervical cap and sponge (Graham et al. 1986; Weiner et al. 1986; Meyskens et al. 1994) or a vaginal suppository (Ruidi et al. 1997). The investigators using a cervical cap and sponge reported a successful and complete response rate approaching 50% in subjects who had mild to moderate forms of cervical dysplasia. However, patients with severe dysplasia did not benefit from the therapy. Graham et al. (1986) concluded that topical application of vitamin A appeared to be effective only in mild to moderate cases of cervical dysplasia. In a similar study, Meyskens et al. (1994) concluded that "a short course of locally applied RA can reverse CINII, but not more advanced dysplasia, with acceptable local side effect." However, because RA can reverse or suppress epithelial preneoplasia, Meyskens et al. (1994) suggested that chemoprevention of human cancer is feasible.

Beta-Carotene

Beta-carotene is a precursor (a substance that is the source of another substance) of vitamin A. In addition to being an important antioxidant in its own right, beta-carotene is converted to vitamin A in our body. From a large study (four countries) of 387 women and 670 controls in Latin America, Potischman et al. 1991 reported a trend of decreased risk of disease of invasive cervical cancer associated with higher levels of beta-carotene. In another study (Palan et al. 1992), the objective was to measure beta-carotene levels in exfoliated epithelial cervicovaginal cells in normal women and in women with histopathologically diagnosed neoplasia and cancer. Cross-sampling was done in 105 women. In addition, beta-carotene levels were measured in women (24) who were participating in an ongoing oral beta-carotene supplementation clinical trial. Palan et al. (1992) found that cervicovaginal cells and plasma beta-carotene levels were significantly decreased in women with CIN and cervical cancer when compared with controls. However, after oral supplementation with beta-carotene, the levels of beta-carotene in cervicovaginal cells increased markedly in a majority of patients (79%). Palan et al. (1992) concluded that their findings support the hypothesis that "beta-carotene deficiency may have an etiologic role in the pathogenesis of cervical intraepithelial neoplasia and/or cervical cancer."

Vitamin B$_6$

Oral contraceptives deplete vitamin B$_6$, which increases the risk of cervical dysplasia (Simpson 1980; Salih et al. 1986). If a woman has diabetes or is overweight and takes oral contraceptives, her need for vitamin B$_6$ is increased. Vitamin B$_6$ plays an important role in protein synthesis, carbohydrate metabolism, and glucose tolerance. Life Extension recommends taking 50–250 mg of vitamin B$_6$ a day, if you use oral contraceptives.

Vitamin C

Vitamin C has been reported to be an independent risk factor for dysplasia (Ho et al. 1998). Nutritional levels of vitamin C that are less than the recommended daily allowance (RDA) levels have been shown to increase the odds of developing cervical dysplasia. As early as 1981, Wassertheil-Smoller et al. reported that a dietary survey estimated that 68% of women in the United States who are of reproductive age receive inadequate levels of vitamin C.

Demonstrating the need for adequate vitamin C levels, another controlled case study looked at the impact of vitamin C on the risk of contracting dysplasia (Romney et al. 1985). The study examined women with completely normal Pap smears and no gynecological problems, as well as women who had two consecutive abnormal Pap smears. These test subjects were evaluated for vitamin C blood plasma levels. Those women with normal Pap smears had twice the vitamin C blood plasma levels than those with abnormal smears.

Vitamin E

In addition to depleting levels of vitamin B$_6$, the use of oral contraceptives can also deplete vitamin E levels, increasing the risk of cervical dysplasia. There have been a number of studies where low levels of tocopherols (vitamin E) were noted in women with cervical dysplasia and cancer. Investigators have reported an inverse relationship between vitamin E levels and increased risk and the severity of the disorder.

Indole-3-carbinol (I3C)

As noted earlier, a diet that contains high levels of fruits and vegetables reduces the risk of cervical dysplasia. Fruits and vegetables contain many anticancer agents including indole-3-carbinol (I3C). I3C, found in the cruciferous vegetables (e.g., broccoli, brussels sprouts, cabbage, cauliflower, bok choy), has been found to play a positive role in preventing or stopping various types of cancer (Grubbs et al. 1995). I3C was shown to prevent the development of vaginal and cervical cancers in HPV-16 transgenic mice (Jin et al. 1999). According to Sepkovic et al. (1995), women with cervical intraepithelial neoplasia II and III (CINII and CINIII) have lower estrogen metabolites ratios than normal women. Through its action on cytochrome P-450 1A1/1A2, I3C is known to alter the pathway of estrogen in both men and women in a manner that decreases the risk of certain tumors (Telang et al. 1992; Stoewsand et al. 1988; Zeligs 1998). The P-450 family of enzymes is known for detoxifying and metabolizing a variety of substances that have been found to be carcinogenic, which may explain the cancer-preventive actions of I3C in humans and animals (Telang et al. 1992).

An interesting study by Bell et al. (2000) was published in *Gynecologic Oncology*. The study included 30 women who had biopsy-proven CINII or CINIII. The women were also assessed for HPV status, and all three groups were similarly matched. The test subjects were randomized to receive either 200 mg or 400 mg of I3C or a placebo orally for 12 weeks. Bell et al. (2002) also tested for urinary 2-hydroxyestrone/16-a-hydroxyestrone ratios at the beginning of the trial and then 4 weeks later. After 12 weeks, the women were biopsied. In the two groups receiving I3C, the researchers found that there was an increase in the 2-hydroxyestrone/16-a-hydroxyestrone ratios, whereas in the placebo group, the ratios were reversed.

Metabolizing of estradiol to 16-a-hydroxyestrone has been shown to be a potent estrogen, whereas 2-hydroxyestrone is considered antiestrogenic. It was hypothesized that the primary mechanism by which I3C works is by altering the 2-hydroxyestrone/16-a-hydroxyestrone ratio. The results of the study were that none (0 of 10) of the women in the placebo group had complete regression of CIN. However, four of eight patients in the 200 mg a day group and four of nine patients in the 4300 mg a day group had complete regression of CIN based on their 12-week biopsy. Bell et al. (2000) concluded that "there was a statistically significant regression of CIN in patients treated with I3C orally compared with the placebo. The 2/16-a-hydroxyestrone ratio changed in a dose-dependent fashion."

All of the positive reports cited concerning the beneficial role of I3C in treatment of cervical dysplasia appear to be reason enough for women to look further into using I3C in the treatment of cervical dysplasia. Please note that the recommended dose of I3C is 200 mg taken two to three times a day depending on body weight.

Folic Acid, Lycopene, and Alpha-Carotene

Folic acid is involved in red blood cell health, as well as other functions in maintaining healthy tissues. Folic acid has also been shown to prevent neural tube defects, both indirectly in the synthesis of transfer RNA and through its function as a methyl donor to create methylcobalamin, which is used in the remethylation of homocysteine to methionine (Butterworth 1993).

In several studies in oral contraceptive users, researchers demonstrated that folate levels are decreased by oral contraceptives (Streiff 1970; Whitehead et al. 1973; Kornberg et al. 1989). Oral contraceptives appear to have a role in disrupting normal folate metabolisms, and supplementation with folic acid can reverse this problem. Use of folic acid daily would appear to be extremely prudent for oral contraceptive users (Ziegler 1986).

Folic acid is also important for healthy cervical tissue. Folic acid has been reported to play a therapeutic role in preventing cervical dysplasia and in reducing the risks of neoplasia in ulcerative colitis (Butterworth et al. 1992a; 1992b; Zarcone et al. 1996). Additional studies demonstrated that folic acid supplementation arrested progression of dysplasia in oral contraceptive users who had mild to moderate dysplasia. In some cases, folic acid supplementation was reported to have reversed dysplasia (Butterworth 1982).

A study by Kanetsky et al. (1998) reported the importance of lycopene relative to the risk and treatment of cervical dysplasia. Another study also reported the association of plasma micronutrients with the risk of cervical dysplasia (Goodman et al. 1998).

Nagata et al. (1999b) reported in the *British Journal of Cancer* that alpha-carotene levels are associated with a decreased risk for cervical dysplasia. The study was conducted in 156 women who had newly histologically confirmed cervical dysplasia and age-matched controls from women who had normal Pap smears. When their cervical tissue and blood samples were compared, the researchers found a decreased risk for cervical dysplasia with the highest serum levels of alpha-carotene (after other factors, such as smoking and HPV, were removed). Decreased risk with lycopene was marginally significant. A nonsignificant decrease in risk was found with zeaxanthin/lutein (Nagata et al. 1999b).

Selenium

Numerous studies on cervical and uterine cancers have found that low selenium levels are associated with risk. These studies show that patients who do not have dysplasia (controls) have higher levels of tissue selenium compared to patients who do have cervical dysplasia. Therefore, low selenium intake and low selenium levels increase the risk of cervical and uterine neoplasia (Sundstrom et al. 1984; Hussain et al. 1992; Lou et al. 1995).

Zinc

Zinc is well-known for its immunity-enhancing function. Although zinc has not yet been studied conclusively for its independent effects on cervical dysplasia, zinc should be included in a woman's supplement program to improve general health and reduce the risk of disease. However, worth mentioning is a study by Liu et al. (1995). These researchers related high levels of retinol to the regression of cervical dysplasia and also observed the protective effects of zinc.

IF YOU HAVE BEEN DIAGNOSED WITH CERVICAL DYSPLASIA

Communicate with your physician. Learn as much as you can about your specific condition and possible treatment options. Help your physician to understand that you want a long-term positive outcome, but with as little surgical intervention as possible. Focus on risk factors that you can change or avoid (e.g., lifestyle choices) rather than those that you cannot. Improve your diet by ensuring that you maintain high levels of fruits and vegetables. Also consider adding supplements, taken orally, as well as delivered topically, as part of an effective integrated treatment approach for cervical dysplasia.

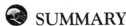 **SUMMARY**

Traditional and integrated medical treatments work best when there is focus on all of the cofactors of cervical dysplasia. Although using a condom may somewhat lower the risk of contracting HPV (associated with almost all cervical dysplasia), HPV can be transmitted between sexual partners even if a condom is used. Eat a well-balanced diet, including adequate protein and fruits and vegetables. If you are a smoker, take all vitamins in higher optimal dosages. If you are taking oral contraceptives, supplement with vitamin E and an additional B-complex vitamin that is high in B_6. Select a physician who is willing to consider treatment that is less aggressive (vaginal inserts, topical preparations) if that is appropriate for your condition. However, more aggressive treatment (chemoprevention, surgery) is often the prudent treatment for more advanced forms of cervical dysplasia.

Supplement Recommendations:

1. Take a multivitamin supplement, such as Life Extension Mix, that is high in B vitamins, zinc, selenium, beta-carotene, lycopene, vitamin E, and vitamin C.

2. Whey protein is an immune booster and can help fulfill necessary protein requirements for a balanced diet. One scoop a day.

3. Vitamin A, 5000–25,000 IU a day. Discuss with your doctor the advisability of vitamin A suppositories. (Avoid extra vitamin A if you might become pregnant. Extra vitamin A can cause birth defects.)

4. Beta-carotene, 25,000 IU a day, and indole-3-carbinol, (I3C) 400–600 mg a day, are important supplements for women who do not consume recommended amounts of fruits and vegetables.

5. Vitamin B_6, 50–250 mg a day, and vitamin E, 400–800 IU a day, are especially important to women on birth control pills. (Life Extension Mix provides 100 mg a day of vitamin B_6 and 400 IU of vitamin E.)

6. Low levels of vitamin C are associated with abnormal Pap smears. Supplement with 2000–6000 mg a day. (Life Extension Mix provides about 2500 mg of vitamin C a day.)

7. Folic acid, 800–10,000 mcg a day, and lycopene, 10–30 mg a day, to maintain healthy cervical tissue.

8. Zinc, 15–50 mg a day, is recommended, especially for women taking oral contraceptives. (Life Extension Mix provides 35 mg a day of zinc.)

9. Selenium has been shown to prevent cancer. Recommended dosage is 200–400 mcg a day. (Life Extension Mix provides 200 mcg a day of selenium.)

 FOR MORE INFORMATION

For more about the effects of drug-induced vitamin depletion, read a book on the subject entitled *The Drug-Induced Nutrient Depletion Handbook, Second Edition* (Pelton et al. 2001).

If you have been diagnosed with cervical dysplasia and would like to contact *A Woman's Time*, the telephone number is (503) 222–2322. *A Woman's Time* specializes in women's conditions and also provides telephone consulting, ranging in price from $40–$80 an hour. *A Woman's Time* can provide information on Vag-Pak (a product by Bezwecken, Germany). Vag-Pak includes topical vitamin A, proteolytic enzymes with zinc, and other nutrient-based treatments for cervical dysplasia.

PRODUCT AVAILABILITY

Life Extension Mix, Enhanced Whey Protein, vitamin A, beta-carotene, indole-3-carbinol (I3C), vitamin B_6, folic acid, vitamin C, vitamin E, lycopene extract, selenium, and zinc can be ordered by telephoning (800) 544-4440 or by ordering online at www.lef.org.

Colorectal Cancer

According to the Centers for Disease Control and Prevention, cancer of the colon and rectum affects nearly 160,000 Americans each year, with one out of every 20 individuals at risk for developing colorectal cancer at some point in their lifetime. It is the second most frequently diagnosed malignancy in the United States, with 85,600 new cases detected causing approximately 62,070 deaths annually. It ranks fourth in global cancer incidence and deaths (Shibuya et al. 2002) because it has a better prognosis than most common cancers.

The lifetime risk of developing colorectal cancer, which is higher in developed countries, appears to be 4.6% for men and 3.2% for women (Chu et al. 1994). Its occurrence is higher in males versus females and in African American versus Caucasian populations. Approximately 50% of colorectal cancers are diagnosed at regional or distant stage (Weir et al. 2003). However, early detection of colorectal cancer dramatically increases survival. For example, 90% of patients who receive early treatment are still alive after 5 years compared to 64% survival when adjacent organs or lymph nodes are affected. With traditional colorectal cancer treatments only 10% of patients are alive after 5 years if the cancer is carried to distant organs (Dashwood 1999). The peak age of onset of colorectal cancer in the United States is at age 65 years (Khan et al. 2002).

ANATOMY

The colon and rectum are organs of the digestive system located in the abdomen and pelvis between the small intestine and the anal canal. Together, the colon and rectum make up the large intestine or colon. Because of their close proximity, cancers of the two organs are often discussed together under the term *colorectal cancer*. The treatment and pattern of recurrence of colon and rectal cancer are affected by the location of the primary tumor and its relationship to the surrounding structures.

The colon initiates at the juncture between the small intestine and the large intestine, called the ileocecal sphincter (valve). The first part of the colon is the cecum, with the appendix lying at the lower edge. The ascending colon travels up vertically on the right

side of the abdomen to the hepatic flexure, and then the transverse colon, which is often not transverse, extends across the abdomen and normally hangs down in a loop which may be as low as the pelvis. Finally, the descending colon leads down vertically on the left side of the body and terminates in the sigmoid colon, which is the narrowest part of the large bowel, and it terminates with the upper rectum. The rectum is the last section of the gastrointestinal tract and leads to the anus.

Functions

The function of the colon is storage and concentration of undigested matter by absorption of salt and water. The colon also mixes and propels its contents by muscular contraction towards the sigmoid colon and rectum for defecation. The rectum stores fecal matter until it is eliminated from the body by defecating, this is often termed a "bowel movement" and the reflex is initiated by distension.

ETIOLOGY

The exact cause of colorectal cancer is a process of genetic change in the epithelial cells of the colonic lining (mucosa). Epidemiological studies have provided specific factors that initiate the process of cancer development in the large bowel mucosa. The main factors that can initiate colorectal cancer development are meat intake, altered vitamin and mineral intake, bile acids, fecal mutagens, fecal pH, and a predisposition to the effects of mutagens (Winawer et al. 1992).

A mutagen is an agent that can cause an increase in the rate of DNA mutation. Differences in protection from the effects of mutagen-induced DNA damage depends on an individual's detoxification enzymes. An example is an enzyme that catalyzes the formation of mutagenic products from heterocyclic amines, which are formed in cooked meats and play a role in colorectal cancer development. Differences in the activity of this enzyme, N-acetyltransferase, classify individuals as slow or fast acetylators. The level of red meat consumption in fast but not slow acetylators is associated with a risk for colorectal cancer development (Welfare et al. 1997).

The mutagenic heterocyclic amines in the stool may be produced by the interaction of digestion and food products, particularly meat (Reddy et al. 1987). Fecal mutagens can be produced by certain diets; for example changing a lacto-vegetarian diet to a diet with increased fiber caused a reduction in the changes that a normal cell undergoes as it becomes malignant

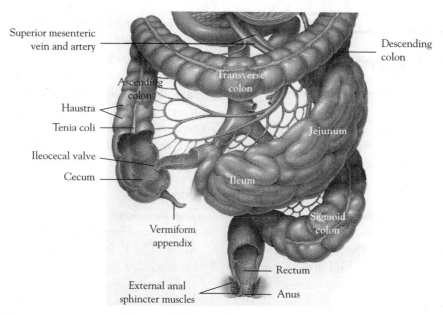

The large intestine is about 1.5 meters (5 ft) in length, with a much larger diameter than the small intestine. The subdivisions of the large intestine are (1) cecum, (2) ascending colon, (3) transverse colon, (4) descending colon, (5) sigmoid colon, (6) rectum, (7) anal canal. This listing indicates the order in which food passes through the large intestine. (Anatomical Chart Company 2002®, Lippincott Williams & Wilkins)

within the stool (Johansson et al. 1997). Intake of antioxidants reduces the mutagenic activity of compounds within the stool. Fiber intake alters the intestinal transit time which in turn affects the exposure of the colorectal lining to mutagens.

There is a high correlation between red meat intake, and the compounds that result from cooking meat at high temperatures, and death from colorectal cancer (Armstrong et al. 1975; Bingham et al. 1996). The association between red meat and colorectal cancer is due, at least in part, to the heterocyclic amines (compounds that can cause mutations in DNA) present in cooked meat (Gerhardsson de Verdier et al. 1991). The frequency of red meat intake and the method of cooking can be correlated with the prevalence of distal colorectal adenomas. Fried meat is the main source of exposure to heterocyclic amines. People who eat fried, browned, red meat more than once per week are 2.2 times more likely to develop colorectal adenomas, as compared to those who eat lightly browned red meat once per week or less frequently.

There is also a strong association between the risk of colon cancer and the consumption of saturated animal fat, a lipid-rich diet containing omega-6 fatty acids (Jones et al. 2003) and total energy intake, which are thought to break down into carcinogens (cancer-causing compounds) in the gut (Pierre et al. 2003). In industrialized Western societies, both polyps as well as colon cancer occur

more frequently due in part to diets low in fruits (Evans et al. 2002), vegetables, vegetable protein, and fiber (Satia-Aboutaj et al. 2003).

Fat consumption is a known risk factor for colorectal cancer (Stadler et al. 1988). The digestion of fats requires the activity of normal bile acids which irritate and damage the epithelial cells of the colon. Consequently, bile acids can cause abnormal increased growth rate of cells lining the intestines (intestinal mucosa) resulting in increased risk for colorectal cancer (Suzuki et al. 1986). Bile acids have been shown to activate factors associated with the promotion of colorectal cancer development (Glinghammar et al. 1999). The ratio between the secondary bile acid deoxycholic acid and cholic acid may be an indicator of colorectal cancer risk (Kamano et al. 1999).

Alkaline environments in the stool (pH >7.0) sustain higher concentrations of potential *carcinogens* (substances that increase the risk of cancer) such as free bile acids (McKeown-Eyssen et al. 1986). This alkaline pH may affect the solubility of bile acid and carcinogens and make them more genotoxic (damaging to DNA) to the lubricated lining of intestinal cells. Epidemiological studies show that higher rates of colon carcinoma are found in individuals with a more alkaline stool pH (i.e., a stool pH >7.0) (Malhotra et al. 1982).

THE BENEFIT OF DIETARY INTERVENTION

Oral calcium supplementation has been proposed as a dietary intervention for individuals at high risk of colorectal cancer because calcium can reduce the growth rate of rectal and colonic epithelial cells both directly and by binding bile acids and fatty acids in the stool, resulting in compounds that are less likely to adversely affect the colon (Rozen et al. 1989). Calcium reduces the risk of colorectal cancer but its effects may occur only in individuals who have a low level of fat intake and may also be site-specific within the colon (Cats et al. 1995). However, oral calcium supplementation reduced benign epithelial tumor (adenoma) formation by 19% (Baron et al. 1999) and was shown to cause a minor nonstatistically significant reduction of epithelial cell proliferation in the rectum (Cats et al. 1995).

Folate is a potentially protective agent against colorectal cancer. Folate depletion in experimental studies increases the risk of tumor formation and also reduces DNA methylation by reducing methyl group availability. Low folate intake, especially when combined with alcohol consumption and a low-protein diet, has been implicated in increased colorectal cancer risk (Kato et al. 1999). Alcohol consumption increases the need for folate intake. Dietary folate influences DNA methylation, synthesis, and repair. Abnormalities in these DNA processes may enhance carcinogenesis, particularly in rapidly growing tissues such as the colorectal mucosa. DNA methylation abnormalities may influence the expression of cancer-related genes, and inadequate levels of folate may lead to uracil misincorporation into DNA and to DNA damage (chromosomal breaks) (Feinberg et al. 1983; Lengauer et al. 1997). An increasing number of epidemiologic studies indicate that higher intakes of folate either from dietary sources or from supplements may lower the risk of colorectal adenoma and cancer (Giovanucci 2002). After supplementing with folate-containing multivitamins for 15 years a reduced risk of colon cancer was observed (Giovannuci et al. 1998) whereas the contribution of dietary folate was modest.

Increased vitamin D intake has been associated with reduced risk for colon carcinoma (Garland et al. 1999). Vitamin D3 causes *differentiation* of colon cancer cells. Cancer cells that are *well differentiated* are close to the original normal healthy colon cells in nature and are usually less aggressive cancer cells. *Poorly differentiated* cells have changed more from the normal healthy cells and are usually more aggressive cancer cells. Total vitamin D intake was *inversely* related to colorectal cancer incidence (Martinez et al. 1996), meaning the higher an individual's intake of vitamin D the lower the rate of colorectal cancer.

In high-risk individuals, the use of multivitamins has been shown to reduce the risk of adenoma formation (Whelan et al. 1999). A reduced risk of colon cancer is associated with the use of vitamin C (Howe et al. 1992). Vitamins C, E, and A showed protection against the risk of developing colorectal cancer (Newberne et al. 1990). Low levels of selenium correlated with the presence of adenomas (benign tumors), whereas increased levels were associated with reduced risk of adenomas (Russo et al. 1997). Intervention trials have found a beneficial effect of selenium supplementation. There is an association between iron exposure and colorectal polyps (Bird et al. 1996a).

RISK FACTORS

Primary Prevention

Identifying and eradicating the causative factors responsible for the development of colorectal cancer is of the utmost importance to those individuals who are at high-risk for developing the disease and to those who have been diagnosed with colorectal cancer. These factors include diet, lifestyle, exercise, tobacco and alcohol use, parity, hormone use, energy intake, and nonsteroidal anti-inflammatory drug (NSAID) use.

Fiber, particularly bran and cellulose appear to be effective in reducing the risk of colorectal *carcinogenesis* (the generation of cancer from normal cells) (Greenwald et al. 1986). Fruit fiber consumption, as opposed to vegetable fiber, reduced the risk of colorectal adenomas (Platz et al. 1997).

There is a direct relationship suggested by epidemiological studies between total fat intake in the diet and increased risk of cancer in the colon and rectum. Animal fat, particularly dairy products, and red meat are associated with colon cancer risk, whereas there is no association with vegetable fats, and fish oils appear to have a protective effect (Schloss et al. 1997). Lower cholesterol levels have been shown in patients diagnosed with colorectal cancer (Forones et al. 1998). Conversely, elevated levels of serum triglycerides have been associated with a higher risk of adenomatous polyps (Bird et al. 1996b).

The risk factor associated with alcohol consumption and cigarette smoking is startling. Daily alcohol intake has been associated with a twofold increase in colon carcinoma (Giovannuci et al. 1998). Smoking is an independent risk factor and long-term smoking is particularly damaging, increasing the relative risk by 1.6–4.5 fold for adenoma formation (Nagata et al. 1999). Smoking more than 20 cigarettes a day increases the likelihood of having polyps by more then 250%, while alcohol consumption increases likelihood by 87%. When combined, smoking and alcohol consumption increase the likelihood by an astonishing 400% (Martinez et al. 1995; Lieberman et al. 2003).

Obesity, particularly abdominal obesity, is associated with an increased risk (Martinez et al. 1999; Russo et al. 1998) whereas physical activity is associated with a decreased risk of colorectal cancer (Giovanucci et al. 1996). There is also an association between diabetes mellitus and colorectal cancer risk; the risk is increased with a high fasting glucose level, high insulin levels, and obesity (Ma et al. 1999; Schoen et al. 1999).

Human colon tumors contain increased amounts of prostaglandin E2 (PGE-2), which is thought to participate in colon cancer development (Rigas et al. 1993). Cyclooxygenase 2 (COX-2) appears to be responsible for the increased production of PGE-2, in response to growth factors in colon tumors (Sheehan et al. 1999). Blocking the production of COX-2, therefore, may assist in the prevention of colon cancer. Indeed, regular NSAID use was associated with a lower risk of colorectal cancer diagnosis than nonuse of NSAIDs (Reeves et al. 1996). Sulindac is an NSAID that reduced polyps by 56% in the setting of familial adenomatous polyposis (FAP) (Giardiello et al. 1993).

Secondary Prevention

Secondary prevention involves identifying individuals at high-risk of developing colorectal cancer or those at increased risk of death from colorectal cancer owing to the existence of a premalignant lesion. High-risk individuals can be identified by their age (older than 40 years), genetic factors such as familial polyposis syndromes, hereditary nonpolyposis colon cancer, inherited colorectal cancer in Ashkenazi Jews, attenuated familial adenomatous polyposis syndrome, or a family history of colon carcinoma or polyps, and predisposing diseases such as inflammatory bowel disease (IBD), granulomatous colitis, history of colorectal carcinoma or polyps or previous cancers, pelvic irradiation, and noncancer surgery. Interventions that can prevent the development of colorectal cancer include screening for adenomas, treatment of adenomatous polyps by endoscopic polypectomy, or excision of the large bowel (in FAP) (Watson et al. 1998; Munkholm 2003).

GENETIC RISK FACTORS

Familial Polyposis Syndromes

Familial Adenomatous Polyposis (FAP) syndromes involve early onset of multiple polyps and virtually 100% risk of colorectal cancer development (Bussey 1990). However, this is a relatively rare disease affecting approximately 1 in 8000 individuals who have a predisposition to develop colon cancer without intervention. The condition is characterized by 500 to 2500 colonic adenomatous polyps, with a minimum of 100 needed for diagnosis of FAP. The polyps are not present at birth but develop over time. Gardner's syndrome is a variant of FAP, in which the entire large bowel may be affected by adenomatous polyposis associated with lipomas (benign fatty tumors), fibromas (benign fibrous tumors), and desmoid tumors (Arvanitis et al. 1990). Oldfield's syndrome and Turcot's syndrome are very rare polyposis diseases in which there is also a genetic defect in the adenomatous polyposis coli (APC) gene (located at 5q21). Polyps arise within 10 to 20 years and cancer follows after 10 to15 years.

Hereditary Nonpolyposis Colon Cancer (HNPCC) Syndromes

HNPCC is inherited as an autosomal dominant trait. Thus, individuals are classified as HNPCC when there is a strong family history of developing colorectal cancer at an early age (average age, 46 years) (Peltomaki et al. 1997). This syndrome accounts for approximately 1 to 6% of colorectal cancers (Marra et al. 1995). Microsatellite instability is present in the tumor of patients (90%) with HNPCC (Akiyama et al. 1997).

Family History of Polyps or Colon Carcinoma

There is a three- to fourfold increased risk of colorectal cancer and an 8% risk of large adenomas among those who have first-degree relatives (sibling, child, or parent) with polyps or colon carcinoma (Boutron et al. 1995; Grossman et al. 1988). Adenomatous polyps (often referred to as *polyps*) are benign epithelial tumors (noncancerous growths) arising as a mass of tissue that bulges outward from the normal surface of the inner mucus lining of the colon or rectum. Polyps can occur at any age, although people over age 50 have a significant risk of developing colon polyps (Foutch et al. 1991).

Polyps of the colon or rectum may be single or multiple adenomas and are almost always benign, usually producing no symptoms but can also become precancerous. The presence of these polyps however, carries a risk of carcinoma within the polyp itself as well as for additional sites within the colon. The probability of any singular polyp becoming cancerous is dependent on several factors: gross appearance, histological features, and size. Polyps larger than 1 cm have an increased risk of progressing to colon cancer, as do polyps with atypical cells or dysplasia (O'Brien et al. 1990). Hyperplastic polyps, as well as adenomas, may serve to identify individuals with a high risk of colorectal cancer (Liljegren et al. 2003).

The cumulative risk of cancer developing in an unremoved polyp is 2.5% at 5 years; 8% at 10 years; and 24% at 20 years after the diagnosis. Removing polyps significantly reduces the relative risk of developing colon cancer to 2.3%, compared to a relative risk of 8.0% for those not removed (Donovan et al. 1998; Winawer et al. 1993). Polyps may cause painless rectal bleeding or internal bleeding, which in turn may cause anemia.

Colorectal carcinomas may occur anywhere in the large intestine. A colorectal carcinoma is a malignant new growth that arises from epithelium in the lining of the bowel. Carcinomas tend to infiltrate into adjacent tissue and spread (metastasize) to distant organs, for example: to the liver, lungs, bone, and the brain.

Medical conditions that predispose (increase susceptibility) an individual to colorectal cancer were previously discussed, and include inflammatory bowel disease (IBD) (particularly ulcerative colitis) (Karlen et al. 1999), Crohn's disease (granulomatous colitis), a history of colorectal carcinoma or polyps (Collett et al. 1999), pelvic radiation, and noncancer surgery such as cholecystectomy (Neugut et al. 1991).

Adenocarcinoma

Adenocarcinoma of the colon and rectum develops in the glands of the inner lining or mucosa of the intestine and makes up 95% of colorectal cancer cases. *Subtypes of adenocarcinoma of the colon include:*

- **Mucinous (colloid):** Mucinous adenocarcinomas are adenocarcinomas that produce mucus and may arise from several primary sites including the colon and ovaries.

- **Signet ring:** A signet ring is an adenocarcinoma whose nuclei are often pushed to the side of the cells. These signet ring tumors often have a propensity to metastasize to the ovary.

- **Other types include:** Neuroendocrine tumors, lymphomas, melanomas, squamous cell, sarcomas, and carcinoids.

SCREENING

Screening involves testing asymptomatic individuals to assess the likelihood that they may have colorectal cancer. Screening achieves two goals: the detection of early-stage nonmetastatic cancers that are surgically curable and the identification and removal of benign adenomatous polyps, the precursor lesions of nearly all adenocarcinomas. Patients who present with symptoms are not appropriate candidates for screening examination, as they require a total colonic examination. Screening tests that can detect early curable colorectal disease and do not involve excessive risk are available.

Those in whom symptoms are compatible with the diagnosis of colorectal cancer, such as those with rectal bleeding, iron-deficiency anemia, alteration in bowel habits, bowel obstruction, or abdominal pain and distension, should undergo total colonic examination. The benefits of early diagnosis are improvements in treatment effectiveness and increased survival. In the general population, the risk of development of colorectal adenoma is approximately 19% and it is estimated that 2 to 5% of sporadic polyps will develop into an invasive carcinoma (Markowitz et al. 1997). Screening of high-risk groups includes:

- Familial Adenomatous Polyposis (FAP): start during adolescence, then colonoscopy after age 24 every 2 years until age 34, then every 3 years until age 44, then revert to general population screening.

- Hereditary Nonpolyposis Colon Cancer (HNPCC): Colonoscopy every 1 to 3 years starting at age 25.

- Family or personal history of colorectal cancer or adenomatous polyps: Beginning at age 40 instead of 50; individuals who have a relative with early-onset disease should start 3 to 10 years prior to the age of onset of their relative's disease.

- Inflammatory bowel disease: Colonoscopy after 8 years of disease in cases of pan-colitis or after 15 years with colitis (Provenzale et al. 1995).

It is recommended that individuals in whom colorectal cancer has been surgically removed undergo complete examination of the colon within 1 year after resection. If the results are normal then the individual can undergo evaluation in 3 years (Winawer et al. 1990).

Screening of average-risk groups includes the general population, particularly older individuals in whom colorectal cancer is much more common. For average-risk groups, the screening consists of digital rectal examination (DRE), fecal occult blood test (FOBT), and endoscopic examination; less invasive virtual colonoscopy may be considered. Asymptomatic individuals with no history of colorectal cancer should begin screening at 50 years of age with DRE and FOBT annually and flexible sigmoidoscopy every 5 years (Simmang et al. 1999). Alternatively, a double-contrast barium enema every 5 to 10 years or a total colonoscopy every 10 years may be considered (Byers et al. 1997). A patient with findings of neoplastic polyps on flexible sigmoidoscopy should undergo complete colonic examination, because the presence of polyps is an indicator of other malignant (cancerous) growths.

Digital Rectal Exam

The digital rectal examination (DRE) is part of a routine physical examination and is not painful or time-consuming to the patient. Approximately 5% to 10% of colorectal cancers may be palpable (perceptible to touch), therefore this examination must be used along with other screening tests. In this examination, a doctor puts a gloved finger into the patient's rectum to find any growths. Physicians usually recommend DRE for all adults beginning at 50 years of age.

Fecal Occult Blood Testing (FOBT)

A fecal occult blood test (FOBT) depends on the presence of occult blood in the stool (not visible to the naked eye and only detectable by chemical means) to indicate an abnormal growth in the large bowel. This occult blood may occur anywhere along the digestive tract, but it is most likely to originate in the colon. Not all rectal cancers bleed and not all blood in the gastrointestinal tract is due to cancer. Physicians usually recommend a FOBT for all adults beginning at 50 years of age. Individuals who are at higher risk because of age, genetics, or a family history of colorectal cancer or polyps may require FOBT prior to 50 years of age.

The FOBT is a simple chemical test of three consecutive stool samples. However, the test has poor sensitivity and this can lead to missed lesions. The test can be positive in many different situations including colorectal cancer, colon or rectum cancer, esophagitis, gastritis, stomach cancer, ulcerative colitis, and hemorrhoids. It is not recommended that red meat or fish be consumed prior to this test (because of heme and peroxidase content) as this can cause a false-positive reading for blood. Other substances which can also cause a false-positive reading include anticoagulants (blood thinners), aspirin, anti-inflammatory and arthritis medication, due to leakage of blood into the intestinal tract; oxidizing drugs such as topical iodine, bromides, boric acid, and reserpine, and vegetables (because of their peroxidase activity) including horseradish, broccoli, turnips, and cauliflower can also cause erroneous results. Vitamin C and salicylates can cause either a false-positive or false-negative test result. If a patient has a positive test a complete colon examination (barium enema and colonoscopy) will be required.

Note: *It is important to discuss all drugs, supplements, and dietary regimens with your physician prior to a FOBT.*

Barium Enema

A barium enema is an x-ray test used to examine the colon and rectum of the lower digestive tract. Because these internal organs are normally not visible on x-rays, barium is inserted by enema into the rectum and colon to enhance visibility. The barium will temporarily coat the inside lining of the rectum and colon, allowing the outline of these organs to be visible on the x-ray pictures. This test is useful for diagnosing cancers and diverticula (small pouches that may form in the intestinal wall).

The x-ray for this test is actually taken as a video by a large camera, positioned over the abdomen, immediately after the enema has been administered. Usually, the room will be darkened during the procedure so that the physician can observe the x-rays on a monitor and pick out photographs for further examination.

The use of the double contrast barium enema has declined in recent years in favor of colonoscopy, despite the lower cost of the barium enema. There are several reasons for the decreased use of the barium enema as a diagnostic tool: reduced sensitivity of this test in detecting polyps of less than 1 cm, reduced sensitivity in detecting polyps in areas where a single lumen is not detectable (i.e., sigmoid, rectosigmoid, hepatic, and splenic flexures), patient comfort and compliance issues and the large amount of radiation needed to view the lower abdominal region of the body. Radiation damages DNA, which could cause mutations that may lead to cancer later in life.

Despite these limitations, when a colonoscopy is not possible, the double contrast barium enema combined with a flexible sigmoidoscopy is an acceptable alternative. A barium enema cannot be used for the surveillance of familial polyps, familial colon cancer, and inflammatory bowel disease, when attention to small details of the colonic mucosa is required and the likelihood of biopsy or polyp removal is high.

As with sigmoidoscopy and colonoscopy, the barium enema requires the colon and rectum to be completely empty. Therefore, before the procedure, the patient will be instructed to drink only clear liquids. Milk or milk products should not be consumed.

Endoscopy

Endoscopic intervention can effectively manage adenomatous polyps, which are the precursor lesions of invasive colorectal cancer (Winawer 1977). Early stage polyps are typically asymptomatic; therefore a screening examination performed as part of a regular health evaluation is the best way to detect polyps in their early stages. The different types of endoscopy include:

- Proctoscopy: examines the rectum.
- Flexible sigmoidoscopy: examines the rectum and lower part of the colon.
- Colonoscopy: examines the entire colon.
- Virtual Colonoscopy: Computed Tomography or Magnetic Resonance Imaging examines the entire colon virtually.

Proctoscopy

Proctoscopy involves an endoscopic examination of the rectum using a lighted scope. It is used to localize, identify, and photograph pathologic changes, to obtain biopsy specimens and perform other surgical procedures, and for medication.

Because a physician cannot determine which polyps will become cancerous by simply looking at them, all polyps should be removed through a polypectomy, which allows the physician to remove polyps without performing surgery and opening the abdominal cavity (Thiis-Evensen et al. 1999). Biopsy of polyps is not recommended because the results may be misleading. Once polyps are removed, they are sent for histological analysis to determine if the polyps are cancerous. Colorectal cancer found in this early stage, before symptoms develop, is the most curable form, and it is for this reason that screening in asymptomatic individuals is so important.

In later stages, colorectal cancer can cause symptoms such as blood in the stool, changes in normal bowel habits, narrowing of the stool, abdominal pain, weight loss, or constant fatigue. Symptoms associated in right-sided, ascending colon tumors include fatigue, weakness, anemia, or iron deficiency of unknown origin. These lesions can become very large without causing any obstructive symptoms because stool in the ascending colon is relatively liquid and can continue to pass through even significantly narrowed lumens. Ascending colon lesions often project into the lumen and ulcerate, causing chronic blood loss and resulting in symptoms of palpitations and possible angina pectoris, as well as fatigue. Any adult with chronic iron deficiency of unknown origin should have a thorough visualization of the entire bowel via colonoscopy.

Symptoms of an obstruction are often the first indication of cancer located in the left descending colon. Since stool in this location is more solidly formed, its passage can become blocked from moving into the rectum by a growing tumor. Such symptoms include changes in bowel habits (constipation and/or diarrhea), and cramping left lower quadrant (abdomen/pelvis) pain. When a patient presents with such symptoms the physician may perform x-rays of the colon and rectum via a barium enema or a colonoscopy to look for tumors. Barium enema x-rays of left-sided lesions often reveal characteristic annular constricting lesions. The physician will take tissue samples of any growths that are found and these samples are examined in a pathology laboratory to determine if they are cancerous.

Flexible Sigmoidoscopy

Flexible sigmoidoscopy can allow detection of up to one-half to two-thirds of colorectal adenomas and cancers (Wilking et al. 1986). It can also detect about 65-75% of polyps and 40-65% of colorectal cancers (Okamoto et al. 2002). It is expected to detect abnormal masses in the distal colon (portion nearest to the rectum) and rectum in approximately 8% of asymptomatic individuals older than age 40 years. Screening by this method is recommended for low- and average-risk individuals older than 50 years of age (Simmang et al. 1999). A flexible sigmoidoscopy has been proven to reduce the incidence and mortality of colon cancer through early detection. A flexible sigmoidoscopy, however, is not an adequate method of screening in hereditary colon cancer, as two-thirds of lesions develop beyond the colorectal area viewed by sigmoidoscopy; in these cases colonoscopy should be considered.

Physicians may use flexible sigmoidoscopy to find the cause of diarrhea, abdominal pain or distension, constipation, bleeding, or inflammation. Early signs of abnormal growths or polyps in the descending colon and rectum but not in the ascending or transverse colon (two-thirds of the colon) may be detected by this technique.

A flexible sigmoidoscope is a short, flexible, lighted tube connected to a tiny video camera, and enables a physician to examine the inside of the large intestine through the sigmoid or descending colon from the rectum. The scope inflates the large intestine by blowing air into the rectum and colon providing a clear image of the inside lining of the colorectal area, which is then transmitted back to a monitor for viewing. Usually a sigmoidoscopy can be performed by a trained, primary care physician without sedation in the practitioner's office.

The colon and rectum must be completely empty for flexible sigmoidoscopy to be thorough and safe. Therefore, 12-24 hours before the procedure, the patient will be instructed to drink only clear liquids. A liquid diet is one containing fat-free bouillon or broth, gelatin, strained fruit juice, plain coffee, plain tea, or water. Prior to the procedure the patient may also be given an enema, which is a liquid solution injected via the rectum to wash out the intestines.

Flexible sigmoidoscopy takes 10-20 minutes. During the procedure, a feeling of pressure and slight cramping may occur in the lower abdomen. Once the air leaves the colon these symptoms will dissipate. A patient with findings of abnormal polyp growth should undergo complete colonic examination. Bleeding and puncture of the colon are possible complications of sigmoidoscopy; however, such complications are very uncommon.

The American Cancer Society recommends the use of sigmoidoscopic evaluation together with annual FOBT for average-risk, asymptomatic individuals every 3 to 5 years, beginning at 50 years of age (USPSTS 2002).

Colonoscopy

Colonoscopy has become the established method of evaluating and treating disease of the large intestine. Abnormal findings on barium enema are an important indication for colonoscopy in order to determine the precise nature of the lesion, either by removing it or by biopsy. Asymptomatic patients with a positive FOBT should also undergo colonoscopy, as approximately 50% may have an abnormal colonic lesion, of which 12% may be cancerous (Winawer et al. 1991).

A colonoscopy is similar to flexible sigmoidoscopy; it enables a physician to see inflamed tissue, abnormal growths, ulcers, and bleeding. However, colonoscopy provides a means of visually examining the entire large intestine, from the rectum all the way up through the colon to the lower end of the small intestine, whereas sigmoidoscopy only allows for a partial examination of the large intestine (35 cm to 60 cm).

As with flexible sigmoidoscopy, colonoscopy requires the colon and rectum to be completely empty. Therefore, 24 hours before the procedure, the patient will be instructed to drink only clear liquids. During this 24-hour period, strong saline-based laxatives are administered to thoroughly clean the lining of the colon. In some instances, a patient may also be given an enema, a liquid solution injected into the rectum which washes out the intestines.

Colonoscopy consists of the insertion of a long, flexible, lighted tube connected to a tiny video camera, called a colonoscope, into the rectum. The colonoscope is slowly guided into the colon. The scope bends and also blows air into the colon, which inflates the colon, allowing enhanced visibility. An image of the inside of the colon is transmitted to a monitor for examination of the colon lining. Pain medication and a mild sedative may be administered to ensure comfort and relaxation during the examination.

If there are any abnormal findings, such as a polyp or colonic masses, they may be completely removed by small instruments passed through the colonoscope. If bleeding is found in the colon, the physician can pass a laser or electrical probe or inject special medications through the scope to stop the bleeding. Most colonoscopies are performed on an outpatient basis with minimal inconvenience and discomfort. Bleeding and puncture of the colon are possible complications of colonoscopy; however, such complications are uncommon.

Virtual Colonoscopy

Virtual colonoscopy uses computer-generated images of the colon constructed from data obtained during an abdominal computed tomographic examination. A CT scan is a special radiographic technique that uses a computer to put together several x-ray images into a 2 dimensional cross-sectional image. Using the same dose of radiation as that of the conventional X-ray machine, an entire slice of the body is made visible with about 100 times more clarity. Sometimes magnetic resonance imaging (MRI) is substituted for CT scan in virtual colonoscopy, as an MRI image is often superior to a normal X-ray image. In an MRI, the patient passes through a tunnel surrounded by a magnet which polarizes hydrogen atoms in the tissues and then monitors the summation of the energies within living cells. A computer tracks the magnetism and produces a clear picture of the tissues, particularly soft tissues.

In virtual colonoscopy the images generated by either CT or MRI scan simulate the effect of a conventional colonoscopy. As with conventional colonoscopy, patients must take laxatives before the procedure, and the colon is insufflated with air just prior to the radiographic examination. The risk with a CT virtual colonoscopy is the large amount of radiation delivered to the body.

Another disadvantage of virtual colonoscopy is that if a polyp or other suspicious lesion is detected, then flexible tube colonoscopy has to be performed anyway. If flexible tube colonoscopy is chosen in the first place, polyps and lesions can be immediately removed and a biopsy done to ascertain if the mass is cancerous.

A recent study compared the accuracy of conventional colonoscopy (flexible tube) to virtual colonoscopy (computer generated image) in detecting polyps. The sensitivity of virtual colonoscopy was only 39% and 55% for detecting lesions sized at least 6 mm and 10 mm, repectively. These results were significantly lower than those for conventional colonoscopy, with sensitivities of 99% and 100% for detecting lesions at least 6 mm and 10 mm, respectively. In this study, virtual colonoscopy missed two of eight cancers. The doctors who conducted the study concluded that virtual colonoscopy "is not yet ready for widespread clinical application. Techniques and training need to be improved" (Cotton et al. 2004).

Based this data, those concerned about preventing colon cancer should choose flexible tube (conventional) colonoscopy every 3 to 5 years as opposed to virtual colonoscopy.

Genetic Tests

New methods of screening patients for colorectal cancer depend on the identification of mutated DNA in stool samples. Stool-based assays for mutated DNA associated with colorectal cancer may significantly increase the identification of patients with potentially premalignant colonic polyps. For example, mutations in the adenomatous polyposis coli (APC) gene that initiates colorectal tumors could potentially provide an optimal marker for detecting colorectal tumors (Traverso et al. 2002).

DIAGNOSIS

When diagnosing cancer, blood and pieces of tumor tissue are tested. These tests help to determine the characteristics of the tumor (aggressiveness, rate of growth, and degree of abnormality). A tumor may be benign (noncancerous) or malignant (cancerous). If a patient is diagnosed with cancer (malignant tumor), professionals will form a treatment team to determine the best course of action. This team may include medical and radiation oncologists (physicians who specialize in diagnosing and treating cancer), a surgeon, and a gastroenterologist (a physician who specializes in treating the digestive system).

The workup of a symptomatic patient can lead to a diagnosis of colorectal cancer. In the 10% to 15% of patients who present with advanced (metastatic) disease, signs and symptoms are usually present. Pathological examination of the tumor should include the gross appearance, as size alone is not predictive of outcome, histological examination, (adenocarcinomas represent 90% to 95% of all colorectal tumors), degree of differentiation and local invasion (potential for cancer spread), lymph node pathology and molecular detection of micrometastases.

Colorectal cancer can spread locally or distantly via the lymphatic and venous systems. The capability of a tumor to invade and spread (metastasize) is the leading cause of death in cancer patients. Local spread can involve the tumor narrowing and constricting the bowel wall. In rectal cancer, the surrounding fat and adjacent organs are most commonly invaded directly through the bowel wall. Tumors limited to the bowel wall can have a lower incidence of spread to lymph nodes. If the lymphatic vessels become blocked by tumor, then lymph nodes at a great distance from the original tumor site can be affected. The liver is by far the most common site of colorectal cancer metastasis because the colon is drained by a large vein that carries blood from the intestines to the liver (portal venous system). Metastasis to other sites without liver or lung involvement is rare. However, colorectal cancer has been observed to spread to the vertebrae, pelvis, and lumbosacral spine (Giess et al. 1998).

Unlike normal healthy cells, which are in constant contact with a surface in the body, cancer cells can survive without attachment to a surface. The ability of cancer cells to detach from the primary tumor and either penetrate into the blood circulation or to implant in a different surface away from the original site is called implantation. Implantation is related to changes in the surface molecules on the tumor cells called cell adhesion molecules. Implantation may occur when cancer cells are shed by surgical manipulation (Zeng et al. 1992). The risk of colorectal cancer spread caused by surgical manipulation is well-recognized.

Staging and Prognostic Factors

The number of factors which have an impact on the overall survival of patients with colorectal cancer continues to grow. The growing number of prognostic factors used in the analysis of colorectal cancer include: age and gender, tumor grade and type, the presence of symptoms versus asymptomatic, the presence of obstruction or perforation, blood vessel or lymph vessel invasion, low Bcl-2 expression, low apoptosis rate, vascular endothelial growth factor (VEGF) levels, and DNA content.

The most reliable prognostic factor in colorectal cancer is the staging of disease at the time that treatment is initiated, for example information obtained during surgery. Imaging techniques, such as CT scan and conventional MRI scan, used prior to surgery have not been successful in reliably staging colorectal cancer (Thoeni 1997). However, 18-Fluorodeoxyglucose Positron Emission Tomography (18-FDG-PET) in the routine staging of colorectal cancer correctly detected 95% of primary tumors. 18-FDG PET is currently the best pre-operative method for the staging of colorectal cancer.

Positron Emission Tomography (PET) should be performed as a first examination after diagnosis of colorectal cancer despite a high rate of false-negative results in patients with lymph node involvement. A PET/CT hybrid system has recently been proposed as optimal in the staging of colorectal cancer (Kantorova et al. 2003). In a retrospective study of relapsed colorectal cancer patients, it was concluded that the 3-year survival rate following surgery would have exceeded 70% if the selection of patients had included an additional PET examination (Dietlein et al. 2003).

Endoscopic ultrasonography is another technique which is accurate in the diagnosis and preoperative staging of colorectal cancer and is not significantly different than conventional histological staging (statistically $p > 0.05$). Endoscopic ultrasonography is a technique in which high frequency sound waves are bounced off organs inside the body and the echo pattern is converted into a 2-dimensional picture of the structures below the transducer. Endoscopic ultrasonography presented 100% sensitivity in cancer detection versus 60% for computed tomography ($p < 0.001$). Endoscopic ultrasonography sensitivity in colorectal cancer staging (T, N, M, and TNM) was 93.8%, 93.8%, 92.5% and 82.5% with corresponding specificities of 99.2%, 97.9%, 92.5% and 94.2% (Kalantzis et al. 2002).

There are three staging systems for colorectal cancer: Duke's classification, The Jass System, and Tumor, Node, Metastasis (TNM) Classification. The TNM classification is the preferred system for colorectal cancer patients, thus treatment decisions should be made with reference to this classification (Yarbro et al. 1999). Colorectal cancers are usually staged after surgical exploration and pathological evaluation of the tissue sample removed during surgery. In contrast to most other cancers, the size of the primary tumor is not considered important in the staging of the disease, however depth of tumor penetration through the bowel wall and local lymphnode involvement may worsen the prognosis.

TNM definitions (AJCC 1997): T = Tumor, N = Node, M = Metastasis

- T: Primary tumor
- TX: Primary tumor cannot be assessed
- T0: No evidence of primary tumor
- Tis: Carcinoma *in situ*, intraepithelial or invasion of the lamina propria*
- T1: Tumor invades submucosa
- T2: Tumor invades muscularis propria
- T3: Tumor invades through the muscularis propria into the subserosa or into nonperitonealized pericolic or perirectal tissues
- T4: Tumor directly invades other organs or structures and/or perforates visceral peritoneum**

Tis includes cancer cells confined within the glandular basement membrane (intraepithelial) or lamina propria (intramucosal) with no extension through the muscularis mucosae into the submucosa.

**Direct invasion in T4 includes invasion of other segments of the colorectum by way of the serosa, for example, invasion of the sigmoid colon by a carcinoma of the cecum.*

Regional lymph nodes (N) - at least 12 lymph nodes should be analyzed

- NX: Regional lymph nodes cannot be assessed
- N0: No regional lymph node metastasis
- N1: Metastasis in 1 to 3 regional lymph nodes
- N2: Metastasis in 4 or more regional lymph nodes

Distant metastasis (M)

- MX: Distant metastasis cannot be assessed
- M0: No distant metastasis
- M1: Distant metastasis

Stage 0

- Tis, N0, M0

Stage 1

- T1, N0, M0
- T2, N0, M0

Stage II

- T3, N0, M0
- T4, N0, M0

Stage III

- Any T, N1, M0
- Any T, N2, M0

Stage IV

Any T, Any N, M1 Poor prognostic indicators include:

- Five or more lymph nodes involved
- Tumor spread to regional lymph nodes
- Tumor penetration through the bowel wall
- Perforation of colon
- Tumor adherence to adjacent organs
- Metastasis to distant organs

Prognostic indicators listed above put the patient in a more advanced staging category. Some other poor prognostic signs not reflected directly by staging are:

- Poorly differentiated histology
- Venous invasion of tumor
- Preoperative elevation of CEA titer greater than 5.0 nanograms/mL
- p53 mutation in tumor cells
- DNA aneuploidy

ADDITIONAL PROGNOSTIC FACTORS

Vascular Endothelial Growth Factor (VEGF)

As a tumor grows, it elicits new blood vessel growth from surrounding normal tissues. This process is called tumor *angiogenesis* (*angio* – blood vessel, and *genesis* – beginning) and diverts the blood supply away from the normal healthy tissue to supply the tumor cells. Unregulated tumor angiogenesis can facilitate the growth of cancer throughout the body.

Vascular endothelial growth factor (VEGF), is a factor that stimulates the growth of blood vessel cells (vascular endothelial cells) and it has been established as one of the most potent factors in the process of *angiogenesis*. Angiogenesis is essential for tumor growth and spread (metastasis) and has been associated with colon cancer progression and metastasis thereby significantly affecting patient survival (Stoeltzing et al. 2003).

Metastasis is the transfer of cancer cells from one organ or area of the body to another not directly connected to it. Cancer cells have the ability to leave the original tumor site, travel to distant locations, and recolonize into new tumors in a different location

than the original primary tumor. The liver is by far the most common site of colorectal cancer metastasis; however, metastasis can also occur in organs such as the lungs, spine, bones, and the brain. Both the bloodstream and lymphatic system (the network connecting lymph nodes throughout the body) serve as vehicles for traveling cancer cells. If vital organs such as the liver, lungs or brain are invaded and destroyed by metastatic cancer the patient may eventually die of the disease.

VEGF is an important factor in the process of colorectal cancer metastasis, particularly those to the liver. The presence (expression) of VEGF correlates with the number of blood vessels in the tumor, which may be useful in predicting distant recurrence in patients who do not have cancer in their lymph nodes (node-negative colon cancer) (Takahashi et al. 1997). Higher serum levels of VEGF have been found in colorectal cancer patients in contrast to healthy individuals. Furthermore, colorectal cancer patients with metastases have been shown to have higher serum levels of VEGF compared to patients without distant metastases (Broll et al. 1998).

The highest levels of VEGF correlate with the advancement of colorectal cancer, especially when metastases are present at the same time. The higher the levels of VEGF the poorer the outcome of survival (worse prognosis) (Kos et al. 2002). Interestingly, increased levels of VEGF expression in normal tissues collected from a site distant from the primary tumor were found to indicate changes in the surrounding tumor environment that may enhance the subsequent spread of tumor cells (Hanrahan et al. 2003).

Various strategies have been utilized to inhibit VEGF activity so as to reduce growth and metastasis of colorectal cancer. For the first time in a well-performed Phase III trial, a targeted therapy was shown impressively to prolong survival for patients with metastatic colorectal cancer that could not be removed by surgery (unresectable). The targeted antiangiogenic agent is bevacizumab (Avastin®), a humanized monoclonal antibody targeting the circulating VEGF (O'Neil et al. 2003).

Bevacizumab is an antiangiogenesis drug, used in molecular targeted therapy to stop tumors from making new blood vessels. This antibody to VEGF fits like a lock and key into a receptor on the cell surface. It stops VEGF from starting the growth of new blood vessels. Without new blood vessels, the tumor cannot grow. Bevacizumab is being studied for the treatment of many different cancers.

Patients with newly diagnosed metastatic colon cancer who received the therapeutic agent bevacizumab

(Avastin®) along with a chemotherapy combination (known as IFL) had substantially longer overall survival times than patients who received the chemotherapy but with a placebo instead of bevacizumab.

A randomized Phase III trial to compare the effectiveness of two combination chemotherapy regimens with or without bevacizumab in treating patients who have locally advanced, metastatic, or recurrent colorectal cancer is underway via the National Institutes of Health (NIH). A Phase I trial to study the effectiveness of bevacizumab combined with fluorouracil and external-beam radiation therapy in treating patients who have stage II or stage III rectal cancer is also ongoing via the NIH. Avastatin® is now an approved drug to treat colon cancer.

Lymphatic and Blood Vessel Invasion

The lymph nodes store special cells that can trap cancer cells that are traveling through the body in lymph. Lymph is an almost colorless fluid that bathes body tissues and carries white blood cells that have entered the lymph nodes from the blood. Lymph is found in the lymphatic vessels that drain the tissues of the fluid that filters across the blood vessel walls from the blood.

When colon cancer spreads, the first place it usually travels is to regional lymph nodes located proximally to the large intestine in the abdomen. Regional lymph node involvement is determined after surgery by a pathologist, who will microscopically examine the nodes (a least 12 nodes) to determine whether or not they contain cancer. The best prognosis is when the cancer remains localized within the colorectal area. The presence of lymphatic vessel involvement is a poor prognostic factor for the outcome of the colorectal cancer patient.

Blood vessel invasion means the invasion of the veins by tumor cells, as opposed to arterial invasion, which is rare. The invasion of blood vessels by cancer cells results in a significant decrease in the 5-year survival rate, as it indicates tumor metastasis.

Tumor Markers

Tumor markers are substances that may be produced by the tumor itself, or by the body in response to the presence of cancer and can be detected in higher than normal amounts in the blood, urine, or body tissues of colorectal cancer patients. Tumor markers may be proteins, antigens, or hormones. Tests for tumor markers may be used in conjunction with a complete medical history and other diagnostic tests (e.g., x-rays) to detect and diagnose many cancers. Tumor marker tests are not used alone in the diagnosis of cancer because most tumor markers can be elevated in people who have benign (noncancerous) conditions, and because tumor markers may not be specific to a particular cancer.

Not every tumor will cause an elevation in tumor marker levels, especially in the early stages of cancer. Physicians can use changes in tumor marker levels to follow the course of the disease, to measure the effect of treatment, and to check for recurrence or relapse. Certain tumor markers are simply more accurate than others in their sensitivity and specificity to detection of cancer.

Serum tumor markers including carcinoembryonic antigen (CEA), carbohydrate antigen 19-9 (CA 19-9), alpha-fetoprotein (AFP), and tissue polypeptide-specific antigen (TPS) may be helpful in the early diagnosis of colorectal cancer, in the initial assessment of the extent of the disease (aggressiveness, metastases), and in monitoring of tumor growth or tumor volume reduction once cancer has been diagnosed and treatment started (Lawicki et al. 2002).

Carcinoembryonic Antigen

Carcinoembryonic Antigen (CEA) is the most reliable and frequently used tumor marker in the detection of colorectal cancer. It is recommended as a monitoring tool for patients who have been treated with curative intent (the intent to overcome colorectal cancer and promote recovery). If a patient's CEA level is raised prior to surgery and does not decrease to normal levels following the surgery, it is an indication that recurrence of the tumor may occur. An elevated CEA level may be a sign of a more advanced colorectal cancer. Carcinoembryonic-secreting tumors (such as colon cancers) induce the production of IL-6 which in turn stimulates tumor cell growth at metastatic sites (Belluco et al. 2000). Measurement of CEA prior to colorectal cancer surgery is desirable as this may provide information which will predict the outcome of the surgery, and may also help with surgical management and provide a baseline level for subsequent determinations.

For patients with stage II and III colorectal cancer who may be candidates for liver resection, CEA levels should be measured every 2-3 months for at least 3 years after diagnosis. For monitoring treatment of advanced disease (Stage IV) CEA should be tested every 2-3 months (Duffy et al. 2003). Although the specificity of the carcinoembryonic antigen test in its present form is high, the sensitivity is disappointingly low, prohibiting the use of the carcinoembryonic antigen test for population screening. Elevated carcino-

colonic carcinoma. However, in one study where patients were supplemented with 1.4 g EPA and 1.0 g DHA per day for approximately 12 days, the growth rate of colorectal cancer was unchanged (Gee et al. 1999).

Large doses of fish oil can inhibit cell proliferation and tumor growth through a free-radical-mediated mechanism, while at more moderate doses, omega-3 fatty acids inhibit inflammation, angiogenesis, and Ras protein activity (McCarty 1996; Collett et al. 2001; Grimm et al. 2002).

Alpha-linolenic acid (ALA) found in vegetarian food sources is usually broken down into the biologically active EPA and DHA fraction in the body. Vegetarian sources of ALA include flaxseed, wheat germ, perilla oil, walnuts, soybeans, black currant seeds, and green leafy vegetables.

The recommendation to eat cold-water fish is based on the EPA present in oily fish, including salmon, mackerel, herring, blue fin tuna, sardines, and trout. A more efficient and consistent way of obtaining high concentrations of EPA and DHA is to consume a standardized fish oil supplement. Cancer patients often ingest a minimum of 3200 mg of EPA and 2400 mg of DHA a day from a standardized fish oil supplement.

Minor side effects of fish oil include mild gastrointestinal symptoms such as belching, bloating, gas, and a fish-oil aftertaste (Bruera et al. 2003).

Vitamins A, D, and E

Several epidemiological investigations have demonstrated that a diet rich in carotenoids could prevent the development of precancerous and cancerous lesions of the digestive tract. Indeed, there are close and inverse correlations between the serum level of carotenoids and colorectal polyps with different histological grades. Serum levels of vitamin A were found to be significantly lower in all patients with polyps than in healthy controls. The lowest levels were found in patients with focal adenocarcinoma in the polyp. The low mean carotenoid levels in patients with adenocarcinoma in the polyp indicate that deficiency of carotenoids may be an important factor in the development of colorectal cancer (Rumi et al. 1999).

In a population-based case-control study of 105 cases of colorectal adenoma, serum concentrations of vitamin A were significantly inversely related to the risk of colorectal adenoma when cases were compared with the control group. The risk of developing colorectal adenomas was found to be reduced in those with high vitamin A levels (Breuer-Katschinski et al. 2001).

Retinol, retinoic acid, and beta-carotene (in nanomolar concentrations) block stimulation of protein kinase C (PKC), which when stimulated has been shown to increase tumor activity in the colon. It has been suggested that beta-carotene could be useful in the prevention and treatment of colorectal cancer (Kahl-Rainer et al. 1994), as beta-carotene has been shown to down-regulate growth factors which contribute towards proliferation of pre-malignant cells. Combined, vitamin A and vitamin D3 have been shown to inhibit tumor-induced angiogenesis (Majewski et al. 1996).

Convincing evidence is available showing that dietary calcium and vitamin D impede the development of colonic carcinogenesis (Lamprecht et al. 2001). Calcium supplementation and vitamin D both appear to have anti-neoplastic effects in the large bowel; they appear to act together to reduce the risk of colorectal adenoma recurrence (Grau et al. 2003). Additionally, dietary vitamin D3 impedes the neoplastic process in murine large intestine (Mokady et al. 2000) and vitamin D3 has demonstrated the ability to inhibit liver cancer cell growth (Alvarez-Dolado et al. 1999; Majewski et al. 1996).

The role of dietary and supplemental sources of calcium and vitamin D in the causation of adenoma recurrence was investigated among 1304 male and female participants in the Wheat Bran Fiber (WBF) trial of adenoma recurrence. Results of this study indicate that a higher intake of calcium decreases the risk of adenoma recurrence by approximately 45%, whereas vitamin D has no significant effect on recurrence rates (Martinez et al. 2002).

Suggested dosage: A suggested dose of vitamin D3 is 4000-6000 IU every day on an empty stomach. When taking doses of vitamin D3 in excess of 1400 IU a day, blood chemistry tests should be performed regularly to monitor kidney and liver function and serum calcium metabolism. Water-soluble vitamin A can be taken in doses of 100,000-300,000 IU every day. Monthly blood tests are necessary to ensure toxicity does not occur in response to these high daily doses of vitamin A and D3. After 4-6 months, the doses of vitamin D3 and vitamin A can be reduced. Refer to the symptoms of vitamin A toxicity in *Appendix A: Avoiding Vitamin A Toxicity.*

Vitamin E is the term used to describe eight naturally occurring essential fat-soluble nutrients: alpha, beta, delta, and gamma tocopherols plus a class of compounds related to vitamin E called alpha, beta, delta, and gamma tocotrienols. Vitamin E in the

American diet is primarily available in plant-oil rich foods such as vegetable oils, seeds and nuts and these foods vary widely in their content of tocopherols. Many epidemiological studies have suggested that vitamin E may help prevent colon cancer. The mechanism of the anticancer activity of vitamin E may involve decreasing the formation of mutagens arising from the oxidation of fecal lipids, and also decreasing oxidative stress in the epithelial cells of the colon and rectum (Campbell et al. 2003).

Vitamin E succinate (d-alpha tocopheryl succinate) has been shown to inhibit tumor cell growth *in vitro* and *in vivo*. For instance, in mice with colon cancer xenografts, vitamin E succinate suppressed tumor growth by 80%. This study epitomizes the cancer cell killing effects of this form of vitamin E which has no known side effects (Neuzil et al. 2001). Furthermore, men with a high intake of vitamin E are 65% less likely to develop colorectal adenomas (precursors to colon cancer) compared to men with low vitamin E intake (Tseng et al. 1996).

A study was conducted on 12 advanced colorectal cancer patients to ascertain if supplementation with vitamin E could enhance immune functions. Colorectal cancer patients (Dukes' C and D) received a daily dose of 750 mg of vitamin E beginning 2 weeks prior to intervention with chemotherapy or radiation treatment. The results showed that short-term supplementation with vitamin E led to increased immune function, specifically, increased CD4:CD8 ratios and enhanced capacity of their T-cells to produce the T helper-1 cytokines, interleukin 2, and IFN-gamma (Malmberg et al. 2002).

It is critically important that cancer patients use the alpha-tocopheryl succinate form of vitamin E as opposed to standard vitamin E preparations (Neuzil 2003). A study compared two different forms of vitamin E using nude mice with colon cancer xenografts. While standard vitamin E (alpha-tocopherol) exerted modest antitumor activity, tocopheryl succinate showed a more profound antitumor effect, at both the level of reducing tumor cell growth and increasing tumor cell death. Vitamin E succinate is a potent and highly specific anticancer agent and/or adjuvant of considerable therapeutic potential (Neuzil 2003; Weber et al. 2002).

Suggested dosage: The suggested dose of d-alpha tocopheryl succinate is 800-1200 IU daily in addition to at least 200 mg of gamma tocopherol.

Tocotrienols

Tocotrienols possess the ability to reduce cancer cell proliferation, while leaving normal cells unaffected (Kline et al. 2001). One of the mechanisms by which tocotrienols are thought to suppress cancer is related to the isoprenoid side chain. Isoprenoids are plant compounds that have suppressed the initiation, growth, and progression of many types of cancer in experimental studies (Block et al. 1992). Isoprenoids are common in fruits and vegetables, which may explain why diets rich in these foods have consistently been shown to reduce the incidence of colon cancer.

The anti-proliferative effect of isoprenoids is thought to be due to suppression of the mevalonate pathway. The mevalonate pathway escapes regulatory control in tumor tissue but remains highly sensitive to regulation by tocotrienols. Tocotrienols are at least 5 times more powerful than farnesol, the body's regulator of the mevalonate pathway (Elson et al. 1994; Yu et al. 1999).

While healthy people normally take about 60 mg a day of palm-oil tocotrienols, cancer patients may consider taking 240 mg daily for a period of 3-6 months.

Calcium

Calcium has been hypothesized to reduce the risk of colon cancer, and in a randomized trial, calcium supplementation was associated with reduction in the risk of recurrent colorectal adenomas (Grau et al. 2003). High calcium intake or calcium supplementation may reduce the risk colorectal cancer.

Accumulating evidence shows that calcium supplementation regulates the growth pattern of colonic epithelium in the individual at high risk for colon cancer (Wargovich et al. 1992). An inverse association between dietary calcium intake and colorectal cancer risk was found in a study of 61,463 women (an average 11.3 years of follow-up). Women with the highest calcium intake (median 914 mg/day) had a reduced risk of colorectal cancer compared with women with the lowest intake (median 486 mg/day). Furthermore, the inverse association was found to be strongest in relation to distal cancers and among older women (Terry et al. 2002).

Calcium supplementation reduces colonic cell proliferation, in part, by decreasing the level of diacylglycerol (DAG). A high luminal level of DAG, a key factor in cell growth control, enhances colonic cell proliferation. Bacterial DAG production is increased by bile acids and phospholipids, both of which may be precipitated by calcium. Calcium was shown to alter fecal lipid composition and to reduce cell proliferation. Oral elemental calcium therapy, 2.4 or 3.6 g/day, for three months markedly reduced fecal DAG concentration and output without enhancing DAG production (Steinbach et al. 1994).

Twenty-two individuals with a history of resected adenocarcinoma of the colon, but free of cancer, were supplemented with 2000 or 3000 mg of calcium for 16 weeks. Calcium supplementation significantly decreased the primary bile acids concentration resulting in a healthier bile acid profile suggesting a protective effect of calcium on colon cancer (Lupton et al. 1996).

Long-term (1-year) calcium supplementation (3.75 g calcium carbonate (1.5 g Ca^{2+}) daily) significantly suppressed rectal epithelial proliferation in adenoma patients, and long-term dietary habits contributed to this effect (Rozen et al. 2001). In a randomized, controlled, crossover, intervention trial, involving 15 patients with right hemicolectomy, 1000 mg of elemental calcium per day for 2 months had a protective effect against colorectal cancer risk (van Gorkom et al. 2002).

Modified Citrus Pectin

Modified citrus pectin (MCP), also known as fractionated pectin, is a complex polysaccharide (sugar) found in the cell wall of plants and the peel and pulp of citrus fruits.

Modified citrus pectin is rich in galactoside residues, giving it an affinity for certain types of tumor cells. Metastasis is one of the most life-threatening aspects of cancer and the lack of effective anti-metastatic therapies has prompted research on MCP's effectiveness in blocking metastasis of certain types of cancers, including colorectal cancers.

Modified citrus pectin, given orally, inhibits carbohydrate-mediated tumor growth, angiogenesis, and metastasis in athymic mice injected with human colon carcinoma cells (LSLiM6) into the cecum, presumably via its effects on galectin-3 function (Nangia-Makker et al. 2002).

The adhesion molecule called E-selectin is present on blood vessel endothelial cells. Several types of cancer cells use surface carbohydrate groups called Lewis antigens (Lewis X and Lewis A.4) to bind to E-selectin. Once the Lewis antigens on the cancer cell bind to the E-selectin adhesion molecule on the blood vessel endothelial cell, the initiation of a metastatic tumor is established.

Modified citrus pectin is a *free sugar* that has been demonstrated to inhibit metastasis by binding to the E-selectin adhesion molecules, thus, preventing cancer cells from attaching to E-selectin on the blood vessel endothelial cells.

Note: *Free sugar is not to be confused with dietary sugars, which will be discussed later.*

Research has demonstrated that if all E-selectin sugar-binding sites are filled with free sugars, the E-selectin is not able to bind to other cells, specifically cancer cells. This would reduce the initial binding of tumor cells to the vascular wall as they circulate. MCP can reduce the growth of solid primary tumors. High-dose orally administered MCP significantly reduced tumor size (by 70%, p < 0.001) in colon-25 tumors implanted in balb-c mice (both) (Hayashi et al. 2000).

Citrus pectin and oligofructose can significantly increase indices of folate status, as was recently demonstrated in rats (Thoma et al. 2003). Based on these findings, 15 grams of modified citrus pectin is recommended daily in three divided doses.

DIET

Dietary habits and nutritional status play important roles in the prevention and promotion of colorectal cancer. Overall, a diet habitually high in fresh fruits and vegetables, modest in calories and alcohol, and low in red meat and animal fat is cancer-protective. Foods high in fat and animal proteins should be consumed moderately. Studies have found that dietary beef *induces* and dietary rye bran *prevents* formation of intestinal polyps (Mutanen et al. 2000). The consumption of meat, particularly organic, hormone-free white meat (poultry, fowl) as part of a balanced and varied diet is permissible. Ingesting a sensible amount of calories and maintaining a desirable weight also play important roles in prevention of colorectal cancer (Mason 2002). Studies suggest that obesity, rather than fat intake per se, predisposes an individual to colon cancer (Stemmermann et al. 1985).

The consumption of cruciferous vegetables has a protective effect on the development of colorectal cancer. The phytochemical sulforaphane is an isothiocyanate found almost exclusively in cruciferous vegetables. The proliferation of colon cancer cells was significantly reduced by sulforaphane at concentrations of greater than or equal to ($\geq$) 0.02 mmol (Frydoonfar et al. 2004). Calcium, folate, selenium, fish oil, and phytochemicals are the leading components in the diet that convey protection from colorectal cancer.

Recent epidemiological studies have indicated that a lipid-rich diet containing omega-6 fatty acids (i.e., linoleic acid, arachidonic acid) may be related with the disease process of colorectal cancer. Arachidonic acid (AA) is an essential, unsaturated, 20-carbon fatty acid that humans use to synthesize regulatory molecules such as prostaglandins and thromboxanes. Arachidonic acid is produced when mast cells activate the membrane enzyme called phospholipase A2 (PLA2), which breaks down membrane components to arachidonic acid. Arachidonic acid is further metabolized by one of two enzyme pathways into various prostaglandins (by cyclooxygenase) or leukotrienes (by lipooxygenase). Both prostaglandins and leukotrienes are highly pro-inflammatory. Therefore, excess amounts of linoleic acid and arachidonic acid are unhealthy because they promote inflammation. Linoleic acid (LA) is an omega-6 fatty acid, that once consumed is converted to gamma-linolenic acid (GLA) in the body. In turn, GLA is further broken down to arachidonic acid.

Rapid metabolism of arachidonic acid, increases activities of phospholipases (PLA2), and elevates levels of cyclooxygenase (COX) and lipooxygenase (LOX) in colonic cells. These events occur in various stages of the malignancy, suggesting a possible link between dietary lipids and the incidence of colorectal cancer (Jones et al. 2003). Based upon these findings, and for reasons previously discussed, a diet low in omega-6 fatty acids should be maintained. Omega-6 fatty acids are found primarily in vegetable oils. Linoleic acid is the primary oil ingredient added to most processed foods and is found in commonly used cooking oils, including sunflower, safflower, corn, and cottonseed. Arachidonic acid is found in egg yolks, meats, (especially organ meats), and other animal-based foods.

While gamma-linolenic acid (GLA) can convert to arachidonic acid, much of the GLA taken as a supplement may actually reduce inflammation by converting to a substance called dihomogamma-linolenic acid (DGLA). DGLA competes with arachidonic acid and prevents the negative inflammatory effects that arachidonic acid would otherwise cause in the body. Having adequate amounts of certain nutrients in the body (including magnesium, zinc, and vitamins C, B3, and B6) helps promote the conversion of GLA to DGLA rather than arachidonic acid. GLA can be obtained from several plant-based oils including evening primrose oil, borage oil, and black currant seed oil.

Tumor cells use glucose from the breakdown of sugar as their primary energy source. Sugars play an active role in reducing the immune response and provoke an increase in insulin that further induces cancer cell division. There is a relationship between lactic acid, insulin, and angiogenesis. In tumors, hypoxic conditions occur through inflammation, which reduces blood flow, promotes anemia, and induces the development of chaotic blood vessels within tumors.

These hypoxic conditions alter the pathways by which tumor cells burn fuel (glucose) for energy. This creates excessive buildup of toxic lactic acid.

In an oxygen-rich (aerobic) environment, glucose is burned in an efficient process that produces a maximum amount of energy and a minimal amount of lactic acid. However, tumor cells in chronic hypoxic conditions produce excessive lactic acid and inefficient utilization of glucose. Thus, there is a vicious cycle in which the reduced energy output stimulates the tumor cells to burn more glucose which in turn produces more lactic acid. Tumor cells consume glucose at a rate 3-5 times higher than normal cells, creating a highly stimulated glycolysis (glucose-burning) pathway.

Based on cancer's sugar dependency, a sugar deprivation diet is strongly recommended. An effective tool in eliminating sugar is to become familiar with using the glycemic index of foods. The glycemic index is a list that rates the speed at which different foods are digested and consequently raise blood sugar levels. The ratings are based on the rate at which a measured amount of pure glucose affects the body's blood sugar curve. Glucose itself has a rating of 100, and the closer a food item is to a rating of 100, the more rapidly it raises blood glucose levels, which in turn increases insulin levels.

Insulin plays an active role in promoting tumor growth via angiogenesis. Insulin is a growth factor that stimulates glycolysis and the proliferation of many cancer cell lines. Insulin is thought to facilitate angiogenesis by increasing lactic acid production in hypoxic tumor cells and by stimulating the proliferation of vascular cells. In cancer patients, elevated levels of insulin are common in cancerous tissue and blood plasma. It is therefore suggested that both a low sugar and a low saturated fat diet be followed.

Foods with very low glycemic index such as vegetables, protein, whole grains, and pulse vegetables are suggested (refer to the Obesity protocol for specific information about low glycemic foods).

Depleting sugar from one's diet can be achieved, in part, by adopting the following guidelines:

- Avoid all white foods including but not limited to sugar, flour, rice, pasta, breads, crackers, and cookies, and sodas.

- Read labels. Sugar has many names, including brown sugar, corn syrup, honey, molasses, maple syrup, high-fructose corn syrup, dextrin, raw sugar, fructose, polyols, dextrose, hydrogenated starch, galactose, glucose, sorbitol, fruit juice concentrate, lactose, brown rice syrup, xylitol, sucrose, mannitol, sorghum, maltose, and turbinado.

• Limit fruit juices. Per glass, fruit juices contain the juice of many pieces of fruit, is high in fructose (fruit sugar), but low in fiber. Instead, infrequently eat low-glycemic index fruit in small portions.

Natural compounds have been reported to inhibit cancer-promoting effects of insulin. For example, vitamin C has been reported to increase oxygen consumption and reduce lactic acid production in tumor cells. In addition, some natural compounds may help reduce insulin production by reducing insulin resistance. Insulin resistance occurs when cells are no longer sensitive to insulin and thus more insulin is produced in an effort to reduce glucose levels.

Insulin resistance has been implicated as a risk factor for cancer, and diets high in saturated fats and omega-6 fatty acids promote insulin resistance. Although the exact pathway is unknown, it is thought that the mechanism of action is via chronic activation of protein kinase C (PKC). Some of the known natural compounds that can reduce insulin resistance include omega-3 fatty acids, curcumin, flavonoids, selenium, and vitamin E.

Dietary risk factors for colorectal cancer must be managed including restriction of dietary sugars and alcohol. A high intake of alcohol is associated with an increased risk of colorectal adenoma. The carcinogenic influence of alcohol in the large bowel is most likely mediated through low folate status (Giovannucci et al. 2003). Alcohol interacts with a folate-related gene, methionine synthase, and the interaction between alcohol and this gene is stronger among those with a low folate intake. An increased occurrence of colorectal cancer and its adenoma precursor is observed among individuals with high alcohol intake and low circulating levels of folate. Individuals at risk of colorectal cancer who consume alcohol should eat an adequate amount of dietary folate sources (dark green leafy vegetables and fruits) and/or consider supplementing with folic acid.

Multivitamins contain several nutrients, including folic acid, that are hypothesized to reduce the risk of colorectal cancer. Previous studies suggest that multivitamin use may reduce colorectal cancer risk but only after a long latency period. A cohort study examined the association between regular multivitamin use (four or more times per week) and colorectal cancer incidence among 145,260 men and women in the Cancer Prevention Study II Nutrition Cohort. The results of this 10-year study were consistent with the hypothesis that past, but not recent, multivitamin use may be associated with modestly reduced risk of colorectal cancer (Jacobs et al. 2003).

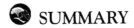 SUMMARY

When considering colorectal cancer treatment options, physicians and patients alike have to sort through much information. This article attempts to simplify and consolidate complicated scientific research into a multimodality protocol. It discusses the integration of surgery, chemotherapy, radiation, biological-response modifiers, supplementation, and dietary changes into a comprehensive approach to fight colorectal cancer.

As discussed in this article, the growth of cancer is based on many interactions occurring via numerous physiological pathways within the body. And despite huge strides in gaining molecular knowledge, there are still many unanswered questions regarding cancer's growth and development. What we do know is that the scientific literature supports an integrated approach to the treatment of cancer. The information put forth within this article reflects that research.

A number of published reports indicate that off-label drugs (such as cimetidine) and certain dietary supplements may improve survival in patients who have undergone conventional therapy. Please read this entire protocol before initiating the various recommendations because there are certain cautions to consider that should be discussed with your physician.

The following is a summary of what an individual with colorectal cancer (either colon cancer or rectal cancer should consider and discuss with their physician, as an adjuvant approach to conventional colorectal cancer therapy:

1. Cimetidine, 800 mg each night for 12 continuous months.

2. Curcumin, 10,800 mg, in divided doses of four 900-mg capsules 3 times a day.

3. Lightly caffeinated green tea extract, 5,250 mg in divided doses of five 350-mg capsules 3 times daily with meals. If caffeine interferes with sleep, take decaffeinated capsules in the evening. Each capsule should contain at least 100 mg of epigallocatechin gallate (EGCG).

4. Se-methylselenocysteine, 200-400 mcg daily in divided doses.

5. Fish oil, 8 capsules of a supplement called Mega EPA supply 3200 mg of EPA and 2400 mg of DHA.

6. Vitamin E succinate, 800-1200 IU daily.

7. Gamma E Tocopherol/Tocotrienols, 200 mg daily.

8. Vitamin D$_3$, 4000-6000 IU, taken daily on an empty stomach with monthly blood testing to monitor for toxicity. Reduce dosage at 6 months.

9. Water-soluble vitamin A, 100,000-300,000 IU daily, with monthly blood testing to monitor for toxicity. Reduce dosage at 6 months (refer to *Appendix A: Vitamin A Precautions*).

10. Modified citrus pectin, 15 grams daily in 3 divided doses.

11. Whey protein concentrate isolate, 10-20 grams three times daily.

12. Resveratrol, 20 mg daily.

13. Vitamin C, 4000-12,000 mg in divided doses throughout the day.

14. CoQ10, 100-300 mg daily.

15. Life Extension Mix, 3 tablets 3 times daily. (Certain patients with advanced colon cancer may want to avoid Life Extension Mix and other multivitamins since they all contain folic acid. While folic acid may be the most effective nutrient to prevent colon cancer, in advanced stages, or in combinations with certain chemotherapy drugs, folic acid may be detrimental because it may facilitate hypermethylation in colon cancer cells).

Note: *If chemotherapy and/or radiation are being considered, refer to the* Cancer Chemotherapy *and* Cancer Radiation *protocols in this book. Some experts do not believe that curcumin, CoQ10, or even high-potency antioxidants should be taken during active chemotherapy or radiation therapy.*

Also refer to the protocol entitled *Cancer Treatment: The Critical Factors*, with special emphasis placed on the use of COX-2 inhibitors and statin drugs in cancer treatment.

FOR MORE INFORMATION

American Cancer Society
http://www.cancer.org/
(800) ACS-2345

National Cancer Institute:
Cancer Information Service Toll-free:
(800) 4-CANCER, (800) 422-6237

NCI Online/Internet
Use http://cancer.gov to reach NCI's Web site.

CancerMail Service
To obtain a contents list, send e-mail
tocancermail@cips.nci.nih.gov with the word "help"
in the body of the message.

 ## PRODUCT AVAILABILITY

Curcumin, green tea, SeMSC (Se-methylselenocysteine), coenzyme Q10, Mega EPA, Pecta-Sol, vitamin D3 caps, water-soluble vitamin A liquid, vitamin E succinate, Gamma E Tocopherol/Tocotrienols, Enhanced Life Extension Protein, vitamin C, enhanced whey protein, and Life Extension Mix can be ordered by calling (800) 544-4440 or by ordering online. Cimetidine can be purchased over the counter at pharmacies in 200 mg tablets, alternatively request a higher potency prescription from your physician.

STAYING INFORMED

The information published in this protocol is only as current as the day the manuscript was sent to the printer. This protocol raises many issues that are subject to change as new data emerges. Furthermore, cancer is a disease with unacceptably high mortality rates, and none of the suggestions contained in this protocol can guarantee a cure.

The Life Extension Foundation is constantly uncovering information to provide the cancer patient with more ammunition to battle their disease. A special website has been established for the purpose of updating new findings that directly pertain to the cancer protocols published in this protocol. Whenever Life Extension discovers information of value to those with cancer, it will be posted on the website www.lefcancer.org.

Before utilizing this cancer protocols, we suggest that you check www.lefcancer.org to see if any substantial changes have been made to the recommendations described in this protocol. Based on the sheer number of newly published findings, there could be significant alterations to the information you have just read.

DISCLAIMER

This information (and any accompanying printed material) is not intended to replace the attention or advice of a physician or other health care professional. Anyone who wishes to embark on any dietary, drug, exercise, or other lifestyle change intended to prevent or treat a specific disease or condition should first consult with and seek clearance from a qualified health care professional. The information published in the protocols is only as current as the day the manuscript was sent to the printer. This protocol raises many issues that are subject to change as new data emerge. None of our suggested protocol regimens can guarantee a cure.

Common Cold

The common cold is caused by more than 300 serologically distinct viruses. Since there are so many different types, it is impossible to develop a single vaccine effective against them all.

The common cold is spread by airborne droplets from an infected person breathing, coughing, or sneezing. Viruses generally will not stay alive long enough on inanimate objects to be a problem, as on a telephone, for instance. The droplets must be inhaled. However, when considering any infection, one must keep in mind a number of things. Infection is by no means automatic. Just because a person is exposed to an infection does not mean that an infection will ensue. Infection is dependent on three important aspects: (1) virulence of the organism, (2) inoculation size of the organism, and (3) the host resistance.

Virulence refers to the inherent ability of a particular organism to cause infection. Some strains may have a low infectivity rate while others have a higher one. Inoculation size refers to the number of biological agents to which the host (the person exposed) is exposed. Host resistance refers to the immunological state of the person exposed. In other words, if two people are standing side-by-side when an infected person sneezes directly into their faces and they both receive the same number of organisms into their airways, it is possible that one or both of them may not get sick. How can this be? One or both of the two people may have a weakened immune system as a result of stress or recent illness, making them more susceptible.

Most people are all too familiar with the symptoms of the common cold: headache, nasal congestion, watery rhinorrhea (runny nose), sneezing, and a scratchy throat accompanied by general malaise (body aches). Because the common cold is virus-borne, antibiotics that treat bacterial-borne infections are ineffective.

The majority of the infections adults have throughout the healthy time of their lives are viral in origin. Having a common cold with congested sinuses is *not* sinusitis. Patients may even have greenish nasal discharge with sinus congestion due to a common cold. Sinusitis is a *bacterial* infection of the sinuses that is very painful and is associated with fever, moderate sinus pressure, and nausea. Only with bacterial sinusitis is an antibiotic necessary.

The same can also be said for a cold associated with a bad cough producing sputum. Usually, this represents a viral infection for which antibiotics are of no use. The only caveat from a clinical perspective is that many physicians will give antibiotics prophylactically to smokers and patients whose immune function may be impaired by other illnesses such as diabetes or asthma.

TREATMENT

Stress is a factor that can increase susceptibility to the common cold. This was shown in a study conducted at Carnegie Mellon University in Pittsburgh and reported by Cohen et al. (1999). Researchers measured the severity of respiratory symptoms, mucus production, and interleukin-6 (IL-6) in test subjects injected with influenza A virus. Volunteers who reported greater psychological stress before inoculation reacted to infection with more intense symptoms, increased mucus production, and higher concentrations of interleukin-6 (Cohen et al. 1999). The same researchers further believe that interleukin-6, a protein produced in the body, may be a biological link between psychological stress and the severity of upper respiratory infections such as cold and flu. The hormone DHEA (dehydroepiandrosterone) suppresses elevated IL-6 levels.

Rest and relaxation while recovering enables the individual to strengthen immune function and enhance detoxification. Avoiding contact with others will help to prevent spreading the infection. While there is no cure for the common cold, there are certain steps that can be taken to relieve symptoms and discomfort.

- Eating properly may help to shorten duration or make the symptoms less severe

- Drink a minimum of 8–10 glasses of fluids a day to avoid dehydration, keep mucous membranes moist, and loosen phlegm

- Abstain from alcohol because it reduces the body's ability to fight infection

- Avoid smoking and smoky places

- To relieve aches and fever, take an aspirin substitute

- Use saline-based, over-the-counter nose drops to relieve a stuffy nose

- To keep nasal passages moist, use a cool-mist humidifier

- Certain dietary supplements as described below have been shown to lessen the discomfort and duration of a cold

People often wonder if they should go to work while they are sick with a cold. The answer is simple—do what your body tells you to do. If you are sick, tired, and feel that you would be more comfortable at home under the covers resting, that is probably what you should do. You can't "catch" a cold from being out in the cold. However, if your body is already under stress, being out in the cold may be the additional stress that lowers your immune threshold to the point that you become ill.

Over-the-Counter and Prescription Medications

Many over-the-counter cold medications provide far more ingredients than are needed to ease symptoms of the common cold. Physicians generally recommend one-ingredient generic brands over expensive mega formulas that attempt to treat several symptoms at once. A simple cough suppressant or oral decongestant should provide satisfactory relief. If a cold formula is necessary, read packaging information carefully for drug interactions to avoid.

A unique therapy to treat the common cold involves the one-time injection of 500,000–3 million IU of interferon (interferon alfa-2a), combined with 40 mg of melatonin every night. Studies document the ability of interferon to kill many common-cold viruses. Interferon is a component of the immune system that kills viruses (and cancer cells). Since it is a prescription drug, a doctor must prescribe and inject the one-time dose of interferon (for additional suggestions, refer to the Immune Enhancement protocol). Getting the average family physician to prescribe interferon for a cold may be difficult. Most physicians are not familiar with it. Various interferons are generally used to treat leukemia and hepatitis C, among other diseases. Long-term use carries with it certain side effects. However, using interferon alfa-2a one time is generally safe. Those interested in this type of therapy should find a physician who practices complementary medicine. Presenting him or her with this book may make them more open to the idea.

Ribavirin (often combined with interferon alfa-2a) is a broad-spectrum antiviral-approved drug for hepatitis C in the United States. There is evidence that some cold virus strains can be stopped from replicating with ribavirin at a dose of 800 mg a day (Bernstein et al. 1989). The brand name of ribavirin sold in the United States is Rebetol.

Ipratropium bromide nasal spray (Atrovent) is a prescription medication that is prescribed for perennial rhinitis. Although this medication would not be appropriate for a simple common cold, if you are plagued with a constant runny nose from allergies or a chronic low-grade infection, Atrovent may help to provide relief. In a multicenter study of 411 volunteers, two sprays of ipratropium bromide per nostril administered three times a day for 4 days caused a 26–34% reduction in rhinorrhea (nasal discharge) compared with people who were taking a placebo (saline spray) and people receiving no treatment at all. Sneeze severity scores were also reduced in people taking the nasal spray (Hayden et al. 1996).

Natural Supplements for Treatment and Prevention

Vitamin C

Vitamin C in doses of 5,000–20,000 mg has been used by many people as a natural antihistamine and antiviral therapy to treat common colds. In 1971, Linus Pauling carried out a meta-analysis of four placebo-controlled trials, concluding that it was highly unlikely that the decrease of common cold symptoms in vitamin C groups was caused by chance alone. Studies carried out since then have found that high doses of vitamin C alleviate common cold symptoms, indicating that the vitamin does indeed have physiologic effects on colds (Hemila 1997a,b). However, despite the large number of placebo-controlled studies showing that vitamin C supplementation alleviates the symptoms of the common cold, widespread skepticism about vitamin C persists.

In a review of six large studies on vitamin C supplementation of 1000 mg a day or less, it was shown that common-cold incidence is not reduced in people taking these relatively low doses (1000 mg a day or less). A further analysis of these studies, however, reveals that some groups do benefit from low-dose vitamin C supplementation. In four studies with British male school children, a statistically significant reduction in common-cold incidence was found in groups supplemented with low-dose vitamin C (Hemila 1997a). One study showed that those who engaged in heavy exercise were 50% less likely to get a common cold if they took only 600–1000 mg a day of vitamin C (Hemila 1996).

As vitamin C has an individually based maximum dose prior to the development of diarrhea, some complementary physicians give patients with bad colds 20–30 grams of IV vitamin C every other day for three treatments. While there may be few studies to date proving efficacy for this treatment, anecdotal clinical experience suggests that it is indeed quite helpful. Holistic physicians have suggested taking 1000 mg of ascorbic acid (vitamin C) every hour if tolerated by the bowel and then reducing the daily dosing based on the dose taken prior to getting diarrhea. Bowel tolerance is the maximum dosage of vitamin C that can be consumed by an individual before they get diarrhea. Once diarrhea occurs, the cells are saturated with vitamin C, and it is spilling over into the colon. At that point, the patient has reached "bowel tolerance" and should take a dosage that preceded the onset of diarrhea. The sicker one is, the more vitamin C they can usually consume before reaching bowel tolerance. The vitamin C assists the cells of the body to fight the infection. (*Remember:* cells make up tissues which comprise the organs of the human body so every organ contains thousands of cells.) A cup of hot tea taken 1 hour before consuming vitamin C as well as an immune-boosting formula containing thymic extracts may help at the very first sign of a cold.

In addition to vitamin C, oxidative therapy with intravenous hydrogen peroxide 0.03%, popularized by Dr. Charles Farr, may be helpful. Ultraviolet blood irradiation has been described anecdotally by some alternative practitioners. Using this therapy, a small sample of blood is drawn from a patient's arm and then irradiated with UV light. Proponents of this treatment suggest that the cold-causing viruses and the cells containing them are identified and killed. When the irradiated blood is returned to the body, the immune system creates a natural defense against active organisms comprised of the dead virus and carrier cells. There are, however, no studies in the scientific literature to document this treatment.

Zinc Gluconate

A randomized, double-blind, placebo-controlled clinical trial has shown that zinc gluconate lozenges produce a reduction in the duration of cold symptoms. In this study, patients received zinc lozenges or placebo lozenges every 2 hours for the duration of cold symptoms. The median time to complete resolution of cold symptoms was 4.4 days in the zinc group, compared with 7.6 days in the placebo group (Anon. 1997).

Another study to test the benefits of zinc gluconate lozenges showed that the time to complete resolution of symptoms was significantly shorter in the zinc group than in the placebo group. The zinc group had significantly fewer days with coughing, headache, hoarseness, nasal congestion, nasal drainage, and sore throat (Mossad et al. 1996). By dissolving two zinc lozenges in the mouth every few hours, the zinc will help inactivate cold viruses multiplying in the throat.

Echinacea

In the past 50 years echinacea has achieved worldwide fame for its antiviral, antifungal, and antibacterial properties (Stimpel et al. 1984; Luettig et al. 1989; Roesler et al. 1991). Four to six 250-mg capsules standardized to 4% echinosides should be taken at onset and then two capsules every 4 hours thereafter, until symptoms are gone for more than 2 days.

Goldenseal

Although goldenseal which comes from the plant *Hydrastis canadensis*, has been touted as an herb that fights against infections such as the common cold, significant studies that support its use for this purpose are not published in the current literature. The plant contains alkaloids which are the active medicinal compounds. The medical literature does contain a study which supported its effect against oral pathogens (Hwang et al. 2003) along with one study about its effect against *Helicobacter pylori*, a bacterium associated with peptic ulcers (Mahady et al. 2003). Consequently, goldenseal is not recommended for the treatment of the common cold at this point in time.

Astralagus

This herb brings support to all deep immune functions and activates cellular immunity (Yang et al. 1987; Yang et al. 1990; Liang et al. 1994; Guo et al. 1995; Peng et al. 1995). Astralagus herbal extract at 300 mg a day can boost immune function and produce direct antiviral effects.

N-Acetyl-Cysteine (NAC)

The amino acid *N*-acetyl-cysteine (NAC) helps to break up excessive mucus and can have a direct antiviral effect. If you get a cold, it is suggested that 600–1200 mg of NAC be taken with at least 2000 mg of vitamin C 3 times a day.

Sambucol

Sambucol (black elderberry) has been shown to have antiviral properties in various strains of influenza, including A and B. One study showed that the Sambucol group had improvement in symptoms in 2 days whereas recovery took at least 6 days in the control group (Zakay-Rones et al. 1995). Sambucol extract is used as an herbal remedy for colds and flu. Although the bottle suggests that the formula be taken in doses of 1 tbsp. 4 times per day, some clinicians have advised that it is more effective if taken every 3 hours within the first 48 to 72 hours of onset of flu-like symptoms until the bottle is finished. (The herb is more effective at inhibiting viral replication if the virus has not multiplied excessively). Similarly, antiviral flu prescription medications mandate that the drug be taken within the first 48 to 72 hours for the same reason.

Digestive Enzymes

Certain combinations of digestive enzymes such as Wobenzyme or Vitalzym exert an anti-inflammatory effect when taken without food. If taken with food, the enzymes will aid digestion but the anti-inflammatory effect will be voided. The best anti-inflammatory effect is achieved when taken in-between meals or at least an hour before a meal. The anti-inflammatory effect can assist the natural processes of the body to more effectively fight the infection.

Samento

Samento is a biologically more potent variety of the medicinal plant called *Uncaria tomentosa* or Cat's Claw. Ordinary Cat's Claw contains an alkaloid called the pentacyclic oxindole alkaloid (POA) which exerts favorable effects on the immune system of those who take it. Cat's Claw contains another alkaloid called the tetracyclic oxindole alkaloid (TOA), which appears to inhibit the effectiveness of POA. The samento type of Cat's Claw is free of TOA, allowing it to exert a potent restorative effect on the human immune system, which includes anti-inflammatory and antioxidant activities. Samento is best found by selecting the wildly grown plant for harvesting at a particular TOA-free time. The product has been used in Europe and is now available over-the-counter in health food stores.

Medicinal Mushrooms

Medicinal mushrooms such as maitake, shiitake and reishi have powerful immune boosting properties which have been used as metabolic activators of the immune system for the common cold, HIV, cancer and other conditions that affect the immune system. Shiitake extracts contain a beta-glucan called lentinan, which stimulates the activity and production of T lymphocytes, macrophages and other immune mediators. The beta-glucans found in shiitake mushrooms (LEM) and maitake mushrooms (maitake-D) exert potent stimulatory effects on the immune system.

Studies have demonstrated that the D-fraction of maitake exerts a powerful immune enhancing effect in cancer patients. The triterpenes found in the very bitter reishi mushrooms have demonstrated anti-viral activity in HIV patients and have been useful in cancer therapy according to scientific studies (see related chapters). Preparations of any of these three mushroom extracts can be found in the local health food store. Some preparations contain a mixture of two to three of these extracts to achieve an optimal balance of immune enhancement. The beta-glucans from these mushrooms have been useful in the common cold and flu to stimulate the body's natural immune defenses to more effectively fight against the infection (Price and Konno 2002; Tenney 1997).

Sodium Chloride Nasal Spray or Drops

Sodium chloride nasal preparations naturally assist with removal of mucus and relief of congestion. This sterile salt water mixture offers some relief to those who prefer not to use antihistamines or decongestants.

Zicam Cold Remedy Nasal Gel

Zicam Cold Remedy Nasal Gel is an over-the-counter preparation that effectively inhibits viral replication when applied topically inside the nostrils as directed on the bottle. It should be taken within the first 48 hours as directed, for optimal results.

Melatonin

An interesting supplement that can assist in both providing a good night's sleep and boosting antiviral function is the pineal hormone, melatonin. Its ability to regulate the circadian cycle and aid sleeping can be most beneficial during times of illness. Melatonin is also the most effective hormone therapy to protect and improve immune function. One of its functions is to stimulate the production of T-helper cells, necessary to identify cancer cells, viruses, fungi, and bacteria. Melatonin has been shown to enhance the production of other immune components, including natural killer cells, IL-2, IL-4, IL-10, gamma-interferon, and eosinophils (Lissoni et al. 1989; 1994; 1995; Maestroni et al. 1993; 1995; Bubenik et al. 1998; Kostogloy-Athanassiou 1998).

Published evidence also suggests that melatonin is highly effective in suppressing immune cell-killing free radicals. The recommended dose for healthy people is 300 mcg–6 mg daily. Therapeutically, doses of 3–20 mg daily may be taken when fighting a cold to help get to sleep and boost antiviral immune function.

Garlic

Scientific research shows that garlic is a source of phytochemicals that protects against infection and inflammation, lowers the risk of heart disease, and has anticancer effects. Garlic is rich in antioxidants that include organosulfur compounds and flavonoids, capable of scavenging free radicals. Garlic also contains selenium, which is required for the antioxidant enzyme glutathione peroxidase. These properties help to enhance the immune system in fighting off infections caused by bacteria, viruses, and fungi.

Human studies (Abdullah 1989) confirm immune stimulation by garlic. Subjects receiving aged garlic extract at 1800 mg a day for 3 weeks showed a 155.5% increase in immune cell activity. Garlic and garlic preparations increase the activity of immune cells, including macrophages that kill infectious invaders.

Scientific studies also show that garlic does not have to be eaten raw or fresh to be effective. While there is much agreement on the efficacy of garlic, a debate continues on whether high-allicin garlic extract (Pure-Gar) is better than aged-garlic extract (Kyolic). Pure-Gar is standardized to 10,000 ppm allicin, a key ingredient involved in disease prevention. Kyolic uses organically grown garlic and through an ambient temperature aging process removes the irritating (and odor causing) components to produce an extract standardized to S-allyl cysteine, a potent antioxidant. The potent odor of garlic may not be necessary for its health benefits. Research shows that aged, deodorized garlic extract sometimes works better than fresh garlic without causing digestive disorders and "garlic breath" that may haunt the fresh garlic eater.

Shark Liver Oil

Shark liver oil has been used for years in the Scandinavian countries as an antibacterial, antiviral, antifungal, and antiparasitic agent. The alkylglycerols in shark liver oil are beneficial because they are known to increase the production of certain cytokines that attack viruses. According to some researchers, viral infections, such as influenza or the common cold, can be prevented or reduced significantly by taking shark liver oil at the first sign of symptoms. For immune system stimulation and prevention of disease, 1 or 2 capsules, formulated to contain 200 mg of the active alkylglycerols, daily is sufficient for most individuals.

Andrographis Paniculata

Andrographis is a traditional herbal remedy used in India and Asia as a broad-spectrum natural antibiotic and immune system stimulator for bacterial, viral, and parasitic conditions. Research conducted by the Max Planck Institute of Germany (Caceres et al. 1999) found 70% improvement of cold symptoms in a group using this herb. This was reconfirmed in Sweden where a study found the rate of improvement at 71% (Melchior et al. 1997). At the onset of a cold, a typical dosage of 400 mg (standardized at 4–6% andrographolide) taken 3 times a day has been proven effective at quickly reducing headache pain, fever, irritation, congestion, and fatigue without toxic side effects.

Lactoferrin

Lactoferrin is a subfraction of whey with well-documented antiviral, antimicrobial, anticancer, and immune modulating/enhancing effects. It has a strong affinity to bind iron and is considered a potent antioxidant. Lactoferrin is composed of over 700 different amino acids and is found in all secretions that bathe mucus membranes. Lactoferrin has been found to directly and indirectly inhibit viruses such as human HIV, cytomegalovirus (CMV), and herpes simplex Type I infection (HSV1) (Puddu et al. 1998; Superti et al. 1997; Harmsen et al. 1995; Swart et al. 1996, 1998). Because of its multifunctional role, lactoferrin is a common-sense prophylactic for bacterial and viral based infections.

SIGNS OF A MORE SERIOUS INFECTION

Most common colds do not require a visit to the doctor or a prescription medication. However, certain symptoms may indicate that a more serious infection is present. Consult a physician if you experience one or more of the following:

- A sustained fever of 100°F or higher for more than 4 days
- Chills and rigors (shakes)
- Facial swelling and/or pain in the ears
- A severe sore throat with a white or yellow coating
- A severe cough with thick discolored mucus; a cough that lasts more than 10 days
- Headache with pain in the face, sensitivity in the upper jaw, yellow or green mucus being expelled from the nose or throat

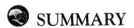 SUMMARY

To achieve fast recovery when beset with the common cold, it is important to take immediate steps to boost immune function and interfere with viral replication. Antiviral drugs are limited because they only work via one mechanism and do not boost immune function.

A simple approach is to take 2 zinc lozenges (24 mg elemental zinc a lozenge) every 2 waking hours. To take a more aggressive approach, a common cold sufferer might consider the following aggressive program in addition to zinc lozenges:

Morning dosing:

- 200 mg of the hormone DHEA (dehydroepiandrosterone)
- 5 capsules of Kyolic Garlic Formula Number 105
- 300 mg of lactoferrin
- 500 mg of echinacea (standardized to provide 20 mg of echinosides)
- 5 tablets of Life Extension Mix
- 500 mg of alpha-lipoic acid
- 2 tbsp of whey protein (if tolerable)
- Five 350-mg green tea extract (95%) capsules
- Four 1000-mg capsules of vitamin C

Afternoon dosing:

- 200 mg of DHEA
- 300 mg of lactoferrin
- 500 mg of echinacea
- 5 tablets of Life Extension Mix
- 500 mg of alpha-lipoic acid
- 5 capsules of Kyloic Garlic Formula Number 105
- 2 tbsp of whey protein (if tolerable)
- Five 350-mg green tea extract (95%) capsules
- Four 1000-mg capsules of vitamin C

Nighttime dosing:

- Ten 900-mg capsules of Pure-Gar (high-allicin garlic) (Take with some food because this can cause temporary burning in stomach and will cause pungent odor.)
- 3–20 mg of melatonin (higher dosing better as long as morning drowsiness is not too severe)
- 300 mg of lactoferrin
- 500 mg of echinacea
- 5 capsules of Kyolic Garlic Formula Number 105
- Four 900-mg capsules of curcumin with bioperine
- Four 1000-mg capsules of vitamin C

DHEA is an adrenal hormone that has shown antiviral and immune-boosting benefits. When flu symptoms occur, 200 mg of DHEA taken 2 times a day until flu symptoms subside can boost the immune system (*refer to the DHEA Replacement Therapy protocol before taking DHEA*).

Life Extension Mix is a broad-spectrum multivitamin formula that contains ingredients that have been shown to boost the immune system. Life Extension Mix contains *N*-acetyl-cysteine, selenium, and other antiviral nutrients. Suggested dose is 9 tablets daily. An additional 600 mg daily of N-acetyl-cysteine may be taken along with the 600 mg contained in Life Extension Mix if there is a need to break up pulmonary mucus.

The potency of the zinc gluconate lozenges that should be taken every 2 hours is 24 mg of elemental zinc per lozenge. The herb *Andrographis paniculata* can be taken at the onset of a cold to lessen its severity, 400 mg (standardized at 4–6% andrographolide) taken 3 times daily. Shark liver oil may be taken every day to stimulate the immune system in the dose of 4 capsules a day for no more than 30 days.

Sambucol extract may be taken in doses of 1 tbsp. 4 times a day, or as some clinicians advise, every 2 to 3 hours and if taken within the first 48 to 72 hours of onset of flu-like symptoms until the bottle is finished.

Medicinal mushrooms (such as maitake) have shown effectiveness against viral pathogens that attack the immune system. A preventive dose of a product such as 10 Mushroom Formula by EcoNugenics is 1 to 4 capsules 2 to 3 times a day or as directed by a healthcare professional.

The medicinal herb samento is a potent immune enhancer that has shown to be more effective than ordinary cat's claw. The suggested daily dose of Life Extension's Samento Formula is 1 capsule daily, or as directed by a health professional.

Digestive enzymes if taken between meals can provide an anti-inflammatory effect for the cold sufferer. Wobenzym M is enterically coated so that the enzymic action is not deactivated by stomach acids. Take 3 tablets, 3 times daily between meals.

Saline & Aloe Nasal Spray by Naturade may help remove mucus and relieve congestion. This product may be used as often as needed or as directed by a health care professional.

Zicam Cold Remedy Nasal Gel can be applied to inside the nostrils as directed on the bottle to inhibit viral replication. This medicine can be found over the counter in most drugstores and should be taken within the first 48 hours of the onset of symptoms for optimal results.

For refractory cold, consider 1.5 million–3 million IU of interferon alfa-2a (subcutaneous injection) one time; IV vitamin C, 30–50 grams 3 times a week for 1 week; or 800 mg of ribavirin daily as prescribed by a physician. Those interested in this type of therapy should find a physician who practices complementary medicine. Ipratropium nasal spray (Atrovent) may be indicated for chronic rhinitis. Atrovent must be prescribed by a physician.

See the *Influenza protocol* for more information on supplements that boost immune function and fight viral pathogens.

 FOR MORE INFORMATION

For the location and telephone number of a physician in your area who specializes in complementary medicine, call the American College for the Advancement of Medicine, (800) 532-3688.

 PRODUCT AVAILABILITY

Zinc lozenges, Life Extension Mix, *N*-acetyl-cysteine, echinacea, astralagus, vitamin C, Sambucol, shark liver oil, lactoferrin, Kyolic Formula 105 and Pure-Gar, melatonin, Saline & Aloe Nasal Spray, Wobenzym N, samento, 10 Mushroom Formula, and other supplements discussed in this protocol are available by calling (800) 544-4440 or by ordering online at www.lef.org. Ribavirin (Rebetol) and alpha-interferon are prescription drugs.

Constipation

Chronic constipation is the number one gastrointestinal complaint in the United States, particularly among the elderly. Constipation accounts for more than 2.5 million physician visits a year and is among the most frequent reasons for patient self-medication (Sweeney 1997).

The *American Family Physician* reported in 1998 that constipation affects as many as 26% of elderly men and 34% of elderly women (Schaefer et al. 1998). Constipation is a health problem that has been related to diminished perception of quality of life. The good news is that there are conventional and alternative treatments that can provide immediate relief.

COMMON SYMPTOMS

Normal evacuation should occur 1–2 times daily. The movement should be formed, but not hard, with a slightly sweet odor. Movements that are hard or small and occur only every other day signify constipation. Any sudden change in a person's ability to move their bowels should be treated with suspicion, particularly in the elderly (constipation can be a first sign of colon cancer due to obstruction). Constipation associated with fatigue can also be an indication of hypothyroidism. More often than not, however, constipation is purely a functional problem unrelated to an underlying disease. Most individuals with uncontrolled constipation develop a variety of symptoms, ranging from large bowel pain, rectal discomfort, abdominal fullness and bloating, nausea, and anorexia to a general feeling of malaise. These individuals feel as if they never completely evacuate their bowels. Severe chronic constipation may be accompanied by fecal impaction.

FIBER IS NOT THE SOLUTION FOR SOME PEOPLE

Studies show that some chronically constipated people do not find relief from fiber supplements.

An example of fiber not working was the report of a trial showing that 80% of patients with slow transit and 63% of patients with a disorder of defecation did not respond to dietary fiber treatment. In 85% of patients *without* these disorders, fiber was effective. This study showed that slow gastrointestinal transit

and/or a disorder of defecation might explain a poor outcome of dietary fiber therapy in some patients with chronic constipation and why nutritional laxative therapy may be important (Vonderholzer et al. 1997).

Another study evaluated whether laxatives and fiber therapies improve symptoms and bowel movement frequency in adults with chronic constipation. Fiber and laxatives decreased abdominal pain and improved stool consistency compared with a placebo. The conclusions were that both fiber and laxatives *modestly* improved bowel movement frequency in adults with chronic constipation. The results of this study showed that there was inadequate evidence to establish whether fiber was superior to laxatives or whether one laxative class was superior to another (Tramonte et al. 1997). Clearly, fiber is not the solution to chronic constipation for many people, despite the endless television commercials and physician recommendations that tout the benefits of fiber.

AGGRESSIVE ALTERNATIVE THERAPIES

Dietary modifications can help most people, but some cases of constipation are caused by insufficient peristalsis, which means there is not enough colon contractile activity to completely evacuate the bowel. However, there are specific nutrients that, if taken at the right time, can induce healthy colon peristaltic action without producing side effects. Although pharmaceutical laxatives have been linked to the development of cancer, nutritional laxatives have many health benefits.

On an empty stomach, certain nutrients have been shown to induce healthy colon peristalsis. One combination is 4–8 grams of vitamin C powder and 1500 mg of magnesium oxide powder taken with the juice of a freshly squeezed grapefruit. A convenient product sold by several vitamin companies is a buffered vitamin C powder product that contains magnesium and potassium salts mixed with ascorbic acid. Depending on the individual, a few teaspoons or, in some cases, 1–2 tbsp of this buffered vitamin C powder produce a powerful but safe laxative effect within 45 minutes. This therapy has to be individually adjusted so it will not cause day-long diarrhea.

Vitamin B5 (pantothenic acid) in a dose of 2000–3000 mg, on an empty stomach, will produce a rapid evacuation of bowel contents. Vitamin B5 powder is unpalatable, but there are many health benefits attributed to it—in addition to its ability to stimulate peristalsis (Mancinella et al. 1982). One way of taking vitamin B5 and other peristalsis-inducing nutrients is to use a multinutrient formula, such as Powermaker II. This better-tasting powder contains vitamin B$_5$, vitamin C, choline, and L-arginine, all of which induce significant peristaltic action when 1–2 tbsp are taken on an empty stomach.

Nutritional laxatives such as magnesium, ascorbic acid, and pantothenic acid are becoming more popular in persons with constipation that is resistant to fiber therapies.

Fiber and Constipation

Dr. Dennis Burkitt (a well-known British surgeon practicing in Africa after World War II) noticed that very few people in Africa suffered from constipation. His epidemiological surveys and studies led to the now well-known fact that dietary fiber in North America is sadly lacking. Burkitt connected low dietary fiber to many illnesses, such as hemorrhoids, diabetes, varicose veins, heart disease, and appendicitis (Jones et al. 1985; Trowell et al. 1986).

Constipation also means that the stool is in contact with the surface of the large bowel wall for a longer time than in the person whose bowels move regularly. Some have suggested that this increased contact between the stool and the bowel wall may increase our exposure to toxins and carcinogens.

Fiber

There are two kinds of fiber: soluble and insoluble (each indigestible by humans). Soluble fiber attracts water and turns to gel during digestion. This slows digestion and the rate of nutrient absorption from the stomach and intestine. *Soluble* fiber is found in oat bran, barley, nuts, seeds, beans, lentils, peas, and some fruits and vegetables. *Insoluble* fiber is found in foods such as wheat bran, vegetables, fruits, and whole grains. Insoluble fiber appears to speed the passage of foods through the stomach and intestines and to add bulk to the stool. The average American now eats 10–15 grams of fiber daily. The recommendation for older children, adolescents, and adults is 20–35 grams daily. Fiber is excellent for overall intestinal health as well as for its benefits in alleviating chronic constipation in some people. Although human beings cannot digest fiber, the 5 lbs or so of intestinal bacteria known as "friendly bacteria" will use fiber for fermentation purposes and for the production of useful short-chain fatty acids that the cells of the intestinal tract can use for their energy source. The following table lists food sources of fiber. Most foods contain a mixture of soluble and insoluble fiber.

Table 1: *Food Sources of Fiber*

Food	Serving size	Total fiber (grams)	Insoluble (grams)	Soluble (grams)
English muffin	1	2.0	0.5	1.5
Spaghetti, cooked	1 cup	2.0	0.5	1.5
Whole-wheat bread	1 slice	2.5	0.5	2.0
White rice, cooked	1/2 cup	0.5	0	0.5
Bran flake cereal	3/4 cup	5.5	0.5	5.0
Corn flake cereal	1 cup	1.0	0	1.0
Oatmeal, cooked	3/4 cup	3.0	1.0	2.0
Banana	1 medium	2.0	0.5	1.5
Apple, with skin	1 medium	3.0	0.5	2.5
Orange	1 medium	2.0	0.5	1.5
Pear, with skin	1 medium	4.5	0.5	4.0
Strawberry	1/2 cup	1.0	0	1.0
Broccoli	1/2 cup	2.0	0	2.0
Corn	1/2 cup	1.5	0	1.5
Potato, baked with skin	1 medium	4.0	1.0	3.0
Spinach	1/2 cup	2.0	0.5	1.5
Kidney bean	1/2 cup	4.5	1.0	3.5
Popcorn	1 cup	1.0	0	1.0
Peanut butter, chunky	2 tbsp	1.5	0	1.5

Ispaghula Husk (Psyllium)

In a multicenter trial, psyllium fiber was compared with lactulose and other laxatives in 381 patients who were constipated. After 4 weeks, Ispaghula (psyllium) husk was rated as superior compared to lactulose and other laxatives because bowel movements were more frequent and of greater bulk. There was a lower incidence of side effects as well (Dettmar et al. 1998). However, an article in *The Lancet* suggested that Ispaghula husk could increase the probability of developing benign tumors on the colon in persons who had a previous history of these tumors (known as adenomas) (Bonithon-Kopp et al. 2000).

Lifestyle Changes

There are a number of factors that contribute to constipation: poor dietary practices, including lack of dietary fiber; not drinking enough water; lack of exercise; improper laxative use; hypercalcemia; inflammatory bowel disorders; and some neurological disorders. Additionally, taking antacids containing aluminum or calcium, as well as reactions to taking medications (e.g., painkillers containing codeine, antidepressants, antiparkinsonism drugs, and diuretics) may cause constipation. In many people, anxiety, depression, and grief (even a routine pregnancy) may also precipitate constipation.

In addition, aging itself can increase the incidence of constipation. As a person ages, the colon wall thickens. When this thickening is combined with a lifetime diet that is low in fiber, constipation can result.

As noted earlier, dietary content can have a significant effect on constipation. People may become constipated if they begin to eat fewer vegetables, fruits, and whole grains. In addition, eating high-fat meats, dairy products, eggs, and sweets high in refined sugars can also lead to constipation.

Unfortunately, many elderly people who live alone lose interest in cooking and eating. As a result, they often turn to eating convenience foods. These foods tend to be low in fiber and high in fat and may contribute to the problem. Furthermore, bad teeth often cause older people to choose soft, processed foods that contain little, if any, fiber.

Constipation can contribute to a loss of bladder control by weakening the pelvic floor muscles as a result of straining. A full bowel pressing on the bladder, causing it to empty prematurely or block the outflow of urine, is a common effect of constipation. People with bladder control problems often do not drink enough fluids for fear of incontinence, which can result in constipation or worsen it, causing more discomfort and anxiety.

Many other people also do not drink enough fluids, especially if they do not eat regular meals. As already noted, water and other liquids add bulk to stools, making bowel movements easier (Krugan 1996).

WHAT THE EUROPEANS ARE DOING

The most popular digestive aid sold in Europe is called Digest RC. This product was introduced in Europe over 45 years ago, and today more than 100 million doses of the product are sold annually, primarily in Eastern Europe.

The mechanism of action of the formula is to stimulate peristalsis of the intestines, speed digestion of fats, and prevent stagnation of food in the digestive tract. Benefits for the user are a reduction in esophageal acid reflux; alleviation of the feeling of fullness and bloating after eating; decreased digestive tract tension; alkalinization of gastric contents; constipation relief; and normalized elimination.

Black radish juice extract is the primary active ingredient in Digest RC. Virtually unknown in the United States, radishes contain a variety of chemicals that increase the flow of digestive juices. The most important function of black radish extract is that it encourages the liver to produce fat- and protein-digesting bile and lowers the tension of the bile ducts. It also improves peristaltic movement. Constipation is one problem benefiting from radish consumption. Rich in fiber and digestive stimulants, regular consumption of radishes helps regulate the bowels. Because dehydration is a major cause of constipation, radishes help hydrate and lubricate the intestines and encourage relaxed bowel movements. The root juice extract of the black radish used in Digest RC is the most potent part of the plant.

A bonus is the ability of the radish to assist the immune system because it contains a variety of chemicals that possess natural antimicrobial actions (Terras et al. 1992). Regular consumption of radishes may lead to a significant improvement in resistance against common microbial infections such as colds, sore throats, ear infections, and the flu. A French study in which liquid radish extract was administered to mice before they were inoculated with influenza virus demonstrated protection against the influenza infection. There was a significant decrease in the mortality rate and a significant increase in the rate of survival as compared to the untreated controls (Esanu et al. 1985).

A second constituent of Digest RC is artichoke, which acts directly on the liver, further increasing production of bile and causing it to flow through bile ducts. It is used in cases of low food tolerance, troubled digestion, and assimilation.

Peppermint, another ingredient of Digest RC, helps relax gastrointestinal smooth muscle (Hills et al. 1991).

The charcoal in Digest RC is particularly useful in absorbing toxins. Charcoal is commonly used for gastrointestinal decontamination by a majority of North American poison control centers (Juurlink et al. 2000). It also calms a stressed digestive system, allowing digestive enzymes to be produced and released. Indigestion and nervous vomiting are also treated with this ingredient. The charcoal in Digest RC is actually a special herbal preparation of linden tree bark, traditionally used in Europe as a digestive aid. This special preparation has antibacterial properties, which when used as directed helps balance the digestive tract and support the creation of the proper intestinal flora. At the same time, it creates an inhospitable environment for parasitic infestation.

Another key ingredient in Digest RC is cholic acid (or pure processed ox bile), a liver enzyme used for digestion. Cholic acid is particularly helpful in digesting fats and meat protein.

Independent clinical research was conducted on Digest RC to analyze the therapeutic effectiveness of the product among patients with chronic digestive problems. Results showed statistically significant improvement in patients' symptoms during treatment. Digest RC was most successful in eliminating the most frequently occurring symptoms such as gas in over 95% of the cases. Symptoms such as constipation, intestinal pains and cramps, heartburn (reflux), and stomach pains and cramps were helped or completely eliminated in over 90% of the cases. Bloating ceased in over 80%, diarrhea in about 75%, and nausea and vomiting in approximately 65% of the cases.

Digest RC was found to minimize the assimilation of undigested toxic products which often stay in the gut for a prolonged period of time. Due to its bile-stimulating abilities, Digest RC was particularly effective in preventing stasis of food and bloating in those patients whose diet was rich in animal protein and fat. Because there are no specific contraindications, Digest RC can be taken together with any medication and can be taken by patients who have various respiratory, cardiovascular, and musculoskeletal disorders. The only people who should avoid Digest RC are those with biliary tract obstruction or gall bladder disease because of the bile-stimulating effects of the black radish and artichoke extracts. It is not known how this product would affect persons who have had their gall bladder removed.

Suggested dosage: Take 2–3 tablets of Digest RC with every heavy meal for the first 2–3 weeks. The dose may then be reduced as symptoms of digestion discomfort are alleviated (Anon. 1999).

ADDITIONAL SUGGESTIONS

As previously discussed, fiber supplements frequently fail to correct chronic constipation. However, one fiber that may work when all others fail is chitosan. Chitosan is a fiber composed of chitin, which is a component of the shell of shellfish that is used for weight and cholesterol reduction. Chitosan has unique properties in its ability to bind fat from food in the stomach and the intestines. When fat content in the bowel increases, it makes the feces soft and smooth (Rossner et al. 1995). If you do not obtain results from other commonly used fiber sources, six 500-mg capsules of chitosan along with 1000 mg of vitamin C before each meal may help alleviate constipation. Ascorbic acid (vitamin C) helps activate chitosan in the stomach and intestine into a fat-absorbing gel. When ascorbic acid was given with chitosan to rats, far more fat was trapped and excreted in the feces than when chitosan was given without ascorbic acid (Kanauchi et al. 1995).

Constipation is a common childhood condition, estimated to occur in 5–10% of children. In most cases, the cause is functional. However, constipation may occasionally indicate a significant organic disorder which can usually be determined by a thorough history and physical examination. Constipation that is present from birth or that begins in the neonatal period is most likely to be congenital in origin. Acute constipation usually has an *organic* cause, although chronic constipation usually has a *functional* cause.

A trial on functional constipation in children showed that most children with fecal incontinence benefit from a strict treatment plan that includes defecation trials, a fiber-rich diet, and laxative medications. Surgery followed by medical treatment was required in patients with Hirschsprung's disease (congenital colon defect) and in some patients with anal stenosis (Loening-Baucke 1997).

Chronic constipation at any age can be a disabling condition that may require removal of part of the colon (colostomy). However, one study showed fiber, cathartic laxatives, or biofeedback therapy to be successful in 65% of patients. Among the remaining patients, two-thirds underwent surgery, of which 83% was successful (Rantis et al. 1997).

Laxative use was significantly reduced in a long-term care facility when an interdisciplinary program was implemented based on a philosophy of prevention and health promotion. Specifically, increased fluid and fiber intake, timely toileting habits, and regular activity or exercise led to a 50% reduction in the number of patients receiving laxatives that were required relative to pre-program levels and in a control unit not receiving the program (Benton et al. 1997).

Constipation is a problem frequently encountered during pregnancy, as is excessive weight gain. Treatment commonly used to control constipation has some drawbacks and often does not help control weight. However, a preparation of lactulose and glucomannan was shown to be effective and well tolerated in pregnant women with constipation and was also shown to be effective in controlling excessive food intake. Fifty pregnant females with constipation were treated with a preparation of glucomannan (3–6 grams) and lactulose (8–16 grams) twice a day for 1–3 months. This preparation resulted in a return to normal frequency of weekly number of evacuations and a parallel control of weight gain (Signorelli et al. 1996).

DRUG THERAPIES

For many persons with chronic constipation that does not improve with fiber or laxatives, a new drug called prucalopride has been shown to help relieve chronic constipation. Prucalopride is a novel, selective, and specific serotonin receptor agonist (5-HT4) that belongs to a new class of medications known as the benzofurancarboxamides. The latest studies report that prucalopride may increase the frequency of bowel movements and improve colonic transit (the time it takes for food to move through the colon), both of which are key factors in the effective treatment of chronic constipation (Slootes et al. 2002). One study involving 10 healthy subjects found when taking prucalopride, stool frequency increased, consistency decreased, and subjects strained less (De Schryver et al. 2002). In all studies, prucalopride was safe and well tolerated.

SOME CONVENTIONAL THERAPIES

Physicians often recommend fiber supplements (bulk producers) to prevent constipation. They also recommend eating more fresh fruits and vegetables, either cooked or raw, and more whole grain cereals and breads. Dried fruit such as apricots, prunes, and figs are especially high in fiber. Some physicians suggest adding small amounts of unprocessed bran ("miller's bran") to baked goods, cereals, and fruit. However, some persons experience bloating and gas for several weeks after adding bran to their diets. Gradually adding bran to the diet is advised to allow the digestive system to adapt. Remember, if your diet is well balanced and contains a variety of foods high in natural fiber, it may not be necessary to add bran to other foods.

Therapies may include:

- **Bulk producers,** such as psyllium, are natural or semisynthetic polysaccharides and cellulose, which hold water, soften the stool, and increase the occurrence of the passage of a stool. They are the most physiologic of the laxatives. Bulk producers are generally recommended for managing irritable bowel syndrome. Results occur within 12–24 hours (may be delayed up to 72 hours).

- **Saline laxatives** are in the hyperosmotic family, meaning their mode of action is to attract water into the lumen of the intestines. The fluid buildup alters the stool consistency, expands the bowel, and encourages peristaltic movement. They are used mostly as a bowel preparation to clear the bowels for rectal or bowel examinations and are not recommended for long-term use. Results occur rapidly (within 0.5–3 hours). Examples include magnesium citrate and magnesium oxide.

- **Stimulant laxatives,** such as sennacides, increase motor activity of the bowels by direct action on the intestines. They are used to evacuate the bowel for rectal or bowel examinations. Most of these laxatives act on the colon; castor oil acts on the small intestine. Results occur in 6–10 hours.

- **Lubricant laxatives,** such as mineral oil, lubricate intestinal mucosa and soften stools. They are used prophylactically to prevent straining in patients for whom it would be dangerous to strain. Generally, mineral oil is recommended at 5–30 mL at bedtime. Results vary. Chronic mineral oil ingestion can result in malabsorption of fat-soluble vitamins and minerals and is not recommended for continuous treatment.

- **Fecal softeners** or emollients (Docusate) promote water retention in the fecal mass, thus softening the stool. They are generally used to prevent straining and are most beneficial when the stool is hard. However, it may require 3 days before results are experienced. Stool softeners and emollient laxatives have limited use because of their resorption of water from the forming stool. Fecal softeners should not be used exclusively but may be useful when given in combination with stimulant laxatives.

- **Lactulose** is an undigestible sugar that is broken down into acids in the colon. Lactulose is used to clear the bowel with minimal water and sodium loss or gain. When it is broken down in the colon, lactulose produces lactic acid, formic acid, acetic acid, and carbon dioxide. These products increase the amount of water in the stool which softens the stool and increases the frequency. Results generally occur in 24–48 hours. The metabolism of lactulose requires the presence of "friendly bacteria" known as *Lactobacillus acidophilus*. The consumption of *Lactobacillus acidophilus* together with lactulose will help to normalize intestinal friendly bacteria content and will eliminate pathogenic bacteria such as *Clostridium*, which are frequently present in the normal bowel. Lactulose is available only by prescription.

- **Golytely** (Colyte) is an electrolyte solution available by prescription and used to clear the bowel with minimal water and sodium loss or gain. It is typically prescribed before a colonoscopy.

☻ SUMMARY

Constipation is a universal affliction of Western civilization. In the United States, Americans spend more than $725 million annually on over-the-counter laxatives in an attempt to self-treat constipation, which is the most common gastrointestinal complaint. There are alternative therapies that are safer and more effective than conventional laxatives and they work better for more people than fiber supplements.

For the most part, chronic constipation is amenable to changes in lifestyle. Begin by increasing exercise or general activity during the day. This can be as little as 20 minutes of walking briskly on a regular basis. Remove as many processed foods as possible from your diet and replace them with fiber-rich foods such as fruits, vegetables, and whole-grain cereals. The addition of 1 tbsp of wheat bran, ground flaxseed, or oat bran to your diet will speed up the process. In most cases, over days or perhaps weeks, your bowels will begin to move more frequently and more easily as a result of these changes. If these changes do not produce the desired effect, and you have ruled out the possibility of underlying disease with your health-care provider, then the suggestions below may be helpful.

For relieving *acute* constipation, one of the following techniques may be tried to induce peristaltic action within 45–60 minutes:

1. Mix 4000–8000 mg of ascorbic acid powder with 1500 mg of magnesium oxide powder and take with the juice of a freshly squeezed grapefruit or orange (best taken on an empty stomach).

2. Mix 1–6 tsp of a "buffered vitamin C powder" that contains magnesium and potassium salts along with ascorbic acid (vitamin C) and take on an empty stomach using room-temperature water.

3. Mix 1–2 tbsp of Power Maker II Sugar-Free Powder in water or juice and take on an empty stomach.

4. Take 2000–3000 mg of pantothenic acid (vitamin B₅) powder on an empty stomach. Pantothenic acid powder is unpalatable.

Note: *Drinking several cups of green tea will enhance the bowel-evacuating effects of the previous four suggestions. Decaffeinated green tea may be taken late in the day to prevent insomnia. Persons with gastritis or stomach ulcers may not be able to tolerate these aggressive peristalsis-inducing approaches.*

For relieving *chronic* constipation, one or all of the following may be used:

1. Chitosan: Take six 1000-mg capsules of chitosan before each meal with one 1000-mg capsule of vitamin C.

2. Digest RC: For 3 weeks, take 2–3 tablets with every meal that contains fat or protein. Dosage may be reduced after symptomatic relief occurs.

3. Fiber Food is a bulk-producing soluble fiber that provides a blend of guar gum, apple and/ or citrus pectin, and psyllium seed husk. Six capsules or 1 tsp should be taken with each meal; 1–2 tbsp of flaxseed may also be helpful. Flaxseed can be sprinkled on cereal at breakfast time. The flaxseed should be purchased fresh and should be ground in a coffee grinder daily. The omega-3 oils present in flaxseed offer an additional benefit.

4. Castor oil: 3 tbsp mixed with a liquid.

5. Follow the dietary and lifestyle changes discussed in this protocol.

Refer to the *Digestive Disorders protocol* for additional information.

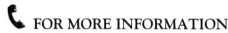 **FOR MORE INFORMATION**

Contact the Consumer Nutrition Hotline of the National Center for Nutrition and Dietetics, (800) 366-1655.

 PRODUCT AVAILABILITY

Ascorbic acid powder, magnesium oxide powder, buffered vitamin C, vitamin B₅ powder, Power Maker II Sugar-Free Powder, chitosan capsules, Digest RC, Fiber Food, and green tea leaves (regular and decaf) are available by calling (800) 544-4440 or by ordering online at www.lef.org.

Crohn's Disease

Crohn's disease is a long-term, chronic disorder of the intestine. The etiology (underlying cause) is unknown. In persons who have Crohn's disease, the gastrointestinal tract becomes inflamed and weak, making digestion difficult and leading to general physical debility. It is a relatively rare disease, occurring in approximately 1–5 people in every 10,000. Clustering of Crohn's disease has been shown in families. In the United States, the annual incidence of the disease is about two out of 100,000 persons, with a slight predominance among females. The incidence of Crohn's disease appears to be increasing in the Western world, leading one to suspect lifestyle factors as a promoter or cause. Crohn's disease is more common among Jews of middle European origin than among non-Jews, and it develops in twins and siblings at a much higher rate than would be predicted by chance.

The symptoms of Crohn's disease are similar to ulcerative colitis, and both conditions are categorized as inflammatory bowel diseases. To distinguish between them, your physician may need to examine a sample of intestinal tissue. As noted earlier, although the etiology of Crohn's disease is obscure, it is thought that certain antigens may activate immune cells in the intestinal wall. These immune cells then secrete proinflammatory agents (cytokines), such as tumor necrosis factor-alpha (TNF-alpha), interleukin-6 (IL-6), and interleukin-1b (IL1b), that can further aggravate the inflammatory cascade. The result is thinning of the bowel wall (McDermott 1990). Since a large percentage of immune cells reside in the gastrointestinal tract, activation of these cells at this level is almost certain to cause gastrointestinal symptoms.

Crohn's disease can attack any part of the digestive system from the mouth to the anus, but it most commonly affects the ileum (lower portion of the small intestine) or the colon (large intestine). Ulcers form on the inner intestinal lining, and they eventually spread through the intestinal wall. As the affected part of the intestine becomes scarred and thick, the passage narrows, disrupting nutrient absorption and normal bowel function.

SYMPTOMS AND DIAGNOSIS

Crohn's disease is typically diagnosed among people in their 20s and 30s, but the disease also occurs in infants and children. More common in women than in men, Crohn's disease is rare in persons of Asian or African descent who live outside the United States. The disease is a lifelong ailment that can be controlled, but at present there is no cure or even a definitive cause. Crohn's disease patients usually experience excruciatingly painful attacks of abdominal pain and diarrhea followed by weeks, months, or even years of remission.

Development of abscesses or fistulas, or tubes that form a connection between two organs and allow the passage of fluid and stool, is a common complication of Crohn's disease. These connections can happen between the intestinal loops, the intestines, and the bladder or between the intestines and the skin. They often occur near the anus. Surgery may be required to close fistulas. Some Crohn's disease patients also have a tendency to manifest nonintestinal disorders, such as inflammation of the eyes; skin eruptions or rashes; kidney stones; or arthritis of the knees, ankles, and wrists. People who have had Crohn's disease for 10 years or more are at risk of developing colorectal cancer. Therefore, if you have Crohn's disease and are over age 30, you should have regular checkups, including screening for colorectal cancer.

The following are the most prevalent symptoms of Crohn's disease:

- Severe abdominal pain and diarrhea that is occasionally mixed with blood (Unlike ulcerative colitis, in which patients may have episodes of diarrhea as often as 10–15 times a day, people with Crohn's may have fewer episodes, although each episode may be extraordinarily painful. However, as with many other elements of the disease, it is difficult to make sweeping generalizations.)

- Cramps or pain after eating, especially in the lower right side of the abdomen

- Chronic low-grade fever, loss of appetite, fatigue or weight loss, especially if accompanied by persistent nausea and vomiting

- Arthritis flare-ups in the arms or legs with the above symptoms

- In young children, any of the symptoms above, plus failure to thrive; in older children, failure to grow at a normal rate

- Anemia

Although the actual cause of Crohn's disease is unknown, it may be an autoimmune disorder. Inflammation apparently occurs when the body's own immune system—for reasons not yet understood—attacks a part of the intestine.

In a published article in the June 2000 issue of *Digestive Diseases and Sciences*, the authors suggest the possibility that various degrees of function and types of neutrophil impairment may manifest into specific genetic syndromes. This proposed theory differs from the current suggested course of the disease, in which genetic syndromes are believed to be responsible for progression of Crohn's into a disease state (Korzenik and Dieckorgraepe 2000). However, researchers and physicians concur that Crohn's disease is an immune response that causes inflammation. It is the suppression of inflammation that can decrease the injurious effects that the immune system inflicts on the Crohn's patient. However, according to the study researchers, it is those critical early events that may initiate Crohn's disease.

Furthermore, the researchers cite recent data that implicate bone marrow as playing a key role in the genesis of Crohn's disease and that instead of Crohn's disease being considered a disease of primary intestinal dysfunction, it may be a consequence of an interaction between bone marrow constituents and intestinal factors. Interestingly, a diverse number of syndromes in which intestinal manifestations are almost indistinguishable from Crohn's disease all share a unifying feature. Each has a distinct deficiency in quantitative or qualitative neutrophil function, providing strong evidence that a functional neutrophil deficiency can result in a common intestinal phenotype of Crohn's disease (Korzenik and Dieckorgraepe 2000).

While the progression from neutrophil dysfunction to the generation of Crohn's disease is speculative, Korzenik and Dieckorgraepe conclude that a common pathway has been observed in neutrophil disorders associated with Crohn's disease. Neutrophils function as a first-time defense when microbes invade the mucosal lining of the intestine. Normally, neutrophils would mediate the rapid clearance of mucosal microbes. However, if the neutrophils are dysfunctional, monocytes-macrophages are recruited and activated, in turn triggering lymphocyte activation of the T cells. Neutrophils and macrophages produce pro-inflammatory cytokines, including tumor-necrosis factor alpha (TNF-a), which contributes to an immune response resulting in inflammation. The scientists point out that current therapy referred to as anti-tumor-necrosis factor therapy has been successful but does not address the underlying etiology of the disease.

The authors indicate that the impairment of neutrophil function may result from a combination of genetic and environmental influences. Smoking, NSAID use, and specific microbial flora are some of the environmental influences that can potentiate neutrophil dysfunction. While this report has promising implications, further research is required. The drug Leukine, which helps correct impaired neutrophil function, is described later in this protocol.

There has been other research indicating the possibility of viral factors causing or contributing to Crohn's disease. Some scientists are exploring this theory. However, no specific viral agent has been identified.

Crohn's disease can usually be diagnosed by a variety of methods. In some cases, it is difficult to distinguish Crohn's disease from ulcerative colitis; therefore physicians may employ more than one diagnostic method. Common diagnostic tools include:

- X-rays of the large and small intestines
- Sigmoidoscopy
- Colonoscopy, usually including tissue biopsy
- Barium enema

Once Crohn's disease is diagnosed, routine blood tests for liver function and iron levels, as well as other blood tests, may be ordered, depending on the treatment being considered, to ensure that other existing health conditions do not interfere with the healing process.

The American Society of Gastroenterologists has provided the following guidelines for gauging the severity of Crohn's disease:

- Mild-moderate Crohn's disease applies to ambulatory patients who are able to tolerate food by mouth without manifestations of dehydration, toxicity (high fevers, rigors, prostration), abdominal tenderness, painful mass, obstruction, or >10% weight loss.
- Moderate-severe disease applies to patients who have failed to respond to treatment for mild-moderate disease or those with more prominent symptoms of fevers, significant weight loss, abdominal pain or tenderness, intermittent nausea or vomiting (without obstructive findings), or significant anemia.
- Severe-fulminant disease applies to patients with persisting symptoms despite the introduction of outpatient steroids or individuals who present with high fever, persistent vomiting, evidence of intestinal obstruction, rebound tenderness, cachexia, or evidence of an abscess.

- Remission refers to patients who are asymptomatic or without inflammatory sequelae and includes patients who have responded to acute medical intervention or have undergone surgical resection without gross evidence of residual disease. Patients requiring steroids to maintain their well-being are considered to be "steroid-dependent" and are usually not considered to be "in remission" (Hanauer et al. 2001).

CONVENTIONAL TREATMENTS

As noted earlier, Crohn's disease is not curable at this time. Depending on severity of the symptoms, medical treatment typically involves a three-pronged approach to controlling the disease: First, drug therapy and a restricted diet are explored; then if necessary, hospital treatment is initiated; the last resort is surgery.

Because there is no cure for Crohn's disease, patients and their physicians try to take steps to avoid recurring attacks for as long as possible. In cases of active disease, if that is not possible, achieving remission is pursued as quickly as possible. Some patients remain on maintenance medications even when there are no symptoms present. Children with Crohn's disease may require high-protein, high-calorie liquid supplements to keep their growth on track because the disease is particularly devastating in children.

Aminosalicylates, such as sulfasalazine, mesalamine, Asacol, Pentasa, and Rowasa, are intestinal anti-inflammatory agents that are the cornerstone of conventional medical treatment. These drugs may be prescribed for many years without interruption and are given in varying dosages depending on the severity of the symptoms.

Aminosalicylates are given orally or as a rectal suppository. They interrupt colonic inflammation. Without inflammation, the symptoms of diarrhea, bleeding, and abdominal pain are greatly diminished. However, many people find that they are allergic to aminosalicylates, which is sometimes manifested by vomiting and headaches or with even more severe symptoms. When a patient starts taking aminosalicylates, if new symptoms occur, particularly of this type, it is important to contact the prescribing physician immediately and advise him of all symptoms.

In cases of active Crohn's disease, steroids such as prednisone are commonly prescribed alone or with aminosalicylates to reduce inflammation of the intestines. Use of steroids can be problematic because of the potential for difficulties associated with the severe side effects of steroids. Side effects of steroids can include:

- Cushing's syndrome
- Muscle disorders
- Hair loss
- Weight gain
- Suppressed immune system and the accompanying risks
- Osteoporosis
- Hypertension
- Hormone imbalance

Even with the associated risks, steroids such as prednisone are often used during the acute stage to help get the symptoms under control. Prednisone mimics the effects of the body's natural corticosteroid hormones by suppressing the release of inflammatory cytokines. Once under control, aminosalicylates are taken for maintenance therapy. Tapering off the use of steroids represents a critical time during disease treatment. Many patients find themselves precariously trying to remain in remission while also weaning themselves from steroids.

To reduce the need for steroids, immunosuppressants such as azathioprine, 6-mercaptopurine (also used in the treatment of some cancers), or cyclosporine may be substituted. Various chemotherapy agents and organ transplant antirejection drugs are also used. Again, these medications have their own problematic or dangerous side effects. Therefore, thoughtful consideration of a treatment plan coordinated by the patient's physician is required. All aspects of the treatment plan must be effectively communicated to the patient. Antidiarrheal agents may be taken for mild bouts of diarrhea, as well as antispasmodics for cramping. When patients have arthritis-like symptoms, antiarthritis medications may also be taken. In cases of severe disease, patients often require a bland, well-balanced diet.

Reducing Levels of Pro-Inflammatory TNF-alpha

First introduced in 1995, a new treatment with a monoclonal antibody known as Infliximab (Enbrel) was used with success when other conventional treatments had failed (van Dullemen et al. 1995; Mortimore et al. 2001). Infliximab functions by reducing intestinal inflammation caused by TNF-alpha and destroying TNF-alpha producing cells. This treatment has been extremely effective in patients who have been resistant to other forms of treatment, even steroids. It can create remission in up to 80% of those in whom it is used. Improvement at 4 weeks was observed in more than 80% of patients treated with 5 mg/kg, and more than 50% achieved a clinical remission (Feagan et al. 2001). Fistulas also healed quickly. After treatment with Infliximab, compared to baseline, patients with Crohn's disease have decreased levels of serum IL-6 (an inflammatory immune factor) and C-reactive protein (Agnholt et al. 2001). Elevated concentrations of TNF-alpha have been found in the stools of Crohn's disease patients, correlating with elevated disease activity. Treatment with Infliximab reduces infiltration of inflammatory cells and the production of TNF-alpha in inflamed areas of the intestine.

Retreatment with Infliximab is likely to be necessary on an ongoing basis to prevent relapse. The long-term side effects are unknown. In addition, initially there can be severe side effects, including transfusion-type reactions, because Infliximab is an antibody that is being introduced into the patient intravenously. Infliximab infusions have been associated with both acute and delayed infusion reactions, including delayed hypersensitivity (serum sickness-like) reactions, particularly after prolonged intervals (>12 weeks) subsequent to an initial treatment. The use of this drug requires long-term planning due to the presumed requirement for repeated infusions over time (Lugering et al. 2001; Martorana et al. 2001; Miller et al. 2001; Mortimore et al. 2001; Sandborn et al. 2001; Hove et al. 2002).

Granulocyte-Macrophage Colony-Stimulating Factor

As stated previously, treatment for Crohn's disease is aimed at immunosuppression. Yet, as Dieckgraefe and Korzenik point out in *Lancet* (2002), inherited disorders associated with defective innate immunity often lead to the development of Crohn's-like disease. Based upon this theory, the researchers performed an open-label dose-escalation trial (4–8 mcg/kg/day) to investigate the safety and possible benefit of granulocyte-macrophage colony–stimulating factor (GM-CSF) on 15 patients with moderate to severe Crohn's disease (Dieckgraefe and Korzenik 2002).

The results were promising. None of the patients was found to have any worsening of the disease while under treatment, and adverse events were negligible. Further, the researchers reported that patients had a significant decrease in mean Crohn's disease activity index (CDAI) score during treatment. After 8 weeks of treatment, mean CDAI had fallen by 190 points, and overall 12 patients had a decrease in CDAI of more than 100 points, while 8 patients achieved clinical remission. Retreatment was effective, and

overall the treatment was associated with increased quality-of-life measures (Dieckgraefe and Korzenik 2002).

While GM-CSF may offer an alternative to the traditional immunosuppression treatment of Crohn's disease, it is important to note that the authors conclude that their findings warrant further validation. They cite the small study size, the very subjective self-report format, and the fact that it was an uncontrolled study as the reasons for ongoing follow-up studies to be performed. GM-CSF is sold under the trade name Leukine and is typically used to restore immune function in cancer patients who have undergone bone marrow–depleting chemotherapy.

Total Parenteral Nutrition

If a patient becomes severely ill and has diarrhea and weight loss, intravenous (IV) nutrition administered in a hospital setting can allow the intestines to have a "resting" period. Total parenteral nutrition (TPN) is also used to rest the intestinal tract. Usually TPN nutrition is administered via a tube directly into the bloodstream by an infusion system. After stabilization, some patients may require continuation of IV nutrition at home with the aid of a visiting nurse service.

Surgery

If Crohn's disease does not respond to treatment with drugs and diet, surgery may be recommended. Because Crohn's disease can affect the entire digestive tract from the mouth to the anus, surgery is directed at removing only the severely inflamed part of the intestine. The goal of surgery is to preserve as much of the intestine as possible. Surgery commonly involves the colon or small intestine. Occasionally, the end of the intestine that has been left in place will need to be brought to the skin's surface. When this procedure involves the small intestine, it is called an ileostomy. If the procedure involves the colon, it is called a colostomy. Although Crohn's disease may recur after surgery, the symptoms are likely to be less severe and less debilitating than they were previously. However, when the disease does recur, it usually does so at the site of the last surgery.

Growth Hormone Research

A study published in the *New England Journal of Medicine* suggested that administering growth hormone (GH) to patients with Crohn's disease may help to resolve many of their associated symptoms (Slonim et al. 2000). In a 4-month study, 19 adults with moderate to severe Crohn's disease were put on a regimen of daily self-injections of GH (5 mg a day for the first week, then

1.5 mg a day). Headaches and edema were reported by 10 and 5 patients, respectively; however, these symptoms dissipated within 2–3 weeks. Marked improvement in symptoms within the first month of self-administered treatment with increasing benefits over the next 3 months was seen. Specifically, the GH group showed significant improvement in three areas of disease activity by the end of the study, which included the number of liquid or very soft stools a day, severity of abdominal pain, and increased feeling of well-being. In addition, half of the patients in the GH group who were on other medications were able to reduce their dosages. The researchers also noted that supplemental protein intake was further enhanced in the intestinal tract when growth hormone was administered (Slonim et al. 2000).

NUTRITION, DIET, AND VITAMIN SUPPLEMENTATION

Because most medications for Crohn's disease have an abundance of side effects, many patients understandably focus on nutrition and diet as a means of staving off active disease or helping to induce remission. There is substantial evidence that intolerance to certain foods and other nutritional factors play a large role in the practical management of Crohn's disease through nutritional modification. Early studies have shown that Crohn's patients tend to consume high amounts of simple sugars, either at the time of diagnosis or following it (Mayberry et al. 1981; Jarnerot et al. 1983; Persson et al. 1992). The propensity to consume simple carbohydrates, which often continues in the main phase of the disease, indicates that many Crohn's patients have not been counseled correctly to reduce their consumption of refined carbohydrates (Kruis et al. 1987).

Indeed, early research also suggested that consumption of highly refined foods may be involved in the etiology itself (Grimes 1976). In another early study, 80% of patients who were on a low carbohydrate diet that excluded all refined sugar had significant symptom relief within 18 months, whereas 40% of patients on a high carbohydrate diet that was high in refined sugar had to discontinue the diet because of flare-ups (Brandes et al. 1981).

Nutritional management of Crohn's disease has the potential for a larger, more beneficial role than methods that primarily use anti-inflammatories and steroids as a first line of treatment. As early as 1990, there were studies reporting that the use of an elemental diet can induce a remission equal to, if not better than, prednisone (Giaffer et al. 1990; O'Keefe 1996). An elemental diet contains the essential elements of good nutrition, usually in a liquid form and usually with hypoallergenic protein contents. In patients who were already taking prednisone, the drug could be reduced or eliminated in 50% or more of patients who followed an elemental diet (Verma et al. 2001). In addition, while on an elemental diet, inflammatory parameters and intestinal permeability tended to decrease (Teahon et al. 1991).

Because many Crohn's patients are often nutritionally deprived at diagnosis, using nutrition to induce remission in confirmed Crohn's disease provides an opportunity for the patient to become nutritionally replete, possibly for the first time in many years. Unfortunately, the elemental diets used by conventional practitioners are often unpalatable. However, detoxification programs do exist in the armamentarium of nutritional physicians that are quite palatable and can introduce concentrated vitamins and minerals needed by the patient for recovery. Nutritional biochemist and researcher Dr. Jeffery Bland has popularized the notion of the 4-R program for managing intestinal disorders of this nature. The R's stand for (1) remove, (2) replace, (3) reinoculate, and (4) repair (Liska et al. 2001).

The protocol would proceed as follows:

1. **Remove** Remove all suspicious foods from the patient's diet that precipitate inflammation. The following have been found to be the most likely to be troublesome: dairy, eggs, nuts, fruit, tomatoes, corn, wheat or gluten, and red meat. All refined carbohydrates should be removed. Also, all fats except for essential fatty acids should be eliminated because hard or trans fats, in particular, have been found to be detrimental for persons with Crohn's disease (Heckers et al. 1988; Lorenz-Meyer et al. 1996). Products such as Vivonex, UltraMaintain, or UltraClear can be used at the outset. UltraClear is preferable because it contains sufficient fiber to maintain regular evacuation of the bowel. Additionally, removal of gastrointestinal parasites, undesirable bacteria, or fungal elements that may be present and contribute to symptoms is important. Removal of yeast overgrowth by using an antifungal drug (e.g., oral nystatin) may also be required.

2. **Replace** By the time Crohn's disease is diagnosed, most patients are already in nutritional imbalance. Replacement of vital nutrients may consist of a good multivitamin and mineral complex, together with minerals that have been found to be lacking. Minerals often lacking are iron, magnesium, selenium, and zinc. Vitamins found to be most lacking

are the B-complex vitamins, including folic acid, vitamin B_6, and particularly vitamin B_{12}, which is absorbed from the end portion of the small intestine. A German study in 1998 examined deficiencies of vitamins and trace elements in patients with inflammatory bowel disease. The records from 392 outpatients, 279 with Crohn's disease and 113 with ulcerative colitis, were analyzed. Deficiencies were found in 85% of patients with Crohn's disease, predominantly deficiencies of iron and calcium. Less frequently, deficiencies of zinc, protein, cyanocobalamin (B_{12}), and folic acid were found (Rath et al. 1998).

Note: *Long-term use of steroids warrants the inclusion of supplemental calcium and vitamin D to prevent the risk of osteoporosis (Hoffmann 2002). Patients with Crohn's disease usually have a moderate anemia that is often caused by several factors: iron deficiency; vitamin B_{12} deficiency related to extensive disease of the terminal ileum; folate deficiency produced by anorexia and the consequent poor intake of dietary folic acid; or by inhibition of folate absorption by sulfasalazine, one of the common drugs used to reduce inflammation. Other nutritional factors may need to be added at a later time. See* **Repair.**

3. **Reinoculate** A normal healthy intestine contains about 5–7 lbs of "friendly bacteria" that are responsible for manufacturing some vitamins and gut cell food. In a diseased intestine, these bacteria are out of balance and are often absent, having been replaced by pathogenic organisms, including yeast overgrowth. Reinoculation consists of taking mixtures of *Lactobacillus acidophilus* and *Lactobacillus bulgaricus* with fructose oligosaccharides (FOS). *L. bulgaricus* is found in Jerusalem artichoke and other vegetables. It is a substrate or food for the *Lactobacillus* species. Stool samples provide clinicians with information regarding these overgrowth factors, pH of the stool, and the balance of fatty acids required for health.

4. **Repair** Frequently in Crohn's disease it is found that the lining of the small intestine has become permeable. The once-protective layer now permits antigens and other incomplete digestive products to pass through the bowel wall. Repair of the protective layer consists of adding nutrients such as glutamine, pantothenic acid (vitamin B_5), zinc, fructose oligosaccharides, and vitamin C to build up the integrity of the intestinal wall itself. This can be done with oligo-antigenic products such as UltraSustain. Measuring intestinal permeability can indicate if a patient's GI function has recovered or if it continues to cause functional abnormalities in the rest of the body through the gastrointestinal lymphoid-associated tissue (GALT), where it increases release of proinflammatory mediators.

At least one study reported that patients who did not have restoration of their small bowel mucosal integrity at discharge from the hospital (i.e., those who still had a "leaky gut" when they left the hospital) had a very high probability of relapse (76–81%) within 1 year. Crohn's disease patients with normal gut mucosal integrity and healing of the gut at release from the hospital had a less than 5% probability of relapse within 1 year. Relapse rate depended greatly on the patients' GI mucosal integrity (evaluated by lactulose/mannitol challenge) on discharge (Wyatt et al. 1993).

Specific Nutritional Components

Significant research has focused on specific nutrients such as essential fats and antioxidants. Humans evolved by consuming a diet that contained about equal amounts of n-3 and n-6 (also known as omega-3 and omega-6) essential fatty acids (named by referring to the carbon double bond position). Omega-3 fatty acids are found in nuts (especially walnuts), seeds, and fish oil, whereas omega-6 is generally found in animal fats such as beef and poultry, as well as in some processed oils (e.g., corn, sunflower seed, safflower seed, cottonseed, and soybean).

Over the past 100–150 years, there has been an enormous increase in the consumption of n-6 fatty acids as a result of the increased intake of vegetable oils. In Western diets today, the ratio of n-6 to n-3 fatty acids ranges from approximately 20:1 to 30:1 instead of the traditional range of 1:1 to 2:1. It is thought that a high intake of n-6 fatty acids shifts the physiologic state to one that is primarily inflammatory by producing inflammatory hormone-like molecules known as prostaglandin E2 series. However, the downstream products of n-3 fatty acids, known as prostaglandin E1 and E3 series, have anti-inflammatory properties. The beneficial effects of n-3 fatty acids have been shown to have an additional benefit in the secondary prevention of coronary heart disease, hypertension, Type-II diabetes, and ulcerative colitis and Crohn's disease in some patients (Simopoulos 1999).

In an article entitled "Modulation of Intestinal Immune System by Dietary Fat Intake: Relevance to Crohn's Disease," Miura and colleagues stated: "Both the amount and type of dietary fat modulate intestinal immune function" (Miura et al. 1998).

DHEA Replacement Therapy

Youthful hormone balance is critical to maintaining health and preventing disease in men and women over the age of 40. One hormone that is deficient in almost everyone over 35 is DHEA (dehydroepiandrosterone), normally the most abundant steroid in the human body.

A wealth of data indicates that DHEA is a vitally important hormone. DHEA appears to protect every part of the body against the ravages of aging. In fact, published studies link low levels of DHEA to aging and diseased states. Specifically, a deficiency of DHEA has been found to correlate with:

- Chronic inflammation
- Immune dysfunction
- Depression
- Rheumatoid arthritis
- Type-II diabetic complications
- Greater risk for certain cancers
- Excess body fat
- Cognitive decline
- Heart disease in men
- Osteoporosis

In 1981, the Life Extension Foundation introduced DHEA in an article that described the multiple anti-aging effects this hormone might produce.

DHEA did not establish scientific credibility until 1996, when the *New York Academy of Sciences* published a book entitled *DHEA and Aging* and summarized the concept of DHEA replacement in their journal *Aging* (Bellino et al. 1995). These highly technical publications provided scientific validation for the many life extension effects of DHEA replacement therapy. Despite the findings from thousands of peer-reviewed studies, the benefits of DHEA are still not recognized by mainstream medicine. DHEA replacement therapy involves the supplementation of the hormone to restore serum levels to those of a 21-year-old. DHEA is a precursory building block that allows our bodies to more easily create hormones that may be in decline because of age, disease, prescription medications, or other factors. Hormones, such as testosterone and estrogen, as well as serum DHEA levels, begin to decline from 25–30 years of age and may be reduced by 95% of youthful peak levels by age 85.

DHEA SUPPRESSES INFLAMMATORY CYTOKINES

Chronic inflammation is an epidemic disease of aging. Advancing age results in an increase of inflammatory cytokines (destructive cell-signaling chemicals) that contribute to many degenerative diseases. Rheumatoid arthritis is a classic autoimmune disorder in which excess levels of cytokines, such as tumor necrosis factor-alpha (TNF-alpha), interleukin-6 (IL-6), interleukin 1(b) [IL-1(b)], and/or leukotriene B4 (LTB4), are known to cause or contribute to the inflammatory syndrome.

Studies have found that adrenal hormones, including DHEA, are of special importance in the treatment of rheumatoid arthritis (Cutolo 2000). There is some evidence pointing to adrenal hypofunction before the onset of rheumatoid arthritis, especially in female patients, who constitute the overwhelming majority of rheumatoid arthritis victims and whose serum DHEA levels are low (male rheumatoid arthritis patients show low plasma and synovial fluid testosterone). Androgens, in general, appear to be protective against the development of autoimmune diseases, and DHEA is an important precursor of various androgens. DHEA replacement appears to be especially important for female rheumatoid arthritis patients.

Chronic inflammation is also involved in diseases as diverse as atherosclerosis, cancer, heart valve dysfunction, diabetes, congestive heart failure, and Alzheimer's disease. In aged people with multiple degenerative diseases, C-reactive protein is often sharply elevated, indicating the presence of an underlying inflammatory disorder. Excess levels of one or more of the inflammatory cytokines [TNF-alpha, IL-6, IL-1 (b), LTB(4)] are usually found when a cytokine blood profile is conducted. DHEA has been shown to lower these proinflammatory cytokines and protect against their toxic effects (Kipper-Galperin et al. 1999; Haden et al. 2000).

Thus, DHEA plays an important role in preventing chronic inflammation and also provides signals needed to maintain healthy immune function.

Of special interest is DHEA's ability to inhibit interleukin 6 (IL-6) and tumor necrosis factor (TNF) (Straub et al. 1998; Kipper-Galperin et al. 1999). These proinflammatory cytokines rise with age and are especially high in patients with inflammatory diseases.

IL-6 is known to play a role in promoting bone loss and possibly also joint destruction (Ferraccioli et al. 1996; Haden et al. 2000). In addition, IL-6 promotes the production of certain immune cells, which attack the body's own tissue in autoimmune conditions, such as rheumatoid arthritis (Wellby et al. 2000). Besides rheumatoid arthritis, the conditions associated with abnormally high IL-6 include atherosclerosis, osteoporosis, Alzheimer's disease, and certain cancers.

The deficiency of DHEA in inflammatory diseases also implies a deficiency in peripheral tissue of various sex hormones for which DHEA serves as a precursor. These hormones, both estrogenic and androgenic, are known to have beneficial effects on muscle, bone, and blood vessels. The mainstream therapy with corticosteroids is itself known to lower androgen levels. Consequently, the researchers argue that hormone replacement for patients with chronic inflammatory diseases should include not only corticosteroids, but also DHEA (Straub et al. 2000) (see the Inflammation: Chronic protocol for additional supplement recommendations on controlling inflammation).

DHEA AS A VIRUS AND INFECTION FIGHTER

Some experts think that a state of inflammation is actually required for the activation of HIV (human immunodeficiency virus) and progression to full-blown AIDS (acquired immune deficiency syndrome). If DHEA has potent anti-inflammatory properties, then it should be of great interest to HIV-infected patients because high levels of DHEA might help prevent the activation of the virus. Even if based on only partial evidence, the advice that HIV patients should maintain DHEA levels as high as possible appears to be sound.

Indeed, it has been shown that DHEA and its synthetic analogs are able to produce partial inhibition of HIV replication. A study discovered that one particular analog of DHEA, IM28, had a somewhat higher activity against HIV replication than DHEA, but at a price: it was more toxic than DHEA (Diallo et al. 2000). The mechanism of DHEA's antiviral action is not fully understood, but its antioxidant properties and its impact on metabolic enzymes are probably part of the explanation.

Another important aspect involves the close relationship between DHEA, cortisol, and the types of cytokines produced (Christeff et al. 2000). As AIDS progresses, we see a deficiency of Type-I cytokines (including interferon gamma and interleukin-2) and an excess of Type-II cytokines,

including interleukin-6 (IL-6). This is accompanied by a rise in cortisol and a drop in DHEA levels. Effective therapy with protease inhibitors has been shown to increase DHEA levels.

In addition, DHEA's ability to help the body fight infection (Araghi-Niknam et al. 1998; Oberbeck et al. 2001) and infection-caused inflammation may be a part of its cardioprotective mechanism. Many holistic experts believe that infection is a significant causal factor in atherosclerosis because infection increases inflammation (Folsom et al. 2002; Futterman et al. 2002). Part of the cardioprotective role of DHEA may stem from its ability to thwart viruses by inhibiting free-radical generation and NF-kappa-B activation, thus reducing inflammation and viral replication (Straub et al. 2000; Du et al. 2001). Therefore, DHEA helps the body lower the pathogen load and use its resources to maintain healthy tissue, including a healthy cardiovascular system.

DHEA'S ANTIAGING PROPERTIES

DHEA has been shown to improve neurological function (including memory, mood enhancement, and EEG readings), immune surveillance, and stress disorders. DHEA replacement therapy has become popular as an antiaging therapy and offers aging patients help in preventing the ravages of advanced age.

The most remarkable finding about DHEA came from a human study by S.S.C. Yen and associates at the University of California (San Diego), in which 50 mg a day of DHEA over a 6-month period restored youthful serum levels of DHEA in both men and women. Dr. Yen showed that DHEA replacement was associated with an increase in perceived physical and psychological well-being for both men (67%) and women (84%). Increases in lean body mass and muscle strength were reported in men taking 100 mg a day, but this dose appeared to be excessive in women (Morales et al. 1994).

DHEA (50–100 mg a day) was also shown to significantly elevate insulin growth factor (IGF) (Morales et al. 1998). Aging causes a decline in IGF levels that contribute to the loss of lean body mass, as well as to excess fat accumulation, neurological impairment, and age-associated immune dysfunction.

DHEA has been shown to protect against heart disease and atherosclerosis. A study using coronary artery angiography showed that low DHEA levels predispose people to more significant coronary artery blockage

(Herrington 1995). Another study showed that DHEA inhibits abnormal blood platelet aggregation, a factor in the development of sudden heart attack and stroke (Jesse et al. 1995). In contrast, some studies on DHEA do not show the cardiovascular disease protection.

In the journal *Drugs and Aging*, an analysis of studies on DHEA showed that (Watson et al. 1996):

- In both humans and animals, the decline of DHEA production with aging is associated with immune depression, increased risk of several different cancers, loss of sleep, decreased feelings of well-being, and increased mortality.

- DHEA replacement in aged mice significantly improved immune function to a more youthful state.

- DHEA replacement has shown a favorable effect on osteoclasts and lymphoid cells, an effect that may delay osteoporosis. (*Note:* DHEA has been shown in other studies to promote the activity of bone-forming osteoblasts.)

- Low levels of DHEA inhibit energy metabolism, thus increasing the risk of heart disease and diabetes mellitus.

- Studies in humans show essentially no toxicity at doses that restore DHEA to youthful levels.

- DHEA deficiency may expedite the development of some diseases that are common in the elderly.

DHEA AND DEPRESSION

Depression is a broad term for a host of unpleasant symptoms, including emotional numbness, lack of energy, little motivation, feeling like one is a failure, and feelings of being undesirable. These feelings frequently show up for the first time in middle-aged people who feel like they are "over the hill." Elderly people also frequently become depressed and are particularly at risk of suicide. Depression is a growing problem among teenagers as well.

Physicians have long known that giving estrogen to women and testosterone to men during midlife can avert symptoms of depression, although the effects have never been phenomenal. Reports are stacking up that DHEA works better. DHEA turns into both estrogen and testosterone. (And it just so happens that DHEA decreases about the time people start thinking about being "over the hill.")

DHEA is especially abundant in the human brain. Not only does the brain utilize DHEA, but DHEA is manufactured by the brain. Although researchers do not know what it is supposed to do yet, they do know

that giving a person 500 mg of DHEA will cause them to have more REM (rapid eye movement or dream) sleep (Friess et al. 1995). This indicates a major role in brain chemistry.

DHEA is the only hormone besides cortisol that has consistently been linked with depression. DHEA was studied as far back as the 1950s as an antidepressant. At that time, researchers reported that it gave people energy and confidence and made them less depressed. Although it seemed to work well, no one followed up on the studies.

DHEA emerged on the scene again in the 1980s when interest in antiaging hormones geared up. It was noted then that antidepressant activity was part of DHEA's overall antiaging benefits. Then, in 1996, a report suggested that DHEA's antidepressant effects might be direct and not just a result of its antiaging benefits in older people. Researchers at Cambridge University discovered that young children with major depression have abnormally low levels of DHEA and abnormally high levels of cortisol (Goodyer et al. 1996).

In the late 1990s, this phenomenon was confirmed in a larger study. Researchers at the University of California at San Diego went back and analyzed old data from a large study that had been done on 699 older women living in Rancho Bernardo, CA. That analysis is the largest study ever done on the association between levels of DHEA and depression. Nine different hormones had been measured during the study that took place during the 1970s and 1980s. Included in the measurements were such things as bioavailable testosterone and sex hormone binding globulin. When the results were in, of all the hormones, only DHEA was associated with depression. Low testosterone levels have been correlated with depression in men (Barrett-Connor et al. 1999).

Women at the lowest end of DHEA were far more likely to be depressed. This coincides with an earlier study in which the percentage of women with depression was 21.7% if they had no detectable DHEA versus 4.6% if DHEA could be detected in their blood. Interestingly, levels of DHEA in the Rancho Study correlate with mood even within the normal range. In other words, the lower the DHEA was, the worse the mood was. And DHEA correlated with mood, irrespective of whether a person was taking antidepressants or not.

A group at the University of California (San Francisco) approached the DHEA/depression question in another way. They decided to give DHEA to people with depression and see if it would help. In the first double-blind, placebo-controlled study on the potential of DHEA as an antidepressant, 11 patients with major depression were given up to 90 mg a day of DHEA for six weeks; 11 were given a placebo. One week before the study actually started, all patients were given a placebo to weed out people who would respond to a sugar pill. The remaining study subjects were then given 30 mg a day of DHEA for the first two weeks; 60 mg for the second two weeks; and 90 mg for the last two weeks. The idea of the graduated dose was to bring patients up to the DHEA levels they had when they were 20–30 years old (DHEA declines with age).

Although the amount of DHEA was not adjusted individually, as it should have been, the graduated dose approximates what it takes to reach a "youthful" level in most people, according to Dr. Owen Wolkowitz, the principle investigator on the study. Some of the participants were taking antidepressants. For these people, the antidepressants were either working partially or not working at all. Only people who had been on the same antidepressant for at least 6 weeks without changing were allowed in the study, and no changes could be made in anyone's medication during the study. After 6 weeks, psychological tests indicated that about half of the participants responded to DHEA therapy, with an overall enhancement of mood scores by 30.5%. This is close to the response rate of antidepressant drugs (Wolko-witz et al. 1999).

An even better response was seen in another study conducted by researchers at the National Institute of Mental Health. In this study, participants were middle-aged people with dysthymia, a chronic, low-grade depression. They were given 90 mg of DHEA a day for three weeks and then 450 mg a day for three weeks more. Batteries of psychological tests were administered, including the Hamilton Depression Rating Scale, the Beck Depression Inventory, a visual analogue scale, and the Cornell Dysthymia Scale. None of the patients were taking any prescription drugs whatsoever except for one man who was taking a hypertension drug. The study was set up in a very rigorous way: all participants received the drug or the placebo for six weeks, and then they were all secretly switched. All people involved in the study were "blind" to who was getting what.

DHEA significantly alleviated the participants' depression. Seven depressive symptoms in particular improved: lack of pleasure, low energy, low motivation, emotional numbness, sadness, inability to cope, and excessive worry. DHEA worked for most people within 10 days. If the supplement was stopped, the symptoms came back. Overall, the response rate was 60% (better than usual results with antidepressants

and dysthymia). A DHEA dose of 90 mg a day was sufficient. No extra benefit was provided by the 450-mg dose (Bloch et al. 1999).

Researchers have different theories about how DHEA alleviates depression. Both DHEA and dehydroepiandrosterone sulfate (DHEA-S) can cross the blood-brain barrier and interact with the brain directly. DHEA can affect serotonin, GABA receptors, and other brain factors. One study indicated it might modulate the serotonin-signaling pathway (Inagaki et al. 1999). In addition, DHEA is the precursor for estrogen and testosterone, which have been reported to enhance mood. DHEA also has antistress effects that may be part of its antidepressant action. Research shows that cortisol, the stress hormone, is elevated in major depression. DHEA counteracts cortisol. Calmness appears to be associated with higher levels of DHEA. People who practice transcendental meditation have higher levels of DHEA than those who do not (Glaser et al. 1992). People who took part in a stress-reduction program were able to increase their DHEA by 100%. At the same time, they reduced their stress hormone by 23% (McCraty et al. 1998).

Another study on the role of DHEA deficiency in depression focused on recovering alcoholics, a group especially susceptible to depression and hence to relapse into drinking. The authors found that abstinent alcoholics showed a deficiency of noradrenaline and a low DHEA-to-cortisol ratio, indicating lower ability to deal with stress (Heinz et al. 1999). Hypothetically, DHEA might prove a useful adjunct therapy for recovering alcoholics.

Exercise has been reported to enhance mood. This mood-enhancing effect may be due to DHEA. Exercise raises levels of DHEA, which also positively affect the heart. In a study in the *American Journal of Cardiology*, depression and heart attack went together: women with depression are at greater risk of heart attack and vice-versa (Lavie et al. 1999).

DHEA INHIBITS CANCER CELL PROLIFERATION

DHEA may be effective in preventing and treating cancer. In one study, DHEA inhibited tumor proliferation of rat liver cells by blocking the cancer cell promoting enzyme glucose 6-phosphate dehydrogenase (G6PDH). The human equivalent dose of 600 mg a day suppressed breast tumors in mice by 70%; yet these scientists showed that even human equivalent doses of 25–120 mg showed striking cancer prevention benefits with no evidence of toxicity (Simile et al. 1995).

DHEA has been shown to inhibit chemically induced cancers in the colon, lung, breast, and skin (Schwartz et al. 1995). When applied directly to the skin, DHEA prevents chemically induced skin cancer (Pashko et al. 1985). DHEA has this effect by blocking the binding of carcinogens to skin cells and by inhibiting the enzyme G6PDH.

One study showed that patients with adult T-cell leukemia (ATL) had significantly decreased levels of DHEA compared to healthy controls (Uozumi et al. 1996). This has led some doctors to speculate that DHEA might be beneficial in treating this form of leukemia because DHEA has already been shown effective in treating hairy cell leukemia. Other cancer studies show DHEA inhibits cancer cell thymidine incorporation needed for cellular propagation and disrupts the oxidizing effects of chemical carcinogens (Schwartz et al. 1986; Hastings et al. 1988; Kim et al. 1999). Scientists point out that DHEA functions not as an antioxidant, but as a modulator of the effects of chemical carcinogens on cells.

DHEA PROTECTS AGAINST BRAIN AGING

Acetylcholine is a neurotransmitter that transmits nerve impulses from one brain cell to another. Acetylcholine is crucial for short-term memory and to protect brain cells against age-associated atrophy. Aging causes a decline in the release of acetylcholine into regions of the brain where it is needed for learning and memory.

In a study published in *Brain Research*, DHEA was administered to rats in order to measure the effect it produced on acetylcholine release into the hippocampus region of the brain. DHEA significantly increased acetylcholine release above pretreatment levels in all doses tested. At the highest dose, DHEA caused a fourfold increase in the release of acetylcholine compared to the control group. The scientists concluded that this was the first study to demonstrate a direct effect of DHEA in promoting the release of acetylcholine from brain cells in the hippocampus (a critical area for the storage of memory) (Rhodes et al. 1996).

In a study published in *Behavioral Brain Research*, DHEA interacted with certain neuronal receptors involved in short- and long-term memory storage. The results showed an improvement in memory in the Y-maze spatial learning test that measures short-term memory and the step-down passive avoidance test that measures long-term memory in mice (Maurice et al. 1997).

A study in *Life Sciences* showed that DHEA could protect against the precursor changes in brain cells that result in the pathological alterations associated with Alzheimer's disease (Danenboerg et al. 1996).

The ability of DHEA to protect the hippocampus and enhance its activity is important in regard to Alzheimer's disease. Studies have generally found increased cortisol and lower DHEA in Alzheimer's disease patients. It is known that excess cortisol damages the hippocampus and potentiates beta-amyloid toxicity. DHEA is believed to be able to antagonize the destructive effects of excess cortisol. The authors of a study have concluded that dementia is correlated with low DHEA more so than with high cortisol (Murialdo et al. 2000).

DHEA SAVES SKIN

DHEA has powerful skin protective effects. A study published in the *Journal of Surgical Research* demonstrates that topically applied DHEA protects the skin's delicate blood vessels. Researchers found that if DHEA were applied after a serious burn, the blood vessels underlying the burned area were protected (Araneo et al. 1995). Protecting the blood vessels saves the skin. Skin and blood vessels that would otherwise die and peel off can be saved by DHEA. No one knows for sure how DHEA saves skin in this way, but its anti-inflammatory action must have something to do with it. DHEA prevents destructive white blood cells and their biochemical cousins from gearing up. In particular, DHEA affects the blood vessel killer known as tumor necrosis factor (TNF). At the same time it is inhibiting the destructive process, it appears to be prolonging the healing process: DHEA causes edema (swelling) to last longer. This apparently helps save tissue.

Estrogen's skin-enhancing effects are well-known. It provokes collagen and a moisture factor known as hyaluronic acid. Aging decreases both estrogen and collagen. Enzymes that convert DHEA to estrogen also decline. Not surprisingly, women who take synthetic estrogen have scientifically proven thicker skin. Women who take both estrogen and testosterone have really thick skin—48% thicker than women who do not take either hormone (Brincat et al. 1983). DHEA is converted to both estrogen and testosterone, providing the benefits of both hormones. DHEA is converted into estrogen and androgen-type metabolites found only in skin.

Studies show that DHEA is absorbed by skin when applied topically. A study from CHUL Research Center (in Canada) shows that the skin activity of DHEA applied topically is 85–90% greater than when taken orally (at least in rodents) (Labrie et al. 1996). No special carriers are needed to get DHEA into skin. A properly formulated topical preparation of DHEA will contain just enough of the hormone to benefit skin without providing enough to escape into circulation. It makes sense to apply the hormones directly to the skin if skin protection is the goal because ingested hormones may end up everywhere but the skin.

DHEA acts against everyday damage as well. By maintaining skin immunity, DHEA preserves the ability of skin to react to cancer-causing, skin-destroying pollutants in air, food, and water (Hastings et al. 1988; Pashko et al. 1992).

DHEA AND IMMUNE FUNCTION

DHEA levels decline 80–90% by age 70 or later. DHEA has demonstrated a striking ability to maintain immune system synchronization. Oral supplementation with low doses of DHEA in aged animals restored immunocompetence to a reasonable level within days of administration. DHEA supplementation in aged rodents resulted in almost complete restoration of immune function (Danenberg et al. 1996).

DHEA has been shown in numerous animal studies to boost immune function via several different mechanisms. Only limited human studies have been done to measure DHEA's effect on the immune system.

In one study that focused on men, scientists proposed that the oral administration of DHEA to elderly men would result in activation of their immune system: nine healthy men averaging 63 years of age were treated with a placebo for two weeks followed by 20 weeks of DHEA (50 mg a day). After two weeks on oral DHEA, serum DHEA levels increased by 3–4 times. These levels were sustained throughout the study. Compared to the placebo, DHEA administration resulted in:

- An increase of 20% in IGF-1. Many people are taking expensive growth hormone injections for the purpose of boosting IGF (insulin-like growth factor) levels. IGF is thought to be responsible for some of the antiaging, anabolic effects that DHEA has produced in previous human studies.

- An increase of 35% in the number of monocyte immune cells.

- An increase of 29% in the number of B immune cells and a 62% increase in B-cell activity.

- A 40% increase in T-cell activity even though the total number of T-cells was not affected.

- An increase of 50% in interleukin-2.

- An increase of 22–37% in natural killer cell (NK) numbers and an increase of 45% in NK cell activity.

- No adverse effects were noted with DHEA administration.

The scientists concluded: "While extended studies are required, our findings suggest potential therapeutic benefits of DHEA in immunodeficient states" (Khorram et al. 1997).

A study published in the *Journal of Clinical Endocrine Metabolism* showed that when old female mice were treated with DHEA, melatonin, or DHEA and melatonin, splenocytes (macrophages) were significantly higher as compared to young mice. B-cell proliferation in young and in old mice significantly increased. DHEA, melatonin, and DHEA and melatonin helped to regulate immune function in aged female mice by significantly increasing the cytokines' interleukin-2 and interferon-gamma and significantly decreasing the cytokines' interleukin-6 and interleukin-10, thus regulating cytokine production (Inserra et al. 1998).

Interleukin-6 (IL-6) is one of the pathogenic elements in inflammatory and age-related diseases, such as rheumatoid arthritis, osteoporosis, atherosclerosis, and late-onset B-cell neoplasia. According to a report in the June 1999 issue of the *Journal of the American Geriatrics Society*, "higher circulating levels of IL-6 predict disability onset in older persons." The authors suggest that IL-6 may cause a reduction in muscle strength or contribute to specific diseases such as congestive heart failure, osteoporosis, arthritis, and dementia, which cause disability (Ferrucci et al. 1999).

DHEA has consistently been shown to boost beneficial interleukin-2 and suppress damaging interleukin-6 (IL-6) levels. Interleukin-6 is overproduced in the aged, which contributes to autoimmune disease, immune dysfunction, osteoporosis, depressions in healing, breast cancer, B-cell lymphoma, and anemia. Continuous DHEA administration maintained immunocompetence in aged animals (by boosting interleukin-2 and other beneficial immune components and suppressing interleukin-6 and other detrimental immune components). Suppression of interleukin-6 with 200 mg a day of DHEA was shown to be effective against systemic lupus erythematosus (Van Vollenhoven et al. 1998).

Researchers compared levels of IL-6 in 283 subjects with a mobility or functional disability with IL-6 levels in 350 adults without a disability. The investigators found that adults in the highest third of values of IL-6 had a 76% higher rate for mobility disabilities and a 62% higher rate for inability to perform daily activities than subjects in the lowest third of values. "These data suggest that IL-6 is a global marker of impending deterioration in health status in older adults," wrote a team led by Dr. Luigi Ferrucci at the National Institute on Aging in Bethesda, MD (Ferrucci et al. 1999).

In a study in the *Proceedings of the Society for Experimental Biology and Medicine*, DHEA has been shown to restore normal cytokine production in immune system dysfunction induced by aging by suppressing the excessive production of cytokines (IL-6) by 75%, although increasing IL-2 secretion by nearly 50%, during a leukemia virus infection in old mice (Inserra et al. 1998).

Another study in normal healthy individuals over the age of 40 found an opposite relationship between plasma DHEA levels and the presence of detectable levels of IL-6. Studies also revealed that low doses of DHEA and DHEA-S inhibited the production of IL-6 in unstimulated human spleen cell suspension cultures and enhanced its release by cultures transferred from organs of the same tissue (James et al. 1997).

The age-related increase in circulating IL-6 levels in humans, which has been attributed to decline in DHEA production by the adrenal gland, is currently attracting attention because of its possible relevance to the etiology and management of a number of age-related clinical disorders. The potential importance of these observations and suggestions has prompted us to perform more detailed studies on the relationship between IL-6 and DHEA. Using immunoassay techniques, scientists found in normal healthy individuals over the age of 40 that low levels of plasma DHEA levels predicted levels of IL-6 (James et al. 1997).

DHEA FOR POSTMENOPAUSAL WOMEN

The importance of DHEA, a precursor of estrogen and testosterone, in psychological and sexual health has been underlined in a number of studies. For example, a German study found that DHEA-deficient women supplementing with 50 mg of DHEA daily for four months had decreased symptoms of depression and anxiety and improved libido (Arlt et al. 1999).

A study by an Italian team of investigators suggests that DHEA may be an effective option for preserving health in postmenopausal women. The study concluded that oral administration of 50 mg of DHEA daily for six months mimics the benefits of traditional hormone replacement therapy (HRT), namely, estrogen-progestin

in terms of its effects on the GHRH-GH-IGF-1 (growth hormone-releasing) axis (Genazzani et al. 2001). The axis oversees the control of several endocrine functions, including the stimulation of osteoblasts (bone cells) to stimulate skeletal growth in children and maintain bone integrity in adults. During menopause, however, the drop in estrogenic activity reduces the secretion of the hormones of this axis and slowly the bone reduces the amount of calcium and osteoporosis begins.

The study by the Italian team involved 31 postmenopausal women, who were divided according to their age into two groups (50–55 and 60–65 years). They were tested for hormonal levels at three months and then six months of therapy and were subjected to a GHRH test before and after the study. Researchers measured the effects of DHEA with ultrasound and bone mass density (BMD) examinations before and after the study. Results showed that the levels of all DHEA-derived steroids and osteocalcin, as well as GH and IGF-1, were increased in plasma under DHEA supplementation (Genazzani et al. 2001).

DHEA DOSING AND SAFETY PRECAUTIONS

Properly managed DHEA therapy can be useful for most older men and women to increase energy, vitality, and foster an overall youthful feeling. However, there are guidelines that should be followed for safe long-term use of DHEA.

When taking oral supplements of DHEA, it is important that antioxidants are available to the liver because DHEA can promote free radicals in liver cells. Animal studies have shown that extremely high doses (from 2000–10,000 mg DHEA daily in human terms) caused liver damage in mice and rats (Metzger et al. 1995). When antioxidants were given along with the DHEA, liver damage did not occur despite the massive doses of DHEA being administered to these animals (Swierczynski et al. 1997). It should be noted that the amount of DHEA shown to cause liver damage is 20 times more than is necessary to produce antiaging benefits. Green tea, vitamin E, and N-acetyl-cysteine (NAC) are antioxidants that have been shown to be especially effective in suppressing free radicals in the liver.

The Life Extension Foundation has evaluated thousands of DHEA blood tests to determine the ideal dose of DHEA for both men and women. The Foundation's findings indicate that the optimal dosage range for DHEA varies considerably between individuals. Prior recommendations to take DHEA 3 times a day are now being replaced with a general recommendation that men and women should consider taking between 15–75 mg a day in 1 morning dose. Most human studies use one daily dose of 50 mg, and this is the typical daily dose that the majority of people use to restore serum DHEA to youthful levels. DHEA can be taken with or without food, although some believe that fat helps DHEA to assimilate better. Some people absorb DHEA better by taking it 20–30 minutes before meals.

A DHEA-S blood test should be taken 3–6 weeks after beginning DHEA therapy to help determine optimal dosing. Some people neglect to test their blood levels of DHEA and wind up chronically taking the wrong dose. When having your blood tested for DHEA, blood should be drawn 3–4 hours after the last dose. DHEA testing can save you money if testing shows that less DHEA can be taken to maintain youthful DHEA serum levels.

The standard blood test to evaluate DHEA status is one that measures DHEA-S. The DHEA-S is calculated in micrograms per deciliter (mcg/dL) of blood. The youthful ranges of DHEA are as follows:

Men	Women
400–560	350–430

People over age 40 who do not supplement with DHEA usually have serum levels below 200 and many are below 100. Chronic DHEA deficiency is a risk factor for developing the degenerative diseases of aging according to the preponderance of evidence existing in the scientific literature.

Some people obtain a baseline DHEA-S blood test before beginning DHEA replacement therapy. However, based upon numerous DHEA blood tests evaluated by the Life Extension Foundation, anyone over age 40 who does not supplement DHEA is already deficient in serum DHEA. Therefore, it may be more economical to have the first DHEA blood test 3–6 weeks after initiating DHEA replacement therapy. There are precautions that should be observed that are different for men and women.

DHEA Precautions for Men

Before initiating DHEA therapy, men should know their serum PSA (prostate-specific antigen) level and have passed a digital rectal exam. Men with prostate cancer or severe benign prostate disease are advised to avoid DHEA because DHEA can be converted into testosterone (and estrogen). These sex hormones and their metabolites can promote benign and malignant prostate cell proliferation. It is important to understand, however, that well-controlled studies show that

serum DHEA levels are usually lower in men with malignant prostate disease compared to healthy control subjects. Therefore, men are advised to have a PSA and digital rectal exam before initiating DHEA therapy to rule out existing prostate disease, not because DHEA causes the disease. On the contrary, there is evidence indicating that maintaining youthful levels of DHEA may protect against prostate cancer. To reduce the risk that hormone modulation with DHEA could contribute to a prostate problem, men taking DHEA are also advised to take:

Vitamin E	400–800 UI a day
Selenium	200–400 mcg a day
Gamma E Tocopherol	200 mg a day
Lycopene Extract	20–40 mg a day
Saw Palmetto Extract	160 mg 2 times a day
Pygeum Extract	50 mg 2 times a day
Nettle Extract	120 mg 2 times a day

Aging men often have high levels of estrogen (estradiol) and dihydrotestosterone (DHT). If a blood test reveals estradiol levels above 30 (pg/mL), an *aromatase inhibitor* should be taken. This can either be in the form of a prescription drug, such as *Arimidex* (0.5 mg taken twice a week), or a dietary supplement called *Super Mira Forte* (6 capsules a day). If serum DHT levels are too high, taking 5 mg a day of the prescription drug Proscar can lower them to safe ranges.

Men over 40 should consider checking their PSA and DHEA-S serum levels every 6–12 months thereafter. Men should also periodically check their blood levels of free testosterone and estrogen to make sure that DHEA is following a youthful metabolic pathway. Men taking DHEA should refer to the *Male Hormone Modulation protocol* to learn about additional hormone balance testing that can be done at the same time serum DHEA and PSA levels are being tested.

DHEA Precautions for Women

DHEA can increase serum estrogen levels in women and eliminate the need for estrogen replacement therapy in some women. To help protect cells (especially breast cells) from excessive proliferation in response to estrogen, women taking DHEA should also take:

Melatonin	300 mcg–3 mg every night
Vitamin E	400–800 IU a day
Gamma E Tocopherol	200 mg a day
Indole-3-carbinol	200 mg twice a day
Vitamin D$_3$	1000–1400 IU a day

Women should consider estrogen and free testosterone testing when they take their DHEA blood test in order to evaluate DHEA's effect on their blood levels of estrogens.

Women who have been diagnosed with an estrogen-dependent cancer should consult their physicians before beginning DHEA therapy. Some studies indicate that higher serum DHEA protects against breast cancer, but no adequate studies have been done to evaluate the effects of DHEA in breast cancer patients. If DHEA were to elevate estrogen too much, this could theoretically increase the risk of breast cancer. Women taking DHEA should refer to the *Female Hormone Replacement* protocol for information about restoring complete youthful hormone balance.

Liver Disease

Men or women with existing liver disease (such as viral hepatitis or cirrhosis) should consider taking DHEA sublingually (under your tongue) or using a topical DHEA cream to reduce the amount of DHEA entering the liver. DHEA is converted by the liver into DHEA-S. Those with liver disease should carefully monitor liver enzyme levels to be certain that DHEA therapy is not making existing liver disease worse.

DHEA is best taken early in the day or possible insomnia could result. DHEA is normally produced by the adrenal glands early in the day and then converted by the liver to DHEA-S by midday when the DHEA/DHEA-S ratio is usually stabilized (10% DHEA/90% DHEA-S).

We again recommend that those already taking DHEA should have a DHEA blood test to make sure they are taking the precise dose to suit their individual biochemistry.

Some people only need to take a small amount of DHEA to restore blood levels to that of a 21-year-old, although others need to take higher levels of DHEA. Those with existing prostate or breast cancers should not take DHEA unless closely supervised by a knowledgeable physician who understands DHEA's metabolic pathways.

Some people supplement with the hormone pregnenolone in lieu of or in addition to DHEA. Because pregnenolone naturally converts into many of the same hormones as DHEA, some of the precautions we advise for DHEA may apply to pregnenolone.

DHEA tests often cost more than $100 at local laboratories, but the Life Extension Foundation offers low-cost DHEA-S and PSA (prostate-specific antigen) testing to members by mail order. For complete information about the availability of discount blood testing in your area, refer to the *Medical Testing* protocol or call (800) 208-3444.

If DHEA replacement sounds complicated, it is, compared to other preventive supplement programs. We suggest weighing the documented antiaging benefits of maintaining youthful serum DHEA levels when deciding whether to embark on a DHEA replacement regimen, or stated differently, review the degenerative effects of chronic DHEA deficiency to decide whether this program is worth your time and money.

 PRODUCT AVAILABILITY

DHEA, melatonin, Natural Prostate Formula (containing saw palmetto, nettle root, and pygeum extracts), selenium, Indole-3-Carbinol (I3C), Super Mira Forte, Gamma E Tocopherol/Tocotrienols, and vitamins D_3 and E (succinate) can be ordered by calling (800) 544-4440 or by ordering online at www.lef.org.

Diabetes Type II and the Syndrome X Connection

Approximately 8% of the population in the United States has diabetes. This computes to nearly 16 million people being diagnosed with the disease, based only on national statistics.

The American Diabetes Association announced that diabetes accounts for 178,000 deaths, 54,000 amputees, and 12,000–24,000 cases of blindness annually. Blindness is 25 times more common among diabetic patients compared to nondiabetics. It is proposed that by the year 2010, diabetes will exceed both heart disease and cancer as the leading cause of death through its many complications.

Considering these startling numbers, an insightful internist recently commented that physicians are losing more patients to diabetes than they are diagnosing. Additionally, it is estimated that 5.4 million people have the disease and are not aware of it. Minorities are at particular risk. Compared with Caucasians, blacks have a 60% higher risk of developing diabetes and Hispanics have a 90% increased risk.

AUTOIMMUNE (TYPE I) DIABETES

This type of diabetes has also been called Juvenile Onset Diabetes Mellitus, Insulin Dependent Diabetes, or Type I diabetes. For reasons we do not clearly understand, the body attacks its own insulin-producing tissue, the beta cells of the islets of Langerhans in the pancreas. When so many of these cells are destroyed that not enough are active to meet the body's need for insulin, the patient becomes diabetic and must take insulin injections.

At one time, we thought that this condition was only found in childhood, and so it was assumed that any young person who started showing signs of disturbed glucose metabolism was insulin deficient. Conversely, we concluded that patients who did not become diabetic until they were adults were not insulin deficient. Today, we know that young people can be metabolically diabetic and that adults can become autoimmune diabetic.

Autoimmune diabetes can be definitively diagnosed with blood testing.

1. Blood insulin and glucose levels, drawn together, will show a deficiency of insulin or an excess of glucose.
2. Anti-insulin antibodies/anti-islet cell antibodies are usually present in autoimmune diabetes (Type I).

Conventional treatment for this condition is not satisfactory. Replacement of insulin by injection can be used to keep blood sugar under control but will not prevent development of all of the dreaded complications of diabetes: loss of sexual function, diabetic retinopathy (blindness), peripheral neuropathy (approximately 10% of diabetics develop neuropathic symptoms, such as throbbing, aching, or numbness of the lower extremities), and peripheral vascular disease (diminished circulation, intermittent claudication, difficult wound healing, and the propensity for gangrenous body parts and eventual amputation). Typically, tight control of blood glucose levels prolongs the onset and progression of symptoms.

However, there is evidence that protecting cells against the adverse effects of unstable serum insulin and serum glucose can mitigate these complications. Therefore, while many of the supplements in this protocol have documented benefits in protecting against Type II diabetic complications, they can also prevent diseases commonly associated with Type I diabetes.

THE DIFFERENCE BETWEEN TYPE I AND TYPE II DIABETES

Type I diabetes, sometimes referred to as insulin-dependent diabetes mellitus (IDDM), has both similar and dissimilar manifestations as compared to Type II diabetes mellitus. Although both Type I and Type II diabetes often result in similar disabilities, that is, neurological disorders, cardiovascular disease, and sometimes organ failure, the causal factors are quite different. For example, Type I diabetes reflects an inability to metabolize carbohydrates caused by an *absolute* insulin deficiency. This type of diabetes occurs most often in children and young adults as a result of inadequate insulin production in the beta cells of the pancreas.

Type II diabetes generally occurs because of a *metabolic failure* at the cellular level, a condition spurred by poor diet, obesity, environmental factors, and genetics. Body tissues, such as cell receptor sites, lose their sensitivity. As insulin attempts to deliver glucose into the cell, the "key no longer fits the lock." Blood glucose, barricaded from the

Pancreas

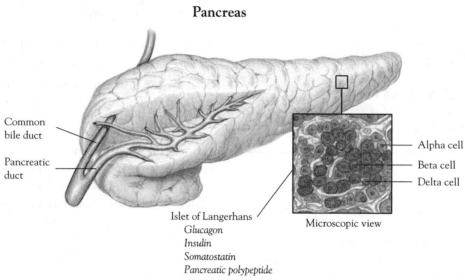

The islets of Langerhans are microscopic structures within the pancreas that are composed of various cell types. The alpha cells secrete glucagon, which accelerates release of stored glucose in the liver (glycogenolysis). The beta cells are most abundant and secrete insulin. The delta cells secrete somatostatin, which regulates release of both glucagon and insulin, among others. (Anatomical Chart Company 2002®, Lippincott Williams & Wilkins)

cell, accumulates in the bloodstream. Unlike Type I diabetes, insulin therapy is usually not indicated in Type II diabetes because typically these individuals already have too much insulin in their bloodstream. However, after an extended period of excess insulin secretion, the pancreas may lose its ability to produce insulin and a Type II diabetic may then become insulin dependent.

In Type II diabetes, the onset is usually after 40 years of age, but the onset can occur at any age. In fact, the incidence of Type II diabetes among 30-year-olds has gone up over 70% in the last decade. Physicians are increasingly reporting the diagnosis of Type II diabetes in teenagers, as well. The number of teenagers (an age group not normally targeted) being diagnosed with Type II diabetes indicates that a diet structured around high glycemic carbohydrates causes chronic states of hyperinsulinemia. A poorly selected diet, along with a lack of exercise, increases the risk of diabetes and premature cardiovascular disease.

Dr. Alan R. Sinaiko (University of Minnesota) in 2001 announced an association between insulin resistance and an elevation in blood pressure among teenage boys. The teenagers were tested when they were 13 years old and again when they were 15 years of age. By the second test, there was a definite association between the teenage boys' insulin resistance and their blood pressure (Smith 2001). (The reason this did not apply to the girls may be due to the fact that males have a higher overall early risk than females.)

SIGNS AND SYMPTOMS OF DIABETES

The symptoms of Type II diabetes can be so subtle that they may be overlooked. But, extreme fatigue (particularly 2–4 hours after a meal), a change in weight, blurred vision, drowsiness, tingling or numbness in hands and feet, slow wound healing, unwarranted hunger (polyphagia), frequent urination (polyuria), and excessive thirst (polydipsia) can be warning signs of abnormal blood glucose levels. *Note:* Polydipsia and polyuria are homeostatic mechanisms that the body uses to extract sugar from the system.

Diagnostic standards for diabetes have been fasting plasma glucose levels greater than 140 mg/dL on two occasions and plasma glucose greater than 200 mg/dL following a 75-gram glucose load. More recently, the American Diabetes Association lowered the criteria for a diabetes diagnosis to fasting plasma glucose levels equal to or greater than 126 mg/dL. Fasting plasma levels outside the normal boundaries require additional testing, usually by repeating the fasting plasma glucose test and (if indicated) undergoing an oral glucose tolerance test.

Glucosuria (sugar in the urine) usually occurs when blood glucose levels reach 160–180 mg per 100 mL of blood. However, this does not confirm diabetes

supplement is examined by itself. Antioxidants (as CoQ10) should be taken with other antioxidants, rather than emphasizing a single factor. Many commercial CoQ10 products are complexed with other antioxidants to balance the effects of CoQ10 at the cellular level.

On the other hand, Japanese researchers gave a favorable nod to CoQ_{10}, citing (among CoQ_{10}'s virtues) its ability to enhance beta cell function and improve glycemic control (McCarty 1999). Recall that the Helicon Foundation (San Diego, CA) selected CoQ_{10} as one of four nutrients (the others are biotin, chromium, and conjugated linoleic acid) as a part of a wholly nutritional therapy against Type II diabetes. A suggested CoQ_{10} dosage is 100 mg/day. Take higher doses if you have neurological or cardiac impairment.

Conjugated Linoleic Acid—aids in weight management, improves insulin sensitivity, and reduces blood glucose levels

According to information released at the national meeting of the American Chemical Society (ACS) in August 2000, the long-awaited first results of human studies evaluating conjugated linoleic acid (CLA), a naturally occurring fatty acid, indicate that the supplement may help overweight adults lose weight and maintain the loss.

Animal studies have for the past 10 years affirmed CLA's importance in weight management, but human studies were lacking. More recently, human studies (conducted in Norway and the United States) substantiated animal studies, confirming that overweight individuals experienced a statistically significant reduction in body fat while supplementing with CLA. The trial participants did not alter eating habits, and no adverse side effects accompanied supplementation.

It is also speculated that CLA may reduce body fat by increasing energy expenditure. Researchers at the Pennington Biomedical Research Center (Baton Rouge, LA) observed that CLA-fed mice (after only 1 week of dosing) experienced increased energy output, a perk that was sustained 6-weeks postsupplementation (DeLany et al. 2001).

The University of Wisconsin (Madison) released results of a 6-month study involving 89 overweight people. Michael Pariza, Ph.D., one of the researchers, determined that exercise and food restriction initially caused a weight loss but noted that the loss was difficult to maintain. Typically, individuals regained their lost weight at a ratio of 75% fat to 25% lean. Individuals supplementing with CLA were better able to

maintain goal weight, with less fat regained and more muscle mass retained (ACS 2000; Pariza 2000).

A team from Purdue University and Pennsylvania State University announced that CLA appears to reduce blood glucose levels and prevent diabetes, at least for the short-term. Animal studies demonstrated that CLA worked as well as a new class of diabetes-fighting drugs, the thiazolidinediones (TZDs).

Karen Houseknecht (assistant professor of animal studies) at Purdue says that CLA may have advantages over current drug therapies considering overall health benefits. When Zucker Diabetic Fatty rats (those specially bred to become obese and develop glucose intolerance) are given TZD, they become fatter. Conversely, when laboratory animals are given CLA, they become leaner. (During the course of the CLA study, obese animals lost 10% of body fat and lean animals lost 25%.) After 2 weeks, the CLA-supplemented rats were diabetes free; all of the unsupplemented rats had developed diabetes (Houseknecht et al. 1998).

Among 22 individuals enrolled in an 8-week CLA/diabetes study, 64% experienced improved insulin sensitivity (the premier focus in reversing Type II diabetes) while taking 6.0 grams a day of CLA (ACS 2000). Maureen Charron (diabetes researcher and associate professor of biochemistry at the Albert Einstein College of Medicine at Yeshiva University in New York), although excited about CLA as an antidiabetic agent, is tempering her enthusiasm until more studies are completed. In the interim, the Purdue team is considering feeding CLA to hogs to see if the CLA content of pork can be increased. The researchers jest that the ramifications of a pork chop that fights both cancer and diabetes is "emotionally overwhelming" (Houseknecht et al. 1998). A suggested CLA daily dose is 3000–4000 mg, usually four to five 1000-mg (76%) capsules.

Food sources of CLA. The polyunsaturated fat is found in meats and cheeses and in lesser amounts in milk, yogurt, poultry, eggs, and cooking oil. (According to Purdue researchers, CLA looks like corn oil, just a little clearer. Note that the CLA content of dairy products and meat is lower than what it used to be because cows primarily eat in feedlots as opposed to eating grass. As a result, CLA supplements have become a popular adjunct weight-loss approach.)

DHEA (Dehydroepiandrosterone)—is beneficial to diabetic and obese individuals, reduces IL-6 levels, and eventually converts to testosterone in some individuals

Although not universally accepted, some studies suggest that high serum insulin predisposes one to low levels of DHEA (Yamaguchi et al. 1998). A fall in serum levels of DHEA is associated with a higher incidence of atherosclerosis and obesity. An association has now been made with diabetes. These observations suggest that DHEA may play a protective role in diseases that gain a stronghold when DHEA levels become low (Lukaczer 1999).

A lack of DHEA appears to be a primary cause of insulin resistance (likely because a DHEA shortage interferes with insulin's ability to regulate blood glucose). Since insulin is one of the hormones that affect fatty acid metabolism, insulin resistance is often observed when fatty acid metabolism is abnormal. Illustrative of this, rats fed a diet containing 0.3% DHEA (ages 5–25 months) had about 25% less body fat than animals not supplemented. Concurrently, the rate of glucose disposal was 30% higher in the DHEA-treated group due to greater insulin responsiveness (Han et al. 1998).

More recently, the dangers of C-reactive protein (CRP), a newer risk factor associated with heart disease, have expanded to include diabetes, with researchers referring to it as a predictive factor for the disease (Pradhan et al. 2001). Since individuals who are obese and insulin resistant often present with higher levels of CRP, addressing CRP levels has become even more relevant for diabetic patients. In addition, elevations in interleukin-6 (IL-6), an inflammatory cytokine, has emerged as another prognostic evaluation for diabetes. Israeli researchers showed that DHEA, an intrinsic neurosteroid, inhibited IL-6 by 95% (Kipper-Galperin et al. 1999).

The kidneys are of significant concern in nonresponsive hyperglycemia. DHEA, a major secretory product of the human adrenal gland, has been shown to possess multitargeted antioxidant activity, including effectiveness against glucose-induced lipid peroxidation. This adaptation protects the kidneys against oxidative damage and impairment of cell growth, suggesting effectiveness in overcoming chronic renal complications associated with diabetes (Brignardello et al. 2000).

Suggested DHEA dosage and caveats. A suggested dosage is 15–75 mg, taken early in the day (50 mg represents a typical daily dose.) Blood tests are valuable 3–6 weeks into therapy to assist in assigning appropriate dosages. Optimal DHEA levels for men are between 400–560 mcg/dL; for women, the range is considered ideal at 350–430 mcg/dL.

Because DHEA invigorates hormonal systems, it is not recommended for men with prostate cancer or for women with estrogen-dependent cancer, without physician approval. (DHEA can be converted into testosterone and estrogen.) Before starting DHEA therapy, men should know their serum PSA (prostate specific antigen) level and have passed a digital rectal examination (DRE). DHEA does not cause prostate cancer, but because DHEA can cause an increase in testosterone levels, the presence of an undetected cancer should be ruled out before initiating the therapy.

For a comprehensive review of the natural products capable of reducing proinflammatory cytokines, please consult the *Inflammation: Chronic protocol*. The *Cardiovascular Disease protocol* contains valuable information regarding the risks imposed by elevated CRP and natural measures to counter it.

Essential Fatty Acids—*promote release of prostacyclin, help maintain cell membrane insulin responsiveness, are beneficial to dieters, and lower CRP*

Omega-3 fatty acids (alpha-linolenic acid), the parent of eicosapentaenoic acid (EPA) and docosahexaenoic acid (DHA), help maintain healthy cell membranes. This means that the membranes are flexible and contain larger numbers of insulin receptors that are more receptive and responsive to insulin (Lukaczer 1999). Researchers have shown that eating a diet that emphasizes omega-3 fatty acids (herring, mackerel, sea bass, salmon, cod, sardines, fresh tuna, whitefish, cold-water halibut, anchovy, and walnuts) along with monounsaturated fats (olives, almonds, pecans, cashews, filberts, and macadamias) is effective medicine against membrane alterations.

Japanese researchers recently showed that EPA reduced plasma lipids and abdominal fat deposits and increased glucose disposal. Results indicate that long-term feeding of EPA appears effective in preventing insulin resistance in diabetic-prone laboratory animals (in part) by improving blood lipid levels (Minami et al. 2002).

Depressed levels of prostacyclin, a major vasoprotective molecule, are central to the pathogenesis of diabetic neuropathy. Because of inadequate amounts of prostacyclin among diabetics, red blood cells (responsible for oxygen carriage) become brittle and rigid. This prevents oxygen from freely entering the cells, a process that most damages small capillaries and the tissues they serve. Gamma-linolenic acid (GLA), an omega-6 fatty acid, promotes the release of prostacyclin. This function (in turn) adds flexibility to blood cells, regenerates capillaries, and stabilizes nerves (Guivernau et al. 1994; Angilley 2001). Using evening primrose oil (EPO), a good source of GLA, resulted in a 22% increase in endoneural (nerve sheath) capillary density (Cameron 1990). Persons beginning EPO therapy should allow 8-10 weeks to realize a significant effect (Fang 1997; Angilley 2001).

Studies have shown that genetically obese people also profit from essential fatty acid supplementation. The weight loss in these individuals is gradual but reliable, even among those considered intractably obese.

GLA appears to stimulate brown fat cells by producing prostaglandin E1 (PGE1). Brown fat is of particular advantage in maintaining a desirable weight because it uses extra calories to provide heat, preventing the deposit of unsightly white fat. Brown fat's energy-use capacity accounts for major differences between brown fat and white fat. Mitochondria are abundantly dispersed throughout brown fat cells (Braly 1985).

Type II diabetics should supplement with at least 900 mg of GLA a day from borage oil, along with 500 mg of EPA and 1300 mg of DHA from fish oil. Research suggests the DHA fraction of fish oil is particularly effective in reducing CRP (Madsen et al. 2001; Pradhan et al. 2001). This quantity of fatty acids GLA, EPA, and DHA can be obtained in 8 capsules by using highly concentrated borage and fish oil supplements.

Fiber—lowers blood glucose levels

It is difficult to overstate the benefits garnered from fiber in regard to blood glucose control. Eating a diet rich in high fiber foods has spared countless individuals the risks imposed by chronically elevated blood glucose and the rigors of aggressive antidiabetic therapy.

A high fiber diet offers many health benefits, some of which accrue whether the appropriate fiber is selected or not (Hayes 2001). However, therapeutically speaking, fibers are not equal; they have different metabolic dispositions.

The two types of fiber are *insoluble* (does not disperse in water) and *soluble* (does dissolve in water). Insoluble fibers are identified as cellulose and many hemicelluloses and lignins; soluble fibers include pectin, gums, mucilages, and some hemicelluloses.

Fibers target different metabolic disturbances. For example, the benefits gleaned from insoluble fibers usually involve the gastrointestinal (GI) tract, promoting bowel regularity, while slowing the breakdown of starch and delaying glucose absorption into the blood. Soluble fibers (the type popularized since the 1980s) slow gastric emptying and the transit of chyme (the semifluid material produced by gastric digestion of food) through the intestines. This function forestalls the quick entry of glucose into the bloodstream. Soluble fibers appear to improve insulin sensitivity

and reduce hyperinsulinemia as well. Many of the conditions surrounding Syndrome X, including poor lipid levels and disrupted coagulation factors, are favorably impacted by fiber.

Some people associate fiber with bran products, but dietary fiber also includes the nondigestible portion of plant foods found in whole grains, fruits, vegetables, and dried beans and peas, as well as nuts and seeds. Although fiber cannot be digested and does not supply calories or nutrients, it is far from a purposeless food factor. In addition to direct impact upon various forms of ill health, soluble fibers provide short-chain fatty acids. Bacteria in the human digestive tract ferment fiber, that is, they digest fibers in the absence of oxygen. This process generates water and short-chain fatty acids. The short-chain fatty acids are absorbed in the colon and yield energy when metabolized (depending upon the extent to which they are broken down and absorbed) (Murray 1996). The short-chain fatty acids produced by GI bacteria are primarily acetic acid, propionic acid, and butyric acid (Whitney 1998).

The American Diabetes Association (ADA) recommends that individuals with diabetes consume the same amount of fiber (both soluble and insoluble) as that recommended for the general population: 20–35 grams a day. This recommendation may not be sufficient to stabilize blood glucose levels. The ADA's guidelines for fiber consumption were based on the rationale that 20–35 grams of fiber were a reasonable amount to expect individuals to obtain from dietary sources. (Considering the amount of fast and convenience foods consumed, it is estimated many people consume only 5–17 grams of fiber a day.)

A study reported in the *New England Journal of Medicine* involved diabetic patients consuming a diet supplying 25 grams of soluble fiber and 25 grams of insoluble. (This amount is about double the amount that is currently recommended by the ADA.) The fiber was derived from foodstuffs, with no emphasis placed on special or unusual fiber-fortified foods or fiber supplements. After 6 weeks, tests revealed that the high fiber diet had reduced blood glucose levels by an average of 10%; equally important, levels of circulating insulin were also reduced (Chandalia et al. 2000).

Fiber is also valuable to persons on diets because it produces a feeling of satiety, negating the desire to overeat. Apart from getting an early sense of fullness, fibrous foods require more chewing; by extending mealtime, the person on a diet is satisfied both physically and emotionally. Because high-fiber foods are digested more slowly, hunger pangs are forestalled. For the most part, fibrous foods represent healthy food (nutrient-dense and low-fat), additional perks for weight watchers.

Fiber should be added slowly, gradually substituting low-fiber foods with high-fiber alternatives. This is necessary for the following reasons: (1) insulin and prescription drugs may have to be adjusted to accommodate lower blood glucose levels, and (2) without a gradual introduction of the new material, gastric distress could occur.

Some individuals prefer to bolster fiber volume by adding supplemental pectin, gums, and mucilages to each meal. Calculate the amount of fiber gained from foodstuffs and supplement with enough to compensate for shortfalls. Recall that successful trials used soluble and insoluble fibers (a total of 50 grams a day). Monitor blood glucose levels closely to assess gains and to adjust oral or injectable hypoglycemic agents.

High-fiber foods follow (those emphasized in the study in the *New England Journal of Medicine*), with soluble fiber identified by (S) and insoluble identified by (I) and expressed in grams per serving (Chandalia et al. 2000). (Fiber content of foods was collected from sources apart from the published study.)

Cantaloupe (one-quarter):	(S) 0.13, (I) 0.80
Grapefruit (one-half):	(S) 0.9, (I) 0.4
Raisins (1/4 cup):	(S) 0.22), (I) 1.30
Orange (1 medium):	(S) 0.79, (I) 1.70
Papaya (1 cup):	2 grams total of fiber
Lima beans (1/2 cup):	(S) 0.2, (I) 1.2
Okra (8 pods):	3 grams total of fiber
Sweet potato (one, 5 in. 2 in.):	3 grams total of fiber
Winter squash (1 cup):	6 grams total of fiber
Zucchini (1/2 cup):	(S) 1.1, (I) 1.4
Oat bran (1/2 cup):	(S) 2.2, (I) 2.2
Oatmeal (1 cup):	(S) 1.64, (I) 2.81

Magnesium—lowers blood glucose levels, increases insulin sensitivity, and calms the sympathetic nervous system

Although the relationship between magnesium and diabetes has been studied for decades, it is still poorly understood. However, what is known about diabetes and magnesium embodies a persuasive list encouraging supplementation:

- Low magnesium levels are common findings in noninsulin-dependent diabetic patients (Paolisso et al. 1989). In fact, diabetes is a frequent cause of secondary hypomagnesemia (lower blood levels of magnesium). Poorly controlled diabetics excrete more magnesium than do nondiabetics.

- Magnesium assists in the maintenance of functional beta cells (insulin factories) (Kowluru et al. 2001). Scientists believe that a magnesium deficiency interrupts insulin secretion and its activity. Magnesium, by enhancing the action of insulin, improves insulin's ability to transport glucose into the cell.

- Magnesium increases the number and sensitivity of insulin receptors (Waterfall 2000).

- An increase in red blood cell magnesium significantly and positively correlated with an increase in both insulin secretion and action. Correction of low erythrocyte magnesium concentrations may allow for improved glucose handling, particularly in elderly diabetic patients (Paolisso et al. 1992, 1993a).

- As magnesium levels plummet, the incidence of diabetic complications escalates. Of particular concern is the association between low magnesium levels and ischemic heart disease and retinopathy. It appears that magnesium may prevent and retard the development of vascular complications common to diabetic patients (Elamin et al. 1990).

- Magnesium not only plays a role in insulin resistance and hypertension, but also plays a role in the correction of carbohydrate intolerance (Murray 1996).

Magnesium is the mineral of choice to reduce hyper-responsiveness occurring in the sympathetic nervous system (SNS). This is important to the diabetic because when the SNS is alerted, blood glucose levels tend to be higher. The SNS is also associated with fostering greater levels of stress and anxiety, earning its reputation as the "flight or fight" division. Since diabetes is considered to be a disease promulgated by stress, supplementation that favors an inner calm is of significant advantage.

Serum magnesium levels are relatively insensitive assessments of magnesium status. Magnesium deficiency is far better detected by measuring mononuclear blood cell magnesium, as opposed to serum levels. A suggested magnesium dosage is 500 mg of elemental magnesium daily along with a diet favoring magnesium-rich foods, for example, whole grain cereals, nuts, legumes, and green vegetables. Since vitamin B_6 is intricately involved in magnesium absorption, at least 30–50 mg of vitamin B_6 should accompany magnesium supplementation.

N-Acetyl-L-Cysteine—protects beta cells against free-radical destruction

Free radicals flourish when blood glucose levels are high, causing various forms of tissue destruction in patients. A study examined the involvement of free radicals in the progression of pancreatic cell dysfunction and evaluated the usefulness of N-acetyl-L-cysteine (NAC), a potent antioxidant, to counter the attack (Kaneto et al. 1999). The study was reported in the journal *Diabetes* and the conclusion was that NAC exerts beneficial effects by preserving beta cell function. This finding supports the implication that free radicals promote beta cell dysfunction and that antioxidant therapy is a useful adjunct in diabetes management.

During NAC therapy, the following observations were made:

- Pancreatic beta cells appeared to be protected against glucose toxicity (Kaneto et al. 1999).

- The insulin-producing beta cell mass was larger in diabetic mice treated with NAC compared to untreated mice (Kaneto et al. 1999).

- Beta cell death was suppressed. The journal *Diabetes* reported that high levels of glucose appeared to directly upregulate the cell death receptor Fas on human pancreatic beta cells. This finding may explain the loss of beta cell mass observed in Type II diabetes (Donath et al. 2001).

- Glucose-stimulated insulin secretion continued, followed by a modest decrease in blood glucose levels with NAC supplementation (Kaneto et al. 1999).

A suggested NAC dosage is 600 mg a day on an empty stomach for optimal absorption.

Note: *When taking NAC, it is recommended that two to three times as much vitamin C be taken conjunctively because of the prolonged presence of the oxidized form of L-cysteine.*

Silymarin—improves liver function and blood glucose control and reduces free-radical activity

The liver performs more than 500 functions, including the regulation of blood glucose. According to information released from the Diabetes Forum (Gopi Memorial Hospital), the liver is the first and most important tissue involved in insulin utilization. In fact, if the liver becomes damaged, secondary diabetes can result. An injured liver is unable to respond to insulin normally and essential blood glucose regulatory systems become less functional. If glycogenolysis (the breakdown of glycogen to supply glucose), gluconeogenesis (the hepatic synthesis of glucose from noncarbohydrate sources), or glycogenesis (the synthesis of glycogen from glucose) is depreciated, tight blood glucose control becomes impossible.

A group of 60 patients with type II diabetes and alcohol-induced liver damage were divided into two groups: for 12 months, 30 received 600 mg per day of silymarin (an antioxidant flavonoid derived from the herb milk thistle) while 30 received a placebo. All subjects were classed as very ill at the onset of the study (Velussi et al. 1997; Challem et al. 2000).

Those receiving silymarin evidenced a significant reduction in fasting blood glucose levels (an improvement also mirrored in urine glucose). Initially, average glucosuria (glucose in urine) was 37 grams, dropping to 22 grams during therapy. Fasting glucose levels rose slightly during the first month of supplementation but declined thereafter from an average of 190 mg/dL to 174 mg/dL. As daily glucose levels dropped (from an average of 202 mg/dL to 172 mg/dL), HbA1c also substantially decreased. Throughout the course of treatment, fasting insulin levels declined by almost one-half and daily insulin requirements decreased by about 24%. Liver enzymes (SGOT and SGPT) modulated, reflecting improved liver function. A lack of hypoglycemic episodes suggests silymarin not only lowers blood glucose levels, but also stabilizes them as well. Glucosuria, fasting insulin, and glucose levels, as well as HbA1c, remained unchanged in the nonsupplemented group.

In an 8-day, cell-culture study, German researchers found that a specific silymarin flavonoid, silibinin, prevented the accumulation of fibronectin protein in kidney cells. (Fibronectin is one of the principal causes of kidney damage in diabetics.) Simone Wenzel, Ph.D., incubated human mesangial cells (a type of kidney cell) in high concentrations of glucose or in a combination of glucose and silibinin. An accumulation of fibronectin was prevented, with protection attributed to silibinin's antioxidant properties (Wenzel et al. 1996).

Silibinin is the most active constituent of silymarin and is sold as a drug in Germany to treat hepatic disorders. Standardized milk thistle extract usually consists of 35% silibinin, whereas the silymarin concentrate used in Europe contains a minimum of 80% silibinin. A suggested silymarin dosage for Syndrome X patients (those not yet diagnosed with diabetes) is a supplement that provides 250 mg a day of silibinin and 60 mg of silymarin. Diabetic patients often take 2–3 silibinin/silymarin capsules providing the same amounts.

Vitamin C—lowers blood glucose and CRP levels, inhibits glycation, prevents accumulation of sorbitol, and protects against free radicals

An exchange occurring between hormones and nutrients maintains health at the cellular level. For example, insulin (by facilitating the transport of vitamin C into cells) decreases capillary permeability and aids in wound healing. Diabetics are often deficient in intracellular vitamin C; this deficiency deprives a diabetic of the protection this important nutrient delivers (Sinclair 1994).

- Vitamin C, an antioxidant, protects against free-radical activity, which is notoriously aggressive in diabetic patients.
- Vitamin C makes blood glucose management easier. Vitamin C deficiencies increase HbA1c (an average measurement of blood glucose levels over the last several weeks) (Sargeant 2000).
- Vitamin C inhibits glycation, a destructive process that occurs when glucose reacts with a protein (Emekli 1996; Vincent 1999). The glycosylation of proteins in red blood cells, the lens of the eye, and nerve cells causes abnormal structure and function of cells and tissues. This untoward sequence contributes to many of the complications common to diabetes (Brownlee et al. 1984).
- C-reactive protein (CRP) is higher in individuals with clinical evidence of insulin resistance. It appears some of the increase in winter cardiovascular mortality may be related not only to a rise in fibrinogen, but also to an increase in other inflammatory markers, such as CRP. This cycle may be spurred as winter infections increase and vitamin C intake decreases because of less availability of fruits and vegetables (Khaw et al. 1997). Vitamin C might be able to influence cardiovascular and diabetic risks by modulating the inflammatory response to infection.
- Vitamin C reduces sorbitol accumulating within the cell and the risk of diabetic complications, including cataracts (Murray 1996).

Administering vitamin C in amounts of 1000–3000 mg daily (in divided doses) has been shown to significantly improve a diabetic's prognosis.

Food sources of vitamin C, enhancers, and antagonists. Fresh vegetables and fruits (particularly citrus) are excellent sources of vitamin C. Bioflavonoids are vitamin C enhancers. Antibiotics, antihistamines, steroid drugs, birth control pills, tobacco, stress, and aspirin are vitamin C antagonists.

Vitamin E—reduces C-reactive protein (CRP) and oxidative stress, enhances insulin sensitivity and glucose transport, and prevents complications arising from inflammation

Vitamin E's antioxidant properties and its ability to enhance insulin's responsiveness are but a few of the reasons the nutrient should be included in a diabetic protocol. This was clearly evidenced in a 4-month study reported in the *American Journal of Clinical Nutrition* with subjects receiving (approximately) 900 mg of vitamin E a day. The researchers assessed how well 15 Type II diabetics and 10 healthy controls tolerated glucose before and after vitamin E supplementation. In healthy subjects, glucose removal from the blood increased 17%. In diabetics, total glucose removal increased 47% and nonoxidative glucose metabolism increased 63%. The study established that pharmacologic doses of vitamin E in Type II diabetes improve insulin's action and reduce free-radical activity (Paolisso 1993b).

Vascular endothelial dysfunction (an early marker of atherosclerosis) has been demonstrated in Type II diabetes mellitus. It appears hyperglycemia is particularly destructive to endothelial cells because it increases oxidative stress and impairs the activity of nitric oxide, the endothelial derived relaxing factor (Giugliano et al. 1995). Oxidative injury may be increased in diabetes mellitus because of a weakened defense due to reduced endogenous antioxidants (vitamin E and reduced glutathione). With compromised nitric oxide activity, diabetic-cardiovascular complications (smooth muscle proliferation, platelet activation/aggregation, and leukocyte adherence to the endothelium) are compounded.

Some of the strongest recent evidence of a vitamin E-diabetes benefit comes from researchers at the University of Texas Southwestern Medical Center in Dallas. Scientists found that vitamin E (1200 IU daily) reduced the risk of heart failure in 75 diabetics by curtailing vascular inflammation in the heart. Left unchecked, inflammation can cause cardiac vessels to swell, promoting cardiovascular disease. Dr. Sridevi Devaraj, assistant professor of pathology and lead researcher, termed the end results of the study very encouraging (Devaraj 2001).

Last, elevated levels of CRP, an inflammatory marker, have recently been found to predict the development of Type II diabetes. A newer finding relating to the functions of vitamin E is that high dose vitamin E lowers CRP. Administering 1200 IU of alpha-tocopherol (daily for 3 months) lowered CRP levels by 30%. CRP levels remained reduced 2 months postsupplementation. By preventing vascular inflammation, many of the complications arising from diabetes are overcome (Devaraj et al. 2000). A suggested vitamin E dosage is 400–1200 IU of vitamin E per day along with at least 200 mg of gamma tocopherol.

Vitamin K—may play a role in insulin's response to glucose

To evaluate the effects of vitamin K on pancreatic function, 25 healthy young male volunteers were evaluated as to plasma-glucose vitamin K levels at baseline and after an oral glucose load. Concurrently, a 1-week food diary estimated mean daily vitamin K intake.

Individuals consuming a vitamin K-rich diet tended to have higher blood vitamin K status then those participants who had less vitamin K in their diet (conclusion reached by examining an average of five blood samples). Fasting plasma glucose levels were not markedly different between the groups, showing about 86 mg/dL among all subjects. However, 30 minutes after a glucose load, the group with the higher vitamin K status had a plasma glucose level of 145 mg/dL; the group with the lower vitamin K levels presented with a plasma glucose level of 160 mg/dL. According to researchers, the results suggest that vitamin K may play an important role on the acute insulin response to glucose tolerance (Nishiike et al. 1999).

Elevated levels of C-reactive protein (CRP) and interleukin-6 (IL-6) have recently been found to predict the development of Type II diabetes mellitus. Since Vitamin K reduces levels of IL-6, it appears equally probable that vitamin K may also be effective in attenuating elevations in CRP. A suggested vitamin K dosage is 10 mg per day.

Note: *Persons on anticoagulant drugs such as Coumadin cannot take vitamin K.*

Vitamin K-rich food sources and antagonists. Although friendly bacteria in the intestines synthesize the majority of vitamin K, the total requirement cannot be met by bacterial synthesis alone. Vitamin K-rich foodstuffs are liver and green leafy vegetables (especially broccoli, turnip greens, lettuce, and cabbage). Antibiotics increase the need for vitamin K, and vitamin E (doses less than 600 IU) antagonizes vitamin K activity.

WHY CONVENTIONAL TREATMENT FOR DIABETES CAN BE WORRISOME

By now, the reader is keenly aware that insulin *in excess* is dangerous. Too often, Type II diabetes patients are treated with insulin as the treatment of choice to control blood glucose levels. Most Type II diabetics have copious levels of insulin, at least before the disease becomes chronic and the pancreas exhausted. Injecting insulin into an already expanded insulin pool is a difficult rationale to justify. Once the pancreas fails, insulin therapy becomes essential.

When Type II diabetes is diagnosed, patients are often treated with antidiabetic drugs that lower blood glucose by stimulating the pancreas to secrete more insulin. These insulin-stimulating agents are classified as sulfonylureas drugs. Conventional medicine also recommends dieting to control obesity (should it exist).

The problem with these conventional treatments is that the vast majority of diets fail to induce long-term weight control. While sulfonylureas drugs temporarily lower blood glucose, they saturate the blood with insulin and worsen the long-term prognosis. Examples of popular sulfonylureas medications and their mode of operation follow:

- Glimepiride (Amaryl) lowers blood glucose by stimulating the pancreas to produce more insulin.
- Glipizide (Glucatrol) controls diabetes by goading the pancreas into secreting more insulin.
- Glyburide (Micronase) controls blood glucose by stimulating the pancreas to produce more insulin and by helping insulin work more efficiently.

Drugs that continuously "whip" the pancreas into producing more insulin appear to be a shortsighted approach to treating the problem. This mechanism weakens the beta cells of the pancreas much quicker, plus the body must deal with the toxic effects of the additional insulin load. Chronically elevated levels of insulin raise the risk of degenerative disease (such as cancer and heart attack) and exacerbate the effect of diabetes.

When profiling many of the sulfonylureas drugs, the *Physician's Desk Reference* includes a perceptive comment: "It is possible that some oral diabetic drugs may lead to more heart problems than diet treatment alone, or diet plus insulin." (Recall that heart disease is regarded as the major complication arising from diabetes.)

Relying upon a sulfonylurea drug to correct a condition, often amendable through discipline, is asking more of a drug than we are asking of ourselves. If attempts at lifestyle modification fail to ameliorate hyperglycemia, oral agents may become necessary but are by no means desirable.

Too often the antidiabetic diet endorsed by orthodox physicians allows far too many carbohydrates to be effective. Recall that Dr. Steven Whiting, Ph.D., believes that chronic adherence to a high carbohydrate diet ensures that the diabetic individual will be a patient for life.

A Safer Oral Drug to Lower Blood Glucose Levels

Note: Because metformin (Glucophage) works from a different prospective in that it does not increase insulin production, it was selected for singular review.

The drug metformin (Glucophage) lowers the amount of sugar in the bloodstream by decreasing sugar production and absorption and by helping the body respond to its own insulin. Many American physicians now prescribe metformin as the first drug of choice. It was safely used in Europe decades before gaining FDA approval.

Metformin lowers fasting blood sugar levels in individuals at risk for Type II diabetes without causing a significant risk of becoming hypoglycemic. However, metformin-induced hypoglycemia is possible in older, weak, and undernourished people as well as those with kidney, liver, adrenal, or pituitary gland problems. If meals are missed, alcohol is consumed, or exercise becomes excessive, hypoglycemia could occur (PDR 1999).

Metformin increases insulin sensitivity, lowers serum insulin levels, and induces moderate weight loss. Metformin causes the number of insulin receptors in muscle and adipocyte cells (fat cells) to increase. Studies have demonstrated that metformin reduces fasting plasma glucose concentrations by 60–70 mg/dL in patients with Type II diabetes as well as HbA1c (Ketz 2001; Life Extension Foundation 2001).

Individuals who need support in maintaining diet-induced weight loss may find additional benefit from metformin therapy. Along with better weight management, some individuals experience a decrease in the incidence of diabetes-associated infections. Some metformin users experience reductions in total and LDL cholesterol, free fatty acids, and two markers reflecting endothelial damage (tissue plasminogen activator antigen and von Willebrand factor) (Charles et al. 1999).

Metformin has better tolerability than many other antidiabetic prescription drugs, but individuals with congestive heart failure or kidney and liver disease are not candidates for metformin therapy. The restriction extends to include those who use alcohol to excess. A benchmark assessment of kidney function followed by an annual renal evaluation is essential (PDR 1999). Vitamin B_{12} levels should also be regularly checked because chronic use of metformin could cause a deficiency in both folic acid and vitamin B_{12}, resulting in neurological impairment and disruption in homocysteine clearance.

A rare side effect associated with metformin is lactic acidosis, an accumulation of lactic acid in the bloodstream, resulting in a lower pH in muscles and serum (Klow et al. 2001). Almost all reported lactic acidosis cases occurred when metformin and a contrast medium were used in patients with preexisting poor renal function. Metformin should not be used for 2 days before or after having an x-ray procedure with an injectable contrast agent (radioactive iodine).

A number of food and drug interactions could occur with metformin therapy, but from natural medicine, high-dose niacin is the only dietary supplement that appears contraindicated. It is important to note that metformin (or any other antidiabetic drug) is only an aid to better glucose control, not a substitute for a good diet and a health-centered lifestyle with emphasis on exercise and stress reduction.

Many physicians report success when prescribing 500 mg of metformin 2–3 times a day to patients over 40, without extenuating health issues that preclude its usage.

🌑 SUMMARY

Diabetes mellitus is a disease characterized by disturbance in the body's use of glucose.

In Type I diabetes mellitus, the body *does not make enough* of the hormone *insulin*, which is needed for most tissues to be able to access and use glucose.

In Type II diabetes mellitus, the patient actually *overproduces* insulin and experiences a systemic metabolic disorder that precludes the efficient utilization of glucose. Type II diabetes is the most commonly seen form of the disease. Everyone who is overweight is at risk of developing this disease.

In the later stages of Type II diabetes, the beta cells in the pancreas become dysfunctional and insulin-enhancement therapy becomes necessary. One of the objectives of this protocol is to keep Type II diabetics from progressing to the point where damaging insulin-enhancing therapies become necessary to suppress elevated blood glucose.

For the majority of Type II diabetics, the most important therapy to prevent or reverse the disease is to reduce excess body fat. The reader is asked to refer to the *Obesity* protocol to learn about novel methods of suppressing excess serum insulin, removing fat from storage and keeping new fat from accumulating in the body. Introducing physical activity into a sedentary lifestyle is also a critical therapeutic component.

The following list summarizes the nutrients profiled in the *Therapeutic Section*:

- Alpha-lipoic acid protects LDL against oxidation and is beneficial in preventing and treating Syndrome X and diabetic complications such as neuropathy. As little as 250–500 mg daily of alpha-lipoic acid may be sufficient in healthy individuals. Diabetics usually take 250–500 mg of alpha-lipoic acid 3 times daily. For the last 30 years, German practitioners have used high doses of lipoic acid to improve insulin sensitivity and diabetic conditions.

- Carnosine interferes with the toxic glycation process, thereby preventing the formation of nonfunctioning structures in the body known as AGEs. Diabetics have greatly accelerated rates of glycation compared to nondiabetics. A suggested dosage is 1000 mg daily.

- Essential fatty acids protect the plasma membrane insulin receptors and reduce CRP. Type II diabetics should supplement with at least 900 mg of GLA a day from borage oil, along with 500 mg of EPA and 1300 mg of DHA from fish oil. By using highly concentrated borage and fish oil supplements, this quantity of fatty acids (GLA, EPA, and DHA) can be obtained in 8 capsules.

- Carnitine improves blood glucose management and increases insulin sensitivity and glucose storage, essential for fat and carbohydrate metabolism. Deficiencies correlate with diabetic neuropathy. A suggested acetyl-L-carnitine dosage is 500–1000 mg twice daily.

- Chromium regulates blood glucose levels, fights insulin resistance, lowers HbA1c, aids in weight loss, and inhibits glycation. A suggested dosage is 200–600 mcg daily.

- DHEA deficiency is associated with a higher rate of insulin resistance and diabetes. A suggested dosage is 15–75 mg, taken early in the day (50 mg represents a typical daily dose). For a discussion relating to caveats surrounding DHEA supplementation, refer to the *Therapeutic Section* of this protocol.

- CLA aids weight loss and may improve insulin sensitivity. A suggested CLA daily dose is 3000–4000 mg (usually four to five 1000-mg (76%) CLA capsules).

- Magnesium lowers blood glucose levels, increases insulin sensitivity, and calms the SNS. Use at least 500 mg of elemental magnesium daily.

- Silymarin improves hepatic glucose control and reduces free-radical activity. A suggested dosage for Syndrome X patients (those not yet diagnosed with diabetes) is a supplement that provides 250 mg a day of silibinin and 60 mg of silymarin. Diabetic patients often take 2–3 of these silibinin/silymarin capsules each day.

- N-acetyl-L-cysteine (NAC) protects beta cells against free-radical destruction. A suggested dosage is 600 mg daily.

- CoQ10 enhances beta cell function and glycemic control and protects against heart disease. A suggested dosage is 100–300 mg a day.

- Vitamin C lowers blood glucose levels, inhibits glycation, prevents accumulation of sorbitol, strengthens capillaries, aids wound healing, and protects against free radicals. A suggested dosage is 1–3 grams daily in divided doses.

- Vitamin E reduces oxidative stress, enhances insulin sensitivity and glucose transport, and prevents complications arising from inflammation. Antidiabetic value has been observed using from 400–1200 IU of alpha tocopherol vitamin E daily along with a supplement that provides at least 200 mg of gamma tocopherol.

- Bilberry reduces blood glucose levels. A suggested dosage is 100–200 mg 3 times daily. (The bilberry extract should be standardized to contain 25% anthocyanidins.)

- Biotin aids in metabolism of macronutrients, enhances glucose utilization, and is beneficial in diabetic neuropathy. A suggested antidiabetic dosage is 8000–16,000 mcg daily.

- Vitamin K appears to play a role in insulin's response to glucose. Vitamin K is nontoxic at the recommended 10-mg daily dose.

A convenient way to obtain many of the nutrients listed is to take the following formulas:

Life Extension Mix
Life Extension Super Booster
ChronoForte
Super GLA/DHA

Some of the nutrients listed are to be taken individually.

Drug considerations:

In addition to diet modification, increased physical activity, and nutrient supplementation, Type II diabetics should consider low-dose aspirin (81 mg per day) to reduce their risk of heart attack and stroke.

The most effective prescription drug to treat many pathological mechanisms of Type II diabetes is metformin sold under the trade name Glucophage. Metformin is also available in generic form. Typical doses of metformin prescribed are 500 mg 2–3 times a day.

Aminoguanidine assists in controlling AGEs, a process that advances diabetic complications. Since aminoguanidine is not readily available, natural alternatives (alpha-lipoic acid, aspirin, carnosine, chromium, and vitamin C) become particularly attractive options.

Drugs to avoid:

If at all possible, avoid the sulfonylurea class of drugs that work by stimulating pancreatic secretion of insulin. While these drugs can lower elevated blood glucose for the short-term, they increase the risk of severe diabetic complications in the future. Insulin injections also increase the likelihood of diabetic complications. Persons with advanced diabetes may need insulin-enhancement therapy, but the objective is to control the disease state so that the body does not require huge amounts of insulin to maintain glycemic control.

Note: *Although fiber improves insulin sensitivity and reduces hyperinsulinemia, fiber should be slowly added to the diet, allowing time for digestive adjustments. Calculate the amount of fiber gained from foodstuffs and supplement to compensate for shortfalls. Successful trials used 50 grams of soluble and insoluble fibers a day. Monitor blood glucose levels closely to assess gains and to adjust either oral or injectable hypoglycemic agents. It is important that prediabetic and diabetic patients be evaluated regarding hemochromatosis, periodontal disease, and CRP levels. These conditions can hasten the onset of diabetes or worsen blood glucose control in confirmed cases; conversely, the correction of these anomalies can culminate in remarkable gains.*

Refer to the *Obesity protocol* for critical information about suppressing excess serum insulin and reducing the percentage of body fat.

 FOR MORE INFORMATION

Contact the American Diabetes Association, (800) 232-3472.

 PRODUCT AVAILABILITY

Alpha-lipoic acid, Life Extension Mix, ChronoForte, Life Extension Super Booster, bilberry extract, Biotin caps and powder, acetyl-*L*-carnitine, Super Carnosine, chromium capsules, CoQ$_{10}$, conjugated linolenic acid, DHEA, Kyolic garlic, Fiber Food caps and powder, Super GLA/DHA, magnesium, NAC, Silibinin Plus, and vitamins C, E, and K are available by calling (800) 544-4440 or by ordering online at www.lef.org.

Digestive Disorders

It is estimated that some form of digestive disorder affects more than 100 million people in America. That is more than half of the U.S. population.

For some people, digestive disorders are a source of irritation and discomfort that may cause them to drastically limit their lifestyles and to frequently miss work. For others, the disorders may be extremely crippling and even fatal.

THE GASTROINTESTINAL TRACT

The gastrointestinal tract (GIT) is a long muscular tube that functions as the food processor for the human body. The digestive system includes the following organs: mouth and salivary glands, stomach, small and large intestines, colon, liver and pancreas, and the gallbladder.

Irritations or inflammation of the various sections of the GIT are identified as gastritis (stomach), colitis (colon), ileitis (ileum or small intestines), hepatitis (liver), and cholecystitis (gallbladder).

The GIT is not a passive system. Rather, it has the capability to sense and react to the materials that are passed through it. For a healthy digestive system, every person requires different food selections that match their GIT capacity.

THE DIGESTIVE PROCESS

The GIT breaks down foods by first using mechanical means such as chewing and then by the application of a host of complex chemical processes. These chemical processes include everything from saliva to colon microbes. Since the GIT is the point of entry for the human body, everything eaten has an impact on the body. The food eaten and passed through the GIT contains nutrients as well as toxins. Toxins can be anything from food additives and pesticides to specific foods that induce a reaction from the GIT.

The process of digestion is accomplished via the surface of the GIT using secretions from accessory glands. The two glands providing the majority of digestive chemicals utilized by the GIT are the liver and the pancreas. The function of the liver is to control the food supply for the rest of the body by further processing the food molecules absorbed through the intestines. The liver does this by dispensing those food molecules in a controlled manner and by filtering out toxins that may have passed through the GIT wall.

Another very important function of the GIT is as a sensory organ. By rejecting foods through objectionable taste, vomiting, and diarrhea, or any combination of these symptoms, the sensing capacity of the GIT can protect the body. The surface of the GIT has a complex system of nerves and other cells of the immune system. The surface of the GIT, or mucosa, is part of a complex sensing system called the MALT (mucosa-associated lymphatic tissue). The immune sensors in MALT trigger responses such as nausea, vomiting, pain, and swelling. Vomiting and diarrhea are abrupt defensive responses by MALT when it senses foods with a strong allergic or toxic component. This kind of food intolerance is responsible for many digestive problems. The GIT is "hard-wired" to the brain via hormonal, neurotransmitter-mediator chemical communication.

The GIT is a muscular tube that contracts in a controlled rhythm to move food through the different sections (peristalsis). Strength and timing variations in the contractions can cause cramping (very strong contractions) and diarrhea (contractions are very frequent). When the contractions are slow and irregular, constipation may occur. *Motility disorder* is the general term used to describe problems with peristalsis.

Food allergy is sometimes the primary cause of GIT problems. Chronic diseases can have their origin in food allergies. The dysfunction, discomfort, and disease associated with GIT can be the result of local immune responses to food selections or combinations of foods. Food selections are a result of personal tastes, social fads, ethnic culture, religion, and, to a larger degree, local or seasonal availability. The food selections made in modern affluent society are based on a developed taste for a rich diet centered on meats and dairy products that are loaded with fats, high concentrations of proteins, and fat-soluble toxins. Advertising and misinformation about healthy diets have overshadowed human nutritional needs.

DIETARY SHIFTS AND DIGESTIVE DISORDERS

Human evolutionary history clearly shows that we are primarily herbivores. Human saliva contains alpha-amylase, an enzyme specifically designed to break down complex carbohydrates into sugar compounds. Our teeth are designed to cut vegetable matter and to grind grains. The so-called canine teeth of humans

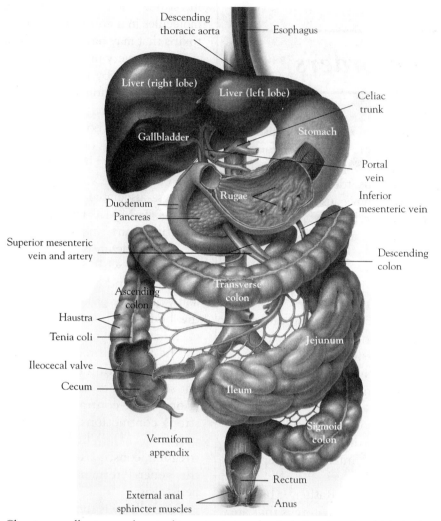

Chewing, swallowing, and peristalsis comprise mechanical digestion, in which food is broken down into tiny particles, mixed with digestive juices, and moved through the digestive tract. Digestive enzymes break down large food molecules into small molecules that can be absorbed into the blood or lymph in the process of chemical digestion. (Anatomical Chart Company® 2002, Lippincott Williams & Wilkins.)

bear no resemblance to the canines of even a domestic house cat. The human digestive system is long, and the food is processed slowly to extract all the nutrients from plant material. Conversely, carnivores have short digestive tracts that digest flesh very quickly. The digestive systems of carnivores are able to eliminate the large amount of cholesterol consumed in their diets, and carnivores do not have alpha-amylase present in their saliva.

The effect of the shift in our diets during the past 100 years has resulted in 44% of Americans and Canadians being afflicted with heartburn, 5% of the population suffering from peptic ulcer disease, and 20–40% of Americans plagued with nonulcer dyspepsia. Over-the-counter medications for these ailments are a multibillion-dollar industry. Nearly every hour on television, there is at least one commercial selling an antacid or similar product.

GASTROINTESTINAL SYMPTOMS

There are five basic symptoms indicating a GIT problem. These symptoms are generally associated with dietary problems or specific food allergies. It is critical that anyone suffering from serious GIT problems work closely with a physician to test for the more developed and serious GIT diseases. The physician should also be experienced in working with dietary factors and food allergies.

Nausea and Vomiting

Nausea and vomiting can vary from an unsettled feeling in the stomach to the violent action of immediate vomiting. Patients with nausea and vomiting symptoms should assume the ingestion of a reactive food (i.e., food containing toxins) or poisoning with a pathogen such as salmonella. Vomiting immediately after eating is usually proceeded by excessive watery salivation. Some chronic low-intensity nausea can occur for a protracted time due to sustained low-level food allergies or problems with food combinations. Patients with low-level nausea usually have their symptoms disappear with diet revision. Nausea and vomiting are also linked with migraines caused by food allergies (*see the Migraine protocol*).

Bloating

Bloating can result from excessive gas in the digestive system, failure of the digestive tract to sustain youthful peristaltic contractions, or a lack of sufficient quantities of digestive enzymes and bile acids to rapidly break down food. Intestinal gas results from food fermentation and from swallowing air while eating. The bloating from intestinal gas is different from that which occurs in the colon.

Constipation

Constipation is the decreased frequency, or slowing, of peristalsis, resulting in harder stools. When the GIT is slowed down, feces can accumulate in the colon with attending pain and toxic reactions. A *spastic colon* results when the colon contracts out of rhythm in painful spasms blocking movement of the stool. Some patients experience painful days of constipation followed by forceful diarrhea and watery stool, often accompanied with abdominal cramps.

Diarrhea

Diarrhea is the increased frequency of bowel movements that is also loose or watery. If diarrhea increases, the possibility of celiac disease is considered. Celiac disease is a serious disease that allows certain macromolecules to pass through the intestinal wall. If blood appears in the stool, ulcerative colitis is likely. Protracted bouts with diarrhea can result in nutritional deficiencies due to the poor absorption of essential nutrients.

Abdominal Pain

Abdominal pain appears in different patterns and with varying intensities. Cramping occurs because of muscle spasms in the abdominal organs. Severe cramping pain, often called *colic*, usually occurs from problems with strong allergic response to food. Abdominal cramping near the navel is typically from the small intestine, and near the sides, top, and bottom of the lower abdomen, the pain is associated with the colon.

Diseases associated with central GIT disorders and diagnoses include depression, migraine, asthma, sinusitis, and fibromyalgia. These diseases have been identified with specific patterns of food allergy response. All of these diseases also have links to Irritable Bowel Syndrome (IBS) (*see the IBS protocol*). (IBS is more accurately referred to as RBS—reactive bowel syndrome.)

STEPS TO A HEALTHIER DIGESTIVE SYSTEM

Elimination diets are a good method of determining what foods cause an allergic reaction in the GIT lining in a patient. Planning and following such diets are a safe starting point for anyone desiring to track their GIT response to food. Interview physicians to learn who may be most qualified to assist in planning an elimination diet. A very good indicator of a healthy GIT is a regular transit time for complete food digestion. Patients who are regular are usually in optimum health.

Aging causes many people to experience problems with digestion. It is estimated that after age 40 there is an approximate decrease in the body's ability to produce enzymes by 20–30%. The use of specific enzymes can help to improve the efficiency of digestion. Enzymes can be used to enhance the proper breakdown of foods in order to more properly digest, absorb, and utilize nutrients.

Enzymes Are a Vital Component of the Digestive Process

Enzymes are essential to the body's absorption and full use of food. The capacity of the living organism to make enzymes diminishes with age, and some scientists believe that humans could live longer and be healthier by guarding against the loss of our precious enzymes.

Enzymes are responsible for every activity of life. Even thinking requires enzyme activity. There are two primary classes of enzymes responsible for maintaining life functions: digestive and metabolic. The primary digestive enzymes are proteases (to digest proteins), amylases (to digest carbohydrates), and lipases (to digest fats). These enzymes function as a biological catalyst to help break down food. Raw foods also provide enzymes that naturally break down food for proper absorption. Metabolic enzymes are responsible for the structuring, repairing, and remodeling of every cell, and the body is under a great daily burden to supply sufficient enzymes for optimal health. Metabolic enzymes operate in every cell, every organ, and every tissue, and they need constant replenishment.

Digestion of food takes a high priority and has a high demand for enzymes. When we eat, enzymatic activity begins in the mouth, where salivary amylase, lingual lipase, and ptyalin initiate starch and fat digestion. In the stomach, hydrochloric acid activates pepsinogen to pepsin, which breaks down protein, and gastric lipase begins the hydrolysis of fats. Without proper enzyme production, the body has a difficult time digesting food, often resulting in a variety of chronic disorders.

Poor eating habits, including inadequate chewing and eating on the run, may result in inadequate enzyme production and, hence, malabsorption of food, which is exacerbated by aging because this is a time of decreased hydrochloric acid production, as well as a general decline in digestive enzyme secretion.

Saliva is rich in amylase, while gastric juice contains protease. The pancreas secretes digestive juices containing high concentrations of amylase and protease, as well as a smaller concentration of lipase. It also secretes a small concentration of maltase, which reduces to dextrose. Animals eating raw food often have no enzymes at all in saliva, unlike humans. However, dogs fed a high carbohydrate, heat-treated diet have been found to develop enzymes in their saliva within a week in response to enzyme-depleting foods.

One of America's pioneering biochemists and nutrition researchers, Dr. Edward Howell (1986), cites numerous animal studies showing that animals fed diets that are deficient in enzymes have an enlargement of the pancreas, as huge amounts of pancreatic enzymes are squandered in digesting foods that are devoid of natural enzymes. The result of this wasteful outpouring of pancreatic digestive enzymes is a decrease in the supply of crucial metabolic enzymes and impaired health.

How significant is an enzyme deficiency to overall health? For starters, organs that are overworked will enlarge in order to perform the increased workload. Those with congestive heart failure or aortic valvular disease often suffer from an enlarged heart, an unhealthy condition. When the pancreas enlarges in order to produce more digestive enzymes, there results a deficiency in the production of life-sustaining metabolic enzymes, as available enzyme-producing capacity is used in digesting food instead of supporting cellular enzymatic functions. The tremendous impact that the wastage of pancreatic enzymes can have on health, and even life itself, has been established in animal studies. The critical question is how this applies to human health.

For much of the 20th century, European oncologists have included enzyme therapy as a natural, nontoxic therapy against cancer, and almost all leading alternative cancer specialists treating Americans prescribe both food enzymes and concentrated enzyme supplements as primary or adjuvant cancer therapies. A New York City cancer specialist, Nicholas Gonzalez, M.D., uses very high doses of supplemental pancreatic enzymes as a primary antitumor therapy. His clinical successes have led conventional drug companies to seek to duplicate these natural therapies and offer them as adjuvant drug therapies. If pancreatic enzymes are effective in treating existing cancers, one might assume that maintaining a large pool of these enzymes in the body should help to prevent cancer from developing. Studies have shown that persons who eat fresh fruits and vegetables with high levels of natural enzymes have significantly reduced levels of cancer and other diseases. It has not been proven that the high enzyme content of these foods is partially responsible for their anticancer effect, but the evidence is compelling.

The pancreas and liver are digestive organs that produce most of the body's digestive enzymes. The remainder should come from uncooked foods, such as fresh fruits and vegetables, raw sprouted grains, seeds and nuts, unpasteurized dairy products, and enzyme supplements.

Food in its natural, unprocessed state is vital to the maintenance of good health. The lack of it in the modern diet is thought to be responsible for degenerative diseases. Cooking food, particularly for long periods of time and at more than 118°F, destroys enzymes in food and leaves what is often consumed in today's enzyme-less diet. This is one reason why, by middle age, we may become metabolically depleted of enzymes. Our glands and major organs suffer most from this deficiency. The brain may actually shrink as a result of an overcooked, overly refined diet that is devoid of enzymes desperately needed by the body. In an effort to meet the deficiency, the pancreas may swell. Laboratory mice fed heat-processed, enzyme-less foods develop a pancreas two or three times heavier than that of wild mice eating an enzyme-containing natural diet of raw food.

When food is consumed uncooked, fewer digestive enzymes are required to perform the digestive function. The body will adapt to the plentiful, external supply by secreting fewer of its own enzymes, preserving them to assist in vital cellular metabolic functions. One of the worst cooking methods is frying, since frying results in much higher temperatures than boiling. Frying damages protein as well as destroying enzymes.

Enzymes can also be wasted by lifestyle factors. Enzymes work harder with increasing temperatures and are used up faster. A fever, for example, induces faster enzyme action and is therefore unfavorable for bacterial activity. Enzymes can be found in urine after a fever and also may be found after strenuous athletic activity.

A natural behavior of animals is to harness the power of enzymes in food by burying or covering their food, allowing enzyme activity to start predigesting the food. By this natural behavior, animals instinctively preserve their own enzyme supply. Similarly, people of some native cultures also preserve their enzyme supply and prevent disease through efficient use of enzymes. Whales have up to 6 inches of fat to keep them warm, but their arteries are not clogged. Eskimos, who frequently consume large quantities of fat, are often not obese. Both of these groups eat the fat-digesting enzyme lipase in the form of raw foods.

Studies (both *in vitro* and controlled *in vivo*) using internal and parenteral routes have examined the effectiveness of many different types and sources of plant enzymes in several conditions, including poor digestion, poor absorption, pancreatic insufficiency, steatorrhea, lactose intolerance, celiac disease, obstruction of arteries, and thrombotic disease.

Enzymes from the *Aspergillus oryzae* fungus were subjected to numerous studies, evaluating their role in supporting healthy digestion. Additionally, human studies suggest the proteolytic enzymes derived from *A. oryzae* fungus may play a role in anti-inflammatory and fibrinolytic therapies. The enzymes appear to be relatively stable in heat, and they are also active throughout a wide pH range. This is important because most enzymes are deactivated in stomach acid. These enzymes are synthesized from fungus but contain no fungal residue even though that is their derivation. Modern filtration techniques and technology enable these fungal enzymes to be well suited for human consumption.

According to Dr. Mark Percival (1985), the oral supplementation of digestive enzymes taken just before or at mealtime can assist digestion. Even though most supplemental enzymes are labile and will deactivate when exposed to stomach acid, Dr. Percival believes some of the enzymes will remain active if they are taken with a meal or just before. Percival says, "The enzymes are physically protected" by the meal and allow some enzymatic activity to occur in the stomach. The enzymes that get through to the small intestine may help with digestion there as well. pH plays a major role in enzymatic activity, therefore, the enzymes derived from *Aspergillus* "may be highly

useful as they appear to be remarkably stable, even when subjected to an acidic environment." Dr. Edward Howell (1986) adds that he chews an enzyme capsule with his food in order to start the digestive process as soon as the food is consumed since enzyme activity has been shown to begin even before the food is swallowed.

As early as 1947, Dr. Arnold Renshaw (Manchester, England) reported in *Annals of Rheumatic Disease* that he had obtained good results with enzyme treatment of more than 700 patients with rheumatoid arthritis, osteoarthritis, or fibrositis: "Some intractable cases of ankylosing spondylitis and Still's disease have also responded to this therapy." He said that of 556 people with various types of arthritis, 283 were much improved, and 219 were improved to a less marked extent; of 292 people who had rheumatoid arthritis, 264 of them showed several degrees of improvement. More time was required before improvement was seen when the duration of the disease had been long-term, although most people started to show some improvement after only 2 or 3 months of enzyme therapy. In spite of these favorable findings, digestive enzyme therapy has been reserved for diseases that directly result in a pathological deficiency of pancreas-derived digestive enzymes.

According to Schneider et al. (1985), common digestive disorders may benefit from enzyme replacement. Oral intake of exocrine pancreatic enzymes is of key importance in the treatment of maldigestion in chronic pancreatitis with pancreatic insufficiency. Schneider studied the therapeutic effectiveness of a conventional and an acid-protected enzyme preparation and an acid-stable fungal enzyme preparation in the treatment of severe pancreatogenic steatorrhea. The results showed that a supplemental enzyme preparation is best for patients with chronic pancreatitis and those who underwent Whipple's procedure (a surgical procedure performed on pancreatic cancer patients), while patients with an intact upper GIT do best with an acid-protected porcine pancreatic enzyme preparation.

Rachman (1997) reported that 58% of the population has some type of digestive disorder and that lack of optimal digestive function associated with enzyme inadequacy may lead to malabsorption and other related conditions. In the elderly, the problem is often exacerbated because the elderly may have suboptimal production of gastric hydrocholoric acid. "This can be a significant factor that can impact nutrient absorption along with the creation of maldigestive-type symptoms. Bacterial production of hydrogen and methane are determined after a carbohydrate challenge. Excessive levels of these gases reflect over-growth of bacteria in the upper gut." Rachman suggests there may be improvement with enzyme replacement. He also adds that enzymes taken orally at meals may improve the digestion of dietary protein, thereby decreasing the quantity of antigenic macro-molecules that leak across the intestinal wall into the bloodstream. Such leaking may trigger the body's defenses against what it perceives to be foreign protein or polypeptide invaders, producing the symptoms of allergies.

Howell (1986) also agrees that allergies can respond to adding enzymes to the diet. He also says excessive cholesterol levels can respond to dietary enzymes as well. Howell quoted a 1962 study by three British doctors (C.W. Adams, O.B. Bayliss, and M.Z. Ibrahim), who set out to discover why cholesterol clogs arteries, ultimately manifesting in heart disease. They found that all enzymes studied became progressively weaker in the arteries as people aged and the hardening became more severe. They suggested a shortage of enzymes is part of the mechanism that allows cholesterol deposits to accumulate in the inner part of arterial walls. As early as 1958, researcher L.O. Pilgeram conducted blood tests at Stanford University and demonstrated a progressive decline of lipase in the blood of atherosclerotic patients in advancing middle and old age.

About the same time, researchers at Michael Reese Hospital in Chicago found that enzymes in the saliva, pancreas, and blood became weaker with advancing age and speculated that fat may be absorbed in the unhydrolyzed state in atherosclerosis. They also found definite improvement in the character of fat utilization following the use of enzymes.

Intravenous (IV) administration of brinase, a proteolytic enzyme prepared from A. oryzae, was found by FitzGerald et al. (1979) to be beneficial in treating chronic arterial obstruction. Patients were observed for 3 months before they were given six IV infusions of either saline or brinase for more than 2 weeks. No changes were observed during the observation period. After infusion, resumed blood flow was found in 17 of 27 obstructed arterial segments. The number of patent segments increased from 11 to 27. No improvements were observed in the patients who were treated with placebos.

Pancreatin is secreted from the pancreas. It provides potent concentrations of the digestive enzymes protease, amylase, and lipase and is sold as a drug to treat those with pancreatic insufficiency. Pancreatin efficacy was demonstrated in a study conducted on patients taking pancreatin to maintain postoperative

digestion. The effects of supplementation were determined by measuring the postoperative intestinal absorption and nutritional status in a randomized trial. The patients received pancreatin or a placebo. Before the trial, patients showed abnormal digestion of fats and protein. Total energy was low at baseline and at 3 weeks after surgery. Supplementation with pancreatin improved fat and protein absorption as well as improving nitrogen balance. However, those patients taking a placebo had worsened absorption after surgery. These data suggest that long-term, postoperative pancreatic enzyme supplementation is both effective and necessary in surgery patients who had pancreatitis.

Considerable evidence exists in support of the beneficial effects of enzymes, both natural and supplemental. Plant enzymes have shown obvious benefit for specific conditions. Research with intact absorption of food substrates has shown that nondigested food substrates enter the blood and that plant enzymes break down different food substrates that would otherwise have been passed into the blood partially digested.

Youth is the time of life when our normal ability to produce enzymes is greatest. It is also a time of rapid growth and often a time with no serious illness. As people age and their food enzymes become depleted, they often begin to suffer a broad range of health complaints.

According to Howell (1986), how long we live and our state of health are determined by our enzyme potential. Howell referred to a study by Meyer and associates at Michael Reese Hospital in Chicago that reported that the presence of enzymes in the saliva of young adults is 30 times higher than that in people over 69 years of age.

Therefore, humans consuming an enzyme-less diet use vast quantities of their enzyme potential from secretions from the pancreas and other digestive organs, perhaps resulting in shortened lifespan, illness, and lowered resistance to all types of stress.

In the early 1970s, G.A. Leveille, a University of Illinois researcher, discovered that enzyme activities in the tissues become weaker with age. Leveille conducted experiments on rats and found that at the age of 18 months—considered to be old for rats—when on enzyme-free fabricated diets, enzyme activity shrunk to less than 20% of its level at one month of age. Howell (1986) agrees: "The more lavishly a young body gives up its enzymes, the sooner the state of enzyme poverty, or old age, is reached."

The answer is to substitute raw foods for cooked foods as much as possible. Howell (1986) recommends that we eat foods with their enzymes intact and supplement cooked foods with enzyme capsules. He suggests we can stop abnormal and pathological aging processes. Howell singles out raw milk, bananas, avocados, seeds, nuts, grapes, and other natural foods as rich in food enzymes. He also suggests that an enzyme supplement be taken with all cooked food. Under medical supervision, Howell suggests large doses of enzyme therapy to treat certain diseases.

Few would disagree with the old adage that "we are what we eat," but it is not quite that simple. Enzymes make the digestion of food possible. This means we must make maximum use of enzyme activity, both internal enzymes and those consumed either in food or as supplements.

Benefits of Artichoke for Digestive Disorders

The artichoke plant is best known for its heart, the bottom part of its spiky flower bud that many of us have learned to appreciate as both a delicacy and a nutritious vegetable. However, other parts of this tall thistle-like plant, which never reach the dinner table, have proven to be even more beneficial for our health. Clinical studies show its large basal leaves to be effective for improving digestion and liver function, as well as cholesterol levels.

Since ancient times, humans have looked to nature for help to cure diseases. Up until modern times, most remedies were derived from the plant kingdom, and even today a large percentage of our current pharmaceutical drugs are based on plant extracts from various parts of the world. Many old herbal remedies, however, have fallen into oblivion with the development of modern medicine.

Artichoke extract is one of the few phytopharmaceuticals whose experiential and clinical effects have been confirmed to a great extent by biomedical research. Its major active components have been identified, as have some of its mechanisms of action in the human body. In particular, antioxidant, liver-protective, bile-enhancing, and lipid-lowering effects have been demonstrated, which correspond well with the historical use of the plant. More research is needed to determine in detail the mechanisms of action for these effects. However, there appears to be enough evidence to suggest a potential role for artichoke extract in some areas where modern medicine does not have much to offer.

Used as a food and a medical remedy as early as 400 BC, the artichoke plant has a long history. At the time, a pupil of Aristotle by the name of Theophrastus was one of the first to describe the plant in detail. Enjoyed as a delicacy, an appetizer, and a digestive aid by the aristocracy of the Roman Empire, it later seemed to fall into oblivion until the 1500s, when medicinal use of the artichoke for liver problems and jaundice was recorded. In 1850 a French physician successfully used extract of artichoke leaves in the treatment of a boy who had been sick with jaundice for a month and had made no improvement from the drugs used at that time. This accomplishment inspired researchers to find out more about the effects of this extract, and their research resulted in the knowledge we have today about the extract and its mechanisms of action.

Artichoke leaf extract is made from the long, deeply serrated basal leaves of the artichoke plant. This part is chosen for medicinal use because the concentration of the biologically active compounds is higher here than in the rest of the plant. The most active of these compounds have been discovered to be the flavonoids and caffeoylquinic acids. These substances belong to the polyphenol group and include chlorogenic acid, caffeoylquinic acid derivatives (cynarin is one of them), luteolin, scolymoside, and cynaroside.

Cynarin was the first constituent of the extract to be isolated in 1934. Interestingly, it is found only in trace amounts of fresh leaves but is formed by natural chemical changes that take place during drying and extraction of the plant material. Cynarin was originally believed to be the one active component of the extract. Today the whole complex of compounds is considered important, since it has not yet been completely clarified which component is responsible for each effect. It is claimed that neither cynarin alone, nor fresh plant material achieves the potency of the dried total extract (Kirchhoff et al. 1994).

Chlorogenic acid, another major component of the artichoke leaf extract, has recently become known as a powerful antioxidant with exciting potential in many applications. Laboratory investigations are ongoing all over the world with promising findings for future clinical application in areas such as HIV, cancer, and diabetes.

Most of the modern research on artichoke has been done with the German artichoke extract *Hepar SL Forte*, standardized to contain 3% caffeoylquinic acids. A new, even more potent extract, standardized at 15% caffeoylquinic acids—calculated as chlorogenic acid—is now available on the American market.

Biological Effects

The original uses of artichoke since ancient times have been as an aid for indigestion and insufficient liver function. The mechanism of action, however, has been essentially unknown. Recent findings have provided a new foundation for our understanding and discovered additional benefits of the extract, such as antioxidant and lipid-lowering effects.

Effects on the Gastrointestinal System

The importance of effective liver function for overall health in general, and proper gastrointestinal function in particular, is rarely emphasized in health discussions in the United States. One reason might be that there is neither laboratory evidence, nor specific physical symptoms to reveal an overburdened liver in the beginning stages. The symptoms may be nonspecific, such as general malaise, fatigue, headache, epigastric pain, bloating, nausea, or constipation. Discomfort following meals and intolerance of fat are also notable indications of disturbances in the biliary system.

It is estimated that at least 50% of patients with dyspeptic complaints have no verifiable disease. Because of the liver's essential role in detoxification, even minor impairment of liver function can have profound effects. It is therefore important to take such chronic complaints seriously. In Germany and France, for example, physicians frequently prescribe herbal liver remedies, such as artichoke extract, with good results when presented with these chronic but nonspecific symptoms. We may have something to learn here.

The proven basis for the beneficial effects of artichoke leaf extract on the gastrointestinal system is the promotion of bile flow. Bile is an extremely important digestive substance that is produced by the liver and stored in the gallbladder. The liver manufactures about 1 quart a day of bile to meet digestive requirements. It is secreted into the small intestine, where it emulsifies fats and fat-soluble vitamins and improves their absorption. Any interference with healthy bile flow can create a myriad of immediate digestive disorders, such as bloating.

Good bile flow is also essential for detoxification, which is one of the major tasks of the liver. The liver is constantly bombarded with toxic chemicals from the environment: the food we eat, the water we drink, and the air we breathe.

Bile serves as a carrier for these toxic substances, delivering them into the intestine for further elimination from the body. This is the major route for excretion of cholesterol. Yet another feature of the bile is helpful here: its promotion of intestinal peristalsis, which helps prevent constipation.

When the excretion of bile is inhibited for various reasons (gallstones or gallbladder disease), toxins and cholesterol stay in the liver longer with damaging effects. One of the causes of inhibited bile flow is

obstruction of the bile ducts by the presence of gallstones. Other common reasons for impairment of the bile flow within the liver itself are, for example, alcohol ingestion, viral hepatitis, and certain chemicals and drugs. In the initial stages of liver dysfunctions, laboratory tests, such as serum bilirubin, alkaline phosphatase, SGOT, LDH, and GGTP, often remain normal. It is not adequate to rely on these tests alone. Symptoms that may indicate reduced liver function are general malaise, fatigue, digestive disturbances, and sometimes increasing allergies and chemical sensitivities.

Excessive alcohol consumption is by far the most common cause of impaired liver function in the United States. It stimulates fat infiltration into the liver cells, causing the so-called *fatty liver*. Some livers are very sensitive to even minute amounts of alcohol; others are more tolerant. Research suggests that fatty liver condition is more serious than previously believed. It may develop to more advanced liver disease, such as inflammation, fibrosis, and cirrhosis.

Because of its long historical use for liver conditions, it seemed reasonable to investigate the artichoke plant scientifically. The first clinical studies were conducted in the 1930s with encouraging results. In the 1990s the interest has been intensified, and several excellent clinical studies have been conducted during the past few years.

Realizing the importance of adequate bile flow for health, German researchers set out to confirm the earlier findings of bile-promoting effect of the artichoke plant in a controlled, double-blind study on healthy volunteers (Kirchhoff et al. 1994). The participants were given a 1-time dose of artichoke extract or placebo, and their bile secretion was measured over the following hours, using special techniques. The bile secretion was found to be significantly higher in the group that received the artichoke extract.

Another clinical study showed an improvement of symptoms in 50% of patients with dyspeptic syndrome after 14 days of treatment with artichoke leaf extract. The study involved 60 patients with nonspecific symptoms such as upper abdominal pain, heartburn, bloating, constipation, diarrhea, nausea, and vomiting. In the placebo group, as a comparison, improvements of less distinct quality were noticed in 38% of the participants (Kupke et al. 1991).

Interesting results were also demonstrated in a large open label study of 417 participants with liver or bile duct disease. Most of these patients had long-standing symptoms, some of them for many years. They suffered from upper abdominal pain, bloating, constipation, lack of appetite, and nausea. These patients were treated with artichoke leaf extract for 4 weeks. After 1

Table 1: *Medical experts agree that individual variation is common and matching doses to patients is essential.*

Goth's Medical Pharmacology (Clark et al. 1992)	"Many adverse reactions probably arise from failure to tailor the dosage of drugs to widely different individual needs."
Goodman and Gilman's The Pharmacological Basis of Therapeutics (Gilman et al. 1990)	"Therapists of every type have long recognized that individual patients show wide variability in response to the same drug or treatment method."
Hazards of Medication (Martin 1978)	"The ultimate hazard is variability of patient response."
American Medical Association Drug Evaluations (AMA 1994)	"Almost all drugs cause reasonably predictable toxic reactions when given in excessive doses."
British Medical Journal (Herxheimer 2001)	"Many drugs have been introduced at doses that later were found to be too high; and usually years have passed, with unnecessary toxicity, before action was taken."
Pharmacoepidemiology and Drug Safety (Heerdink et al. 2002)	"Optimal drug therapy requires appropriate dosing in order to obtain the desired therapeutic effects at minimum risk."
Variability in Drug Therapy— A Sandoz Workshop (Rowland et al. 1985)	"Even if we try to forget, we are constantly reminded, by one experience or another, that patients differ in their responses to drugs."
Goth's Medical Pharmacology (Clark et al. 1992)	"Biologic variation in drug effect is an important reason to individualize dosage and adjust treatment to the requirements of a given patient."
Paracelsus (1493-1541): (Gilman et al. 1990)	"All substances are poisons; there is none which is not a poison. The right dose differentiates a poison and a remedy." ("Principles of Toxicology and Treatment of Poisoning").

LISTENING TO PROZAC

When I began treating patients in 1970, I quickly noticed how differently people responded to medications and began adjusting doses accordingly. Although this occurred with every drug I used, I didn't realize the depth of the problem until Prozac arrived in 1988.

As I did with all new drugs, I waited awhile before prescribing Prozac. New drugs, like new model cars, often manifest unexpected problems. But I heard only good things about Prozac, so I began prescribing it. I saw two distinct patterns. Half of my patients did extremely well. Prozac was clearly a breakthrough drug, far better than any earlier antidepressant.

But the other half of my patients had side effects, some severe. One woman became so agitated it incapacitated her. Another became completely psychotic after just three Prozac doses. The problem? The recommended, one-size-fits-all initial dose, 20 mg, was too strong. I would have started patients with lower doses, but Prozac was marketed in only one size, a 20-mg capsule. After these reactions occurred, I had patients open the capsules, mix the powder in juice and start lower. Most did fine at 5 mg to 10 mg daily, and the severe, dose-related reactions ceased.

Meanwhile, troubled by the reactions I saw, I searched the medical literature for explanations. I found more than I anticipated. A study published before Prozac's approval showed that just 5 mg helped 54% of patients, while 20 mg—the recommended dose—helped 64% (Wernicke et al. 1988). In other words, quadrupling the dose only improved efficacy 10%. To me, this meant that 5 mg was a reasonable starting dose, yet doctors were told to start everyone at 20 mg, even the 54% who needed only 5 mg! I was shocked and appalled.

Meanwhile, other doctors began reporting severe reactions to Prozac and that lower doses worked better (Table 2). Yet today, the standard starting dose of Prozac remains 20 mg, and there's still scant information in the package insert or *Physicians' Desk Reference* (PDR) about the effectiveness of the 5-mg dose (*Physicians' Desk Reference* 2003). Prozac and other selective serotonin reuptake inhibitors (SSRIs) continue to cause high incidences of dose-related side effects such as headaches, nausea, weight gain, irritability, sexual dysfunctions (impaired orgasm, reduced libido), low energy, dry mouth, and tremor. Insomnia or anxiety occur frequently, too, which doctors handle not by reducing the dose, but by adding a dependency-causing sleep or anxiety remedy.

Dosage Problems with Other Antidepressants

Doctors follow the guidelines in the drug company-written PDR. The PDR still advises 75 mg initially for Elavil (amitriptyline), yet 10 mg or 25 mg is frequently enough for mild depressions or pain syndromes. Effexor is recommended at 75 mg, but 37.5 mg or 50 mg often is enough initially. Zoloft is recommended at 50 mg, but 25 mg works well for many mild depressions. Serzone is recommended at 100 mg twice-daily, but 50 mg once or twice daily is usually plenty initially.

Similar strategies apply to Paxil, Wellbutrin, Celexa, Norpramin, Pamelor, imipramine, doxepin and just

Table 2: *Low-Dose Prozac*

Studies before and shortly after Prozac's approval revealed that 5 mg—one-quarter the standard 20-mg initial dose—was highly effective and less toxic for many people.

J. Clin. Psychopharmacol. (Schatzberg et al. 1987)	"Clinically, we have observed fluoxetine (Prozac) to be effective over a wide range with many patients requiring very low dosages..."
Psychopharmacol. Bull. (Wernicke et al. 1988)	5 mg helped 54% with major depression; 20 mg helped 64%. Fewer adverse effects with the 5 mg dose. Conclusion: "No lower limit for an effective dose of this potent serotonin uptake inhibitor has been demonstrated in moderately depressed outpatients."
J Clin. Psychiatry (Salzman 1990)	"A single daily dose of 20 mg may overmedicate some older depressed patients. Experienced geriatric clinicians sometimes advise older patients to open the capsule and sprinkle small amounts of fluoxetine in a flavored beverage such as orange juice. Alternatively, the contents of an entire capsule may be dissolved in a beverage, but only a part (such as one quarter or one half) is consumed each day."
J Clin. Psychiatry (Schatzberg 1991)	"Today, it is clear, however, that the precept of pushing the depressed patient quickly to a high dosage of antidepressant medication is not the optimal strategy for serotonergic agents. 'Start low and stay low' may be the new watchword, particularly with... compounds such as fluoxetine [Prozac]."
J Clin. Psychiatry (Cain 1992)	"In the 5 mg, 20 mg, and 40 mg fixed-dose study, there were no differences in effectiveness between the active treatment groups, all of which were superior to placebo. Side effect dropouts increased significantly with dosage....With endpoint analysis, numerically, 5 mg/day outperformed 40 mg/day which outperformed 20 mg/day...These data point to 5 mg/day as optimal, although there is no evidence that doses below 5 mg/day are not equally effective."
J Clin. Psychiatry (Louie et al. 1993)	"We conclude that starting fluoxetine at doses lower than 20 mg is a useful strategy because of the substantial fraction of patients who cannot tolerate a 20-mg dose but appear to benefit from lower doses.... Patients often benefitted clinically from treatment at lower doses, and failure to tolerate 20 mg/day of fluoxetine should not be taken as evidence that the agent cannot be used efficaciously in these patients."
Conn's Current Therapy (Rakel 1993)	"Many patients respond to the starting dose of 20 mg per day, but a substantial proportion need lower doses (e.g., 2.5 to 10/day)"
N. Engl. J. Med. (Gram 1994)	"The results of three dose-effect studies... [demonstrated that] a dose of 5 mg per day was effective as any of the higher doses."

about every other antidepressant. "The sales representatives for most antidepressants are now giving out sample packs starting with half-strength doses," Dr. Anthony Weisenberger, a top psychopharmacologist, recently said. "They lose so many sales because patients get side effects and quit treatment, the drug companies have finally caught on that the dose makes a big difference."

Why is this happening with drug after drug? One reason is that the standard doses of antidepressants are based on studies of major depression—a severe disorder that requires strong treatment. In contrast, the great majority of office patients with depression have mild disorders. Yet, no distinction is made about treating mild and severe disorders in the dosage guidelines of most antidepressants, so doctors prescribe the same doses to everyone.

DRUGS FOR ELEVATED CHOLESTEROL AND C-REACTIVE PROTEIN

The statins—Lipitor, Zocor, Pravachol, Mevacor, Lescol—were the best-selling group of drugs in America in 2001. There's no doubt that statins help millions by reducing heart attacks, strokes and overall cardiac mortality. But statins harm thousands, perhaps millions more, often unnecessarily.

Duane Graveline's first dose of Lipitor caused amnesia "so severe that I landed in the emergency room of a hospital near my Vermont home. I didn't remember any of it." Dr. Graveline, a retired family doctor, flight surgeon and astronaut (www.spacedoc.net), was perplexed. After all, he wasn't usually sensitive to medications, and he'd taken only 10 mg, the lowest dose recommended and marketed by the manufacturer.

Yet, 10 mg of Lipitor is very strong, much stronger than many people need. It was much stronger than Dr. Graveline needed, because he needed only 2.5 mg of Lipitor—75% less medication than he got. How do we know? Experts advise doctors to select statin doses based on the reduction in LDL-C (the bad, low-density-lipoprotein cholesterol) that each person needs (NCEP 2001). Ten milligrams of Lipitor reduces LDL-C 39%, a strong response needed by cardiac patients and people with severely elevated cholesterol.

But most people with high cholesterol have mild-to-moderate elevations and no cardiac history, and they require only 20% to 30% reductions in LDL-C. This can be attained with only 2.5 mg or 5 mg of Lipitor (Nowrocki et al. 1995; Wolffen-buttel et al. 1998; Bakker-Arkema et al. 1997; Cilla et al. 1996). Dr. Graveline required a 25% reduction in LDL-C and should have been started at 2.5 mg. Yet, there's no information about 2.5 or 5 mg of Lipitor in the package insert or PDR and no pills in these doses, so doctors start everyone at 10 mg, or even 20 mg or 40 mg.

Excessive Statin Doses, Unnecessary Side Effects

Dr. Graveline received 400% more medication than he needed and got a major dose-related side effect because of it. This is a common story. Cognitive and memory problems, sometimes severe and long lasting, occur far more often with statins than doctors recognize. Muscle pain and abdominal discomfort occur frequently. All of these are dose-related.

Liver disorders occur in 1% of patients taking statins. With statins now recommended for 35 million Americans, that's 350,000 people with liver problems, which include liver toxicity and, rarely, death. Dr. W. C. Roberts, the editor-in-chief of the *American Journal of Cardiology*, states, "With each doubling of the dose, the frequency of liver enzyme elevations also doubles" (Roberts 1997). Liver enzyme elevations signify liver injury. So if you get 10 mg of Lipitor when you only need 2.5 mg, your risk of liver injury is also quadrupled.

Lipitor is the best-selling drug In America. In 2001, patients filled more than 57 million prescriptions for Lipitor, and sales are skyrocketing. Zocor, the third-best-selling drug, presents the same dose problems as Lipitor. Zocor's standard starting dose, 20 mg, reduces LDL-C 38%. Many people need only 10 mg or even 5 mg, which reduce LDL-C 30% and 26%, respectively (*Physicians' Desk Reference* 2003). If the standard doses of such widely advertised, top-selling drugs, are so strong, how can we rely on the standard doses of any drug?

More is not always better with medications. Some people do need strong statins. Often, however, a milder drug that works is preferable to a potent one. "Pravachol is the statin drug I prescribe most often because it is the weakest of the bunch," Dr. Stephen Sinatra writes. "We don't need to prescribe large doses of these statins to get results" (Sinatra 2002). People with mild cholesterol elevations usually don't need high potency doses of Lipitor and Zocor, but doctors prescribe them anyway even when milder statins—Pravachol, Mevacor, Lescol—would do (Table 3).

Table 3: *The Potency of Different Statin Drugs*

The initial dose is generally based on the amount of LDL reduction required. However, these numbers are averages, and you may get a larger or smaller response than listed. Statin therapy should always be combined with a heart-healthy diet.

MEDICATION	AVERAGE LDL REDUCTION
Lescol (fluvastatin)	
20 mg	22%
40 mg	25%
80 mg	36%
Lipitor (atorvastatin)	
2.5 mg	20–25%
5 mg	27–29%
10 mg	39%
20 mg	43%
40 mg	50%
80 mg	60%
Mevacor (lovastatin)	
10 mg	21%
20 mg	27%
40 mg	32%
80 mg	40%
Pravachol (pravastatin)	
10 mg	22%
20 mg	32%
40 mg	34%
Zocor (simvastatin)	
5 mg	26%
10 mg	30%
20 mg	38%
40 mg	41%
80 mg	47%

Adapted from: *Over Dose: The Case Against The Drug Companies. Prescription Drugs, Side Effects, and Your Health.* Tarcher/Putnam, New York: October 2001.

Even with the latter drugs, lower doses work for millions of people. A study conducted by the manufacturer of Pravachol showed that just 10 mg was sufficient for 83% of people with moderate cholesterol elevations (Bristol-Myers Squibb 2000). Four studies by Mevacor's manufacturer showed that just 10 mg, with diet counseling, reduced cholesterol satisfactorily in 69% to 75% of subjects. Indeed, the LDL-C of 17% to 26% of subjects dropped below 100 mg/dL, the level sought for people with cardiac disease (FDA 2000). This isn't surprising; some people get much better LDL-C reductions than the averages in the PDR.

Treating Elevated C-Reactive Protein

Half of all cardiac deaths occur in people with normal cholesterol levels. Something else is going on. New studies suggest that elevated C-reactive protein

(CRP), a test for internal inflammation, may be as important an indicator of cardiovascular risk as cholesterol levels, because inflammation in artery walls plays an important role in the development of atherosclerosis (Ridker et al. 2002).

Mainstream doctors are already prescribing statins to people with elevated C-reactive protein (CRP) levels, often at doses that are unnecessarily high. Meanwhile, other, safer methods such as omega-3 oils, which are known to reduce inflammation and cardiac risk (Carroll et al. 2002; GISSI-Prevenzione Investigators 1999), are being overlooked.

DRUGS FOR HIGH BLOOD PRESSURE

Fifty million Americans have high blood pressure (hypertension), and 90% of us will ultimately develop this potentially deadly disease as we age. Hypertension is a particularly vicious disease, a silent destroyer of blood vessels that causes heart attacks, strokes, kidney disease, peripheral vascular diseases and erectile dysfunctions in men. Much of this is preventable with treatment. Yet half of the people starting treatment for hypertension quit within a year. Most do not last 90 days. Why? Medication side effects.

Wendy reacted to one antihypertensive drug after another. Her side effects were dose-related, usually occurring with the first doses, a sure sign of excessive dosing. Wendy knew her hypertension posed a serious threat because relatives had died prematurely from hypertension-related strokes. Wendy was motivated, but side effects made treatment impossible. "I don't know what I'm going to do," she told me.

Experts acknowledge the problem: "Often, the cure is perceived as being worse than the disease, and when this is the case, the patient is unlikely to remain [in] treatment" (Elliott et al. 2000). People get worn down by side effects such as dizziness, weakness, drowsiness, fatigue, diarrhea, muscle cramps, and sexual impairments, and they give up. Doctors often dismiss so-called "minor" side effects, but minor reactions drive millions from needed treatment—with dire consequences. There's a better solution.

Lower Doses Recommended by Experts

Because most side effects with antihypertensive drugs are dose-related, experts recommend starting with the very lowest effective doses. But what are they? Most doctors turn to the PDR, but the PDR's doses often aren't the lowest. An analysis published in the *Archives of Internal Medicine* in 2001 found that for 23 of 40 top-selling antihypertensive drugs, the initial doses recommended by the drug companies in the PDR were much higher than recommended by the Joint National Committee—the national board of medical experts on hypertension (Cohen 2001).

For example, the manufacturer's initial dose for Norvasc, the fifth-most-prescribed drug in the U.S. in 2001, is 5 mg. The experts recommend 2.5 mg, 50% less medication. The manufacturer of Capoten (captopril) recommends 50 mg to 75 mg/day initially, 100% to 600% more than the 12.5 mg to 25 mg recommended by experts.

When Tenormin (atenolol) was introduced in 1976, the one-size-fits-all dose was 100 mg. It wasn't until 1980 that a 50-mg dose was available and until 1989 that 25 mg was produced. The manufacturer still recommends 50 mg initially, 100% higher than the 25 mg recommended by the national board.

The manufacturer of Lasix (furosemide), a commonly prescribed diuretic, recommends 80 mg initially; the national board, 40 mg. The top-selling diuretic hydrochlorothiazide (HCTZ) was recommended at 100 mg initially, but this dose caused serious metabolic problems that affected millions. Yet it took decades for manufacturers to lower the dose to 25 mg, still 100% higher than the 12.5 mg experts recommend today.

Similar over-dosing is seen with top-sellers Zestril, Prinivil, Altace, Inderal (propanolol), Cardura, Cozaar, and many others (Table 4). Is it any wonder why so many people quit treatment?

Some savvy doctors recognize that starting with the lowest dose not only reduces risks, but allows people time to improve their diets, lose weight, start exercising, and learn stress reduction or meditation. These methods not only lower blood pressure, but can reduce the amount of medication you need. As one specialist put it, "With blood pressure, it's easy to overshoot the mark. That's why I always start low and give people time to make other changes. Very often, their blood vessels relax over a period of time and you wind up ultimately needing less medication. When I start with standard doses, we spend the rest of our lives combating side effects."

Note: *When it comes to antihypertensive drugs, some patients are not taking them frequently enough to maintain continuous blood pressure control. Many antihypertensives are sold in "one-per-day" dosing units, but some people need to take these drugs in two divided doses to achieve all-day blood pressure control. Optimal control of hypertension requires blood pressure checks throughout the day. This is the only way to make sure the antihypertensive drug is not wearing off and endangering the arterial system.)*

Table 4: *Lower Initial Doses of Antihypertensive Drugs*

Anti-Hypertensive Drug	PDR	Proven Lower dose
ACE Inhibitors		
Accupril (quinapril):	10 mg	5 mg
Altace (ramipril):	2.5 mg	1.25 mg
Capoten (captopril):	50-75 mg	25 mg
Prinivil, Zestril (lisinopril):	10 mg	5 mg
Angiotensin Receptor Blockers (ARBs)		
Cozaar (losartan):	50 mg	25 mg
Beta Blockers		
Inderal (propanolol):	80 mg	40 mg
Kerlone (betaxolol):	10 mg	5 mg
Levatol (penbutolol):	20 mg	10 mg
Lopressor (Metoprolol):	100 mg	50 mg
Sectral (acebutolol):	400 mg	200 mg
Tenormin (atenolol):	50 mg	25 mg
Zebeta (bisoprolol):	5 mg	2.5 mg
Calcium Antagonists (Blockers)		
Calan, Isoptin, Verelan (verapamil):	120-180 mg	90 mg
Cardizem, Dilacor (diltiazem):	180-240 mg	120 mg
Norvasc (amlodipine):	5 mg	2.5 mg
Plendil (felodipine):	5 mg	2.5 mg
Diuretics		
Demadex (torsemide):	10 mg	5 mg
Edecrin (ethacrynic acid):	50 mg	25 mg
HCTZ (Hydrochlorothiazide):	25 mg	12.5 mg
Lasix (Furosemide):	80 mg	40 mg
Spironolactone:	50 mg	25 mg
Thalitone (Chlorthalidone):	15 mg	12.5 mg
Triamterene:	200 mg	25 mg

Adapted from: *Over Dose: The Case Against The Drug Companies. Prescription Drugs, Side Effects and Your Health.* Tarcher/Putnam, New York: October 2001.

And from: Cohen, JS. Adverse Drug Effects, Compliance, and the Initial Doses of Antihypertensive Drugs Recommended by the Joint National Committee (JNC) vs. the *Physicians' Desk Reference. Archives of Internal Medicine* 2001;161:880-85.

ANTI-INFLAMMATORY DRUGS

In package inserts and PDR descriptions of nonsteroidal anti-inflammatory drugs (NSAIDs) such as Motrin, Voltaren, Celebrex and Vioxx, the FDA specifically requires drug companies to tell doctors to use "the lowest dose for each patient." Why? Because gastrointestinal hemorrhaging and kidney damage from NSAIDs have caused more than 16,000 deaths and 100,000 hospitalizations annually. In 1999, the *New England Journal of Medicine* reported that NSAIDs were the 15th leading cause of death in the U.S.: "Yet these toxic effects remain largely a 'silent epidemic,' with many physicians and most patients unaware of the magnitude of the problem" (Wolfe et al. 1999). And they are unaware that these reactions can occur without any warning signs.

These and other NSAIDs side effects are dose-related, yet doctors and patients often aren't informed about the very lowest effective doses, so overdosing is common.

Motrin and Voltaren

When Motrin (ibuprofen) was introduced in America in 1974, the lowest dose was 300 mg and the most prescribed dose was (and still is) 400 mg. Yet, studies had already proven that 200 mg was effective for osteoarthritis (degenerative arthritis) and rheumatoid arthritis (Chalmers 1969; Brooks et al. 1970; Thompson et al. 1970; Hingorani 1970). Yet, low-dose Motrin wasn't available for 10 years until over-the-counter Motrin arrived in 1984. Most doctors still don't know about its effectiveness and instead usually prescribe 400 mg when half as much will do.

The standard dosage of Voltaren (diclofenac) for osteoarthritis is 50 mg twice or three times daily. Yet, studies before Voltaren's approval showed that 25 mg three times daily is enough for many patients (Durrigl et al. 1975; Mutru et al. 1978; Ciccolunghi et al. 1978, 1979).

Celebrex and Bextra

Dosing with new drugs like Celebrex and Bextra is even worse. Both drugs are one-size-fits-all for osteoarthritis, their most common use. This means that an identical amount is prescribed to football players with injury-induced arthritis and to osteoarthritic 90-year-olds weighing 95 pounds and taking nine other drugs.

The standard dose of Celebrex for osteoarthritis is 100 mg, twice daily. A Mayo Clinic study showed that 50 mg twice daily works for many people with severe osteoarthritis. Moreover, compared with higher doses, the 50-mg dose not only caused fewer side effects, but wasn't associated with kidney problems (Bensen et al. 1999). Starting at this lower, safer dose would make sense, but the package insert and PDR don't say a word about it, and the smallest Celebrex pill is a 100-mg capsule. Bextra was effective at half (5 mg) and quarter (2.5 mg) doses in early studies, but this was ignored and only 10 mg is offered for osteoarthritis.

OTHER DRUGS

A half dose of the antihistamine Allegra is effective, but because the drug is one-size-fits-all and the pill is a capsule, a half dose is difficult to get. Half doses of Claritin, especially Claritin-D, work for some people, but for others even full-dose Claritin isn't enough. In fact, the FDA wanted Claritin produced at 20 mg, but this dose could cause sedation, which would hamper advertising. So doctors and patients are stuck with a one-size-fits-all 10 mg dose that is inadequate for as many as 50% of patients (Hall 2001).

Half doses of Zantac, Axid and Pepcid were proven effective long before they were first marketed in the 1980s. It was only a decade later, when the drugs were marketed over-the-counter, that lower doses became available. Until then, people with mild heartburn got the same strong doses as people with bleeding ulcers.

Prilosec is effective at a half dose of 10 mg, but there's scant information about it in the PDR, so doctors rarely prescribe it. Over-the-counter 10-mg Prilosec will finally allow people to take a lower, safer dose for mild conditions.

Viagra has been linked with more than 500 deaths and 1,500 heart attacks, strokes, and other vascular events (Azarbal et al. 2000). The manufacturer and FDA blame this on patients' age, health, or sexual activity, but many deaths have occurred in men with no major medical problems and before they even had sex. Suspicion remains that Viagra may affect blood pressure or cause a cardiac arrhythmia in rare individuals. The standard starting dose is 50 mg for all men ages 18 to 65, but starting with a half dose is suggested, especially in middle-age men (Cohen 2000), the group in which many reactions have occurred. A half dose works for some men; if it isn't enough, it can be easily increased.

Lotronex generated a controversy that did not have to happen. Lotronex is effective for irritable bowel syndrome, a nasty disorder that limits people's lives, but the condition isn't an emergency requiring immediate powerful dosing. Yet Lotronex was released one-size-fits-all, and after causing hospitalizations and deaths, was withdrawn. As reported to the FDA, one-size-fits-all drugs tie doctors' hands by keeping them from matching doses to patients' needs or reducing doses when side effects emerge. Belatedly, after unnecessary harm and a public furor, Lotronex was re-released in 2002—at a half dose.

Dosage is key with the widely used heart drug digoxin because excessive doses can cause cardiac arrhythmias. For years, the recommended starting dose was 0.25 mg. However, a half dose works. A 1997 study showed that 0.125 mg of digoxin improved congestive heart failure, whereas higher doses produced diminishing improvement and greater toxicity (Slatton et al. 1997).

Sleep medicines such as Ambien and Halcion (triazolam) are often effective at half doses. Halcion is another drug released at excessive doses that, after undue harm, widespread controversy, and being banned in many countries, had its dose lowered.

The neuroleptic Risperdal was marketed in 1993 at 2 mg/day, which was rapidly increased to 6 mg within three days. Doctors quickly learned—from patients' adverse reactions—that these doses were excessive, and the manufacturer now recommends 1 mg the first day, increasing to 3 mg in three days. That's 50% less medication. Still, doctors start some patients at 0.25 mg or 0.5 mg. Similar patterns have occurred with Haldol and other drugs.

Because Xenical, a weight-loss drug, works by blocking fat absorption, it can cause embarrassing side effects. Dosage is key, yet whether you are slightly overweight or massively obese, whether you eat a little or a lot, you get the same dose of one-size-fits-all Xenical: 120 mg three times a day. A half dose was proven effective in studies, but the manufacturer does not market it.

Zyban, widely advertised for smoking cessation, is started at 150 mg, then doubled to 300 mg in three days, but even at this strong dose long-term cessation rates aren't impressive. Some people taking Zyban can tolerate only 150 mg, and others tolerate even less. In 2001, British regulators issued warnings about seizures

with Zyban at the standard dosage (Reuters Health 2002). To obtain lower doses, some doctors prescribe Wellbutrin, an antidepressant that's identical to Zyban but comes in lower doses.

In 2001, users of inhaled steroids for asthma or allergies learned that these drugs had been discovered to cause bone loss. "The message really is, we need to use inhaled corticosteroids at the lowest doses that we can," Dr. Elliott Israel told the *San Diego Union-Tribune* (Associated Press 2001). But why weren't they doing so from the start?

The list goes on and on (Table 5). Repeated discoveries of dose-related toxicities years after people have started medications is not satisfactory. We know that most side effects are dose-related, which means that many are preventable by defining the lowest, safest doses initially, not years or decades later after problems inevitably emerge or drugs go over-the-counter.

Table 5: *Lower, Safer, Effective Doses for 36 Other Frequently Prescribed Drugs That You Won't Find in the PDR or Most Other Drug References*

Even if a drug isn't listed here, a lower dose may still work. Many drugs are never tested at lower doses or the research isn't published, but a lower initial dose may be appropriate in some situations. Work with your doctor. Do not change doses without medical direction; undertreatment can be harmful.

Medication	Drug Company Initial Dose	Effective, Lower Initial Dosing
ALLEGRA (FEXOFENADINE)	60 mg twice daily	20 mg 3 times a day, or 40 mg twice daily (Tinkelman et al. 1996)
AMBIEN (ZOLPIDEM)	10 mg	5 or 7.5 mg at bedtime (Merlotti et al. 1989)
AXID (NIZATIDINE)	150 mg twice daily or 300 mg at bedtime	25–75 mg twice daily 100 mg at bedtime (Cloud et al. 1989)
CELEBREX (CELECOXIB)	100 mg twice daily	50 mg twice daily
COLCHICINE	0.6 mg twice daily	0.3 mg twice daily
CYTOTEC (MISOPROSTOL)	200 mcg 4 times a day	50 or 100 mcg 4 times a day (Cohen et al. 1985)
DALMANE (FLURAZEPAM)	30 mg at bedtime	15 mg at bedtime (Salkind et al. 1975)
DESYREL (TRAZODONE)	150 mg/day	25–100 mg/day (Schatzberg et al. 1987)
EFFEXOR (VENLAFAXINE)	75 mg/day	37.5 or 50 mg/day (Mendels et al. 1993)
ELAVIL (AMITRIPTYLINE)	50–75 mg/day	10–25 mg/day (Roy et al. 1987)
ESTRACE (ORAL ESTRADIOL)	1–2 mg/day	0.5 mg/day (Ettinger 1999)
ESTRADERM (TRANSDERMAL ESTRADIOL)	0.05–0.1 mg/day	0.02–0.025 mg/day (De Aloysio et al. 2000)
ESTRATAB (ESTERIFIED ESTROGENS)	1.25 mg/day	0.3–0.625 mg/day (American Society of Hospital Pharmacists 1999)
LIPITOR (ATORVASTATIN)	10 mg/day	2.5 or 5 mg/day
MEVACOR (LOVASTATIN)	20 mg/day	10 mg/day
MOTRIN (IBUPROFEN)	300–400 mg 3 or 4 times a day	200 mg 3 times a day
NORPRAMIN (DESIPRAMINE)	100 mg/day*	10 or 25 mg/day
PAMELOR (NORTRIPTYLINE)	50–75 mg/day	10 or 25 mg/day (Schatzberg 1991; Sjoqvist et al. 1984)

Table 5: *Lower, Safer, Effective Doses for 36 Other Frequently Prescribed Drugs That You Won't Find in the PDR or Most Other Drug References (continued)*

Medication	Drug Company Initial Dose	Effective, Lower Initial Dosing
PEPCID (FAMOTIDINE)	20 mg twice daily or 40 mg at bedtime	10 mg twice daily or 20 mg at bedtime (Savarino et al. 1989)
PRAVACHOL (PRAVASTATIN)	10–20 mg/day	5–10 mg/day
PREMARIN (CONJUGATED ESTROGENS), for vasomotor symptoms or osteoporosis:	0.625 mg/day	0.3 mg/day
PRILOSEC (OMEPRAZOLE)	20 mg/day	10 mg/day (Lauritsen et al. 1991)
PROZAC (FLUOXETINE)	20 mg/day	2.5, 5, or 10 mg/day
RISPERDAL (RISPERIDONE)	1–2 mg/day	0.5 mg/day (Rainer et al. 2001)
SERZONE (NEFAZODONE)	100 mg twice daily	50 mg once or twice daily (Elliott et al. 1996; Rickels et al. 1994)
SINEQUAN (DOXEPIN)	75 mg/day	10, 25, or 50 mg/day (McCue 1992)
TAGAMET (CIMETIDINE)	800 mg at bedtime	400 mg at bedtime
TOFRANIL (IMIPRAMINE)	75 mg/day	10–25 mg/day (Preskorn 1993)
VASOTEC (ENALAPRIL)	5 mg/day	2.5 mg/day** (JNC V 1993)
VOLTAREN (DICLOFENAC)	50 mg 2, 3, or 4 times a day	25 mg 3 times a day
WELLBUTRIN (BUPROPION)	100 mg twice daily	50 mg twice daily (Kirksey et al. 1983)
XENICAL (ORLISTAT)	120 mg 3 times daily	60 mg 3 times daily (Rossner et al. 2000)
ZANTAC (RANITIDINE)	150 mg twice daily or 300 mg at bedtime	100 mg twice daily (Dobrilla et al. 1981)
ZOCOR (SIMVASTATIN)	10–20 mg/day	2.5, 5, or 10 mg/day (Steinhagen-Thiessen 1994; Tuomilehto et al. 1994)
ZOFRAN (ONDANSETRON)	8 mg twice daily	1–4 mg 3 times a day (Beck et al. 1993)
ZOLOFT (SETRALINE)	50 mg/day	25 mg/day

*The manufacturer recommends starting with a lower dose, but doesn't specify.

**The manufacturer does recommend 2.5 mg for people on a diuretic, but this lower initial dose may also be useful for small, elderly, or other people.

Adapted from: Cohen, JS. *Over Dose: The Case Against The Drug Companies. Prescription Drugs, Side Effects, and Your Health.* Tarcher/Putnam, New York: October 2001.

EXCEPTIONS

There are some drugs for which the low-dose approach does not apply. For example, antibiotics, antifungal, and anticancer drugs should be used at full doses. These drugs are not targeting you, but invaders that can be made stronger if inadequate doses are used.

The Elderly

"The overall incidence of adverse drugs reactions in the elderly is two to three times that found in young adults," states the *New England Journal of Medicine* (Montamat et al. 1989). Although people over age 60 comprise 19% of the population, they account for 39% of all hospitalizations and 51% of all deaths related to medication reactions (Smucker et al. 1990).

Seniors metabolize drugs more slowly than younger people, so they are frequently more sensitive to their effects. That's why gerontologists recommend extra caution in treating seniors and starting with low doses (Table 6). Yet, for scores of top-selling drugs, drug company guidelines tell doctors to use the same strong doses for young and old. Even when we know that blood levels of drugs rise much higher in seniors, doctors are told to ignore this fact and prescribe the same doses.

Table 6: *Lower Medication Doses for Older People*

Experts consistently recommend lower doses for seniors.

J. Am. Geriatrics Soc. (Rochon et al. 1999)	"Choosing the correct dose of a drug therapy is Geriatrics critical when prescribing for older people because adverse effects are often dose-related. The conventional wisdom has been to start low and go slow."
Goth's Medical Pharmacology (Clark et al. 1992)	"In general the best approach is to start with lower doses and to increase dosage slowly and in small increments."
Public Citizen's Worst Pills, Best Pills II (Wolfe et al. 1993)	"If drug therapy is indicated, in most cases it is safer to start with the dose which is lower than the usual adult dose."
Drug Safety (Brawn et al. 1990)	"Starting doses can often be reduced in the elderly."
FDA Consumer Magazine (Williams 1997)	"There is evidence that older adults tend to be more sensitive to drugs than younger adults, due to their generally slower metabolisms and organ functions. . . The old adage, 'Start low and go slow,' applies especially to the elderly."
Archives of Internal Medicine (Everitt et al. 1986)	"The elderly are especially sensitive to both the intended pharmacologic effects of drugs and their undesirable adverse reactions."
BMJ (British Medical Journal) (Rochon et al. 1997)	"If drug treatment is necessary, the lowest feasible dose of the drug should be used."
United States Pharmacopeia, Drug Information (USP DI 1994)	"Some clinicians recommend that geriatric patients, especially those 70 years of age or older, be given one-half of the usual adult dose initially."
Australian Family Physician (Gibian 1992)	Article title, "Rational drug therapy in the elderly, or, How not to poison your elderly patients." Recommends: "The starting dose should be lower than that recommended for younger adults; the maximum tolerated dose may well be lower than for younger individuals." "Select the minimum dose of the safest medication. . . . Start low and go slow."

For example, Allegra blood levels rise 99% higher in seniors versus younger adults. Claritin rises 50% higher. Blood levels of top-selling antihypertensives Zestril and Prinivil rise 100% higher. Blood levels of Prilosec and Nexium are higher in the elderly. Yet, the recommended doses of all these drugs are the same for young and old (*Physicians' Desk Reference* 2003).

The Celebrex package insert tells us "the incidence of adverse experiences tended to be higher in elderly patients," yet no dosage adjustment is recommended. Blood levels of Lipitor, Zocor and Mevacor rise higher in seniors (Cheng et al. 1992). In fact, the Lipitor package insert tells of "a greater degree of LDL-lowering at any dose in the elderly patient population compared to younger adults" (*Physicians' Desk Reference* 2003). So seniors should need less Lipitor, but they are dosed the same as younger people. Could this be why so many reports of cognitive and memory problems in older people taking statins are being reported?

The FDA itself states, "There is evidence that older adults tend to be more sensitive to drugs than younger adults, due to their generally slower metabolisms and organ functions. The old adage, 'Start low and go slow,' applies especially to the elderly" (Williams 1997). Yet the FDA keeps approving drugs at identical doses for young and old. Perhaps this explains why 9% of all hospital admissions for seniors are related to side effects from standard doses of prescription drugs (Montamat et al. 1989).

Women

In the summer of 2002, two studies caused alarm by revealing increased risks of cancer and heart disease with Premarin and Prempro, the top-selling hormone replacement therapies (HRT) for menopausal women (Writing Group 2002; Lacey et al. 2002). The dose of estrogens in these drugs: 0.625 mg. But we've known for years that lower doses of Premarin (0.3 mg) and other estrogens are often effective and cause fewer risks (Ettinger 1999; Weinstein 1987; Greendale et al. 1998; McNagny et al. 1999). Might these doses be safe enough today? Quite possibly, but the studies ignored this obvious question, leaving women in the lurch.

The studies also didn't mention that from 1964 through 1999, the recommended dose of Premarin for hot flashes was 1.25 mg. How much cancer did this double dose cause? Why was such a strong dose approved in the first place? These questions weren't answered. A similar pattern was seen with birth control pills. The hormone doses in the first pills were 300% to 1000% higher than in

Table 7: *Which Hormones Are Natural?*

Premarin is advertised as "natural" because it's derived from horses. For decades, doctors continued making Premarin a best-seller while truly human-identical hormones were available.

Manufactured/Compounded Formulas	Type Of Estrogen	Identical To Human Estrogens
ESTROGENS		
DRUG COMPANY PRODUCTS		
PREMARIN (0.3, 0.625, 0.9, 1.25, 2.5 mg) (Premarin contains 3 different estrogens)	Equilin, Estrogens and Estrone	No Yes
ESTRATAB (0.3, 0.625, 1.25, 2.5 mg) (Estratab contains 2 different estrogens)	Equilin and Estrone	No Yes
OGEN, ORTHO-EST (0.75, 1.5, 3, 6 mg)	Estropipate	No
ESTINYL (0.02, 0.05 mg)	Ethinyl Estradiol	No
ESTRACE (0.05, 1, 2 mg)	Estradiol (Oral)	Yes
ESTRADERM, CLIMARA 0.05 and 0.1 mg/day	Estradiol (Transdermal)	Yes
COMPOUNDING PHARMACY PRODUCTS*		
NATURAL ESTRIOL Estriol: 1, 2 mg twice daily	Estriol	Yes
TRIPLE NATURAL ESTROGEN 80% Estriol, 10% Estradiol, 10% Estrone (0.625, 1.25, 2.5, or 5 mg twice daily)	All 3 Estrogens	Yes
DUAL NATURAL ESTROGEN 80% Estriol, 20% Estradiol (0.625, 1.25, 2.5, 5 mg twice daily)	Estriol/Estradiol	Yes
PROGESTERONES		
DRUG COMPANY PRODUCTS		
MEDROXYPROGESTERONE Provera, others: 2.5, 5, 10 mg		No
COMPOUNDING PHARMACY PRODUCTS		
NATURAL MICRONIZED PROGESTERONE Progesterone: 50, 100, 200 mg twice-daily		Yes
COMBINATION PILLS**		
DRUG COMPANY PRODUCTS		
CONJUGATED ESTROGENS & MEDROXYPROGESTERONE Prempro, Premphase: Premarin 0.625 mg and Provera 2.5, 5 mg		No
COMPOUNDING PHARMACY PRODUCTS		
MIXTURES OF THE ABOVE NATURAL ESTROGENS AND PROGESTERONES ARE INDIVIDUALIZED		Yes

* Not generally available in regular pharmacies. These nonpatented products are made by compounding pharmacies, which upon receiving physicians' orders will mail prescriptions to patients. These products are not generally available in regular pharmacies. For a compounding pharmacy near you, call the Professional Compounding Centers of America, 800-331-2498.

** Although a combination pill is slightly more convenient, a wider choice of hormones and more precise dosing can be accomplished with separate estrogen and progesterone products.

Adapted from: *Over Dose: The Case Against The Drug Companies. Prescription Drugs, Side Effects, and Your Health*. Tarcher/Putnam, New York: October 2001.

today's pills (Snider 2002; Marks 1999; Vessey et al. 1973; Bottiger et al. 1980), yet it took decades—and hundreds of women's lives—before high-dose pills were withdrawn and replaced with today's lower doses.

Similar problems are seen with other medications. A study of ibuprofen for menstrual pain showed that 44% of women did just fine with the 200 mg over-the-counter dose, but the researchers still recommended 400 mg for all women (Shapiro et al. 1981). Studies of cholesterol-lowering drugs show that many women respond to lower doses (Wierzbicki et al. 2000; Ose et al. 1999; Peters et al. 1994; Leitersdorf 1994), but they are routinely prescribed the same doses as men.

Side effects with antihypertensive drugs occur more often in women (Lewis 1996; Israili et al. 1992), which, according to the *American Journal of the Medical Sciences,* "could be due to the fact that women are treated with antihypertensives using the dosage and schedule established with men, even though it is well known that body size, fat distribution and coronary artery size differ in women and men" (Lewis 1996).

Not all women require lower doses, but many do, especially small women. Why aren't doses developed for them? A 2001 report of the U.S. General Accounting Office found not only that women are underrepresented in the dose studies, but even when dose differences are identified, they usually aren't reflected in the final dosage guidelines (GAO 2001). A 2001 report by the National Academy of Sciences recommended additional attention to differences between men and women in diseases and treatments (Wizemann et al. 2001). The panel's report added that medical researchers often view men as the norm while underreporting rather than highlighting sex differences. Commenting on this report, Dr. Woosley added that many drug studies he sees "don't consider sex differences at all" (Kritz 2001).

Is this important? In the United States, 55% of women versus 37% of men take a prescription drug daily (Bowman 2001). And of the 11 drugs withdrawn in recent years, eight (maybe nine) affected women more than men (Table 8).

ENTRENCHED PROBLEMS WITH THE MEDICAL-PHARMACEUTICAL COMPLEX

"It's long been known that for individual subjects the dosage listed on a drug label is not necessarily the right one," Dr. Carl Peck, the highly respected director of Georgetown's Center of Drug Development Science and a former division director at the FDA, stated in September 2002 (Zuger 2002). This is a chilling, and accurate, comment. Yet, the medical-pharmaceutical complex—drug companies, FDA, and mainstream doctors—maintain that our medications are as safe as possible. Clearly, this isn't the case.

Compare the situation to the automobile industry in 1960, when auto executives insisted that our cars were as safe as possible. Then we learned that safety could be greatly enhanced with seat belts, air bags, bumpers that didn't fall off, side panels that didn't cave in, dashboards not made of metal, gas tanks positioned more safely, and other improvements. Similarly, there's much that can be done to increase drug safety and end the side-effect epidemic now, and it begins with identifying and marketing the lowest, safest doses of all drugs.

Problems in Drug Industry Research

Why isn't this done now? Why aren't drug doses designed to fit individuals and to prevent side effects? Don't drug manufacturers care? They do care. "More and more senior executives are concerned that so many patients are dropping out of therapy prematurely,"

Table 8: *Eight of the 11 Drugs Withdrawn by the FDA*

Since January 1997 Posed Greater Risks for Women*				
Drug	Usage	Date Approved	Date Withdrawn	Risk
Pondimin (Fenfluramine)	Appetite suppressant	6/14/73	9/15/97	Heart valve disease
Redux (Dexfenfluramine)	Appetite suppressant	4/29/96	9/15/97	Heart valve disease
Seldane (Terfenadine)	Antihistamine	5/8/85	2/27/98	Cardiac arrhythmias
Posicor (Mibefradil)	Cardiovascular Drug	6/20/97	6/8/98	Low heart rate in elderly, multiple drug interactions
Hismanal (Astemizole)	Antihistamine	12/19/88	6/18/99	Cardiac arrhythmias
Rezulin (Troglitazone)	Diabetes	1/29/97	3/21/00	Liver failure
Propulsid (Cisapride)	Gastrointestinal	7/29/93	7/14/00	Cardiac arrhythmias
Lotronex** (Alosetron)	Gastrointestinal	2/9/00	11/28/00	Impaired intestinal blood flow

* Baycol, withdrawn in 8/01, may also have affected women more.

** Lotronex has been reintroduced at a lower starting dose.

Adapted from: Heinrich, J., Director, Health Care–Public Health Issues, United States General Accounting Office. "Drug Safety: Most Drugs Withdrawn in Recent Years Had Greater Health Risks for Women." Letter to Senators Harkin, Snowe, Mikulski. GAO-01-286R Drugs Withdrawn from Market, Jan. 19, 2001.

declared *DTC [Direct to Consumer] In Perspective* magazine in 2002. "So many are asking, 'What can I do to increase patient retention?'" (Smith 2002). Each year, patients driven from treatment by side effects cost the drug industry billions in sales.

Yet, many economic factors keep the system from changing (Table 9). Drug companies are profit-driven entities, so marketing issues weigh very heavily. Manufacturers feel great pressure to keep costs down while hastening new drugs to market. And drug companies aren't held responsible for the huge costs of dose-related side effects to the healthcare system. The result is that marketing issues frequently outweigh medical science in drug company decisions.

Indeed, marketing influences affect science so severely that even the medical journals, which depend on drug company advertising, rebelled against them. In September 2001, Reuters Health reported: "Seeking to curb the growing influence exerted by drug firms over research findings, the world's top medical journals announced steps on how to prevent firms that fund studies from manipulating results to favor their drugs and bury studies that are unfavorable" (Reuters Health 2001). The editors of *JAMA*, *Lancet*, the *New England Journal of Medicine*, and ten others declared: "We are concerned that the current environment in which some clinical research is [conducted] may threaten medical objectivity...The use of clinical trials primarily for marketing makes a mockery of clinical investigation...." (Davidoff et al. 2001). The journals implemented new guidelines to ensure the integrity of clinical studies, but a year later few medical schools had adopted them (Schulman et al. 2002).

Drug marketing is geared toward doctors' preferences, and doctors like drugs that can be dosed simply and quickly. No time is required to match doses to individual patients if drugs are one-size-fits-all. Expediency sells. So does pumped-up effectiveness. Strong doses produce higher efficacy numbers, which are essential for introducing a new drug into a competitive market. Dr. Thomas Bodenheimer of the University of California, San Francisco, reported: "Drug company studies are often done in younger, healthier populations—providing better rates of effectiveness and fewer adverse reactions—than those who will actually receive the drug" (Bodenheimer 2000).

Dr. Alexander Herxheimer, Professor Emeritus at the Cochrane Center in Britain, concurred in *Lancet*. "For quick market penetration, a drug must be simple to use and effective in the greatest number of people. Drugs are often introduced at a dose that will be effective in around 90% of the target population, because this helps market penetration. The 25% of patients who are most sensitive to the drug get much more

Table 9: Why Don't Drug Companies Produce Doses That Fit Individuals?

1. Cost:	Good dose studies cost a little more.
2. Time:	Good dose studies take a little more time, placing a company at a disadvantage versus its less diligent competitors.
3. Unrepresentative:	Women and seniors are often underrepresented in dose studies. A *Populations: 2001* GAO analysis found that 78% of subjects in dose trials are male.
4. Study designs:	Drug companies prefer to study serious disorders because they are more stable and measurable. Serious disorders usually require potent doses. When marketed, these same doses are often prescribed for milder disorders that don't usually require such potent doses.
5. Less inventory:	Fewer doses cost less to manufacture.
6. Effective advertising:	Higher doses produce higher efficacy rates, which makes great advertising that influences doctors.
7. Effective marketing:	Simplicity sells. Doctors like one-size-fits-all drugs because they are easy and quick to use.
8. Weak FDA regulations:	FDA definitions of "effective and safe" do not ensure that the lowest, safest doses are marketed.
9. FDA analysis:	Fearing long delays if a drug is denied, drug companies use strong doses to ensure that the efficacy passes FDA analysis.
10. No public pressure:	The public isn't aware of the side effect epidemic or that most side effects are dose-related, so it doesn't demand change.
11. No accountability:	The drug industry isn't required to pay the billions for the extra doctors' visits, prescriptions, ER visits, and hospitalizations from dose-related side effects.
12. Basic economics:	With record profits and weak regulation, the drug industry has little incentive to change.

than they need" (Herxheimer 1991). With nearly 100 million Americans taking a prescription drug daily, that's 25 million people.

The FDA's Role

As of November 2002, there were many scientists at the FDA concerned about these dose issues, but also some who weren't. Overall, the FDA has not pushed the drug industry to provide better dose studies or a range of doses to match patients' differences.

The FDA's decisions about drug doses have been criticized even from within the FDA itself. Based on his recent study showing that dozens of drugs ultimately require dosage reductions years after approval, FDA officer James Cross stated in September 2002, "We've seen a lot of situations where drugs are approved by the FDA and subsequent important information about their optimal dose is not determined until afterward" (Zuger 2002).

Even if the FDA wanted to push the matter, could it? The pharmaceutical industry has the biggest lobby in Washington and is a top contributor to elected officials. With Congress pressuring the FDA to approve drugs faster and faster over the past decade, and the new commissioner vowing to speed approvals even more, the FDA isn't likely to reject drugs for better dose studies. "Making sure the dosages that are used best serve the patients should be near the top of the agenda for regulators and the prescribing community," Dr. Herxheimer insists. "Right now this item seems to be nowhere on the agenda" (Herxheimer 2001).

Consequences of a Flawed System

The failure of the system is revealed by disaster after disaster. "Discovery of new dangers of drugs after marketing is common," a 1998 study in JAMA declared. "Overall, 51% of approved drugs have serious adverse effects not detected prior to approval" (Moore et al. 1998).

Another study disclosed that 20% of all new drugs ultimately require a new "black box" warning, indicating serious or fatal reactions. The study noted: "Serious adverse drug reactions commonly emerge after FDA approval. The safety of new agents cannot be known with certainty until a drug has been on the market for many years" (Lasser et al. 2002).

How can long-term side effects be minimized? By using the lowest, safest doses. For example, the jury is still out on the long-term safety of statin drugs, but already serious nerve injuries are being reported. A 2002 study found that "people who had taken statins were 4 to 14 times more likely" to develop peripheral nerve injuries (tingling, numbness, shooting or electrical pain, muscle weakness)

(Gaist et al. 2002). These reactions occur in one in 2,000 users of statin drugs per year. With 35 million Americans projected to take statins, that's 17,500 cases of peripheral neuropathies each year. Discontinuation doesn't always bring reversal. Most important, the risk is cumulative: the higher the dose, the greater the risk.

Doctors and the Drug Industry

Some doctors are terrific. Some aren't. But even good doctors often don't have all of the information you'd like in order to make good dose decisions. Doctors ultimately decide which drugs are successful, so doctors are in a position to demand better drug information, a wider range of drug doses to fit patients and better information about nondrug alternatives. Doctors can play a pivotal role, but so far they haven't demanded anything. Many doctors aren't even aware that a problem exists.

"There is an informational void about pharmaceuticals in the training of most doctors, despite the importance of the prescription in medical care," stated Harvard physician Jerry Avorn. "Most of those who have looked thoughtfully at this process have been appalled at its inadequacy" (Avorn 1995).

The result is that doctors' knowledge of medications is less than ideal, which is directly linked to the high rate of side effects. "Much of the morbidity and mortality currently associated with drug therapy is due to well-recognized adverse effects and reflects our inability as health professionals to implement current knowledge fully," Dr. Alastair Wood, Vice Chancellor of Medical Affairs at Vanderbilt, wrote in 1998 (Wood et al. 1998).

Experience shows that specialists are usually more knowledgeable about drugs than general physicians, but many specialists don't even understand the importance of precision prescribing. One heart specialist said, "Most doctors don't think about dose-response. They think you either get side effects or you don't." Dr. Herxheimer agrees: "Clinicians rarely think critically about the dose–response relations of the drugs they use" (Herxheimer 2001).

Marlene had a serious reaction to Lipitor, so her doctor switched her to Zocor. When another reaction occurred, he switched her to Pravachol. After another reaction, she quit treatment. "If a medication doesn't work or causes side effects," a pharmacist said years ago, "most physicians just switch from one to another, then another, then another, until they either find a drug that works, or they or the patient give up. Very few physicians go to the trouble of adjusting drug dosages to fit their patients. Most don't deviate from the drug companies' recommendations."

Marlene was 64 and obviously sensitive to statin drugs, but the doctor never considered simply reducing the dose. Why? Dr. Woosley, who develops medical training programs, said "Only about fifteen of the medical schools today teach formal courses in clinical pharmacology, which is the discipline that emphasizes individual variability in response to drugs. This small effort will never counter the overwhelming message from the drug industry that one dosage is all that is needed and everyone will respond nicely without side effects."

The result is that most doctors accept drug company information uncritically. They assume that the drug companies and the FDA have chosen doses carefully and that the recommended doses are right for everyone. They accept incomplete side-effect lists in the PDR as the final word, even when published studies repeatedly say otherwise.

Most doctors get their drug information from the drug company-written PDR, the 80,000 drug representatives dispatched to doctors' offices, the drug advertising that fills medical journals, drug company-designed studies, and drug company-underwritten conferences. Many doctors don't hesitate to accept $500 stipends and fancy dinners to receive drug company-paid presentations.

One concerned doctor wrote to the *New England Journal of Medicine*: "The conflicts are obvious to everyone in the field. Who hasn't sat through a company-sponsored presentation by a well-known colleague without squirming a little at the obvious bias in the discussion?" (Young 2000). A doctor visiting from Germany, appalled at the overt willingness of doctors to accept drug company goodies, wrote to JAMA, "In the long run this behavior will undermine the respect and trust of physicians and the standing of the entire medical profession" (Vollmann 2000).

Dr. Marcia Angell, former Editor-in-Chief of the *New England Journal of Medicine*, chided doctors, "It is well to remember that the costs of the industry-sponsored trips, meals, gifts, conferences, symposiums and honorariums, consulting fees, and research grants are simply added to the prices of drugs and devices" (Angell 2000). But many doctors eagerly accept these freebies. As one doctor wrote, "Physicians as a group have an amazing capacity to rationalize their own greed."

Some doctors are rightfully concerned, but not nearly enough. "Many physicians have grown accustomed to industry-subsidized education and now resist paying even modest amounts to attend classes" offered

by unbiased medical centers, the *Wall Street Journal* reported in 2002 (Hensley 2002). Yet, if you bring your own ideas about drugs and doses to your doctor, don't expect a warm reception. Many doctors get defensive, even hostile, when patients question their methods. If there's any area that defines doctors, it's their ability to prescribe drugs. They are the experts, and too often they choose to defend their turf rather than expand their minds.

"Doctors don't like to be challenged," a pharmacist wrote. "One doctor was prescribing Paxil well above the highest recommended dosage. When I asked him about it, he said, 'Are you a doctor? Who are you to be telling me what to do!' Indeed, some doctors have difficulty admitting even common side effects listed in the PDR. Being defensive doesn't strengthen doctor-patient relationships. More and more, doctors are perceived as pill pushers and as defenders of the medical-pharmaceutical machine instead of their own patients.

This perception is enhanced when drug companies can so easily convince doctors to prescribe new drugs even when older, better-known drugs are equally effective. For years, the FDA has warned doctors against using new drugs unless a patient has a specific need. Dr. Janet Woodcock, Director of the FDA Center for Drug Evaluation and Research, has stated, "The sad truth is that, even after all the clinical development that occurs with every drug and even after drugs have been approved for a time, we only have a crude idea of what they do in people" (Cimons 1999). With the FDA approving drugs faster than ever, the American public is frequently the world's first population to try out new drugs.

Yet doctors repeatedly make new drugs bestsellers within months. Drug reps fill doctors' cabinets with "free" samples, knowing that if patients do well on them, they won't want to switch. Drug advertising seizes upon any difference, no matter how trivial, to sway doctors to prescribe expensive new drugs with no track records, and doctors readily oblige. You'd think that after recent disasters with Baycol, Rezulin, Lotronex, Duract, Redux and Fen-Phen, doctors would learn, but they keep prescribing new drugs like Clarinex, Nexium, and Bextra at greater risk and cost. These repeated problems compelled Drs. Marcia Angell and Arnold Relman, another former editor of the *New England Journal of Medicine*, to warn, "Few Americans appreciate the full scope and consequences of the pharmaceutical industry's hold on our health care system" (Angell et al. 2001).

One healthcare observer wrote, "The root cause is the physician, his lack of knowledge or intellectual curiosity.

The pharmaceutical companies are trying to make a buck any way they can, and it is up to the physician to have the fortitude to resist." He has a point. Doctors can't have it both ways. They can't be objective advisors to patients while being so reliant on drug company data and accepting of drug company influences.

Such reliance explains why people today make more visits to alternative practitioners than to mainstream doctors. It explains why mainstream doctors remain largely unaware of proven-effective alternatives like omega-3 oils for reducing inflammation and sudden cardiac death, policosanol and inositol hexanicotinate for reducing cholesterol, or the importance of coenzyme Q_{10} for people taking statins. It explains why mainstream doctors continued to make Premarin, with its conjugated horse estrogens, a top-seller for decades although many types of human estrogens (estradiol, estriol) were available.

It explains why, despite hundreds of studies in medical journals, most doctors don't know anything about magnesium's essential role for normal blood vessel functioning, or that 80% of westerners are deficient in magnesium. By balancing calcium, magnesium is a safer, natural, much less expensive way to help reduce blood pressure than the prescription calcium blockers for which doctors write $4 billion in prescriptions each year, yet few mainstream doctors know about it.

Without drug-company backing, vital information about lower drug doses and nondrug alternatives can take years or decades to permeate mainstream medicine. That's why *Over Dose: The Case Against The Drug Companies* was written to expose the problems in the medical-pharmaceutical complex, while providing low-dose and other important self-help information to patients and doctors. That's why, despite its revelations about the drug industry and mainstream medicine, the *Journal of the American Medical Association, Publishers Weekly, Booklist, Mensa Bulletin,* and everyone else have strongly recommended the book (see reviews at www.amazon.com).

To begin bridging the information gap in mainstream medicine, a free electronic newsletter and a series of inexpensive booklets with evidence-based information for patients and their doctors are being made available. You can sign up for the newsletter or obtain the first booklets (*Magnesium for High Blood Pressure* and *Magnesium for Migraine Headaches*) at www.MedAlternatives.com. If we are to improve our medical care and end the side effect epidemic, we have to make all doctors integrative practitioners. To do so, we have to develop new mechanisms for getting good drug and nondrug information to mainstream doctors.

What You Can Do

If you are doing well on a medication, that's good. That's the goal: receiving benefit without side effects. But if medications are causing problems, or if the next time you need a medication you want to minimize the risk, you need to inform yourself about the lowest, safest doses. Do not reduce doses without your doctor's guidance. Undertreatment can have serious medical consequences.

Hopefully, you have a doctor who recognizes the importance of precision prescribing. Some do. Following a 1999 article in *Newsweek* (Cohen 1999), one doctor wrote, "I have always found that patients do well on low, 'subtherapeutic' doses, which are not just placebos." Another wrote, "As a physician who is a patient with a chronic illness, I can tell you from my vast experience that the doses in the PDR are often way off."

If your doctor, like most doctors, isn't aware of the low-dose alternatives, what can you do? Inform yourself. The day when you could rely on doctors to provide all of the important drug information is long gone. Doctors have less time than ever to read medical journals or to search the medical literature. You can access it yourself at www.PubMed.org, established by the National Institutes of Health. People spend a lot of time researching an auto or stereo purchase; they need to do the same for their own bodies.

YOU HAVE A RIGHT TO BE INFORMED

The American Medical Association's Code of Medical Ethics states: "The patient's right of self-decision can be effectively exercised only if the patient possesses enough information to enable an intelligent choice" (American Medical Association 1999).

What is "enough information?" Surely, if a lower dose is effective, you have a right to know about it. If you are prescribed a standard dose of a drug without being told about an effective lower dose, you haven't received informed consent. If the standard dose has done major harm, you may have grounds to sue.

Higher doses are certainly appropriate sometimes. Emergencies and acute situations demand immediate relief. However, 90% of office visits aren't for acute problems, but for minor or chronic conditions. There's time to match doses to individuals. There's time to start with a lower, safer dose and then to adjust upward, if necessary. You are paying the bill

Table 10: *Are You Sensitive to Medications?*

For You And Your Doctor When Deciding On Medications*
[Enlarge and fill out, and ask your doctor to place a copy on your chart.]

1. Are you sensitive to any prescription or nonprescription drugs?
    o Y o N If yes, please list and describe: _____
_____
_____

2. How are you affected by alcohol? Check one and describe:
    o Easily affected o Moderately affected o Not affected
_____
_____

3. Do some drugs make you tired or sleepy? If so, please list and describe:

Cold or allergy remedies or antihistamines: _____
(such as Benadryl, Claritin, Contac, Tavist, Zyrtec, etc.)
_____

Benzodiazepines: _____
(tranquilizers or anticonvulsants, such as Ativan, Klonopin, Valium, Xanax):
_____

Others: _____
(such as motion sickness remedies Dramamine or Bonine, or anti-nausea agents Phenergan or Compazine):
_____

4. Do some drugs give you energy, or cause anxiety or insomnia?
    o Y o N If yes, please list and describe: _____
_____

Coffee, tea, chocolate or other caffeine-like substances: _____
_____

Appetite suppressants (prescription or nonprescription): _____
_____

Cold or allergy remedies or decongestants (such as Sudafed): _____
_____

Others: _____

5. Have you ever had a reaction to epinephrine (adrenaline chloride, often injected by dentists with pain-numbing medication)? Typical reactions include palpitations, sweating, anxiety, and headaches:
_____
_____
_____

6. Have you had any side effects from any other prescription or nonprescription drugs (such as impaired memory or coordination, blurred vision, headaches, indigestion, diarrhea, constipation, dizziness, palpitations, rashes, swelling, ringing in the ears, other reactions)? If so, please list the drugs and prescribed side effects:
_____
_____
_____

7. Overall, how would you describe yourself with regard to medications?
o Very sensitive
o Not particularly sensitive to medications
o Very tolerant; usually require high doses
_____
_____
_____
_____

*Adapted from: *Over Dose: The Case Against The Drug Companies. Prescription Drugs, Side Effects, and Your Health.* Tarcher/Putnam, New York: October 2001.

and taking the risk, so you have a right to be fully informed about the options.

The low-dose method is especially fitting for:

• Older people

• Small people

• People with multiple medical conditions

• People taking multiple medications

• People with histories of medication sensitivities

• People wanting to minimize costs

• People wanting to minimize risks

The "start low, go slow" approach may take a little more time initially, but it saves a lot of time (and money) in the long run. Some people will get surprisingly good results with a low dose and never need higher doses. Some won't, and the dose will need to be increased. Even then, they are assured that they are getting exactly what their bodies need.

Not everyone opts for the low-dose approach. Some people know that they aren't sensitive to medications. With such people, starting with standard doses is valid. Indeed, some people seem resistant to drugs and require very high doses. The key is to match the dose with the person. Ultimately it doesn't matter whether you need a low dose or a high dose—what matters is that you get the right dose for you.

Doing so requires good dose information and a range of drug doses. If anything, the drug industry is providing less of each. The irony is that other industries not only recognize the differences among people, they capitalize on it. They produce cars, clothes, cosmetics, and all kinds of commodities in vast arrays to match individual sizes and needs. But with its monopolistic patents and sway over doctors, the drug industry can do what it likes and charge what it wants.

In 2001, 3.2 billion prescriptions were filled in America—12 prescriptions for each man, woman, and child. Forty-six percent of adult Americans take a prescription drug every day. Each year, drug sales increase 25% (*Pharmacy Times* 2002), and medication side effects remain a top killer. How can we restore sanity to this system? It will have to begin with you.

You are paying the bill and taking the risk, so you have a right to ask questions and to request better information. You have a right to ask your doctor why he's selecting a specific drug at a specific dose. Are there lower doses that work? What is his source of information? We must require doctors to explain their decisions, to think about their choices, and to consider other sources of information.

Most people don't like taking medication. If they must take it, they want to use as little as possible. When the low-dose approach has been offered to patients, most have opted for it, side effects have dropped dramatically, success rates have climbed, patients are pleased, and so is the doctor. Most side effects are avoidable. The side effect epidemic can be halted, and everybody wins. But the current system is entrenched, so change is going to have to begin with us.

☎ FOR MORE INFORMATION

Much of the information contained in this chapter was excerpted from an article written for *Life Extension* magazine by Jay Cohen, M.D. The following books and booklets by Dr. Cohen are available and highly recommended:

• *Over Dose: The Case Against The Drug Companies. Prescription Drugs, Side Effects, and Your Health.* Tarcher/Putnam, New York: October 2001.

• *Magnesium For High Blood Pressure (Hypertension): The Complete Guide To Using Magnesium To Help Prevent and Treat High Blood Pressure Naturally.* Del Mar, CA: 2002. Books available at: www.medalternatives.com

• *Magnesium for Migraine and Cluster Headaches: The Complete Guide To Using Magnesium To Prevent and Treat Migraines and Cluster Headaches Naturally.* Del Mar, CA: 2002.

These books can be ordered by calling 1-800-544-4440.

61,000 cases of newly diagnosed epilepsy in the elderly. In general, the disease is secondary to cardiovascular or cerebrovascular conditions (Epilepsy Association 2001a; Epilepsy Foundation 1999; 2002a,b). Epilepsy in the elderly poses special problems (Kilpatrick et al. 2002). Many elderly already take numerous drugs which can negatively interact with AEDs; resistance is decreased; and susceptibility to serious injury from seizure-related falls and accidents is increased (Epilepsy Foundation 2003d). Monotherapy is preferred in the elderly. Typically, elderly individuals with epilepsy take lower doses of AEDs (the first-line choice is often Dilantin).

OUTCOME

Monotherapy vs. Polytherapy

Seizures can be well controlled with modern drugs and medical techniques in about 80% of individuals who have been diagnosed with epilepsy (NINDS 2001). The optimal balance between seizure control and undesirable side effects is obtained with monotherapy, using one *first-line* anti-epileptic drug recommended for its effectiveness to control the specific seizure with the fewest side effects.

Although seizures are well-controlled with a single anticonvulsant in individuals with some types of epilepsy, approximately 20% of patients with primary generalized epilepsy and 35% of patients with focal epilepsy have medically intractable seizures (Cascino 1990; Nair 2002). If seizure activity is not controlled by an initial dose of a first-line AED, and there is no drug toxicity, the dose of the drug should be systematically increased. If seizures continue, another first-line drug can be tried, or another first-line drug can be added to the first AED regimen (polytherapy or polypharmacy).

The rationale behind polytherapy is to use two (or more) AEDs that have different modes of action, but do not cause an increase in adverse side effects (Ochoa et al. 2002). If a third or fourth AED is tried at appropriate therapeutic levels and seizure activity continues, the likelihood of finding an AED that will enable a patient to be seizure-free drops to as low as 5%. Patients who are intractable to medical therapy should be referred to an epilepsy surgery center to determine if they are candidates for some other form of treatment (surgical, electrical, dietary) (Nair 2002).

AED Withdrawal

After a seizure-free interval of 2 years of continuous use, consideration can be given to withdrawing the AED (Fischer 1998; Nair 2002). The risk of seizures recurring after AED discontinuation is 25% in patients without risk factors and 50% in patients with risk factors (age at onset; structural lesion; abnormal EEG; number of AED drugs taken; history of intractable epilepsy) (Medical Research Council 1993; Berg et al. 1994; Nair 2002). The decision to stop AEDs is highly individualized. If an AED is discontinued, it should be reduced (tapered off) gradually (e.g., by 25% every 2–4 weeks) over several days to several weeks depending on the individual and characteristics of the AED (Fischer 1998; Nair 2002).

Gradual tapering minimizes withdrawal seizures. The tapering off procedure should be slower with some AEDs (carbamazepine, phenobarbital, benzodiazepines). If seizure activity is exacerbated by withdrawing the drug, the dose should be increased to the previous level. After seizure control is regained, the tapering off procedure can be tried again, reducing the dose by smaller amounts and increasing the time interval between decreases (Fischer 1998). Risk of seizure recurrence decreases as the time without seizures increases (Medical Research Council 1993).

SUMMARY

While it can be a debilitating disease, there are many treatment options for epilepsy (Richard et al. 1995). Conventional treatments include antiepileptic drugs, surgery, and electric therapies. Diet plays an important role in treating the disease. Sugar intake should be monitored, and triggers such as alcohol and caffeine should be avoided. Additionally, allergy testing should be performed to rule out additional food triggers.

The ketogenic diet is also an option, though its efficacy for adults remains questionable. Stress level is also crucial. Promoting a relaxed state, through exercise, diet, and nutrient supplements, is beneficial. The ability to recognize an aura is also helpful, and can lead to the development of behaviors designed to interrupt the brain's seizure activity. Women and people over 50 with epilepsy should be aware of special considerations, and discuss these with their doctor. Finally, use of nutrient supplements can increase seizure control.

1. Amino acids taken on an empty stomach may be helpful: taurine, 1–4 grams daily (begin at lower end); glycine, 600 mg, one to three times daily; alanine, 600 mg, one to three times daily.

2. For a more relaxed state and to counteract the effects of certain antiepileptic drugs: calcium, 150 mg daily (may be increased to 3 grams if well tolerated).

3. For those not receiving enough sunlight: vitamin D, 400 mg daily.

4. For seizure reduction in some people: vitamin E, begin at 150 IU daily and increase to 400–800 IU daily.

5. To control electrical discharge in the brain: magnesium, 450–900 mg daily, taken on an empty stomach.

6. To aid in sugar metabolism: manganese, 10–30 mg daily.

7. For glutathione peroxidase deficiency: selenium, 10–100 mcg daily.

8. To protect brain cells, especially in children: zinc, 25–80 mg daily, in the form of zinc gluconate lozenges.

9. Several herbs have beneficial effects for seizure control: *Coleus forskohlii*, hyssop, black cohosh, blue cohosh, lobelia, and Saiko-Keishi-To (follow instructions of formulary for dosage).

CAUTION B vitamins may be of value to some individuals with epilepsy by aiding the conversion of glutamic acid to GABA; however, in other individuals it might be risky. If taken long term, the full vitamin B complex should be used: 100 mg, three times a day, is recommended (physician-supervised injections are preferable). To help improve circulation, additional vitamin B_3 in a dose of 50 mg daily may be taken. For non-sensitive individuals, vitamin B_6 in a dose of 80–400 mg daily may be taken.

Note: *Large doses of vitamin B6 can cause peripheral neuropathy.*

 FOR MORE INFORMATION

Epilepsy.com
(http://www.epilepsy.com/epilepsy/medicine_lines.html)

Citizens United for Research in Epilepsy (CURE)
(312) 923-9117

Epilepsy Foundation
(301) 459-3700; (800) 332-1000

Epilepsy Institute
(212) 677-8550

National Council on Patient Information and Education
(301) 656-8565

The National Institute of Neurological Disorders and Stroke
(301) 496-5751; (800) 352-9424

Parents Against Childhood Epilepsy (PACE)
(212) 665-7223

 PRODUCT AVAILABILITY

Vitamin B complex, vitamins B_1, B_3, B_6, B_{12}, folic acid, taurine, glycine, GABA, calcium, evening primrose oil, vitamin D, vitamin E, Gamma E Tocopherol/Tocotrienols complex, black cohosh, forskolin, magnesium, manganese, SMSC (selenium), and zinc can be ordered by telephone at (800) 544-4440 or online at www.lef.org.

Esophageal Reflux

Esophagus: from the Greek word, *oisophagos*, meaning throat

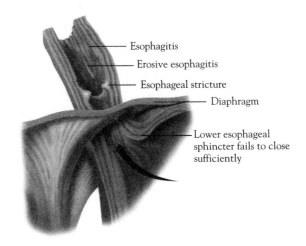

Esophagitis

Erosive esophagitis

Esophageal stricture

Diaphragm

Lower esophageal sphincter fails to close sufficiently

Gastrointestinal Reflux Disease (GERD) is caused by irritation of the esophageal mucosa by acidic stomach contents that reenter the esophagus. Inflammation and discomfort can be caused by very small quantities of acidic material. (Anatomical Chart Company 2002®, Lippincott Williams & Wilkins)

What the English have called dyspepsia—or heartburn—is actually esophageal reflux. The discomfort of esophageal reflux is caused by the *upward* backflow of stomach acid, bile, pepsin, ingested liquids, and foods into the esophagus. The esophagus makes no contribution to digestion. Its sole function is to squeeze food down into the stomach. In normal digestion, the valve that separates the esophagus and stomach (the lower esophageal sphincter) opens to allow food to pass into the stomach. Then it closes to prevent food and stomach (gastric) contents from flowing back up. Esophageal reflux occurs when the esophageal sphincter relaxes more often than it should or at inappropriate times, allowing the stomach contents to back up.

The stomach has a lining that protects it from the effects of acid and other digestive juices. Because the esophagus lacks this type of lining, the stomach contents that reflux will cause pain, inflammation (esophagitis), and damage. Excessive backflow of stomach contents into the esophagus causes gastroesophageal reflux disease (GERD). Untreated GERD can result in precancerous changes called Barrett's esophagus and can eventually progress to esophageal cancer. The prevalence of adenocarcinoma of the esophagus is increasing in Western nations at a rate greater than any other form of cancer.

There are serious misconceptions about esophageal reflux. Most laypeople and physicians attribute reflux and heartburn only to stomach acid backing up into the esophagus. This is further drilled into patients and consumers by a barrage of advertisements for drugs and antacids that function to reduce stomach juice acidity. While acid reflux is a major cause of heartburn, there are other constituents of stomach juice that can induce long-term damage to the esophageal lining. For example, some people experience alkaline reflux damage to the esophagus that emanates from *pancreatic* secretions in the duodenum (upper small intestine). For these people, acid suppression therapy using antacids (Tums), histamine 2 (H2) receptor antagonists (Tagamet), and proton-pump inhibitors (Prilosec) is only a partial solution.

In this protocol, the terms GERD (gastroesophageal reflux) and esophageal reflux will be used interchangeably.

CAUSES OF GERD

The underlying cause of GERD is an incompetent lower esophageal sphincter. The condition is aggravated in persons who are smokers, overweight, or pregnant. A person who eats fried, fatty, or spicy food; eats chocolate, peppermint, and citrus fruits; or drinks coffee, tea, alcohol, and carbonated drinks can also experience reflux because these substances can increase the tendency of the esophageal sphincter to relax. The most important admonition is to avoid lying down within 3 hours of eating. This means persons with GERD should avoid eating food for 2–3 hours before bedtime.

Gastritis (inflammation of the stomach itself), ulcer disease, and excess consumption of nonsteroidal anti-inflammatory drugs (NSAIDs) such as aspirin and ibuprofen can result in reflux. Sometimes, particularly in obese people, the opening through the diaphragm that allows the esophagus to pass from the chest to the abdomen becomes enlarged. This condition is called a hiatal hernia and can result in esophageal reflux.

One estimate is that 40% of the population in the United States has some degree of esophageal reflux, with 20% of adults complaining of weekly episodes of heartburn and 7–10% complaining of daily symptoms.

SYMPTOMS OF GERD

The most obvious symptom of esophageal reflux is heartburn. Heartburn occurs after eating and can last from a few minutes to a few hours.

Heartburn feels like a burning sensation that can begin in the pit of the stomach or lower breastbone region. It can then move upward into the chest and throat, causing a bitter acid taste. Heartburn is also called acid regurgitation, acid indigestion, or sour belching. A person can also experience heartburn from bending over or lying down. Sometimes belching can be a symptom of heartburn. When esophageal inflammation is present, symptoms may manifest as a sharp, stabbing pain in the center of the chest that can take as long as a week to subside, even after acid-suppressing therapy has been initiated.

Persons with GERD can have long-term complications. GERD can cause esophageal scarring or Barrett's syndrome, a chronic irritation from acid-bile reflux that causes the normal esophageal lining cells to be replaced by dysplastic (precancerous) cells. When dysplastic cells are present in the esophagus, there is an increased risk for development of cancer.

Pain during swallowing and slight bleeding can be caused by the inflammation of the esophagus. Peptic esophageal ulcers are open sores on the esophageal lining, with the pain occurring behind or just below the breastbone. The pain can be relieved by antacids, taken 40 minutes to 1 hour after eating. Peptic ulcers can be healed by using drugs to reduce stomach acid over a 4- to 12-week period. Peptic ulcers heal slowly and tend to recur. The esophagus can become more narrow, making swallowing solid food painful.

A number of tests can be used in persons with esophageal reflux, including x-rays; endoscopy; manometry of the lower esophageal sphincter; or the Bernstein test. Before an x-ray is taken, the patient drinks a barium solution and then lies on an incline with the head lower than the feet, causing reflux of the barium from the stomach into the esophagus. X-rays will also reveal any esophageal ulcers or a narrowed esophagus. *Esophagoscopy* (endoscopy) involves examining the esophagus through a flexible viewing tube which can also take a biopsy to correctly identify acid reflux. *Manometry* is a pressure measurement taken of the esophageal sphincter that will indicate its strength and will distinguish a normal sphincter from one that has poor function. The *Bernstein test* involves placing an acid solution into the lower esophagus. If the symptoms appear quickly and then disappear when a salt solution

is placed in the lower esophagus, the problem is acid reflux. If diagnosis of esophageal reflux is difficult, the physician may consider measuring the acid levels inside the esophagus using a pH test.

CAUTION X-rays to evaluate upper digestive tract disease expose patients to tremendous amounts of radiation. Ask your physician for a non-radiation diagnostic, such as endoscopy, rather than CAT scans which use x-rays.

CONVENTIONAL TREATMENT

The reason for treating esophageal reflux is to prevent gastric contents from entering the esophagus, allowing this area to heal and preventing further damage. Fortunately, there are a number of lifestyle modifications that people can make on their own. Although it will be difficult to follow all of the recommendations, eliminating just some of these underlying causes of reflux could help reduce the severity of GERD. Here are the most commonly recommended lifestyle modifications:

1. Maintain a reasonable weight.

2. Avoid eating tomatoes, garlic, and onions; chocolate and peppermint; citrus fruits; and fatty and oily foods.

3. Avoid coffee, tea, alcohol, and any carbonated drinks.

4. Instead of eating three large meals each day, eat smaller meals more frequently (perhaps four or five daily). Do *not* lie down after meals.

5. Do not eat for at least 2–3 hours before bedtime. When going to bed, elevate the head of the bed about 6 inches to facilitate keeping gastric contents in the stomach. Also, sleeping on the right side causes less pressure on the esophageal sphincter, helping to keep gastric contents from backing up.

Note: *Elevating the head of the person's bed 6 inches (use a few telephone books, foam, or wood blocks) is much more effective than elevating only the patient's head with an extra pillow. When a person sleeps at an angle with the entire upper part of the body elevated, gravity helps keep the stomach contents out of the esophagus.*

6. Get plenty of exercise and rest.

7. Do not smoke because nicotine relaxes the esophageal sphincter.

8. Do not take excessive amounts of aspirin, ibuprofen, and other NSAIDs. People who take prescribed aspirin to prevent heart attack and stroke should take aspirin early in the day.

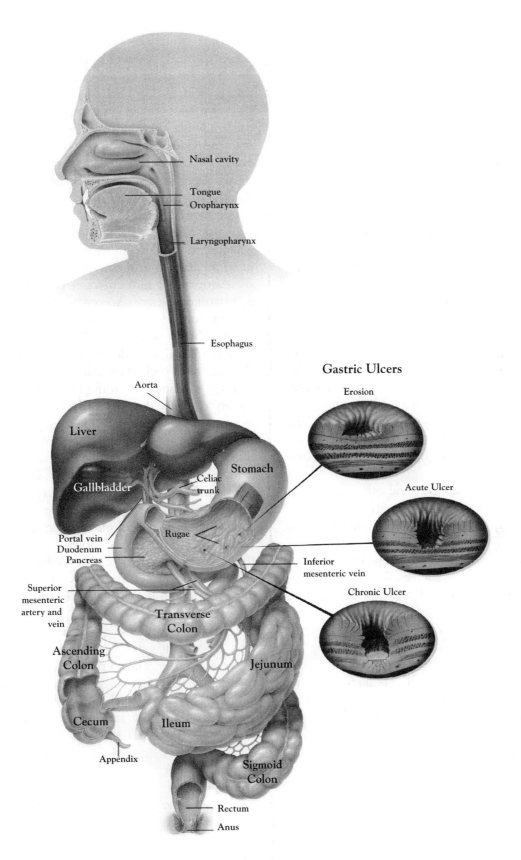

The esophagus is a muscular mucus-lined tube (about 10 inches long) that connects the pharynx to the stomach. Ulcers are open wounds in the stomach or duodenum caused by acidic gastric juice. Frequent use of NSAIDs and infection from the *H. pylori* bacterium are associated with the development of ulcers. (Anatomical Chart Company 2002®, Lippincott Williams & Wilkins)

Conventional management of GERD symptoms in patients with mild to moderate esophageal reflux without erosive esophagitis (in which the lining of the esophagus breaks down) requires a systematic approach beginning with lifestyle modification plus *over-the-counter* preparations, such as H2 antagonists (Tagamet, Pepcid, Zantac, Axid) and antacids (Tums, Maalox, etc.). If these measures do not suppress heartburn, then *prescription* pharmacologic management with proton-pump inhibitor drugs (Nexium or Prevacid) has become standard therapy. Many physicians now prescribe proton-pump inhibitor drugs as a first-line therapy. Prilosec is now available over-the-counter. Its generic name is omeprazole.

For people who have GERD, long-term therapy might be required. It should be individualized according to severity of symptoms; degree of esophagitis; and presence of other reflux complications. In most patients, maintenance therapy is vital. In the last decade, the proton-pump inhibiting drugs, omeprazole (Prilosec) and lansoprazole (Prevacid), are taken by people who were previously unresponsive to other medications. Omeprazole and lansoprazole completely suppress acid production, normally providing relief after 1 week. The benefits, safety, and costs of the available therapeutic alternatives must be considered in choosing acute and long-term therapy.

Appropriate use of *endoscopy* and other diagnostic tests is important in ruling out erosive esophagitis, Barrett's syndrome, esophageal cancer, stomach ulcers, or stomach cancer. For those who are at high risk for developing esophageal cancer (Barrett's syndrome), the long-term use of drugs, such as Nexium, Prilosec, or Prevacid, may reduce the risk of esophageal cancer, but as you will read later, taking these proton-pump inhibiting drugs for more than 6–12 continuous months could cause serious problems, including an increased risk of esophageal cancer.

People who do not respond well to or do not want to take medication might opt for a *surgical procedure* known as Nissen fundoplication. This procedure wraps the stomach around the esophagus, creating a new valve to prevent acid from refluxing from the stomach. A laparoscope is used in this minimally invasive surgery, dramatically reducing the discomfort and recuperative time, with the patient being hospitalized for 2 nights and returning to full activity in 1–2 weeks.

ALTERNATIVE TREATMENT

One of the difficulties associated with chronic or long-term administration of H2 blockers (Tagamet) or proton-pump inhibitors (Nexium) is that the stomach is not intended to have a weak acid environment. One of the functions of hydrochloric acid in the stomach is to break down proteins for digestion. The failure of the stomach to perform this task may result in improper digestion and the absorption of so-called digestive remnants into the blood through the wall of the intestine. Normally, proteins are broken down into individual amino acids. If the proteins are not entirely broken down and get into the blood, this can set up allergies mediated by certain white cells called T-cells, resulting in a host of other problems, such as autoimmune disease.

Yet, as noted earlier, the constant irritation of stomach contents on the lining of the esophagus can result in an increased risk of esophageal cancer and esophagitis. Antioxidant nutrients can protect against esophageal inflammation. According to published studies, antioxidant nutrients may lower the risk of esophageal cancer (Taylor et al. 1994; Zhang et. al. 1995). If you have heartburn, consider taking 3 tablets of Life Extension Mix with each meal. Life Extension Mix is a high-potency, multinutrient formula that contains nutrients shown to reduce the risk of esophagitis and gastric and esophageal cancers. (More about esophageal cancer risk reduction will appear later in the protocol.)

Digestion of food is a high priority and has a high demand for enzymes. When we eat, enzymatic activity begins in the mouth, where salivary amylase, lingual lipase, and ptyalin initiate starch and fat digestion. In the stomach, hydrochloric acid activates pepsinogen to pepsin (which breaks down protein) and gastric lipase begins the hydrolysis of fats. Without proper enzyme production, the body has a difficult time digesting food, often resulting in a variety of chronic disorders.

Digestive enzyme supplements should be considered to aid digestion and help prevent heartburn. Enzymes are essential to the body to absorb and fully use food. The primary digestive enzymes are proteases (to digest protein); amylases (to digest carbohydrate); and lipases (to digest fat). These enzymes function as a biological catalyst to help break down food. Raw foods also provide enzymes that naturally break down food for proper absorption.

People with GERD should take digestive enzyme products at the beginning of each meal to facilitate rapid breakdown of ingested food. A digestive enzyme supplement rich in protease, lipase, and amylase—which are all naturally produced in the body—can also aid in digestion in aged or diseased individuals.

Propulsid is a pro-motility drug that improved some of the motility defects present in GERD by increasing peristaltic movement and moving food out of the stomach faster. After its approval in 1993, this drug later showed lethal cardiac side effects and was withdrawn from the market on July 14, 2000. (Propulsid is available by prescription through a limited-access program regulated by the manufacturer and the FDA.) Interestingly, a completely natural supplement called Digest RC also functions to enhance peristaltic movement, facilitating digestion of fats and proteins and moving them out of the stomach faster. Digest RC was used for 45 years in Europe before being introduced to the United States. The only precaution associated with Digest RC is that persons whose gall bladder has been removed should not take Digest RC because it can cause a temporary increase in biliary secretion.

Take 2–4 tablets of Digest RC 5 minutes before a meal. Digest RC can also be taken following a meal. Do not take Digest RC within 3 hours of bedtime because it has a temporary effect of increasing bile secretion (*refer to the Digestive Disorders protocol for more information about the use of digestive enzymes and Digest RC*).

LICORICE EXTRACT

Glycyrrhizin, an extract of licorice root (*Glycyrrhiza glabra*), exhibits various anti-inflammatory, anti-allergic, anti-gastric ulcer, anti-hepatitis, and anti-hepatotoxic activities. Because glycyrrhizinic acid, a constituent of licorice, has been linked to high blood pressure, a process was developed to remove it, resulting in deglycyrrhizinated licorice or DGL, a beneficial product with no known side effects. DGL protects the digestive tract from corrosive stomach acids by increasing the number of mucus-secreting cells from glands in the upper portion of the stomach known as the fundus. This mechanism of action stimulates and/or accelerates the differentiation to glandular cells as well as mucus formation secretion leading to an improved stomach environment (van Marle et al. 1981).

In 20 patients with aphthous ulcers who were taking DGL, 15 experienced improvement the first day followed by complete healing by the third day (Das et al. 1989). A clinical double-blind trial of DGL on ulcer patients demonstrated a statistically significant reduction in ulcer size (Turpie et al. 1969). Therefore, because of its ability to accelerate healing of the stomach, esophagus, and mucous membranes, DGL would be a useful adjunct to any treatment for gastroesophageal reflux disease.

For reflux and support of the lining of the stomach and intestinal tract, chew two 380-mg tablets 3 or 4 times daily between meals.

DANGERS OF DRUGS USED TO TREAT REFLUX

The long-term use of histamine 2 (H2) receptor antagonist drugs such as Tagamet, Pepcid, Zantac, and Axid could be dangerous to persons who have GERD. One reason is that although these agents help suppress heartburn pain, they do not prevent damage done to the esophagus by acid, enzymes, bile, and other stomach contents. Some physicians are concerned that suppressing heartburn pain with H2 receptor antagonist drugs might result in patients not making the lifestyle changes needed to control chronic esophageal reflux (Suleiman et al. 2000). As discussed earlier in this protocol, failure to adequately control GERD can result in esophagitis and esophageal cancer.

A growing trend in treating reflux-induced heartburn is the long-term prescribing of proton-pump inhibitors, such as Nexium, Prilosec, and Prevacid. These drugs are heavily advertised for relief of heartburn and have become huge moneymakers for pharmaceutical companies. Some patients like taking these drugs because the drugs often relieve the symptoms of heartburn without any apparent side effects.

The short-term use of proton-pump inhibitors cures 90% of esophagitis cases. Increasingly, physicians are prescribing these drugs for long-term use to prevent heartburn and to keep esophagitis from returning. There is a theory that these acid-suppressing drugs will reduce esophageal cancer risk by preventing acid irritation. Evidence, however, shows that long-term use of proton-pump suppressing drugs may not only increase esophageal cancer risk, but other digestive tract cancers as well.

Therefore, although proton-pump-inhibiting is highly effective and safe in providing *short-term* relief from heartburn and esophagitis, there is an underlying cancer risk in their *long-term* use. The problem is that proton-pump inhibitors alleviate acid reflux, but the total number of reflux episodes remains unchanged, meaning that in certain people, the esophagus continues to be exposed to bile, pepsin, and other contents of the stomach. The solution is to find agents that reduce the number of reflux episodes, thus sparing the esophagus from chronic exposure to irritating agents that should stay in the stomach. Blocking reflux episodes would protect the esophagus against excess regurgitation of all stomach contents including acid and bile (Boeckxstaens et al. 2002). This is important because bile reflux has also been implicated in cellular dysplasia that can lead to esophageal cancer.

However, far more frightening is the fact that long-term use of proton-pump inhibitors may increase the risk of pancreatic, stomach, and other cancers via an overlooked mechanism. The culprit in cancers related to proton-pump inhibitors is a hormone called "gastrin." When stomach acid is low, the stomach secretes gastrin in an attempt to induce acid secretion. Because proton-pump inhibitors virtually eliminate stomach acid, large amounts of gastrin are continuously secreted in a futile attempt to produce stomach acid. Excess levels of gastrin are associated with a host of digestive tract cancers.

Adenocarcinoma cells of the esophagus are loaded with gastrin receptor sites (Moore et al.). One study showed that gastrin binds to the receptor sites of these cancer cells and increases the proliferation rate by 50–100% in a dose-dependent manner (Corsetti et al.). The scientists who conducted this study pointed to the grim statistic that adenocarcinoma of the esophagus is increasing in the Western world at a rate greater than any other malignancy. This epidemic of esophageal adenocarcinoma might be correlated with the increased use of proton-pump inhibiting drugs. Numerous studies show that gastrin stimulates the growth of other adenocarcinoma cells in the digestive tract.

Thus, a logical question is: How much excess gastrin do proton-pump-inhibiting drugs induce? One study showed that Prilosec increased gastrin levels by 46% after 4 weeks at 20 mg a day (Pilotto et al. 1995). In another study, long-term administration of Prilosec was associated with a two- to fourfold increase in gastrin levels over baseline in one-third of the patients (McCloy et al. 1995).

A mechanism by which gastrin stimulates cancer cell proliferation is through activation of nuclear factor-kappa beta (NF-KB) (Toyota et al.). Pancreatic (Liptay et al.), gastric (Todisco et al.), lung (Chen et al. 2002), and colon cancer cells often over-express NF-KB on their receptor sites and use this as a growth vehicle to escape cell regulatory control (Thorburn et al. 1998). Gastrin has been shown to over-express NF-KB through the protein kinase C pathway.

The good news is that nutrients, such as curcumin, green tea, and soy genistein help suppress over-expression of NF-KB. However, this does not mean that one should take proton-pump inhibitors over the long-term and expect dietary supplements to provide complete protection.

We want to emphasize that there is *no* evidence of any increased cancer risk in the short-term use (6–12 months) of proton-pump inhibiting drugs to treat esophagitis. However, persons with existing cancer (adenocarcinoma) may want to avoid proton-pump inhibiting drugs altogether because increased gastrin could fuel rapid propagation of gastrin receptor- and NF-KB receptor-positive cancer cells.

Because the concern with long-term use of proton-pump inhibitors (as well as H2 receptor antagonists) is that chronically elevated gastrin levels could increase the risk for developing a deadly adenocarcinoma, the challenge is to find another method of treating GERD. We have already discussed lifestyle changes that have proven to be highly effective. Additionally, our research has uncovered an FDA-approved drug (baclofen) that may be more effective in the comprehensive treatment of esophageal reflux than proton pump inhibitors. Baclofen (generic for Lioresal) is a skeletal relaxant used for disorders that are associated with muscle spasms (multiple sclerosis and spinal cord injuries), as well as for other nervous system conditions including hiccups.

Baclofen has been shown to reduce the number of esophageal sphincter relaxations. In a study of 20 patients with moderate to severe esophagitis, 40 mg of baclofen reduced the number of reflux episodes by 43% (Zhang et al. 2002). In another study, baclofen was given to 10 GERD patients for 30 days at a dose of 10 mg 4 times daily (four patients received a placebo). Several measurements of reflux were measured including esophageal pH; frequency and intensity of bitter taste; regurgitation; and pain at various times of the day. The number of reflux episodes was significantly lower in the baclofen group (265 before baclofen; 54 after baclofen). The percentage of time with esophageal ph below 4 was also significantly lower. Baclofen reduced the intensity of symptoms such as pain by 76%, and reduced the frequency of symptoms by 90%. There were no improvements in the placebo group. The researchers concluded that "baclofen given for one month reduces esophageal acid reflux and significantly improves symptoms in people with GERD" (Giccaglione et al.).

For those with severe GERD, a dose of 10 mg of baclofen taken 4 times a day should be considered. The starting dose of baclofen should be 5 mg 4 times per day for the first two weeks. Rare side effects include constipation, nausea, dizziness, and hypotension. Baclofen has been around for 30 years and side effects usually occur only in persons with underlying health problems.

Note: *Baclofen should not be taken by persons with cerebral palsy, stroke, or Parkinson's disease because its benefits have not been proven in these conditions. Persons with epilepsy or psychotic disorders may worsen while taking baclofen.*

Female Hormone Replacement Therapy

Women should be concerned about their levels of sex steroid hormones at two critical times in their life. The first interval is from the onset of menses until menopause and the second interval is from menopause to death. Hormonal changes occurring during these life phases can significantly influence a woman's feelings of health and well-being.

Menopausal symptoms parallel the declining production of estrogen, progesterone, testosterone, and DHEA. These changes in the levels of hormones and the associated symptoms begin to affect many women around age 45. Restoration of hormonal balance can relieve menopausal symptoms, enabling women to feel normal again. A youthful balance of hormones protects against osteoporosis, mental depression, thinning of the skin, immune dysfunction, and other age-related diseases and discomforts.

This protocol will discuss state-of-the-art options for managing menopause. See the *Premenstrual Syndrome and Menstrual Irregularities* protocol for information on properly managing hormone levels during child-bearing years.

HOW WIDESPREAD IS THE PROBLEM?

According to the North American Menopause Society, no data exist on the number of women in the United States that are menopausal. The 2000 Census estimated 41.8 million women are over age 50 (the average age of spontaneous menopause). Estimates are that another 1.8 million women reached menopause in the year 2000, or 4200 per day (Pinn et al. 2002). A large population of female baby boomers is now approaching menopause. There is growing concern about how to treat "the change of life" issues associated with menopause which is growing exponentially.

Concern about the life-threatening side effects of synthetic hormone drugs has caused many women to deny themselves the benefits of safer, natural hormone replacement therapy. Proper hormone replacement can prevent degenerative disease and improve physical and emotional functioning at the beginning of menopause and thereafter. Many of the sexual dys-

functions, including lack of libido, can be mitigated when hormone levels are restored to youthful levels. Menopause might also be delayed and be less traumatic if hormonal adjustments are made in a timely manner. A number of female health problems have been linked to altered hormonal balance. Life expectancy trends suggest that women may spend the last one third to one half of their lives with a less than optimal hormonal balance. Quality and quantity of life for these women will be determined by how well they (and their doctors) understand and manage hormone replacement.

THE ESTROGEN DILEMMA

Between the ages of the early forties to mid-fifties, the amount of a woman's primary estrogen dwindles. This deficiency can cause menopausal symptoms, including hot flashes, depression, vaginal dryness, anxiety, and forgetfulness. The decline in production of many hormones, including estrogens, is a direct cause of premature aging and increased osteoporosis.

Estrogen replacement therapy (ERT) remains controversial. FDA-approved estrogen drugs have been documented to cause cancer and increase the risk of cardiovascular disease. The first conclusive report showed that women taking estrogen and a synthetic progesterone-like drug (known as a "progestin") showed a 32–46% increase in breast cancer (Colditz et al. 1995). Another study showed a 29% increase in breast cancer, along with a higher risk of heart attack, stroke, and pulmonary embolism in women taking a popular estrogen/progestin drug combination for only 5.2 years (Rossouw et al. 2002).

Colditz et al. (1995) showed that the carcinogenic risk of estrogen/progestin replacement therapy becomes most pronounced when used for 10 or more years. Other data have suggested that the relative risk is increased by 20% after only four years of estrogen use, and that there is a 40% increase in the risk of breast cancer when estrogen and a progestin are combined (Smart et al. 1997). The hormone combination of estrogen and the progestin used was Premarin®, which contains mostly estrone (a strong estrogen), along with a synthetic form of progesterone (a progestin) called medroxyprogesterone. (The combination product is sold as Prempro®). Most of the studies used Premarin® as the estrogen and medroxyprogesterone as the progestin. Premarin® is derived from the urine of pregnant mares and contains cancer promoting estrogens, whereas medroxyprogesterone is a synthetic form of progesterone. These hormones are not identical to the sex hormones found in humans.

Rodriguez et al. (1995) showed that long-term estrogen replacement therapy increased the risk of ovarian cancer. Women who used estrogen drugs for 6–8 years had a 40% higher risk of ovarian tumors, while women who used estrogen drugs for 11 or more years had a 70% higher risk of dying from ovarian cancer. The increased carcinogenic risk from estrogen is a serious concern. Cancers of the breast, uterus, and ovaries account for 41% of the incidence of cancer in U.S. women. Breast cancer is at epidemic levels, affecting 1 in 8 women, up from 1 in 30 women in 1960. Conventional ERT and estrogen-based oral contraceptives have been used extensively since 1960. An alternative is needed to provide the anti-aging and health-enhancing benefits of estrogen, while protecting against the risks of cancer and cardiovascular disease.

Why Estrogen Drugs Have a Bad Reputation

Traditionally, the estrogen prescribed by physicians was either a synthetic form of estradiol or Premarin®, a preparation containing mostly estrone. Estradiol and estrone are very potent estrogens. Most innovative doctors believe that all of the hormones, including the three main estrogens (estradiol, estriol, and estrone) along with progesterone, pregnenolone, and the androgens (testosterone and DHEA) should be balanced in the post-menopausal years to optimize overall well-being and minimize side effects.

The cause of the increased incidence of breast, ovarian, and uterine cancer may relate to the imbalance of the hormones used to replace the declining hormones that occur during menopause. Too much estradiol and progestins were prescribed in the past and the doses were not individualized. The hormones were not given in a natural cyclic manner when they were first used many decades ago. This common practice was simply the "standard of care" of that time.

Another cause of the increased incidence in cancer may relate to the fact that most physicians were not taught to follow hormone levels after menopause. Once the diagnosis of menopause was made, the patient was placed on a generous standard dose of estrogens with or without a standard dose of a progestin. (Progestin was prescribed only if the woman had an intact uterus, i.e., didn't have a hysterectomy, in order to protect the uterus from developing cancer.) If symptoms persisted, the doses would be adjusted accordingly. The hormone drugs were only available in a few, limited dosages. A synthetic testosterone would be added to the regimen if symptoms had not improved substantially. Blood levels of hormones were not monitored, but if they had been, physicians would have been surprised by the large amounts of estrogens

that were found in women given standard doses and by the excess of testosterone in some women who were given more than necessary. Physicians simply weren't taught to check blood levels of hormones to monitor therapy. It wasn't the standard of care.

The standard starting dose of Premarin® was 0.625 mg daily. This dose was adjusted by halving or doubling that amount as determined by the patient's symptoms. Most of the hormones previously prescribed were either synthetic or extracted from pregnant mare's urine. They were not formulations that were bio-identical to the natural hormones in the human body. Estrace®, a prescription drug containing estradiol derived from soybeans, was sometimes prescribed at a starting dose of 0.5 mg.

The newer methodology prescribes compounded, human hormone preparations that are applied topically as creams, gels, or patches, or delivered sublingually or orally. The goal is to achieve a minimal dose of each hormone to meet an individual's needs, based on hormone levels and symptoms. Other routes of administration are possible, including intra-vaginal creams or suppositories, or rectal suppositories.

Dietary factors must be considered before initiating hormone replacement therapy. A woman who consumes large amounts of soy might have higher serum levels of estrogens and would require less or no supplemental estrogens. Some women receive sufficient benefits from using soy isoflavone extracts and other natural supplements such as DHEA, a hormone precursor.

A small percentage of women will continue to make adequate amounts of hormones even in the post-menopausal years, regardless of diet. These women might only need replacement of either estrogen, testosterone, progesterone, or nothing at all. Hormone status can change with time, so symptoms should be monitored and hormone levels should be checked if symptoms occur.

Dangerous Estrogen Drugs

The most popular estrogen drug in the United States has been Premarin®, which contains estrogens derived from the urine of pregnant mares. This is a mixture of "conjugated" estrogens (mostly estrone), which are foreign to the human body and can promote cancer. Other popular estrogen drugs that are sold under the names Estrace® and Estraderm® are pure natural estradiol. Estrace® is usually derived from soybeans. Provera® is the name of a popular synthetic progestin often given with Premarin® to help prevent estrogen-induced uterine cancer. Unfortunately the standardized combination of Provera® and Premarin®

(Rossouw et al. 2002) may actually increase the risk of estrogen-induced breast cancer and cardiovascular disease (Weiss et al. 2002).

Estrogen and progestin drugs have side effects that cause many women to avoid using them. In addition to increased risk of cancer, some other risks of estrogen/progestin drugs include:

- Weight gain
- Abnormal blood clot formation (thrombosis)
- Increased risk of gallstones, fibroid tumors, and headaches
- Premenstrual-type symptoms (irritability, fluid retention)

In 2002, the largest randomized, controlled trial on hormone replacement therapy conducted on healthy women with an intact uterus was halted (Rossouw et al. 2002). The study was called the Women's Health Initiative (WHI). The trial was stopped because there was a significant difference between the placebo group and the treatment group receiving Prempro®, a drug combination containing both conjugated equine estrogens (Premarin®) and a progestin called medroxyprogesterone acetate (Provera®), which mimics the action of the human hormone progesterone.

The risk of coronary heart disease, stroke, venous thromboembolic (blood clots in the legs) disease, cancer of the breast, and events related to coronary heart disease (such as a heart attack) was increased by 29% in women taking estrogens plus medroxyprogesterone. The rate of stroke was 41% higher in women receiving estrogen plus medroxyprogesterone. Women in the estrogens plus medroxyprogesterone group also had a twofold increase in the rate of venous thromboembolism, deep vein thrombosis, and pulmonary embolism (Rossouw et al. 2002).

Although previous studies of Premarin® with or without a progestin suggested that Premarin® can protect against coronary heart disease, these studies usually reported results following less than 10 years of therapy. In the WHI study, which was halted after 5 1/2 years, the risk of developing coronary heart disease and pulmonary embolism clearly began within the first year of use and continued for at least 5 1/2 years. The risk of stroke and invasive breast cancer only rose significantly after 3–5 years of medicating with these synthetic hormones. The WHI study involved a large number of women who were randomized from the beginning into the two groups. On a positive note, there was a reduction in osteoporotic fractures by 25%. The authors of the study reported:

Results from the WHI indicate that the combined post-menopausal hormones CEE (Conjugated Equine Estrogen which is Premarin®), 0.625 mg/day, plus medroxyprogesterone which is Provera®, should not be initiated or continued for the primary prevention of coronary heart disease (CHD). The substantial risks for cardiovascular disease and breast cancer must be weighed against the benefit for fracture reduction in selecting from available agents to prevent osteoporosis (Rossouw et al. 2002).

A strong association between estrogen-only therapy and ovarian cancer has been reported, especially in those who have taken the replacement hormone for more than 10 years (Lacey et al. 2002). Considering these latest developments in the research of hormone replacement therapy, our advice to women who are already taking Premarin® and Provera® is to visit your physician, wean off the hormones, and find another means of controlling menopausal symptoms.

Why Women Still Choose Synthetic Estrogen

Despite unpleasant and sometimes lethal side effects, many women use estrogen drugs because estrogen reduces the side effects of menopause and because of the anti-aging properties of estrogen. Estrogens are steroid hormones that promote youthful cell growth in organs of the body. The anti-aging benefits of estrogen replacement therapy include:

- Enhanced skin smoothness, firmness, and elasticity (Castelo-Branco et al. 1998)
- Enhanced moistness of skin and mucous membranes
- Enhanced muscle tone
- Reduced genital atrophy and enhanced sex drive (Head 1998)
- Reduced menopausal miseries such as hot flashes and anxiety (Vincent 2000)
- Reduced risk of osteoporosis (Sites 1998)
- Reduced risk of colon cancer
- Improved memory and neurological function (Sherwin 1994; Jacobs et al. 1998)
- Greater feelings of well-being

The benefits of estrogen make it desirable for most menopausal women to maintain youthful levels of this hormone. The question is: can the anti-aging benefits of estrogen be obtained without increasing the risk of cancer and arterial blood clots? One alternative to potent hormonal drugs is natural estrogen supplements produced from plant sources. These estrogens are known as "phytoestrogens," have been studied extensively, and may be safer. The literature reveals some interesting findings about plant-derived estrogens. Phytoestrogens from soy reduce hot flashes and protect against age-related diseases such as osteoporosis, heart disease, and cancer (Vincent et al. 2000).

NATURAL DIETARY APPROACHES TO MENOPAUSE

Before we go into the specifics of plant-derived natural hormone replacement, it is important to understand that plant-derived natural hormones are weaker than synthetic hormones. Natural plant-derived hormones require a nutritionally supportive environment for optimal function. A balanced nutritional program will optimize any natural therapy that you undertake. The concept of natural hormone replacement therapy originated from observations that many of the menopausal disorders of Western civilization were absent in the East. The Asian diet contains a significant amount of soybean products consumed with a low intake of fat. It is likely these factors contribute to a very low incidence of menopausal disorders in Asia.

Hormones are messengers, carrying a signal from one organ to another or from one organ to a group of specialized cells. Estrogens are hormones that create growth of the endometrium (lining of the uterus). Steroid hormones like estrogens send their message by combining with receptors inside the cell of the target organ. The hormone-receptor complex then causes changes in the cellular metabolism of the cell by turning on or turning off certain genes that code for the manufacture of specific proteins. These changes in proteins produce a biological effect. Estrogens, for example, causes growth of the uterine lining to prepare for implantation of a fertilized egg.

Aside from affecting the uterus, estrogens play different roles in other organs. Estrogens help maintain bone mineral density. To exert these effects on the genes, the structure of the estrogen receptor must be such that it efficiently combines with the hormone molecule. The structure of the hormone receptor is dependent upon the kind of food that we eat, particularly the kind of fat. Imbalances of dietary fat cause changes in the three-dimensional structure of the cell membranes that interact with the estrogen receptors such that the receptor site's configuration (or shape) is changed. Thus, when the hormone comes along to transmit a message, it may not properly fit into the receptor or interact with the cell membranes correctly, and the message is either changed, delayed, or not sent. Think of the receptor site as a lock and the hormone as a key. If the fit is off, then the lock is harder to open, if at all. By taking in a good balance of saturated and unsaturated fats (which include omega-3 oils), and eliminating trans fatty acids will help ensure that receptor sites operate optimally.

After most hormones have transmitted a message they are typically deactivated by being metabolized, so that they are deactivated and excreted. Estrogen metabolism occurs in the liver by a process called glucuronidation or conjugation. If this process is not working efficiently, active estrogen may continue to circulate and overstimulate the genes. Any chronic digestive or liver condition and any imbalance of healthy bowel bacteria can potentially lead to this situation. Keeping our digestive system in a healthy state may seem very remote from menopausal hormones and hot flashes; however, it is an integral part of the whole process.

What should your diet be like as you enter menopause? Like any other healthy diet, it should be moderate in protein and complex carbohydrates, with less than 30% of the calories coming from fat. Saturated fat from animal products should be low, and unsaturated fats should come from cold water fish (salmon, mackerel, sardines, halibut, and herring), with a good portion of the diet containing fresh fruits and vegetables. Keeping the bowel bacteria in balance by taking probiotics such as Lactobacillus acidophilus on a regular basis can be helpful.

Soy Estrogens Versus Estrogen Drugs

Based upon records of dietary soy consumption in Japan, where breast cancer incidence is very low, daily soy isoflavone intake has been estimated to be about 50 mg a day. The typical Western diet provides only 1–5 mg per day of soy isoflavones to possibly protect against several forms of cancer.

Clinical studies show that soy phytoestrogens in doses ranging from 40–160 mg per day produced rapid and significant reductions in menopausal symptoms. Other studies reported that in countries where soy is a major constituent of the diet, women do not experience uncomfortable menopausal symptoms like Western women (Ostman 1997). Soy phytoestrogens may be safer and almost as effective as FDA-approved estrogen drugs. Soy isoflavones protect against menopausal disorders that are normally treated by FDA-approved estrogen drugs. Unlike these synthetic drugs, phytoestrogens from soy have been shown to:

• Prevent cancer at multiple sites

• Prevent gallstones

• Protect kidney function

• Stimulate bone formation

- Lower cholesterol levels
- Inhibit the oxidation of LDL cholesterol
- Inhibit the development or progression of atherosclerosis

Unlike estrogen drugs, phytoestrogens have a balancing effect on the body. When estrogen levels are too low, their very mild estrogenic effect raises total estrogenic activity. When estrogen levels are too high, they compete with estrogen at cellular receptor sites, thus lowering total estrogenic activity. Women given 80 mg daily of soy phytoestrogens for two months demonstrated greater estrogenic activity and reduced hot flashes (Cassidy et al. 1994).

Not all studies support the positive effects of phytoestrogens, but most studies agree that soy intake greater than 50 mg/day increases bone mass and lowers low-density lipoprotein cholesterol and triglycerides (Wagner et al. 1997; St. Germain et al. 2001), but has no estrogenic effect on vaginal and uterine epithelium. There have been frequent positive anecdotal reports on the effect of soy on menopausal symptoms such as hot flashes, which are not supported by clinical studies.

Phytoestrogens Prevent Osteoporosis

Genistein is one of the active components soy that prevents bone loss in ovariectomized rats. The mechanism of action of genistein (the most abundant soy phytoestrogen) differs from that of estrogens (Fanti et al. 1998). Post-menopausal women received daily either soy protein containing phytoestrogens or milk-derived protein that contained no phytoestrogens. Significant increases in bone density and bone mineral content of the lumbar spine in the women receiving the higher dose of phytoestrogens derived from soy protein diets (which provided 2.25 mg of isoflavones) resulted, but not after milk-derived protein. Soy isoflavones show potential for maintaining bone health (Potter et al. 1998).

Studies on post-menopausal Japanese women consuming at least 50 mg/day of soy isoflavones confirmed the positive effect on bone density (Horiuchi et al. 2000); the lowering of low density lipoprotein cholesterol; and amelioration of the adverse cognitive effects of menopause (Somekawa et. al. 2001). An adequate amount of soy must be consumed to have any impact on bone density and soy may not be sufficient when given alone to improve bone density of the hip, an important bone to protect against fractures in the elderly. The long-term effect of soy on bone density has not been established. Women who are at high risk for osteoporosis should not rely only on soy phytoestrogens to maintain their bone density. (Refer to the

Osteoporosis protocol for complete information about maintaining healthy bone integrity.)

More Benefits of Soy Estrogens

The widespread use of insecticides, fungicides, chemicals used in manufacturing, and chlorine-based substances that mimic or mutate estrogen might be a major cause of the breast cancer epidemic. These fat-soluble substances called "hormone modulating pollutants" accumulate in the body over time and are contributing factors in the development of hormone-related cancers. Women with breast cancer have high levels of estrogen-altering pesticide residues in the fat cells of their breasts, compared to women who do not have breast cancer. Soy contains "friendly estrogens" that block estrogen-receptor sites on cells that are vulnerable to stimulation or blockade by carcinogenic "mutated" estrogens.

The estrogenic activity of the principal soy isoflavones daidzein, genistein, and glycitein has been confirmed (Setchell et al. 2001). Consumption of modest amounts of soy protein results in relatively high blood concentrations of phytoestrogens that could have a significant hormonal effect in individuals (Setchel 1998). Considering the increased risk of breast cancer and uterine cancer in women using estrogen drugs, one alternative for women might be to include more phytoestrogens in the diet, such as soy-based products containing isoflavones, daidzein, or genistein, which have been shown to protect against breast cancer, uterine cancer, and cardiovascular disease (Hawrylewicz et al. 1995; Goodman et al. 1997; Anthony et al. 1998; Cline et al. 1998).

The amount of soy isoflavones needed to provide positive hormonal effects is approximately 40–60 mg/day. Just four ounces per day of a fermented soy product such as natto or tempe provides this. Fermented soy products are preferred over other soy food preparations because they are more easily digested and absorbed. If soy food products do not appeal to your palate, soy isoflavones and soy protein concentrate can also be taken as a supplement in capsule form.

Cynomolgus female monkeys without ovaries simulate the hormonal situation of the post-menopausal woman. When given soy protein isolate, the monkeys showed a significant improvement in lipoprotein concentrations and plasma lipids, with improvements in insulin sensitivity and glucose tolerance. There was a significant interaction between soy and E2 (β-estradiol), such that animals consuming soy protein and E2 had the lowest content of cholesterol in the arteries. This suggests that ERT combined with dietary soybean protein has beneficial effects on cardiovascular risk factors (Wagner et al. 1997). Life Extension believes that additional agents are needed to protect against the increase in cardiovascular risk caused by estrogen drugs.

In another study with male and female Cynomolgus monkeys, it was shown that isoflavone-intact soy protein significantly improved LDL and HDL cholesterol and displayed the least amount of atherosclerosis. The researchers concluded: "Potential mechanisms by which soy isoflavones might prevent atherosclerosis include a beneficial effect on plasma lipid concentrations, antioxidant effects, antiproliferative and antimigratory effects on smooth muscle cells, effects on thrombus formation, and maintenance of normal vascular reactivity" (Anthony et al. 1998). (For more information about soy, in general, and cholesterol reduction, see the *Cardiovascular Disease: Comprehensive Analysis* chapter).

Soy Estrogens Are Readily Available

While the health benefits of soy are well-documented, it has been difficult and expensive in the past to obtain the amount of genistein and other soy isoflavones that scientists suggest to treat menopausal symptoms. In October 1997, a soy extract concentrate was introduced that contained enough phytoestrogens from soy to provide the amount of genistein, daidzein, and glycitein found in the typical Japanese diet. This soy extract is so concentrated that only a small amount is needed to obtain enough phytoestrogens to provide effective estrogen replacement for many women. This concentrated soy extract is now available in several commercial formulations. Thomas et al. (2001) found that bioavailability for soy isoflavones in supplement form is similar to that observed in people on Asian diets.

Ipriflavone and Bone Loss

Early reports on the synthetic isoflavone known as ipriflavone were positive for the prevention of bone loss, certainly in early menopause. This synthetic isoflavone is synthesized from daidzein and has generated considerable attention in the research community interested in hormone and bone loss (Gennari et al. 1998). A 2-year trial tested women that were post-menopausal by less than five years who had low vertebral bone density: 56 women received 200 mg of ipriflavone three times a day with meals or one gram of calcium daily. After two years, vertebral bone density did not change in those receiving ipriflavone. By comparison, women receiving the calcium showed limited bone loss during the treatment.

In another 2-year study, 198 post-menopausal women (50–65 years of age) were randomly allocated to treatment with oral ipriflavone. All subjects received one gram of calcium carbonate. The ipriflavone-treated women showed a significant increase of vertebral bone density, whereas the placebo group showed a significant decrease of vertebral bone density. Urinary hydroxyproline (HOP)/creatinine (Cr) ratios, a measure of bone loss, were significantly decreased, suggesting a reduction in the turnover of bone. There was a reduction in vertebral fractures in the ipriflavone-treated group compared to placebo (Agnusdei et al. 1997a).

Osteoporotic women (65–79 years of age) with prevalent vertebral fractures received ipriflavone, plus one gram of oral calcium daily. A significant increase in forearm bone mineral density occurred after ipriflavone treatment. The placebo group showed limited bone loss, probably due to the calcium supplement. Urinary HOP, a measure of bone loss, was decreased in the ipriflavone-treated group, suggesting a reduction in bone turnover. There was a reduction in vertebral fractures in the ipriflavone-treated group (Agnusdei et al. 1997b). Almost 3000 patients were treated with ipriflavone for a total of over 3000 patient-years in three countries. The incidence of adverse reactions in the ipriflavone-treated patients was similar to placebo, suggesting that long-term treatment with ipriflavone may be considered safe, may increase bone density, and may possibly prevent fractures in elderly patients with established osteoporosis (Agnusdei et al. 1997b).

Halpner et al. (2000) found that urinary N-linked teleopeptides, another marker of bone breakdown, declined by 29% in those receiving ipriflavone supplements. Nozaki et al. (1998) tested conjugated estrogens and ipriflavone together and reported that in ovariectomized women, bone mineral density was reduced 48 weeks after treatment by the use of placebo, conjugated estrogen alone, and ipriflavone alone. However, a combination of conjugated estrogen and ipriflavone resulted in much less bone loss following ovariectomy. The reason for using a potent estrogen drug and ipriflavone was to prevent acute short term bone loss following ovariectomy.

Contrary to the majority of trials, a recent trial with 474 post-menopausal osteoporotic participants showed no changes versus placebo in bone loss or biochemical markers of bone metabolism. Ipriflavone caused lymphocytopenia (a decrease in the number of lymphocytes) in a significant number of women, although this effect was reversible. This latter side effect has not been reported before and needs to be monitored when considering treatment (Alexandersen et al. 2001). Research on ipriflavone is in its early stages and further studies are warranted before considering ipriflavone as a viable alternative or adjunct to other hormonal treatments for the prevention of bone loss.

Black Cohosh Alleviates Menopausal Discomforts

An important and widely studied plant component used to treat menopause is a standardized extract from the black cohosh plant, which is also known as

Cimicu-fuga racemosa. Black cohosh extract is approved by the German Ministry of Health for the treatment of menopausal symptoms related to estrogen deficiency. Standardized black cohosh has been trademarked under the name Remifemin® for sale as a drug in countries throughout the world. More than 1.7 million women in Europe and Australia have used this natural herbal extract to treat menopausal symptoms. Clinical studies show that Remifemin® alleviates hot flashes, depression, anxiety, vaginal atrophy, and other menopause-related disorders (Liske 1998).

Women who were given standardized black cohosh extract, Valium®, or Premarin® for menopausal symptoms revealed that the women in the black cohosh group were relieved of their depression and anxiety more effectively than the women receiving Valium® or Premarin® (Warnecke 1985).

When black cohosh extract was given to women under age 40 who produced very little natural estrogen or progesterone due to a total hysterectomy, it was observed that supplemental estrogens had differing effects. Estriol (a weak, but safer estrogen compound), Premarin®, Premarin® and a progestin drug, black cohosh extract, and placebo were given. The women were rated according to symptoms of hot flashes, irritability, and heart palpitations. Women in all groups receiving different forms of estrogen-progestin and black cohosh extract experienced a 30% improvement. The majority of women receiving the estrogen drugs or black cohosh extract were symptom free. Most importantly, the women receiving the black cohosh extract reported fewer side effects. This study showed that phytotherapy with standardized black cohosh worked as well as estrogen drugs at relieving menopausal symptoms, but produced fewer uncomfortable and dangerous side effects (Lehmann-Willenbrock et al. 1988).

The most impressive early study on black cohosh was carried out in 629 menopausal women. Black cohosh extract produced clear improvement in over 80% of patients within 6–8 weeks. Both physical and psychological symptoms improved. The results of the changes in specific menopausal symptoms were as follows:

Symptom	Percent who became symptom-free	Percent who showed improvement
Hot flashes	43.3	86.6
Profuse perspiration	49.9	88.5
Headache	45.7	81.9
Vertigo	51.6	86.8
Heart palpitation	54.6	90.4
Tinnitus	54.8	92.9
Nervousness/irritability	42.4	85.6
Sleep disturbances	46.1	76.8
Depressive moods	46.0	82.5

Most of these patients reported benefits within four weeks. After 6–8 weeks, complete resolution of symptoms was reported in a high number of patients (Stolze 1982).

Duker et al. (1991) investigated the hormonal mechanisms by which black cohosh alleviates menopausal symptoms. Hot flashes corresponded closely with a surge of luteinizing hormone (LH) released from the pituitary gland in response to estrogen deficiency. The weak estrogen-like effects of black cohosh suppressed increased luteinizing hormone secretion in menopausal women and was specifically linked with a reduction in hot flashes (Duker et al. 1991).

Black cohosh extract has shown estrogenic effects within the body in several studies, but it does not elevate estrogen levels in the blood. It appears to bind to estrogen receptors and mimic the hormonal effects of a weak estrogen, like estriol. Estriol protects against the types of cancers that more potent forms of estrogen (estradiol and estrone) may cause. Black cohosh has an "estriol-like" effect. This weak estriol-like effect of black cohosh has not been shown to have a significant effect on bone density. Because bone density decreases substantially during the first seven years after menopause, osteoporosis is one of the long-term risk factors resulting from a prolonged deficiency of hormones or an imbalance of these hormones in the menopausal and post-menopausal period.

Liske (1998) states that black cohosh shows good therapeutic efficacy and tolerability. Because of the impressive safety record of standardized black cohosh extract, it is has become a popular natural alternative to FDA-approved estrogen drugs. This phytoestrogen has no effect on the prevention of osteoporosis. It should be used in conjunction with other agents that protect against bone loss.

MORE ESTROGENIC PLANTS

There are other important plant-derived hormone modulators that are used by alternative physicians to treat menopausal symptoms. Estrogens are continually being modified (metabolized) as they circulate in the body. They are converted from one form to another which causes their biological activity to vary considerably. While the combination of soy phytoestrogens and standardized black cohosh may provide a nearly complete estrogen replacement, there are other hormonal factors to adjust for if the metabolism of youth is to be maintained (or restored).

Licorice Root Extract

An extract from the licorice root called glycyrrhetic acid (GA) stimulates the natural conversion of testosterone to estrogen in the body (Takeuchi 1988). Glycyrrhetic acid is an antioxidant that is often used to protect the liver and suppress viral activity in hepatitis patients (Abe et al. 1994). Some alternative cancer clinics prescribe high doses of GA in injectable form to patients because studies show that GA modulates immune function and suppresses cancer cell replication. Note that while FDA-approved estrogen drugs can cause abnormal blood clotting, the GA contained in licorice root inhibits the clotting factor thrombin (Francischetti et al. 1997), thus reducing the risk of a heart attack or stroke. Licorice root extracts have many disease-fighting applications, but for menopausal women, the most important factor is that glycyrrhetic acid extracted from licorice may be a safer source of natural estrogen (Rafi et al. 2000; Tamir et al. 2000). Numerous studies indicate that GA is an effective estrogen replacement therapy in humans, and the Chinese have used licorice extracts for over 3000 years to treat menopausal disorders.

CAUTION Chronic licorice consumption induces hyperaldosteronism, which changes sodium, potassium, and fluid balance, causing high blood pressure. The Dutch Nutrition Council advises adult intake of glycyrrhizic acid of less than 200 mg per day for an average size person. Do not take this product if you are hypertensive, on ACE inhibitors, or angiotensin receptor blockers (van Gelderen et al. 2000).

Dong Quai

Dong Quai extract is a female tonic in traditional Chinese medicine. It has been used successfully to alleviate PMS (premenstrual syndrome) and menopausal symptoms (Hardy 2000). Dong Quai extract has been shown to have a muscle relaxant effect and has been used as an analgesic and anti-inflammatory agent. Scientists believe that one mechanism of action of Dong Quai is to promote natural progesterone synthesis.

Beware of commercial Dong Quai root supplements that contain too much active ingredient (i.e., 250–535 mg of Dong Quai per capsule). This dose is too high and not necessary when taking other hormone-modulating plant extracts such as black cohosh, soy phytoestrogens, and glycyrrhetic acid, because it can be toxic. A balanced herbal formula should not contain more than 50 mg of Dong Quai as the recommended daily dose.

Progesterone (to be discussed further in this chapter) is another hormone whose production declines at menopause. Progesterone may be more important than estrogen for preventing and treating osteoporosis because progesterone is directly involved in the production of bone-forming cells called osteoblasts. Many menopausal women use a topical natural progesterone cream allowing direct absorption of progesterone into the bloodstream.

Vitex Extract

Another hormone imbalance that women encounter with age is excessive prolactin secretion from the pituitary gland. Prolactin interferes with the beneficial effect of estrogen and may promote the development of estrogen-induced cancers. The primary clinical symptom of excessive prolactin secretion is a modest amount of breast milk production in a non-pregnant woman, noted by a milky discharge from the nipples of the breast (galactorrhea). The diagnosis is confirmed by a serum blood test for prolactin which may be followed by a brain scan to search for a prolactin-secreting adenoma (tumor) of the pituitary gland.

Prolactin secretion may be suppressed by a natural extract called vitex agnus castus (Chaste tree berry). Milewicz et al. (1993) noted that vitex agnus castus extract (abbreviated as vitex) suppressed excessive prolactin secretion and promoted natural progesterone synthesis over a 3-month period with no side effects. Vitex acts on the pituitary gland to decrease prolactin secretion. This increases progesterone production because excess prolactin suppresses progesterone. This herb is primarily used to control premenstrual symptoms (PMS) rather than the symptoms of menopause; however, vitex can be used together with other natural agents during the menopausal period.

WARNING Prolactin is so dangerous in patients with hormone-dependent cancers that the Life Extension Foundation advocates prolactin suppression drug therapy (Dostinex®, 0.5 mg twice a week) for breast and prostate cancer patients who have excess prolactin in their blood.

A PHYTOESTROGEN NATURAL ESTROGEN REPLACEMENT APPROACH

When choosing a natural estrogen replacement program, one should be certain that the ingredients are standardized to achieve pharmaceutical purity and potency. An investigation conducted in 1998 of natural estrogen products sold in health food stores showed that many companies were not using the standardized plant extracts that had been used in the published studies to treat menopausal symptoms. Telephone calls to these companies confirmed that many extracts were "one-to-one" ratios, meaning that less of the active ingredient was present. This investigation also found that respected brand-name supplement companies were using good pharmaceutical-grade standardized extracts in their

Intraductal Papillomas

Small, wart-like, benign growths that project into the breast ducts near the nipple are intraductal papillomas (National Cancer Institute 2001b). They usually occur singly, but can also appear as multiple lesions. The smaller nodules are difficult to palpate. The primary sign of intraductal papilloma is nipple discharge, either clear or bloody. Breast pain and tenderness may occur.

NODULES WITH POTENTIAL FOR CANCER

Complex Cysts

Complex cysts have more than one compartment within the cyst. Ultrasonography is valuable in differentiating simple cysts from complex cysts or solid masses (Bassett et al. 1991). Complex cysts are somewhat more likely to be cancerous, so doctors will often order further tests, beginning with fine needle aspiration and perhaps a biopsy, to be certain the cyst is not cancerous or pre-cancerous.

Fibroadenomas

Fibroadenomas (sometimes called adenofibromas) are smooth, firm, benign tumors that are extremely mobile, feel slippery, and move around easily in the breast. They consist of structural (fibro) and glandular (adenoma) tissue (Anon. 2000, National Cancer Institute 2001b). Fibroadenomas feel round with well-defined margins and vary from pinhead in size to very large. They grow rapidly and usually occur near the nipple or on the outside of the upper quadrant. Fibroadenomas occur most often in women in their 20s and 30s and occur twice as often in African-American women as in other American women (National Cancer Institute 2001b). When aspirated, if there is no fluid in the lump, it is most likely a fibroadenoma. Fibroadenomas do not cause pain or tenderness. A "complex" fibroadenoma contains abnormal growths or exhibits abnormal cell changes. Although fibroadenomas themselves do not become cancerous (National Cancer Institute 2001b), they can act as *markers* for the disease. Women with a family history of breast cancer who also develop complex fibroadenomas might be at a higher risk for developing cancer than other women. Fibroadenomas are not difficult to remove and rarely recur.

Paget's Disease

A slow-growing intraductal carcinoma that begins as a scaling, eczema-like lesion on the nipple is called Paget's disease (Anon. 2000). The nipple becomes red and irritated and the lesion extends along the skin and into the ducts. The lesion can progress to a mass located deep in the breast.

Phyllodes Tumor

Phyllodes tumor is a breast tumor that might be malignant (Mazy et al. 1999). Phyllodes tumor is a rare type of breast tumor, similar to a fibroadenoma, but it is composed of an overgrowth of fibrous connective breast tissue that can become quite large. If malignancy is discovered (rare) through biopsy, the tumor and a margin of normal breast tissue are removed surgically.

FACTORS AFFECTING INCREASED RISK OF BREAST CANCER

When a woman finds a breast nodule, the first concern is that it might be cancerous. Most of the time, breast nodules are not cancerous (benign). According to Hurley et al. (1997), there are three basic, agreed-upon classifications of benign breast disease: nonproliferative, proliferative without atypia, and atypical hyperplasia. However, there can be an association with benign changes in the breast in young women and an increased risk of breast cancer with age, particularly later in life. Therefore, pathologists sometimes add comments to the pathology report indicating whether or not benign changes are relevant to an increased risk of cancer. One study followed 644 women with breast nodules between 1976 and 1982. The researchers found a relationship between subsequent cancer in women with multiple cysts and in 15 of the women whose cysts had been aspirated. The authors concluded that women with multiple breast cysts that have been aspirated have an increased risk of breast cancer. These women should perform more breast self-examinations and have follow-ups accordingly (Bundred et al. 1991).

Benign breast conditions are more often found in premenopausal women (Ernster 1981; Bodian 1993a). Breast cancer occurs more often in postmenopausal women (75% of cases) (NBCC 1999). Estimating the risk for future breast cancer from a benign condition is difficult: the extent of mammography screening differs in the population and often, significant time passes between diagnosis of benign disease in a younger woman and the increased risk for breast cancer development in older women. Because benign breast disease is difficult to distinguish from malignant disease, diagnostic biopsy is required for a definitive diagnosis (NBCC 1999).

Women with biopsy-confirmed benign disease do appear to have an overall modest increase in risk for subsequent development of breast cancer, particularly for more hyperplastic or epithelial (the covering or lining) proliferative forms. However, the evidence regarding the risk of breast cancer for nonproliferative conditions is conflicting. Some research found that the risk of breast cancer for women with nonproliferative disease is about double that of women without benign disease (Bodian et al. 1993b), while others find that lesions with no proliferative changes were not associated with an increased risk (Oza et al. 1993; Henderson et al. 1996; NBCC 1999). According to Hurley et al. (1997) atypical hyperplasia is a risk factor, but it is not with certainty followed by breast cancer; risk applies to both breasts, with greater risk on the affected side. There is no means to predict which women will go on to develop breast cancer and the effectiveness of current screening and management methods is unknown. Further complicating a physician's ability to predict a woman's risk for breast cancer is that most women do not have a history of biopsy for a benign lesion. Additionally, at the time of this writing there is no generally agreed upon classification of mammography patterns of breast tissue that is a predictive measure of which conditions are indicative of increased risk (Bodian et al. 1993c; NBCC 1999).

HORMONE REPLACEMENT AND BREAST CANCER

In the July 17, 2002 edition of the *Journal of the American Medical Association*, after decades of accumulated *observational* evidence, the Women's Health Initiative Investigators group raised concerns about the balance of risks and benefits for hormone use in healthy postmenopausal women. The concerns resulted from a randomized controlled primary prevention trial. The trial recruited 16,608 postmenopausal women (50–79 years of age) with an intact uterus at age 40 to United States clinical centers from 1993–1998. The study was designed to last 8.5 years. Participants in the study received placebo (8102 subjects) or conjugated equine estrogen (0.625 mg daily) plus medroxyprogesterone acetate (2.5 mg daily) in a single tablet (8506 subjects), commonly known as Prempro. The study monitored coronary heart disease, invasive breast cancer, stroke, pulmonary embolism, endometrial cancer, colorectal cancer, hip fracture, and death due to other causes.

After 5.2 years, the data and safety monitoring board recommended stopping the trial because one statistic (for invasive breast cancer) had exceeded the stopping boundary for an adverse effect and the global index statistic supported risks exceeding benefits. Although the *absolute risk* was still low, investigators stopped the estrogen plus progestin part of the study. They concluded: "Overall health risks exceeded benefits from use of combined estrogen plus progestin for an average 5.2-year follow-up among healthy postmenopausal U.S. women." Women in the other groups in the study (women taking estrogen alone, on a low-fat diet, taking calcium and vitamin D supplements, and women in the observation-only group) were advised to continue with their assigned treatment regime. However, prescribing the combination of estrogen and progestin was not recommended for long-term use or for prevention of chronic diseases (Women's Health Initiative Investigators 2002). Theories abound about why there appear to be complications with combination HRT, with one being that the progestin part of the therapy may have an antagonistic action on the estrogen part. Other co-factors include obesity, diabetes, and influence of family health history.

Another much smaller study in 2001 (158 women: 58 using HRT with Prempro (conjugated equine estrogen, 0.625 mg, plus medroxyprogesterone acetate, 5 mg); 51 using low-dose oral estrogen alone (estriol), 2 mg daily; and 55 using transdermal estrogen via a patch with estradiol, 50 mcg each 24 hours) evaluated the impact of different HRT regimens on mammographic breast density. Independent radiologists were unaware of the HRT and analyzed coded mammography films. The research indicated that an increase in mammographic density was more common in women taking continuous combined HRT (40%) than in those using oral low-dose estrogen (6%) or transdermal (2%) treatment (Lundstrom et al. 2001). The researchers reported that increased density was already apparent at the first visit after beginning HRT. During long-term follow-up, there was very little change in mammographic status, leading Lundstrom et al. (2001) to conclude that there was an "urgent need to clarify the biological nature and significance of a change in mammographic density during treatment and, in particular, its relation to symptoms and breast cancer risk."

Scientists, environmentalists, physicians, and governmental agencies have all produced reports in support of their particular stance on hormones: are they safe or not and should they be used or not? Therefore, in light of continuing concerns about the safety of using HRT, particularly HRT containing estrogen plus a progestin component, decisions concerning hormone use and modulation are personal ones related to each woman's particular risk factors and her reasons to consider using HRT. It is more important than ever to consult your physician for guidance concerning the decision to use any hormone therapy (*also see the Female Hormone Modulation Therapy protocol*).

Signs of Breast Cancer

Nodules that are hard, poorly delineated, and fixed to the skin or to underlying tissue are *suggestive* of breast cancer. Cancerous nodules can cause dimpling, nipple deviation, or nipple retraction. They usually occur singly and often are *not* painful. There may be nipple discharge that is clear or bloody. Bloody discharge is more *suggestive* of breast cancer. Ulceration may occur in later stages (Anon. 2000). (Further discussion of breast cancer is beyond the scope of this protocol. See the *Breast Cancer protocol* for a discussion of additional information.)

OTHER CAUSES OF BREAST NODULES

Mastitis or postpartum mastitis is an infection in women who are breastfeeding in which a milk duct becomes blocked, causing milk to pool, permitting a bacterial infection, and resulting in inflammation (AMA 1989). The breast appears red and feels warm and may also be tender. Mastitis can be accompanied by chills, fever, and cracking of the nipple.

Mammary Duct Ectasia

Mammary duct ectasia causes ducts beneath the nipple to become clogged and inflamed, particularly in women nearing menopause or in postmenopausal women (National Cancer Institute 2001b). The condition can be itchy and tender, with transient pain, and it may produce a thick, sticky multicolored discharge. The skin over the nodule may even be a blue-green color. Nearby lymph nodes can also be inflamed.

Pseudolumps

Pseudolumps are normal lumpy areas of breast tissue. This type of lumpiness will often disappear or vary with cyclic hormonal levels. Pseudolumps also result from silicone injections to enlarge the breasts or as a consequence of breast surgery or radiation therapy.

Fat Necrosis

Fat necrosis produces painless, round, firm lumps that form from damaged and disintegrating fatty tissue (National Cancer Institute 2001b). Fat necrosis is more likely to occur in obese women with large breasts. It may also develop in response to a bruise or blow to the breast. Sometimes the skin around these lumps looks red or bruised.

Breast Pain

Mastalgia refers to breast pain that is severe enough to cause a woman to seek medical treatment. Mastalgia can occur at rest or during movement, intermittently, cyclically, or constantly and can be sharp or dull and radiate to the back, arms, or neck. Pain can be aggravated by palpation (such as during physical examination). However, mastalgia is an *unreliable* indicator of a serious condition such as cancer (Anon. 2000). Although many women experience uncomfortable tenderness and swelling, pain characterized as severe occurs only about 15% of the time.

Breast pain not related to the menstrual cycle is called non-cyclical breast pain. Non-cyclical breast pain is rare and much more difficult to treat. Non-cyclical breast pain can be caused by old trauma to the breast (such as a blow to the breast, a biopsy, or surgery), infection, or some other condition completely unrelated to the breast (Anon. 2000). Arthritis is a possible cause of breast pain. Arthritis pain is usually felt in the breastbone, at the center of the chest. Women with arthritic breast pain also may experience increased discomfort when they breathe deeply.

An early study showed that there were significant abnormalities in pituitary function (via prolactin mechanisms) seen in severe *cyclical* mastalgia and nodular breast disease, but not in women with *noncyclical* mastalgia (Kumar et al. 1984).

DIAGNOSING FIBROCYSTIC BREAST DISEASE

A healthcare provider who is experienced in diagnosing breast conditions should examine *any* new breast mass or lump. Additionally, if there is any skin irritation, dimpling, nipple pain or retraction, redness or scaling of the nipple or breast skin, or nipple discharge other than breast milk in lactating women, see a physician for an evaluation. Breast conditions usually can be diagnosed by an examination by a physician. It is not unusual for a physician to recommend a mammogram, ultrasound, or biopsy procedure to assist or confirm the diagnosis (National Cancer Institute 2000b).

A mammogram, the most frequently used diagnostic tool for breast lumps, is a type of x-ray examination. If the mammogram suggests that abnormal tissue is benign, follow the physician's recommendations and recheck the lump (in perhaps 4 to 6 months) (National Cancer Institute 2000b). If the mammogram is inconclusive or if it indicates the need for further examination, your physician may recommend a computer-aided diagnosis procedure using ultrasound. This additional diagnostic procedure is designed to improve identification of a potentially malignant lesion.

Ultrasound uses high-frequency waves to outline a part of the body and is useful to further evaluate possible abnormalities found during mammograms or physical examinations. Besides aspiration, ultrasound is the only way to determine if the lump is a fluid-filled cyst. Fluid-filled cysts have a distinctive appearance on an ultrasound screen.

Fine-needle aspiration biopsy (FNAB) is used if the physician is almost certain that the lump is a cyst. Aspiration is also used to extract a material from a lump for further analysis (National Cancer Institute 2001b). A very thin needle is inserted into the breast tissue as the doctor palpates the lump. The procedure is essentially painless because nerves are located primarily in the skin, not in the breast tissue itself. Ultrasound is used to guide the needle when a lump is difficult to palpate or is very small. FNAB has decreased the need for surgical biopsy.

Core-needle biopsy uses a needle larger than the type employed with FNAB. The procedure is performed in a physician's office with local anesthesia of the breast area to be biopsied. Core-needle biopsy removes a small cylinder of tissue for examination.

Stereotactic biopsy is a newer approach that relies on a three-dimensional x-ray to guide the needle biopsy of non-palpable mass (National Cancer Institute 2001b). The breast is x-rayed from two different angles and a computer plots the position of the suspicious area. Once the area is precisely identified, the radiologist uses a needle to biopsy the lesion.

Surgical biopsy may also be necessary to remove all or part of a lump for examination (National Cancer Institute 2001b). This procedure is done either in a physician's office or in an outpatient hospital facility under intravenous sedation or local anesthesia.

There are newer methods, such as vacuum-assisted biopsy, which remove even more tissue, but so far there is no universal agreement about when these procedures should be used, even though current studies show consistent reliable results (Fine 2001; Maganini et al. 2001; Ohsumi et al. 2001; Jackman et al. 2002; Perlet et al. 2002).

TREATING FIBROCYSTIC BREAST DISEASE

Although some physicians consider FBD to be more correctly termed a condition, its symptoms cause significant pain and discomfort for many women. Women who have FBD may find relief from any of several conventional and natural treatments. Some procedures (FNAB) for the conventional treatment of FBD can often be performed in a physician's office. Other procedures (such as a biopsy) are usually performed in an ambulatory or hospital surgical facility.

Breast *cysts* are relatively simple to treat. Simple breast cysts are aspirated by a physician with a needle and syringe (National Cancer Institute 2001b). A biopsy is often *not* necessary. Fluid aspirated from a cyst is rarely tested unless it is bloody or the woman is older than 55 years of age. Gross breast cysts that are benign disappear after aspiration. (However, a cancerous lump remains even after fluid is withdrawn.) Following imaging by mammography and ultrasonography, complex cysts require laboratory investigation usually beginning with fine needle aspiration and perhaps biopsy.

Intraductal Papilloma

In intraductal papilloma, the diseased ducts can be removed surgically if discharge becomes bothersome (National Cancer Institute 2001a; 2001b). The appearance of the breast is usually unchanged.

Mastitis

Mastitis or postpartum mastitis is an infection that is treated with antibiotics (Anon. 1998). Pus-filled abscesses may need to be drained or removed. Lactating women with mastitis should use a breast pump to prevent additional pooling of breast milk and discard the milk. Breast milk should not be used until the infection has responded to antibiotic treatment.

Mammary Duct Ectasia

Mammary duct ectasia is treated with antibiotics, warm compresses, and sometimes surgery (National Cancer Institute 2001b).

HORMONE AND DRUG THERAPY

The anterior pituitary gland secretes follicle-stimulating hormone (FSH) which in turn causes follicle cells in the ovaries to secrete estrogens. The anterior pituitary also secretes luteinizing hormone (LH) which causes the corpus luteum to secrete progesterone and a small amount of estrogens, including estradiol (E2). LH and FSH work together to bring about ovulation and menstruation. The corpus luteum produces progesterone for about 11 days (the luteal phase) after ovulation. About 3 days later, when levels of estrogen and progesterone are at their lowest, menstruation begins.

In an early study comparing women with normal breast tissue to women with benign breast disease, there was a significant imbalance of progesterone over estradiol during the luteal phase in women with benign breast disease (Sitruk-Ware et al. 1979). When the women were grouped according to the type of breast lesion, there was elevated or normal estradiol in women with adenosis tumors and increased nodularity of both breasts. Plasma progesterone was also consistently lower in all groups as compared to the normal women. The authors concluded: "From these results it may be postulated that an imbalance in the secretion of E2 and progesterone by the corpus luteum is a constant finding in women with benign breast disease" (Sitruk-Ware et al. 1979).

Oral Contraceptives

Sometimes physicians treat breast pain and swelling associated with FBD by prescribing oral contraceptives which tend to stabilize (or level out) hormone levels. Results of studies indicate that oral contraceptives have positive benefits by decreasing the symptoms of FBD, particularly in younger women (Mishell 1993; Rohan et al. 1999; Scott 1993).

Hormone Replacement Therapy (HRT)

HRT, often recommended to post-menopausal women, may actually increase the symptoms of FBD depending on the hormone combination used. As with any type of hormone administration, however, the results and effects differed widely among women studied. When on HRT, it is important to monitor *any* changes in breast tissue and to evaluate these changes with your physician as they relate to the positive benefits (cardiovascular, bone density) versus the risks (increased density of breast nodules) of continuing HRT (Lundstrom et al. 2001; Ozdemir et al. 1999). (*See the protocol on Female Hormone Modulation Therapy.*)

In a 1997 study, doctors treated women with painful FBD by giving them estroprogestins (estrogen-progesterone compounds) for 3 months. They found that 60% of the women reported reduced or improved symptoms (Leonardi 1997). However, like HRT, estrogen replacement therapy (ERT) has also been linked to higher rates of FBD among post-menopausal women; in fact, they are twice as likely to develop FBD as women who have not used estrogen replacement (Pastides et al. 1987). Women on ERT also experience more fibroadenomas. The risk seems to increase the longer the therapy is employed.

Powerful drugs with hormonal effects are also available and are prescribed with caution when pain from FBD is severe. However, physicians are hesitant to use them because of potential side effects and interactions with other drugs or conditions (such as tamoxifen and danazol).

Tamoxifen

A medicine that blocks the effects of the estrogen hormone in the body, Tamoxifen, is primarily used to treat breast cancer that is estrogen receptor positive (Chatterji 2001/2002). It has also been used in some women who do not have breast cancer, but who are at high risk to develop it. Tamoxifen has been used to relieve *significant* breast pain associated with FBD. An early double-blind controlled study was done with tamoxifen in 60 patients who had severe mastalgia lasting more than 6 months. The patients were treated with a placebo or 20 mg of tamoxifen for 3 months. There was relief of pain in 71% of the patients receiving tamoxifen, demonstrating that tamoxifen was valuable in the treatment of severe cyclical and non-cyclical mastalgia and that treatment can be achieved with few side effects (Fentiman et al. 1986). How tamoxifen works and its long-term effects are not precisely known. However, the use of tamoxifen requires careful monitoring by a physician to assess side effects, blood levels, and so forth.

Indole-3-carbinol (I3C) is a phytonutrient with similar properties to tamoxifen: I3C partially inactivates estrogen (Bradlow et al. 1994); fights free radicals (Arnao et al. 1996); and interferes with tumor cell production (Bradlow et al. 1999a). See the detailed description below on I3C and how it may be used as an adjunct or an alternative to tamoxifen.

Danazol

Danazol is a synthetic steroid that is prescribed for pain and infertility caused by endometriosis and for the pain and tenderness of FBD. When prescribed for FBD, danazol may produce partial or complete disappearance of nodules and relief from pain and tenderness (Greenblatt et al. 1982; Mansel et al. 1982; Lopez et al. 1996). However, danazol has undesirable side effects such as allergic reactions (particularly for persons who are allergic to preservatives or anabolic steroids) and drug interactions. For example, danazol may increase the anticoagulant effect of warfarin, a drug frequently prescribed as a blood-thinning agent, increase blood sugar levels in diabetes mellitus, and increase the occurrence of migraine headaches (Meeks et al. 1992). Additionally, this synthetic testosterone derivative may cause women to develop male sexual characteristics such as facial hair (Peress et al. 1982). Danazol is not recommended for pregnant women or women who are breast feeding because of undesirable effects on the infant. However, danazol does help alleviate breast pain. As early as 1985, a study found that the drug eased pain in 70% of women with cyclical pain and in 31% of women with noncyclical pain (Pye et al. 1985). Symptoms often recur after treatment with danazol is stopped.

Bromocriptine

Another drug, bromocriptine, also helped 20% of women with non-cyclical pain and 47% of women with cyclical pain (Pye et al. 1985). Bromocriptine is a drug that affects the pituitary gland (blocks the release of the hormone prolactin) and is prescribed for menstrual problems and to stop milk production in some women. It is also used to treat other conditions such as infertility, Parkinson's disease, and acromegaly (overproduction of growth hormone). Bromocriptine has side effects, including significant nausea, allergic reactions, and interactions with drugs taken for other conditions (hypertension, mental illness, and liver conditions).

Lisuride

Lisuride (used in Parkinson's disease), a drug with endocrine effects similar to those of bromocriptine, reduced FBD symptoms in 63% of the women studied. Estrogen levels in those patients were reduced and progesterone levels were increased (Lopez-Rosales et al. 1991).

DHEA

Dehydroepiandrosterone (DHEA) is a steroid hormone chemically related to testosterone and estrogen. It is made by the adrenal glands from cholesterol. DHEA levels in the human body peak in the mid-20s and steadily decline beginning about the mid-30s (Leowattana 2001). Researchers have studied the actions of DHEA for over 20 years and have found that it may have beneficial implications in many areas, such as improving immunity; reducing menopausal symptoms; preventing cancer, heart disease, Alzheimer's disease, and chronic inflammation; improving longevity; and aiding weight loss (Kimura et al. 1998; Kurzman et al. 1998; Murialdo et al. 2000; Leowattana 2001; Corsini et al. 2002; Polleri et al. 2002; Simpson 2002; Takayanagi 2002; Yang et al. 2002). DHEA should only be taken under the supervision of a physician who can monitor blood levels of steroids and cholesterol and existing health conditions (Nestler et al. 1988; Barrett-Connor et al. 1995; Yen et al. 1995). DHEA is contraindicated in both men and women who have hormone-related cancer. (*See the DHEA Replacement Therapy Protocol.* Life Extension recommends specific dosing and blood testing schedules for all persons desiring to take DHEA safely.)

NUTRITIONAL RECOMMENDATIONS

There are a number of natural treatments that may help women with FBD. These therapies may be employed alone or in combination with conventional treatments.

Nutritionists make several general recommendations concerning FBD and diet:

- Reduce fat to less than 20% of your diet, particularly saturated fats (animal products).
- Include more foods that are high in fiber. (Fiber is important in aiding bowel transit time.)
- Limit eggs, chicken, and dairy products.
- Include soy protein products (tofu).
- Reduce caffeine intake or consider avoiding coffee, tea, soft drinks, and chocolate (caffeine and methylxanthine) altogether.
- Reduce or eliminate sugar, white flour, and refined foods.
- Take vitamins (beta-carotene, vitamin C, vitamin E, vitamin B-complex, vitamin B_6).
- Take minerals (selenium, zinc, copper, calcium, magnesium, iodine).
- Consume omega-3 fatty acids from cold-water fish, fish oil supplements, or Perilla-seed oil supplements.

In addition, some form of daily exercise (walking, bicycle riding, yoga, weight training) and not smoking are strongly recommended.

As with any nutritional issue, studies concerning dietary recommendations seem to often be contradictory. Therefore, many choices concerning a type of diet to follow or foods to be included or avoided will be personal ones based on each individual's particular circumstance and experience. Consult with your physician with any concerns before making nutritional changes to control or treat FBD.

Dietary Fat

Beginning as early as 1980, numerous studies have examined the relationship between FBD and dietary fat. Obesity tends to increase estrogens, free fatty acids, and triglycerides (Leijd 1980; Clarke 1981; Bates et al. 1982; Siiteri et al. 1987; Blum et al. 1988; Zumoff 1988; Kaplan 1989; Hunt et al. 1995; Singh et al. 1995; Vanhala et al. 1998; Inukai et al. 1999; Despres et al. 2000; Hudgins et al. 2000). The typical Western diet provides about 40% of its calories from fat. However, nutritionists recommend that a healthy diet should include 30% of calories from fat with only 10% of these calories coming from saturated fat. Some researchers suggest that additional lowering of dietary fat levels (to 15%) may help stabilize hormonal imbalances that can lead to FBD (Mishra et al. 1994). In an early two-part study reported by Rose et al. (1987), investigators put 16 women on a diet with fat comprising 20% of total calories. After 3 months, the investigators found significant reductions in circulating estrogens, while levels of serum progesterone remained stable.

In another early study, researchers studied women who had had severe cyclical FBD for at least 5 years (Boyd et al. 1988). These women were advised to limit their dietary fat to 15% of calories consumed, while increasing complex carbohydrate consumption. After 6 months, the women reported significant reduction in the severity of premenstrual breast tenderness and swelling (Boyd et al. 1988). In a follow-up study in 1997, 817 women were randomly assigned to two groups (an intervention group to reduce intake of dietary fat and increase carbohydrates and a control group) and followed for two years. In all subjects, baseline mammography images were taken and compared with images that were taken two years later. After two years, there was a reduction in breast mass, leading the authors to conclude that "a low-fat high-carbohydrate diet reduced the area of mammographic density, a radiographic feature of the breast that is a risk factor for breast cancer." The authors suggested that longer follow-up of a larger number of subjects is required to determine if these effects are associated with changes in the risk for breast cancer (Boyd et al. 1997).

A study conducted at Harvard University followed more than 300,000 women (Huang et al. 1999). Their data suggested that "greater waist circumference increases risk of breast cancer, especially among women who are otherwise at lower risk because of never having used estrogen replacement hormones."

Conversely, mounting evidence also suggests that some dietary fat is desirable and provides protection for the breast (Kaizer 1989; Franceschi et al. 1996; Maillard et al. 2002). Women experienced better breast health if their diet included moderate levels of fat. However, women desiring to add some dietary fat should not do so by merely increasing their consumption of meat, dairy products, and products with vegetable oils that contain saturated fat (palm and coconut oil). Better sources of dietary fat are from unsaturated fats such as fish; olive, peanut, and sunflower oils; olives; and avocados.

Beneficial Fatty Acids

Beneficial or *essential fatty acids* (EFAs) are vital nutrients for good health just like other vitamins and minerals. EFAs are polyunsaturated fats ("good" fats) and contribute to healthy functioning of cell membranes, the skin, the immune system, and the cardiovascular system. Although fatty acids are essential for overall health, our body does not manufacture them. We need to obtain them through our diet.

Conjugated Linoleic Acid

Conjugated linoleic acid (or CLA) is a source of natural dietary fat. CLA is an essential fatty acid occurring in dairy and other products such as whole milk, cheese, and red meats from ruminant animals. CLA is considered to be "a healthy fat" because it is polyunsaturated (liquid at room temperature). Because the CLA content in dairy products is directly related to the fat content, CLA levels are greatest in higher fat (rather than lower fat) products. Good dietary sources of CLA are homogenized milk, butter, plain yogurt, cheese, and ground beef. Interestingly, the CLA content of milk and other dairy products is highest in pasture- or range-fed cows (McBean/National Dairy Council 1999). Skim milk does not contain CLA (Roloff 1997). As stated earlier, CLA is found in dairy products; however, it occurs at relatively low levels in these dietary sources. Therefore, we probably cannot get adequate CLA from food alone. (Life Extension suggests 3000–4000 mg of a 76% CLA supplement be taken daily.)

Studies in animals have documented a number of potential health benefits of CLA: an anti-carcinogenic effect, lowered total and LDL cholesterol, a reduction of body fat, increased rate of bone formation, and improved glucose utilization (McBean/National Dairy Council 1999). Although FBD is often a benign condition, there are important tumor-modulating, anti-cancer, and anti-inflammatory effects associated with CLA that are beneficial and perhaps preventative. In studies conducted using laboratory rats, CLA was found to confer lifelong protection against mammary cancer and to also reduce the density of mammary glands.

Banni et al. (1999) continued earlier research suggesting that CLA fed during mammary gland development resulted in diminished mammary epithelial branching, which might possibly result in reduced mammary cancer risk. Data showed a "graded and parallel reduction of terminal end bud density and mammary tumor yield produced by 0.5 and 1% CLA. No further decrease in either parameter was observed when CLA in the diet was raised to 1.5–2%." Banni et al.

(1999) concluded: "optimal CLA nutrition during pubescence could conceivably control the population of cancer-sensitive target sites in the mammary gland." Ip et al. (1999a,b) also conducted studies in laboratory rats to investigate the role of CLA in inhibiting mammary carcinogenesis. They found that CLA "can act directly to inhibit growth and induce apoptosis of normal mammary epithelial cell organoids and may thus prevent breast cancer by its ability to reduce mammary epithelial density" (Ip et al. 1999a). (Apoptosis is the normal, healthy programmed death of cells.) CLA is therefore recommended because of its anti-tumor effects (three to four capsules of CLA-76% supplement daily for healthy people).

Omega-3 and Omega-6 Fatty Acids

The omega-3 and omega-6 fatty acids are important members of the EFA family. Omega-3 and omega-6 are scientific names derived from the chemical composition of their fatty acid molecules. Each one contains different fatty acids. Although the names are scientifically useful, most people just need to know that both of them are essential fatty acids and the body needs both of them in balance.

Omega-6 fatty acids are generally available in adequate amounts from the grains and vegetable oils that are commonly present in the processed foods in our diet unless lifestyle (consumption of alcohol, excessive sugar, and saturated fats) or health conditions are a factor. Dried beans, including inexpensive northern beans and soybeans, are an excellent source of omega-6 fatty acids. Omega-6 fatty acids are also found in linoleic acid from safflower, sunflower, corn, and soybean oils.

Greater effort is often required to ensure that adequate omega-3 EFAs are available from our daily diet. Omega-3 fatty acids are abundant in fish oils from mackerel, salmon, halibut, and herring. Soybeans, flaxseed, and green leafy vegetables also contain omega-3 fatty acids.

Women with severe mastalgia and FBD appear to have abnormal fatty-acid levels that may lead to endocrinologic hypersensitivity (imbalance of proper hormonal ratios and the resultant affect on other systems) (Ayers 1983; Mansel et al. 1990c). FBD seems to be associated with exaggerated estrogen-progesterone ratios and increased levels of prolactin (Kumar et al. 1985; BeLieu 1994). Thus, increasing omega-6 fatty acids may reduce FBD symptoms (Mansel et al. 1990a). The correct balance of omega-6 and omega-3 fatty acids will also help to inhibit the inflammatory cascade that may precede the onset of fibrous tissue.

Evening Primrose Oil

Several European studies support using evening primrose oil to treat breast pain and cysts (Pye et al. 1985; Gateley 1990; Mansel et al. 1990b; Gateley et al. 1991; McFayden et al. 1992; Cheung 1999; Norlock 2002). Evening primrose oil is a good source of beneficial gamma-linolenic acid and linoleic acid. In a 1990 survey, as many as 13% of surgeons and 30% of breast surgeons in Great Britain recommended evening primrose oil, particularly for cyclic mastalgia (Pain et al. 1990; BeLieu 1994). Evening primrose oil significantly improved the fatty-acid profiles of women with FBD (Gateley et al. 1992) and improved pain symptoms.

Borage and Flax Seed Oils

These two oils modulate inflammatory prostaglandins (Mancuso et al. 1997; Belch et al. 2000), often giving considerable relief to FBD symptoms. It may take 4–6 weeks before there is noticeable improvement. Nonetheless, treatment should be continued for 4–8 months.

Fruits, Vegetables, and Dietary Fiber

A diet that emphasizes fruits and vegetables also includes benefits for women with FBD. Natural, beneficial chemicals present in fruits and vegetables assist enzymes in the body to detoxify potentially harmful compounds (called carcinogens) (BCERF 1998). In fact, women who maintain a vegetarian diet are actually able to excrete two to three times more estrogen than omnivorous women. This could be part of the explanation for why vegetarian women have a lower incidence of breast cancer (Goldin 1981, 1982).

In addition, some of the chemical components of fruits and vegetables benefit the function of (switch on) the parasympathetic nervous system, thus minimizing development of tumors and cysts. Increasing fiber consumption appears to be a component in reducing the symptoms of FBD in some women. Fiber assists elimination of waste from the system, decreasing levels of circulating estrogens (BCERF 1998). Obtain plenty of fiber from your diet. Good sources of dietary fiber are legumes (kidney and pinto beans, peas, and lentils), vegetables (Brussels sprouts, broccoli, and carrots), raw fruits (apples, oranges, and bananas), and grains (particularly bran and oats) (Anderson et al. 1988; Van Horn 1997). Additional fiber may be obtained from dietary supplements in the form of powders or capsules. (Life Extension recommends Fiber Food Caps, Fiber Food Powder, and Apple Pectin Powder.)

Indole-3-Carbinol

Indole-3-carbinol (I3C) is a naturally occurring dietary compound (a phytochemical) that is found in some fruits and the cruciferous vegetables such as broccoli, cauliflower, brussels sprouts, cabbage, turnips, kohlrabi, bok choy, and radishes. Phytochemicals are also natural anti-cancer compounds. Indole-3-carbinol appears to work in several ways: partially inactivating estrogen (Michnovicz 1997; Bradlow et al. 1994; Wong et al. 1997); fighting free radicals (Arnao et al. 1996); and directly interfering with tumor cell reproduction (Bradlow et al. 1999a). Indole-3-carbinol triggers the release of enzymes that help break down estrogen precursors into a harmless form rather than the form that is linked to breast cancer (Michnovicz et al. 1997; Bradlow et al. 1999b; Meng et al. 2000; Terry et al. 2001). Cabbage and broccoli also contain sulforaphane, another phytonutrient that has been shown to stimulate the release of enzymes that attach to cancer-causing substances and transport them from the body (Mowatt 1998).

The National Cancer Institute and the U.S. Department of Agriculture have said that by eating five servings of vegetables and fruit a day, a person can cut the risk of cancer by more than 50%. Most people do not come close to meeting this guideline, particularly the recommendation for vegetables, because they do not like cruciferous vegetables, the vegetables are not readily available, or they cannot eat the quantity required each day to meet recommended dietary guidelines for phytonutrients. Sometimes raw vegetables are not easy for the system to digest. Storage and processing by the supplier or overcooking in the home contributes to loss of phytonutrients. Often, only half the phytonutrients in any serving of raw vegetables ultimately becomes available for absorption—the other half is quickly eliminated from the body. Concentrated vegetables (particularly those with the water content removed and which are ground to the consistency of powdered sugar) are more digestible. In this form, it is estimated that 90 to 100% of phytonutrients, and all of their cancer-fighting properties, become available for absorption into the body (Mowatt 1998). (Indole-3-carbinol is available from Life Extension in capsule form.)

Studies in animals indicate that I3C is safe at recommended doses (NIEHS 2000). Trials in humans have also found no significant side effects (Wong et al. 1997). A study by Cover et al. (1999) found that the naturally occurring chemical I3C found in vegetables of the *Brassica* genus, is "a promising anticancer agent that we have shown previously to induce a G1 cycle arrest of human breast cancer cell lines, independent

of estrogen receptor signaling." According to Cover et al. (1999), a combination of I3C and anti-estrogen tamoxifen cooperated to inhibit growth of the estrogen-dependent human MCF-7 breast cancer cell line more effectively than either agent used alone. They suggested that "I3C works through a mechanism distinct from tamoxifen." Cover et al. (1999) concluded that "these results demonstrate that I3C and tamoxifen work through different signal pathways to suppress the growth of human breast cancer cells and may represent a potential combinatorial therapy for estrogen-responsive breast cancer."

CAUTION Some recommend that pregnant women should not take indole-3-carbinol. Research is continuing on indole-3-carbinol and at this time there are no well-known drug interactions. Do not attempt to treat breast nodules with indole-3-carbinol without first consulting with your physician.

Note: *The Life Extension Foundation suggests indole-3-carbinol to persons seeking an alternative to tamoxifen. See the protocol on Breast Cancer for more information.*

Soy

Soy has been the subject of research for overall breast health. Some studies indicate that soy foods containing phytoestrogens (natural estrogens from plants) may offer some protective benefit. Researchers also believe that soy may play a role in balancing hormone levels in premenopausal women and perhaps in relieving premenstrual syndrome and menopausal symptoms (Imaginis 2001). Good dietary sources of soy are canned soybeans, tofu, soy protein bars, and tempeh. Life Extension suggests a supplement called Natural Estrogen (containing phytoestrogens from soy extract and other phyto extracts).

Researchers speculate that some of the anti-tumor activity of soy compounds may result from production of enzymes that attack free radicals (Molteni et al. 1995). However, as with other nutrients, agreement is impossible and many authorities are reluctant to give soy universal endorsement. Others suggest that soy can modulate hormonal activity and even act as an antioxidant. If using soy, carefully monitor your breasts to assess the response of breast tissue to soy products.

CAUTION Soy extract or soy products should not be used by persons with estrogen-receptor-positive cancer.

Simple and Complex Carbohydrates

Carbohydrates, whether simple or complex, might be an even greater concern in FBD than fat. Italian researchers found that heavy consumption of starchy foods, including pasta and white bread, increased breast cancer risk (Franceschi et al. 1996; Augustin et al. 2001). Carbohydrates are of two types: *simple* and *complex*. Both types are composed of sugar units. *Simple* carbohydrates are composed of one or two sugar units. Simple carbohydrates are found in fruit and vegetable juices, candy, soft drinks, and foods with added sugar. The problem with simple carbohydrates is that they induce an insulin spike upon ingestion. Insulin can promote cancer cell division which is why consumption of starchy foods might increase cancer risk. *Complex* carbohydrates are made from many sugar units that would structurally look like beads in a bracelet. Foods such as whole grain products, fruits, vegetables, and legumes (dried beans and peas) are good sources of complex carbohydrates that do not induce a sharp insulin spike because they release sugar more slowly into the bloodstream. Both simple and complex carbohydrates are converted to blood sugar by the body to use as energy or fat storage. However, complex carbohydrates are a much better nutritional value because they include vitamins, minerals, and fiber (Quagliani 1997).

Vitamins

Vitamin E

Since 1965, using vitamin E has been recommended by some researchers for treatment of FBD (Abrams 1965). However, researchers are not unified concerning the use of vitamin E to successfully treat or manage FBD and evidence has been inconclusive. Vitamin E in the form of alpha tocopherol has corrected abnormal estrogen-progesterone ratios in some patients with mammary dysplasia (London et al. 1981). Results of that study, however, were not replicated in 1985 (London et al. 1985). Another study of 105 women with FBD found that 600 mg of vitamin E for 3 months had no effect on symptoms (Meyer et al. 1990).

Vitamin E should be taken in doses of 600–800 IU daily. However, women with hypertension should start with about 400 IU. If you take a blood-thinning medication, consult your physician before taking vitamin E and monitor your usage carefully since vitamin E is known to enhance blood thinning. Vitamin E containing both alpha and gamma tocopherols may produce the most desirable results. It may be necessary to use vitamin E for several months before noticeable improvement is realized.

Folic Acid

Many physicians also recommend taking folic acid along with vitamin E. In some women, combining the two seems to have a more beneficial effect than either one taken alone. Folic acid is abundant in green, leafy vegetables, but is often deficient in the standard American diet. Women of child-bearing age are particularly encouraged to include folic acid in their diet. (Life Extension recommends at least 800 mcg of folic acid along with at least 300 mcg of vitamin B_{12} daily.)

Vitamin A

Studies have shown that vitamin A has been able to inhibit the growth of breast cancer cells (Fontana et al. 1992; Wu et al. 1997; Yang et al. 1999; Widschwendter et al. 2001). Therefore, there is some justification for women with FBD to take vitamin A. In one of only a few studies (Band et al. 1984), 12 women with FBD were given 150,000 IUs of vitamin A daily for 3 months. Nine of the women reported marked pain reduction.

However, large doses of vitamin A can also be toxic. Therefore, beta-carotene may be a more practical treatment. In one study, 25 women who had moderate to severe pain before their menstrual periods were given daily supplements of beta-carotene and retinol. After 6 months, most of the women reported marked reduction in breast pain with no side effects (Santamaria et al. 1989). A diet high in yellow and orange fruits and vegetables will raise beta-carotene levels. You may also wish to use a beta-carotene supplement.

Vitamin C

The immune system requires vitamin C for proper function, tissue repair, diuretic action, anti-inflammatory responses, and adrenal hormone balance. Try 2.5–6 grams daily. If using buffered ascorbate, take it with magnesium or potassium.

Detoxifying Herbs

The liver supports many mechanisms including providing a detoxifying and filtering system for all body wastes as well as binding and eliminating extra hormones (including estrogen clearance). If the liver does not adequately perform its detoxifying and binding functions, estrogen stores may increase. As noted earlier, increased fiber in the diet improves removal of toxins and waste from the system. Nutrients that support the liver include choline, S-adenosyl-methionine (SAMe), green tea, and N-acetyl-cysteine. If you have FBD, consider using these supplements daily. *Detoxifying* your system by aiding cleansing of the liver may also improve symptoms of FBD.

Herbs that support detoxification include echinacea (*Echinacea purpurea*) and goldenseal (*Hydrastis canadensis*). These herbs should be started about a week before menstruation begins, used for 7–10 days, and then discontinued for 4–7 days. Goldenseal should be followed by a probiotic that contains *acidophilus* and *Bifido* bacteria to replace good bacteria in the gut. Life Flora provides beneficial intestinal bacteria (flora) to recolonize the gastrointestinal (GI) tract when normal GI bacteria have been destroyed by disease, digestive conditions, poor absorption of nutrients, infections, and toxins. (Life Flora contains *Bifidobacterium longum* and *bifidum*, *Lactobacillus acidophilus*, *Streptococcus faecium*, and *Lactobacillus casei*.)

Supplements and Herbs to Relieve Cyclical Pain and Reduce Inflammation

Dandelion (Taraxacum Officinale) and Milk Thistle (Silibinin Marianum)

Dandelion and milk thistle will help to detoxify your system (Maliakal et al. 2001; Saller et al. 2001; Cho et al. 2002; Hagymasi et al. 2002; Kosina et al. 2002). Dandelion has also been used to treat painful breasts and relieve impacted milk glands. Drink up to two cups of dandelion tea daily (or take a 500-mg capsule two to three times daily). In large doses, dandelion can provoke hypoglycemia in some people. High potency silibinin extract from milk thistle may also be taken at a dosage of about 500 mg daily.

Saw Palmetto

Saw palmetto (*Serenoa repens*) is used to treat prostate problems, but its anti-estrogenic characteristics also make it useful as a treatment for hormonal disturbances. Saw palmetto should be standardized to contain 85–95% fatty acids and sterols. (One capsule containing saw palmetto extract at a dosage of 320 mg daily is recommended.)

Violet Leaf

Poultices made from violet leaf may be used for pain and inflammation. Two or more cups made of 500 mL daily may bring dramatic relief for cyclical swelling and tenderness.

Castor Oil Packs

Warm castor oil packs may help dissolve lumps and relieve pain. Sometimes lumps will shrink after only a few applications. Warm castor oil packs over the liver not only invigorate, but also reduce inflammation. Some herbalists recommend alternating castor oil packs with ginger packs.

Chasteberry

Chasteberry (*Vitex agnus-castus*) has been used to relieve FBD. Chasteberry may decrease prolactin, leading to increased progesterone production during the menstrual cycle, and it seems to result in a shift in the estrogen-progesterone balance, regulating hormones and inhibiting release of FSH and LH. This results in less estrogen to stimulate breast tissue. Eat the equivalent of 20–40 mg of fresh chasteberry berries daily or take 175–225 mg daily of a preparation that is standardized to contain 0.5% agnuside.

CAUTION Avoid chasteberry if you take oral contraceptives or are pregnant.

Caffeine and Breast Conditions

Some women find that reducing or even eliminating caffeine intake by avoiding coffee, tea, chocolate, and soft drinks significantly decreases breast discomfort (Russell 1989). However, the topic is controversial because studies linking caffeine and FBD have had inconsistent results or have been inconclusive (Allen et al. 1985, 1987; Horner et al. 2000; Imaginis 2000).

An early study by Minton et al. (1981) was widely publicized because it claimed that abstaining totally from caffeine lessened symptoms and resolved FBD completely. According to Minton, abstinence from consuming methylxanthine (a chemical present in foods and beverages that contain caffeine) decreased the need for major breast surgery and breast biopsies because of benign disease (Minton 1979, 1981, 1989).

A 2002 study of the literature on causes of breast pain found that some investigations did find an association between caffeine intake and FBD and breast pain (Norlock 2002). However, other studies over the past 20 years have examined the relationship of caffeine to breast conditions and have reported inconclusive or even the opposite conclusions (Boyle et al. 1984; La Vecchia et al. 1985; Rosenberg et al. 1985; Horner et al. 2000). One study of more than 2000 women reported by Rosenberg et al. (1985) concluded that coffee consumption was not associated with an increase of breast cancer among women with a history of FBD. Another study, reported by La Vecchia et al. (1985), even found "slight" evidence that the more coffee a woman consumed, the less likely she was to have breast cancer.

Even though the evidence of a direct link between caffeine and FBD is inconclusive, many clinicians do recommend a low caffeine intake in women with FBD. Some women report significant relief from FBD symptoms after eliminating caffeine from their diets. If you suspect caffeine might have a role in your FBD symptoms, eliminate sources of caffeine (chocolate, coffee, tea, soft drinks) from your diet for 3 months to see if your symptoms improve.

As noted above, methylxanthine is a chemical present in foods and beverages that contain caffeine. Methylxanthines increase circulating catecholamines (chemicals which are present in responses to stress). There is some evidence that women with FBD have an increased sensitivity to catecholamines. However, as with caffeine, the studies are inconclusive. Both the National Cancer Institute and the American Medical Association's Council on Scientific Affairs state that there is *no* association between methylxanthine intake and FBD at this time (AMA 1984; Schairer et al. 1986).

OTHER CONSIDERATIONS

Thyroid Deficiency

According to some alternative-care practitioners, a malfunctioning thyroid gland may be a precursor to many disorders in females. With hypothyroidism, hormones such as LH, FSH, and prolactin may be overly stimulated. Researchers have linked breast abnormalities, including FBD, to repeated hormonal arousal (Lark 1996). An early study of 19 women with breast pain (mastodynia) and nodularity caused by FBD reported that almost half (47%) the women had total relief after daily treatment with 0.1 mg of levothyroxine (Synthroid). Three patients had elevated serum prolactin levels. Their prolactin levels became normal and they experienced dramatic pain relief after treatment with levothyroxine (Estes 1981).

A review of three clinical studies using sodium iodide, protein-bound iodide, and molecular iodine showed clinical improvements in FBD of 70%, 40%, and 72%, respectively (Ghent et al. 1993). The review concluded that molecular iodine was non-thyrotropic (did not alter) and was the most beneficial. Thus, some suggest that treating thyroid problems might reduce the risk or incidence of FBD and improve the symptoms (Ghent et al. 1993).

Another study looked at thyroid hormones and FBD. The data suggested that free T3 had an important role in the physiology of FBD (Martinez et al. 1995). To further examine this theory, a study looked at the levels of triiodothyroxine (T3), thyroxin (T4), thyroid stimulating hormone (TSH), and prolactin (Prl) in FBD (Zych et al. 1996). The authors found that the T4 levels were significantly lower in women with FBD than in controls. They concluded that there seemed to be a connection between FBD and thyroid function (Zych et al. 1996).

Taking daily iodine will help support a healthy thyroid. Kelp may also be beneficial. However, be certain that the seaweed is harvested from clean water. A simple, convenient source of iodine is table salt containing iodine.

Pancreatic Enzymes

According to researchers from Germany, pancreatic enzymes may reduce tumors and cysts, inflammation, and soreness. In a study of 96 patients, cyst size was reduced significantly after women took an enzyme preparation for 6 weeks. Additionally, the women reported significant improvement and less pain. A preparation containing lipase, protease, and amylase was recommended at a dosage of 10X strength (Ditmar et al. 1993)

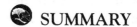 ## SUMMARY

More than 50% of all women experience symptoms of FBD at some time in their lives. In some women, the symptoms improve after a menstrual cycle. Symptoms may also cease or improve after menopause. It is not unusual for FBD to continue in postmenopausal women who use hormone replacement therapy (HRT). There is no conclusive evidence that FBD is associated with an increased risk of breast cancer.

Practice monthly breast self-examination. If a new or an unusual change is detected, contact your health care practitioner promptly for an evaluation. Have a yearly breast examination from your health care practitioner. Also have a mammogram yearly or as recommended by your physician.

Dietary Recommendations

Take preventive measures to lessen your chances of developing or intensifying FBD. Eat whole foods, emphasizing fruits and vegetables, and support your immune and hormonal systems with supplements. While there is little evidence that caffeine causes FBD, some women report that FBD improves after eliminating caffeine from their diets.

Supplements

Consider Indole-3-Carbinol: 1 capsule twice daily for those weighing under 120 pounds; 1 capsule 3 times daily for those weighing 120–180 pounds; and 1 capsule 4 times daily for those over 180 pounds.

1. If you have FBD, try natural therapies (diet and nutritional supplements) for three months and monitor your symptoms. If you choose conventional medical therapy, consult your physician for advice about the options for treating FBD. Proceed to hormonal or drug treatments *only* with the advice of a physician or if you still experience no relief (*see the protocol on Breast Cancer*).

CAUTION Some believe that pregnant women should avoid indole-3-carbinol.)

2. Consider Natural Estrogen (a soy-based phytoestrogen), one caplet morning and evening taken cyclically: 3 weeks on and 1 week off, beginning on day 5 of the menstrual cycle for premenopausal women and every day for postmenopausal women.

3. Consider Pro Fem, natural progesterone cream from soy, applied according to label instructions.

4. DHEA should be considered in women over the age of 40. The usual dose ranges from 15–50 mg. *Refer to the DHEA Replacement Therapy protocol for specific directions.*

5. CLA 76% may be taken for anti-cancer, anti-inflammatory effects: three to four 1000-mg capsules daily for healthy people.

6. A balanced formula of the essential omega-3 and omega-6 fatty acids is available in Super GLA/DHA; 6 softgels daily are recommended.

7. Take Fiber Food Caps (6 capsules with each meal), Fiber Food Powder (1 tsp with each meal), or Apple Pectin Powder (1 tsp before meals).

Note: *Do not take fiber supplements with oil-based products such as CLA.*

8. Consider taking Life Flora. Six 300-mg capsules taken daily with NutraFlora ($^1/_2$ to 1 tsp daily) are suggested for initial GI tract loading. One to four capsules of Life Flora are suggested for maintenance of healthy GI tract bacteria. Life Flora is most effectively used when taken between meals in divided doses, either dissolved in the mouth or taken with water.

9. Take folic acid (800 mcg) + B$_{12}$ (300 mcg), 1 capsule daily for healthy people. Folic acid is especially important for women of child-bearing age.

10. Vitamin A (beta-carotene), 1 or 2 capsules (25,000–50,000 IU) daily, may inhibit the growth of breast cancer cells.

11. Vitamin C is required for all tissue repair; 2.5–6 grams daily are suggested (includes dietary *and* supplemental sources). (Vitamin C Caps from Life Extension contain 1000 mg per capsule.)

12. Gamma E Tocopherol/Tocotrienols is a balanced vitamin E supplement that acts as an antioxidant and may also help balance hormone levels; 1 capsule daily is suggested.

13. Support the pancreas with pancreatic enzymes. Pancreatin (4X enzymes), 1–3 (500-mg) capsules taken on an empty stomach between meals, is suggested.

14. Echinacea is a detoxifying herb. For healthy people, take 1–2 capsules daily for 10–14 days, then 4–7 days off. Smaller doses, such as in Life Extension Herbal Mix, may be taken continuously.

15. Goldenseal may be taken as a substitute for Echinacea: 1–3 capsules daily for healthy people in divided doses for 1–2 weeks. Smaller doses, such as in Life Extension Herbal Mix, may be taken continuously.

16. Saw palmetto may relieve cyclical pain and reduce inflammation; 160–320 mg daily, standardized to contain 85–95% fatty acids and sterols, is suggested. (Super Saw Palmetto softgel from Life Extension contains 320 mg per capsule.)

17. Consider the herb chasteberry for anti-inflammatory properties: 20–40 mg of fresh berries or 175–225 mg daily.

CAUTION Women taking oral contraceptives or pregnant women should not take chasteberry.)

18. Drink up to 2 cups of dandelion tea daily (or take a 500-mg capsule 2–3 times daily).

19. Apply warm castor oil packs.

20. Apply violet leaf poultices: 2 or more cups made from 500 mL.

21. Support a healthy thyroid by taking 200–250 mcg of iodine daily. Kelp, 1500–2000 mg in divided doses, may also be beneficial.

FOR MORE INFORMATION

For more information about research studies, contact the American Cancer Society, (800) 227-2345.

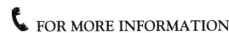 PRODUCT AVAILABILITY

Indole-3-Carbinol, Natural Estrogen, Pro Fem, Super Soy Extract Powder, DHEA, Fiber Food Caps, Fiber Food Powder, Life Flora, NutraFlora, CLA 76%, Folic Acid + B$_{12}$, Vitamin A, Vitamin C Caps, Super GLA/DHA, Gamma E Tocopherol/Tocotrienols, Pancreatin (4X enzymes), Echinacea, Goldenseal, Super Saw Palmetto, and green tea extract, may be ordered by calling (800) 544-4440 or by ordering online at www.lef.org.

Gulf War Syndrome

Gulf War syndrome (GWS), affecting a number of men and women who served in the Persian Gulf War, represents a group of medical and psychological complaints, including fatigue, respiratory illness, muscular pain, spasms, skin rash, memory loss, dizziness, peripheral numbness, and sleep disturbances. A 1996 VA study (Kang et al. 1996) reported that Gulf War veterans were 50% more likely to die in a motor vehicle accident than military personnel not sent to the Gulf War. Robert W. Haley, University of Texas Southwestern Medical Center, Dallas, reported similar findings but added in an article published by the Associated Press that the Gulf War veteran also has a higher rate of depression and suicide. Haley correlated these findings medically with individuals who have sustained brain injuries (Haley 1997; 1998; Haley et al. 1997a; 1997b).

Between August 1990 and March 1991, the U.S. deployed more than 697,000 troops in Operation Desert Shield and Operation Desert Storm. The majority of the troops were stationed in Saudi Arabia, Kuwait, or aboard ships in the Red Sea. Of these, more than 100,000 (one in seven) have reported serious health concerns to the Department of Veterans Affairs or the Department of Defense. Unfortunately, some family members of those stricken gradually display signs and symptoms of the syndrome as well, suggesting an infectious explanation of the illness.

SPECULATIVE CAUSES OF GWS

When causative factors are obscure and not unilaterally accepted, as in GWS, speculation oftentimes overrides a precise explanation. This appears true in GWS. Suppositions are many in regard to the contributory sequence that terminated in the physical and psychological symptoms familiar to veterans diagnosed with GWS.

The postulations being most scrutinized are exposure to toxins in the environment (such as oil fires), chemical and biological weapons, low-level uranium exposure, an immune reaction to a drug administered to protect against attacks of Soman (a nerve gas), dust, and even the immunizations (specifically, the anthrax vaccine and polio booster) given to the troops prior to deployment. Any of these theories could explain a state of unwellness when imposed upon a vulnerable host.

Nutritionally oriented clinicians subscribe to the rationale, "If you can't eat it, don't smell it." This caveat was not possible to heed in the Gulf War environment. More than 500 oil well fires were burning in Kuwait during June 1991, emitting extremely high levels of particulate matter. Detections of sarin, a potentially fatal nerve gas, tabun, a neuroparalytic toxic agent, and sulfur mustard gas were reported during the period of January 19–21, 1991. Troops responsible for cleaning up Iraqi ammunition dumps may have been exposed to depleted uranium, a form of uranium used in munitions because of its density and metallurgical properties. Korenyi-Both et al. (1992) reported that the combination of Saudi dust and pigeon droppings ignited an acute hyperallergic reaction that has come to be known as Desert Storm pneumonitis or Al Eskan disease. There are those who question whether the very preventative measures—drugs and vaccinations—employed to protect the troops from chemical or biological warfare may be the agents provoking the illness. Confounding the inquest, manifestations of the syndrome are unpredictable. Just as cancer can occur long after exposure to the causative factor, the complications arising from GWS can be just as unpredictable.

EXTENDED HEALTH CONCERNS

The illnesses apparent in the Gulf War veterans are not just nuisance complaints, but represent concern for vulnerability to catastrophic disease. Thousands of U.S. soldiers have died of infectious diseases, chemical exposure, and other causes resulting from Operation Desert Storm.

On April 6, 2000, the Associated Press reported that the VA announced a year-long study to determine whether there is a higher incidence of Lou Gehrig's disease—amyotrophic lateral sclerosis or ALS—among the veterans of the Gulf War. It appears that at least 28 Gulf War veterans have been diagnosed with this deadly disease. Researchers are interested in locating other veterans diagnosed with ALS or other motor neuron diseases who were actively serving duty between August 2, 1990, and July 31, 1991, regardless of location. Those who did not go to the gulf area will serve as part of the control group. Eligible veterans may call (877) 342-5257.

Antisqualene Antibodies

Dr. Bob Garry of Tulane University tested 400 veterans for antibodies to squalene and found that

95% of those individuals with GWS had high levels of the antibody (Asa et al. 2000). Though a participant in metabolic processes, squalene, found in shark liver oil, some vegetable oils, and the human liver, can also be incorporated into a vaccine to accelerate, enhance, or prolong a specific immune response. Mystifying the sleuthing process, information currently available states that squalene, though once considered an immunologic potentiator, was never used as an adjuvant in the vaccines administered to the Gulf War veterans. Because the antibody to squalene is commonly found in individuals plagued by GWS, applying the Antisqualene Antibody Assay to stricken veterans may prove a valuable tool in diagnosis. It has been hypothesized that GWS is a result of an autoimmune reaction, in which the immune system inappropriately turns on its own natural supply of squalene. The assay is available through Autoimmune Technologies, LLC, of New Orleans, LA.

Mycoplasmal Infections and GWS

Rare germs called mycoplasmas are often evidenced in individuals with GWS. Mycoplasmas are bacteria-like organisms that cause atypical pneumonia in confined groups, such as military personnel. They are small, free-living, self-replicating organisms that can cause a respiratory, flu-like illness that can progress to systemic chronic fatigue syndrome-like or fibromyalgia syndrome-like illness, sometimes advancing to multiple sclerosis-like, amyotrophic lateral sclerosis-like, and arthritis-like symptoms. Researchers found that slightly less than half of very ill Gulf War veterans with signs of chronic fatigue-immune deficiency syndrome (CFIDS) or fibromyalgia syndrome (FMS)—that is, fatigue, depression, joint pain, cognitive disturbances, burning muscles, faltering speech, headache, incontinence, alimentary disorders, sore throat, tinnitus, or loss of libido—involved mycoplasma infections. Although these microorganisms do not directly cause CFIDS, FMS, GWS, or rheumatoid arthritis (RA), mycoplasmas appear to encourage their progression and exacerbation.

Most microorganisms like mycoplasmas are not considered important human pathogens when they are found at superficial sites, such as the oral cavity or intestines, as symbiotic gut flora, but some species, such as M. fermentans, M. penetrans, M. pneumoniae, M. genitalium, M. pirum, and M. hominis, have the capability to penetrate blood circulation and colonize various tissues. The study was reported by Rawadi et al. (1996).

Sexual Impairments and Birth Defects

Whether Gulf War personnel have an increased incidence of infants born with birth defects compared to nondeployed personnel is unclear. Of the 75,414 infants born in military hospitals during the study period, seven presented with some of the ocular, aural, or cardiac impairments associated with a condition commonly referred to as Goldenhar syndrome. Only five of the seven babies, however, were born to Gulf War veterans (34,069 births), although the remaining two infants were born to nondeployed military personnel. Some affirm that birth defects are not alarmingly disproportionate among Gulf War veterans; others angrily argue that the incidence is much higher than among the nonmilitary population, with some incidences of infantile defect not being appropriately recorded. Sexual malperformance, such as impotence, has been reported among service personnel participating in the Gulf War.

WHY NOT EVERYONE?

Researchers observed illnesses resembling GWS in laboratory animals exposed to a mixture of cholinesterase inhibitor insecticides and pyridostigmine; soldiers in the Persian Gulf War have been exposed to both agents.

Before addressing the impact that such toxins could have upon exposed individuals, it is important that the autonomic nervous system be briefly explained to the reader. The autonomic nervous system, regulating involuntary functions, consists of two divisions, referred to as the sympathetic and the parasympathetic nervous system. Each division performs functions within the body that influence cardiac muscle, smooth muscle, and glandular activity.

Individuals are born with a sympathetic, parasympathetic, or balanced nervous system, referred to as a metabolic type. Our metabolic type identifies us individually and contributes to the personality that we display to society. Passivity, aggression, right brain/left brain preeminence, sleep patterns, etc., are but a few of the characteristics metabolic dominance influences. But, diet, exercise, supplements, exposure to toxic materials, and stress can make more virulent the responsiveness of the already dominant division. The body is healthiest when neither of the two divisions holds supremacy, but rather when balance prevails.

Cholinesterase inhibitors can turn the volume up on the parasympathetic nervous system by allowing acetylcholine, a neurotransmitter, to accumulate at the cholinergic receptor, thus producing effects similar to excessive stimulation of cholinergic receptors throughout the central and peripheral nervous systems. An already parasympathetic dominant individual could, after sufficient exposure to cholinesterase inhibitors, display a heightened parasympathetic expression.

Dr. Nicholas Gonzalez (www.dr-gonzalez.com), a New York physician, specializing in cancer treatment, has many times insightfully explained the disease-promoting role of the autonomic nervous system, when the two divisions become unbalanced. Dr. Gonzalez explains that the protective closure around a cell and the nucleus that controls the exchange of materials between the cell and its environment is referred to as the membrane. The membrane protects the contents of the cell with the same fervor that a solicitous parent extends to a child. It is when the membrane loses its worthiness, a process enacted by excessive calcium loss, that the cell becomes flimsy and unprotected. If toxic materials gain entry into the nucleus, the genetic control center of the cell, damage to the cell's DNA can occur quite rapidly. Should this happen, serious destruction has befallen the host.

The membrane of the cell is different in the sympathetic and the parasympathetic individual. The sympathetic dominant individual tends toward a tighter membrane that stores waste accumulations quite well. It takes longer for toxic materials to migrate into the nucleus because the tightness of the nuclear membrane is embracing and, thereby, protective. But when the maximum load in the nuclear area has been reached, anomalies, such as tumors, may become apparent.

By contrast, the cellular and nuclear membrane, according to the work of Dr. Gonzalez, in a parasympathetic individual tends to be weak and leaky, allowing noxious materials *ad libitum* entry into cells. The entry of contaminants is met with slight opposition, as the cell membrane exercises sparse resistance against the invader. Noxious materials, as well as viruses, find little hindrance passing through the membrane and gaining entry into the cell.

This bit of neurophysiology may best explain the poisoning that appears to have occurred in several of the Gulf War veterans. Which of the theories, i.e., exposures to low-level uranium, oil fires, chemicals of warfare, etc., is accurate when defining the causative factor in GWS? It may not matter, because, in reality, any of the theories or all of the theories may be accurate. Any noxious exposure was too much for some of the veterans. Metabolic dominance may have made some more immediately vulnerable to the exposures; for others, the appearance of Gulf War illnesses may be longer in appearing. The effects of the exposure may take several twists before full understanding of the depth of the devastation is reached, but the cell membrane appears to be a principal player in all of the scenarios.

Chronic Toxicity

Dr. Jeffery Bland, Ph.D., of the Institute for Functional Medicine, reported that the first signs of chronic toxicity may appear as neuro- and immunotoxicity. Dr. Michael R. Lyon, M.D., of the Oceanside Functional Medicine Research Institute, Nanaimo, British Columbia, stated that the nervous and immune systems are highly sensitive to oxidative stress and xenobiotics, that is, drugs and organic poisons. He points out that both the nervous and immune systems have a powerful memory, which means they have tremendous capacity for recalling exposure to substances to which they have become sensitive. They become increasingly sensitized to these agents as their immune system builds antigenic memory.

Classic studies involving rats showed that exposure to a poison and a simultaneous whiff of camphor later produced serum sickness or autoimmune crisis when the animals were exposed to only a sniff of camphor. The immune system was so hypervigilant in protecting against the poison that even the scent of the camphor signaled an alert. Too many of us have, either by neglect or happenstance, been exposed to environmental pollutants that may be damaging either to the nervous or the immune system. Dr. Lyon warns that attention deficit disorder, FMS, and CFIDS are going to force society into looking at these disorders from a toxicological perspective.

Hair analysis, if properly conducted, can be a dependable assessment tool in determining toxicity from heavy metals. Detection of chemical toxicity can be made by urinary organic acid analysis and by measuring blood and fatty tissue for suspected chemicals. Concurrently, the liver should be tested in regard to serum bilirubin and enzyme levels.

DETOXIFICATION . . . WHAT IS IT?

The detoxification process is an elaborate mechanism conducted chiefly by the liver to eliminate both exogenous and endogenous toxins. The liver participates in the detoxification process, largely by the action of two sequential steps referred to as Phase I and Phase II systems. Phase I reactions involve blood filtration, bile excretion, and the interaction of enzymatic processes acting upon the toxin. Bile excretion is most efficient, in regard to the detoxification process, if adequate amounts of dietary fiber are simultaneously available to escort the toxin from the intestines.

Phase I detoxification involves a group of enzymes, referred to as the cytochrome P450 family. Some 50–100 enzymes make up the cytochrome P450 systems, with each enzyme working more efficiently at neutralizing certain classes of chemicals. Phase I enzymes can directly neutralize some chemicals, but most toxins are converted to an intermediate form of the toxin. The intermediate form is considered more toxic than the original and requires the action of Phase II detoxification to complete the cycle.

Ideally, Phase I and Phase II detoxification mechanisms work synergistically. If Phase I detoxification is highly active and Phase II detoxification is lethargic, the individual is referred to as a "pathological detoxifier," a condition which increases sensitivities to environmental poisons.

Phase II reactions include sulfation and glucuronidation, which are key to human detoxification, along with glutathione conjugation, methylation, amino acid conjugation, and acetylation. Phase II detoxification typically involves biochemical conjugation, in which various enzymes in the liver attach small chemical moieties to the toxin. The conjugation reaction neutralizes toxins and reactive intermediates left over from Phase I detoxification. Both Phase I and Phase II detoxification require assistance from a healthy supply of enzymes. Enzyme quantity can be influenced by dietary components. Green tea and products found in red wine grapes encourage glucuronidation and glutathione conjugation enzymes, respectively.

Glucuronidation, a significant pathway in the Phase II detoxification mechanism, is the combining of glucuronic acid with toxins, a process that requires the enzyme UDP, glucuronyl transferase (UDPGT). Foods rich in limonene, a monoterpene found in citrus peel, dill weed oil, and caraway oil, can increase UDPGT activity and encourage the glucuronidation mechanism.

Many commonly used substances—for example, aspirin, menthol, synthetic vanilla, acetaminophen, morphine, diazepam, digitalis, benzoates, and some hormones—are detoxified through the glucuronidation pathway. Beta-glucuronidase, regarded as a dangerous enzyme, interferes with the glucuronidation process, allowing toxic levels of drugs and contaminants to accumulate. Older individuals appear particularly susceptible to increased beta-glucuronidase formation because of long-term exposure to toxic agents.

A phytoextract, D-glucarate, has been shown to support the glucuronidation pathway by inhibiting the activity of beta-glucuronidase. D-glucarate may be obtained naturally by emphasizing apples, grapefruit, broccoli, and brussels sprouts in the diet and by supplementing with calcium-D-glucarate and vegetable concentrates. According to data released from the University of Texas M.D. Anderson Cancer Center, D-glucarate inhibited beta-glucuronidase by 57% in the blood, 44% in the liver, 39% in the intestines, and 37% in the lungs, thus protecting the action of the glucuronidation pathway (Dwivedi et al. 1990).

Murray et al. (1998) report that the glucuronidation pathway is also impaired in the 5% of the population with Gilbert's syndrome. Gilbert's syndrome is a benign hereditary condition characterized by hyperbilirubinemia (serum bilirubin level 1.2–3.0 mg/dL) and jaundice. The Gilbert's syndrome patient typically complains of loss of appetite, malaise, and fatigue, symptoms often identifiable with liver dysfunction.

If entry of noxious materials is not controlled, detoxification, a cleansing ritual, can no longer keep pace, and alternative measures to encourage detoxification should be employed. Many nutrients and therapies assist in detoxification but glutathione is particularly important since it contributes to both Phase I and Phase II detoxification mechanisms. According to Eric R. Braverman, M.D., glutathione lessens the toxicity of heavy metals, automobile exhaust, cigarette smoke, fungicides, herbicides, nitrates, solvents, plastics, detergents, insecticides, and drugs. Furthermore, repeated exposure to any of these toxins can deplete glutathione faster than it can be produced or absorbed. Vitamin C appears to be an excellent nutrient to increase glutathione stores by stimulating the rate of glutathione synthesis. Glutathione supplementation is also available for individuals not wishing to rely upon vitamin C for glutathione enhancement. Glutathione in 250-mg capsules, taken on an empty stomach 1 or 2 times daily, is the recommended dosage.

Fasting

At one time, Paavo Airola, N.D., Ph.D. referred to fasting as the royal road to health and long life. Fasting is a popular method of detoxification because the body can begin extricating the noxious materials rather quickly, allowing the body to commence the healing process. Literally, fasting means to deprive oneself of food for a specific period, usually for therapeutic or religious purposes. Medical journals have presented articles that support fasting as a therapeutic means of ridding hazardous materials from the body (Imamura et al. 1984).

If there is a down side to fasting, apart from dietary abstinence, it would be the caution required as pollutants are released from internal caches. During a fast, the concentration of toxins in the urine can be 10 times higher than normal. After the toxic load is decreased, the body has greater latitude to concentrate upon the healing process.

A professional who understands the detoxification process best implements a fast. Many practitioners prefer juice fasting to water fasting, believing the juices expedite the process of detoxification and impose less stress upon the individual. (It is recommended that juices be diluted with distilled water.) Also, a professional will know how to deal with a Herxheimer's reaction, which alludes to symptoms initially appearing more intensified as toxins are freed. The nervous system is particularly vulnerable to the release of fat-soluble toxins.

Some individuals who fast report being energized, but this usually occurs after repeated short fasts have eliminated many of the toxins and the internal milieu is cleaner.

The initial fasting experience in a toxic individual most often produces a feeling of fatigue, as the body does battle with the poisons. For this reason, working individuals may wish to plan a short fast (with the aid of their healthcare professional) over a weekend when the workload is lighter. The body is extremely engaged as noxious materials are being extracted. Conversely, the digestion of foodstuffs requires a tremendous work effort; therefore, a sabbatical from food allows the body the energy for detoxification.

Starting a fast and breaking a fast require special guidance, so that the cleansing effort is not lost by inappropriate binge eating. Fasting is not for everyone; a hypoglycemic often finds it extremely difficult to fast, even for short periods of time. A guided fast may, however, prove a valid therapy for some individuals wishing to expedite the detoxification process.

Detoxifying Herbs

Many practitioners believe that the best approach to detoxification is a gradual, but ongoing process. There are a number of herbs that historically have had an impressive reputation as detoxifying and blood purifying agents. A popular term that an herbalist might use for agents that clean up the bloodstream is an "alterative," meaning the constituents of the blood are gradually being changed from a state of poor health to one of wellness. The herbs facilitate the filtration of

toxins and wastes while killing poisons and balancing nutrients and plasma substances.

A number of herbs have a similar purpose in the blood purification and liver detoxification process. Often, herbalists combine herbs of similar likeness into a complex, believing the synergistic value of the herbs delivers greater efficacy than a single herbal. A list of these "clean-up herbs" and a brief description of their contribution to the detoxification mechanism follow.

Hepatics, Alteratives, Diuretics, Laxatives, and Diaphoretics

Dandelion root (Taraxacum officinalis), an excellent blood purifier, assists in many ways to boost the detoxification process. While dandelion root enhances the performance of the liver, dandelion leaves have a diuretic action, pulling toxins and excess water from the body.

Licorice (Glycyrrhiza glabra), though from a different herbal family than dandelion (licorice from Leguminosae and dandelion from Compositae), is also regarded as an alterative. Licorice protects the blood supply by defending the liver, the detoxification plant of the body. In fact, so strong is licorice's contribution toward detoxification that Mowrey (1986) reminded us that the Chinese have dubbed it the "The Great Detoxifier." Licorice is best used as part of a complex containing various other herbs and is usually well tolerated in this application. Licorice contains estrogenic properties and could elevate blood pressure or heighten adrenal expression, if administered in large amounts.

Pau D'Arco (Tabebuia heptaphylla) is an effective blood purifier, extracting toxins that lead to blood toxicity. Pau D'Arco also protects the liver while the liver is aggressively involved in neutralizing poisons.

Yellow dock (Rumex crispus) primarily affects liver function, enhancing the detoxification mechanism and increasing straining of contaminants and purification of the bloodstream. Ritchason (1995) reports that yellow dock is regarded as a favorite alterative among many individuals, sometimes using it against arsenic poisoning. Yellow dock attains tonic status by increasing energy and vitality throughout the body with particular emphasis upon the muscular, nervous, and digestive systems. Eclectics commonly used yellow dock when they perceived that blood-borne toxins instigated the appearance of skin diseases, for example, a rash.

Sarsaparilla root (Smilax officinalis) attacks and neutralizes microbial substances in the bloodstream through its antibiotic activity. By acting as a diuretic and diaphoretic (promotes perspiration), sarsaparilla encourages excretion of toxins and waste materials and acts as an antidote for various poisons. Heavy metallic contaminants in the blood can be extracted from the system with the judicious use of sarsaparilla. Sarsaparilla exerts strong power over fibers and tissues of the nervous system that may be particularly beneficial to the Gulf War veteran.

Stillingia root (*Stillingia sylvatica*) has the nature of an alterative and is beneficial in disease states that affect the skin, for example, psoriasis and eczema. Stillingia, though extremely beneficial in blood purification, is best used in small amounts, complexed with other herbs such as prickly ash (*Zanthoxylum americanum*). Prickly ash bark is a diaphoretic, assisting in the discharge of toxins.

Burdock root (*Arctium lappa*), according to Santillo (1984), is a traditional blood purifier, or alterative, with diuretic and diaphoretic activity. Burdock is considered an appropriate herb for eliminating long-term impurities from the bloodstream. It can neutralize most poisons, relieving kidney and lymphatic systems. Hepatic functions are influenced by burdock, *barberry* (*Berberis vulgaris*), and *Oregon grape root* (*Berberis aquifolium*), preparing the liver for more efficient detoxification.

Cascara Sagrada bark (*Ramnus purshiana*) is regarded as a reliable laxative herb, contributing to the elimination of toxic debris from the colon. It usually accomplishes this task without the miseries associated with laxatives. *Buckthorn bark* (*Rhamnus frangula*) is also considered a laxative, having an energetic, evacuative effect and stimulating bile production from the liver. Buckthorn is regarded as a bitter herb, capable of expelling impurities.

Ritchason (1995) regards *echinacea* (*Echinacea augustifolia*) as one of the premier alteratives, echinacea having been called the "King of Blood Purifiers." It appears to stimulate the elimination of waste products by stabilizing the relative percentage of neutrophils to other leukocytes in the blood. Historically, echinacea has been used to purify the blood after noxious exposures, for example, venomous wounds and blood poisoning, by improving lymphatic filtration and drainage. Echinacea often benefits a toxic headache with vertigo and a confused mental state when the condition is predisposed by toxemia.

Kelp and *algin* appear important adjuncts to any cleansing program since they bind radioactive barium, cadmium and zinc in the gastrointestinal tract, hindering absorption. Kelp appears to reduce the risk of environmental poisoning by acting as a nondigestible fiber, increasing fecal bulk while enhancing the immune response. A factor found in kelp, sodium alginate, binds with radioactive strontium-90 in the intestines and carries it out of the body. (Findings reported at the Gastrointestinal Research Laboratories of McGill University in Montreal.) (*Note:* Some herbalists regard Norwegian kelp freer of impurities and, by various standards, the preferred form to use.)

McCaleb et al. (2000) report that *red clover* (*Trifolium pratense*) has a long history of usage as a blood-cleansing herb that thins the blood, aids digestion, and stimulates detoxification through the liver and gall bladder. It has merit when used as a single herb, or if complexed with other purifying herbs. The user should be aware, however, that red clover possesses estrogenic activity, and since it thins the blood, it may be inappropriate for some supplemental regimes.

Cayenne (*Capsicum annum*) is added as a catalyst in many herbal complexes to enhance the effectiveness and delivery of other herbs. It also has a diaphoretic action, encouraging the expulsion of toxins through perspiration.

Many variations of these herbs are available through either health food stores or the supplier.

Milk Thistle (Silybum Marianum) Complexed with Phosphatidylcholine

The tradition involving milk thistle (*Silybum marianum*) as an herbal medicinal dates back over 2000 years, with Dioscordes using the extract to treat mushroom poisoning and snake bite (1st century CE). The modern use of milk thistle, according to Ogletree et al. (1997), began in 1949 when animal studies confirmed that it could protect the liver from the toxic effects of carbon tetrachloride. In 1968, an active ingredient was isolated and named silymarin. Milk thistle has been the subject of over 100 clinical trials, primarily for liver disease. More recently, milk thistle has emerged as a staple in emergency procedures throughout Europe to treat amanita mushroom poisoning and as a protectant against toxins found in acetaminophen.

Highly polluted areas, like the Gulf War arena, exacerbate the production and activity of free radicals, the harbinger of most degenerative disease. Ogletree et al. (1997) state that the hepatoprotective effects of milk thistle are accomplished via three main pathways: (1) antioxidant activity, (2) protection of the hepatocellular membrane, and (3) stimulation of hepatocytes.

A human study evaluated the effectiveness of milk thistle on occupational exposure to liver toxins, primarily solvents, paints, and glues. The study was placebo controlled, with 35 participants receiving 420 mg a day of milk thistle, while 20 subjects received a placebo. At the end of the treatment period (15–20 days), there was a meaningful decrease in liver enzymes (aspartate aminotransferase, alanine aminotransferase, gamma-glutamyl transpeptidase, alkaline phosphatase) and bilirubin in the milk thistle group. There were no improvements observed in liver function in the placebo group (Boari et al. 1981). Complexing silymarin with phosphatidylcholine (PC) enhances the bioavailability of the herb, while PC itself is highly regarded as a hepatoprotective agent.

Chelation Therapy: A Means of Extracting Heavy Metals

Chelation therapy refers to a treatment in which certain synthetic chemicals and body proteins bind metal molecules, extracting them from the system. Literally, chelation therapy is derived from the Greek word *chele*, which alludes to a claw-like action imposed upon unwanted materials accumulating in the body. Chelation is currently best associated with the clearance of plaque from the arteries, establishing normal blood flow to the vasculature.

Historically, chelation therapy has been used for other objectives apart from cardiovascular health. As early as 1941, Providence Hospital in Detroit used chelation, employing intravenously administered ethylenediaminetetraacetic acid (EDTA), a synthetic amino acid, to extract lead. EDTA, a nontoxic chelator, also clears mercury, cadmium, nickel, copper, calcium, and other metals from the body. Even physicians who are not proponents of chelation therapy admit that evidence in regard to extracting heavy metals appears convincing. Chelation therapy has been useful in treating schizophrenia and Lou Gehrig's disease as well.

For the 25% of the U.S. population who have varying levels of heavy metal poisoning, the dangers are manifold. Illustrative of this, molecularly, some metals closely resemble the chemical structure of enzymes, with a small amount of the metal chelated into the enzyme's structure (Walker 1990). If an excess of the metals replaces the normal mineral content of the enzyme, the enzyme can become chemically altered and nonfunctional, hindering metabolic activity. Because enzymes ignite detoxification, the process suffers when enzymes are in short supply. The Gulf War veteran who was exposed to unreasonable amounts of environmental metallic poisons could be shutting down enzymatic systems vital to detoxification processes.

The signs of heavy metal poisoning closely resemble the complaints of the service personnel of the Gulf War, for example, headache, fatigue, muscle aches and pains, tremors, anemia, mental confusion, mental illness, depression, tingling in the extremities, abnormal nerve reflexes, insomnia and/or drowsiness, dizziness, irritability, disorientation, decreased male fertility, spontaneous abortions in women, and poor circulation. Virtually every organ system responds adversely to heavy metal accumulations, including the respiratory, cardiovascular, muscular, integumentary (skin, hair, nails), nervous, endocrine, skeletal, urinary, and digestive systems.

Walker (1990) believes that chelation therapy is 3.5 times safer than taking an aspirin tablet for a headache. LD-50 refers to the pharmaceutical term "lethal dose 50," the dose of a substance that is fatal to 50% of test animals. Aspirin has a LD-50 at only 558 mg per kilogram in humans, while EDTA's LD-50 is 2000 mg/kg.

A crucial phase of chelation is re-establishing the beneficial minerals that were extracted, along with the heavy metals. This may be accomplished either orally or intravenously. It would be to the patient's advantage were the physicians using autonomic balancing as the premise for refusion of the minerals. The selection of appropriate minerals to normalize imbalances occurring in the autonomic nervous system appears an integral phase of the success or failure of chelation therapy.

An individual wishing to obtain chelation therapy may want to contact a physician who follows the standard chelation protocol of the American College of Advancement in Medicine. The number of sessions required to enact a change cannot be presupposed, but the recommended maximum dosage is currently about 3 grams of EDTA, dosage usually calculated by body weight, given by IV infusion 1–3 times weekly, as a drip for 3–4 hours. Initially, the dosage may be as small as 1/2–1 gram of EDTA.

Can What You Eat Make a Difference?

According to Dr. Steven Whiting of the Institute of Nutritional Science, supplemental fiber, as well as fibrous food choices, not only protects the digestive system from concentrated toxins, but it also serves as a cleansing factor for many poisons accumulating in the body. Certain foods, such as bran, whole grain wheat, oats, corn, cereals, lentils, beans, peas, peanuts, figs, dates, and apples, are natural chelators. Supplementing with psyllium seed husks, oat, and wheat bran (if not allergic to wheat), and acacia gum, plus emphasizing high-fiber food choices assists in binding noxious materials in the digestive tract and expelling them in fecal material.

OTHER TREATMENTS FOR GWS

Mycoplasma Forecast

Nicolson et al. (1998) have released the heartening news, gathered from their research at the Institute for Molecular Medicine, Huntington Beach, CA, that thousands of soldiers are being helped when mycoplasma infections are identified and killed.

The presence of mycoplasma infections in the blood of fractions of patients with CFIDS, FMS, GWS, or RA enable health care professionals to rule out psychological or psychiatric based illness as a causative factor in the above-mentioned conditions and instead direct their efforts toward correction of medical anomalies. Administering antibiotic therapy is sometimes a chosen treatment modality. Appropriate cyclic treatments with antibiotics or other medications that suppress chronic infections have resulted in improvement and even recovery in most of the individuals treated. If blood infections are diagnosed, patients receive continuous antibiotics for at least 6 months before beginning a 6-week cyclic treatment. The recommended treatments for mycoplasmal blood infections require long-term antibiotic therapy, usually multiple 6-week cycles of doxycycline (200–300 mg a day), ciprofloxacin (Cipro) (1500 mg a day), azithromycin (Zithromax) (500 mg a day), or clarithromycin (Biaxin) (750–1000 mg a day). (*Note*: Administering some antibiotics produces no favorable clinical response; in fact, penicillin results in patients becoming more symptomatic.)

Multiple antibiotic cycles are required because few patients recover after only a few cycles or even within the first year of therapy if the illness is chronic, possibly because of the intracellular locations of the infections and the slow-growing nature of the microorganisms. As with other treatments used to rid infiltrations of noxious materials or microorganisms, a Herxheimer's reaction usually occurs, meaning the patient feels poorer than before beginning the curative. This reaction occurs as die-off or release of toxic materials from damaged microorganisms is increased. As die-off decreases, stabilization occurs, and the patient slowly moves nearer recovery.

Confounding the treatment, some patients recover only to a certain point and then fail to continue to respond to the antibiotics, suggesting that other problems, such as viral infections, environmental exposures, and other toxic events, are working synergistically with the microorganism to produce a state of ill health.

A 3-year follow-up of antibiotic therapy by the SHASTA CFIDS Association of Northern California reported that a majority (about 80%) of the patients with confirmed mycoplasmal infections who participated in the antibiotic therapy recovered from 50–100% of their preillness health, within the 3 years.

Antibiotics are not without their dark side. Apart from an ugly list of side effects that commonly accompany antibiotic therapy, antibiotics can disrupt the friendly flora that resides symbiotically in the gut. Gut flora represents several pounds of highly sensitive material that is regarded as immune modulating. Disturbance of "friendly flora" can antagonize the immune and inflammatory process. Reinoculation of the gut with cultures of *Lactobacillus acidophilus*, *Lactobacillus rhamnosus*, *Bifidobacterium longum*, and *Bifidobacterium breve* is vital to recovery. Selection of a probiotic that is touted to be antibiotic resistant is recommended.

To be successful, each patient must comply with a complementary health approach that employs the best of orthodox and natural medicine. Gulf War veterans presenting with mycoplasmas typically display nutritional deficiencies and poor absorption that must be corrected. Mega vitamin/mineral therapy is warranted, and sublingual or liquid supplements should be considered. Vitamin C, which detoxifies most heavy metals (5–15 grams daily, in divided doses), vitamin E (600–1000 IU daily), CoQ_{10} (50–150 mg daily), bioflavonoids (200 mg 3 times a day), choline (1000 mg daily, in divided doses), inositol (750 mg daily), vitamin B_5 (500–1500 mg daily), PABA (500–1000 mg daily), sublingual vitamin B_{12} (1000 mcg daily dose), and flaxseed or fish oils (1 tbsp daily), along with minerals, such as zinc (50 mg daily), calcium (1000 mg a day), and selenium (up to 300 mcg a day), may be used. Minerals should be taken apart from antibiotics because minerals can affect antibiotic absorption. Garlic (*Allium sativum*) is a potent detoxifier. Use 2 capsules (300 mg each) 3 times a day with meals. Use 500 mg of *L*-cysteine, *L*-tyrosine, *L*-glutamine, and *L*-carnitine daily on an empty stomach.

Interest has been keen in regard to patients wishing to be tested for mycoplasmas, though additional volunteers are welcomed into the clinical trials conducted by the VA. The Institute for Molecular Medicine can test patients for evidence of mycoplasmal infections and other infections of the types that worsen human diseases, such as chronic fatigue immune deficiency syndrome, fibromyalgia syndrome, Gulf War syndrome, and rheumatoid arthritis. Blood sample can be sent to:

Prof. Garth L. Nicolson
The Institute for Molecular Medicine
15162 Triton Lane
Huntington Beach, CA 92649-1401
Tel: 714-903-2900
Fax: 714-379-2082
E-mail:gnicimm@ix.netcom.com

Dioxychlor

Dr. Robert W. Bradford, president of Bradford Research Institute, states that Dioxychlor is the major oxidant of demonstrated effectiveness, capable of ridding the system of pathogenic organisms. An inorganic compound composed of chlorine and two atoms of nascent oxygen covalently bonded, Dioxychlor is currently being used to treat individuals suffering with GWS, Epstein-Barr virus, and cytomegalovirus. Nicolson (1998) reported the usefulness of this therapy.

Broad-spectrum antibiotics bring short-term relief of infections, but the positive effect of antibiotics may be countered by long-term negativity. The Bradford Institute has determined that environmental diseases are typically characterized by systemic Candida, numerous allergies, autoimmune disorders, and compromised antigen kill. Largely, these disorders are iatrogenic in nature, meaning they are caused by either diagnostic or treatment procedures. Chronic or haphazard administering of antibiotics participates in this decadent cascade.

Dioxychlor, a homeopathic substance displaying low toxicity, offers an alternative to this quandary. Dioxychlor appears to destroy mycoplasmas while reducing sensitivity reactions and improving the status of gravely ill patients, such as those suffering from ALS.

An oral dose of Dioxychlor is 5–20 drops in 2 oz of water (4 tbsp), 1–3 times daily, based on patient tolerance. Should "die off" of foreign materials intensify symptoms, reduce the dosage. Dioxychlor can also be administered by slow drip with the assistance of a qualified physician.

A Single Herbal that Appears Helpful in Gulf War Syndrome Complaints

James Duke Ph.D., botanist and humanitarian, illustrates that yellow sweet clover (*Melilotus officinalis*) contains herbal activity that may prove beneficial in regard to symptoms apparent in those stricken with GWS, for example, headache, myalgia, spasms, mycoplasmosis, ischemia, rheumatism, nervousness, sores, and cardiopathy (1997).

Yellow sweet clover contains 0.9–2% coumarin, which may be the substance that elicits the benefit. Coumarin should, however, be used cautiously, for high doses can cause symptoms, such as headache, stupor, thinning of blood, and elevated liver enzymes, which appear transient upon discontinuance.

Individuals wishing to purchase yellow sweet clover may do so by contacting the following two suppliers:

Dragon River Herbals
P.O. Box 74
Ojo Caliente, NM 87549
Tel: (800) 813-2118

Mark's Drugs Roselle
384 E. Irving Park Rd.
Roselle, Illinois 60172
Tel: (630) 529-3400

Use 1/2 tsp (30 drops), taken 2–3 times a day, for 7–10 days. It is advisable to observe a 3–5-day respite from yellow sweet clover before repeating the herbal therapy.

Oxygenation Therapy

Oxidative therapy can be useful in suppressing a variety of anaerobic infections when administered at 1.5 ATM for 60 minutes. Hyperbaric oxygen therapy (HBO) refers to a monoplace chamber, in which only one patient is entirely enclosed in a pressure chamber, breathing oxygen at a pressure greater than atmospheric pressure. HBO is regarded as a therapeutic modality because significant physiological mechanisms are activated as a result. HBO delivers 10–15 times the oxygen to tissues as normal breathing. Popularly, HBO is used in the formation of new capillaries around a wound area and to treat anemia, ischemia, and some poisonings.

The flooding of the body with oxygen, as in hyperbaric therapy, tends to remove other gases, such as carbon monoxide and acute cyanide poisoning. HBO inhibits the growth of a number of anaerobic, as well as aerobic, organisms by enhancing phagocytic activity. This effect complements the improved action of host disease-fighting factors and is useful in disorders involving immunosuppression. Studies have demonstrated a prolonged postantibiotic effect when hyperbaric oxygen is combined with therapeutic dosages of antibiotics.

Exercise Intolerance

Deeper understanding of the energy processes involved in human physiology and the role of the mitochondria, the powerhouse of the cell, may help in managing chronic disease processes. According to Bland (2000), an intermittent or sporadic form of mitochondrial myopathy, in which exercise intolerance is the predominant symptom, has been observed in individuals suffering from FMS, GWS, and encephalomyopathies.

The nucleus and the mitochondria each possess genetic information contained in DNA, a trait not shared with other organelles. Mitochondria can be damaged in such a way that communication with fellow mitochondria or other cellular organelles becomes faulty. Bland lists factors suspected as contributory events in malfunctioning mitochondria. Among them are the following:

1. Oxidative stress is associated with low oxygen tension or ischemia, which contributes to mitochondrial oxidation and can result in injury to mitochondrial DNA. According to Bruce Kristal, Ph.D., of the department of biochemistry at Cornell University Medical College, about 90% of oxygen supply is used by the mitochondria for oxidative phosphorylation, a process that produces ATP, an energy molecule. Electron leakage, perhaps less than 1–4%, occurs during oxidative phosphorylation and becomes a harbinger for free radicals. Free radicals perform a cyclic dance, as one radical may be neutralized only to produce another. An aggressive complex of antioxidants increases protection against oxidative stress. Consider traditional antioxidants, such as vitamin C, vitamin E, vitamin A, selenium, garlic, glutathione, green tea, grape seed extract, and lipoic acid.

2. Glucose intolerance or increased concentrations of glucose reportedly potentiate injury to mitochondrial DNA. Individuals suffering dysinsulinism and dysglycemia, with increased glycosylated hemoglobin levels, may have a greater propensity for mitochondrial DNA damage.

3. Sleep debt appears associated with impaired metabolic and endocrine performance, which may have physiopathologic consequences over time.

4. Dietary factors, such as calorie restriction in animals, have lessened the incidence of mitochondrial injury and mutation.

5. Environmental injury imposed by persistent or exaggerated contact with noxious agents may overwhelm the ability of the natural antioxidant systems to accommodate the exposure, and cellular damage results. The susceptibility of mitochondrial DNA to environmental mutagens appears even greater than the vulnerability of the nucleus, according to Johns (1995).

6. Medications, such as an antiretroviral nucleoside analogue like AZT, specific antibiotics, nucleoside-analogue reverse-transcriptase inhibitors, and the fibrate drugs, that is, antihyperlipoproteinemic drugs, appear to increase mitochondrial oxidative injury.

7. Chronic inflammation is associated with increased release of cell messengers, for example, tumor necrosis factor alpha, or interleukin-1 and interleukin-6, which may have effects on the mitochondria.

Exercise intolerance hearkens back to the work of Dr. Nicholas Gonzalez. Exercise may intensify parasympathetic expression and further tame the sympathetic nervous system by "burning off" epinephrine and norepinephrine hormones released by the adrenal medulla. Recall that cholinesterase inhibitor insecticides, to which the Gulf War veterans were exposed, may amplify parasympathetic expression, a metabolic type that may have been dominant from birth in individuals more vulnerable to GWS. It is possible that exercise tolerance will increase, if choices are made to balance the autonomic nervous system.

Elite athletes have benefited from large doses (20 grams) of creatine supplements when compromised ATP production was suspected. The benefits observed in muscular performance among athletes may extend to individuals suffering the pain and fatigue of myalgia. Use 5 grams of creatine, 4 times a day for 5 days. Thereafter, use 1 gram of creatine, following exercise. Though creatine is considered remarkably safe, individuals with kidney impairment may find it advisable to avoid creatine supplements.

Dioxychlor increases oxygen supply throughout the body and may be of benefit in preserving mitochondrial integrity.

Exercise Conclusion

Air travel, excessive exercise, and a lack of sleep worsen symptoms of GWS. Flying lowers oxygen tension and can stimulate borderline anaerobes. Exercise, though essential in moderation, should not be aggressive, for a relapse due to overexertion can occur.

Dry saunas help rid the system of chemicals. Saunas may be considered 3 times a week, followed by 15–20 minutes of dry sauna and a tepid shower. Repeat saunas no more than 2 times a day. Work up a sweat, eliminating chemicals, without goading the body into stressful activity. Always replace body fluids during and after each session.

Should individuals choose to incorporate walking into their rehabilitation program, select the exercise arena carefully. Roadside exercise, because of contaminants, negates the value of the activity. Become good environmental stewards, screening the entry of pollutants and allergens into an already challenged biochemistry. For recovery, after light exercise and to decrease muscle soreness, use a Jacuzzi or hot tub, adding 2 cups of Epsom salt, after a sufficient cool down period. The final caution in regard to exercise is to keep it simple, without taxing or exhausting the system.

⬤ SUMMARY

1. Implementation of detoxification techniques to stimulate extraction of noxious materials from the system is highly recommended. Fasting, if employed as a detox mechanism, should be performed under the supervision of a qualified professional, who will fully structure the fast and assist in ridding poisons from the system.

2. Herbs that are often complexed to assist in blood purification and detoxification include dandelion root, yellow dock root, sarsaparilla root, echinacea, licorice root, stillingia root, burdock root, buckthorn, barberry, Cascara Sagrada bark, prickly ash bark, Pau D'Arco, red clover, kelp, Oregon grape, and cayenne.

The following dosages represent general guidelines only for individual herbs. Drug interactions and contraindications regarding long-term use and specific medical conditions must first be evaluated. An herbal detoxification program should be considered only under the supervision of an experienced healthcare provider.

- Dandelion root (*Taraxacum officinale*): A typical dosage of dandelion root is 2–8 grams 3 times daily of dried root; 250 mg 3–4 times daily of a 5:1 extract; or 5–10 mL 3 times daily of a 1:5 tincture in 45% alcohol. The leaves may be eaten in salad or cooked.

- Licorice (*Glycyrrhiza glabra*): For supportive treatment of ulcer pain along with conventional medical care, the standard dose of deglycyrrhizinated licorice (DGL) is two to four 380-mg tablets of DGL taken before meals and at bedtime. A typical dose of whole licorice is 5–15 grams daily. However, doses this high are not recommended for longer than a few weeks. For long-term consumption, about 0.3 grams of licorice root daily can safely be taken by most adults.

- Pau D'Arco or Lapacho (*Tabebuia impestiginosa, T. avellanedae*)(also known as Pau d'Arco and Taheebo): Pau D'arco contains many components that don't dissolve in water, so making an herbal tea is difficult. As a capsulized powdered bark, the typical dose is 300–500 mg 3 times daily. The inner bark of the lapacho tree is believed to be the most effective part of the plant.

- Yellow dock (*Rumex crispus*): Typical doses of yellow dock root are 2–4 grams of the dried root, 2–4 mL of the liquid extract, or 1–2 mL of the tincture.

- Sarsaparilla root (*Sarsaparillae radix*—sarsaparilla root derived from *Smilax* species): Dried root, 2–4 grams 2–3 times daily as a decoction; liquid extract (1:1, 50% ethanol), 2–4 mL 2–3 times daily.

- Stillingia root (*Stillingia sylvatica*): Tincture (Fresh root, 1:2, Recent Dry root, 1:5, 50% alcohol) 10–30 drops, preferably in small frequent doses.

- Burdock root (*Arctium lappa*): A typical dosage of burdock is 1–2 grams of powdered dry root 3 times a day.

- Barberry (*Berberis vulgaris*): Powdered bark, 1/4 tsp several times daily. Fluid extract (1:1, 1:5), 20-40 drops daily. Solid extract, 5–10 grains.

- Oregon grape root (*Mahonia aquifolium*) (also known as Mountain grape): Available in homeopathic formulations.

- Cascara Sagrada bark (*Rhamnus purshiana*): Cut bark, powder or dry extracts for teas, decoction, cold maceration, or elixir. One 450-mg capsule daily or 2 grams of finely cut drug strained in hot water as a tea.

- Buckthorn bark (*Rhamnus frangula*): Cut bark, powder or dried extracts for teas, decoction, cold maceration, or elixir. The daily dosage is 2–5 grams corresponding to 20–30 mg hydroxyanthracene derivatives, calculated as glycofrangulin A. A tea may be made of 4 grams of cut drug strained in hot water.

- Echinacea (*Echinacea augustifolia*): The typical dosage of echinacea powdered extract is 300 mg 3 times a day. Alcohol tincture (1:5) is usually taken at a dosage of 3–4 mL 3 times daily, echinacea juice at a dosage of 2–3 mL 3 times daily, and whole dried root at 1–2 grams 3 times daily. Long-term use of echinacea is not recommended.

- Kelp: There is no appropriate therapeutic dosage of kelp because it is not yet known whether kelp is truly therapeutic for any conditions. However, because of its high iodine content, it is important not to overdo your use of kelp. The iodine content in 17 different kelp supplements studied by one group of researchers varied from 45 to 57,000 mcg a tablet or capsule (*Food Addit. Contam.* 1988; 5: 103–109). The recommended daily intake for iodine is 150 mcg a day for people over the age 4, and taking a great deal more than this can cause thyroid problems.

- Algin: Algin is any hydrophilic, colloidal substance found in or obtained from various kelps. Algin prevents living tissue from absorbing radioactive materials and encourages the action of dietary fiber, by supplying nutrients and normalizing bowel functions. Dosage not available.
- Cayenne (*Capsicum frutescens, Capsicum annuum*): Two 500-mg capsules daily may be taken.

3. Silibinin, 500 mg along with 1800 mg of phosphatidylcholine is particularly valuable as a hepatoprotective.

4. It is extremely important to reinoculate the gut after antibiotic therapy. Select a probiotic touted to survive through antibiotic therapy and that contains *Lactobacillus acidophilus, Lactobacillus rhamnosus, Bifidobacterium longum*, and *Bifidobacterium breve*. *L. acidophilus* has a wide variance of live-culture activity, ranging from 20 million/cap to 4 billion/cap to 10 billion/gram. During the course of antibiotic therapy, *L. acidophilus* should be taken about 2 hours after the medication. The antibiotic will destroy the beneficial cultures if taken together; only some of the activity will be obliterated if taken separately from the antibiotic. After the course of antibiotic therapy is completed, probiotic therapy should be doubled or tripled for 2 weeks, depending upon the quantity of the cultures present in the formulary.

5. Chelation therapy may be valuable to the Gulf War veteran. In chelation, heavy metals and contaminants are pulled from the system by intravenous administration of ethylenediaminetetraacetic acid (EDTA). It is best administered by a physician following the Chelation Protocol, subscribed to by the American College of Advancement in Medicine.

6. Selecting foodstuffs with high fiber content and supplementing with additional fiber, such as psyllium, acacia, apple pectin, and oat and wheat bran, assist in ridding poisons from the body. Fiber complexes, containing a variety of soluble and insoluble materials, can be added (1 heaping tsp) to a full glass of liquid and used 1–3 times a day. The smaller dose should be used until the system adjusts to the fiber. Should gas or bloating occur, reduce the dose size until tolerance is achieved.

7. "If you cannot eat it, don't smell it." Chronic exposure to noxious materials may overwhelm the body's natural antioxidant system, and a generation of endogenous toxins may allow cellular damage to occur. For many individuals, the process of detoxification is maximally amplified just cleaning up from everyday pollutants. For the Gulf War veteran, whose detoxification mechanism has been inordinately stressed, it reflects good judgment to avoid exposure to pollutants and chemicals that further frazzle this essential process. Avoid yard and garden sprays, household cleansers, emissions from gas and diesel engines, industrial pollutants appearing in water and the atmosphere, freshly dry-cleaned garments (air before wearing), paint, varnishes, stains, creosote and wood emissions from a fireplace, dust, insulation, insecticides, and foods exposed to sprays of uncertain safety. The list is endless in our society; prudent persons work toward improving their health status by continuously monitoring their exposure to hazardous substances.

8. Antibiotic therapy has proven to be of advantage in reducing the population of mycoplasmas. Administering antibiotic therapy requires prescriptions and monitoring by a qualified medical professional. A regime representing natural medicine should also be administered. Consider vitamin C (5–15 grams daily, in divided doses), vitamin E (400–1000 IU daily), CoQ$_{10}$ (100–300 mg daily), bioflavonoids (200 mg 3 times a day), choline (1000 mg daily, in divided doses), inositol (750 mg daily), vitamin B$_5$ (500–1500 mg a day), PABA (500–1000 mg daily), vitamin B$_{12}$ (a 1000 mcg sublingual daily dose), and fish oil (2–3 grams daily), along with minerals such as zinc (50 mg daily), calcium (1000 mg a day), and selenium (up to 300 mcg a day). Minerals should be taken apart from antibiotics because minerals can affect antibiotic absorption. Garlic (*Allium sativum*) is a potent detoxifier. Use 2 300-mg capsules 3 times a day with meals. Use *L*-cysteine, *L*-tyrosine, *L*-glutamine, and *L*-carnitine (500 mg each, daily) on an empty stomach.

9. Yellow sweet clover, *Melilotus officinalis*, has analgesic, anti-inflammatory, digestive, diuretic, hepatoprotective, immunostimulant, myorelaxant, proteolytic, sedative, spasmolytic, and mycoplasmotic activity (*see the section entitled A Single Herb that Appears Helpful in Gulf War Syndrome Complaints for the names of suppliers and dosing instructions*).

10. A hyperbaric oxygen chamber kills both anaerobic and aerobic bacteria while improving immune function and displacing noxious gases. HBO is well seeded as a primary therapy in the treatment of medical disorders such as carbon monoxide poisoning and gas gangrene. HBO therapy is

increasingly being used as an adjunctive process in the management of a variety of refractory disorders such as GWS.

11. Dioxychlor may assist in the control of sensitivities observed in GWS and also in the ridding of mycoplasmas. By increasing oxygenation, Dioxychlor may help preserve mitochondrial integrity. An oral dose of 5–20 drops dissolved in 2 oz of water, 1–3 times a day, may be appropriate. Should symptoms intensify, the dosage should be reduced until the body "catches up" with the die-off. Dioxychlor can be administered intravenously with the assistance of a qualified physician.

12. Administering an aggressive complex of antioxidants increases protection against oxidative stress. Consider a combination of traditional antioxidants such as vitamin C, vitamin E, vitamin A, selenium, garlic, glutathione, green tea, grape seed extract, zinc, N-acetyl-cysteine, and lipoic acid. An approximate dosage is 3 capsules daily, depending upon the strength of the antioxidants complexed.

13. Creatine may be of benefit if impaired ATP production is suspected. Use 5 grams of creatine, 4 times a day for 5 days. Thereafter, use 1 gram of creatine following exercise. Creatine, though regarded as exceptionally safe, may not be appropriate for individuals with kidney disease.

14. Working with a physician trained in autonomic balancing appears vital to full resolution of GWS.

15. Exercise should be approached cautiously, for activity will further encourage parasympathetic nervous system expression, which may already be abrasively dominant. Perspiration will, however, promote toxin excretion. A sauna may provide the better means of encouraging expulsion of contaminants through pores. Even in this environment, caution should be taken. Replace fluids, as internal stores are lost.

 ## FOR MORE INFORMATION

Call the VA Gulf War Veterans Information Helpline at (800) PGW-VETS. The Special Assistant for Gulf War Illnesses can be reached at (800)497-6261.

 ## PRODUCT AVAILABILITY

Life Extension Mix, GastroPro (containing phosphatidylcholine), silymarin, Silibinin Plus (silibinin is the most active extract of silymarin), echinacea, Life Flora (probiotic), Fiber Food, Pure Gar w/EDTA, green tea extract, grape-seed-skin extract, N-acetyl-cysteine (NAC), alpha-lipoic acid, creatine, vitamin C, vitamin E, liquid emulsified vitamin A, vitamin B5, CoQ10, choline bitartrate powder, inositol, PABA, methylcobalamin, Super GLA/DHA, flaxseed oil, Udo's Choice Oil, calcium citrate, zinc, selenium, glutathione, L-cysteine, L-tyrosine, L-glutamine, and L-carnitine are available by telephoning (800) 544-4440, or order online at www.lef.org.

Hearing Loss

Nearly 16 million Americans are affected by hearing loss, ranging from temporary to permanent or from partial to complete (Bertoni et al. 2001). Hearing loss affects about 30% of all adults ages of 65–74. The percentage increases to 50% for adults by the time they reach age 75–79. Hearing loss is classified as conductive (external or middle ear disorders that block the transmission of sound); sensorineural (disorders of the inner ear or the eighth cranial nerve); mixed (a combination of conductive and sensorineural disorders); and functional (resulting from psychological factors and with no identifiable organic damage). Hearing loss may result from the dysfunction of any part of the auditory system. Possible causes of hearing loss include disease (genetic or infectious), allergies, exposure to noise (either chronic or a single event), ototoxic drugs, polyps, tumors, brain injury, and injury to the cochlear nerve. The most common type of hearing loss in elderly persons is called *presbycusis*, a term used to describe sensorineural hearing loss that affects people over the age of 50 (i.e., hearing loss generally attributed to the aging process). The specific cause of age-related hearing loss is unknown (Bertoni et al. 2001).

DETECTING HEARING LOSS

Screening for hearing loss is the first step in determining the type and degree of hearing loss. Today's technology allows hearing screening in a physician's office to be a quick procedure. In a matter of a few minutes, a screening audiometer can identify patients who need to be referred to an otolaryngologist or audiologist for further examination.

Many elderly patients are reluctant to admit a loss of hearing because of embarrassment or fear. Often, if the hearing loss does not affect speech frequencies, the patient may not be aware of it (Bertoni et al. 2001). It is extremely important that adults over the age of 65 be screened regularly. A study of elderly patients has shown that untreated hearing loss increases psychosocial difficulties and reduces functional health. These physical and psychological problems might be easily avoided by treating the problem of hearing loss properly (Anon. 2000).

TREATMENT

Hearing Aids

Amplification provided by a hearing aid is the best rehabilitative strategy for some types of hearing loss that cannot be treated medically or surgically. Many hearing-impaired patients can be significantly helped through hearing aids, assistive listening devices, and rehabilitation. Hearing aids have evolved from cumbersome, highly visible devices to amazingly sophisticated, discreet minicomputers (AMA 1989). There are more than 1000 models of hearing aids available. An audiologist or hearing-instrument specialist can help with selection of the hearing aid that is right for you based on your preferences and degree of hearing loss.

Cochlear Implants

For a minority of patients who have profound hearing loss, surgery is an indicated treatment. The cochlear implant is an option for those patients who derive no benefit from the most powerful hearing aids. A cochlear implant is a mechanical device implanted surgically on the inside or outside of the cochlea. The cochlea is the part of the inner ear that transforms sound vibrations into nerve impulses that will be transmitted to the brain. During the surgery, a tiny receiver is implanted under the skin, either behind the ear or in the chest, with a wire that connects it to the device on the cochlea. The patient will also need to wear an external transmitter that is connected to a sound processor and a microphone. A cochlear implant does not restore normal hearing, but it may improve the patient's understanding of speech and facilitate lip-reading. Implantation of this device involves mastoid surgery and brief hospitalization (AMA 1989). Cochlear implants are only recommended to a limited number of patients who would be totally deaf otherwise. Because individual compliance in learning to use a cochlear implant is essential, the usefulness of the implant for any particular person cannot be reliably predicted, but for some patients, the cochlear implant makes a tremendous difference in hearing capacity.

ALTERNATIVE TREATMENTS

Alpha-lipoic acid

There is evidence that agents such as alpha-lipoic acid, which reduce free-radical formation, play an important role in (1) reducing presbycusis and improving cochlear function (Seidman et al. 2000) and (2) reducing the auditory toxicity caused by aminoglycosides (Conlon et al. 1999), cisplatin (Rybak et al. 1999a; 1999b; 1999c), and noise (Armstrong et al. 1998). Studies show that alpha-lipoic acid, lessens nerve damage induced by ototoxic aminoglycoside antibiotics (Conlon et al. 1999). According to Conlon, the studies "highlight a potential clinical therapeutic use of alpha-lipoic acid in patients undergoing aminoglycoside treatment." Alpha-lipoic acid has also been shown to provide very good protection against cisplatin auditory toxicity in several studies by Rybak et al. (1999a; 1999b; 1999c). Patients undergoing treatment with drugs that have ototoxic side effects may benefit from a dose of 500 mg of alpha-lipoic acid twice daily.

Hydergine

The drug Hydergine is considered to be an all-purpose "brain booster" and may help improve hearing (Jimenez-Cervantes et al. 1990). Although the FDA has approved doses of only 3 mg a day of Hydergine, doses of 12–20 mg a day may be required to help improve hearing. Hydergine is nontoxic and relatively safe. Its potential side effects include mild nausea and some gastric disturbance. It is not recommended for people with psychosis, low blood pressure, or an abnormally low heartbeat.

Hydergine was originally produced and distributed by Sandoz Pharmaceuticals. The original patent has since expired and generic versions are now available in various strengths by prescription. However, many people choose to obtain low-cost 5-mg Hydergine from overseas pharmacies.

Ginkgo biloba

Ginkgo biloba has helped some people with various hearing disorders, including tinnitus (ringing in the ears) (Dubreuil 1986; Hoffmann et al 1994; Holstein 2001). Ginkgo also provides a wide range of health benefits, including improved neurological function (Soholm 1998), and has been shown to have a protective effect against gentamicin-induced cochlear damage (Jung et al. 1998).

Vitamins

Vitamin A

For many years, researchers have investigated the potential benefits of vitamin A for persons with hearing loss. As early as 25 years ago, hearing loss was observed in volunteers who participated in a study on the effects of hypovitaminosis A (low vitamin A) (Chole et al. 1976). Research results have sometimes been contradictory, but they did show that vitamin A is essential in inner-ear morphogenesis (Chole 1978; Lohle 1982; Biesalski 1984). According to Romeo

(1985), several researchers reported an improvement of 5–15 decibels in the tone threshold of patients with presbycusis. Biesalski et al. (1990) studied the effects of vitamin A deficiency and noise-induced hearing loss. Although their study was conducted with guinea pigs, they concluded "that vitamin A deficiency increased the sensitivity of the inner ear to noise and that this increased sensitivity increases the probability of noise-induced hearing loss" (Biesalski et al. 1990).

Vitamin B

Several of the B vitamins have been shown to have positive benefits for persons with hearing loss, including B_1 (thiamine), B_6 (pyridoxine), B_{12} (cyanocobalamin), biotin, and the vitamin B complex. In a study of 51 subjects with sudden deafness (hearing levels worse than 100 decibels) who were treated with vitamin B as part of their treatment regimen, hearing recovery began between days 2–28. Only seven subjects showed ultimate hearing levels worse than 100 decibels. Most were in the 55- to 80-decibel range. Two subjects achieved complete recovery (hearing levels better than 20 decibels).

Note: *A normal hearing level is 20 decibels; profound hearing loss is over 90 decibels.*

The subjects who recovered hearing within the first 14 days had a better ultimate outcome (Sano et al. 1998). As part of their treatment regimen, another group of patients with tinnitus were given the vitamin B complex. After 5 weeks, 54% of them reported that the treatment had been effective. Long-term effectiveness was not investigated in this study (Ohsaki et al. 1998).

Vitamin B_1 deficiency has been associated with delayed auditory brainstem responses. In a study on animals, the delayed response was corrected in 2–4 days after beginning vitamin B_1 (Shigematsu et al. 1990). Biotin deficiency is also thought to affect development of the auditory nerves. Diagnosis and treatment of biotin deficiency is essential in the first year of life (Taitz et al. 1985; Wallace 1985; Bressman et al. 1986; Wastell et al. 1988). Vitamin B_{12} is often deficient in vegetarian diets. Deficiency has been associated with chronic tinnitus and noise-induced hearing loss (Shemesh et al. 1993). A study of 55 women conducted by Houston et al. (1999) examined the association of age-related auditory dysfunction and vitamin B_{12} deficiency. In both of these studies, subjects with hearing dysfunction exhibited low blood levels of vitamin B_{12}. This led these researchers to recommend that serum levels of vitamin B_{12} be evaluated in persons with tinnitus, noise-induced hearing loss, or age-related hearing loss.

Vitamin C

Although the studies were conducted with animals, researchers found beneficial effects of vitamin C, particularly in the areas of aiding overall nutritional status and protection from or lowering damage to cochlear hair cells and hearing caused by exposure to noise (Branis et al. 1988; Lautermann et al. 1995).

Vitamin D

The possible role of vitamin D deficiency in otosclerosis (abnormal bone growth in the inner ear), unexplained cochlear deafness, presbycusis, bilateral cochlear deafness, and bilateral sensorineural hearing loss has been the subject of scientific studies (Brookes 1983, 1985a,b; Ikeda et al. 1989). These researchers concluded that vitamin D deficiency is likely one of the causal factors in some cases of otosclerosis, cochlear deafness, and presbycusis. According to Brookes (1983; 1985a,b) and Ikeda et al. (1989), vitamin D deficiency should be considered in persons with hearing loss. The studies by Brookes indicated that vitamin D replacement therapy resulted in significant hearing improvement in two of four patients (1983) and three of 16 patients (1985b). The encouraging conclusion was that cochlear deafness and progressive hearing loss may be partly reversible by replacement vitamin D therapy.

Minerals

Zinc

The relationship between zinc deficiency and tinnitus, cochlear damage, and hearing damage has been studied in both humans (Shambaugh 1989; Podoshin et al. 1997) and animals (Gunther et al. 1989; Rubio et al. 1998; McFadden et al. 1999b). Results in both of the human studies (Shambaugh 1989; Podoshin et al. 1997) and one animal study (McFadden et al. 1999b) indicated that zinc deficiencies increase the vulnerability of the cochlea to damage associated with normal aging. Shambaugh (1989) reported that zinc supplementation improved tinnitus and sensorineural hearing loss in a third of elderly patients who were marginally deficient in zinc and stated: "We believe zinc deficiency is one causation of presbycusis; by recognizing and correcting it, a progressive hearing loss can be arrested." According to Podoshin et al. (1997), the incidence of tinnitus in presbycusis is 11% and not gender related, but it is correlated with exposure to noise. Interestingly, they stated that tinnitus occurred in 13% of children who passed audiometric screening texts, in 23 to 60% of children with hearing loss, and in 44% of children with secretory otitis media. Only 3% of children complain about tinnitus, because they do not consider it to be abnormal. According to Podoshin et al. (1997), tinnitus might be a factor in behavioral problems in children.

Magnesium

Magnesium deficiency and its possible role in noise-induced hearing loss has been the subject of numerous studies in both humans (Altura et al. 1992; Joachims et al. 1993; Attias et al. 1994;) and animals (Ising et al. 1982; Cevette et al. 1989; Gunther et al. 1989; Joachims et al. 1983, 1989; Spasov et al. 1999; Scheibe et al. 2000a; 2000b). In animals, magnesium had positive beneficial effects: faster recovery from hearing threshold shift (Scheibe et al. 2000a); significant reduction of trauma caused by high levels of noise exposure (Ising et al. 1982; Joachims et al. 1983; 1989; Scheibe et al. 2000 a); reduced ischemia-induced hearing loss (Spasov et al. 1999; Scheibe et al. 2000b); and a protective effect for ear hair cells (Gunther et al. 1989; Spasov et al. 1999).

Beneficial effects were also found in the human studies. Using double-blind, placebo-controlled methods, Joachims et al. (1993) and Attias et al. (1994) studied military recruits (320 and 300 respectively) who had normal hearing. The recruits were studied for 2 months during basic military training, which included repeated exposure to high levels of firearm noise. All of the recruits wore earplugs. Noise-induced hearing loss was significantly higher in the placebo group than in the group receiving magnesium in both studies. According to Attias et al. (1994), "This study may introduce a significant natural agent for the reduction of hearing damage in the noise-exposed population."

Copper

Most people receive adequate amounts of copper from their diet. However, copper deficiency has been associated with auditory system disorders (Farms et al. 1993; Prohaska et al. 1996) and age-related hearing loss (McFadden et al. 1999). In one study in animals, McFadden et al. (1999a) concluded that "the results indicate that copper/zinc superoxide dismutase deficiency potentiates cochlear hair cell degeneration, presumably through metabolic pathways involving the superoxide radical." In a case reported by Hamano et al. (1997), a female patient with copper deficiency as a result of gastrointestinal tract disturbance developed severe neurological symptoms, including hearing loss. Hamano et al. (1997) recommended treating gastrointestinal tract conditions that affect absorption and administration of copper to prevent progression of neurological disease.

Trace Elements

Iodine

Although iodine deficiency is most commonly associated with endemic goiter (overgrowth of the thyroid gland caused by lack of iodine in the diet), studies in animals and humans find that iodine deficiency also has a role in sensorineural hearing loss (Meyerhoff 1979; Wang et al. 1985; Delange et al. 1989; Valeix et al. 1992, 1994; DeLong 1993), including middle ear changes, cochlear lesions, congenital deaf-mutism and bilateral hearing deficits, and high hearing thresholds in children. Adequate maternal iodine status is critical for brain development of the fetus, beginning about the 14th week and continuing perhaps into the third trimester (DeLong 1993). Iodine is available from household salt. However, levels of iodine content are deliberately low in some types of table salt in an effort to compensate for the excessive use of table salt by many persons (Delange et al. 1989). Certain medical conditions also require strict limitation of dietary salt, further reducing intake of iodine.

Iron

Iron deficiency can result from too little dietary iron, poor absorption of iron, or chronic or acute bleeding. The effects of iron deficiency have been studied in animals (Sun et al. 1987; 1990; 1991). These studies indicated that iron deficiency resulted in several hearing abnormalities, including damage to the inner ear cells and sensorineural hearing loss, elevated auditory thresholds, and a basis for noise-induced hearing loss and cochlear deafness. Conversely, some of the research in animals has focused on the role of iron in gentamicin-induced ototoxicity. Gentamicin and other similar drugs are commonly used antibiotics worldwide, despite their known toxicity to the inner ear (Song et al. 1996; 1997; 1998; Sha et al. 1999; Conlon et al. 1998; Song et al. 1998). In these studies, gentamicin combined with iron actually produces free radicals and ototoxicity. Iron supplementation for anemia-related hearing loss should be discussed with your physician. The Life Extension Foundation does not recommend iron supplements unless blood testing reveals iron-deficiency anemia.

Amino Acids

Arginine

Arginine is one of the essential amino acids. In addition to the benefits often associated with arginine (e.g., in hypertension, age-related protein synthesis, and wound healing), studies indicate that arginine is also protective against sensorineural hearing loss and cochlear damage caused by the toxins that are produced by Streptococcus pneumoniae infections (Amaee et al. 1995). Pretreatment with arginine was found to provide marked protection to the cochlea.

CAUTION Diabetics and borderline diabetics should use arginine with care; children, teenagers, and pregnant and lactating women should not use arginine except under a physician's supervision; persons who have had ocular or brain herpes should not use arginine; and persons with certain psychoses may experience worsened symptoms. Always take antioxidants with arginine.

Carnitine

Carnitine is an amino acid recognized as an effective antiaging therapy to maintain youthful cellular energy metabolism. However, the results of a study suggest that carnitine can have beneficial effects on the central neuropathy associated with diabetes (Yildiz et al. 1996). The diabetes-induced brain stem auditory evoked potentials (BAEP) deficits were improved after carnitine treatment. Acetyl-L-Carnitine is the preferential form of carnitine because of its superior absorption. A daily dose of 1000–2000 mg is suggested.

Methionine

Methionine is an antioxidant amino acid found in meat and dairy products. It has been found to have important protective benefits from various types of ototoxic hearing loss:

- Aminoglycoside-induced hearing loss (Sha et al. 2000)

- Ionic platinum compounds, the therapy most commonly used to treat metastic tumors (Reser et al. 1999)

- Cisplatin, an effective agent used in the treatment of squamous cell cancer of the head and neck (Campbell et al. 1996; Gabaizadeh et al. 1997)

- An epidemic outbreak of peripheral neuropathy (Cuba 1992–1993), affecting over 50,000 people (Roman 1994), some with sensorineural deafness. The deafness produced high-frequency hearing loss. Obvious malnutrition was not present, but a deficit in micronutrients including methionine appeared to be a primary determinant of the epidemic (Roman 1994).

CAUTION Methionine is the precursor to homocysteine in the body. Always take folic acid and vitamins B_{12} and B_6 supplements with methionine to protect against excess accumulation of homocysteine.

Glutathione

Glutathione is another amino acid that has been shown to have protective benefits against hearing loss caused by acoustic overstimulation (Yamasoba et al. 1998a). A depleted glutathione state increased noise-induced hearing loss, whereas replenishment of glutathione reduced the damage (Yamasoba et al. 1998a; 1998b). Another protective benefit of glutathione was protection from gentamicin ototoxicity, particularly when the diet was low in protein (Lautermann et al. 1995). More benefit was attained in subjects with the lower-protein diets. Alpha-lipoic acid, selenium, whey protein, and cysteine supplements boost glutathione levels in the cells.

Taurine

Taurine is described as one of the "conditionally essential" amino acids. Absence of a conditionally essential nutrient may not produce an immediate deficiency disease, but deficiency can cause problems in the long term, particularly in preterm and term infants (Gaull 1989; Tyson et al. 1989; Chesney et al. 1998; Dhillon et al. 1998). Infants with inadequate dietary taurine had shorter auditory brain stem responses (Dhillon et al. 1998). In animal studies, taurine-supplemented diets resulted in earlier maturation of the brainstem auditory response, leading Vallecalle-Sandoval et al. (1991) to suggest that taurine plays "an important role in the anatomical and functional development of the auditory system." Because taurine is defined as a "conditionally essential" amino acid, the clinical consequences that result from taurine deficiency are reversible with taurine supplementation, particularly in infants (Chesney et al. 1998).

Coenzyme Q_{10} (CoQ_{10})

CoQ_{10} is an antioxidant that has already received favorable evaluation in the clinical treatment of heart disease. However, animal studies by Sato (1988) have reported that CoQ_{10} is also effective in promoting recovery from acute sudden deafness resulting from hypoxia. Sato's results also indicated that CoQ_{10} was effective in promoting the recovery of damaged auditory hairs and in preventing respiratory metabolic impairment of the hair cells caused by hypoxia. Another interesting study by Suzuki et al. (1998) investigated the effect of CoQ_{10} on neurosensory deafness resulting from maternally inherited diabetes mellitus and deafness (MIDD): 50 patients (29 with MIDD, 7 with impaired glucose tolerance, and 15 with normal glucose tolerance) were treated daily with 150 mg of CoQ_{10} for 3 years. The control group consisted of 28 patients (16 with MIDD, 5 with impaired glucose tolerance, and 5 with normal glucose tolerance). Each group received yearly examinations. Suzuki et al. (1998) found that CoQ_{10} prevented progressive hearing loss and improved blood lactate after exercise in patients with MIDD without affecting other diabetic complications or clinical symptoms. CoQ_{10} did not affect the insulin secretory capacity of the other subjects (those with impaired glucose tolerance or normal glucose tolerance), and there were no side effects during the therapy.

Oxygen

Hyperbaric oxygen treatment has been used as part of multistep therapy for sudden hearing loss of unknown cause (Wolf et al. 1991; Sano et al. 1999); acute noise trauma from a car airbag (Stankiewicz et al. 2000); Meniere's disease (Fattori et al. 2001a); and rapid-onset hearing loss of unknown cause that can progress or severe deafness (Fattori et al. 2001b). The hyperbaric oxygen treatment varied: several short treatments, lasting 15 minutes (Wolf et al. 1991); daily treatment for 10 days in a row, with maintenance treatments for 5 days in a row each month in the first year and then treatments 5 days in a row every 3 months for the second, third, and fourth years (Fattori et al. 2001a); and daily treatment for 10 days in a row only (Fattori et al. 2001b).

Wolf et al. (1991) and Fattori et al. (2001a, b) reported positive results, leading Fattori et al. (2001b) to state: "Patients in the hyperbaric oxygen treatment group experienced a significantly greater response to treatment than did those in the vasodilator group, regardless of age and sex variables. Significantly more patients in the hyperbaric oxygen treatment group experience a good or significant response. Based on our finding, coupled with the fact that oxygen therapy is well tolerated and produces no side effect, we conclude that hyperbaric oxygen treatment should be considered the preferred treatment for patients with rapid onset hearing loss of unknown origin." Hyperbaric oxygen treatment and vasodilator therapy were not effective in the case of hearing damage (tinnitus and hearing loss in one ear) caused by noise trauma from a car airbag. However, the patient was not treated for 5 months. The airbag mechanism was presented as the cause of the noise trauma (Stankiewicz et al. 2000).

⬤ SUMMARY

Hearing loss is most common in adults over 65 years of age. To determine the degree of hearing loss and appropriate treatment, your physician will administer a hearing test and make the necessary referrals to an otolaryngologist or audiologist for further examination.

Many patients experiencing hearing loss can be treated effectively through use of a hearing aid. For others with more profound hearing loss, surgery involving cochlear implants may be an option. Cochlear implants may be recommended for patients with profound deafness who derive no benefit from hearing aids.

Alternative treatments that may help in preventing age-related hearing loss and provide protection from ototoxicity include:

1. Alpha-lipoic acid, 500 mg twice daily, has been shown to reduce hearing loss from ototoxic drugs. After the ototoxic drugs are discontinued, the dose of alpha-lipoic acid can be reduced to 250 mg twice a day.

2. Hydergine, 12–20 mg a day, may help improve hearing.

3. People with hearing loss should consider taking 120 mg of Ginkgo biloba extract daily.

4. Vitamin A deficiency has been shown to be a factor in hearing loss, including noise-induced hearing loss. A supplement supplying 10,000 IU daily of vitamin A is suggested.

5. The B vitamins have shown positive benefits for persons with hearing loss. A high potency complete B complex is recommended. Alternatives are to take 500 mg of vitamin B_1, 250 mg of B_6, and 500 mcg of vitamin B_{12}.

6. Vitamin C is particularly beneficial in aiding overall nutritional status and protecting cochlear cells from damage caused by noise. About 2500 mg a day is suggested.

7. Vitamin D deficiency has been shown to be a causal factor in several hearing disorders, including age-related hearing loss. Daily doses of 400–1400 IU are suggested.

8. Zinc deficiency increases the vulnerability of the cochlea to hearing loss associated with normal aging; 30–80 mg of zinc are suggested. (If more than 50 mg of zinc is taken daily, also take 2 mg of copper.)

9. Magnesium has been shown to have protective benefits against noise-induced hearing loss. Take 500–1000 mg of elemental magnesium a day.

10. Copper plays an important role in overall neurological health, including hearing. Copper deficiency has been associated with hearing loss. One 2-mg copper capsule every *other* day is suggested. (If taking zinc, 1 capsule daily is recommended.)

11. Ensure adequate dietary consumption of iodine.

12. Ensure adequate dietary consumption of iron. If blood testing reveals iron deficiency anemia, Iron Protein Plus (15 mg a capsule) may be taken to restore normal iron levels.

13. Arginine is an essential amino acid that is protective against sensorineural hearing loss and damage to the cochlea by toxins produced by infection. Take 2700 mg daily. Always take antioxidants with arginine.

Note: *Diabetics, borderline diabetics, children, teenagers, pregnant women, lactating women, or persons who have had ocular or brain herpes or who have certain psychoses should not take arginine without the supervision of a physician.*

14. Methionine has protective benefits for aminoglycoside-induced hearing loss. A suggested dose is 700 mg daily or 1/4 tsp of *L*-methionine powder. Always take folic acid, B_{12}, and B_6 with methionine.

15. Taurine is a "conditionally essential" amino acid that plays a role in anatomical and functional development of the auditory system. A daily dose of 500–1000 mg is suggested.

16. Coenzyme Q_{10} has been shown to be effective in preventing progressive hearing loss in diabetics, without affecting other diabetic complications or clinical symptoms. The daily dose is 100–200 mg of an oil-based CoQ_{10} supplement.

17. Hyperbaric oxygen therapy has been shown to be an effective therapy. It is well-tolerated with no side effects.

Note: *Many of the nutrients recommended above can be obtained in a high-potency multinutrient supplement called Life Extension Mix. The nutrients found in Life Extension Mix are a high-potency vitamin B complex, taurine, vitamin C, vitamin D_3, copper, zinc, iodine, and vitamin A.*

potentially expose other persons, particularly children in the home. At home, raise your awareness of potential sources of exposure to toxic materials. Take measures to limit access to toxic products. Whenever possible, replace toxic products with less dangerous alternatives. Properly dispose of those that are no longer needed. Learn to recognize the symptoms of ingested toxic substances. Learn first aid procedures. Display emergency contact numbers by the telephone.

Strive to achieve proper, balanced nutrition by choosing fresh (organic when possible) fruits, vegetables, grains, lean meat, and cold-water fish.

Consider taking supplemental antioxidants, herbs, minerals, amino acids, phytoextracts, detoxifying agents, protective agents, and fiber as adjuncts to a healthy diet to enhance vital organ functioning and to aid in your body's natural detoxifying actions. The dosage recommendations listed below are for healthy persons.

1. Life Extension Mix provides a convenient source of vitamins, trace minerals, amino acids, and herb extracts. The recommended dose of Life Extension Mix is 3 tablets taken 3 times daily.

2. Life Extension Herbal Mix incorporates 27 different herbs into a powder designed to make 1 daily drink. The suggested daily dose of Life Extension Herbal Mix is 1 tbsp taken first thing each morning.

3. Life Extension Booster contains three forms of selenium, vitamin E, and other important nutrients. The suggested dose is 1 capsule daily with any meal.

4. Vitamin C is an antioxidant known for its immune and oxidative benefits. A prophylactic dose of 2.5–6 grams daily from all of the various forms of vitamin C (including dietary sources) is recommended. Vitamin C may cause gastric upset for some people. Taking vitamin C with meals may alleviate gastric upset, as might using an antacid, buffering agent, or a buffered form of vitamin C.

5. Vitamin E has known antioxidant, immune enhancement, and cardiovascular benefits. The suggested dose is one 400-IU capsule daily. For therapeutic use, a dose of 1–5 capsules taken with meals is suggested.

6. Vitamin A has important antioxidant properties and proven benefits for cancer and heart disease prevention. A daily dose of one to two 25,000-IU capsules is recommended.

7. Glutathione is one of the body's most powerful antioxidants. A daily dose of two to six 750-mg capsules daily is recommended.

8. Selenium is an essential micronutrient that is important in immune and antioxidant functions. A recommended daily dose is one 200-mcg capsule of selenium.

9. Zinc is another essential micronutrient that is important in immune and antioxidant functions. One 30-mg capsule of zinc daily is suggested.

10. Lactoferrin is known for its ability to have an affinity for iron. One 300-mg capsule of Lactoferrin daily is recommended as a dietary supplement.

11. Garlic has been used for centuries for medicinal purposes and has proven protective benefits from pollutants, heavy metals, and cancer-causing substances. A recommended dose is two 200-mg capsules taken with meals.

12. Consider using cilantro. Cilantro is readily available from high-quality produce sources or as oil that can be rubbed into the skin. Steep 1–15 drops in hot water 2 times daily (5 days on, 2 days off). During mercury chelation therapy, stop using cilantro after 2 weeks or on the day therapy begins during the third week.

CAUTION   Keep cilantro out of the reach of children. If you have any discomfort after taking cilantro, discontinue using it orally and try using cilantro oil on your skin (1 drop on the wrist twice daily).

13. Green tea has been demonstrated to be a powerful antioxidant. For protective purposes, one 350-mg capsule daily is suggested. For therapeutic purposes, consider taking 2–4 capsules.

14. Calcium is an essential mineral for maintaining healthy bones as well as having properties that block the absorption of free radical-generating iron into the bloodstream. Depending on individual requirements, 1000 mg is a beginning dose of supplemental calcium. A daily dose of one to two 1000-mg capsules is suggested. For those who have a low calcium-content diet or who do not take other calcium supplements, consider taking more. Calcium absorption and utilization is enhanced by also taking vitamin D_3. It is recommended that calcium be taken daily in divided doses.

15. *L*-cysteine, *N*-acetyl-cysteine, and glutathione are important antioxidants. When taking *L*-cysteine, *N*-acetyl-cysteine, or glutathione, it is recommended

that vitamin C also be taken to help maintain their powerful free radical-suppressing effects. Take 2–6 capsules of the supplement *L-Glutathione, L-Cysteine, & C* daily.

16. Alfalfa sprouts are available as a food product in most health food stores and may be added to salads or blended into a juice. Dried herbs from alfalfa leaves and sprouts may be brewed into a tea—1 oz steeped in 1 pint of water for 20 minutes—2 cups daily. Dried powder capsules may also be taken at a dose of 4–6 capsules a day. Due to its high iron content, alfalfa should not be taken by individuals with toxic or chronic iron overload.

17. Include citrus fruit and foods containing buckwheat flour in your diet as natural sources of rutin. A convenient source of supplemental rutin is 1/4 tsp of Rutin Powder taken 2–3 times daily with a beverage.

18. Consider taking MSM, alpha-lipoic acid, glycine, and chlorella for their natural detoxifying benefits. MSM has anti-inflammatory benefits. A daily dose of one to three 1000-mg capsules is suggested. MSM is most effectively utilized when taken with meals. Alpha-lipoic acid is a universal antioxidant and meets all antioxidant evaluation criteria. For healthy people, take one to two 250-mg capsules daily. Glycine is a chemically simple and abundant conditionally essential amino acid. It combines with many toxic substances and converts them to harmless forms, which are then excreted. One tsp. of glycine powder provides 2.8 grams of pure glycine (1 gram or more may be taken because glycine is nontoxic). Glycine powder is easily soluble in juice or water and is not unpleasant tasting.

Note: *Chlorella causes diarrhea in some persons. Start with a small dose (i.e., two 500-mg tablets daily) and consider adding cellulose enzyme.*

19. Include daily dietary fiber from natural sources such as carbohydrates, fruits, vegetables, whole grain products, wheat bran, and beans, when possible. Supplemental fiber from Fiber Food Caps is another good source of natural, soluble fiber. Take 6 capsules with each meal and at least 10 oz of water. If necessary, use smaller doses at first until your digestive system adjusts to the added fiber. If gas or bloating occurs, reduce the dose until tolerance is achieved.

20. On an empty stomach, take one to four 200-mg capsules of SAMe daily with water. Take folic acid, B_{12}, and B_6 when taking SAMe.

WARNING SAMe should not be taken with antidepressants except under a physician's care.

21. Consider silibinin and silymarin for their liver protective benefits. A suggested dose of Silibinin Plus is one 326-mg capsule taken 2 times daily. An alternative is one 100-mg capsule of Silymarin taken 4 times daily. Silymarin contains milk thistle standardized at 80%.

 ## FOR MORE INFORMATION

American Board of Chelation Therapy, (312) 266-7246; American College of Advancement in Medicine, www.acam.org; American College of Nutrition, (727) 446-6086; American Association of Naturopathic Physicians, (877)969-2267; National Institutes of Health, (301) 496-4000; Food and Drug Administration, (888) 463-6332; Agency for Toxic Substances and Disease Registry, (888) 422-8737.

PRODUCT AVAILABILITY

Life Extension Mix, Life Extension Herbal Mix, Life Extension Booster, selenium, OptiZinc, Lactoferrin, vitamin E succinate, Gamma E Tocopherol Complex, Vitamin C Caps, Beta-Carotene, Liquid Emulsified Vitamin A, Kyolic Garlic Formula, Pure-Gar Caps, Super Green Tea Extract, green tea leaves, Long Life Organic Green Tea Bags, L-Cysteine Capsules, N-Acetyl-Cysteine Capsules, L-Glutathione, L-Cysteine & C, rutin powder, MSM, Super Alpha-Lipoic Acid w/Biotin, glycine powder, Fiber Food Caps, Fiber Food Powder, apple pectin powder, SAMe, Silibinin Plus, and silymarin are available from Life Extension by telephoning (800) 544-4440 or by ordering online at www.lef.org.

increase the absorption of iron from the digestive tract into the bloodstream. Therefore, hemochromatosis patients should take one 500-mg *buffered* vitamin C capsule 3 times a day between meals. Published findings demonstrate that in iron-overloaded plasma, vitamin C acts as a potent antioxidant against lipid peroxidation. On the other hand, some doctors suggest that hemochromatosis patients should avoid vitamin C altogether.

To combat liver damage, vitamin E is an important weapon. Vitamin E is a vital lipid-soluble antioxidant that has been shown to be decreased in patients with hereditary hemochromatosis and in experimental iron overload. Iron loading has been shown to significantly decrease hepatic and plasma vitamin E which can be overcome by vitamin E supplementation. Free-radical index markers increase three- to fivefold in the iron-loaded livers, but supplementation with vitamin E has been shown to reduce these levels of free-radical activity by at least 50% (Brown et al. 1997).

Iron-overload disease causes severe depletion of liver glutathione. Glutathione is an important antioxidant, and its depletion in iron overload causes additional free-radical damage. (It should be noted that copper overload induces free radical-induced damage that is similar to iron overload.)

We therefore recommend that hemochromatosis patients take the following in divided doses 2 or 3 times a day with meals:

- 400 IU of vitamin E (alpha tocopherol) with at least 200 mg of gamma tocopherol
- 200 mcg of selenium
- A complete vitamin B complex
- 800 mcg of folic acid
- 30 mg of zinc
- 300 mg of grape seed-skin extract
- 120 mg of ginkgo extract
- 1000 mg of aged-garlic extract
- 500 mg of alpha-lipoic acid
- 60 mg of palm-oil tocotrienols
- 600 mg of N-acetyl-cysteine (NAC)
- 300 mg of elemental calcium with each meal
- 500 mg of elemental magnesium
- 500 mg of a silymarin extract containing a high percentage of silbinin
- 1200 mg of a green tea extract (95%) with most meals

In addition, patients should take 300 mcg–3 mg of melatonin at bedtime.

ALTERNATIVE TREATMENTS

Hemochromatosis patients may also consider intravenous (IV) chelation therapy administered by a knowledgeable physician. Chelation therapy refers to a treatment in which certain synthetic chemicals and body proteins bind metal molecules, extracting them from the system. Literally, chelation therapy is derived from the Greek word *chele*, which alludes to a claw-like action imposed upon unwanted materials accumulating in the body. Chelation is currently best associated with the clearance of plaque from the arteries, establishing normal blood flow to the vasculature. However, it is also an effective tool in treating heavy metal toxicity.

As early as 1941, Providence Hospital (Detroit) used chelation, employing intravenously administered ethylenediaminetetraacetic acid (EDTA), a synthetic amino acid, to extract lead. EDTA, a nontoxic chelator, also clears cadmium, nickel, copper, calcium, and some other metals from the body.

An individual wishing to obtain chelation therapy may want to contact a physician who follows the standard chelation protocol of the American College of Advancement in Medicine. The number of sessions required to enact a change cannot be presupposed, but the recommended maximum dosage is currently about 3 grams of EDTA (dosage usually calculated by body weight) given by IV infusion 1–3 times weekly, as a 3- to 4-hour drip. Initially, the dosage may be as small as 1/2–1 gram of EDTA.

Desferal (deferoxamine) is the preferred agent for iron chelation in cases of secondary iron overload from transfusion-dependent anemias or as an adjunct in acute iron intoxication. Desferal is not administered for primary hemochromatosis because phlebotomy is the current standard procedure. Desferal is given by intramuscular or subcutaneous infusion.

One interesting antiaging and immune-boosting therapy involves freezing one's phlebotomized blood and storing it for future administration during a debilitated state. Having access to one's own youthful blood during a state of disease or severe aging could be of benefit.

Nutritionist Carmen Fusco has successfully helped patients with the most severe form of hemochromatosis. Her regimen includes tea with every meal (for the tannins that bind iron) and extra calcium because calcium competes with iron and prevents some of its absorption. If a glass of wine is desired once the condition of the liver improves, red wine with the tannins and chromium found in the grape skins is preferable to white wine.

SUMMARY

The most important step is locating a physician with specialized knowledge of hemochromatosis who will treat the disease as a life-threatening disorder. In too many cases, patients are not aggressively treated with phlebotomies, and liver iron overload reaches lethal levels.

In addition to conventional treatment, the following lifestyle changes and supplements are suggested:

1. Adopt a diet high in fruit and vegetables; avoid food fortified with iron, red meat, alcohol, and other recreational drugs. Coffee and tea are fine; after recovery, some red wine is permissible.

2. Vitamin C, one 500-mg *buffered* capsule 3 times daily in between meals.

3. Take the following in divided doses, 2 or 3 times a day, with meals:

    • 400 IU of vitamin E with 200 mg of gamma tocopherol
    • 200 mcg of selenium
    • A complete vitamin B complex
    • 800 mcg of folic acid
    • 30 mg of zinc
    • 100 mg of grape seed-skin extract
    • 120 mg of ginkgo extract
    • 1000 mg of garlic
    • 500 mg of alpha-lipoic acid
    • 200 IU of gamma-tocopherol
    • 600 mg of N-acetyl-cysteine (NAC)

4. Lecithin granules, 1 tsp mixed with meals.

5. Life Flora, high-potency cultures of acidophilus and bifido bacteria, 1–3 capsules before meals.

6. If there is continuing weakness in advanced conditions, try vitamin B_{12} by injection or 1000 mcg of methylcobalamin absorbed under the tongue once a day.

7. Take the following to reduce iron absorption with each meal that contains iron:

    • 300 mg of elemental calcium.
    • 4 grams of Fiber Food (psyllium, guar gum, and pectin fiber)

8. Melatonin, 300 mcg–3 mg taken nightly at bedtime.

9. Silibinin Plus, derived from the herb milk thistle, will help detoxify and protect the liver, three 260-mg capsules daily.

10. Green tea extract, 4 capsules with each meal. Each capsule should provide at least 300 mg of a 95% polyphenol extract.

Note: *This nutritional program should be combined with phlebotomies and regular physician follow-up to be certain that stored iron does not reach dangerous levels.*

If liver damage has occurred, refer to the *Liver Cirrhosis* and *Liver Degenerative Disease* protocols in this book. Refer to *Appendix A* below for additional suggestions.

FOR MORE INFORMATION

Visit http://hemochromatose.tripod.com/linkseng.html

PRODUCT AVAILABILITY

Calcium citrate, green tea extract, buffered vitamin C capsules, vitamin E, selenium, lecithin granules, melatonin, Life Flora, ginko biloba, magnesium, Vitamin B complex, zinc, folic acid, grape seed-skin extract, aged garlic extract capsules, alpha-lipoic acid, Gamma E Tocopherol/Tocotrienols, NAC, Silibinin Plus, and Fiber Food caps and powder can be ordered by calling (800) 544-4440 or by ordering online at www.lef.org.

APPENDIX A

Hemochromatosis: A Novel Case Study
by WALTER LAST

This unorthodox case study is presented for the interest of our readers. The hemochromatosis patient who wishes to follow Mr. Last's high antioxidant recommendations, especially in regard to vitamin C intake, should first discuss it with his or her physician.

I had two patients with hemochromatosis. Both had normal ferritin levels within weeks of starting nutritional therapy, without any further need for phlebotomies. I was able to monitor one of these patients for 12 years as described in the following case history.

Case History
My patient was a 51-year-old male. He had collapsed at work 3 years earlier. His main symptoms were dizziness, tachycardia, profuse sweating, difficulty breathing, and extreme weakness. He was discharged from an Intensive Care Unit without diagnosis and his

weight loss and weakness continued. The diagnosis of hemochromatosis was made 15 months later with a serum ferritin level of 3200 ng/mL and a liver biopsy that showed extremely high iron levels. With weekly phlebotomies, this was reduced to 1585 ng/mL before using fortnightly and later monthly phlebotomies, each time removing 1 liter of blood.

Phlebotomies continued for 20 months without reducing the ferritin to normal levels. The lowest level reached was 440 ng/mL. During all of this time, the patient was very weak, and as an additional complication, a specialist diagnosed Meniere's disease. In December 1990, he stopped having phlebotomies and started nutritional therapy. His liver was very hard and enlarged, he was grossly underweight, and his doctor had given him 5 weeks to live. The ferritin level at this time was still at 458 ng/mL. Normal ferritin levels for males are under 400 ng/mL.

Three weeks after starting nutritional therapy, his ferritin was 393 ng/mL (within the normal range for the first time since diagnosis). At the same time, he started gaining weight, his strength rapidly improved, and the symptoms of Meniere's disease (progressive deafness, dizziness, ringing in the ears, headache, and nausea) disappeared as well.

The red blood cell count, which had remained below normal during the period of phlebotomies, became normal and hemoglobin improved to the middle of the normal range. He continued to have blood tests, initially monthly, then at 3 months, and later at 6 months. On two occasions during the first year the ferritin level went slightly above the normal range.

The main aspects of the initial therapy were a vegetarian raw-food diet, combined with 20 g of vitamin C in divided doses before meals and at bedtime, in addition to 1000 mg of natural vitamin E, vitamin A, and vitamin B complex, sublingual vitamin B_{12}, Kyolic garlic, lecithin, acidophilus culture, and trace minerals except iron. After 3 weeks, when the ferritin level had normalized, dietary restrictions were eased by adding cooked food, including fish and white meat. Vitamin C was reduced to 10 grams and later to a maintenance amount of 5 grams in divided doses. However, whenever a ferritin test was slightly above normal, vitamin C was increased to 10 grams until the next test, which then showed a normal ferritin level. Because he could not tolerate ascorbic acid, vitamin C was used in the form of sodium ascorbate.

For about 10 years, his ferritin remained within the normal range without any further phlebotomies. However, in the year 2000, he adopted the high-protein *Zone Diet* and his next test was 429 ng/mL. After increasing vitamin C to 10 grams and returning to his previous diet,

the next ferritin test 6 weeks later was down to 300 ng/mL and again in the normal range. Subsequent tests remained normal up to the present time.

Genetic tests confirmed that his hemochromatosis is the hereditary form. A recent liver scan did not show any abnormalities. His overall health is above average for his age. In comparison, several other patients with advanced hemochromatosis—but in a less serious condition—who were diagnosed at about the same time as my patient and treated in the medically accepted way, have all since died of liver-related diseases. Another indication of the very advanced original condition of my patient is the fact that his ferritin level could not be normalized after 20 months of phlebotomies (generally regarded as a very poor prognosis).

Discussion

This case was first published over 10 years ago in the *International Clinical Nutrition Review* (Last 1991), but has been completely ignored by hemochromatosis specialists and researchers. The reason for this may be the prevailing dogma that 90 mg of vitamin C is sufficient for everyone to remain healthy (slightly more for smokers) and that vitamin C supplements may be dangerous, especially with hemochromatosis. I do not need to discuss here the merits of vitamin C supplementation as William Faloon has covered this subject extensively in his article A *Critical Analysis of The National Academy of Sciences' Attack on Dietary Supplements* at www.lef.org.

The main reasons for the common advice to avoid vitamin C with hemochromatosis are twofold. It is generally acknowledged that vitamin C can improve the absorption of iron, especially in iron-deficient individuals and from vegetarian diets. However, I believe that the body does not normally absorb more than it needs, and the increased absorption by hemochromatosis patients from meals high in vitamin C is mainly the result of an internal deficiency of bivalent iron.

The second reason is that small amounts of vitamin C supplements, in the order of 500 mg, may mobilize stored iron, and this may cause oxidative tissue damage to membrane lipids. This is really not surprising, as it is well known that high concentrations of ferric ions oxidize protective antioxidants, notably the vitamins C and E. This means that with low antioxidant intakes, we can expect pronounced antioxidant tissue deficiencies in iron overload diseases. In this case, low levels of supplemented vitamin C are likely to be present mainly in oxidized form as reversible dehydroascorbate or as irreversible oxidation products.

Similarly, any liberated iron would be in the form of ferric dehydroascorbate and other oxidized products, and it is these that cause the peroxidative membrane damage.

Also, vitamin A is important for iron metabolism. Supplementation improves the iron status (serum iron, hemoglobin, as well as transferrin saturation) without at the same time increasing ferritin levels, while iron supplements without sufficient vitamin A just increase ferritin levels. Also, vitamin A-deficient subjects may develop anemia despite sufficient dietary iron (Bloem et al. 1990). These effects may be interpreted as a normalizing function of vitamin A in the transport and usage of iron, while iron alone in the presence of vitamin A deficiency will mainly increase iron stores.

A similar normalizing role in iron metabolism may be exhibited by the other antioxidants. Vitamin C not only improves the absorption of iron, but it is also required to move iron in and out of ferritin tissue stores. Without adequate antioxidants, ferric iron stores may build up because iron cannot be liberated from ferritin tissue and transferred onto transferrin plasma, a step that requires a temporary reduction of ferric to ferrous iron.

There are two sites or steps at which antioxidant deficiency might cause or contribute to hemochromatosis. The synthesis of heme requires the reduction of ferric to ferrous ions. While this reduction proceeds enzymatically through ferrochelatase, it is ultimately dependent on the overall redox potential within the cells. In the case of a generalized antioxidant deficiency, the function of this enzyme is likely to be impeded. This then leads to low hemoglobin levels and increased ferritin stores because a cellular deficiency of ferrous ions for the synthesis of heme will stimulate increased absorption of iron.

However, the second possibility appears to be the decisive defect in hemochromatosis. This is a difficulty in recycling iron from the continual breakdown of hemoglobin from old erythrocytes in the spleen and liver. About 25 mg of iron are recycled daily in this way, but this requires a reduction-oxidation step to transfer ferritin iron in the tissue onto plasma transferrin. With antioxidant deficiency there will be only a partial recycling. Most of the unusable iron stores will build up in the liver.

Very high ferric iron stores in the liver also make this organ more antioxidant deficient than other tissue. The highest antioxidant activity can be expected to be in the intestinal mucosa because these have first call on the antioxidants absorbed from food. Therefore, transferrin will preferentially pick up iron from the intestinal mucosa and avoid the liver stores as they are too difficult to convert. Another piece of evidence for this proposed mechanism may be seen in the rapid normalization of ferritin levels in the reported case without any abnormal loss of iron in the urine being detected.

The initial use of very high amounts of vitamin C was designed to rapidly change the total oxidation-reduction or redox potential of the body from one high in oxidizing to one high in reducing abilities. This allowed the rapid mobilization and normalization of excessive iron stores without any danger of tissue damage that might result from mobilizing iron slowly with low-level antioxidant supplements.

The initial defect in hereditary hemochromatosis (HH) may simply be a higher-than-normal antioxidant requirement to maintain healthy liver functions. Any period of increased antioxidant requirement, such as prolonged or severe stress, infections, or chemical exposure, may lead to a deficiency and thus start the accumulation of ferric iron in the liver. This will then make it increasingly more difficult for a low level of antioxidants to penetrate the strongly oxidative liver environment to reduce ferric iron, and additional iron will be absorbed from the intestines instead. The strongly oxidative liver environment may also be seen as the main cause of the commonly developing liver cirrhosis and liver cancer. Conversely, I attribute the normalization of the liver damage of my patient to his high antioxidant intake.

If there would be a fundamental defect that causes genetically predisposed individuals to automatically absorb increased amounts of iron, then nearly everyone would be affected. However, this is not so. Only a small percentage of genetically predisposed individuals accumulate dangerous amounts of iron. Therefore, the main factor clearly is not genetic and must be something else. From the provided case report, it is clear that this decisive factor is antioxidant deficiency.

This discussion shows that in effect at the cellular level, hemochromatosis may be regarded as a bivalent iron deficiency disease due to chronically low antioxidant levels. Unfortunately, I cannot offer any references from the medical literature to support my case history because a therapy with very high vitamin C levels has not been tried before. However, my theoretical assessment should be obvious to any biochemist. If you, as a hemochromatosis patient, are interested in proof for the efficacy of the proposed vitamin C treatment, then I suggest that you lobby for a clinical trial.

Recommended Therapy

The diet should be high in organic or unsprayed fruits and vegetables with an emphasis on sprouted seeds and fresh vegetable juices. Initially, a vegetarian raw-food diet is recommended, lasting for several days with mild conditions and for several weeks in advanced conditions and suspected liver damage. After this cleansing period, reintroduce other foods individually and with self-observation. Avoid any food that causes an unpleasant reaction or that increases the pulse rate more than most other foods. Check your pulse before and 30–60 minutes after meals.

Highly recommended are the so-called "purple foods" for their high antioxidant value. These produce a purple juice when pressed and include red beets, black and purple grapes, blackberries, black currants, and blueberries. You may use a moderate amount of white meat, such as poultry, fish, and other seafood. However, with a damaged liver, try to obtain organic meat and low-mercury fish. Use extra-virgin olive oil as the main oil or fat.

Initially, avoid and later minimize red meat, gluten-grains (mainly wheat and oats, to a lesser degree rye and barley), cow's milk products, nonfermented soy products, sugar and sweetened food, processed food, and food with added non-biological chemicals. Continue to avoid iron-fortified food, alcohol, nicotine, and other recreational drugs. Moderate amounts of coffee or tea and also a glass of red wine with meals, except with apparent liver damage, are acceptable.

The mainstay of this therapy is a high vitamin C intake. With high ferritin levels and suspected high iron stores in the liver, start with 10 grams in four to six divided doses and if that is well tolerated, increase to 20 grams the next day. If high vitamin C intake causes problems, such as diarrhea, cut back to the amount that can be tolerated. Otherwise stay with 20 grams until ferritin drops to the normal range. Then continue with 10 grams until general health and any liver problems have sufficiently improved. Finally, continue with a maintenance intake of about 5 grams daily. However, whenever a ferritin test is higher than normal, temporarily increase vitamin C again to 10 grams until ferritin returns to the normal range.

With these high intakes, sodium ascorbate or mixed ascorbates (buffered vitamin C powder) are generally easiest to tolerate, but with high blood pressure, additional ascorbic acid is beneficial as well. For a maintenance program, use buffered vitamin C powder, but if your blood pressure is elevated, use ascorbic acid instead. Try to take the vitamin C in liquid form about 30 minutes before meals and at bedtime. However, if that causes digestive problems, then take it with food that is low in iron. With impaired kidney functions, high doses of vitamin C can cause edema.

In this case, greatly increase the intake of water and other fluids and reduce vitamin C intake to a level that does not cause problems; also avoid salt.

As the basis of the supplement program, take 4 capsules (or 3 tablets) of the Life Extension Mix 3 times daily. This is free of iron and contains high but balanced amounts of all vitamins, minerals, and other essential nutrients. It is also high in antioxidants with about 2.5 grams of vitamin C, so that for the maintenance program, only an additional 2.5 grams are needed to obtain a total of 5 grams a day of vitamin C. However, initially, until ferritin is in the normal range or if you have continuing difficulty controlling ferritin levels, you may take the capsules half an hour before meals with some fruit or juice.

Until the iron metabolism appears to be normalized, take 10,000 or 20,000 IU of liquid emulsified vitamin A once a day. Many individuals find it difficult to absorb beta-carotene and convert it into vitamin A. As a maintenance dose, the vitamin A in 12 capsules of Life Extension Mix (approximately 4300 IU) should be sufficient.

If weakness remains in advanced conditions try vitamin B_{12} by injection or 1000-mcg (10-mg) tablets (methylcobalamin) absorbed under the tongue once a day.

To normalize the intestinal tract, take cultures with acidophilus and bifido bacteria, such as high-potency Life Flora capsules. Initially take 2 or 3 capsules before each meal. After sufficient improvement, reduce that to 1 capsule per meal and later 1 a day. Generally, take 1 tsp of lecithin granules mixed with meals.

With indications of liver damage, remain on a program high in antioxidants for an extended period. Also see the other protocols on *Liver Cirrhosis* and *Liver Degenerative Disease* for further treatment suggestions.

Combining Nutritional with Conventional Therapy

With a moderately high ferritin level, there is no problem in combining this antioxidant therapy with a series of phlebotomies. On the contrary, repeated phlebotomies are often less than successful because patients deficient in antioxidants have difficulty mobilizing iron stores. With concomitant antioxidant therapy, more iron may be removed with each unit of blood.

However, we do not yet know if antioxidant therapy with very high ferritin levels would pose any problems. Therefore, if the initial ferritin level is very high, it may be advisable to have a series of weekly phlebotomies until ferritin is in the moderately high range or starts leveling off before starting antioxidant therapy. Phlebotomies may then be continued together with antioxidant therapy until ferritin is in the middle of the normal range. From this point on, antioxidant therapy alone should be sufficient to prevent a relapse. However, if you are so inclined, you may make periodic or occasional blood donations even after full recovery.

The main beneficiaries of antioxidant therapy are patients with advanced hemochromatosis and liver damage who until now had a very poor prognosis. These individuals should now have a normal life expectancy by combining nutritional with conventional therapy. Furthermore, individuals who are genetically predisposed to developing hemochromatosis can now easily protect themselves with antioxidant supplements. I assume that 2–5 grams of vitamin C a day will be sufficient, especially if other antioxidants, and especially vitamin E, are used in addition or if the diet is high in antioxidant nutrients. However, during stressful periods, including infections, these amounts may be doubled.

Present nutritional therapies focus on reducing the absorption of iron with special supplements and foods. Commonly used sources are calcium, tea, and soluble fiber. High-dose fiber is not recommended if you choose to follow the high antioxidant therapy proposed above because along with iron, essential trace minerals and even vitamins may be reduced. These alternatives are recommended if you choose conventional treatment with phlebotomies.

In summary, it is postulated that the basic biochemical defect that leads to the development of hemochromatosis is a tissue deficiency of antioxidants. This has two effects. One effect is that it inhibits the recycling of iron from old erythrocytes in the liver and leads to a gradual accumulation of ferritin. The second effect is a deficiency of bivalent iron. This in turn induces increased intestinal iron absorption for the necessary synthesis of heme. Accordingly, hemochromatosis can be successfully treated or prevented with high levels of vitamin C and other antioxidants. The obvious advantages of antioxidant therapy as compared to the traditional management of hemochromatosis will hopefully stimulate more research in this area.

Walter Last studied chemistry and biochemistry at a German university (Greifswald) from 1952 to 1959 and acquired a degree comparable to a master of science degree in the United States. He worked in medical departments of several German universities and at Bio-Science Laboratories in Los Angeles. After 1975 he worked as a health writer and nutritionist in New Zealand and Australia.

Hepatitis B

CAUSATION AND TRANSMISSION

Hepatitis B (HBV) is a viral illness causing inflammation of the liver, resulting from infection with a DNA-type virus. This virus consists of an inner core surrounded by an outer capsule. The inner core contains the core antigen (HB_cAg) and the antigen (HB_eAg) also known as the "e" antigen. The outer capsule contains the hepatitis B surface antigen (HB_sAg).

Hepatitis B infection is passed via blood products, as in transfusions or in the sharing of contaminated needles. It may also be acquired by exposure to body fluids during sexual intercourse, or transmission from mother to fetus. About 5–10% of volunteer blood donors show evidence of having prior hepatitis B, meaning that they once did have hepatitis B and may or may not still be infectious with the viral agent.

In the United States and Europe, approximately 1.25 million people are chronically infected with the virus (Malik et al. 2000). About 5–10% of those with acute hepatitis B will develop chronic infection. The remainder will recover and develop antibodies to the virus that make them immune from further viral activity. (Lammert et al. 2000; Mayerat et al. 1999). At least 1 million chronically infected individuals die each year of complications due to HBV-related diseases, especially liver cancer and cirrhosis. In the entire world, about 5% of the population, or 350 million people, have chronic hepatitis B (Gumina et al. 2001).

SYMPTOMS AND ASSOCIATED DISEASE STATES

The incubation period, from exposure to the virus to developing acute hepatitis B, is approximately 6 weeks, but can range from 5–13 weeks. The incidence of hepatitis B is increased in dialysis patients, IV drug users, persons with AIDS, transplant recipients, and patients frequently receiving blood transfusions, such as those with leukemia or lymphoma. When acute hepatitis occurs, symptoms include weakness, nausea, vomiting, body aches (myalgias), diarrhea, fever, joint pains (arthralgias), jaundice (yellow discoloration of the skin and whites of the eyes), loss of appetite,

weight loss, loss of interest in tobacco products, and sometimes an itching skin rash. The symptoms of acute hepatitis last on the average from 1–3 months. During the final phase of symptoms, the body begins to build immunity against the hepatitis B infection and does become immune 90% of the time (Lammert et al. 2000). In the other 10% of cases, however, a state of persistent infection occurs for more than 6 months. These persons are designated as having chronic hepatitis B. A liver biopsy is done in those patients having chronic hepatitis B—about one-third of these have chronic active hepatitis and two-thirds have chronic persistent hepatitis. Of these two types, the chronic active hepatitis is more aggressive and has a more rapidly progressing course.

Small groups of people develop chronic hepatitis B without any history of acute infection. In these persons, it is simply not known where the original infection was contracted. They present with signs of chronic hepatitis and in the course of their evaluation, laboratory studies are positive for hepatitis B infection.

The Delta agent is a small RNA virus that is dependent on previously existing hepatitis B infection before it can infect the host. Care should be taken in giving blood transfusions to those already infected with hepatitis B because addition of the Delta agent can provoke fulminant hepatitis and death. Infection with the Delta agent can occur at the same time as with hepatitis B or singly at a later time. Also, if a person with chronic hepatitis B has been doing well and relapses, the Delta agent should be suspected.

Hepatoma, or liver cancer, can develop in the chronically inflamed liver infected with hepatitis B. Hepatoma is to be suspected if a markedly downhill course develops with hepatitis B. Hepatoma occurs in a minority of patients, however.

TESTS FOR DIAGNOSING AND TRACKING HEPATITIS B

Remember that there are several antigens or protein parts of the hepatitis B virus that comprise the hepatitis B virus particle. These include the surface antigen in the outer envelope and the core and e antigens of the inner core. The body, in its attempt to fight the virus, makes antibodies to each of these proteins. The particles and their antibodies are used in monitoring hepatitis B infection, as are actual blood or serum levels of the virus itself. Testing of hepatitis B includes evaluation of the following markers for presence of disease state:

- HB_sAg—Hepatitis B surface antigen. This is the first test to become positive with hepatitis B infection. It rises before symptoms begin and then returns to negative when jaundice disappears. The person is considered to be a carrier of hepatitis B if this antigen persists in the blood beyond 6 months. Rarely, a patient may be a "late seroconverter" of surface antigen, i.e., they may convert from carrier state to immunity.

- Anti-HBs—Antibody against surface antigen. The body makes this antibody to fight the viral infection. Its presence usually indicates immunity against hepatitis B, that is, the person has previously had hepatitis B, recovered, and is now immune, or the person has been vaccinated against hepatitis B and is now immune. Persons positive for this antibody will not develop a hepatitis B infection again. Hepatitis B Immune Globulin (HBIG) becomes detectable about 6 months after acute hepatitis B and will remain in the serum for life, although its level will decrease over many years. Super-concentrated injections of the antibody HBIG are given to those exposed to hepatitis B to prevent the disease.

- HB_eAg—Hepatitis B e antigen. Presence of this antigen indicates the person is highly infectious with hepatitis B and that viral replication is ongoing in the host. It is found during the time of early symptoms of acute hepatitis. If the presence of HB_eAg persists, it indicates chronic infection.

- Anti-HB_eAg—Antibody to e antigen. The presence of Anti-HB_eAg indicates that infectivity is decreasing and that the period of high infectivity is ending.

- Anti-HB_cAg—Antibody to core antigen. This antibody appears about 1 month after acute infection and declines very gradually over many years. It is also present in chronic hepatitis. During the time lag between the disappearance of HB_sAg and the appearance of hepatitis B surface antibody (HB_sAb/Anti-HBs), core antibody is elevated. This may be the only marker indicating a recent hepatitis infection during this time; it is termed the "core window."

- Viral load—In a known hepatitis C virus (HCV) carrier or in chronic hepatitis B, the viral load is measured by a lab test known as "quantitative HCV PCR." PCR refers to the type of assay used in the lab test and the result is reported in number of copies of the virus. Quantitative HCV PCR is used to measure response to treatment.

- Liver function tests—An elevation of some liver function tests, particularly the transaminases, found on routine blood chemistry testing, should prompt the physician to order a hepatitis screening panel, which would include screening tests for hepatitis B, as well as the other forms of viral hepatitis.

VACCINATION FOR HEPATITIS B

Newborn infants are now routinely vaccinated for hepatitis B. Travelers and any other persons at risk for exposure to hepatitis B should also be vaccinated. The series of immunizations consists of three injections of the hepatitis B antigen given over a period of 6 months. When injected into the recipient, the antigen causes the host to make antibodies against it. The host, then having antibodies against hepatitis B surface antigen, will make those antibodies if presented (exposed) with the entire Hepatitis B particle. Thus, the host is immune against infection from Hepatitis B. Immunity is conferred after vaccination in 85–90% of persons and is proven by finding a titer greater than 10 mIU/mL of surface antibody in the vaccine recipient.

The United States Task Force on Adult Immunization recommends that adults receiving hepatitis B vaccination have a titer to check for immunity 1–6 months after completing the series. The vaccine must be given in the deltoid muscle of the upper arm to maximize effectiveness in adults. It is not absorbed as well when administered in the hip in adults. However, the anterolateral thigh is the preferred site for infants. If the titer is below 10 mIU/mL 1–6 months after the initial vaccination series is completed, the individual is not considered to be immune and the Task Force recommends giving an additional dose. The titers should again be measured 6 months later. These additional doses of Hepatitis B Vaccine can be given up to 3 times until the titer rises above 10.

At this point, the U.S. Task Force recommends no further doses even if the titer status remains nonimmune. However, cases of acute hepatitis B and the accompanying risk of chronic hepatitis have been reported in these patients. Patients who do not become immune with the usual series of hepatitis B vaccine have been shown to have a genetic variant involving the way antigen is presented to their immune cells (Desombere et al. 1995; Durupinar et al. 1996).

In Japan and Europe, other protocols have been used in "nonresponders" to hepatitis B vaccine. In Great Britain and some other parts of Europe, a higher dose of 40 mcg of vaccine may be used instead of the usual 10 mcg. In the United States, this is known as a "dialysis dose" of the vaccine and is the dose most commonly used in dialysis patients. In a study reported in the *Journal of Infectious Disease*, 100% of persons given the 40-mcg dose developed immune status (Bertino 1997).

Even though not routinely recommended in the United States, it is worth noting that higher dosing of vaccine has successfully been used abroad to obtain an immune titer that is sufficient to prevent future infection with hepatitis B. This higher dose also provides immunity in "nonresponders" (those who do not become immune after receiving the usual initial dosing regimen in the vaccination series). Many persons now receive hepatitis B vaccine routinely at work (such as health care workers, some police officers, firemen, and others), and many receive it when traveling to protect against infection. If you are not immune after the initial usual series of hepatitis B vaccine (meaning your titer for hepatitis B surface antibody is less than 10 mIU/mL when it is checked with a blood test), you may wish to receive the "dialysis dose" because that has been shown to provide 100% response in all persons, including "nonresponders."

The hepatitis B vaccine is now recommended as part of the routine vaccination schedule for all infants as well as adolescents who have not previously been vaccinated. Some states require this vaccination for entrance to middle school. Although the 3-dose schedule is standard, an optional 2-dose schedule of Recombivax HB for adolescents age 11–15 became available in February 2002. The second dose is given 4–6 months after the first dose. Each of the 2 doses contains 10 mcg of hepatitis B surface antigen compared with 5 mcg a dose in the three series. To date, follow-up data indicate that the rate of decline in antibody titers for the 2-dose schedule is similar to that for the 3-dose schedule. However, long-term follow-up studies will determine whether booster doses will be required. If it is not clear which dose an adolescent was administered at the start of a series, the series should be completed with the 3-dose schedule.

In September 1999, Merck Vaccine Division (Merck & Co., Inc., West Point, Pennsylvania) received approval from the Food and Drug Administration for an optional 2-dose schedule of Recombivax HB to be used as an alternate vaccination for adolescents age 11–15 years. The Advisory Committee on Immunization Practices approved the optional 2-dose schedule in October 1999 and recommended in February 2000 to include this schedule in the Vaccines for Children Program. Using the 2-dose schedule, the adult dose of Recombivax HB (1.0-mL dose containing 10 mcg of hepatitis B surface antigen [HB_sAg]) is administered to adolescents aged 11–15 years, with

the second dose given 4–6 months after the first dose. In immunogenicity studies among adolescents age 11–15 years, antibody concentrations and end-seroprotection rates (10 mIU/mL of antibody to HB_sAg) were similar with the 2-dose schedule (1.0 mL dose containing 10 mcg of HB_sAg) and the currently licensed 3-dose schedule (0.5 mL dose containing 5 mcg of HB_sAg). The overall frequency of adverse events was similar for the 2-dose schedule and the 3-dose schedule.

Short-term (2-year) follow-up data indicate that the rate of decline in antibody levels for the 2-dose schedule was similar to that for the 3-dose schedule. No data are available to assess long-term protection (beyond 2 years) or immune memory following vaccination with the 2-dose schedule, and it is not known whether booster doses of vaccine will be required. As with other hepatitis B vaccination schedules, if administration of the 2-dose schedule is interrupted, it is not necessary to restart the series. Children and adolescents who have begun vaccination with a dose of 5 mcg of Recombivax HB should complete the three-dose series with this dose. If it is not clear which dose an adolescent was administered at the start of a series, the series should be completed with the 3-dose schedule. [The information provided above on the vaccination schedule and dosing of Recombinex HB for adolescents was taken from the CDC MMWR, March 31, 2000/49(12); (http://www.cdc.gov/mmwr/preview/mmwrhtml/mm4912a5.htm)].

TREATMENT

Interferon alpha and lamivudine are two drugs presently approved for treating chronic hepatitis B. Interferon alpha induces seroconversion in 30–40% of patients, but its use is often limited by toxicity. Problems with toxicity include flu-like symptoms, nausea, diarrhea, energy loss, decreased blood cell counts of platelets and white cells, and depression. (See the section on Hepatitis C for a further explanation of interferon alpha.) Lamivudine (3TC, Epivir) is an antiretroviral agent that helps suppress the replication of the virus and delay the progression of the disease. It is also prescribed in the treatment of HIV in combination with AZT. Lamivudine is well tolerated and has seroconversion rates of 15–20% for hepatitis B at one year. If therapy with lamivudine continues for more than one year, the seroconversion rate also rises (Matthews et al. 2001).

Chronic hepatitis B infection is frequently diagnosed within the genitourinary tract. In the UK, sexual transmission is the most common route of acquisition. Only 3–5% of adults who contract acute hepatitis B will progress to chronic infection, and these individuals can be identified by the presence of HB_sAg in the bloodstream 6 months after infection. Individuals at highest risk of long-term complications, such as cirrhosis and hepatocellular carcinoma, carry HB_eAg and have high levels of circulating hepatitis B virus (HBV) deoxyribonucleic acid (DNA). Therapy should be targeted toward this group of patients.

Two forms of therapy are now licensed for use in chronic hepatitis B infection: interferon-alpha and lamivudine (Epivir). Seroconversion occurs in 30–40% of patients treated with interferon, and treatment is often limited by toxicity. Lamivudine is well tolerated, with seroconversion rates of 15–20% at one year, rising with increasing duration of therapy. Long-term monotherapy is limited, however, by the development of resistant mutations. Combination nucleoside therapy is likely to become the treatment of choice in the future. Patients with chronic hepatitis B should be counseled regarding transmission, partner vaccination, alcohol intake, and coinfection with other hepatitis viruses (Matthews et al. 2001).

Therapy for hepatitis B with interferon and lamivudine is recommended to continue for 1 year. Interferon works by increasing the body's immune response against the hepatitis B virus. Note that there is now another form of interferon, called pegylated interferon. This is standard interferon that is made into a longer molecule by complexing it with a polyethylene glycol molecule. Modifying the interferon into pegylated interferon (or "peg-interferon") makes it longer acting so that it can be injected once a week instead of 3 times a week, as regular interferon must be.

Pegylated interferon is now used in preference to interferon for treating hepatitis C. The medical literature regarding treatment for hepatitis B is slowly catching up to hepatitis C, meaning that an official recommendation regarding peg-interferon over interferon in the treatment of hepatitis B has not yet been made. This may be due to the fact that more research and funding are provided for hepatitis C. Hepatitis C affects a much larger number of people in the United States, and generally is a much more serious health problem. (Hepatitis C is now the most common cause of liver transplant in the United States and is a huge international public health problem as well.)

Specialists who treat liver disease prefer peg-interferon for hepatitis B and C treatment because it is easier to administer (given once weekly) and has somewhat fewer side effects than interferon. Patient compliance is therefore better in those taking peg-interferon. People needing treatment for hepatitis B would be wise to consult with a gastroenterologist (GI specialist) or hepatologist (liver specialist) who is very familiar with treating both hepatitis B and C and who is affiliated with a university center engaging in research treating these diseases.

Because therapy with one agent only is associated with the development of viral strains resistant to the drug, combination therapy is likely to be the wave of the future. Therapy with lamivudine alone is particularly associated with the development of drug resistance (Delaney et al. 2001). Interferon alpha combined with lamivudine may have an additive or synergistic effect (Mutimer et al. 2000). More research is needed on combination therapy with antiviral agents that will improve response and lessen the problem of drug resistance. Nucleoside agents such as entecavir and nucleotides such as adefovir and dipivoxil are currently being tested (Galan et al. 2001).

A PROMISING NEW THERAPY

A peptide called thymosin alpha-1 has been extensively studied for its beneficial effects on immune response, as well as its therapeutic value. Originally isolated from the thymus gland, thymosin alpha-1 is an amino-terminal acylated peptide of 28 amino acids. It is found in highest concentrations in the thymus but has also been detected in spleen, lung, kidney, brain, blood, and a number of other tissues.

In more than 70 studies involving hepatitis B and C, HIV, influenza, and certain cancers, thymosin alpha-1 has exhibited immunomodulatory activity and demonstrated benefits, whether used alone or in conjunction with a conventional therapy. Many of these effects appear to be synergistic with those of other cytokines (alpha interferon and interleukin-2), and thymosin alpha-1 may work best in combination with other immunomodulators.

Interest in using thymosin alpha-1 for treatment of human hepatitis B is based on the fact that it can trigger maturational events in lymphocytes, augment T-cell function, and promote reconstitution of immune defects.

In clinical studies on hepatitis B patients, thymosin alpha-1 has been primarily investigated as monotherapy, but promising results have also been obtained when thymosin alpha-1 is used in combination with interferon. In addition, thymosin alpha-1 has an excellent safety record. In treatment of more than 3000 patients with a range of diseases including hepatitis B and hepatitis C, thymosin alpha-1 has been well tolerated and is not associated with any significant side effects.

Four randomized controlled studies have investigated the safety and efficacy of thymosin alpha-1 monotherapy for the treatment of chronic hepatitis B. These studies show that thymosin alpha-1 promotes disease remission in 25–75% of the patients treated. Two of the studies resulted in statistically significant findings, and the third trial was statistically significant for the primary treatment center. When all the studies are considered together in a meta-analysis, the results show that six months of treatment with thymosin alpha-1 almost doubles the sustained response rate (36%) compared to controls (19%) (Ancell et al. 2001).

Thymosin alpha-1 is available in more than 20 countries around the world, but it has not yet been approved by the FDA. A large Phase III trial is currently underway in the United States, testing thymosin alpha-1 in combination with pegylated interferon alpha-2a in the treatment of hepatitis C. If the trial is successful, this promising therapy could become available in the United States by 2005.

TREATING ACCIDENTAL EXPOSURE TO HEPATITIS B

If an accidental exposure occurs, such as a needlestick in a healthcare worker, hepatitis B immunoglobulin (HBIG) should be given to prevent infection, and the person should immediately begin the vaccination series for hepatitis B if immunity has not been established. ["Updated U.S. Public Health Service Guidelines for the Management of Occupational Exposures to HBV, HCV, and HIV and Recommendations for Postexposure Prophylaxis" CDC MMWR *Morb Mortal Wkly Rep*, 2001 Jun 29; 50(RR-11); 1-42; http://www.cdc.gov/mmwr/preview/mmwrhtml/rr5011a1.html]

PRECAUTIONARY STEPS TO AVOID INFECTING OTHERS

If you are diagnosed as a hepatitis B carrier, the following precautions will reduce the risk of transmitting the disease to others:

- Remind your doctor, dentist, or healthcare providers that you are an HBV carrier.
- All cuts and open sores should be covered with a bandage. Wipe up your blood spills. Then reclean the area with a solution of 1 part household bleach to 10 parts water.
- Do not share toothbrushes, razors, needles, syringes, nail files, clippers, scissors, or any object that may come into contact with your blood or body fluids.

Do not share food that has been in your mouth, and do not prechew food for babies.

- Do not donate blood, plasma, body organs, tissue, or sperm.
- If pregnant, tell your physician you are an HBV carrier. A child born to a carrier mother needs to receive the hepatitis B immunoglobulin and the first hepatitis vaccine injection within 12 hours of birth.
- Avoid or severely restrict alcohol intake. Your liver may be further damaged by alcohol, particularly if taken with acetaminophen, found in Tylenol or other cold and headache remedies.
- Be careful not to spread the HBV virus to others. Hepatitis B is transmitted by contact with infected blood, serum, semen, and vaginal fluids. Wash your hands with soap after touching your own blood or body fluids. Throw personal items such as tissues, menstrual pads, tampons, or bandages away in a plastic bag. HBV is not spread by sneezing, coughing, or casual contact.
- Tell sexual partners you have hepatitis B. Partners should be tested for HBV, and if they are not immune to the virus, they should receive the vaccination series of three shots. Until protection from HBV has been guaranteed, use a condom.
- People living in the same household as a carrier should see their doctor for hepatitis B testing and vaccination. If anyone is exposed to your blood or body fluids, hepatitis B immunoglobulin given within 2 days–2 weeks can prevent the infection.

NONDRUG THERAPIES TO ENHANCE LIVER FUNCTIONING

Antioxidant Therapy

As with other diseases related to inflammation and tissue damage, oxidative stress is a key mediator that continues and magnifies the ongoing disease process. Markers of cellular oxidative stress, such as malonaldehyde and others, are increased in hepatitis. Minimizing oxidative stress and quenching free radicals is important in optimizing response to treatment. According to a report in the June 1998 issue of the *Journal of Clinical Gastroenterology*, investigators showed that nutritional antioxidants are potential therapeutic and preventive agents for diseases such as hepatitis. Other investigators reported at the same time that oxidative stress (free-radical damage) is often seen in hepatitis B and may contribute to the emergence of a hepatocellular carcinoma, a tumor seen in patients after years of chronic inflammation of the liver. They stated that antioxidants that down-regulate oxidative damage may be a useful complement to specific antiviral drugs in the therapy of viral diseases (Peterhans, 1997).

In a related study, vitamin E (alpha tocopherol) was reported in a randomized, double-blind, placebo-controlled study to be a successful adjunct approach when combined with alpha-interferon therapy in the treatment of hepatitis due to its strong antioxidant activity (von Herbay et al. 1997).

Selenium

The protective role of selenium against hepatitis B viruses was reported in early January of 1997 in the journal *Biological Trace Element Research*. The study reported that, in areas of China with high rates of hepatitis B and primary liver cancer, high levels of dietary selenium reduce liver-cancer incidence and hepatitis B infection. In a 4-year trial on 130,471 Chinese, those who were given selenium-spiked table salt showed a 35.1% reduction in primary liver cancer, compared with the group given salt without selenium. In the same journal report, another clinical study of 226 hepatitis B-positive people showed that a 200-mcg tablet a day of selenium reduced primary liver cancer incidence down to zero. Upon cessation of selenium supplementation, primary liver cancer incidences began to rise, indicating that viral hepatitis patients should take selenium on a continuous basis (Yu et al. 1997).

These human trials have been duplicated in animal studies showing that selenium supplementation reduced hepatitis B infection by 77.2% and precancerous liver lesions by 75.8%.

Another report in the *Journal of Trace Elements and Medical Biology* discussed the role of trace minerals for diseases such as liver disease and hepatitis. The report indicates that, while there is still some debate regarding the specific role of trace minerals, minerals such as selenium and zinc are of benefit to those with diseases such as hepatitis (Loguercio et al. 1997).

A 3-year study investigated whether supplementation of sodium selenite could prevent hepatitis B in a population of 20,847 persons in Jiangsu Province, China. The researchers concluded: "the incidence of virus hepatitis infection in the test population was significantly lower than that of controls provided with no selenium" (Yu et al. 1989).

Polyunsaturated Phosphatidylcholine (PPC)

Phosphatidylcholine is a naturally occurring phospholipid, derived from lecithin, necessary for maintaining the integrity of cell membranes. Oral phosphatidylcholine is incorporated into liver cell membrane to improve functioning (i.e., determining which substances are allowed to enter the liver cell and which are blocked from entry). As also discussed in the hepatitis C protocol, adding phosphatidylcholine to interferon improves the therapeutic value of interferon. Interferon alpha is a mainstay of medical treatment for chronic hepatitis B. Phosphatidylcholine also helps normalize transaminase levels on liver function tests (blood tests of liver functioning).

In chronic active hepatitis C patients, phospholipid therapy has been shown to significantly reduce disease activity and help regenerate liver cells. Phosphatidylcholine has a history of not only being liver protective, but also being able to enhance the bioavailability of various herbs and nutrients. The increased power of milk thistle, vitamin E, and interferon complexed with phosphatidylcholine corroborates this finding. Lessening the liver's work effort, in regard to detoxifying injurious substances, allows the liver the latitude to begin the healing process.

Milk Thistle (Silybum Marinum)

Silymarin and its chief active ingredient, silibinin, are derived from milk thistle, a member of the daisy family. Both substances help prevent toxic liver damage and help the liver regenerate faster if damage is done. Silymarin and silibinin actually accelerate the rate of protein synthesis in the liver, leading to faster cell regeneration (Sonnenbichler 1986, Valenzuela 1994). Silymarin and silibinin act in the ribosomes, special cellular organelles where protein synthesis takes place. It was discovered that silibinin can bind to the receptor for an important enzyme called DNA-dependent RNA polymerase I. This brings an increase in ribosomal RNA, which then leads to more protein synthesis. When milk thistle is added to phosphatidylcholine in the treatment of chronic hepatitis B, markers of oxidative stress such as malonaldehyde are decreased.

S-Adenosylmethionine (SAMe)

SAMe is the product of a biochemical reaction between ATP and methionine. Half of all methionine in the body is used in the liver to make SAMe. SAMe has been compared to ATP in its importance for the body. It is used in many different cellular processes, from replication to biochemical reactions that create melatonin and phosphatidylcholine. SAMe is particularly important for the liver because glutathione, the liver's natural antioxidant, is synthesized from it. Without sufficient glutathione levels in the liver, free radical damage will occur.

The liver contains the third highest amount of SAMe in the body, after the adrenal and pineal glands. SAMe is so important for liver function that it can be considered an essential nutrient for that organ. It has also been shown to be an effective antidepressant as well as playing a leading role in liver regeneration.

Glutathione

Glutathione is a potent antioxidant and is necessary for maintaining a normal redox state in the liver, which is vital to hepatic functioning. Nutrients that enhance glutathione levels in the body are:

1. *N*-acetyl-cysteine (NAC)—NAC is another substance that improves the response rate to interferon. It is necessary for glutathione production and thus decreases oxidative stress.

2. Whey protein—Whey protein will help boost immune function, protect against free radical damage, and improve cellular glutathione levels.

3. Alpha-lipoic acid—Alpha-lipoic acid is a potent antioxidant that helps to increase cellular glutathione levels. In addition, alpha-lipoic acid helps to regenerate other essential antioxidants.

4. Glutamine—Studies have demonstrated that glutamine supplementation increases glutathione stores in hepatic tissue, which protect the liver function.

AVOIDING LIVER TOXICITY

The best possible diet for the individual with hepatitis features chemical-free (organic) foods. Strict attention to optimal bowel evacuation must also be carried out in order to avoid any unnecessary toxic bowel load upon the immune system and the liver. All alcohol should be avoided. As in the case with all liver disease, one must be certain that the body load of iron is not excessive because excessive iron, itself, is a liver toxin. Measurements of serum iron, total iron-binding capacity, percent saturation, complete blood count, blood ferritin, and sometimes bone marrow analysis for iron stores may be needed and should be discussed with your physician. Iron depletion therapy (extracting blood as in blood donation) may be recommended by your physician if testing reveals very high serum iron levels. Iron depletion therapy is contraindicated in the presence of anemia, which is often a consequence of treatment for hepatitis. Close monitoring by a physician is required.

Certain nutritional supplements have shown evidence of reducing serum iron levels. To help keep serum iron levels in the normal range of 30–80 grams/dL, high doses of green tea polyphenols and high-allicin garlic may be beneficial. Lactoferrin, a subfraction of whey protein, may be especially beneficial as an adjunctive treatment for serum iron overload in hepatitis patients. Lactoferrin is a potent antioxidant, antiviral agent, and scavenger of free iron. In addition, lactoferrin is directly involved in the up-regulation of natural killer (NK) cell activity, making it a natural modulator of immune function.

As mentioned earlier in this protocol, the hepatitis B virus induces free radical reactions that damage liver cells. A standardized grape-seed extract providing a high percentage of antioxidant proanthocyanidins can help protect the liver against oxidative stress.

Some herbs can be toxic to the liver, especially in high amounts. The following herbal preparations have shown liver toxicity: germander, comfrey, chapparal leaf, ginbu-1, pennyroyal, skullcap, and mistletoe.

Some hepatitis B patients take 500 mg of licorice root extract 3 times a day. There is a controversy about hepatitis B patients taking high-dose licorice; we therefore suggest it only be taken under the supervision of a knowledgeable health care provider. If high doses of licorice are taken, monitor blood pressure to guard against any untoward increase.

It should also be noted that spoiled peanuts produce a toxin called aflatoxin, which is hepatotoxic and has been associated with the development of hepatoma. Nonspoiled, nonmoldy peanuts do not contain aflatoxin. Corticosteroids are useful in other types of hepatitis but not in viral hepatitis. They may be harmful in the presence of viral hepatitis.

◉ SUMMARY

In addition to conventional drug therapy, broad-spectrum antioxidant supplementation is recommended along with specific supplements to protect and enhance liver functioning. Some hepatitis B patients cannot tolerate beta-carotene, vitamin A, or niacin found in many multinutrient formulas, including Life Extension Mix. Blood tests (ALT, AST, GGTP) that measure liver enzymes can determine patient tolerance to these substances. People who cannot take Life Extension Mix can take individual supplements to provide optimal nutritional support.

The following individual supplements are important in the integrated treatment of hepatitis:

1. Selenium, 200–400 mcg a day.

2. Polyunsaturated phosphatidylcholine (PPC), 1800–2700 mg a day in divided doses. (Sold under the name HepatoPro in the United States as a dietary supplement. In Europe, it is available only as a drug.)

3. SAMe, 200 mg 3 times a day.

4. Silibinin (silymarin milk thistle extract), 260 mg 3 times a day.

5. Vitamin C, 500–10,000 mg a day in divided doses.

6. Vitamin E, 400 IU taken daily with at least 200 mg of gamma tocopherol.

7. *N*-acetyl-cysteine (NAC), 600 mg once a day.

8. Whey protein, 20–30 grams once a day.

9. Alpha-lipoic acid, 250 mg twice a day.

10. Grape seed-skin extract, 100 mg 2 or 3 times a day.

11. Lactoferrin, up to three 300 mg capsules daily.

12. High-allicin garlic, 4000 mg a day in divided doses.

13. Green tea polyphenols, 600–800 mg early in the day, either from green tea extract capsules or from drinking 5–10 cups of green tea (some people cannot tolerate the caffeine in tea beverages and have to use decaffeinated green tea extract capsules). In order to obtain 600–800 mg of polyphenols from green tea extract, it will be necessary to take 2–3 300-mg green tea extract (95%) capsules each day.

14. Glutamine—if given orally, use *L*-glutamine, 500–1000 mg daily. If given IV, use either free glutamine or alanyl glutamine at the same dose.

(*See the Immune Enhancement protocol from Life Extension for more information regarding the possible benefits of supplements and/or an integrated therapy treatment approach. Also see the Hepatitis C protocol for additional suggestions.*)

 FOR MORE INFORMATION

Contact the American Liver Foundation, (800) 223-0179.

 PRODUCT AVAILABILITY

HepatoPro (consisting of polyunsaturated phosphatidylcholine), selenium, Silibinin Plus, Pure-Gar (garlic) Caps, vitamin C, vitamin E, glutathione, Enhanced Whey Protein, alpha-lipoic acid, lactoferrin, NAC, SAMe, grape seed-skin extract, and green tea extract (95%) caps can be ordered by calling (800) 544-4440 or by ordering online at www.lef.org. Interferon and Lamivudine are drugs that must be prescribed, administered, and supervised by a physician experienced and knowledgeable in their use in treating hepatitis B. Thymosin alpha-1 is not yet available in the United States and is extremely expensive if purchased offshore.

Hepatitis C

The incidence of the hepatitis C virus (HCV) has grown into a virtual epidemic. HCV can be transmitted by narcotics use, transfusion of blood, and exposure of medical personnel to infected patients. In some cases, how one contracted HCV cannot be determined.

Hepatitis C was originally called non-A/non-B hepatitis, denoting the fact that this was a viral hepatitis not caused by either the A or B viruses. Hepatitis C is the most common infection transmitted by blood and blood transfusions with up to 200 million persons infected worldwide (Herrera 2001; QMG 2002). In the United States, more than 4 million people are infected with HCV. Most liver transplants in the United States are a result of HCV. Hepatitis C has a frightening tendency to result in chronic hepatitis and the sequelae of cirrhosis and hepatocellular carcinoma (primary liver cancer) (Smith et al. 2001).

HCV is an RNA virus, spherical and enveloped in a lipid (fatty) outer envelope. It is somewhat similar to the viruses causing yellow fever, dengue, and Japanese encephalitis. It was first isolated in 1989, making it a relatively recent challenge for the medical profession to treat.

HOW HEPATITIS C DAMAGES LIVER CELLS

HCV inflicts most of its damage by latching onto molecules of iron, resulting in free-radical damage to liver cells. These free radicals can induce liver inflammation, cirrhosis, and primary liver cancer via oxidative attacks on liver cells. Successful eradication of HCV from the body often requires that iron levels in the liver and blood be very low. In many cases, high stores of iron in the liver preclude successful therapy against HCV. Therefore, it is desirable to reduce iron levels in the body before initiating treatment with conventional (interferon and ribavirin) therapy. Despite substantial scientific evidence, few physicians implement iron-depletion therapy when treating HCV. This partially accounts for the high failure rate to eradicate the virus (Boucher et al. 1997; Martin Vivaldi et al. 1997; Tsai et al. 1997). *Note:* In HCV patients, systemic depletion of glutathione is also observed, especially in the liver. This

depletion may be another factor underlying resistance to interferon therapy (see the section on Boosting Liver Glutathione Levels).

An age-associated decline in immunity also appears to play an important role in HCV. The virus often becomes active in the body after age 40, indicating that there is an association between age-related immune decline and progression of HCV.

In this protocol, we review drug therapies currently used in the treatment of HCV. We then reveal adjuvant approaches that may enhance the safety and efficacy of these conventional treatments. We also discuss natural therapies that have been shown to protect the liver against the damaging effects of HCV.

THE PHASES OF HCV INFECTION

Acute phase infection with HCV develops about 6 weeks after exposure. This stage of illness is usually dismissed by the patient because it passes with very few, if any, signs or symptoms. The acute phase may be thought to be the flu, or it may not be identified with any state of illness whatsoever. If blood tests were to be done at this time, they might show elevated serum ALT (a liver transaminase) (Hoofnagle 1997; Iwasaki et al. 2002) or a slight elevation of bilirubin, but usually not enough to cause noticeable jaundice (yellowing of the skin from bilirubin): Approximately 75% of acute hepatitis C cases have no observable jaundice (Esteban et al. 1990).

An acute phase HCV infection is often discovered during routine blood testing for some other condition or prior to a medical procedure. An elevated ALT would alert a physician to the possibility that HCV infection might be present. If ALT is elevated, a blood test for HCV antibody would be done. If the HCV test is negative, then other causes of ALT elevation should be investigated. It takes 4–6 weeks after exposure for the antibody to be detectable in the bloodstream. Therefore, if there has been a known exposure to HCV, the patient is still at risk, and an HCV antibody test should be repeated in 6 weeks. *Note:* Antibody might continue to be undetectable in immunosuppressed persons such as those infected with HIV. In these patients, a test for HCV-RNA by polymerase chain reaction (PCR) is required to make the diagnosis (Rieske et al. 1998). Other blood tests might show a slight elevation in bilirubin (Esteban et al. 1990).

Unfortunately, early detection of acute phase HCV is unlikely unless a known exposure exists. (*Later in this protocol, the section on Diagnosis, Testing, and Monitoring of Hepatitis C Virus will provide additional information about diagnosing HCV.*)

Almost all patients who have acute hepatitis C enter a chronic phase that continues for decades. In many viral illnesses, the patient is able to develop immunity via the reaction in the immune system against the infecting virus. However, in hepatitis C, the human immune system is usually unable to mount an effective antiviral response. As many as 75–85% of infected individuals are unable to spontaneously clear the virus after the acute stage of infection and go on to develop chronic hepatitis. The exact reason people are unable to develop effective immunity is unknown, but it may relate to the highly variable chain areas on the virus where genetic base substitutions occur, frequently changing the exact composition of the virus. Some sort of immunity does develop after acute hepatitis C infection, as witnessed by positive serologic markers, such as antibodies to hepatitis C; however, this immunity is quite incomplete and incapable of conferring immunity against the virus. (These factors related to immunity also have important implications in the difficulty of developing a vaccine for hepatitis C.)

The disease progresses very slowly and is marked by episodes of acute hepatitis, with liver inflammation and elevation of serum ALT. Blood products from these persons are infectious at this time, but usually the disease itself is still not recognized by the patient until 18–20 years after the acute infection. At that time, nonspecific symptoms such as fatigue usually prompt the patient to visit a physician. Again at this time, symptoms are often very mild and laboratory findings consist of only mild elevations of the liver enzymes ALT and AST. Without an astute practitioner, these laboratory abnormalities could be dismissed as inconsequential.

If HCV is suspected at this time, a hepatitis screen should be ordered, looking for various types of hepatitis, including antibody to hepatitis C, which will be positive. A liver biopsy is indicated for patients having elevated ALT and a positive screen for hepatitis C. The findings of the liver biopsy will help guide treatment. (Furthermore, up to 75% of persons with cirrhosis have no symptoms, again pointing out the usefulness of liver biopsy.) Usually, only this initial single liver biopsy is required throughout the entire management of the disease. It provides the necessary information to assess the present severity of liver damage and guide treatment (Tappe et al. 2002).

The goal of treatment at this stage is to prevent the progression of the disease to cirrhosis, primary liver cancer, and liver failure. After the initial 20-year quiescent period, more advanced liver disease begins to develop, eventually leading to cirrhosis and liver failure (Jankovic 1999; Amarapurkar 2000).

There are two subsets of patients who have a much more rapidly progressive course: people with alcoholic liver disease or those who have concomitant infection with HIV. Hepatitis C in the presence of alcoholic liver disease or HIV tends to be much more severe and progresses more rapidly than hepatitis C infection alone. Patients who continue to use alcohol have a particularly rapid progressive course in general, and for this reason, the cessation of alcohol use is mandatory to optimize outcome and control the progression of disease. Additionally, persons who continue to use alcohol have a poor outcome from chronic hepatitis C in general.

Even in the absence of associated ongoing alcohol use or HIV infection, there are some persons with hepatitis C who do not follow the typical slowly progressing course. Why a more rapid progression occurs in some persons is not known. Therefore, this points to the importance of ongoing observation and obtaining a liver biopsy to assess severity of disease at initial presentation.

The occurrence of hepato-cellular carcinoma (hepatoma) is a late consequence of hepatitis C infection and occurs in 1–6% of patients with chronic hepatitis C (Di Bisceglie 1997). (However, in Japan, where hepatitis C seems to be more severe, hepatoma is more common.) Hepatoma only occurs in patients who have developed cirrhosis and therefore have an ongoing inflammatory process. Hepatoma is to be suspected if the following symptoms develop in an environment of chronic hepatitis C: sudden worsening of the symptoms of cirrhosis, such as pronounced fatigue, jaundice, and ascites (accumulation of fluid in the abdomen) and possibly pain in the right upper quadrant of the abdomen.

Liver enzymes, including alkaline phosphatase, are usually very high and a mass is seen within the liver on ultrasound or CT scan of the abdomen. Liver biopsy of the mass confirms a diagnosis of hepatoma. Patients with hepatoma have a limited lifespan in spite of treatment.

With most types of hepatitis, there is a slight possibility of the development of fulminant hepatitis (a catastrophic hepatitis, leading to liver failure and death). However, with hepatitis C, a fulminant stage has not been recognized, with the possible exception of occurrence of occasional fulminant hepatitis in Japan. Note: Hepatitis C occurring in Japan appears to be generally of a more severe nature. The severity of the Japanese form may be related to a higher prevalence of a certain genetic type of the virus (Type II) and possibly also to genetic differences in the hosts (Pozzato et al. 1994).

HOW HEPATITIS C VIRUS IS ACQUIRED AND TRANSMITTED

The virus is transmitted via exposure to blood or blood products infected with the hepatitis C virus. Blood transfusions occurring before 1992 are a known risk factor for the development of hepatitis C. By far the most common method of infection is the sharing of needles during IV (intravenous) drug abuse. The risk of transmission of HCV in the United States from blood that has tested negative for HCV antibodies is less than 1 in 103,000 transfused units (Lauer et al. 2001).

Occupational exposure via infected needle sticks in health-related professions is another possible exposure route. However, hepatitis C is no more frequent in healthcare workers than in the general population. The rate of transmission of the virus to a healthcare worker from blood known to be infected with HCV ranges between 0–10% (Hernandez et al. 1992; Mitsui et al. 1992). The CDC recommends frequent testing for HCV in hospital personnel exposed via needle sticks because the data suggest that treatment for HCV is more effective when started early (Anon. 2001).

Perinatal transmission during birth is possible, with mixing of blood between mother and baby. This type of transmission is rare, however, and thought only to occur in mothers having very high viral titers, such as those who also have HIV infection. As noted earlier, the presence of HIV is associated with a more severe progression of hepatitis C. The United States Public Health Service has estimated that perinatal transmission is only on the order of about 5–6%. Breastfeeding does not increase the risk of transmission (Dienstag 1997).

Other possible, yet unproven risk factors for transmitting the HCV virus include body piercing, tattooing, and sharing contaminated household items such as toothbrushes, razor blades, and nail clippers. Lock et al. (2002) investigated whether or not HCV is transmitted by sharing the toothbrush of an infected individual. Their results, although inconclusive, suggest that this may be possible.

The Question of Sexual Transmission

Vertical transmission (from parent to child) within families has not been shown to occur (Dienstag 1997). The possibility of horizontal transmission (via sexual partners) has been investigated in the literature extensively. Initially, it was thought that the virus might be sexually transmitted with a very low frequency because some persons living in the same household were both found to be HCV positive. These studies are difficult to interpret, however, because lifestyle factors, such as drug use and possibility of multiple sexual partners, confounded the data. Perhaps the most reliable studies come from Saudi Arabia, where cultural behaviors are more restrictive (al-Faleh et al. 1995). In this study, no spouse of an HCV positive index case was infected.

An Italian study looked at women who had been infected with HCV after blood transfusions (Sachithanandan et al. 1997). The authors concluded that the study suggested a "zero female to male sexual transmission rate of HCV." A similar study using blood products was conducted in Finland (Kolho et al. 1991). According to researchers, the results showed that "even though about 10% of persons with reported cases of acute hepatitis C in the United States report a history of potential sexual exposure, sexual transmission is negligible in sex-partner studies" (Dienstag 1997). However, epidemiological studies suggest that the rate of sexual transmission increases with traumatic intercourse or with the presence of genital ulcers due to breaks in the mucosal barrier. Sexual transmission of HCV is thought to be the method of transmission in less than 3% of cases (Thomas 2001).

In animal studies, a colony of chimpanzees was used to study the potential for sexual transmission of HCV. Nonpercutaneous (not piercing the skin) transmission, including sexual transmission, was not found to be a mode of transmission (Suzuki et al. 1993).

TREATMENT OF HEPATITIS C

Standard therapy for hepatitis C has consisted of ribavirin combined with interferon. However, a combination therapy of peg-interferon alfa-2b and ribavirin is currently the standard of care. Pegylated interferon is standard interferon that has been changed by attaching a polyethylene glycol molecule to the interferon proteins. The polyethylene glycol molecule lengthens the time the drug stays in the bloodstream, hence, the patient needs only one subcutaneous injection a week. There exists another pegylated interferon called alfa-2a, which is administered in a fixed dose rather than the alfa-2b, which is dosed by weight. The alfa-2a has not yet been approved by the FDA for treatment (Molineux 2002). For purposes of this protocol, the terms interferon and pegylated interferon may be used interchangeably. In medical literature published in 2002 or after, the reader may assume that interferon refers to the newer, more advantageous pegylated interferon form.

healthy controls found that "levels of plasma lactoferrin are decreased in HIV-1 infected patients in relation to the progression of the disease" (Defer et al. 1995). Another study found that the lack of lactoferrin (and secretory IGA) found in the oral cavities of people with HIV correlated strongly with the frequent infections in those areas often seen in patients with AIDS (Muller et al. 1992). Lactoferrin was also found to have "potent" antiviral effects against the replication of both human HIV and cytomegalovirus (CMV) in several *in vitro* studies with no cytopathic effects on healthy cells.

An adequate and cost effective dose of lactoferrin for the adjunctive treatment of disease is estimated to be 300 mg daily. There are dietary supplements that provide potent doses of lactoferrin extracted from whey. When using these supplements, it is important to use a form of lactoferrin called "apolactoferrin," which is depleted of iron. In studies, the apolactoferrin form has been shown to provide the benefits of lactoferrin as an antioxidant. Studies also show that the "apo" form may have additional benefits over that of other forms of lactoferrin.

Coenzyme Q_{10}

Coenzyme Q_{10} (CoQ_{10}) is an antioxidant produced in the body and found in small amounts in some foods. HIV-positive people are often deficient in this important substance. CoQ_{10} is found in high concentrations in the healthy heart, where it plays an important role in initiating cell-produced energy. Studies have documented its effectiveness in improving the quality of life in people with advanced heart disease, congestive heart failure, angina, and arrhythmia. It has been found to increase a number of immune parameters, including IgG, T4 cells, and the ratio of T4/T8 lymphocytes (Folkers et al. 1988; 1991; 1993). In a pilot study in AIDS patients, CoQ_{10} supplementation provided significant benefits. It is suggested that HIV patients take at least 200 mg daily of CoQ_{10} (Folkers et al. 1988; 1991; 1993; Yamashita et al. 1997).

L-Glutamine

There are causes of immune suppression that have been proven to create a malabsorption syndrome in the gastrointestinal tract (e.g., diarrhea, metabolic conditions, AIDS wasting, and drug therapies) (*see also the section on Other Causes of Immune Suppression*). Malabsorption syndrome is a significant component in the vicious cycle of immune suppression because it can be considered to be both a *cause* and an *effect* of immune suppression. Therefore not being able to utilize ingested foods and nutrients can be a specific cause of malnutrition in immune-suppressed patients. It is essential to break the cycle of malabsorption, antioxidant depletion, oxidative stress, immunosuppression, and the resulting increase in malabsorption. It is helpful to remember that the majority of immune system components and their activity are located in the gastrointestinal tract. Immune system activity has a particularly dominant influence in the mucosal lining since the mucosal lining is the area of the body that must assimilate material entering the gastrointestinal tract from the environment.

In addition to its important role in the mediation of oxidative stress and free-radical damage, the amino acid glutamine also plays a major role in the overall health and well-being of the gastrointestinal tract and its supportive organs (stomach, small and large intestine, liver, pancreas, and gall bladder). Glutamine is vital to the function of intestinal cells called enterocytes. Enterocytes are located in the fingerlike projections of the mucosal villi. These cells make up the mucosal lining of the small intestines and are some of the most rapidly dividing cells in the body. They have high energy requirements. Glutamine is the primary nutrient for enterocytes. Enterocyte cells break down glutamine to form glutamate, which is then converted to ATP and used as the energy supply for the cells. Studies have confirmed that glucose (sugar) is not utilized as a fuel source for the intestine (Newsholme et al. 1985; Souba et al. 1985; Hartmann et al. 1989; Alverdy 1990).

WARNING

- Glutamine supplementation is clearly not indicated for individuals who have severe cirrhosis of the liver, Reye's syndrome, or any other metabolic disorder that can lead to an accumulation of ammonia in the blood because of an increased risk for encephalopathy or coma. Under these conditions, the body is unable to metabolize excess nitrogen, which converts to ammonia and can cause brain swelling and brain death. When the liver is severely damaged or when hepatic coma is imminent, glutamine is not effective and can actually cause further brain damage.

- Wasting is a life-threatening condition that should not be self-treated. If you have involuntarily lost more than 10% of your body weight, you should suspect that wasting is taking place and seek the care from a knowledgeable physician. Bio Impedance Analysis can determine lean body mass and establish a baseline for you, against which the efficacy of future treatments can be judged. In addition to glutamine, it is also important to review the information about whey protein isolate, which is extremely bioavailable and tissue-sparing. In addition to these treatment recommendations, your physician may wish to include anabolic steroids, such as testosterone, and nandrolone, and growth hormone. Treatments with steroids and growth hormone are very well-grounded and medically prudent in some cases of wasting and should be considered when necessary.

A study in *Nutrition* (Shabert et al. 1999) reported supplementation of both antioxidants and glutamine in 28 patients with at least a 5% weight loss from baseline. The supplementation was found to increase body weight and cell mass and to normalize intracellular water distribution, while providing "a highly cost-effective therapy for the rehabilitation of HIV-positive patients with weight loss."

L-Carnitine

Another nutrient often overlooked by persons with HIV is *L*-carnitine. *L*-carnitine has been shown to boost immune function, via several different mechanisms, in order to protect the heart against AZT toxicity and to enhance essential fatty-acid and glucose uptake. Protease inhibitors (PIs) can raise triglyceride to harmful levels. *L*-carnitine can be an appropriate treatment for this side effect. High doses of *L*-carnitine have also enhanced immunological and metabolic functions in those who were deficient in *L*-carnitine. *L*-carnitine also has positive effects on preserving CD4 cells by affecting apoptosis (De Simone et al. 1993; 1994; Cifone et al. 1997; Di Marzio et al. 1997; Mutomba et al. 2000). The recommended dose is 3–4 grams twice daily on an empty stomach.

Olive Leaf Extract

Olive leaf extract is a nonprescription, over-the-counter food supplement that has been used as a natural treatment of viral, bacterial, fungal, and parasitic infections; skin diseases; arthritis; heart disease; and many other illnesses. The ethnopharmacology of the olive tree has a colorful historical past because it has been thought to be the tree that is referred to as the "Tree of Life" in the Book of Genesis. The ancient Egyptians may have been the first to employ the olive leaf as part of the mummification of their royalty. Hippocrates, the father of medicine, used olive oil to treat ulcers, cholera, and muscle pains more than 2500 years ago. In later cultures, olive oil was used as a popular folk remedy for the treatment of fevers. In the 1850s, the first formal medical documentation of the use of olive leaves to treat severe cases of fever and malaria was made. In 1854, a healing remedy of olive leaves was published in *Pharmaceutical Journal*, England's leading medical journal of that time. Italian researchers also discovered that olive leaf extract could lower blood pressure in animals. It was also confirmed that olive leaf extract increased blood flow to the coronary arteries, relieved arrhythmias, and treated intestinal muscle spasms. In addition, olive leaf extract is thought to have powerful antioxidant properties. Countless studies illustrate that antioxidant activity is crucial to the management of HIV disease.

Olive leaf extract contains a phenolic glucoside, known as oleuropein, which has been shown to be the source of its extremely powerful disease-resistant properties (Renis 1970; Hirschman 1972; Fredrickson 1994; Privitera 1996; Ripka et al. 1996; Gay Men's Health Crisis 1997–1998; Walker 1997). In the late 1960s, olive leaf extract was tested by Upjohn Pharmaceuticals and was found to kill a large number of viruses. According to Jim Van Sweden at Upjohn Pharmaceuticals, Dr. H. E. Renis conducted prolific research on olive leaf extract, working in Upjohn's Department of Virology. His study, "*In Vitro* Antiviral Activity of Calcium Elenolate," published in the peer-reviewed journal *Antimicrobial Agents and Chemotherapy*, revealed calcium elenolate's formidable antiviral activity because it inactivated almost all viruses tested against it (Renis 1970).

Calcium elenolate is a chemical compound of oleuropein found in olive leaves. William Fredrickson, Ph.D. (researcher and CEO of F+S BioGenesis Group, Inc.), has also studied olive leaf extract extensively and believes the compound (+)-2-epienolic acid found in olive leaf extract is a natural reverse transcriptase inhibitor. He cites Hirschman's (1972) study, "Inactivation of DNA Polymerases of Murine Leukemia Viruses by Calcium Elenolate," as documentation of olive leaf extract's reverse transcriptase mechanism of action. He also believes that it is a natural protease inhibitor because he has seen 100% protease inhibition activity *in vitro* while conducting a laboratory screen of oleuropein. However, there is no documentation to support his observation. In 1996, as an alternative to taking toxic pharmaceutical protease inhibitors, the AIDS community discovered this possible natural source of protease inhibitors known as olive leaf extract. It has been shown to be nontoxic in all animal studies, even when given in doses of 3 grams per kilogram of body weight. By functioning as a reverse transcriptase inhibitor and a believed protease inhibitor, it is selectively cytotoxic to virus-infected cells but has never shown any toxicity to human DNA alpha-, beta-, or gamma-polymerases.

Olive leaf extract has been taken by persons with AIDS in doses of one 500-mg capsule or tablet 4 times per day. Olive leaf extract products should have the recommended 23% oleuropein content and be guaranteed fresh.

Olive leaf extract does not have any side effects *per se*, although some people may experience a "die-off" effect (also called the Herxheimer reaction). A "die-off" effect is caused by a rapid increase in volume of waste material and pathogens being brought into the lymph system. Reactions to the die-off effect include extreme fatigue, diarrhea, headaches, muscle and joint achiness, and flu-like symptoms. These reactions are temporary and will pass once the body has expelled the circulating toxins. If these detoxifying symptoms are too uncomfortable, reduce the amount of olive leaf extract taken or discontinue using it temporarily. Upon feeling better, resume the supplement at a lower amount and increase it to your desired dose slowly. Testimonials about olive leaf extract may be obtained from Mark Konlee, Director of Keep Hope Alive, P.O. Box 27041, West Allis, WI 53227, (262)548-4344, or at www.khope@execpc.com.

SPV-30

SPV-30 is an herbal extract derived from the European boxwood tree (*Buxus sempervirens*), a species of evergreen (Durant et al. 1998). The proprietary extract is manufactured by Arkopharma in Nice, France. Arkopharma is the largest phytopharmaceutical company in Europe and is dedicated to natural herbal products. Research scientists have identified 20 active alkaloids in SPV-30 of a total of nearly 100, using HPLC (high performance liquid chromatography) and gas chromatography. The five most active alkaloids are buxtaurine, cyclobuxine D, boxamine, cyclovirobuxine D, and cyclovirobuxine C.

The potential of SPV-30 as a natural antiretroviral was first identified by Jacques Durant, M.D., head of the Infectious Diseases Department of the Hospital de l'Archet in Nice. He learned about SPV-30 from a person with AIDS who took SPV-30 and was able to maintain high CD4 levels over a sustained period of time despite episodic IV drug abuse and bouts of opportunistic infections (OI).

In a double-blind, placebo-controlled Phase I trial in France, patients taking SPV-30 had an average increase of 94 CD4 cells after 30 weeks (Durant et al. 1998). The placebo group saw an average loss of 43 CD4 cells after 30 weeks. No toxicities were noted and no serious side effects were reported. These results encouraged Professor Luc Montagnier, co-discoverer of HIV and one of the world's leading AIDS researchers, to act as scientific adviser and chief virologist for an 18-month, multicenter, Phase II/Phase III study in France (Vandermander et al. 1996). The French Ministry of Health had classified the study as an antiretroviral

trial. Of the 22 trials listed in the Ministry of Health 1995 *Clinical Trials Directory*, SPV-30 is the only natural herbal product listed in an antiretroviral trial.

As early as 1996, an informal, community-based study was conduced in the United States using SPV-30 in 400 HIV-infected subjects who had CD4 cell counts of 0–700 per microliter and plasma HIV RNA levels of $0–10^6$ copies per milliliter. Although there was only mild plasma HIV-RNA activity, and the results were considered inconclusive, Bryson (1996) presented a preliminary analysis of this study to an AIDS conference in Vancouver, Canada.

Later evidence suggested that SPV-30 works primarily as an antiretroviral, as well as an antioxidant, which favorably alters over-expressed cellular transcription factors (Durant et al. 1998). SPV-30 inhibits HIV by targeting the reverse transcriptase enzyme, the same enzyme that AZT and other nucleoside agents target. There is evidence that SPV-30 reduces a cellular messenger, TNF-alpha, which becomes elevated in people with HIV. Many studies have shown that this elevation, associated with an inflammatory response, correlates with increased viral replication and cell loss.

One outcome of a number of SPV-30 studies was a noticeable quality-of-life improvement, experienced by many of the participants. When asked to comment on many factors affecting them, such as energy levels, ability to fall asleep, appetite, digestion, and overall sense of well-being, nearly half of the participants reported "much improved" energy, while other participants believed their energy levels were either much improved or about the same. About half also commented that their overall sense of well-being had greatly improved. These findings are significant enough to warrant consideration by those infected with HIV because so many of the taken-for-granted components related to quality of life begin to slowly erode after HIV diagnosis.

AIDS buyers' clubs around the country have anecdotally reported on a specific SPV-30 treatment regimen that has produced the most beneficial results. It is included here:

- Upon rising, on an empty stomach, take five 500-mg capsules of bitter melon with 2 large glasses of water. Wait 30 minutes before eating.

- Consume the following 3 times daily, with or without food, and with one large glass of water:

  - Glycyrrhizinate Forte (licorice), 300 mg, Jarrow Formulas

Note: *Licorice can elevate blood pressure.*

- 1-SPV-30 (boxwood extract), 330 mg, Arkopharma
- Consume the following at the end of the evening, 2 hours after eating:
  - Bitter melon, five 500-mg capsules with 1 large glass of water

Thymic Immune Factors

Thymic Immune Factors is a synergistic formula that contains herbal activators and a full complement of homeopathic nutrients, in addition to fresh, healthy thymus, lymph, and spleen tissues, which produce white blood cells to fight invading organisms and cancer cells. The immunological tissue extracts in this product are raw, concentrated, toxin-free, and freeze-dried to preserve their biological activity. HIV-infected individuals may consider using a unique product such as Thymic Immune Factors to potentiate white blood cell production and activity.

Silymarin

Milk thistle extract, or silymarin, is a unique type of bioflavonoid that exerts a protective effect on the liver. This is of importance to persons with HIV, because they may be taking hepatotoxic antiviral medications and also because silymarin supports activities of the liver, one being the production of glutathione, which is extremely crucial in correcting immune system functioning. Silibinin is the most active constituent of silymarin, now available in the United States. Please refer to the section on *Boosting Glutathione Levels* for more information concerning products that promote healthy liver function (Flora et al. 1998).

Enzymes

Proper digestion of nutrients is necessary for maintaining good health in all of us. Persons with HIV or AIDS have an elevated necessity for life-sustaining nutrients. In many cases, even the consumption of all the correct nutrients simply does not result in adequate nourishment because of malabsorption. A comprehensive digestive enzymes formula should be used to encourage the greatest possible digestive activity. Some digestive enzymes are also used by the body to dissolve tumors, which can also be a consideration for those who are immunocompromised.

Plant Sterols

Beta-sitosterol and beta-sitosterol glucoside are substances found in plants, which are absorbed in human tissues after ingestion. Plant sterols have been found to have immune modulating activity and antitumor

activity in animal models and human clinical trials (Bouic et al. 1999). These substances may also be obtained as supplements. Beta-sitosterol, taken in sufficient doses, has some antitestosterone activity. This antitestosterone activity should be taken into consideration by males using this therapy if decreased libido or decreased sexual function appears. Testosterone levels should also be monitored, which is usually advisable in ongoing monitoring of persons with AIDS.

Green Tea Extract

A catechin is a bioflavonoid found in tea that has powerful antioxidant properties. The most abundant catechin found in green tea, epigallocatechin gallate (EGCG), has properties that inhibit HIV from infecting human T-cells. A study demonstrated that EGCG can bind to CD4 cells and block the virus from attaching to and infecting human T-cells. This study marks a breakthrough in HIV research. EGCG however, should not be substituted for current conventional HIV therapy since the dosage needed to achieve similar results has not been determined and the amount of EGCG tested in the study was far beyond what could be consumed by drinking green tea.

Nonetheless, this breakthrough information may significantly impact HIV research if future investigation can determine the precise location on the CD4 molecule in which EGCG exerts its effect and whether it is the same location in which the HIV glycoprotein binds to the CD4 cell. If this is the case, EGCG could become a promising form of anti-HIV therapy (Kawai et al. 2003).

HORMONE LEVELS AND HIV

Decline in several important hormones is associated with HIV and, in many cases, has also been associated with progression of severity of disease. Some of the hormones known to be related to HIV will be discussed below.

DHEA

According to researchers, low serum levels of DHEA-sulfate are associated with HIV illness markers, including viral load, and tend to indicate a negative prognosis (Yang 1994; Ferrando et al. 1999). DHEA has been found to decline in patients as they progress from only being HIV-positive, to displaying symptoms, to having the full-blown AIDS (Jacobson 1991; Mulder et al. 1992). These declines in DHEA have been associated with the development of opportunistic infections and malignancies. Interestingly, about 6 months after therapy with a protease inhibitor is begun, DHEA begins to rise.

Because levels of DHEA are also age-related, as well as HIV-illness related, testing of DHEA levels is recommended before beginning supplementation. DHEA is a hormone that progressively declines with age so reliably that it can even be used as a biomarker of aging. However, a 20-year-old with AIDS may have a very low DHEA level and benefit from supplementation, while in the healthy adult, DHEA supplementation is very rarely needed under age 35. Over-supplementation with DHEA and other androgenic substances can contribute to liver disease, which is also often associated with AIDS or with the side effects of AIDS therapy. This must be considered before beginning DHEA supplementation. Liver function tests must be followed regularly, as would be expected with the monitoring of the HIV state itself. This "first pass effect" of the DHEA through the liver may be circumvented by opening the capsule and placing it under the tongue, allowing the contents to be absorbed through the mucosal tissue rather than in the GI tract. If some is swallowed, this amount will be metabolized in the liver. If the remainder is not swallowed (e.g., spit out), the levels may be variable or similar to those compared to an oral dose. Thus, it is again essential to monitor DHEA levels with blood tests.

DHEA helps to maintain healthy functioning of the immune system, while HAART helps to reduce viral load but is "less effective in immune constitution" (Clerici et al. 2000). DHEA is contraindicated in both men and women with hormone-related cancers. Please refer to the *DHEA Replacement Therapy* protocol for more information.

The Cortisol/DHEA Connection

Cortisol is a major hormone produced by the adrenal glands. At normal levels, cortisol assists in the metabolism of glucose, protein, and fats. It also has a strong impact on the immune system. At consistently high levels due to illness or stress, cortisol suppresses immune response and accelerates the aging of major organ systems. Rises in cortisol herald the onset of numerous illnesses. In general, rising levels of cortisol are associated with physical and severe mental stress. Similarly, in HIV, cortisol levels are increased (Clerici et al. 2000). Cortisol induces apoptosis of the CD4 lymphocyte, thereby decreasing CD4 counts.

In several studies, DHEA and cortisol levels have been monitored and expressed as a cortisol/DHEA ratio. With progression of HIV disease, cortisol rises and DHEA decreases; therefore this ratio would increase with disease progression and decrease with improvement in clinical status. A therapeutic goal would be to decrease the ratio. This could be done by decreasing cortisol levels, increasing DHEA, or preferably both. Supplementation with DHEA can be started after blood levels are checked. There are very few measures that decrease cortisol levels. DHEA, vitamin C, and aspirin have been shown to block excess cortisol production. Various techniques in stress reduction do affect cortisol levels favorably. The European procaine drug, Gerovital (or GH3), has been claimed to block the effects of cortisol on the immune system.

Increases in the cortisol/DHEA ratio are seen with the development of malnutrition and lipodystrophy (fat metabolism abnormalities) in AIDS. In regard to the evidence that decreasing the ratio of cortisol/DHEA in the AIDS patient might have clinical significance, Christeff et al. (2000) stated: "These findings have practical clinical implications, since manipulation of this ratio could prevent metabolic (protein and lipid) perturbations." Cortisol should be measured as a fasting level drawn upon waking. There is considerable variability in cortisol levels throughout the day, and variations as well from person to person, making values difficult to interpret. The DHEA level or cortisol/DHEA levels are easier to interpret if fasting blood is consistently drawn.

Growth Hormone

Supplemental growth hormone (GH) is an approved treatment for AIDS wasting. This means the therapy is covered by many health insurance plans. When a person has lost at least 10% of their baseline body weight, a diagnosis of AIDS wasting is considered. In this situation, GH is usually given for a 12-week period. Some studies have also shown that a 2-week course of GH at the time of acute OI is beneficial (Paton et al. 1999). This may be a less expensive option than the longer course of treatment for those who must pay for the therapy themselves.

The dose of GH in AIDS therapy is much higher than the dose used for replacement therapy in the aging adult who does not have HIV. Lipodystrophy (disturbances in fat metabolism) is common in AIDS and also is associated with AIDS drug treatments. The lipodystrophy syndrome includes abnormalities in lipids (cholesterol, LDL cholesterol) and also redistribution of body fat stores to the abdomen and redistribution of body mass from muscle to fat. GH therapy helps counteract these fat abnormalities. GH and its messenger hormone IGF-1 have been shown to enhance immune function (Koo et al. 2001). According to Roubenoff (2000), "randomized, double-blind trials have shown that GH therapy increases total body weight, lean body mass, exercise capacity, and quality of life."

As noted earlier, many insurance companies will underwrite the cost of GH therapy if the treatment is concurrent with the use of antiretroviral drugs. If you do not have insurance or the resources to pay for GH therapy, call the National Organization of Rare Disorders (NORD) at (888) 628-6673. NORD can provide you with the names of compassionate care programs available from several drug manufacturers. NORD also has its own compassionate care program.

Melatonin

Melatonin is a hormone secreted by the pineal gland during sleep. It is considered to be a master hormone because it is a neuroendocrine modulator and can exert a regulatory effect over many different areas in the body. Evidence suggests HIV immune suppression may be slowed by nightly intake of melatonin. Melatonin enhances the production of T-helper cells. It also stimulates the production of other immune system components, including NK cells; interleukin-2, -4, and -10; gamma-interferon; eosinophils; and red blood cells (Lissoni et al. 1995). In addition to enhancing different modalities of the immune system, melatonin is a formidable antioxidant in its own right and can prevent immune system cell loss directly through this mechanism.

Dr. George Maestroni, a pioneer in melatonin immunotherapy, conducted a pilot AIDS study in Italy, wherein 11 people with HIV were given 20 mg of melatonin every night. After a month of treatment, the patients had a 35% increase in T-helper cells, a 57% increase in NK cells, and a 76% increase in lymphocyte production.

In spite of these remarkable findings, this line of research has not been pursued because melatonin cannot be patented and consequently will never generate enormous profits for the pharmaceutical giants. However, melatonin appears to benefit persons with AIDS in many other ways, including providing protection against AZT toxicity and wasting syndrome.

Testosterone

In both men and women, testosterone declines with HIV progression. In a study of men with HIV, the scrotal testosterone patch raised blood levels of testosterone but did not improve the participant's symptoms (Dobs et al. 1999), implying perhaps that the drug should be given by injection. There are also nonscrotal patches that make testosterone replacement therapy easier and enhance patient compliance. Because low testosterone levels are very common in males with HIV, they may also be especially associated with the AIDS wasting syndrome. Furthermore, treatment with HAART at this stage does not reverse the testosterone deficiency, and replacement of testosterone itself is required (Rietschel et al. 2000). Testosterone is one of the rare therapies in HIV that helps depression, as well as improving decreased energy and libido (Rabkin et al. 2000). Testosterone replacement also improves morbidity, such as development of opportunistic infections, dementia, and quality of life (Kopicko et al. 1999).

In women with HIV, between 50–95% have testosterone levels below normal for their age group. A testosterone patch (or some other dermal preparation, such as micronized gel) can maintain normal blood levels (*for additional information, see http://womenshealth.medscape.com/24784.rhtml*).

In addition to total testosterone in the blood, free testosterone levels should also be monitored. The amount of testosterone bound to protein is also frequently measured, although free testosterone is a more important value because it relates to the biologic effects of testosterone.

OTHER PHARMACEUTICALS TO CONSIDER

Naltrexone Hydrochloride

In 1984, naltrexone (ReVia) was approved as a "narcotic antagonist." It was used in the treatment of heroin and other opiate addictions. In 1995, it was approved for the treatment of alcoholism. Naltrexone works by temporarily blocking opiate receptors in the brain. It also has another interesting effect—it increases the amount of endorphins in the brain. Endorphins are hormonal neurotransmitters and immune modulators. Naltrexone increases the natural brain endorphin, metenkephalin, which in turn enhances NK cell function and stimulates cytotoxic lymphocytes. Endorphins also serve as natural "upregulators" of the immune system. High endorphins are believed to reduce the abnormally high level of alpha-interferon found in AIDS patients, which seems to interfere with the normal functioning of the immune system.

Naltrexone for HIV infection is taken in a very low dose (about 3 mg in the evening), enough to sustain the up-regulation of the endorphin system. It appears to have no negative side effects when taken at these low doses. At higher doses, such as those used in the treatment of alcoholism and in obesity trials, there were side effects, such as insomnia, nausea, anxiety, nervousness, abdominal pain and cramps, vomiting, low energy, and joint and muscle pain. Naltrexone is currently available in the United States with a prescription. Call the Life Extension Foundation for a list of physicians who offer this therapy.

Isoprinosine and Diethyldithiocarboliate

Isoprinosine is a drug that has been shown to be capable of slowing down the progression of AIDS. Since 1986, the Foundation has recommended that persons with HIV add this antiviral to their treatment program. Isoprinosine therapy can beneficially boost thymus gland activity. Isoprinosine has been approved by every regulatory agency in the world except the Food and Drug Administration in the United States. A study published in the *New England Journal of Medicine* in 1990 is one of many reporting that isoprinosine can boost immune function in persons with HIV (Pedersen et al. 1990). Isoprinosine has also been shown to boost immune function in cancer patients and even in healthy people (Tsang et al. 1985; Richner 1991).

In 1985, the Foundation recommended that persons with HIV take isoprinosine to slow down the progression of immune suppression, which can lead to full immune system collapse. Isoprinosine and some other immune-boosting drugs work best when taken on an alternating dosing schedule (e.g., 2 months on and 2 months off).

As early as 1985, researchers demonstrated that a reducing agent, diethyldithiocarboliate (Imuthiol), which has been used as an immunomodulator—and has also inhibited tumor production—could be useful to improve the immune response in persons with HIV by preventing and treating AIDS (Pompidou et al. 1985a; Pompidou et al. 1985b; Lang et al. 1988; Brewton et al. 1989; Reisinger et al. 1990; Hadden 1991).

Biostim

A French drug called Biostim was studied with regard to its effect on modulating various immune responses. In response to *Staphylococcus* infection, Biostim therapy significantly increased the critical phagocytic component of immune attack (Scheffer et al. 1991). Biostim also modulated synthesis of human polymorphonuclear granulocytes (Roch-Arveiller et al. 1991).

The immunological effect in aged humans was studied to understand which specific immune components were affected by oral administration of Biostim. The results showed significant restoration of cell-mediated immunity; an increased percentage of $CD3^+$, $CD2^+$, $CD4^+$, and $HNKI^+$ immune cells; and increased phagocytic activity.

Preincubation of immune cells with Biostim resulted in augmentation of natural microbicidal activity. Nonspecific activation of host defenses may have a significant impact on the outcome of infections in the immunocompromised patient. Biostim was shown to be effective in increasing resistance to experimental infections in animals. It also exhibited anti-*Candida* effects.

Alveolar macrophages are issued from circulating monocytes and are the front line defense of the lungs. The effectiveness of Biostim in respiratory infections is due to its action in cells deep in the lungs, in particular, alveolar macrophages. This drug has been shown to stimulate phagocytosis (the ingestion of bacteria by phagocytes), increase enzymatic activities, and promote interleukin-1 secretion and TNF-alpha (Sozzani et al. 1988). These activities have been demonstrated *in vitro*, as well as in animal and human subjects. In one study, Biostim (RU 41740) was found to have a nonspecific enhancing effect on cellular and humoral immune responses and to stimulate phagocytosis in patients with chronic bronchitis (Boissier 1988). In another study on chronic bronchitis, Biostim increased the anti-*Candida* activity of monocytes and enhanced the phagocytosis indexes of both polymorphonuclear and mononuclear phagocytes (Fietta et al. 1988).

Biostim is an immunomodulator of organic origin, acting on cells of the immune system (B-cells, T-cells, phagocytic cells) and on mediators (IL1-CSG). Its mode of action has been explored by means of experimental infections. The types of defenses involved differed according to whether the experimental infection was caused by an extracellular or intracellular microorganism. *Candida albicans* and *Saccharomyces cerevisiae* were used to produce fungal infections, although bacterial infections were produced with *Staphylococcus*, *Escherichia coli*, *Streptococcus*, and other organisms. The influenza virus was used to produce a viral infection. In these experimental models in animals, Biostim increased the survival time of the infected animals and reduced bacterial, fungal, and viral proliferation. These effects were also observed in immunocompromised mice. These studies have demonstrated Biostim as an effective immune adjunct *in vitro* and *in vivo* (el Abbouyi et al. 1988; Joly 1988).

Persons with HIV should consider using Biostim in 3-month dosing schedules as follows: 2 tablets daily for 8 days, then discontinue for 3 weeks; 1 tablet daily for 8 days, then discontinue for 3 weeks; 1 tablet daily for 8 days, then discontinue for 9 months.

Thymosin Alpha-1

Thymosin alpha-1 is a peptide that has been extensively studied for its beneficial effects on immune response and therapeutic value. In more than 70 studies, thymosin alpha-1 exhibited immunomodulatory activity and demonstrated benefits, whether used alone or in conjunction with a conventional therapy. Many effects of thymosin alpha-1 appear to be synergistic with those of other cytokines (alpha interferon and interleukin-2), and thymosin alpha-1 may work best in combination with other immunomodulators.

Originally isolated from the thymus gland, thymosin alpha-1 is an amino-terminal acylated peptide of 28 amino acids. It is found in highest concentrations in the thymus but has also been detected in spleen, lung, kidney, brain, blood, and a number of other tissues.

The immunomodulatory activities of thymosin alpha-1 are centered primarily on the augmentation of T-cell function. Studies demonstrate that thymosin alpha-1 shows promise in the treatment of a wide variety of diseases. Thymosin alpha-1 has been shown to increase production of interferon, interleukin-2 (IL-2), and interleukin-3 (IL-3) (Svedersky et al. 1982; Sztein et al. 1986; 1989; Serrate et al. 1987; Hsia et al. 1989; Leichtling et al. 1990; Mutchnick et al. 1991). Thymosin alpha-1 has been shown to increase NK cell activity (Serrate et al. 1987; Favalli et al. 1989; Di Francesco et al. 1994) and enhance production of CD3, CD4, and CD8 cells in patients with chronic hepatitis B (Mutchnick et al. 1991) and cancer (Salvati et al. 1996). Treatment with thymosin alpha-1 has also been shown to decrease replication of the HIV-1 virus in human peripheral blood cells, and it has been reported to inhibit the *in vitro* growth of various nonsmall-cell lung-cancer cell lines (Moody et al. 1993; 1998).

Stimulation of the immune system, especially in combination with antiviral agents, has received considerable interest as a potential means to treat AIDS and HIV-infected patients. Studies have shown a high degree of immune restoration from the combined administration of thymosin alpha-1 and alpha interferon (IFNa). Thymosin alpha-1 in combination with AZT and IFNa has been investigated for treatment of HIV-infected patients. At the University of Rome, a group of researchers conducted a study to investigate the combination of thymosin alpha-1, IFNa, and AZT for the treatment of HIV-infected patients with CD4 counts of 500 or lower (Garaci et al. 1992). The study included seven patients in each of four treatment groups: thymosin alpha-1 + IFNa + AZT; thymosin alpha-1 + AZT; IFNa + AZT; and AZT.

Treatment was continued for 12 months for the majority of patients, with up to 18 months for a smaller cohort of patients. After 1 year, the thymosin alpha-1 + IFNa + AZT combination therapy resulted in a statistically significant increase in CD4 cells and stimulation of lymphocyte cytotoxic activity against natural killer-sensitive target cells compared with the other three treatment groups (Garaci et al. 1992).

Thymosin alpha-1 is available in many countries outside the United States. FDA approval is pending multicenter Phase III trials that are currently underway. Thymosin alpha-1 should be available in the United States by 2004.

OTHER CAUSES OF IMMUNE SUPPRESSION

The number one cause of immune deficiency in the world is acknowledged to be malnutrition. Those with intestinal diseases often fail to absorb critical nutrients and are at risk from immune-suppressing agents. That is why maintaining intestinal health is such an important aspect of long-term HIV therapy. A second known cause of immune suppression can result from pharmaceutical or recreational drug use, particularly when used in combination.

The immunosuppressive effects of many drugs have been well-documented for many decades. As recorded in the medical literature for more than 50 years, conditions such as pneumonias, mouth sores, fevers, swollen lymph glands, night sweats, and bacterial infections can be indicative of immunosuppression. Antibiotics, steroids, and antiviral drugs (such as AZT, ddI, ddC, 3Tc, and D4T) are also well-known to have damaging effects on the immune and digestive systems. Many HIV/AIDS treatment drugs are immunosuppressive when used on a daily basis. Bactrim and Septra antibiotics (also known as TMP/SMX) are a double chemotherapeutic, folic-acid inhibitor and are very effective at destroying digestive flora. According to the American Medical Association, these drugs may cause a folic-acid deficiency, resulting in anemia, as well as other adverse effects, such as nausea, vomiting, diarrhea, loss of appetite, headache, dizziness, muscle and joint pain, and rash.

Folic acid is a common B vitamin that is present in most normal diets. It is required by several kinds of bacteria that are normally present in a healthy intestinal colony. A perfectly healthy-looking person can actually have a drug-induced, subclinical state of malnutrition as a result of taking antibiotics, thus promoting a potential end result of immune suppression. TMP/SMX is a powerful sulfonamide derivative. When combined with nitrite, such as is found in amyl nitrite and isobutyl nitrite (a recreational drug known as "poppers"), sulfonamide is a very strong electrophilic oxidizing agent. The immunosuppressive effects of recreational drug use have been recorded in the medical literature since the turn of the century. In large urban areas in Western countries, male homosexuals have patterns of behavior that include the use of recreational nitrite drugs along with long-term prophylactic use of antibiotics. Both chemicals—pharmaceutical SMX and recreational nitrites—reduce the oxygen-carrying capacity of red blood cells by oxidizing ferrous iron to ferric iron in the hemoglobin. This results in a condition known as methemoglobulinemia, a progressively life-threatening deficiency of the oxygen supply in the respiration chain of mitochondria (Home 1979; Dixon et al. 1981; Tyler 1992).

CONSIDERATIONS FOR THE FUTURE
Development of an AIDS Vaccine

Development of an effective vaccine does not appear to be likely in the near future. This situation is related to both technical difficulties that are peculiar to HIV and possibly also political reasons. More recent advances in understanding and augmenting the cellular immune response to HIV have perhaps moved us farther along the path of vaccine development. However, to date, only one vaccine, containing the gp120 surface protein of the virus, has continued far enough along the path to reach the status of a large-scale, Phase III clinical trial. In his book, *Shots in the Dark: The Wayward Search for an AIDS Vaccine,* Jon Cohen (2001) stated that the wayward search for an AIDS vaccine could have been shortened considerably via centralization of leadership and unification of direction under a model similar to that of the effective development of the polio vaccine by the March of Dimes. With no similar type of organizational leadership, there has been no master strategy in the development of an AIDS vaccine. Cohen charges that the National Institutes of Health (NIH) has been unable to provide this leadership and that research virologists, interested only in understanding HIV pathogenesis and its reaction with the immune system, have not encouraged the appropriate research necessary to find a vaccine. Cohen is impressed by initiatives taken by the International AIDS Vaccine Initiative and by the formation of the activist organization, the AIDS Vaccine Advocacy Coalition.

Future Research Needs

In contrast to the drug treatments we have at present, more effective therapies are needed that are cost effective, less toxic, and more aggressive to resistance. The philosophy of "hit early and hit hard" is no longer the therapeutic bastion of HIV treatment. Because of the difficulties with present therapies, more "drug holidays" and other nondrug therapies are being considered by patients and practitioners alike before beginning HAART. More research is needed for these and other nondrug treatments of AIDS. Presently, HIV treatment proceeds with inadequate research data regarding large segments of the treatment population. In order for treatment to be effective, practitioners must accumulate conclusive outcome data regarding when to change a drug regimen, what therapy to change to, when to stop therapy, and how to effectively treat the population harboring multiple virologic failures.

SOURCES OF ADDITIONAL ALTERNATIVE INFORMATION
Organizations
The Life Extension Foundation

This nonprofit, medical research foundation is politically motivated to promote freedom of choice in American health care. The Foundation, as the world's strongest critic of the FDA, is the only nonprofit, member-driven organization to successfully sue this government agency, whose main purpose is to protect the financial interests of the pharmaceutical industry. The Foundation is the fastest and easiest source for comprehensive health and nutritional information, longevity research, and pharmaceutical-grade nutritional products and herbals.

Group for the Scientific Reappraisal of the HIV/AIDS Hypothesis

Members of this organization are scientists, researchers, and leaders of the debate about etiology of AIDS from all over the world. They publish a monthly newsletter, *Reappraising AIDS,* which offers readable and highly informative insights.

The Group
7414 Girard Avenue #1-331
La Jolla, CA 92037

HEAL (Health Education AIDS Liaison)

HEAL is a nonprofit, community-based education network with independent chapters located throughout the United States. HEAL was originally founded in 1982 as an AIDS support group under the direction of Dr. Michael Ellner, president and Dr. Frank Buincouckas, science adviser. In 1985 HEAL New York became the inspiration for an international movement challenging the validity of the HIV/AIDS hypothesis and the efficacy of HIV-based treatments. For more than a decade, HEAL New York has been a leading source of comprehensive information on effective, nontoxic, and holistic approaches to recovery from AIDS and has served as a consistent voice that calls for honesty in AIDS issues. There are presently chapters in 20 North American cities and seven countries worldwide.

> HEAL New York
> New York, NY
> Telephone: (212) 873-0780

Continuum

Continuum is a bimonthly magazine published in London. It features extensive articles on alternatives to pharmaceutical therapies and standard AIDS "think" while covering AIDS news and events around the world.

> *Continuum*
> 172 Founding Court
> Brunswick Centre
> London, WC1N 1QE, England
> Telephone: (44)(0)171-713-7071
> Fax: (44)(0)171-713-7072

Internet Sites

www.lef.org

The Life Extension Foundation hosts the fastest and easiest source for comprehensive health and nutritional information, longevity research, and pharmaceutical-grade nutritional products and herbal medicines. Join immediately and add your voice to the 50,000 members of the Life Extension Foundation who have changed the course of medicine in the world by demanding freedom of choice in healthcare.

www.virusmyth.com

The Group for the Scientific Reappraisal of the HIV/AIDS Hypothesis came into existence as a group of signatories in an open letter to the scientific community. This website contains more than 250 Web pages with more than 200 articles.

www.epcnet.com/heal and www.aliveandwell.org

HEAL Los Angeles offers free educational forums to inspire a will to live, participate in life, and cultivate a healthy future. The scientific data HEAL makes available help people separate fear from facts and provide a solid foundation upon which to base important health decisions. HEAL forums emphasize personal independent understanding of medicine and science, and individual responsibility in health management.

www.healsf.org

HEAL San Francisco provides a chapter website. What if everything you thought you knew about AIDS was wrong? This site examines the mounting body of evidence that much of what the general public has been told about AIDS is wrong. If you or a loved one is HIV-positive, this site offers an alternative view.

SUMMARY OF POSSIBLE TREATMENTS FOR HIV/AIDS

1. Antiretroviral drugs in routine use (under physician supervision):
   - NRTIs (nucleoside analog reverse transcriptase inhibitors):
     - Zidovudine (AZT, ZDV)
     - Didanosine (ddI)
     - Zalcitabine (ddC)
     - Lamivudine (3TC)
     - Stavudine (d4T)
     - Abacavir (ABC)
   - NNRTIs (non-nucleoside reverse transcriptase inhibitors):
     - Nevirapine (NVP)
     - Efavirenz (EFV)
     - Delavirdine (DEL)
   - PIs (protease inhibitors):
     - Saquinavir (SQV)
     - Indinavir (IND)
     - Ritonavir (RIT)
     - Nelfinavir (NEL)
     - Amprenavir (AMP)
2. Glutathione boosters:
   - NAC, 600 mg 2 times daily
   - Vitamin C, 1000 mg 3 times daily
   - Alpha-lipoic acid, 250 mg twice daily
   - Whey protein isolate, 30–60 grams daily
   - SAMe, 400–800 mg daily

- Glutathione, 500 mg twice daily
- Silibinin, 250-mg capsules 3 times daily

3. Antioxidants:
   - Vitamin C, see above
   - Beta carotene, 25,000 IU daily
   - Vitamin A, 10,000 IU daily; higher doses with supervision of a physician only
   - Vitamin E, 400 IU daily
   - Green tea extract (95%), five 300-mg capsules, three times a day
   - Life Extension Mix, 3 capsules 3 times daily, may be taken in place of many supplements listed here

4. Immune modulators:
   - Lactoferrin, 900 mg daily
   - CoQ$_{10}$, 200 mg daily
   - Plant sterols such as Moducare, 2 capsules daily

5. Micronutrients:
   - Selenium, 200 mcg 2 times daily
   - Zinc, one 30-mg capsule daily
   - Vitamin B$_{12}$, 5000-mcg sublingual lozenge 1 time daily (methylcobalamin form)

6. Amino acids:
   - *L*-glutamine, 1–2 grams daily
   - *L*-carnitine, 3–4 grams daily in 2 divided doses (acetyl-*L*-carnitine works best)

7. Natural antivirals:
   - Olive leaf extract containing 23% oleuropein, 1 500-mg capsule 4 times daily
   - SPV-30, one 330-mg capsule 3 times daily (*see text for complete treatment recommendations*)
   - Thymic Immune Factors, 2 capsules daily

8. Digestive enzymes:
   - Super Digestive Enzymes, 2 capsules before each meal

9. Hormonal treatments:
   - Growth Hormone, after testing and with supervision of a physician
   - Melatonin, 3–30 mg at bedtime
   - Testosterone, after testing and with supervision of a physician
   - DHEA, after testing and with supervision of a physician (usual dosages are 50–200 mg daily)

10. Other pharmaceuticals being used in the treatment of AIDS:
    - Naltrexone
    - Isoprinosine
    - Diethyldithiocarboliate
    - Biostim
    - Thymosin alpha-1

 PRODUCT AVAILABILITY

Life Extension Mix, vitamin C, NAC, whey protein, alpha-lipoic acid, SAMe, glutathione, *L*-glutamine, acetyl-*L*-carnitine, CoQ$_{10}$, beta carotene, vitamin A, vitamin B$_{12}$, vitamin E (Gamma E Tocopherol/Tocotrienols), methylcobalamin (sublingual), lactoferrin, silymarin, Silibinin Plus, Moducare, DHEA, melatonin, selenium (Se-Methylselenocysteine), magnesium, zinc, Thymic Immune Factors, olive leaf extract, Green Tea Extract (95%), and Super Digestive Enzymes are available by telephoning (800) 544-4440 or ordering online at www.lef.org. Biostim and SPV-30 are available from several on-line pharmacies.

Hypertension and Hypertensive Vascular Disease

OVERVIEW

Hypertension (high blood pressure) is the primary and most important manifesting symptom of *hypertensive vascular disease*. A diseased vasculature predisposes one to further hypertension, and thus, further vascular disease. Hypertension often progresses with the development of various diseases involving the circulatory system, such as *arteriosclerosis, atherosclerosis, coronary heart disease, congestive heart failure,* and disorders of coagulation (*stroke, hemorrhage,* heart attack), immunity (inflammation, infection), and *diabetes*. All of these disorders are both causative and secondary to the development of hypertension.

The purpose of this discussion is to ultimately substantiate and provide a protocol that can be followed that will prevent the development of hypertension, and thus, the development of hypertensive vascular disease and its subsequent and allied disease states. Protocols have been described in other sections of this book that concern the prevention and treatment of most of these other diseases of the cardiovascular system (see *Cardiovascular Disease: Overview* and *Comprehensive Analysis*). Some degree of overlap is inevitable here, however, this section will more specifically focus on understanding the mechanisms behind the development of hypertension; a **symptom** that frequently precedes and further aggravates the progression of a number of common cardiovascular-related diseases.

Hypertension will be defined in terms of the *physiological* and *endocrinological* systems that control blood pressure. The *genetic* and *epidemiological* basis of hypertension will be characterized, particularly with respect to the role of salt intake (as sodium chloride). Physiological and endocrinological systems that control sodium retention are extremely crucial to the maintenance of blood pressure. Accordingly, all of our most effective drug therapies for hypertension impact one or more of the components in these highly complex and highly interrelated organ systems.

At the organ level, sodium intake triggers a well-characterized, coordinated sequence of physiological events that typically causes some degree of hypertension, particularly in those genetically predisposed to the effects of salt, or who, as a result of aging or other nutritional/environmental factors are otherwise sensitized to sodium intake. At the tissue level, there is strong evidence that regulatory processes within *vascular smooth muscle* or *vascular endothelial cells* are dysfunctional and/or compromised by the affects of hypertension, declining testosterone levels, and also accumulated age-related damage or other nutritional and hormone imbalances.

In summary and in general, disorders of electrolyte balance result in chronic hypertension (and then hypertensive vascular disease), which leads to further cardiovascular disease. This section details the physiology of hypertension, the pharmacological approaches used to treat pathophysiologic states that result from hypertension, and the biochemical basis of nutritional approaches useful in the prevention of hypertension, or as adjuvant therapy to ongoing, traditional medical treatment.

EPIDEMIOLOGY

It is estimated that over 50 million Americans have hypertension. Eventually, especially if left untreated, they develop the common cardiovascular disease known as *hypertensive vascular disease*. The disease is primarily a manifestation of elevated arterial pressure (high blood pressure). However, high blood pressure is really a symptom of one or more of the many underlying disease processes that often express the **symptom** of hypertension.

Hypertension is two times more prevalent in Blacks versus Whites, higher in men versus women (until after menopause), and is typically related to many dietary factors, particularly salt intake (Appel et al. 1997). Hypertension is commonly seen in the elderly. Over 70% of women and 50% of men over the age of 70 have hypertension. These latter factors are associated with hypertension because they all are independent risk factors for accelerated atherosclerosis. It is a disorder traditionally characterized by blood pressure persistently exceeding 140/90 mmHg. Current research indicates that an optimal blood pressure is below 120/80 mmHg.

It is important to note that damage to the vasculature can occur when the blood pressure is moderately but chronically elevated. Some individuals may not realize they are hypertensive because symptoms such as epistaxis (nosebleed), tinnitus, dizziness, headache, blurred vision, and arrhythmias are not always present. Other risk factors include high cholesterol levels, smoking, obesity, and diabetes (Calvert 2001). There are newer risk factors including homocysteine and C-reactive protein.

The lifetime risk for hypertension among middle-aged and elderly individuals is 90%; corrective intervention (at an earlier age) could relieve a huge public health burden (Miura et al. 2001; Vasan et al. 2002). Hypertension refers to the high tension levels (or pressure levels) that must be developed in the heart to eject blood into the arterial system. Blood pressure is always the result of cardiac output multiplied by the peripheral vascular resistance. The role of salt (sodium chloride) is particularly important in the development of hypertension and in the understanding of the etiology of the disease. It is noteworthy that the amount of salt in the typical American diet greatly exceeds what is derived from a natural diet. In this respect, this level of sodium chloride intake is pharmacological, with pronounced but insidious adverse side effects. Because the *isotonicity* (salt content) of the blood is very critically regulated by many interconnected systems, elevated retention of sodium chloride and fluid by the body is pathological. This retained salt water expands the volume of the plasma compartment, increases demands on the heart to pump more volume (increased cardiac output), and thus, raises blood pressure.

Healthy blood pressure readings are below 120/80 mmHg. Hypertension that requires medical intervention is generally defined as systolic and/or diastolic blood pressures of 140/90 or higher. Naturally, higher blood pressures are associated with more serious degrees of hypertension. It is noteworthy that individuals with pressures in between these values still show an increased risk of cardiovascular disease. Generally, a higher diastolic pressure presents a more serious risk than a higher systolic pressure. Although the symptom of hypertension is the best indicator of developing hypertensive vascular disease, it is a symptom that is usually only detected by more than one measurement of blood pressure.

The exact cause of hypertension is not clearly understood in approximately 90–95% of those affected, so it is accordingly referred to as essential hypertension, primary hypertension, or idiopathic hypertension. Secondary hypertension results from defined causes and includes roughly 5–10% of people with hypertension. Many of these cases can be treated because we know the cause. A clear understanding of the cause of primary hypertension is critical to properly controlling hypertension, and ultimately treating hypertensive vascular disease and its associated cardiovascular diseases.

By instituting treatment regimens to reduce high blood pressure we significantly arrest the development of related cardiovascular diseases, but we may not correct some of the disease processes that are still present, still progressing, or minimally affected by the level of blood pressure. This is the danger of this silent disease, often only detectable through repeated measurement of blood pressure. It is possible that the underlying disease is still progressing, now even more silently, after blood pressure is controlled (Calvert 2001).

There are numerous processes that have been identified as contributing causes to hypertension or to the diseases that are related to hypertensive vascular disease. Because of the complex relationships associating the symptom of hypertension with the cardiovascular diseases, diseases such as hypertensive vascular disease, congestive heart failure, renal disease, stroke, arteriosclerosis, atherosclerosis, and diabetes are often interrelated. They all can ultimately express the symptom of high blood pressure or develop as a result of high blood pressure. Each disease can both cause hypertension, and in turn, is aggravated by hypertension. Control of hypertension can sometimes prevent the development of some diseases like congestive heart failure, but only modestly slow the progression of diseases like diabetes and atherosclerosis. In the end, uncontrolled hypertension generally leads to death secondary to atherosclerosis (Williams 2001). Most deaths due to hypertension result from myocardial infarction or congestive heart failure.

ETIOLOGY

Essential Hypertension

Hypertension is generally referred to as either essential or secondary. It's not completely known what causes *essential hypertension* that accounts for 90% to 95% of cases. Research indicates that significant factors include a complex interaction between genetic, environmental and other variables. *Secondary hypertension* is caused by known medical conditions, such as kidney disease, pregnancy, hyperthyroidism, or *aldosteronism*.

Otherwise known as primary or idiopathic hypertension, essential hypertension affects a number of physiological systems that regulate (arterial) blood pressure, including the autonomic nervous system, adrenal glands, kidneys, vasculature, and complex hormonal systems that interconnect these systems. It is likely that the causes of essential hypertension are in some ways related to the known causes of secondary hypertension. An understanding of those known causes is useful in hypothesizing and understanding the etiology of essential hypertension.

Genetic Predisposition

The heritability of hypertension supports a genetic basis to hypertensive vascular disease. Given the many different and interrelated physiological systems affected by hypertension and which contribute to hypertension, it is likely that many different genes and genetic mutations contribute to hypertension and other cardiovascular diseases. Many specific gene defects have been linked to susceptibility for hypertension, most of which control the expression of proteins involved in the renin-angiotensin-aldosterone-axis or endothelial cell function. However, the evidence is particularly strong for linkage of the angiotensinogen gene (Williams 2001). This gene, presumably, codes for a collection of different proteins that participate in the regulation of the renin-angiotensin-aldosterone-axis, not simply the protein structure for angiotensinogen present in the plasma.

Environmental Factors

Many environmental factors determine the expression of the degree of hypertension that results in particular individuals. The manipulation of these environmental factors through changes in salt restriction, diet, alcohol intake, and stress, can reduce or eliminate less serious forms of hypertension.

Environmental Salt

"The environmental factor that has received the greatest attention is salt intake. [T]his factor illustrates the heterogeneous nature of the essential hypertensive population, in that the blood pressure in only approximately **60% of hypertensives** is particularly responsive to the level of sodium intake. The cause of this special sensitivity to salt varies, with primary aldosteronism, bilateral renal artery stenosis, renal parenchymal disease, and low-renin essential hypertension accounting for about half the patients. In the remainder, the pathophysiology is still uncertain, but postulated contributing factors include chloride intake, calcium intake, a generalized cellular membrane defect, insulin resistance, and "nonmodulation" [status] (see below)". (Williams 2001).

Because the response to salt is so important to understanding the etiology of hypertension, it is important to know which physiological systems respond to salt intake and how each system influences the function of complementary systems. This understanding is paramount in understanding not only hypertensive vascular disease, but also the other cardiovascular diseases. It is beyond the scope of this writing to provide a detailed understanding of all of these allied diseases; however, some basic understanding of each of the cardiovascular diseases provides insight into the probable etiology of hypertension.

Salt sensitivity tells us more about the disease than other environmental factors like smoking, alcohol, exercise, and obesity. The acute and chronic responses to high sodium chloride intake are well-characterized. Without diminishing the importance of these other environmental factors, it is a fairly straight-forward judgment that smoking most likely affects the vasculature through oxidative stress (as does stress, in general). Similarly, chronic obesity clearly increases the work load on the cardiovascular system, and in the long term, alters lipid metabolism, insulin response, and blood pressure adversely. The high correlation of obesity with diabetes is important in understanding pathological changes in the vascular system relevant to hypertension. Diabetes mellitus is associated with physiological changes that potentiate endothelial dysfunction, including hypertension (Brown and Hu 2001). Alcohol causes many metabolic disturbances, drug effects, and alterations to lipid metabolism. Accordingly, a detailed look into its mechanisms of action would be highly confounded, contributing little to our understanding of hypertension.

The Renin-Angiotensin-Aldosterone-Axis

Drugs that target the renin-angiotensin-aldosterone-axis represent the most effective medications available for hypertensive vascular disease. They are the most selective agents in use that offer the least side effects. This level of drug specificity generally indicates that the critical systems in a given disease are probably being affected. Recall that alterations in the angiotensinogen gene are positively correlated with hypertension and may represent part of the genetic basis for this heritable disease (Williams 2001). The enzyme called renin is secreted by juxta-glomerular cells in the kidney. These cells release the enzyme renin whenever there is increased filtration of sodium (chloride) by the kidney, perhaps secondary to high dietary salt intake.

Renin release is the most important endocrine response of the kidney. It exerts pronounced influences on the cardiovascular system and blood pressure and is primary controlled by three factors:

1. Beta-1 adrenergic agents directly stimulate renin release by acting on the juxta-glomerular cells. This stimulation of the sympathetic nervous system (through noradrenaline release) prepares the body for potential acute emergencies requiring the maintenance of blood volume and pressure (such as dehydration and hemorrhage) or to redirect blood flow to the muscles for "fight or flight" situations.

2. Blood pressure inhibits renin release via the *intra-renal baroreceptor pathway*, which may use prostaglandins as mediators (see the section on *Membrane Biochemistry and Essential Fatty Acids*). Renin secretion and blood pressure has been shown to be selectively reduced by inhibitors of cyclooxygenase-2 (COX-2).

3. The *macula densa* cells, that reabsorb almost all of the filtered sodium, inhibit renin release. These specialized kidney cells "sense" the amount of sodium chloride that is not reabsorbed by the kidney. When significant amounts of sodium chloride are not reabsorbed, prostaglandins (of the series-2, PGI2 and PGE2) are released that stimulate renin release (Williams 2001). Macula densa-induced stimulation of renin release may be mediated by both COX-2 and nitric oxide synthase, which generates nitric oxide (NO) from arginine to promote vasodilation (Williams, 2001).

Once released, renin enzymatically converts circulating angiotensinogen into angiotensin I. Further and usually immediate conversion into angiotensin II by angiotensinogen-converting enzyme produces the most powerful vasoconstricting substance in the body, causing vasoconstriction of smooth muscle cells in the arterial tree, especially in the vascular capillary beds lined with endothelial cells. This action raises blood pressure by increasing total peripheral vascular resistance.

The second primary action of angiotensin II is to stimulate aldosterone release from the adrenal glands, which in turn, acts on the kidney to promote sodium retention in exchange for potassium loss. Water is retained along with sodium in the plasma, volume expands, and the juxta-glomerular cells stop secreting renin. This is an example of a classical negative feedback-loop, typical of all *functional* endocrine systems in the body. Furthermore, this endocrine system interconnects the physiological functions of the circulatory, renal, and adrenal systems in the highly important physiological function of regulating blood pressure and electrolyte balance.

There is a subgroup of people (20%) that have **essential hypertension with low plasma renin activity**. They have expanded fluid volumes (which probably increases their blood pressure), but normal serum potassium levels (suggesting no stimulation of aldosterone release). This condition prevails more commonly in Blacks. They appear to be more sensitive to angiotensin II (which is why renin can remain low), and which probably accounts for their hypertension and (aldosterone-mediated) sodium retention. Normal and high salt diets in this subgroup do not suppress

aldosterone. The subgroup overlaps with people with normal levels of renin and essential hypertension (Williams 2001). These groups are sensitive to salt intake and should eliminate or restrict it.

Another 25–30% of people with essential hypertension demonstrate a reduced adrenal (aldosterone) response to sodium. "[S]odium intake does not modulate either adrenal or renal vascular responses to angiotensin II. Hypertensives in this subset have been termed **nonmodulators** because of the absence of the sodium-mediated modulation of target tissue responses to angiotensin II. These individuals make up 25 to 30% of the hypertensive population, have plasma renin activity levels that are normal to high if measured when the patient is on a low-salt diet, and have hypertension that is salt-sensitive because of a defect in the kidney's ability to excrete sodium appropriately. They also are more insulin-resistant than other hypertensive patients, and the pathophysiologic characteristics can be corrected by the administration of a converting-enzyme inhibitor. Furthermore, the nonmodulation characteristic appears to be genetically determined (associated with a certain allele of the angiotensinogen gene). Thus, nonmodulators are probably the most completely characterized intermediate phenotype in the hypertensive population" (Williams 2001). They are *not* sensitive to dietary intake of salt.

There is final subgroup of individuals possessing high renin levels (15%). However, half of these people are not benefited by the highly effective angiotensin II receptor antagonists and it is hypothesized that hypertension in this subgroup is related to overactivity of the adrenergic system (Brown and Hu 2001; Williams 2001).

Secondary Hypertension

Research into the known causes of secondary hypertension tells us that all forms of hypertension may be related to altered kidney function or hormone secretion, and particularly, to altered renal endocrine function. Again, sodium homeostasis and adrenergic factors are the primary and most important considerations to our understanding of chronic and acute hypertension, respectively.

Renal Hypertension

Activation of the renin-angiotensin-aldosterone-axis is the cause of secondary hypertension caused by "renal hypertension." Renal hypertension generally results when blood flow to one of the kidneys is reduced to less than 30% of normal. Activation of the renin-angiotensin-aldosterone-axis is simply the

Hypoglycemia

Hypoglycemia literally means "low blood sugar" and is often mistaken for a disease when it is actually a symptom. Ingested carbohydrates (sugars and starches) trigger a release of the hormone insulin from the pancreas. Insulin helps the body turn sugars into energy and stored fats. In some people, the amount of insulin released is too high for the amount of carbohydrates ingested, resulting in too much sugar being burned up too quickly. A net loss of blood sugar results. In hypoglycemia attacks, there is too much insulin and not enough blood sugar, causing fatigue, weakness, loss of consciousness, and even death.

There are three general types of hypoglycemia. Two of them are rare organic forms involving the pancreas. The third and most common form is called *functional hypoglycemia* (FH) and is usually caused by an inadequate diet too high in sugar and refined carbohydrates. Hypoglycemia may be better described as *carbohydrate intolerance*: the body is unable to absorb certain carbohydrate loads effectively without adverse consequences. Different people react differently to ingested sugars and **starches**, with some individuals having a higher tolerance level than others.

Although predisposition to FH may be an inherited condition and is most often due to dietary factors, it can also be found in people with such disorders as schizophrenia, alcoholism, drug addiction, juvenile delinquency, hyperactivity, diabetes, and obesity. In some people, severe FH can contribute to other illnesses such as epilepsy, allergies, asthma, ulcers, arthritis, impotence, and mental disorders.

SYMPTOMS

The symptoms of hypoglycemia include:

- Fatigue, dizziness, shakiness, and faintness
- Irritability and depression
- Weakness or cramps in feet or legs
- Numbness or tingling in the hands, feet, or face
- Ringing in the ears
- Swollen feet or legs
- Tightness in chest
- Frequent heart pounding or palpitations
- Anxiety, nightmares, and panic attacks
- Night sweats
- Constant hunger
- Headaches and migraines
- Impaired memory and concentration
- Blurring of vision
- Nasal congestion
- Abdominal cramps, loose stools, or diarrhea

Functional hypoglycemia may be subclinical, meaning that symptoms are subtle, episodic, and difficult to diagnose. Patients may have a low but acceptable blood sugar level that does not drop until the last hours of a prolonged test. Glucose tolerance tests often miss the lowest blood sugar levels that had triggered acute symptoms. Severe regular attacks of hypoglycemia may have diabetes as the underlying cause. If symptoms persist, see your doctor.

Hypoglycemia and Diabetes

Hypoglycemia can also be a common complication of diabetes. Diabetes occurs when the body cannot use glucose for fuel either because the pancreas is not able to make enough insulin or the insulin that is available is not effective. As a result, glucose builds up in the blood instead of getting into body cells. The aim of treatment in diabetes is to lower high blood sugar levels. To do this, people with diabetes may use insulin or oral drugs, depending on the type of diabetes they have or the severity of their condition. (*Refer to the Diabetes protocol for further information.*) Using these medications may lower their blood sugar too much, making them hypoglycemic.

HYPOGLYCEMIA AND DIET

A perfectly regulated diet can help to control hypoglycemia. Usually a regimen high in protein, unrefined carbohydrates (which are slow to be absorbed, such as whole-grain products and vegetables), and moderate fats is recommended. Heavily sugared foods should be avoided, and foods high in natural sugars should be restricted. Alcohol, caffeine, tobacco, and other stimulants should be avoided, because they are capable of precipitating an attack. Small meals taken often during the day are recommended to control the amount of carbohydrates entering the system.

Short-term treatment focuses on raising the blood sugar level without delay. Any substance containing simple sugars, such as fruit juice, soft drinks, or candy—if taken at the onset of a hypoglycemic episode—will help to raise blood sugar quickly and ease the severity of the attack. Sugar combined with a protein source, such as a glass of milk or a piece of cheese, will help slow the absorption of glucose into the system, avoiding the "seesaw" effect caused by rapidly changing blood sugar levels.

NUTRITIONAL SUPPLEMENTATION

Vitamin B$_6$

Hypoglycemia may damage brain cells. When hippocampal brain-cell cultures are deprived of glucose, a massive release of lactate dehydrogenase (LDH) occurs, which is an indicator of neuronal death. The addition of the vitamin B$_6$ metabolite pyridoxal 5-phosphate has been shown to inhibit the LDH release. When pyridoxal 5-phosphate is given before glucose deprivation, a more potent inhibitory effect on LDH release has been observed. Scientists have suggested that pyridoxal 5-phosphate protects neurons from glucose deprivation-induced damage. These scientists recommend that pyridoxal 5-phosphate be used prophylactically to protect against brain-cell death induced by metabolic disorders such as hypoglycemia (Geng et al. 1997).

Chromium

Another possible cause of low blood sugar is the inability to release glycogen (stored sugar in the liver), secondary to vitamin B$_6$ and chromium deficiency. Some hypoglycemics are helped by the daily administration of 100–250 mg of pyridoxal 5-phosphate and 200 mcg of chromium. Chromium is a mineral found in brewer's yeast, whole-grain breads and cereals, molasses, cheese, lean meats, and dietary supplements.

Cysteine

Too much insulin in the blood can be partially neutralized by taking the amino acid cysteine along with vitamin B$_1$ and vitamin C. Hypoglycemics should start in the first week with once-a-day doses of 500 mg of cysteine along with 250 mg of vitamin B$_1$ and 1500 mg of vitamin C. This dose should be administered 2 times a day during the second week and 3 times a day by the third week. The objective is to prevent hypoglycemic attacks by neutralizing excess insulin. Every hypoglycemic is slightly different, so the dosage ranges will vary from person to person (Pearson et al. 1982).

Glutamine

Glutamine plays a vital part in the control of blood sugar. It helps prevent hypoglycemia, because it is easily converted to glucose when blood sugar is low.

Glutamine can enter the Krebs cycle and serve as a noncarbohydrate source of energy for the body. In fact, this is the main way it usually contributes to the production of energy. However, if the blood sugar is low, glutamine is readily catabolized (broken down) in the liver and used to create more glucose. Together with alanine, glycine, serine, and threonine, glutamine is an important "gluconeogenic" (glucose-rebuilding) amino acid, in fact the primary one. Providing abundant glutamine through diet and supplementation means that less muscle tissue (if any) will be broken down to provide glucose.

This production of glucose from glutamine takes place mainly in the liver. Recently, however, it has been discovered that the kidneys can contribute as much as 25% to whole-body glucose production, a phenomenon that occurs only during hypoglycemia (Stumvoll et al. 1999). Actually this is not surprising, because the kidneys are especially equipped to process glutamine owing to its importance in the detoxification of ammonia.

Glucose has recently been shown to be synthesized in the small intestines through the breakdown of glutamine in a fasting or diabetic state. Under these conditions, the small intestine contributes 20–25% of whole-body endogenous glucose production (Mithieux 2001; Croset et al. 2001).

Avocado Sugar

As discussed earlier in this protocol, hypoglycemia often occurs when too much insulin is secreted, thus driving blood glucose down too quickly. A potential method of avoiding hypoglycemic attacks would be to consume a dietary supplement that has proven insulin-suppressing effects.

In the 1960s, research was conducted using a sugar from the avocado called d-manno-heptulose. Scientists were able to demonstrate a specific insulin-suppressing effect when d-manno-heptulose was administered both by intravenous infusion and by oral ingestion. The research showed both safety and efficacy, but it was not possible to provide d-manno-heptulose in a standardized dose at that time.

Since the excess production of insulin is also involved in obesity, scientists became motivated to develop a system that would make d-manno-heptulose consistently available to the bloodstream. There is now a standardized avocado sugar (d-manno-heptulose) extract available as a dietary supplement. While studies have been conducted with this supplement in the treatment of obesity and hyperinsulinemia (excess blood insulin), it has not been tested as a way of avoiding hyperglycemic attacks.

One potential method may be to consume 100–200 mg of d-manno-heptulose after each meal to inhibit excess insulin secretion and the subsequent hypoglycemia that follows. The dosage of d-manno-heptulose will inevitably vary between individuals, but it may represent a breakthrough in controlling hypoglycemic attacks.

For complete information on this avocado sugar extract (d-manno-heptulose), refer to the *Obesity protocol* of this book. Once a formal protocol is developed for using d-manno-heptulose to control hypoglycemia, it will be inserted into the *Hypoglycemia protocol* that can be accessed by logging on to www.lef.org.

 SUMMARY

1. A perfectly regulated diet can help to control hypoglycemia.

2. Fruit juice, soft drinks, or sweets, if taken at the onset of a hypoglycemic episode, help to ease the severity of the attack quickly.

3. Some hypoglycemics are helped by the daily administration of 100–250 mg of the vitamin B_6 metabolite pyridoxal 5-phosphate and 200 mcg of chromium.

4. Hypoglycemics should start in the first week with once-a-day doses of 500 mg of cysteine along with 250 mg of vitamin B_1 and 1500 mg of vitamin C. Increase this dosage regimen to 2 times a day in week 2 and 3 times a day in week 3.

5. Glutamine powder can be added to a protein drink or several 500 mg capsules can be added daily with your regular supplements.

6. Avocado sugar (d-manno-heptulose) in the dose of 100–200 mg after each may be considered. Log on to the *Hypoglycemia* protocol at www.lef.org for updated dosing suggestions.

 FOR MORE INFORMATION

Contact the Hypoglycemia Association, Inc. (HAI), Box 165, Ashton, MD 20861-0165; (202) 544-4044.

PRODUCT AVAILABILITY

The amino acids cysteine and glutamine, and vitamin B_1, vitamin B_6, pyridoxal 5-phosphate, vitamin C capsules, avocado sugar (d-manno-heptulose) tablets, and chromium picolinate are available by calling (800) 544-4440, or by ordering online at www.lef.org.

Immune Enhancement

The Life Extension Foundation's Immune Enhancement Protocol is designed to enhance immune function in aging persons, in patients receiving cancer chemotherapy, and in those with chronic viral or bacterial infections.

The first section is written in highly technical form. If you want to bypass this molecular information, skip down to the next section entitled *The Harmful Role of Free Radicals*.

MOLECULAR IMMUNOLOGY

The immune system is the most diverse and ubiquitous system in the body. If you imagine a fortress, then the immune system consists of the walls outside and the soldiers within. The soldiers have many different functions in the hierarchy of the fort, each having their own job, and yet *interacting with each other as a team* to effectively defend the fort from invaders. The soldiers of the immune system consist of particular cell types, not all of which have been defined by researchers. The cells are divided into two main groups defined by their place of maturation: B-cells, or bursa/bone marrow derived, and T-cell, or thymus derived.

B-cells are responsible for humoral immunity (e.g., formation of specific antibodies), and T-cells are responsible for cell-mediated immunity and the production of chemicals and messenger molecules that kill the invading foreign materials. The "fort walls" of the body consist of the areas that come into contact with the outside environment—the skin, mucous membranes of the mouth, genitals, nose, and eyes, the lung lining, and the whole intestinal system. These are physical barriers, and injury of any kind or even a change in cellular structure of the membrane can allow invasion. In the GI mucosa, for example, a thinning of the cells that line the gut (as in colitis, for example) can result in leakage of toxins into the blood stream (Hunter 1991; 1998). Any crossing of the barrier by what is considered foreign by the immune system will result in activation of the system and the defense forces will rally.

After an organism has gained entry, the first line of defense are nonspecific effector mechanisms of the body, in particular the *phagocytic* (cell-eating) cells, such as *neutrophils*. *Macrophages* (big eaters) also play a role in phagocytosis, but may require activation. Some toxins will activate what is known as the *complement system*. The complement system comprises a set of proteins that are designed to eliminate microorganisms and other antigens from tissues and blood. These proteins are present in plasma, other tissue fluids, and on cell surfaces. It is one of the most intricate and rigorously controlled sets of reactions.

Enzymes, cofactors, receptors, and other molecules act in a symphony to elicit proinflammatory and cell killing reactions in response to toxins. The deposition of fragments of complement proteins (especially C3) on the surface of invasive microorganisms is termed *opsonisation*. This "tags" the cells so that phagocytic cells know to actively ingest and destroy that particular material. Activation of complement will also promote local inflammation at the site of infection, through the release of chemical components—known as *cytokines, interleukins,* and *tumor necrosis factor* (TNF-a). In the case of viral infections, infected cells may synthesize *interferons* and/or be recognized and split apart by natural killer (NK) T-cells. The nonspecific immune mechanisms are particularly important early in infection, because the antigen-specific response takes several days to develop, but the nonspecific mechanisms continue to play a role in the immune response until resolution of the infection and healing of tissue damage.

The second line of defense is antigen processing. When, for example, a macrophage eats bacteria, proteins (antigens) from the bacteria are broken down into short peptide chains and those peptides are then "displayed" on the macrophage cell surface attached to special molecules called Major Histocompatibility Complex Class II (MHC II). Bacterial peptides are similarly processed and displayed on MHC II molecules on the surface of B-lymphocytes. When a T-lymphocyte "sees" the same peptide on the macro-phage and on the B-cell, the T-cell stimulates the B-cell to turn on antibody production.

The stimulated B-cell undergoes repeated cell divisions, enlargement, and differentiation to form a clone of antibody secreting *plasma cells*. Hence, through specific antigen recognition of the invader, clonal expansion, and B-cell differentiation, you acquire an effective number of plasma cells *all secreting the same needed antibody*. That antibody then binds to the bacteria making them easier to ingest by white cells.

Cytotoxic T-lymphocytes (CTL) recognize surface markers on other cells in the body that label those cells for destruction. In this way, CTLs help to keep virus-infected or malignant cells in check.

THE HARMFUL ROLE OF FREE RADICALS

Immune cells are highly reactive metabolically, and they have a high turnover. Proinflammatory cytokines will produce free radicals to kill foreign cells in what is called an *oxidative burst* of activity (Goldsby et al. 2000). Although free radicals kill foreign cells, they can also be deadly to our own cells. Free radicals have been linked to immune system damage that accompanies normal aging. A strong immune system is critical to the prevention of infection by viruses, fungi, and bacteria. It is thought that cancer cells form regularly and that a vigilant immune response is therefore required to kill or deactivate these deformed cells before they become malignant tumors. Members of the Life Extension Foundation have long been encouraged to follow a daily antioxidant regimen that protects against immune-suppressing free radicals.

The incidence of cancer and new infectious diseases increases every year in the United States. In addition, many dangerous bacteria have become resistant to the antibiotics that once kept them in check. These virulent, antibiotic resistant strains of bacteria are increasingly becoming a threat to our well-being. There is strong scientific evidence showing that antioxidants and other natural therapies can play an important role in maintaining and enhancing immune function.

NUTRITIONAL IMMUNOLOGY

The concept that appropriate nutrients can enhance the human immune response is known as nutritional immunology. The foundation of this field of study was laid in the early 1800s when physicians discovered that severe malnutrition led to thymic atrophy. For most of that century, the evidence of a relationship between malnutrition and the immune system was based on anatomical findings. With the discovery of vitamins, it became evident that essential nutrients played a critical role in maintaining immune function (Beisel 1996).

Studies published in the 1980s and 1990s clearly show specific immune-enhancing effects of the proper use of nutritional supplements, proteins, hormones, and certain drugs. Micronutrients are now known to play a key role in many of the metabolic processes that promote survival from critical illnesses (Chandra 1983; Chandra et al. 1986). The paragraphs that follow discuss the correct balance of nutrients, nutrient supplements, proteins, and hormones and examine their role in enhancing the human immune system.

THE ROLE OF VITAMINS

Vitamins are essential for oxidative phosphorylation (the energy generating pathway of the cell) and protection against oxidants. They also act as cofactors in many enzymatic reactions and as signal mechanisms to other cells. Researchers use levels of immune cells, presence of antibody, and response to stimulation by antigens as measures of immune activity *in vitro* and *in vivo*, for example, levels of IgA, IgE, B-cells, T-cells, T4/T8 ratios, and response to phytohemagglutinin to name a few (Chandra et al. 1994).

Over the last 30 years, a large amount of literature supports repeatedly the connection between vitamin and mineral balance and immunity, resistance to infection, and allergy (High 1999). The most consistent nutrients linked to immune dysfunction have been low levels of vitamins A, C, E, and B_6, copper, iron, and zinc (Johnson et al. 1992; Grimble 1997; Shankar et al. 1998; Ravaglia et al. 2000). Interestingly, many of these nutrients are linked to deficiency in the North American population. Kenneth H. Brown, a University of California at Davis nutrition professor, estimated that as much as half of the world population is at risk for zinc deficiency and 40% of children in low-income countries have stunted growth related to zinc deficiency. Infants, young children, and pregnant or nursing women are especially at high risk for zinc deficiency because they have increased needs for this essential nutrient.

Chandra et al. (1983) have repeatedly demonstrated that groups such as atopic, formula-fed children, low-birth-weight infants, obese adolescents, malnourished hospitalized patients, and the elderly have not only increased immune dysfunction but also increased risk for infection and allergic disorders, such as eczema. Many of these studies have actually shown improvement of immune function when supplemented with appropriate nutrients and foods (Chandra 1999). Although actual protein malnutrition is rare in North America, we experience more undernutrition and overconsumption—that is, we eat too much poor-quality food, namely, fat, sugar, and processed foodstuffs.

Another area where immunity suffers in western civilization is at the gut lining—the walls of the fortress. About 60% of the immune system cells are collected around the small intestine in areas known as Peyer's patches or the GALT (gut associated lymphoid tissue). Any thinning of the gut lining, such as in lactose intolerance, food allergy, gluten sensitivity, ulcerative colitis, Crohn's disease, antibiotic-induced colitis, yeast overgrowth, and so forth, will render the gut leaky. This leakiness allows incompletely digested food proteins, which are immune stimulating, to enter the blood stream. The walls of the fort have been invaded and the immune cells respond by mounting an inflammatory response. If the problem is not dealt with at the source (i.e., the thin gut wall and its causes), then the immune response becomes chronic. This chronic activation and negative cycle leads to further damage. Keeping our gut healthy through a high-residue, nutrient-dense diet can help to protect against this misfortune.

From the above, it can be seen that a strong immune system is dependent on a good foundation of nutrition. There is no single nutrient that, by itself, will enhance immunity (Lesourd 1997; Scrimshaw et al. 1997). In fact, too much of one nutrient can do the opposite of what one might want and decrease immunity (Delafuente 1991). Thus, the descriptions that follow, where individual nutrients are identified as being important, should be taken in the context of "a chain is only as strong as its weakest link."

Vitamin A

During the 1920s and 1930s, vitamin A became known as the anti-infective vitamin, and the first attempts were made to use vitamin A therapeutically during the course of infectious illnesses. Abraham E. Axelrod and his students initiated the first systematic studies of immunonutritional interrelationships in laboratory animals in 1947. Human studies soon followed, and by the late 1970s, the field of nutritional immunology was well-established. Newer research into vitamin A shows its importance to overall good health and its protective effects against tumor growth. Specifically vitamin A is a cell-signaling vitamin and supports immunity by helping to maintain the integrity of the body's mucosal surfaces (Villamor et al. 2000). Human sources are from liver. The carotenes from plant foods are converted to vitamin A as needed by the body. Large doses of vitamin A can be toxic, and pregnant women should never take vitamin A above the RDA because it is cancer-causing to the fetus. *Refer to Appendix A: Vitamin A Precautions when taking more than 5000 IU a day of vitamin A.*

Beta-Carotene

Beta-carotene has been shown to have a powerful effect in boosting natural killer (NK) cell activity in elderly men. In a controlled, double-blind study, the effects of 10–12 years of beta-carotene supplementation on NK cell activity were evaluated. Although no significant difference was seen in NK cell activity in the middle-aged groups, elderly men supplemented with beta-carotene had significantly greater NK cell activity than the corresponding control group (of elderly men) who were receiving placebo (Santos et al. 1996).

Results show that long-term beta-carotene supplementation may be beneficial for immune viral and tumoral surveillance. A French study using mice concluded that, although beta-carotene supplementation resulted in a nonsignificant increase in NK cells in the spleen, their killing capacity was significantly enhanced after beta-carotene supplementation. The treatment had no adverse effects (Carlos et al. 1997). It is safer to take large doses of beta-carotene than vitamin A, although a yellowing of the skin that is harmless will occur at higher levels. Because we do not know which carotenes of the many varieties are needed, a supplement of mixed carotenes is advised—or better still, eat red-, orange-, and yellow-colored vegetables, which contain high levels of all the carotenes.

Vitamin E

The best-publicized study of the use of vitamin E to boost immune function appeared in 1997 (Meydani et al. 1997). The double-blind, placebo-controlled study looked at healthy humans at least 65 years of age. Supplementation with vitamin E for 4 months improved certain clinically relevant indices of cell-mediated immunity. These results clearly show that a level of vitamin greater than that currently recommended by the FDA enhances certain clinically relevant *in vivo* indices of T-cell-mediated immune function in healthy elderly persons.

Oral alpha-tocopherol supplementation at the rate of 100 mg/day significantly increased NK cell activity in a 16-month-old Japanese boy with Shwachman syndrome (a syndrome associated with severe vitamin E deficiency). The study showed that severe vitamin E deficiency causes impaired NK cell activity but that the condition is reversible with alpha-tocopherol supplementation (Adachi et al. 1997).

Vitamin C (Ascorbic Acid)

High levels of vitamin C can protect levels of vitamin E in tissue and may contribute to the immune-enhancement of vitamin E (Niki 1987; Chan 1993; Stahl et al. 1997). Being an antioxidant, adequate vitamin C is an essential ingredient for "mopping up" the free radicals left behind after the immune system produces its oxidative burst killing activity. A steady supply of vitamin C is vital to good health. Because the human body can neither manufacture nor store vitamin C, our requirements must be met from dietary sources, such as citrus fruit, vegetables, and supplements. Vitamin C's antioxidant protection is especially important to healthy lungs. Numerous studies have shown that vitamin C protects the airways against inhaled (environmental) and internal oxidants. Individuals with asthma, allergies, and sensitive respiratory systems will receive significant protection from adequate doses of vitamin C.

Vitamin B₆ (Pyridoxine)

Deficiencies are associated with marked immune depression. This vitamin has many functions throughout the human body in addition to its support of the immune system. Chandra et al. (1980, 1986) have reported that deficits of pyridoxine in addition to calories and zinc resulted in a significant lowering of serum thymic factor, a hormone involved in cell-mediated immunity. Others have demonstrated in animal studies that both low and high levels of this vitamin can lead to immune suppression (Rall et al. 1993; Katunuma et al. 2000). Vitamin B₆ is an activator of the enzymes necessary for transferring methyl (-CH₃) groups to other molecules involved in immune function, so this vitamin's impact is not only on immunity but on all body functions. Once again, balance is always important. Although the known obvious side effects of excessive vitamin B₆ should be watched for (tingling and numbness in the extremities at doses of greater than 300 mg a day for some weeks), it is not known at what dose the immune suppressive effects may occur.

TRACE ELEMENTS

It is now understood that trace elements are essential, not only for their direct antioxidant activity, but also for their role as cofactors for a number of antioxidant enzymes. Wound-healing and immune function are highly dependent on adequate levels of trace elements, as well as vitamin levels. Dietary supplements of (some) trace elements are crucial to compensate for mineral-depleted soils providing much of the food we eat. Trace elements are greatly affected by what are called heavy metals—typically aluminum, arsenic, cadmium, lead, and mercury. Zinc is particularly susceptible to the effects of cadmium, a ubiquitous heavy metal.

Chowdhury et al. (1987) showed that in mice relatively low levels of cadmium would decrease NK cell activity and that this could be reversed by zinc. This led Chowdhury et al. to state: "Human civilization and a concomitant increase in industrial activity has gradually redistributed many toxic metals from the earth's crust to the environment and increased the possibility of human exposure. Among the various toxic elements, heavy metals cadmium, lead, and mercury are especially prevalent in nature due to their high industrial use. These metals serve no biological function and their presence in tissues reflects contact of the organism with its environment. They are cumu-

lative poison." Heavy metals are basically poisonous to enzyme systems overall and should be removed from the body if present in excess by chelation or detoxification. Trying to overpower the action of heavy metals by taking extra nutrients to antagonize them is not advised (see Heavy Metal Toxicity protocol).

Zinc

The trace element zinc has many roles in basic cellular function. These include DNA replication, RNA transcription, cell division, and cell activation. Zinc is a specific activator of T-cells, T-cell division, and other immune cells (Prasad et al. 1997). Zinc also functions as an antioxidant and stabilizes membranes. Zinc-deficient patients display reduced resistance to infection, and Scott et al. (2000) found that in the parasite-infected host (in this case mice), any zinc deficiency results in better survival of the parasite. Thus, zinc is known to play a pivotal role in the efficiency of the entire immune system. In our diet, zinc and protein are linked, so that protein deficiency of any kind will inevitably result in zinc deficiency. Zinc is present in high-protein foods such as meat, oysters, nuts, and seeds. Zinc's importance in many aspects of the immune system, from skin barrier to lymphocyte gene regulation, may be based on its importance in cellular function.

Immune dysfunction and susceptibility to infection have been observed in zinc-deficient human subjects. A study investigated the production of cytokines and characterized the T-cell subpopulations in three groups of mildly zinc-deficient subjects (Prasad 2000). These included head and neck cancer patients, healthy volunteers found to have a dietary deficiency of zinc, and healthy volunteers in whom a zinc deficiency was induced by dietary means.

Prasad (2000) demonstrated that zinc status affects cytokine levels, but has no effect on the anti-inflammatory cytokines. Production of interleukin-2 and gamma-interferon was decreased even when the zinc deficiency was mild. Natural killer cell activity was also decreased in zinc-deficient subjects. T-cell formation was decreased even in mildly zinc-deficient subjects. The study demonstrates the crucial role of zinc in promoting specific immune responses.

Zinc is not only seen to be an important regulator of immunity but has also been found clinically to be an excellent mineral to take in the event of viral illness, such as the common cold. There have been contradictory studies in this regard, but a double-blind placebo-controlled trial published by Prasad (2000) was positive. It showed a very significant reduction in overall duration of cold symptoms (50%), cough (50%), and nasal discharge (30%) at a dose of 12.8 mg of zinc in a lozenge taken every 2–3 hours while awake. However, pro-inflammatory cytokine levels did not change significantly in this study. Zinc must be taken as a lozenge at the *start* of the cold symptoms to be effective.

Copper, Manganese, and Selenium

In addition to zinc, copper, manganese, and selenium act as cofactors of antioxidant enzymes to protect against oxygen free radicals produced during oxidative stress (Leung 1998). Although all are essential, selenium is found to be most deficient in traumatized patients. In recent years, the benefits of selenium have been recognized by researchers as an effective protector against certain cancers, such as breast, lung, liver, urogenital, colorectal, prostate, and ovarian cancer, by removing harmful lipids and hydroperoxides from the body. In addition to being a regulator of enzyme reactions, selenium acts with vitamin E, and the two are intricately interwoven as antioxidants in the glutathione regeneration cycle. Cell-mediated immunity is impaired by this pair's deficiency.

A copper deficiency will impair lymphocyte response to antigen stimulants and also impairs cell-mediated immunity. Copper is an important cofactor in many of the body's enzyme reactions, including the antioxidant splitting enzyme superoxide dismutase, and again may be deficient in our diet. Once again, however, an excess of this nutrient may be toxic.

Manganese is also involved in many antioxidant functions, but it has been found in levels that are too high in some patients on home parenteral nutrition. It is also involved in the generation of glutathione, an important antioxidant.

A convenient way of obtaining most of the nutrients needed for healthy immune function is to take 3 tablets 3 times daily of the 89-ingredient Life Extension Mix. One capsule daily of Life Extension Booster provides additional amounts of the nutrients that protect immune system cells against damaging free radicals.

A number of studies have shown that the combination of zinc and selenium enhances immunity in the elderly. A pioneering study published in the *Lancet* (Chandra 1992) found that seniors taking modest doses of a multivitamin/multimineral supplement containing zinc and selenium showed a general reduction in infection and required antibiotics for significantly fewer days annually. A more recent study brings the effect of these two minerals into sharper focus. This well-designed study (randomized, placebo-controlled, double-blind) found that seniors taking zinc and selenium had significantly fewer infections over a 2-year period, but that vitamin supplementation alone did not have a major effect (Girodon et al. 1997). The zinc and selenium supplement cut the number of infections by nearly two-thirds compared to placebo. A follow-up study demonstrates that seniors supplemented with zinc and selenium show improved antibody response to the flu vaccine (Girodon et al. 1999).

PROBIOTICS

Probiotics are natural substances that can be taken by humans to enhance the bacterial flora of the intestinal tract. The better-known probiotic is *Lactobacillus acidophilus* that is found in live yogurt cultures and can be helpful in combating yeast and other organisms that should not be in the GI tract. Arunachalam et al. (2000) have found *Bifidobacterium lactis* (1.5×10^{11} units) in low-lactose milk consumption by healthy elderly subjects improves immune function after 6 weeks as measured by enhanced levels of alpha-interferon and phagocytic cell capacity. In one animal study, Perdigon et al. (1988) showed a strong response to *L. acidophilus, L. bulgaricus, and L. casei* via the oral route. In general, probiotics are known for their ability to create a positive environment in the human GI tract for enhanced immunity, appropriate gut flora balance, and enhanced nutrient formation for enterocytes (cells of the intestinal wall) (Chiang et al. 2000; Gill et al. 2001a; 2001b).

Lactoferrin

Lactoferrin can be considered a prebiotic, that is, a substance that when ingested suppresses the formation of antagonistic bacteria, thereby promoting the production of probiotics, such as acidophilus. Will Brink (2000) wrote an article in *Life Extension Magazine* on lactoferrin that reviews the literature on this substance, which is a fraction of whey protein. Although many of the studies are on animals, lactoferrin is present naturally in many mucous membrane secretions in the human, suggesting an innate human immune enhancing function (Nishiya et al. 1982). Brink suggests that the *apo*-form of lactoferrin is the best. It appears to act partially by increasing the production of probiotics, such as *L. acidophilus*, and, at least in animal studies, inhibits pathogenic bacterial growth, such as *Escherichia coli, Staphylococci*, and *Helicobacter pylori* (Wada et al. 1999).

FATS

The kind of fat that we eat will determine the balance of proinflammatory and anti-inflammatory hormones and messengers. In addition, the structure of all our cells will be determined by the amounts of saturated versus unsaturated fat in our diet. The omega-3 series dietary fatty acids (polyunsaturated or PUFAs) are rapidly incorporated into cell membranes, and profoundly influence biological responses. These lipids influence membrane stability, membrane fluidity, cell mobility, the formation of receptors, binding of ligands to their receptors, activation of intracellular signaling pathways either directly or through the formation of eicosanoids, gene expression, and cell differentiation. For the most part, in the Western world we are oversupplied with saturated fats that lead to the expression of inflammatory messengers, rigid cell walls, and fatty deposits in the arteries.

In terms of immune system function, most studies show that dietary intake of linoleic acid (LA) has a strong growth-promoting effect on many rodent tumors, whereas fatty acids, such as alpha-linolenic and eicosapentaenoic acids (EPAs) are recognized as cancer chemo-preventive (Penturf et al. 1997). However, Sauer et al. (2001), writing on the mechanism for the antitumor and anticachectic effects of n-3 fatty acids, stated: "In general, eicosanoids [prostaglandins] formed from the omega-3 fatty acids are much less potent in causing biological responses than those formed from the omega-6 fatty acids, including stimulation of cytokine production and inflammatory responses. In well-controlled clinical studies, consumption of omega-3 fatty acids has resulted in reduction of cardiovascular diseases including arrhythmias and hypertension, protection from renal disease, improvement in rheumatoid arthritis, improvement in inflammatory bowel diseases, reduced episodes of rejection, and protection from infection."

Teasing out the different effects of fats on the immune system is in a state of transition, no doubt due to the widely differing effects that different fats can have on different cells, and on the membrane structure of all cells.

OTHER FACTORS

Other factors that influence immunity are manifold. Chandra et al. (1991) have identified multiple factors that can predispose to immune dysfunction in the elderly—living alone, physical or mental disability, recent loss of spouse or significant other, use of multiple medications, poverty, and high alcohol consumption. The emotional and social factors should not be taken lightly. We have already discussed the impact of GI integrity and thinning of the bowel wall as a significant factor in immune response.

ECHINACEA

Echinacea is also known as purple coneflower and is a member of the daisy family. Echinacea's ability to fight cold viruses and respiratory infections has long been known. In vitro studies have shown that echinacea increases antibody production, reduces inflammation, and enables white blood cells to migrate to the infection site.

Orally, echinacea is commonly used for treating and preventing the common cold and other upper respiratory infections. Echinacea is also used orally as an immune stimulant and as an anti-infective for a variety of other infections, including urinary tract infections and vaginal yeast infections (Broumand et al. 1997). When used orally for reducing symptoms associated with influenza-like infections, such as the common cold and flu, evidence generally indicates that echinacea preparations can decrease the severity and duration of symptoms associated with these viruses if started when symptoms are first noticed and used for 7–10 days.

Generally, high doses are not recommended to be used as a preventive, and the formulation and species that might offer the most benefit is unclear (Melchart et al. 2000; Percival 2000). Studies to date have used a variety of preparations, including extracts of Echinacea purpurea herb, combination root and herb extracts, and root extracts of Echinacea pallida, Echinacea augustifolia, and Echinacea purpurea. Studies have also used echinacea compound herbal teas (Lindenmuth et al. 2000). Collectively, the data indicate that E. purpurea, at least, and possibly other plant compounds, appear to contain phytochemicals capable of stimulating production of NK cells, as well as augmenting their cell breakdown function in animals of advanced age (Currier et al. 2000).

GRAPE SEED-SKIN EXTRACT

The effects of the proanthocyanidins found in grape seed-skin extract on immune dysfunction were studied in mice. The proanthocyanidin enhanced in vitro interleukin-2 production and natural killer cell cytotoxicity. In vitro, grape seed-skin extract has been shown to have antioxidant action 50 times greater than vitamin E and 20 times greater than vitamin C (Bagchi et al. 1997). The antioxidant protection of grape seed-skin also extends across the blood brain barrier to the brain and spinal nerves (Bagchi et al. 1998).

RICE BRAN EXTRACT (MGN-3)

MGN-3 is a complex containing arabinoxylane as a major component. It is produced by hydrolyzing rice bran using enzymes from mycelia of certain mushrooms.

Some studies suggest it might improve immunity by, among other things, enhancing natural killer cell activity and production of tumor necrosis factor alpha. Some evidence suggests that MGN-3 has activity against HIV. Results from three small studies of healthy individuals and individuals with cancer suggest that MGN-3 also enhances natural killer cell activity. Most studies have been either *in vitro* or small human studies (Ghoneum 1995; 1998; Ghoneum et al. 1996).

In research at the Department of Otolaryngology of Drew University of Medicine and Science, MGN-3 was examined for its effect on human NK cell activity (Ghoneum 1998). During 2 months of supplementation, NK activity was shown to have increased significantly, leading to the conclusion that MGN-3 could be used as a new biological response modifier with possible therapeutic effects against cancer. More research is definitely needed into the benefits of this supplement.

WHEY PROTEIN

Whey protein isolate dramatically raises glutathione levels (Micke et al. 2001). Glutathione protects immune cells and detoxifies harmful compounds in the body and is intimately tied to immunity. Reduced glutathione levels have been associated with AIDS and other viral diseases, and raising glutathione levels appears to be one way of modulating immunity.

In one study, glutathione in animals was raised to higher-than-normal levels by whey protein better than by other proteins, including soy. A study involving HIV-positive men fed whey protein concentrate found dramatic increases in glutathione levels, with most men reaching their ideal body weight (Bounous et al. 1993). Whey protein improves immune function and fights infections. Immune response also was dramatically enhanced in animals fed whey protein concentrate when exposed to immune challenges, such as *Salmonella*, *Streptococcus* pneumonia, and cancer-causing chemicals. Again, this effect on immunity was not seen with other proteins.

Studies have examined the impact of whey protein concentrate on preventing or treating cancer. When different groups of rats were given a powerful carcinogen, those fed whey protein concentrate showed fewer tumors and a reduced pooled area of tumors (tumor mass index). The researchers found that whey protein offered "considerable protection to the host" over that of other proteins (McIntosh et al. 1995). It should be noted that not all whey protein concentrates are created equal. Processing whey protein to remove the lactose and fats without eliminating its biological activity requires special care by the manufacturer. The process must use low temperature and low acid conditions so as not to "denature" the protein. Maintaining the natural state of the protein is essential to its biological activity. Immune-suppressed patients should consider taking 30 grams a day of specially designed whey protein concentrate.

L-CARNITINE

Carnitine is an amino acid complex primarily known for its ability to transport fat across the cellular membrane and for the breakdown of fat within the cell. It is found mainly in meats. A number of papers have described the potential use of carnitine in HIV/AIDS. Carnitine levels are often low in AIDS patients, particularly those on AZT analogues for treatment and prevention of transmission of infection. High-dose carnitine (6 grams a day) seems to have the ability to increase some immune parameters, such as NK cell activity. Its effect on immunity in other diseases has not been researched (De Simone et al. 1982; 1993; 1994; Franceschi et al. 1990).

COENZYME Q_{10}

Coenzyme Q_{10} (CoQ_{10}) is an important antioxidant produced in the body and found in small amounts in some foods. CoQ_{10} is found in high concentrations in the healthy heart, where it plays an important role in initiating cell-produced energy. Studies have documented its effectiveness in improving the quality of life in people with advanced heart disease, congestive heart failure, angina, and arrhythmia. It has been found to increase a number of immune parameters, including IgG, T4 cells, and the ratio of T4/T8 lymphocytes (Folkers et al. 1982, 1985, 1993).

Because of its immuno-stimulatory potential, CoQ_{10} has been used as an adjuvant therapy in patients with various types of cancer. CoQ_{10} has also shown promise in clinical trials on breast cancer patients in which tumor spread and mortality rate were significantly lowered with trial dosages (Lockwood et al. 1994a; 1994b; 1995). Austin (1997) has written an excellent review of the use of CoQ_{10} in the treatment of metastatic disease and has critically evaluated the papers by Lockwood et al. (Austin 1997). Although CoQ_{10} may show indirect anticancer activity through its effect(s) on the immune system, there is evidence to suggest that analogs of this compound are able to suppress cancer growth directly. Additional research is needed to determine long-term toxicity in cancer treatment.

DHEA

Dehydroepiandrosterone, or DHEA, as it is more often called, is a steroid hormone produced in the adrenal gland. DHEA levels are known to fall precipitously with age, falling 90% from ages 20–90. DHEA is like the hub of a wheel and is the central hormone that is a precursor to the numerous steroid sex hormones (including estrogen and testosterone). Although there is an apparent lack of any direct hormone action for DHEA, it has been suggested that it may serve the role of a buffering hormone, which would alter the state-dependency of other steroid hormones. Although the specific mechanisms of action for DHEA are only partially understood, supplemental DHEA has been shown to have antiaging, antiobesity, and anticancer influences, as well as significant immune-enhancing functions. DHEA has demonstrated a striking ability to maintain immune system synchronization. Oral supplementation with low doses of DHEA in aged animals restored immuno-competence to a reasonable level within days of administration. DHEA supplementation in aged rodents resulted in almost complete restoration of immune function.

DHEA has been shown in numerous animal studies to boost immune function via several different mechanisms (Danenberg et al. 1995; Loria et al. 1996; Solerte et al. 1999). Only limited human studies have been done to measure DHEA's effect on the immune system, and there are side effects to this potent hormone.

In a 1997 study, scientists proposed that the oral administration of DHEA to elderly men would result in activation of their immune systems: Nine healthy men with an average age of 63 were treated with a placebo for 2 weeks followed by 20 weeks of DHEA (50 mg a day). After 2 weeks on oral DHEA, serum DHEA levels increased by three- to fourfold. These levels were sustained throughout the study. Compared to the placebo, DHEA administration resulted in:

- An increase of 20% in IGF-1. Many people are taking expensive growth hormone injections for the purpose of boosting IGF levels. IGF stands for insulin-like growth factor and is thought to be responsible for some of the antiaging, anabolic effects that DHEA has produced in previous human studies.

- An increase of 35% in the number of monocyte immune cells

- An increase of 29% in the number of B-cells and a 62% increase in B-cell activity

- A 40% increase in T-cell activity even though the total numbers of T-cells were not affected

- An increase of 50% in interleukin-2 (IL-2)

- An increase of 22–37% in number of NK cells and an increase of 45% in NK cell activity

- No adverse effects were noted with DHEA administration, but this was a short study with few subjects

The scientists concluded: "While extended studies are required, our findings suggest potential therapeutic benefits of DHEA in immunodeficient states" (Khorram et al. 1997).

A study in the *Proceedings of the Society for Experimental Biology and Medicine* demonstrated that when old female mice were treated with DHEA, melatonin, or DHEA plus melatonin, splenocytes (macrophages) were significantly higher as compared to young mice. B-cell proliferation in young and in old mice significantly increased. DHEA, melatonin, and DHEA plus melatonin helped to regulate immune function in aged female mice by significantly increasing Th1 cytokines, interleukin-2 (IL-2), and interferon-gamma and significantly decreasing Th2 cytokines, interleukin-6 (IL-6), and interleukin-10 (IL-10), thus regulating cytokine production (Inserra et al. 1998).

Interleukin-6 (IL-6) is one of the pathogenic elements in inflammatory and age-related diseases such as rheumatoid arthritis, osteoporosis, atherosclerosis, and late-onset B-cell neoplasia. "Higher circulating levels of IL-6 predict disability onset in older persons," according to their report in the June 1999 issue of the *Journal of the American Geriatrics Society*. The authors suggest that IL-6 may cause a reduction in muscle strength or contribute to specific diseases, such as congestive heart failure, osteoporosis, arthritis, and dementia, which cause disability (Ferrucci et al. 1999).

DHEA has consistently been shown to boost beneficial IL-2 and suppress damaging IL-6 levels. IL-6 is overproduced in the aged, which contributes to autoimmune disease, immune dysfunction, osteoporosis, depressions in healing, breast cancer, and B-cell lymphoma and anemia. Chronic DHEA administration maintained immuno-competence in aged animals by boosting IL-2 and other beneficial immune components and by suppressing IL-6 and other detrimental immune components. Suppression of IL-6 with 200 mg a day of DHEA was shown to be effective against systemic lupus erythematosus (van Vollenhoven et al. 1998).

Researchers compared levels of IL-6 in 283 subjects with mobility or functional disability, with IL-6 levels in 350 adults without a disability. The investigators found that adults in the highest third of values of IL-6 had a 76% higher rate for mobility disabilities and 62% higher rate for inability to perform daily activities than subjects in the lowest third of values. "These data suggest that IL-6 is a global marker of impending deterioration in health status in older adults," writes a team led by Dr. Luigi Ferrucci (Ferrucci et al. 1999).

In a study by Inserra et al. (1998), DHEA was shown to restore normal cytokine production in immune system dysfunction induced by aging by suppressing the excessive production of cytokines (IL-6) by 75%, while increasing IL-2 secretion by nearly 50%, during a leukemia virus infection in old mice.

DHEA has potential benefits for the immune system, but caution is urged. Serum or salivary levels should be checked before starting any DHEA supplementation, and dosages should be monitored by your health care practitioner.

For DHEA dosing information and safety precautions, refer to the DHEA Replacement Therapy protocol.

MELATONIN AND KH3

Aging, cancer, AIDS, chemotherapy, and infectious agents can all stimulate excessive cortisol production from the adrenal glands, decimating immune function, and leading to immune system destruction and desynchronization. It is crucial to inhibit excessive cortisol production. (As has been noted in the HIV Infection (AIDS) protocol, there are 17 European studies showing that HIV causes the destruction of the immune system by stimulating excessive cortisol production.)

DHEA and melatonin work together to suppress cortisol levels. High doses of the European procaine drug KH3, taken at least twice a day, are suggested as a potential way of protecting against the effects of elevated cortisol levels so often seen in cancer, AIDS, and stressed-out patients. On an empty stomach, take 1–2 tablets of KH3 first thing in the morning and repeat the dosage 1 hour before dinner. It is difficult to test cortisol levels in the blood because adrenal surges of cortisol can occur erratically throughout the day, which is one reason why this important cause of immune system destruction has been largely ignored by American doctors. KH3 is legal only in the state of Nevada.

The most effective hormone therapy to protect and improve immune function is melatonin, which enhances the production of T-helper cells that are necessary to identify cancer cells, viruses, fungi, and bacteria. Melatonin enhances the production of other immune components, including natural killer cells, IL-2, IL-4, IL-10, gamma-interferon, and eosinophils (Lissoni et al. 1989; 1994; 1995; Maestroni 1993; Bubenik et al. 1998; Kostogloy-Athanassiou 1998).

The latest evidence suggests that melatonin is even more effective than nutrient antioxidants in suppressing immune cell-killing free radicals.

BIOSTIM

Influenza and other infectious diseases tend to be more severe in older patients. Despite immunization, elderly people often lack the immune capacity to generate an antibody response to prevent infection from the influenza virus. As many as 69,000 Americans have died from influenza in a bad epidemic year. Biostim is an immunomodulator extracted from a bacterium called Klebsiella pneumoniae (strain O1:K2). In humans, it is able to reduce the number and duration of infectious exacerbations of chronic bronchitis. This has been demonstrated in many double-blind studies over the last 10 years. An examination of the published literature reveals that if Biostim were available in the United States, thousands of American lives could be saved every year. These studies also indicate that Biostim would dramatically reduce the need for antibiotic therapy, thereby saving untold millions of dollars in prescription drug costs.

A double-blind trial was conducted to evaluate the capacity of Biostim to diminish the frequency of infectious episodes in chronic bronchitis. The study duration was 9 months. Of the 73 subjects selected, 38 received Biostim, and 35 received a placebo. By the 9th month, the duration in days of infectious episodes was 60% lower in the Biostim group compared with the placebo group. The use of antibiotic therapy was reduced by 81% in the Biostim group compared with the placebo group. Prewinter administration of Biostim to subjects significantly diminished the frequency of infectious episodes and thus the consumption of antibiotics (Viallat et al. 1983).

In another study, 314 elderly subjects admitted to hospitals were given either Biostim or a placebo. The subjects were regularly examined every 3 months for 1 year. The incidence of acute infectious episodes was evaluated in both groups. The number of subjects with infection in the group receiving the Biostim was significantly lower than in the placebo group. In the group receiving the Biostim, the number of infectious episodes was reduced throughout the 12 months of the trial. Finally, there was a significant decrease in the duration of antibiotic therapy. Biostim was well-tolerated. This study shows that Biostim is effective in protecting elderly, and therefore fragile, subjects against respiratory infections (Hugonot et al. 1988).

An evaluation of the safety of Biostim given with an antibiotic to treat acute infections was performed in three double-blind, placebo-controlled studies on fragile institutionalized or hospitalized patients. Two of the studies showed that in acute respiratory infections, Biostim was well-tolerated and resulted in a more rapid improvement. The third study showed that Biostim produced a more rapid improvement in the most severely ill patients. It was concluded that Biostim can be initiated safely during acute episodes occurring in subjects with recurrent respiratory infections and that it results in a faster improvement of clinical symptoms (Lacaille 1988; Minonzio et al. 1991; Fietta et al. 1992).

Biostim Therapy (3-Month Dosing Schedule)

Take 2 tablets daily for 8 days, then stop for 3 weeks; 1 tablet daily for 8 days, then stop for 3 weeks; 1 tablet daily for 8 days, then stop for 9 months. Repeat Biostim therapy once a year. It is contraindicated in people with autoimmune disorders.

THYROID-STIMULATING HORMONE

Aging, cancer, and AIDS often generate suboptimal levels of thyroid hormone production. Proper levels of thyroid hormones are crucial for optimal immune function. Blood tests do not always detect a thyroid hormone deficiency. One blood test is the TSH, a pituitary hormone that regulates production of thyroid hormone from the thyroid gland. If your TSH is high, it may indicate a need for thyroid replacement therapy. Popular prescription thyroid replacement drugs are Synthroid (synthetic thyroid hormone, T4) and Cytomel (T3 thyroid hormone). You must be careful not to overdose on thyroid hormones, so the advice of a knowledgeable physician is important when you are considering thyroid hormone therapy.

Note: *As of this writing, the FDA has begun an extensive review of Synthroid due to its history of problems and has ordered Abbott Laboratories to phase down distribution until the FDA review is complete.*

The Life Extension Foundation recommends the use of Cytomel for thyroid underproduction, due to its metabolically active pharmacology. Refer to the *Thyroid Replacement protocol* for more specific details about determining your thyroid status.

THYMIC IMMUNE FACTORS

Thymic Immune Factors is a glandular compound prescribed by many alternative doctors that provides extracts of fresh, healthy tissue from the thymus, lymph, and spleen. These glands produce the disease-fighting cells of our immune system and the white blood cells that engage in life-or-death combat with invading organisms in our bloodstream under instruction of the thymus gland. The primary ingredient is immunologic tissue from the thymus gland.

Thymic Immune Factors has been used to amplify the immune-potentiating effect of DHEA replacement therapy. T-cells mature in response to hormones secreted by the thymus gland. The thymus gland shrinks with age, and the resulting reduction in the production of thymic immune factors could be a cause of the progressive decline in immune function that occurs with aging. By taking 2–4 capsules daily of Thymic Immune Factors, you may replace some of the thymic factors lost to aging.

EXERCISE

Japanese studies show that regular physical activity may enhance NK cell activity (Shinkai et al. 1997). However, too much of a good thing may actually decrease immune effectiveness. A very low fat diet (less than 15%) coupled with a heavy exercise schedule has been shown to decrease immune efficacy (Venkatraman et al. 1996; Konig et al. 1997). Given the many other health benefits, regular, *moderate* exercise should be on everyone's health agenda. There is research evidence that vitamin supplementation becomes increasingly important with exercise because physical activity raises oxygen demand, causing an increase in the formation of oxygen radical species. Many vitamins and cofactors are involved in energy metabolism and free-radical scavenging.

IMMUNITY, STRESS, AND EMOTIONS

For many years, the concept that our emotions can affect immunity has been bandied about. It was Carl Simonton, the radiation oncologist from Fort Worth, TX, who first noticed that meditation and visualization could impact the recovery of cancer patients. Since that time our understanding of how emotion can affect immunity has been increased by the knowledge of how brain cells "talk to" immune cells. Many articles and books have been published on this now accepted idea (Pert 1999). Immune cells carry receptor sites for neuromodulating substances such as dopamine and serotonin and thus are able to receive information about mood change via cell-to-cell signaling.

Salivary IgA, a known immune biomarker, has been found to increase in children given suggestion under hypnosis to simply "increase immune factors in

Unlike in Canada, Europe, and Japan, where melatonin is regulated as a drug, citizens of the United States can buy pharmaceutical-grade melatonin at extraordinarily low prices.

As already stated, the optimal dose of melatonin has considerable individual variability. Many people find as little as 300 mcg is ideal, while others take 3–6 mg of melatonin before bedtime to solve their sleep problems. Too much melatonin can interfere with sleep in some persons, so the lowest effective dose of melatonin needed to get to sleep and stay asleep is often the best course of action to follow.

Melatonin Plus Cofactors

Some people still wake up too frequently during the night or too early in the morning, even after taking melatonin. In order to duplicate the mechanisms by which the young pineal gland induces youthful sleep patterns, a formula called Natural Sleep was developed in 1995, and it has produced a good track record in helping alleviate chronic insomnia problems. This formula contains two different melatonin delivery systems that work together to generate the same kind of secretion of melatonin that occurs naturally in young people.

First, the Natural Sleep capsule bursts open in the stomach within 5 minutes after swallowing to provide immediate-release melatonin. That induces the drowsiness needed to get to sleep. Then, Natural Sleep gradually introduces tiny beadlets of sustained-release melatonin into the digestive tract, to enable the person to stay asleep and avoid the nocturnal tossing and turning characteristic of age-related sleep disturbances.

Each capsule of Natural Sleep contains 2.5 mg of immediate-release melatonin plus 2.5 mg of sustained-release melatonin. Many people find this dose effectively enables them to enjoy a complete night's rest every night. Natural Sleep also contains vitamin B_{12} because of studies that show it can normalize circadian rhythms, thereby enabling people to enter sleep without stress or tension (Chang et al. 1995; Kohsaka 1998; Yamadera et al. 1998). Chromium picolinate and chromium polynicotinate are included in this formula to help lower blood sugar levels that can inhibit the ability to fall asleep. Niacinamide ascorbate, magnesium, calcium, and inositol are included as well in Natural Sleep to help induce a state of relaxation (Tramer et al. 1996; Hornyak et al. 1998).

Natural Sleep does not contain any potentially toxic herbal extracts. Insomnia often is a lifelong affliction, requiring the continuous need for nightly self-medication. The ingredients in Natural Sleep have been investigated for long-term safety and can be taken for an indefinite period of time without any risk of toxicity or tolerance.

Some people who occasionally wake up in the middle of the night will take another dose of melatonin to get back to sleep.

OTHER NATURAL SLEEP-INDUCING THERAPIES

Some people find that commercially available GABA taken before bedtime is helpful. Tryptophan is available at compounding pharmacies and can be taken before bed. 5-Hydroxytryptophan is available at most health food stores and can be taken before bed as well. Avoid taking vitamin B_6 supplements within 6 hours of taking 5-hydroxytryptophan (5-HTP) because vitamin B_6 can cause the conversion of 5-HTP to serotonin in the blood before it has a chance to cross the blood-brain barrier to increase serotonin in the brain. Excessive serotonin in the blood can be dangerous, which is why it may be safer to use tryptophan rather than 5-hydroxytryptophan (5-HTP). Both of these compounds can be converted to serotonin in the brain, which plays a role in sleep (Birdsall 1998). Patients taking SSRI antidepressants, such as Prozac, should consult with their physicians prior to taking these agents because the dose of antidepressant may need to be reduced. This is true for St. John's Wort as well.

Although the long-term administration of valerian is not recommended, passion flower or valerian extract taken in moderation for short- to medium-term treatment of insomnia in conjunction with the other therapies mentioned may be helpful. A study with mice and an aqueous extract of passion flower showed sedative properties (Soulimani et al. 1997). It is available as a tea, in capsules, and as a tincture.

Some people use the herb valerian to fall asleep. Valerian produces a drug-like hypnotic effect within the central nervous system similar to benzodiazepine drugs, such as Valium and Halcion. Because valerian-containing products often are promoted as natural herbal remedies, the public mistakenly believes they are safe to take on a regular basis (Donath et al. 2000). Studies indicate, however, that there is a possible toxicity risk when taking valerian over an extended period of time (Chan et al. 1995). Because a tolerance effect occurs with valerian due to its Valium-like properties, people often need to take greater and greater amounts of it as time goes by in order to continue to obtain the desired hypnotic (sleep-inducing) effect.

USE OF PRESCRIPTION DRUGS

The use of tranquilizing drugs to solve chronic insomnia is not recommended by conventional or alternative medicine. The first problem cited by critics is addiction. It's not that the patient necessarily gets addicted to the drugs themselves. The problem arises when the insomniac becomes accustomed to the good night's sleep the drugs induce and does not want to stop taking the medication. The other problem is tolerance, which means the drug slowly stops working, even when higher doses are taken. The dual problems of addiction and tolerance cause physicians to be extremely cautious when prescribing sleep medications. Other reasons for avoiding these drugs include increasing the risk of sudden death for the following individuals: (1) sleep apnea patients, (2) those who consume alcohol, and (3) some elderly people. Elderly people slowly metabolize sedative drugs, meaning that clearance from their body can take too long, and they experience fatigue the next day. It should also be noted that benzodiazepine drugs frequently used to induce a sedative effect can impair mental function.

Having said all of the above, we want to make the argument that for the chronic insomniac who cannot find relief by safer natural therapies, long-term, prescription drug therapy should be considered.

It is our position that a chronic insomniac should do almost anything to alleviate a sleep problem. We suggest that some insomniacs consider resorting to prescription tranquilizers under the guidance of a cooperating physician if all else fails. One reason for this suggestion is that within the next 10 years, there is a chance that a drug could be developed that will safely help people to sleep without any side effects or tolerance problems. If this were to happen, those chronic insomniacs who avoided prescription sleeping pills would have suffered needlessly because once a "cure" was discovered, they would no longer need their sleep medication. There is also the quality of life issue. If the judicious use of prescription sleeping pills provides a chronic insomniac with 5–10 years of good sleep, it may be worthwhile.

One way of avoiding the tolerance problem is to alternate the type of sleeping pill used. Here is a suggested prescription drug schedule to treat chronic insomnia for the person who has never taken prescription sleeping pills:

1. Valium, 2.5 mg taken *only* at bedtime for 30 days.
2. During the next 30-day cycle, switch to 5–10 mg of Ambien taken *only* at bedtime.
3. During the next 30-day cycle, switch to Klonopin 1–3 mg taken *only* at bedtime.

This cycle may be repeated, using a wide variety of tranquilizing drugs, for many years without the tolerance factor occurring.

At some point, a person may find that they do better by taking the Valium on one night, Ambien on the next night, and Klonopin on the third night. The drug Sonata in the dose of 5–10 mg provides about 5 hours of sleep and can be helpful for occasions when only a limited amount of sleep time is available. If heavy alcohol is ever consumed, these types of drugs should be avoided on that night. It should be noted that chronic alcohol intake in and of itself is a major cause of poor sleep patterns.

An "old" drug frequently prescribed to induce a state of deep sleep is a tricyclic antidepressant drug called Elavil (amitriptyline hydrochloride). This drug normally puts people to sleep fast, but induces many side effects such as severe dry mouth, weight gain, constipation, and a host of other problems. Newer tricyclic antidepressant drugs produce fewer side effects, but do not work as well in inducing deep sleep patterns. A typical dose of Elavil taken a few hours before bedtime is 10–25 mg. Some people use Elavil until the side effects become too pronounced and then discontinue it for months or years.

There are a number of prescription drugs that will induce a state of sleep. Halcion seems to produce the most severe side effects and is not recommended. A person with chronic insomnia must develop a close relationship with a physician who understands that some people need sleep medications on a routine basis or their lives will be miserable and that they are also at a higher risk of contracting a serious degenerative disease.

Low-dose melatonin may help any of these prescription drugs work more effectively.

OTHER SLEEP DISORDERS

Nocturnal myoclonus (an abrupt spasm of a group of muscles) and "restless legs" syndrome are related conditions. "Restless legs" syndrome is exactly what its name suggests. It is a familial disorder characterized by an irresistible urge to kick the legs about, often disturbing sleep. Many patients have both conditions. Patients with a family history are likely to benefit from higher-dose therapy with folic acid, about 5–10 mg per day (Botez et al. 1976). Those taking folic acid should make sure they are receiving at least 500–1000 mcg a day of vitamin B_{12}. Kelly (1998) suggests that insomnia and restless legs syndrome may be secondary to folate deficiency.

Note: If you have epilepsy, consult your physician before taking folic acid. Folic acid interacts with some epilepsy medications and may trigger seizures in some people.

Another consideration of sleep disorder is low blood iron in the presence of anemia. This can be determined by testing the ferritin level, which, if low, reflects low iron. Treatment with 15–30 elemental mg of iron protein succinate should do the trick. However, one must watch for excessively high iron levels because of the free radical promoting nature of iron, which contributes to aging. Magnesium citrate at doses of about 250 mg taken at night, may also be beneficial.

If no abnormality is found to be causing sleeplessness, another test known as a sleep latency study may be conducted. The person is asked to take little naps during the day, and the period of time it takes prior to falling asleep is measured. Narcolepsy, a disorder in which people fall asleep during the day very suddenly despite normal nighttime sleep, may be diagnosed by this test.

Another, less commonly diagnosed disorder is pathological daytime sleepiness. Again, the person sleeps normally during the night but feels sleepy during the day. People who have this disorder may feel sleepy, but they don't fall asleep on the spot like persons with narcolepsy do.

Once a diagnosis is made, treatment options can be sought. Sleep apnea may be corrected with CPAP, which is assisted breathing that prevents collapse of the airway during sleep (Gugger et al. 2000). There are a number of other treatments, including surgery. Central apnea—when breathing is not obstructed, but results from a failure of the brain to tell the person to breathe—is more difficult to treat. We know of no alternative therapies for treating central apnea at this time.

Depression may cause insomnia and insomnia may exacerbate the misery of chronic depression, chronic pain, and aging. A study examined diagnosed depression and suicide rates in Harvard alumni during a follow-up period of 23–27 years. A total of 387 first attacks of depression occurred among 10,201 people who survived through 1988; 129 suicides occurred among 21,569 alumni during a follow-up through the same period. Lower rates of depression were found among the physically active and sports participants. Depression rates were higher among those who had personality traits such as insomnia, exhaustion, cuclothymia, and self-consciousness (Paffenbarger et al. 1994).

Smoking may also play a role in chronic insomnia. The study by Paffenbarger et al. (1994) found depression to be higher in smokers. A more recent study examined the relationship of mood disturbance to cigarette smoking among 252 people with a mood disorder. It was found that insomnia was positively associated with the number of cigarettes smoked a day. The researchers concluded that smokers suffered from higher levels of fatigue and experienced more severe symptoms of insomnia than nonsmokers (Patten et al. 2001).

It is very important to recognize that one of the early signs of depression is a change in sleep pattern. A person may not have all of the classic symptoms of a major depressive illness, but yet have disturbed sleep. When the depression is treated, the sleep normalizes (*please see the Depression protocol*).

Insomnia may also be part of climacteric syndrome, the constellation of symptoms that affect women during and after menopause. In a study of postmenopausal women with climacteric syndrome, the women who had the worst anxiety, insomnia, and depression symptoms were found to have a high cortisol/ dehydoepiandosterone (DHEA) ratio. (Cortisol is a hormone produced when the body is under stress. DHEA is a hormone recognized as being associated with an increase in perceived physical and psychological well-being.) In the study, 20 postmenopausal women (12 with and 8 without climacteric syndrome) were given Korean red ginseng. After 30 days of supplementation with Korean red ginseng, the women with climacteric syndrome had improved cortisol/DHEA ratios, better psychological test results, and improvement in fatigue, insomnia, and depression (Tode et al. 1999). Women who are experiencing insomnia thought to be anxiety- or stress-related may experience relief of their symptoms by taking Korean red ginseng (early in the day).

Another study found that low DHEA-S levels were associated with high degrees of self-rated disability and insomnia in the elderly. Men and women may have differing effects of DHEA supplementation and should therefore closely monitor their own feelings of how effective DHEA is when being used as an aid in relieving insomnia (Morrison et al. 1998). Like ginseng, DHEA should be taken early in the day so that any energy boosting effects occur during waking hours and not upon bedtime.

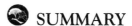 SUMMARY

Consider the following supplements based upon your overall health and physical responsiveness:

1. Try melatonin at the lowest effective dose before sleep.

2. Natural Sleep contains both immediate and timed-release melatonin along with other cofactors that promote sleep, 1–2 capsules before bedtime.

3. GABA helps promote sleep in some people, 1/4 tsp of powder before bedtime.

4. Valerian or passion flower may be taken on a limited basis before bedtime. Follow label dosage directions as extracts may vary in potency.

5. Folic acid at a dose of 5–10 mg daily may help control restless leg syndrome associated with insomnia.

6. Iron deficiency anemia may be a cause of insomnia. Blood testing and a recommendation from your physician are needed before taking an iron supplement.

7. Magnesium citrate may help induce sleep, 250 mg at bedtime.

8. DHEA levels decline with aging. DHEA may help reduce cortisol levels and also produce a feeling of well-being, 25–50 mg daily. Blood serum testing is recommended before starting DHEA therapy to establish baseline levels and eliminate the possibility of hormone-related cancer. Take DHEA early in the day.

9. Korean ginseng has been shown to relieve fatigue, insomnia, and depression, one 200-mg capsule twice daily with meals is recommended.

10. The following lifestyle changes may also relieve insomnia:

    - Avoid caffeine at least 6 hours before bedtime.
    - Avoid alcohol or smoking 2 hours before bedtime.
    - Get regular exercise, but at least 3 hours before bedtime.
    - Establish regular bedtime hours, waking up each morning at the same time.
    - Ensure that your bedtime routine is calming. Read or listen to soft music.
    - Do not use the bedroom to do work.
    - Learn to meditate.
    - Consider using a light sound machine to relax.
    - Consider using cranioelectroneural stimulation.
    - Consider specialized sleep tapes and CDs.

11. When all else fails, consider the judicious use of prescription drugs.

 FOR MORE INFORMATION

Contact the National Sleep Foundation, 1367 Connecticut Ave. NW, Department SCM, Washington, D.C. 20036. *GHB The Natural Mood Enhancer* by Ward Dean, John Morgenthaler, and Steven W. Fowkes is recommended reading.

 PRODUCT AVAILABILITY

To order Natural Sleep or other melatonin products, ginseng, folate products, DHEA, Iron Protein Plus, GABA, tryptophan, or magnesium citrate capsules, call (800) 544-4440 or order online at www.lef.org. Call (800) 456-9887 for specialized Sleep Tapes—Tools for Exploration.

Irritable Bowel Syndrome

Irritable bowel syndrome (IBS) is a functional bowel disorder that is characterized by a change in bowel habits with features of *disordered defecation* and *bowel distention* in the *absence of any demonstrable causes*. Chronic or recurrent gastrointestinal (GI) symptoms associated with this disorder include stool urgency, abdominal fullness, bloating, diarrhea alternating with constipation, and abdominal cramps that are relieved with defecation.

IBS is the most common intestinal disorder seen in physicians' offices today, affecting at least 22 million people in the United States and approximately 10–20% of all adults worldwide with a female predominance (Talley et al. 2002). According to the National Institute for Diabetes, Digestive and Kidney Disease (NIDDK), IBS causes 34,000 hospitalizations each year, 3.5 million physician office visits, and 2.2 million prescriptions; and results in 400,000 people becoming disabled. Reportedly, IBS patients have twice as many healthcare visits per year as age-matched controls (Levy et al. 2000). In the United States, IBS accounts for up to a 75% excess in healthcare visits that are for non-GI somatic (of the body) complaints (Levy et al. 2000). This is because the syndrome is associated with other somatic disorders. As a result, this syndrome alone poses a significant impact on heathcare costs. Individuals with IBS are absent from work three times more than other persons in the work force and they experience an overall impaired quality of life (Sperber et al. 1999; Markowitz et al. 2001). A familial predisposition of the syndrome has also been established (Talley et al. 2002; Gonsalkorale et al. 2003).

Psychiatric disorders such as major depression, anxiety, and somatoform (psychic in origin) disorders also occur in the majority of IBS patients. Whitehead et al. (2002) reported that these disorders occur in up to 94% of patients. Additionally, approximately 49% of patients with *fibromyalgia* were found to have IBS, as well as 51% of *chronic fatigue syndrome* patients; 50% of patients with *chronic pelvic pain*; and 64% of patients with *temporomandibular joint* (TMJ) *dysfunction*, according to special reports assembled by Whitehead et al. (2002). Clinical observation of these patients has found that worsening of IBS symptoms is correlated with an exacerbation of the psychiatric disorder. Other less frequently occurring conditions that have been associated with this disorder are numerous and include back pain, various gynecological disorders, and interstitial cystitis. The incidence of headache also occurs more frequently in patients who have IBS than in the general population. Additionally, patients with IBS often experience urinary dysfunction, sexual dysfunction, and altered sleep patterns (Whitehead et al. 2002).

SYMPTOMS AND DIAGNOSIS

Symptoms of IBS may include abdominal cramps, abdominal bloating, flatulence, belching, feeling of urgency or incomplete evacuation, abnormal stool frequency, diarrhea or constipation, or diarrhea alternating with constipation. In most instances, the IBS is either diarrhea predominant or constipation predominant. A diagnosis of IBS used to be made by ruling out all other causes of the patient's symptoms (a diagnosis of exclusion). Clinically, this still holds true. However, because the disorder is so common, three different criteria to assist in making the diagnosis have evolved during the past 3 decades: the Manning, Rome I, and Rome II criteria. Rome II, the most recent criteria, was created in 1992 as an adaptation of Rome I. Rome II has more stringent parameters. Critics of this newer set of standards argue that many cases of true IBS are left undiagnosed when only the Rome II criteria is used. Therefore, the criteria may be most useful for research purposes and are used clinically as an *aid* to diagnosis rather than as an *absolute*. (*Note:* A committee has been formed to re-evaluate the symptomatic criteria to create a Rome III and is expected to be published in 2006.)

The Rome II Criteria for the diagnosis of IBS include at least 12 or more weeks (which need not be consecutive) of abdominal discomfort or pain that has two of the following three features (Soffer 2003):

- Relieved by defecation
- Onset associated with a change in frequency of stool (greater than 3 times per day or less than three times per week)
- Onset associated with a change in form (appearance) of stool (lumpy/hard or loose/watery)

The following symptoms cumulatively support the diagnosis of IBS:

- Abnormal stool passage (straining, urgency or feeling of incomplete evacuation)

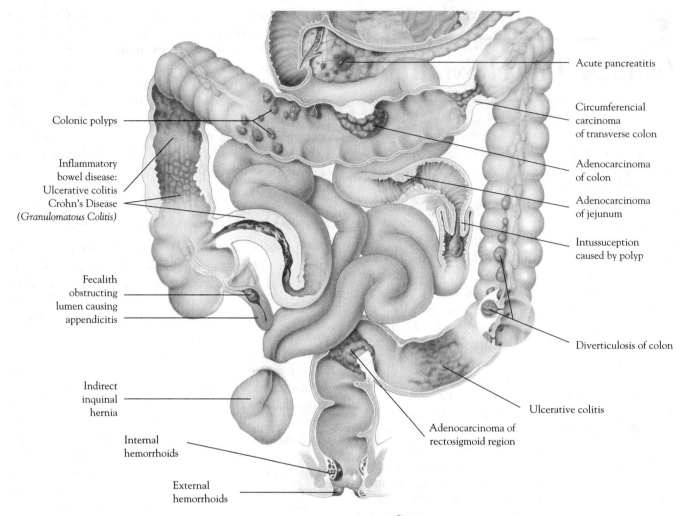

Colonic polyps

Inflammatory
bowel disease:
Ulcerative colitis
Crohn's Disease
(*Granulomatous Colitis*)

Fecalith
obstructing
lumen causing
appendicitis

Indirect
inquinal
hernia

Internal
hemorrhoids

External
hemorrhoids

Acute pancreatitis

Circumferencial
carcinoma
of transverse colon

Adenocarcinoma
of colon

Adenocarcinoma
of jejunum

Intussuception
caused by polyp

Diverticulosis of colon

Ulcerative colitis

Adenocarcinoma of
rectosigmoid region

Diseases and conditions of the lower intestinal tract. (Anatomical Chart Company 2002®, Lippincott Williams & Wilkins)

- Passage of mucus

- Bloating or feeling of abdominal distention

Organic diseases that may cause the symptoms should be considered before making the diagnosis. This is accomplished with a thorough medical history and physical examination by a well-trained physician. Based on the findings of the medical history and physical examination, the physician might consider ruling out infectious causes of the symptoms; malabsorption disorders such as lactose intolerance or lipid intolerance; other irritable bowel diseases such as ulcerative colitis or Crohn's disease, diverticulitis, and *Clostridium dificile* colitis; and endocrinopathies such as diabetes and thyroid disorders. Dietary influences should also be investigated. For example, a diet high in nonabsorbable artificial sweeteners can cause diarrhea. A diet low in fiber and fluids can cause constipation. In some instances, a physician may want to rule out colon cancer as well.

Surveillance with a colonoscopy or a rectosigmoidoscopy with a barium enema may be required to exclude other causes of the symptoms before making a diagnosis of IBS. Blood, stool, and imaging tests may also be indicated. However, a physician must use discretion in each patient to avoid unnecessary testing. Data reported by researchers in November 2002 support this discretion. Patients in the study who met the symptom-based criteria for IBS were *rarely* identified as having organic GI diseases. However, there was an increased incidence of celiac disease among IBS patients in that study (Cash et al. 2002).

ETIOLOGY AND PATHOPHYSIOLOGY

To date, three of the most important mechanisms that contribute to the development of IBS include an altered visceral perception (pain) in the gut, disturbed

GI motility (resulting in cramps, diarrhea, and/or constipation), and psychosocial factors (such as chronic stress, anxiety, and depression). Other significant factors implicated in the etiology of IBS include recent GI infection, inflammation of the GI mucosa, and alteration in the intestinal ecosystem (De Schryver et al. 2000; Talley et al. 2002).

Great strides have been made regarding the pathophysiology of IBS during the past several years. Numerous studies have demonstrated that IBS is characterized by visceral hypersensitivity, suggesting that patients with IBS may have more sensitive pain receptors in the GI tract than age-matched controls. These studies strongly suggest that alteration in communication between the nervous system and the immune system in the GI tract may trigger a series of events that give rise to chronic changes in visceral sensitivity, causing the affected individual to have highly sensitive pain receptors in the GI tract. Animal studies have demonstrated that gas in the bowel stretching the bowel wall causes psychological stress and can also cause an increase in the sensitization of visceral receptors, which results in a lower threshold for pain (Delvaux 1999).

Researchers exploring the causes of IBS, fibromyalgia, and the chronic fatigue syndrome have proposed that the cause may be due to a neuroendocrine-immune system dysfunction that is characterized by a complex integration of pathways that connect the nervous, endocrine, and immune systems to the GI tract (Mayer et al. 2001a, 2001b; Ringel et al. 2001; Chang et al. 2002). This connection is, in part, mediated by the neurotransmitter serotonin (Goldberg et al. 1996). The relationship is particularly interesting because these disorders often coexist, and the likelihood of a common etiology cannot be overlooked (Whitehead et al. 2002).

Monga et al. (1997) discovered that women with IBS have lower bladder and esophageal sensory thresholds, suggesting that there may be an underlying smooth muscle hyperreactivity disorder that is related to the autonomic nervous system. This explains the increased incidence of coexisting IBS with an irritable bladder condition and gastroesophageal reflux disease (GERD). The hypothesis deserves further investigation.

Regardless of whether it is *diarrhea predominant* or *constipation predominant*, IBS is frequently associated with depression and anxiety, and the symptoms of IBS may be exacerbated by stress (Chang et al. 1997). Studies have been inconclusive regarding which comes first, IBS or the psychological stressors. To date, it is believed that either can come first; however, IBS can be exacerbated by psychological stressors in either instance (Yehuda et al. 2002).

A focus of attention among researchers has also been on the pathways that connect the nervous system and the GI tract. It has been established that activities in the GI tract such as inflammation, infection, hypermotility, or changes in visceral sensitivity affect the nervous system. Conversely, psychosocial stressors such as stress, anxiety, and depression that manifest in the central nervous system (CNS) are transmitted to the bowel by various pathways. This gut-brain connection has provided a basis for new therapeutic approaches to IBS (Monnikes et al. 2001).

Several studies have suggested that infection and inflammation in the GI tract cause changes in the intestinal physiology that can persist after the infection and inflammation have resolved. The altered intestinal lining that is left after the inflammation has resolved is believed to trigger a neuroimmune interaction that may be implemented in the pathogenesis of some IBS patients (Yehuda et al. 2002).

Researchers have found that cells that mediate inflammation have been found very close to nerve endings in the intestinal lining of animals (Tornblom et al. 2002). Inflammation in the GI mucosa has been found to coexist with a degeneration of intestinal nerves of IBS patients (Tornblom et al. 2002). These findings have been implemented in the pathogenesis of this syndrome and provide a basis for further investigation.

Another discovery still under investigation is that symptoms are possibly mediated through partial degranulation of mast cells (mediators of inflammation) in the bowel mucosa (Bodemar et al. 2001). Yang et al. (1997) found an increase in mast cells in the bowel mucosa (specifically in the cecum and ileojejunal junction) of animals with IBS. These mast cells were often located very close to unmyelinated nerves, suggesting that mast cell stabilizers or the antagonism of mast cell products may have potential therapeutic applications in IBS (Yang et al. 1997).

The pathways that connect the brain and the gut are mediated by intrinsic neuroreceptors called 5-hydroxytryptamine-3 (5-HT3) and 5-hydroxytryptamine-4 (5-HT4). These serotonin receptors are involved in both the modulation of visceral pain and regulation of GI motility that cause diarrhea, constipation and urgency. Because patients with IBS have both *hypermotility* of the smooth muscle of the bowel and *hypersensitivity* to visceral pain, a new class of therapeutic agents targets the modulation of these serotonin receptors in the bowel

(Goldberg et al. 1996; Sanger et al. 1998; Houghton et al. 1999). This new class of serotonin receptor medications will be discussed later in the protocol.

Over the past 30 years, numerous studies have looked at the overlap between IBS and psychiatric disorders. These studies found that 54–94% of IBS patients meet the diagnostic criteria for at least one psychiatric disorder. Major depression followed by generalized anxiety disorder rank among the most commonly associated psychiatric conditions associated with IBS. Consequently, selective serotonin reuptake inhibitors (SSRIs) that are used to treat depression have been used to treat IBS because serotonin is involved peripherally in the regulation of motility and sensation in the gut and centrally in mood disorders (Whitehead et al. 2002).

Interestingly, a history of sexual abuse and to a lesser degree physical abuse is more common in patients with IBS than in patients with other GI conditions; however, this *does not mean* that a patient with IBS has been sexually abused. The only explanation found so far is that there is an overall increase in somatic complaints among abused persons (Walker et al. 1993; Talley et al. 1995; Blanchard et al. 2002).

TREATMENT OPTIONS

Conventional Drug Treatment

Traditionally, IBS has been treated symptomatically with agents that relax the intestinal smooth muscle to relieve abdominal cramps that are associated with muscle spasms (Bentyl, Levsin, or Levsinex), antidepressants to target associated depression and anxiety (SSRIs such as Prozac or Paxil) in patients who exhibit those co-morbid conditions, antidiarrheal agents in patients who have diarrhea (Lomotil or Immodium), and bulk-forming laxatives and fiber (Metamucil or guar gum) in patients who have constipation. Unfortunately, no panacea has been found to date that consistently relieves the symptoms, and many patients continue to suffer the consequences of poor quality of life. As more information becomes available about the exact etiology of the symptoms, researchers can delve into a potential cure. However, as described earlier in this protocol, the etiology and pathophysiology appear to be a complicated integration of several systems. On a more positive note, breakthroughs regarding how the systems integrate have been enormous in the past decade and it appears that investigators are on the brink of putting together the entire picture in the next decade. More recently, newer classes of agents that modulate the serotonin receptors 5-HT3 and 5-HT4 have been used.

Tegaserod maleate (Zelnorm) was approved for the treatment of IBS in July 2002. Tegaserod is a 5-HT4 receptor partial agonist that increases GI motility. This medication is used for short-term treatment of women with *constipation predominant* IBS. Although the drug is probably just as effective in men as in women, the drug was approved specifically for women because the clinical trials that were used to obtain FDA approval consisted of 2470 women and no men.

This prescriptive medication should only be given to adults who are over the age of 18. It should be taken before meals in a dose of 6 mg twice daily for 4–6 weeks. If the patient responds to this drug therapy, a physician may consider an additional 4- to 6-week course of drug therapy. Contraindications to the use of tegaserod maleate include severe liver impairment, severe kidney impairment, history of bowel obstruction, symptomatic gallbladder disease, suspected sphincter of Oddi dysfunction, and abdominal adhesions. Tegaserod maleate should not be initiated in patients who are currently experiencing or frequently experiencing diarrhea. Common adverse reactions include abdominal pain, diarrhea, nausea, flatulence, and headache and back pain (PDR 2002). (**Note:** Tegaserod meleate will be under close observation by the FDA because medications that affect the serotonin system have historically been associated with side effects.)

Alosetron HCL (Lotrinex), a 5-HT3 antagonist, is indicated for women with severe *diarrhea-predominant* IBS who have had chronic IBS symptoms for more than 6 months, have been refractory to conventional therapy, have been excluded from anatomic or biochemical abnormalities of the GI tract, and who have frequent and severe abdominal pain/discomfort, frequent bowel urgency/fecal incontinence, and severely impaired quality of life and restriction of activities of daily living due the symptoms of IBS.

The FDA initially approved Alosetron in February 2000. Within 8 months of being on the market, numerous reports of ischemic colitis (a potentially lethal condition characterized by a blockage of blood supply to the intestines) were associated with this drug. Alosetron HCL was also responsible for causing severe constipation in many persons who used the drug. Four deaths have been linked to Alosetron HCL. The severity and frequency of these side effects resulted in the drug being withdrawn from the market by its sponsor. On June 7, 2002, the FDA issued a supplemental new drug application that allows Alosetron to be marketed through a prescribing program that specifies the restrictions for its use listed above. This prescribing program requires an attestation and qualification form signed by the prescribing physician and an informed consent form signed by the patient.

An editorial report in the September 2002 issue of *The British Medical Journal* estimates that under this present program, approximately 2 million people in the United States will be approved to take Alosetron. According to previously reported statistics, this would result in 2,000 cases of severe constipation, 5,714 cases of ischemic colitis, 11,090 surgical interventions, and 324 deaths. The decision by the FDA to allow this medication back on the market was made in spite of strong opposition that is still ongoing. Opponents argue that this is a serious and significant public health concern and the risks of using Alosetron may outweigh potential therapeutic benefits. However, Alosetron has proven to be a miracle drug for many who could not obtain relief from other traditional therapies and who did not experience side effects from taking this medication. The FDA will closely monitor reports of adverse events of Alosetron in the future (Lievre 2002).

Drugs on the Horizon

Additional drugs that affect the serotonin receptors similarly to Tegaserod and Alosetron are currently under investigation by competing pharmaceutical companies and may become available in the future.

Other medications that may soon become available to treat *diarrhea predominant* IBS are the more selective antispasmodics—M3-receptor antagonists such as Zamifenacin—and darifenacin in *constipation-predominant* IBS. Clinical trials are ongoing to test these drugs.

In addition, the role of inflammatory cytokines such as tumor necrosis factor alpha, interleukin-6, interleukin 1(b), and leukotriene B(4) in the inflammation of the intestinal tract of IBS patients should be investigated.

Psychosocial factors such as stress reduction and the effect of anxiety and depression should be addressed in every patient with IBS. Additionally, studies have shown that the physician/patient relationship is especially important for IBS patients. Physician/patient support is an essential part of treatment and cannot be overlooked (De Schryver et al. 2000).

Natural Therapies

Peppermint and Caraway Oil in Combination

An enteric-coated peppermint/caraway oil combination (sold under the name Regimint) has been used successfully to treat cramps and abdominal pain associated with IBS. This combination acts locally to relax the smooth muscle of the intestines. The enteric coating allows the oil to bypass digestion in the stomach where the acid environment would otherwise destroy the active ingredient so that it can be delivered to the site where pain and cramping are located. (**Note:** Uncoated peppermint oil ingested orally has an undesirable side effect of relaxing the gastroesophageal sphincter that allows food to enter from the esophagus to the stomach during digestion. Relaxation of this sphincter causes backflow of food and acid from the stomach into the esophagus, a condition called gastroesophageal reflux disorder or GERD. The enteric coating on the fixed combination of peppermint/caraway oil prevents this side effect.)

This fixed peppermint/caraway herbal combination has offered significant relief for many persons who experience the debilitating effects of IBS and cannot get results from traditional medications. The product, when taken as directed, is also considered to be safe and well tolerated. The combination was initially used in Germany where it was approved by a government authority (the German Kommission E) equivalent to the United States FDA.

A *fixed combination* is defined as a formula containing multiple herbal ingredients, prepared consistently in exactly the same proportions. To be approved by the German Kommission E, the combination must show the following: each active component must make a positive contribution to the evaluation of the whole preparation, proof of effectiveness should be established by clinical documentation for each component or for the whole preparation, the components of the fixed combination must have an established dosage for appropriate effectiveness, and the safety of all fixed combinations is to be tested by suitable methods. Approved fixed combinations can be advantageous over single herbs if the therapeutic effectiveness is increased or if the side effects of a single component are lessened or negated. Currently, the largest category of use for approved fixed combinations is for digestive complaints (35 combinations).

Studies conducted over the past 20 years support the use of enteric-coated peppermint oil alone for the treatment of IBS symptoms. As early as 1979, a multi-centered, double-blind, crossover trial conducted by Rees et al. demonstrated that peppermint oil was superior to placebo for relieving symptoms of irritable bowel syndrome. The active ingredient in peppermint oil (menthol) relaxes the intestinal smooth muscle, relieving spasms of the bowel (Dew et al. 1984). Although multiple well-designed studies support the use of enteric-coated peppermint oil for the treatment of IBS, one compelling study using the herbal combination of enteric-coated peppermint oil and caraway oil strongly favored the use of this combination over the use of peppermint oil alone. This is based on a review of the literature, which suggests that it was the most effective treatment, producing the best relief in the shortest duration of time.

In a clinical trial using a fixed combination of peppermint/caraway oil, 45 patients with nonulcer dyspepsia (the majority with IBS) were studied in a double-blind placebo-controlled trial. The test group took 1 capsule, 3 times daily, for a period of 4 weeks. Each capsule contained 90 mg of peppermint oil and 50 mg of caraway oil. While all patients complained of moderate to severe pain before the commencement of therapy, almost one half of the patients (42.1%) in the test group were pain-free in just 2 weeks after taking the combination therapy. Only one patient (5%) in the placebo group reported freedom from pain. After 4 weeks of treatment, 63% of the patients were pain-free; and 89% showed improvement in the test group vs. 25% in the placebo group. With regard to clinical global impression, 95% of the test group showed overall improvement in their condition (May et al. 1996). Similarly, physicians and naturopaths who have used the enteric preparation of peppermint oil and caraway oil for the treatment of IBS symptoms have reported improved clinical outcomes for their patients.

Probiotics

Probiotics are a dietary supplement consisting of beneficial bacterial flora that normally inhabit the small and large intestines. These beneficial bacteria compete with *pathological* bacteria to maintain a balanced ecosystem in the intestines. This balanced ecosystem is responsible for the production of digestive enzymes such as lactase to digest dairy products and is considered a significant part of the immune system that is present in the GI tract. When we consume medications such as antibiotics or steroids, this ecosystem is disrupted. Antibiotics, which are often over-prescribed, destroy not only pathological microorganisms, but also the beneficial ones. This causes an overgrowth of yeast in the intestines, resulting in inflammation of the GI mucosa on the walls of the intestines. This condition adversely affects the absorption of nutrients (such as dairy products) during digestion, causing gas and bloating and sometimes abdominal pain after meals.

In time, the disruption of normal intestinal flora adversely affects the immune system. Steroids, which have potent anti-inflammatory properties, exert negative effects on the immune system in the intestines as well as contributing to the overgrowth of yeast microorganisms. This condition is called leaky gut syndrome or dysbiosis. Lactose intolerance can be created by this syndrome due to a lack of the digestive enzyme lactase that is naturally produced by beneficial gut flora. When flora is diminished, symptoms of lactose (milk sugar) intolerance can develop. Consequently, IBS symptoms can be improved by the ingestion of digestive enzymes that include lactase.

Leaky gut syndrome is believed to be the cause of many of the symptoms in IBS patients. Unfortunately, the evidence-based literature does not support this concept because little research has been done to examine this cause/effect relationship. However, studies have shown that probiotics administered to patients with irritable bowel disease (colitis or Crohn's disease) resulted in improvement in symptoms. If inflammation is part of the pathoetiology of IBS, this process would likely be the culprit in many instances of IBS (Shanahan 2001). **Note:** Research on the subject of irritable bowel disease and prebiotics-probiotics shows that prebiotics increase the numbers of *Lactobacilli acidophilus* and *Bifidobacterium*. *Bifidobacteria* are more likely to reside in the large intestine, with *Lactobacilli acidophilus* residing primarily in the small intestine. The digestive tract primarily contains *Bifidobacteria* until the age of 5; after age 5, *Lactobacillus acidophilus* becomes more prominent in the small intestines and *Bifidobacterium* remains more prevalent in the large intestines. (Prebiotics are most often fiber- or sugar-based nutrients that pass through the stomach and small intestine undigested. In the large intestine, they nurture and promote the growth of beneficial probiotic species by positively affecting the pH balance of the gut.)

Clinical experience in physicians' practices has supported the cause and effect relationship between IBS and inflammation because patients with IBS symptoms frequently improve when they take probiotics (Niedzielin et al. 2001; Marteau 2002; Sach et al. 2002) with digestive enzymes. Some experts in this field claim that probiotics should be taken with prebiotics called fructo-oligosaccharides (FOS). FOS serve as food for the beneficial bacteria to feed on, allowing them to proliferate and adhere to the bowel wall (Sghir et al. 1998).

Other authorities argue that FOS that feed the good bacteria also feed yeast, but there appears to be no support for this argument. A stool digestive analysis for bacterial flora and yeast, performed by the Great Smokies Diagnostics Laboratory (GSDL) can aid in the treatment plan. This is not a standard test and most traditional physicians are not familiar with it. Controversy also exists regarding the type of bacterial flora that one should consume. Most probiotics consist of *Lactobacillus acidophilus* and *Bifidobacterium* species as well as a host of other beneficial bacteria. Some authorities maintain that one type of bacterial species such as *Lactobacillus acidophilus* is preferred so that the organisms do not compete with each other. Others claim that it is best to use a combination of several beneficial strains.

In either case, the supplement should contain at least 3 billion microorganisms of bacteria because the shelf life is limited. The expiration date of the bottle should also be checked. The product often requires refrigeration to preserve the bacteria, but some do not. If yeast is present, a Candida diet can be helpful. This diet may be found in the *Candida* protocol in this book. It can take up to 9 months of daily treatment for leaky gut syndrome for gut flora to be completely restored. In refractory cases where overgrowth of yeast is severe, an antifungal prescription medication such as Nystatin or Diflucan may be necessary to eradicate the yeast.

An example of a remarkable clinical case history demonstrates the benefits of restoring the gut flora in a patient with severe abdominal pain resembling a clinical picture of IBS. For this patient, every test had been performed to rule out the cause of the patient's excruciating, debilitating pain, which came in waves of exacerbations and remissions. All tests were negative. Medications had failed to consistently relieve the symptoms. The patient finally had a surgical procedure (an exploratory laparoscopy) of the abdomen and pelvis to look for a cause. Some adhesions (scars) from a previous surgery were removed and were thought to be the cause. However, a few months later, the symptoms of severe abdominal pain returned. In a desperate attempt to try anything, the physician gave the patient probiotics and digestive enzymes. The symptoms never returned. This clinical case history is one of many seen in physicians' offices.

Without a doubt, more documented research needs to be done to support the use of probiotics in clinical practice. When this research is done, perhaps more physicians will use this functional medicine concept in their clinical approach to IBS and fewer patients will have to suffer as a result.

Enzymes and Laxatives

Digestive enzymes and nutrients that enhance bile flow from the liver may aid in digestion and enhance the transit time of food through the GI tract. Digestive enzyme capsules and artichoke-black radish tablets should be taken five minutes before meals to enhance digestion and improve bowel function.

Bulk-forming laxatives such as psyllium as well as the soluble fiber guar gum have been shown to be effective in some patients with constipation-predominant IBS. In one bulk laxative study, soluble fiber (guar gum) and insoluble fiber (bran) were compared to determine which one was more effective in relieving symptoms with the fewest side effects. Patients preferred guar gum, although bran was also effective. Guar gum was found to be more tolerable and less irritating to the bowel. At least three other studies have shown that bran supplementation either exacerbated symptoms or did nothing other than relieving constipation (Cann et al. 1984; Francis et al. 1994; Snook et al. 1994).

Those suffering from *constipation-predominant* IBS may not benefit from bulk forming laxatives. They may, instead, need to judiciously use natural therapies that can induce rapid peristalsis in order to completely evacuate their bowels. One such therapy is to mix in an eight-ounce glass of water a powdered vitamin C supplement that is buffered with potassium or magnesium and drink this on an empty stomach. There are several natural laxative approaches to enhancing peristalsis that are discussed in the *Constipation* protocol of this book.

Dietary Intervention

Various diets have been proposed for IBS patients and they may be worth trying. For patients who have Candida in the bowel, a "Candida diet" should be used. This diet, which consists of avoiding sugary and starchy foods, can be found in the *Candida* protocol in this book. The best way to determine if Candida is present is by a digestive stool analysis performed by Great Smokies Diagnostics Laboratory, which looks specifically for Candida and other yeast-like organisms. Patients who experience a great deal of gas and bloating should eliminate gas-forming foods such as beans and other legumes, cabbage, cauliflower, broccoli, onions, and garlic. Patients who are allergic may obtain good results by using a diet that eliminates all suspected allergens from food.

Many patients who have IBS-like symptoms may indeed have celiac disease (also known as gluten intolerance or gluten allergy). Gluten is a protein found in wheat and other grains. Gluten intolerance can be diagnosed with specific tests performed in a physician's office. If gluten intolerance is the cause of symptoms, a diet free of gluten is often the prescribed treatment. All foods containing wheat, rye, or barley must be avoided. Avoiding products with oats should also be considered. Specially manufactured substitute foods are available, including gluten-free bread, flour, and pasta. There is no restriction of meat, fish, eggs, and dairy products; vegetables; fruits; and rice and corn.

Additionally, *L*-glutamine can aid in restoring the lining of the colon in patients who have inflammation as part of the etiology of their disorder. However, clinical trials have not been established to date to demonstrate the efficacy of this supplement for the treatment of IBS. Biopsies often show no inflammation of the intestinal mucosa in patients with IBS.

Nondietary Interventions

Certain lifestyle changes may be helpful in relieving IBS symptoms that are related to stress and depression. Massage, meditation, walking, and changes in life routine can be important factors in treatment. Acupuncture has also been helpful to some patients.

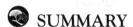 **SUMMARY**

Irritable bowel syndrome (IBS) that affects both the small and large intestines causes impaired quality of life in a significant percentage of the population, with approximately 5% of persons with this syndrome experiencing severe symptoms refractory to current therapies. While significant discoveries have been made about the etiology and pathophysiology of IBS in the past decade, researchers have a long way to go before clearly understanding the complex integrative pathways that link the immune, nervous, and endocrine systems with the GI tract. Additionally, research has suggested that there is a correlation between recent GI inflammation and bowel motility disorder with symptoms of IBS.

Soon these systems may be linked with the inflammation and bowel motility disorder in such a way that a basis for new therapies will be created. Investigators have found the specific receptor sites that are responsible for regulation of GI tract motility and the sensation of pain in the GI tract. With this information, a new class of medication has been created. Unfortunately, side effects are of concern in one of the two approved medications, and the second medication is being carefully watched for reported side effects. Natural supplements, including peppermint and caraway oil combinations, probiotics, and digestive enzymes, have been successfully used to improve symptoms in these patients. These natural remedies are often more effective than currently available prescription medications and have no known side effects when taken in appropriate doses.

IBS is so prevalent that several conventional and alternative approaches are available. The key to finding a solution is to use a daily regimen that addresses your individual needs.

Several prescription drugs have been discussed, but most people prefer to try natural-based therapies first before resorting to drugs that may induce side effects. The following natural therapies were discussed:

1. Enteric-coated peppermint/caraway oil (sold under the name Regimint); 1 capsule, 3 times daily, to relax spastic bowel wall muscle.

2. Super Digestive Enzymes; take 2 capsules 5 minutes before the beginning of each meal to diminish excess gas and bloating caused by a deficiency of digestive enzymes. The deficiency results from diminished bowel flora that make these enzymes. Two tablets of Digest RC® (that contain artichoke, black radish, and other digestive aids) can also be taken 5 minutes before meals to facilitate digestion and transport food through the intestinal tract. Refer to the *Digestive Disorders* protocol for additional information about digestive enzymes and bile-enhancing supplements.

3. Soluble fiber; take psyllium guar gum, 1000–3000 mg, with each meal to aid in constipation. Some people with *constipation-predominant* IBS have insufficient peristalsis and have difficulty eliminating fiber. Those who have insufficient peristalsis should consider the nutritional laxatives discussed in the *Constipation* protocol in this book.

4. *L*-Glutamine; take two 500-mg capsules 3 times daily, with each meal, to rejuvenate the bowel mucosa in IBS associated with inflammation.

5. EPA fish oil capsules; take 2 capsules with each meal 3 times per day to decrease inflammation in the bowel mucosa if inflammation appears to be an apparent cause (i.e., post-infection or if there is some other inflammatory condition present).

6. Probiotics and prebiotics may be taken to decrease inflammation and restore gut ecosystem by replenishing the beneficial bowel flora. Choose from three probiotics: Jarro-Dophilus, 1–2 capsules daily, preferably on an empty stomach; Life Flora Mix, 1 capsule 4 times daily for 5 days, then 1 capsule daily; or Primal Defense, 1 capsule, 3 times per day, increasing to 6–12 capsules daily over a period of 2 months as tolerated or as directed by a physician.

7. Persons with *constipation-predominant* IBS should refer to the *Constipation* protocol in this book for specific recommendations. There are several natural therapies that can induce rapid peristalsis resulting in complete evacuation of the bowels. One of the natural laxative therapies involves mixing several teaspoons of a powder that contains ascorbic acid, potassium, and/or magnesium powder into an 8-oz glass of water and drinking it on an empty stomach. Some people require a second 8-oz glass of water mixed with this buffered vitamin C powder. Rapid evacuation usually occurs within 60 minutes, though there may be a residual diarrhea effect.

8. Dietary recommendations described in this protocol are dependent on the individual needs of a person who has IBS.

Editor's Note: This protocol was researched and written by Michele Morrow, D.O., F.A.A.F.P., Family Physician and Medical Consultant to the Life Extension Foundation.

 PRODUCT AVAILABILITY

Regiment (peppermint/caraway oil combination), Digest RC, buffered vitamin C powder and other nutritional laxatives, probiotics, prebiotics, digestive enzymes, soluble fibers, glutamine, EPA fish oil, and other supplements discussed in this protocol may be ordered by calling (800) 544-4440 or by logging on to www.lef.org. Many conventional therapies require a prescription drug from your physician.

were responsible for the immune system-enhancing effects. Next, they discovered that alkylglycerols are found in the livers of cold-water sharks, such as the Greenland Shark. The shark in general has attracted attention because cancer occurrence is very rare in sharks. The existence of alkylglycerols in the liver of sharks may be one reason for the natural immunity to cancers.

The biologic effects of shark liver oil include stimulation of blood leukocyte and thrombocyte production (Le Blanc et al. 1995), as well as the activation of macrophage and antitumor activity. Other effects include the ability to protect against radiation damage during radiation therapy for various types of cancer. Alkylglycerols act as a powerful immune system booster against infectious disease and help give nursing animals, including breast-fed babies, protection against infection until their own immune systems can fully develop.

In a study published in the *Journal of Cell Physiology* (February 1999), Wang et al. studied the cell differentiation-promoting potential of a particular type of alkylglycerol on human colon cancer cells. The scientists wanted to observe the ability of alkylglycerols to change the biological makeup of human colon cancer cells. Alkylglycerols were shown to ". . . promote a more benign or differentiated phenotype in colon cancer cells." Treatment of the cancer cells with alkylglycerols resulted in a reduction of cellular proliferation and a reduced capacity for cellular invasion. In other words, alkylglycerols led to lowered cancer cell reproduction and a reduced ability of the cancer cells to invade healthy cells. The authors concluded that alkylglycerols possess both cancer preventative properties, as well as cancer treatment effects (Wang et al. 1999).

Shark liver oil has been around for 40 years and has been used as both a preventive and therapeutic agent. Not only have alkylglycerols been used to treat leukemia, as in the case of the children in Sweden, but they have also been used to prevent radiation sickness stemming from radiation cancer treatments. Furthermore, the high level of alkylglycerols that exist naturally within any given tumor cell has led scientists to postulate that this may be an apparent attempt of the body to control cell growth. Protein kinase C, an essential step in cancer cell growth, can actually be stopped or inhibited by alkylglycerols. In addition, it has been suggested that alkylglycerols directly act on the macrophages (large immune cells that "gobble up" cancer cells). Overall, alkylglycerols are able to stimulate the macrophage to secrete more than 50 substances concerned directly or indirectly with the immune system. Some of these substances, the interleukins, are powerful immune system fighters that interact with lymphocytes (Pugliese et al. 1998; 1999).

Resveratrol

Resveratrol, a phytoextract found in grapes and red wine may act as a chemotherapeutic agent and inhibit the growth of various leukemia and melanoma cell lines.

Resveratrol is a plant polyphenol found in grapes and red wine. A study published in the journal *Blood* indicates that resveratrol effectively inhibits acute myelogenous leukemia (AML) cells *in vitro* through several differentiating properties: blocking activation of nuclear transcription factor NF-kB, inhibiting proliferation, causing S-phase arrest, and inducing apoptosis. This suggests that resveratrol may have a role as a therapeutic agent in the treatment of AML (Estrov et al. 2003).

Asou et al. studied the *in vitro* activity of resveratrol on acute myeloid leukemia by examining its effect on proliferation and differentiation in various cell lines and in fresh samples of 17 AML patients. Used alone, resveratrol inhibited the growth of all AML cells. The authors concluded that resveratrol inhibits proliferation and induces differentiation of myeloid leukemia cells (Asov et al. 2002).

Niles et al. examined the effect of resveratrol on the growth of two human melanoma cell lines. They found it inhibited growth and induced apoptosis in both cell lines with one (A375) being more sensitive. The authors concluded that resveratrol may be effective as either a therapeutic or chemopreventive agent (Niles et al. 2003).

From the in vitro studies cited above, an appropriate human dosage cannot be extrapolated.

Monthly Blood Markers

Because all cancer therapies produce individual responses based on factors such as the type of disease, patient's age, and the presence of other diseases, the Foundation recommends monthly blood markers and other diagnostic testing to monitor the benefits of any supplemental therapies. The results of these tests provide critical information to evaluate the effectiveness of nonconventional therapies. If tumor indicators do not decrease after the initiation of any nonconventional therapy, patients should discontinue their use and seek other alternatives immediately.

Inhibiting Protein-Tyrosine Kinase with Gleevec

In the various cancer protocols discussed in this book, references are made to nutrients like curcumin, genistein, and tocopherol succinate that function as protein-tyrosine kinase inhibitors. Because tyrosine kinases induce hyperproliferation of cancer cells, inhibiting these kinases has been shown to slow cancer cell propagation.

A drug called Gleevec (formerly known as STI 571) is a protein-tyrosine kinase inhibitor that specifically interferes with the Bcr-Abl tyrosine kinase—the typical chromosomal abnormality seen in chronic myeloid leukemia (CML). Gleevec inhibits proliferation and induces apoptosis in Bcr-Abl cell lines as well as fresh leukemic cells from "Philadelphia chromosome positive" chronic myeloid leukemia (CML). Gleevec may also inhibit growth of other types of cancer cells.

Gleevec (imatinib mesylate) was first made available to patients with chronic myeloid leukemia (CML) in May 2001 after the results of exciting clinical studies were released in Europe. Gleevec is indicated for the treatment of patients with Philadelphia chromosome positive (Ph+) chronic myeloid leukemia (CML) in blast crisis, accelerated phase, or in chronic phase after failure of interferon-alpha therapy.

The effectiveness of Gleevec is continuously being evaluated for efficacy, though it is now an FDA-approved drug. To read about the latest findings on Gleevec, log on to a special website www.gleevec.com.

It is interesting to note that a drug that functions along a similar mechanism as certain dietary supplements was put on the FDA's "fast-track" for approval.

⬤ CONCLUSION

Leukemia, Hodgkin's lymphoma, and non-Hodgkin's lymphoma generally respond well to conventional therapies. There are many different types of these diseases; therefore, chemotherapy and radiation therapy are individualized. Patients who do not respond well to chemotherapy and radiation therapy may benefit from other treatments such as bone marrow transplantation or a peripheral blood stem-cell transplant. In addition to conventional treatment, there are a number of alternative therapies available. Patients with certain types of leukemia or lymphoma may derive beneficial effects from Vesanoid, vitamin A, vitamin D3, curcumin, green tea, and soy extracts. It is imperative that patients have regular monitoring of tumor markers (or tumor size) to assess the usefulness of any treatment. Consult your hematologist or oncologist prior to initiating alternative treatments.

⬤ SUMMARY

1. Early diagnosis and treatment of leukemias and lymphomas are essential. Symptoms of leukemia and lymphoma are generalized and include fatigue, weight loss, fever, and night sweats. In Hodgkin's and non-Hodgkin's lymphomas, swollen lymph nodes may be present.

2. Diagnosis of the specific disease may include MRI scans, CT scans, and biopsy.

3. Chemotherapy and radiation therapy are usually used in combination to treat these diseases. The actual course of therapy depends on the specific type of disease.

4. Interferon-alpha, a biologic response modifier has been proven effective in the treatment of some leukemias and low-grade lymphomas.

5. Patients who do not respond to chemotherapy and radiation therapy may be considered for peripheral blood stem-cell transplants or bone marrow transplants.

6. Vesanoid, a vitamin A analog, has proven effective in patients with chronic promyelocytic leukemia and may be beneficial for other types of cancers. For chronic myeloid leukemia (CML), ask your doctor about Gleevec.

7. Water-soluble vitamin A may provide a useful alternative to Vesanoid for some cancer patients. The recommended dosage of this vitamin is 100,000–300,000 IU daily.

CAUTION Monthly blood tests are necessary to avoid vitamin A toxicity.

8. Vitamin D3 and its analogs may induce differentiation of cancer cells into normal cells in certain types of lymphomas and leukemias. A high dose to consider is 4000–6000 IU daily.

CAUTION Serum calcium, kidney function, and liver function should be monitored monthly to avoid vitamin D toxicity.

9. Curcumin may induce cancer cell death via a blockade of various signal transduction pathways. The recommended daily dosage is four 900-mg capsules 3 times daily with food, taken 2 hours apart from all medications.

CAUTION Patients with biliary tract obstruction should not take curcumin. High doses of curcumin may induce NSAID-like side effects in the stomach.

10. Green tea extract providing high amounts of epigallocatechin gallate (EGCG) suppress VEGF and other growth factors used by cancer cells to escape regulatory control. An appropriate dose for VEGF blockade would be 5 capsules of the lightly caffeinated Super Green Tea Extract capsules with each meal. Each capsule provides 100 mg of the critical anticancer polyphenol called EGCG. Caffeine has been shown to potentiate tea polyphenols, such as EGCG. Because caffeine can keep some people awake at night, it might be preferable to take 5 decaffeinated Super Green Tea Extract capsules as the evening dose, or use decaffeinated green tea exclusively if hypersensitive to caffeine.

11. Patients who are positive for mutant p53 oncogenes may receive substantial benefits from the use of soy extracts. Soy extract high in genistein, such as Ultra Soy Extract, may inhibit cancer cell growth for a number of types of cancer. Recommended daily dosage of Ultra Soy Extract is five 700-mg 40% isoflavone extract capsules taken four times a day.

12. DHEA replacement therapy may be considered. Blood testing is recommended prior to and during therapy (*refer to DHEA Replacement Therapy for more information*).

13. Alpha-lipoic acid may help activate the enzyme caspase, which kills leukemia cells. It may also suppress the cancer gene c-fos. People on a chemotherapeutic regimen should discuss the use of alpha-lipoic acid with their oncologist before taking this supplement. Typical doses of alpha-lipoic acid for cancer patients are 500 mg twice a day.

14. Shark liver oil functions via several mechanisms to suppress cancer growth, enhance immune function, and protect against radiation damage. We recommend five or six 1000-mg capsules (containing 200 mg of alkylglycerols each) daily for a period not to exceed 30 days.

CAUTION At no time should the maximum recommended dose of shark liver oil be exceeded. In the case of chronic use, more than 30 consecutive days, a possible, albeit rare, side effect known as thrombocythemia (excess thrombocytes) can occur, leading to a tendency for the blood to clot. This condition is easily diagnosed with a blood test and reversed with lower dosages, the addition of a low-dose aspirin (81 mg daily), or omega-3 fatty acid supplementation. Consult with your physician if thrombocythemia is a consideration or if you are using shark liver oil for the treatment of serious disease states. Other than the rare instance of blood clotting at chronic high doses, the alkylglycerols found in shark oil are remarkably nontoxic.

15. GLA/DHA may be taken for the suppression of inflammatory cytokines. Super GLA/DHA is derived from borage oil and marine lipid concentrate. The suggested dose is 6 softgels daily.

16. Resveratrol has been shown to act as a chemotherapeutic agent *in vitro* on certain leukemia cell lines. Although as a therapeutic agent, a dosage has not been established, one 20-mg capsule daily of resveratrol provides multiple health benefits.

Note: *At this juncture, the hormone melatonin is not recommended in the treatment of lymphoma and leukemia. Patients should avoid the use of this product until more information is available. If patients do choose to use melatonin, monthly blood testing for tumor markers should be closely monitored to determine if melatonin is promoting leukemic or lymphatic cell proliferation.*

 FOR MORE INFORMATION

Contact the American Cancer Society, (800) ACS-2345.

 PRODUCT AVAILABILITY

Water-soluble vitamin A liquid, vitamin D3 capsules, vitamin C, alpha-lipoic acid, Ultra Soy Extract, curcumin, green tea extract, Resveratrol, Super GLA/DHA, DHEA, and shark liver oil are available by telephoning (800) 544-4440 or by ordering online. Vesanoid, Gleevec and cerivastatin are prescription drugs and should be prescribed by your oncologist or hematologist.

STAYING INFORMED

The information published in this protocol is only as current as the day the manuscript was sent to the printer. This protocol raises many issues that are subject to change as new data emerge. Furthermore, cancer is still a disease with unacceptably high mortality rates, and none of our suggested regimens can guarantee a cure.

The Life Extension Foundation is constantly uncovering information to provide to cancer patients. A special website has been established for the purpose of updating patients on new findings that directly pertain to the published cancer protocols. Whenever Life Extension discovers information that may benefit cancer patients it will be posted on the website www.lefcancer.org.

Before utilizing the cancer protocols in this book, we suggest that you check www.lefcancer.org to see if any substantive changes have been made to the recommendations described in this protocol. Based on the sheer number of newly published findings, there could be significant alterations to the information you have just read.

Alternatively, call 1-800-226-2370 and ask a Health Advisor if your topic of interest has been updated on the website - www.lefcancer.org

DISCLAIMER

This information (and any accompanying printed material) is not intended to replace the attention or advice of a physician or other health care professional. Anyone who wishes to embark on any dietary, drug, exercise, or other lifestyle change intended to prevent or treat a specific disease or condition should first consult with and seek clearance from a qualified health care professional.

The information published in the protocols is only as current as the day the manuscript was sent to the printer. This protocol raises many issues that are subject to change as new data emerge. None of our suggested protocol regimens can guarantee a cure.

Liver Cirrhosis

In the human, the liver is the second largest organ in the body (skin being the largest). The liver is about the size of a football and it weighs approximately 4 lbs. The liver is responsible for performing more functions than any other organ in the body, including metabolizing the food we eat by breaking it down to useful parts; filtering and detoxifying (neutralizing) poisons in our blood to remove numerous toxic compounds that we are exposed to on a daily basis, producing immune agents to control infection, and regenerating itself when part of it has been damaged (NIDDK 2000). Several times each day, our entire blood supply passes through the liver. At any given time, about a pint of blood is in the liver (or 10% of the total blood volume of an adult).

Another important function of the liver is to produce prothrombin and fibrinogen (two blood-clotting factors) and heparin (a mucopolysaccharide sulfuric acid ester that helps prevent blood from clotting within the circulatory system). The liver also converts sugar into glycogen and stores it until the muscles need energy. The released glycogen becomes glucose in the blood stream. The liver also synthesizes proteins and cholesterol and converts carbohydrates and proteins into fats, which it also stores for later use. Additionally, the liver produces and secretes bile (that is stored in the gallbladder until needed), which is needed to break down and digest fatty acids. It also produces blood protein and hundreds of enzymes needed for digestion and other bodily functions. As the liver breaks down proteins, it produces urea, which it synthesizes from carbon dioxide and ammonia. (Urea is the primary solid component of urine and is eventually excreted by the kidneys.) Essential trace elements, such as iron and copper, as well as vitamins A, D, and B_{12} are also stored in the liver.

Until recently, the most common cause of cirrhosis of the liver in the United States was attributed to alcohol abuse. Hepatitis C is now the number one cause of liver cirrhosis (26%), followed closely by alcohol abuse at 21% (NIDDK 2000). A cofactor such as the hepatitis C virus can increase the risk of cirrhosis in those who also consume alcohol in excess (NIDA 2002).

ETIOLOGY OF CIRRHOSIS

Cirrhosis of the liver is a chronic, diffuse (widely spread throughout the organ), degenerative disease in which the parenchyma (the functional organ tissue) deteriorates; the lobules are infiltrated with fat and structurally altered; dense perilobular connective tissue forms; and often areas of regeneration develop. The surviving cells multiply in an attempt to regenerate and form "islands" of living cells that are separated by scar tissue. These islands of living cells have a reduced blood supply, resulting in impaired liver function. As the cirrhotic process continues, blood flow through the liver becomes blocked; portal hypertension may occur (high blood pressure in the veins connecting the liver with the intestines and spleen); glucose and vitamin absorption decrease; the manufacturing of hormones and stomach and bowel function are affected; and noticeable facial veins may appear. Most patients die from cirrhosis in the fifth or sixth decade of life (Wolf 2001).

Approximately one-third of cirrhosis cases are "compensated," meaning there are no clinical symptoms. Compensated cases are usually discovered during routine tests for other problems or during surgery or autopsy. Cirrhosis is irreversible. Unless the underlying cause of cirrhosis is removed and the person takes measures to treat the condition, the liver will continue to incur damage, eventually leading to liver failure, ammonia toxicity, gastrointestinal hemorrhage, kidney failure, hepatic coma, and death. For some people, the only chance for a long-term cure is a liver transplant.

According the Centers for Disease Control (CDC), in the year 2000, preliminary data compiled by the Division of Vital Statistics revealed that even though cause of death from cirrhosis and chronic liver disease had fallen a rank from 7th to 12th, the number of people who died from liver disease was 26,219, almost the same as when cirrhosis was ranked 7th (Minino et al. 2001).

SYMPTOMS OF CIRRHOSIS

Common symptoms of cirrhosis include nausea or indigestion and vomiting; loss of appetite; weight loss; constipation or diarrhea; flatulence; ascites (the accumulation of serous fluids in the peritoneal cavity); edema (fluid retention in the legs); light-colored stools; weakness or chronic dyspepsia; dull abdominal aching; varicosities; nosebleeds, bleeding gums, or other internal and external bleeding; easy bruising; extreme skin dryness; intense skin itching; and spider angiomas (a central, raised, red dot about the size of a pin head from which small blood vessels radiate).

Cirrhosis

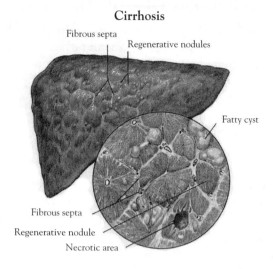

Fibrous septa
Regenerative nodules
Fatty cyst
Fibrous septa
Regenerative nodule
Necrotic area

Infectious diseases, chronic alcohol abuse, and malnutrition can lead to cirrhosis. Fatty and fibrous tissue along with necrosis will result when toxins accumulate faster than the liver can detoxify and regenerate itself. (Anatomical Chart Company 2002®, Lippincott Williams & Wilkins)

In cirrhosis, healthy, functioning liver cells are destroyed, and scarring and distortion of the liver eventually takes place. As fewer liver cells function, smaller amounts of albumin (a protein) are manufactured. Lower albumin levels facilitate water retention (edema) in the legs and abdomen (ascites). Excessive bile product deposits cause intense skin itching, often accompanied by jaundice (yellowed skin). Other symptoms are testicular atrophy, gynecomastia (enlargement of the male breast), and loss of chest and armpit hair.

Psychotic mental changes such as extreme paranoia can also occur in cases of advanced cirrhosis.

SYSTEMIC COMPLICATIONS FROM CIRRHOSIS

In the cirrhotic liver, when blood flow is restricted, blood can back up in the spleen, causing an enlarged spleen and sequestered blood cells. In this situation, the platelet count typically falls and abnormal bleeding results. In extreme cases, blood actually flows backward from the portal circulation to systemic circulation. In addition to esophageal varices, varicose veins can develop in the stomach (gastric varices) and rectum (hemorrhoids). Ruptured varices cause massive bleeding and are often fatal. Bilirubin levels may also build up in the blood, causing jaundice and bright yellow to dark brown urine. Additionally, insulin resistance and diabetes mellitus, kidney dysfunction,

and congestive heart failure, as well as osteomalacia (the adult form of rickets, resulting in bone softening that often leaves them brittle) and osteoporosis (reduction in bone mass) are associated with cirrhosis (NIDDK 2000).

If cirrhosis prevents bile, a green-brown fluid that is produced by the liver, from reaching the gallbladder, a person may develop gallstones (NIDDK 2000). It is then secreted through tiny channels within the liver into a duct to the gallbladder. Bile is stored in the gallbladder until it is needed for digestion of fats. Most gallstones are formed from cholesterol. If the liver is healthy, the bile contains the proper constituents to dissolve cholesterol excreted by the liver, but in a cirrhotic liver, the bile cannot adequately dissolve cholesterol. The cholesterol then forms crystals, which settle to the bottom of the gallbladder and eventually become stones (ALF 2002; MFMER 2002; WebMD 2002).

A cross-sectional study was conducted in 1010 patients with cirrhosis related to alcohol abuse, chronic viral infection, or miscellaneous causes (42%, 48%, and 10%, respectively). Gallstone development was monitored by ultrasound in 618 patients who were free of gallstones at enrollment. The overall prevalence of gallstones was 29.5% and increased significantly with age without differences according to sex or cause of cirrhosis. During a mean ± SD follow-up of 50 months ± 9 months, 141 (22.8%) of 618 patients developed gallstones, with an estimated cumulative probability of 6.5%, 18.6%, 28.2%, and 40.9% at 2, 4, 6, and 8 years, respectively. Multivariate analysis showed that degree of cirrhosis and high body mass index carried a significantly greater risk of gallstone formation, leading the researchers to conclude: "Cirrhosis per se represents a major risk factor for gallstones whose prevalence and incidence were far higher than those reported in a general population from the same area" (Conte et al. 1999).

Note: *Cholesterol in the bile has no relation to the cholesterol in the blood. Therefore cholesterol-lowering drugs do not prevent gallstones.*

Toxins that the liver normally removes build up in the blood, dulling mental function and leading to personality changes. The condition of the liver also affects how drugs are filtered from the body. Drugs the patient is taking that are normally filtered out by the liver and disposed of in the urine may remain in the bloodstream for a much longer period, acting longer than expected or even building up in body tissue. A cirrhotic liver is usually much larger than a healthy liver (Clayman 1989; Glanze 1996; NIDDK 2000; Wolf 2001).

Treating the Complications

In patients who have cirrhosis, complications from the disease must be treated. In particular, acute variceal bleeding is a very serious, life-threatening medical emergency. Infections such as spontaneous bacterial peritonitis must be promptly treated with appropriate antibiotics. Coagulation disorders will sometimes respond to vitamin K. However, drugs that are metabolized in the liver must be used with caution.

Ascites

Mild cases of ascites are treated with a salt-restricted diet (2000 mg of sodium daily or less in some cases). Cirrhosis patients often need guidance in planning a diet that has low sodium content without compromising caloric and nutritional requirements (NIDDK 2000). If salt restriction is not effective, diuretic drugs are the next treatment consideration (e.g., Aldactone or Lasix). In patients who continue to be resistant to drug therapy, peritoneovenous and portosystemic shunts (plastic tubing) are inserted subcutaneously to connect the peritoneal cavity or the portal system to an internal jugular or subclavian vein (Wolf 2001).

Hepatic Encephalopathy

Blood ammonia will be checked because an elevated serum ammonia level is a classic laboratory finding in hepatic encephalopathy. Lactulose is helpful in some patients to assist in removal of ammonia (Wolf 2001). Lactulose is a synthetic sugar that is not absorbed by the body and is used a laxative. Neomycin and other antibiotics are also used to decrease bacteria in the intestine that produce ammonia. Depending on nutritional status, dietary protein may be restricted in patients who are having an acute flare-up of hepatic encephalopathy (Wolf 2001).

Esophageal Varices

Restricted blood flow in the portal vein causes blood from the intestines and spleen to back up into stomach and esophagus blood vessels. These vessels are not intended to carry large amounts of blood and become enlarged. As these veins enlarge (varicose veins or varices), the walls become thin and are likely to burst as pressure increases. Variceal hemorrhaging is very serious and requires immediate medical attention. As part of routine monitoring, a diagnostic endoscopy will be done to determine if a patient has asymptomatic esophageal varices. If varices are present, treatment can include reducing salt intake; taking diuretics to eliminate excess salts and fluids from the body; taking a beta-blocker (propranolol, nadolol); injection of a clotting agent; injection of a scarring chemical (sclerotherapy); or rubber-band ligation (a surgical procedure using a device to compress the varices and stop bleeding) (Pugh et al. 1973; NIDDK 2000; Wolf 2001). In addition, there is a radiological procedure called transjugular intrahepatic protosystemic shunt (TIPS) that shows some promise.

Hepatoma

In the United States, hepatocellular carcinoma is observed in 10–20% of patients who have cirrhosis (Wolf 2001). The liver cells develop a malignant change leading to a type of cancer called hepatocellular carcinoma (HCC). As with other cancers, early detection and number and size of tumors influence survival. Treatment for HCC ranges from surgical removal of the HCC if the patient has good liver function to transplantation (NIDDK 2000; Columbo 2001; Wolf 2001). If the patient cannot have surgery (advanced age, other health conditions, poor liver function, large tumors, or tumors in strategic locations), possible treatment includes ultrasound-guided injection of solutions that cause necrosis of tumor cells in the cancerous area; using a catheter to eliminate blood supply to the tumor; injecting antitumor agents directly into the tumor; systemic chemotherapy; and radiation (Columbo 2001).

Portal Hypertension

A healthy liver can accommodate a wide range of changes in portal blood flow without alteration of portal blood pressure. However, when the portal vein is obstructed, portal hypertension (very high blood pressure) occurs (Clayman 1989; Wolf 2001). Factors causing increased resistance to blood flow are fibrotic changes in the liver caused by cirrhosis, compression of the nodules that are regenerating liver tissue, and increased collagen deposition and levels of chemicals that act to constrict the blood vessels in the liver. Other causes are a blood clot in the portal vein or congenital narrowing (Clayman 1989). Treatment can consist of controlling ascites with salt restriction and diuretics; treating varices; or surgically implanting a shunt to divert blood from the portal vein to another blood vessel to relieve some of the pressure on the portal vein (Clayman 1989).

CIRRHOSIS AND THE HEPATITIS C FACTOR

Until recently, the most common cause of cirrhosis of the liver in the United States was attributed to alcohol abuse. Because of the rapid increase of hepatitis C virus infection, hepatitis C has now taken over first place (26%), with alcohol abuse falling to second place, but only slightly behind at 21% (NIDDK 2000). There are vaccines for some of the hepatitis viruses, but at this time, there is no vaccine to prevent transmission of the hepatitis C virus. Preventive and deterrent practices are the only means to avoid it (Alter et al. 1998; Buggs 2002; NIDA 2002). The most common routes of infection with the hepatitis C virus are via needles, sexual contact, and blood transfusions, and from an infected pregnant female to her newborn (NIDA 2002) (*see the protocol on Hepatitis C for a complete discussion of the hepatitis C virus*).

Hepatitis C is one of six viruses known to cause liver disease (Buggs 2001; NIDA 2002, Strickland 2002). Hepatitis C is very difficult for the immune system to overcome and often becomes chronic, leading to serious and permanent liver damage. Typically hepatitis C infection is mild in the early stages and rarely recognized until it has caused significant damage to the liver. From infection to noticeable or significant liver damage can take 20 years or more. The symptoms of hepatitis C are also very mild in the early stages. Fatigue, the most common symptom, may not appear for many years. Other symptoms are mild fever, muscle and joint aches, nausea and vomiting, poor appetite, and vague abdominal pains. Hepatitis C often goes undiagnosed because the symptoms come and go and are so suggestive of a flu-like illness. Its presence is usually identified during a routine blood test or because the hepatitis C antibody is positive at the time of a blood donation.

A low level of infection with practically no symptoms can continue for years. The hepatitis C infection causes inflammation of the liver, with chronic infection resulting in cirrhotic-like scarring. Unfortunately, more than 80% of infected individuals eventually progress to the chronic stage of hepatitis C which results in cirrhosis (severe scarring of liver tissue). Persons with the late stages of hepatitis C can also develop liver cancer. When the hepatitis C virus is a cofactor, there is an increased risk of cirrhosis in those who also consume alcohol in excess (NIDA 2002).

CIRRHOSIS AND THE ALCOHOL FACTOR

Although alcohol affects many organs in the body, it is especially harmful to the liver. Alcohol is metabolized in the body, and the liver performs most of that work, potentially incurring serious damage in the process. Not only does alcohol destroy liver cells, it also destroys their ability to regenerate, leading to a syndrome of progressive inflammatory injury to the liver.

In the United States, approximately 1% of the population (more than 2 million people) has alcoholic liver disease. Additional cases go undetected because patients are asymptomatic and never seek medical treatment. Alcoholism and alcoholic liver disease are higher in minorities. Women are also more susceptible to the adverse effects of alcohol than men. Women develop alcoholic hepatitis in a shorter time frame and from smaller amounts of alcohol than men (Day 2000). The survival rate after 5 years is also lower for women than for men (30% compared to 70%). There seems to be no single factor to account for increased susceptibility to alcoholic liver damage in females, but the effect of hormones on the metabolism of alcohol may play an important role (Day 2000; Mihas et al. 2002).

Symptoms

Although mild forms of alcoholic liver disease are often completely symptom-free, the symptoms are quite similar to cirrhosis: nausea, generally feeling unwell, a low-grade fever, impaired liver function, altered mental state, gastrointestinal bleeding, abdominal bloating, and seizures (Mihas et al. 2002). As long as consumption of alcohol continues, alcoholic inflammation of the liver will usually continue. Alcoholic inflammation of the liver will often eventually progress to cirrhosis. If use of alcohol ceases, inflammation of the liver generally resolves slowly over several weeks to months to years. Some improvement can continue for several years. Unfortunately, if cirrhotic damage has already occurred, there will be residual cirrhosis (Mihas et al. 2002).

How Much Alcohol Causes Cirrhosis?

When relating alcohol consumption to those persons who will actually go on to develop cirrhosis, the amount of alcohol consumption required varies widely. In less than 10% of drinkers who do develop cirrhosis, many factors that may be causally related to the development of cirrhosis remain unknown (e.g., genetic, malnutrition, toxic effects of ethanol, free radicals generated as byproducts of ethanol, and immune mechanisms) (Day 2000). In fact, in alcoholics there is actually a rather weak relationship between the *amount* of alcohol consumed and the risk of developing cirrhosis, and many alcoholics will not develop severe or progressive liver injury (Mihas et al. 2002).

Is There a Genetic Factor?

Since ancient times, common belief has been that alcoholism runs in families. For decades, researchers have investigated this folk opinion with scientific studies. According to the National Institute on Alcohol Abuse and Alcoholism (NIAAA) and the National Institutes of Health (NIH), as early as the 1970s, studies documented that alcoholism does occur in families. However, studies do not answer questions such as: does alcoholism occur in families because children observe the parents drinking, does the environment in the home play a role, do children inherit genes that create a predisposition for alcoholism, or does alcoholism result from a combination of factors? Continued studies have investigated these questions as well as the possibility that there is an underlying vulnerability to incur organ damage from alcohol that is under genetic control (Gordis 1992, 2000).

Progress has been made using genetic, biochemical, and behavioral characteristics; population, family, and twin studies (male and female; identical and fraternal); and studies of adopted children; however, results have been difficult to interpret because of study variables. It is the opinion of the NIAAA that "more than one gene is likely to be responsible" for the vulnerability to alcoholism and that "it is probable that environmental influences are at least as important, and possibly more important, than genetic influences" (Gordis 1992; 2000).

If research is successful in revealing the genes that are involved in increasing an individual's vulnerability to become an alcoholic, physicians will be better able to identify individuals who are at high risk for alcoholism and perhaps develop more effective treatment for alcohol-related health conditions such as cirrhosis of the liver (Day 2000).

What Role Does Diet Play?

It has been estimated that chronic alcoholics receive at least half of their daily caloric intake in the form of alcohol. Additionally, chronic abusers of alcohol often have vitamin deficiencies caused by self-neglect and poor eating habits, and it is not unusual for them to need significant vitamin supplementation to correct these vitamin deficiencies. Acute thiamin (vitamin B_1) deficiency is typical. Patients with alcoholic inflammation of the liver also have protein/calorie malnutrition. Even though early studies in baboons demonstrated that cirrhosis can develop in subjects with good dietary nutrition, improved nutritional status does have positive effects for patients with alcoholic inflammation of the liver (Lieber et al. 1970). Nutrition should be improved with a healthy diet. Counting calories is a useful method to ensure adequate intake. Nutritional supplements and appetite stimulants should be used when appropriate (Mihas et al. 2002).

Interestingly, obesity can exist even in persons who have poor nutritional status. In alcoholics, the presence of obesity increases the risk of cirrhosis development, probably because obesity also contributes to an earlier development of fatty liver (steatosis), now known to facilitate liver damage and make the liver more susceptible to a variety of insults, including alcohol consumption, infections, toxins, medicines, and so forth. (Day 2000). Fatty liver causes scarring of the liver.

Diagnosing Alcoholic Liver Disease

Tests to confirm a diagnosis of alcoholic inflammation of the liver include a complete blood count (CBC); liver enzyme, liver function, and electrolyte testing; and screening for other health conditions (presence of hepatitis B and C viruses, liver cancer, gallstones). Imaging studies are rarely used for diagnosis. (Sometimes they are used to exclude other potential causes such as gallstones, obstructions, or abnormal tissue or to evaluate the extent of existing conditions.) In some cases, a liver biopsy is used to confirm the diagnosis, the presence or absence of cirrhosis, and to exclude other causes (Mihas et al. 2002).

Treatment

There is no specific treatment paradigm for mild cases of alcoholic hepatitis. The common sense approach is to follow the instructions of your physician; stop all use of alcohol; ensure good dietary nutrition; and take supplements that enhance liver functioning such as N-acetyl-cysteine and lecithin. More severe cases may benefit from hospitalization to stabilize complications of the disease. The most predictive indicators for eventual outcome are willingness of the patient to not drink alcohol, the severity of any encephalopathy, levels of serum bilirubin and albumin, prothrombin time; the patient's age, and existing kidney function (Mihas et al. 2002).

OTHER CAUSES OF CIRRHOSIS

Additional causes or conditions that can lead to cirrhosis are congestive heart failure, genetic disorders such as hemochromatosis (excessive iron accumulation) or Wilson's disease (excessive copper accumulation in the liver), advanced syphilis, exposure to parasitic flatworms or infections, exposure to heavy metals, ingestion of poisons (alcohol, phosphorus, carbon tetrachloride), cystic fibrosis, a severe reaction to an over-the-counter, prescriptive, or "recreational" drug, and injury to the liver from an accident (NIDDK 2000).

from damage due to hepatitis C. The suggested dose of SAMe is 400 mg 3 times daily. Do not take SAMe on an empty stomach.

- Polyenylphosphatidylcholine (PPC) has been shown to prevent the development of fibrosis and cirrhosis and to prevent lipid peroxidation and associated liver damage from alcohol consumption. PPC is sold as a drug in Europe. A product called HepatoPro is one of the few American dietary supplements to provide pharmaceutical-grade polyenylphosphatidylcholine. Take two to three 900-mg capsules daily.

- Silymarin extract from milk thistle can raise glutathione levels and has shown multi-faceted protective benefits to the liver. The most active flavonoid in silymarin is silibinin. A product called Silibinin Plus is formulated to provide the same silibinin extract used in European prescription drugs. One 325-mg capsule taken twice daily is recommended for healthy people. Patients with liver disease may take up to 6 capsules daily.

- Branched-chain amino acids can enhance protein synthesis in the liver and are particularly beneficial in alcoholic cirrhosis. The suggested dose is 2–4 capsules daily between meals with fruit juice or before eating. Each capsule should contain 300 mg of leucine, 150 mg of isoleucine, and 150 mg of valine.

 FOR MORE INFORMATION

More information on conventional therapies is available by contacting the American Liver Foundation, (800) 223-0179.

 PRODUCT AVAILABILITY

HepatoPro (polyenylphosphatidylcholine), Silibinin Plus, branched-chain amino acids, choline capsules, B vitamins, SAMe, vitamin C, vitamin E (tocopheryl succinate and gamma tocopherol), selenium, zinc, coenzyme Q_{10}, acetyl-L-carnitine, alpha-lipoic acid, and N-acetyl-cysteine (NAC) may be ordered by calling (800) 544-4440 or by ordering online at www.lef.org.

Lupus

Lupus is an autoimmune, inflammatory disease with multiple acute and chronic manifestations. In its most common and serious form, *systemic lupus erythematosus* (SLE) is a potentially fatal dysfunction of the autoimmune system. Instead of defending against invading viruses and bacteria, the body's multitude of immune agents mistakenly identify its own tissues as the enemy and they attack the organs, blood, skin, joints, and gastrointestinal tract. In its most life-threatening form, SLE produces kidney, brain, heart, and lung inflammation. Even in milder forms, this inflammatory process leads to arthralgia (joint pain), fever, fatigue, mood changes, and other symptoms that may become disabling.

There are two other forms of this disease: *discoid lupus erythematosus* (DLE), a less serious form primarily causing disc-shaped skin lesions; and *drug-induced lupus erythematosus* (DILE), which is transient and subsides when the causal agent is withdrawn. A further discussion of DILE will be provided later in this protocol.

The epidemiology of lupus reveals it to be primarily a disease of younger women, although men and children are represented as well. Although incidence peaks between ages 15–40 years, as many as 40% of cases may present initially after age 60. SLE affects one in 3000 persons in the United States, striking women 5–9 times more often than men. United States statistics show the disease to be more prevalent in African American and Hispanic women than in white women, but this finding may be influenced by socio-economic factors (Pisetsky 1993).

The Lupus Foundation of America estimates that as many as 2 million United States residents have SLE. Lupus is a many-faceted disease, with a range of impact from minor to life-threatening, and with a multitude of symptomatic areas throughout the entire body. It is an unpredictable disorder, capable of long remissions and sudden unexplained "flare-ups" (sudden activation of apparently quiescent disease states). Fortunately, the recognition and treatment of SLE has improved dramatically in recent years. Once SLE is under reasonable control, many lupus patients have normal life expectancies. The key is to prevent or quickly deal with any inflammatory organ involvement.

The causes of SLE are not entirely clear, but most experts believe there is a genetic predisposition involved, although on a polygenetic level "there doesn't appear to be a single causative gene" (DeHoratius 1999). Because of this, lupus does not often occur in multiple generations of a family. Researchers previously have identified chromosome 6 (the human leukocyte area, HLA) as an important genetic marker, and in 1997, Tsao et al. identified a significant area on chromosome 1 as well. In either case, the low correlation between genetic factors and active lupus indicates that environmental triggers must play a critical role in the development of SLE. These environmental factors may be infections, nutritional deficits, stress, or some unsuspected agent. It is accepted that these same factors (infections, nutrition, and stress) can exacerbate lupus and even induce flare-ups.

The biochemistry of lupus is important in the understanding of how traditional medical and alternative/supportive treatments work. Basically, the body has a vast array of cells at its disposal to deal with infections, depending on the type of invader it detects. Some cells focus on this detection process, telling other cells what to do and what to attack by labeling foreign substances (antigens) as enemies and choosing the appropriate disease-fighting agent from the dozens available. Antibodies produced by the immune system attack labeled antigens. Other groups of cells, including the complement system, are charged with regulating and cleaning up excess antibodies. If antibodies are present in excess while mediating substances are at low levels, inflammation may be excessive and unchecked. A complete description of the body's defense system is beyond the scope of this protocol, but may be found in Wallace (1995).

Depending on which antigens are identified, specific antibodies will be activated to destroy them. In lupus, as in other autoimmune diseases, antibodies misidentify as a foreign invader the body's own self-antigens, causing an inappropriate immune response that can occur in any tissue or organ in the body. In lupus, the question is: which tissues were misidentified? The body's systems become so disrupted that they begin manufacturing "autoantibodies" (antibodies that attack the person's own tissues). The autoantibodies thus produced lead to the multitude of symptoms in SLE and help explain why the disease is so varied. As will be seen, medical tests for lupus search for excessive amounts of different key antibodies and are used to chart the course of the disease.

SYMPTOM AREAS AND DANGERS

The following are brief descriptions of the most common areas of lupus activity:

Joints.   Approximately 90% of patients have some form of musculoskeletal symptoms, typically pain in the hands, wrists, knees, and shoulders (arthralgia).

Kidney.   Nearly 50% of lupus patients have significant renal disease and can experience kidney failure.

Lung.   The most common involvement is pleuritis, an inflammation of the membrane surrounding the lungs, with or without pleural effusion (buildup of fluids).

Cardiac.   As with the lungs, inflammation of the lining of the heart (pericarditis) is the most common symptom.

Blood.   Lupus inflammation may produce anemia and leukopenia (a dangerous reduction in white blood cells which leaves the body easily susceptible to infection).

Central Nervous System.   SLE frequently produces brain dysfunctions, including strokes, seizures, headaches, cognitive dysfunction, and dementia.

Mouth and Nose.   Mucosal ulcers are seen in approximately 30% of patients (Belmont 1998), but rarely are serious threats to overall health.

Skin.   Various dermatological disruptions are extremely common, varying from facial rash (the famous "butterfly" pattern of lupus that is similar to the facial markings of a wolf, giving rise to the name "lupus"), to photosensitivity (which may initiate a system flare-up), to discoid skin lesions, to hair thinning.

Gastrointestinal Tract.   Outbreaks here may be as a direct result of the disease itself or as a consequence of the use of anti-inflammatory medications, especially steroids.

The Vascular System.   Besides the effects on the blood supply of the brain, kidneys, and other organs, SLE causes a specific and dangerous complication for the blood vessels themselves, called vasculitis.

The Immune System.   Despite overreactivity to its own tissues, the immune system in SLE patients is inefficient against external disease-causing organisms. As a result, people with lupus are particularly susceptible to infection.

Bones.   Osteoporosis is seen in lupus both as a direct result of the disease itself (when chronic inflammation and inactivity lead to demineralization) and as a side effect of corticosteroid therapy.

Medical Diagnosis of SLE

Despite its many facets, lupus has been misdiagnosed for many years. Many lupus patients look healthy and even after being obviously ill have brief remissions that make it appear as if they have recovered from whatever they had. Of course, the historic prevalence of SLE in females has produced a lack of research, interest, and funding. Even today, patients may wait for years before an accurate diagnosis is made (Wallace 1995).

In 1971 (revised in 1982), the American College of Rheumatology devised 11 criteria for the presence of SLE. A person with four of the 11 may be diagnosed with lupus. The first four are symptoms of the skin: photosensitivity, mouth sores, butterfly rashes, and discoid (disc-shaped) lesions. The next four criteria describe inflammatory reactions in the joints, the central nervous system, the kidneys, and the linings of the lungs or heart.

The final three criteria are blood test abnormalities:

1. *Positive antinuclear antibody (ANA) testing*—This test is very sensitive, but not specific. A positive ANA result is found in nearly all lupus patients, although some people with positive ANAs do not have lupus (a false-positive). They may have a related disorder, such as arthritis, or they may have no signs of any active disease state. This test measures the presence of immune system agents (antibodies) which falsely identify the nuclei of our own cells as enemies and proceed to attack and inflame them. Physicians can use ANA results as a measure of current lupus activity.

2. *Altered blood count*—Low red or white blood cell levels are common.

3. *Other abnormal antibody counts*—These include a positive LE (lupus erythematosus antibodies), anti-DNA (antibodies that attack genetic material), false-positive syphilis tests, and tests with names such as anti-Sm, complement, antiRo, and rheumatoid factor. Each of these antibodies, when elevated in the blood, produces a specific, different symptom in the body.

It is possible for lupus patients to manifest such symptoms as fatigue and depression without concomitant blood abnormalities. This may be caused by stress, medication, or another group of blood proteins called cytokines which are responsible for the chronic inflammation seen in lupus and other autoimmune disorders.

MEDICAL MANAGEMENT OF SLE

Fortunately for present-day lupus patients, the survival and quality of life statistics continue to improve dramatically as newer, more sophisticated techniques become available. This section of the protocol will describe the primary pharmacological treatments in current usage.

Steroids

Despite their negative consequences, steroids are a critical intervention for lupus, particularly when the disease threatens an organ. Steroids (cortisone, prednisone, Dexamethasone, and their cousins) are hormones that have a number of functions in the body, including the stabilization of inflammatory cells and the decrease of the white blood cells responsible for immunologic memory. Steroids may be administered orally, intravenously, intra-articularly (into the joint), intramuscularly, or locally (for skin involvement).

If there is heart, lung, kidney, liver, or blood involvement, high-dose steroids are necessary. Other severe flare-ups often require a lower dosage. In all cases, whenever it is possible to discontinue steroid treatment, it is preferable to do so. Side effects include palpitations, agitation, tachycardia (rapid heart rate), insomnia, impaired wound healing, impaired response to infection, loss of bone calcium, avascular necrosis (bone death), glucose intolerance (leading to or exacerbating a diabetic state), water retention, hypertension, heartburn, and a number of other unpleasant results.

It should be noted that topical steroid creams do not cause these side effects. Additionally, with oral and injectable administration, some people have only a few side effects, and the impact is dose-dependent. For those with inflammation of the gastrointestinal tract, there is a steroid named Budesonide which offers far fewer side effects. Some natural treatments such as the use of DHEA (see below) can help by lowering the dose required for steroid use, thus decreasing the side effects (van Vollenhoven 2000).

Immunosuppressive Therapies

These treatments typically are used in organ-threatening cases when steroids have failed or are not tolerated by the patient. In truth, these regimens are forms of chemotherapy (also referred to as cytotoxic therapy) and may involve some of the same drugs used in treating cancer. As such, they offer the same powerful positive and negative consequences of most chemotherapy. As with steroids, immunosuppressants, because of their toxicity, should be utilized only when other treatments are ineffective. The most common drugs used are cytoxan and methotrexate.

A survey conducted at the University of Toronto Lupus Clinic has shown that approximately 33% of the patients have received cytotoxic therapy at some point in their course of treatment. These agents were initiated for a variety of manifestations, with renal manifestations being the major indication, accounting for 28.2% of the cytotoxic agents used. Other common indications for initiation of cytotoxic therapy included attempts to reduce steroid dosage (18.4%), global flare-ups (12.5%), neurologic manifestations (11.4%), and musculoskeletal complications (8.6%). Azathioprine, methotrexate, and cyclophosphamide accounted for 98% of all cytotoxic agents used. Azathioprine was the most frequently used cytotoxic drug (70%), followed by methotrexate (21.5%) and cyclophosphamide (9.4%) (Rahman et al. 1997). Pulsing cyclophosphamide may also reduce the side effects of this medication. More recently, cyclosporin (an antirejection drug) has been used with some success in small trials.

Intravenous Immunoglobulins

In Europe and the Middle East, researchers have attempted suppression of the lupus autoantibodies using intravenous immunoglobulins. While no prospective blinded trials have taken place, the case control studies are impressive in their ability to provide long-term remission in a number of studies. Intravenous immunoglobulins do not have such a significant side effect profile as do the immunosuppressive agents mentioned above.

NSAIDs

The nonsteroidal anti-inflammatory drugs (NSAIDs) are an excellent substitute for steroidal medications whenever they provide sufficient suppression of SLE activity. These drugs (from simple aspirin and ibuprofen to Naprosyn, Indocin, Lodine, and Daypro) are less expensive and safer and are often as effective as the previously mentioned therapies. They relieve fever, arthralgias, headaches, fatigue, pain, and various inflammations. NSAIDs have some particular benefits and side effects that make careful selection very important. One concern is the kidney-liver "profile" of each drug. Because they often are taken for long periods of time, kidney and liver complications are cumulative. Although new NSAIDs, supposedly without the same side effects, became available in 1999, they are now being shown to have similar side effects as the earlier forms. Consult a physician for the appropriateness of the new medications regarding your case. In addition, the use of NSAIDs on an ongoing basis can actually affect the intestinal tract in an adverse way by thinning out the lining and increasing inflammation. Thus, some complementary/alternative approaches avoid the use of NSAIDS and work to ensure bowel integrity through diet, cleansing, and supplementation with probiotics (*see the Arthritis protocol for more information on NSAIDs*).

Antimalarials

This class of drugs is remarkable for its effectiveness, safety, and multiple benefits. However, antimalarials are not useful in organ-threatening SLE and they take months to reach their full effectiveness. These medications, most often Plaquenil, may be used in combination with other treatments or in some mild cases may be the only drug required. The antimalarials decrease inflammation, protect the skin from ultraviolet light damage, inhibit blood clotting, provide energy, block cytokines (which promote inflammation), and, as a bonus, lower cholesterol. In addition, the antimalarial hydroxychloroquine appears to protect against osteoporosis in corticosteroid treated patients with SLE (Lakshminarayanan et al. 2001). Aside from a rare buildup in the eyes which can be monitored easily, Plaquenil has no major drawbacks other than possible gastrointestinal intolerance. Choice of medication is important because some other antimalarials (chloroquine) may cause permanent eye damage.

Related Medical Treatments

Some of the lesser-used therapies for SLE include dialysis (for advanced kidney damage); gold (for its antirheumatic properties); cyclosporin A (for inflammatory arthralgia); antileprosy drugs (for skin and joint problems); retinoids (vitamin A derivatives); gamma-globulin (for recurrent infections); dimethyl sulfoxide (DMSO) (for lupus-related urinary tract cystitis); and antidepressants for the frequent emotional disturbances commonly found with SLE patients (Sotolongo et al. 1984).

DRUG-INDUCED LUPUS

Mentioned previously, DILE (drug-induced lupus) requires medical treatment to identify and discontinue the provocative agent. These are some of the drugs capable of causing lupus, according to Callegari et al. (1995) and Wallace (1995):

Atenolol (Tenormin)

Captopril (Capoten)

Carbamazepine

Chlorpromazine HCl (Thorazine)

Clonidine HCl (Catapres)

Danazol (Danocrine)

Diclofenac (Cataflam, Voltaren)

Disopyramide (Norpace)

Ethosuximide (Zarontin)

Gold compounds

Griseofulvin

Hydralazine HCl (Apresoline)

Ibuprofen

Interferon alfa

Isoniazid (Laniazid, Nydrazid)

Labetalol HCl (Normodyne, Trandate)

Leuprolide acetate (Lupron)

Levodopa (Dopar, Larodopa)

Lithium carbonate

Lovastatin (Mevacor)

Mephenytoin (Mesantoin)

Methyldopa (Aldomet)

Methysergide maleate (Sansert)

Minoxidil (Loniten, Rogaine)

Nalidixic acid (NegGram)

Nitrofurantoin (Furadantin, Macrobid, Macrodantin)

Oral contraceptives

Penicillamine (Cuprimine, Depen)

Penicillin

Phenelzine sulfate (Nardil)

Phenytoin sodium (Dilantin)

Prazosin (Minipress)

Primidone (Mysoline)

Procainamide HCl (Procan, Pronestyl)

Promethazine HCl (Anergan, Phenergan)

Propylthiouracil

Psoralen

Quinidine

Spironolactone (Aldactone)

Streptomycin sulfate

Sulindac (Clinoril)

Sulfasalazine (Azulfidine)

Tetracycline

Thioridazine HCl (Mellaril)

Timolol maleate (Betimol, Timoptic)

Tolazamide (Tolinase)

Tolmetin sodium (Tolectin)

Trimethadione (Tridione)

Additionally, the following drugs may exacerbate lupus:

- Antibiotics (particularly sulfa drugs and tetracycline)
- Oral contraceptives
- Oral diabetes drugs
- Cimetidine (Tagamet)
- Sulfa-based medications

The list is far from complete. Any patient with lupus-like symptoms should be removed from potentially causative substances for an adequate period of time to assess their possible role in the disease state.

A report in the *Journal of Rheumatology* suggests that estradiol may increase the production of lupus type T-cells (at least *in vitro*), raising the question of whether hormone replacement therapy (HRT) is advisable in menopausal women with SLE. T-cells are antibodies that indicate increased immune activity (Rider et al. 2001).

NEWER MEDICAL TREATMENTS

Thalidomide

This previously shunned drug has been found to be useful in lupus, specifically for the treatment of ankylosing spondylitis, a related rheumatic syndrome. Research has shown that thalidomide suppresses an important inflammatory agent known as TNF-alpha (Breban et al. 1999). There have been a number of studies to show that it is particularly effective in chronic discoid lupus with severe skin problems. A large percentage of patients respond to the therapy, but once it is discontinued, the symptoms reappear fairly rapidly (Cuadrado et al. 2001). This, together with some severe side effects including a reversible peripheral neuropathy and teratogenic effects, make it much less attractive. It should only be used as a last resort.

Prestara (Formerly GL 701)

This substance is a synthetic hormone similar to DHEA which has undergone Phase II and III clinical trials. Both trials have shown objective and subjective improvement with a response rate greater than placebo. Data were presented at the Clinical Trial Symposium at ENDO 2000 (the 82nd Annual Meeting of The Endocrine Society in Toronto, Canada). Patients treated with Prestara showed a 35% greater response rate than the placebo group: 66% of patients (87/132) responded to treatment with Prestara compared to 49% (65/133) for patients who received placebo. The study showed a trend toward a reduction in

the incidence of disease flare-ups, a serious manifestation of lupus which was more than 24% lower in the Prestara patient group (31/132) compared to patients who received placebo (41/133).

Further evidence from the trial demonstrated that Prestara significantly increased bone density, compared to placebo, in patients receiving chronic corticosteroid therapy. Bone density measurements, using the Dual X-ray Absorptiometry (DXA) test, were taken at 8 of the trial's 27 investigator sites. Thirty-seven SLE patients were evaluated for mean changes in bone density of both the lumbar spine and hip. These patients had been on steroids for at least 6 months prior to entry in the study. In this study, 18 lupus patients on chronic steroid therapy who received Prestara demonstrated a statistically significant increase in mean bone density in lumbar spine, compared to 19 patients receiving placebo. Mean bone density in the spine increased 1.83% in patients on Prestara vs. a decrease of 1.78% in placebo patients. Prestara also demonstrated improved changes in mean bone density of the hip. Total hip mean bone density increased 2.08% in patients receiving Prestara and decreased 0.16% in placebo patients.

Prestara appears to be well tolerated. In this trial, adverse events were reported in both the placebo and the treatment group. Adverse events associated with Prestara were generally mild and expected and included acne, facial hair growth, and hormonal changes, which are typical androgenic hormones side effects. In patients receiving Prestara, there was a statistically significant decrease in high-density lipoprotein (HDL) cholesterol. On the other hand, there was also a statistically significant reduction in triglycerides, a lipid that in high levels may increase risk of heart disease. Underscoring the serious nature of lupus, there were five deaths, including two suicides, among patients in the study. All of the deaths were in the placebo group. The findings from this Phase III trial confirmed the tolerability of Prestara seen in other studies in patients with lupus.

Genelabs, makers of Prestara, received a letter of approval from the FDA in August 2002. If the final approval process goes forward, Prestara will be the first medication introduced in 40 years for the treatment of lupus.

Kiel Synchronization Protocol

This procedure, developed by a German clinic, is a variation on the NIH (National Institutes of Health) protocol for the treatment of severe SLE. The NIH protocol uses Cytoxan (an immunosuppressant chemotherapy drug) and cortisone on a frequent and long-term basis (Gourley et al. 1996). In contrast, the Kiel protocol uses smaller and less frequent doses of the same powerful drugs, but combines them with a blood filtration technique called plasmaphoresis, which removes undesirable proteins and antibodies. This is reported to have achieved a long-term, treatment-free remission in 64% of their 28 patients (Schroder et al. 1997). The Kiel protocol reports are promising and warrant further scrutiny.

Collagen

Research in rheumatoid arthritis (Trentham 1993) pointed to the potential of using oral collagen (a protein that is a major component of joints and skin) to signal the body to reduce inflammation.

Monoclonal Antibodies

Findings regarding these substances also come from arthritis research. One such substance blocks the protein TNF-alpha, an important part of the inflammatory chain reaction mentioned above in thalidomide treatment research.

LIFESTYLE MANAGEMENT OF SLE

An individual lupus patient can play an important role in minimizing the impact of the disease on both longevity and quality of life. The recommendations in this section relate to either reducing the "triggers" of lupus flare-ups or making the body more capable of withstanding the assaults of this complex disease.

1. Environmental triggers—Substances encountered in everyday life may exacerbate SLE:

   - Aromatic amines (commonly used in hair dyes)
   - Silicone and silica dust
   - Alfalfa sprouts
   - Hydrazines (found naturally in some mushrooms and tobacco smoke)
   - Tartrazines (used as preservatives in food dyes such as FD&C yellow #5).

2. Ultraviolet light—Ultraviolet A and B (UVA and UVB) are strongly related to lupus through several biochemical reactions. Although people believe they look healthier with a tan, SLE patients may find that flare-ups are induced by exposure to the sun. Even on cloudy days, ultraviolet light is present in sufficient amounts to provoke a reaction. Not all lupus patients are photosensitive, although some are hyperreactive. Sunscreens help (with at least an SPF of 15), but they only reduce the negative responses, rather than eliminating them. An individual's own history is the best predictor of the effects of the sun.

3. Rest—Lupus is typified by reduced energy levels. Some ways of coping with this problem are to get sufficient sleep, pace yourself as much as possible, and rest when necessary. Failure to rest when tired is a formula for longer periods of exhaustion. It is just as bad to remain in bed too long, which leads to the next recommendation.

4. Exercise—As important as exercise is for the average person, it is even more critical for those with SLE. Aerobic exercises such as walking or swimming build desperately needed endurance and help to deter the muscle atrophy which so easily occurs if a patient doesn't take advantage of those times when energy is available. Most people with lupus have such good periods, particularly if they utilize the peak of medication activity. In addition to aerobic exercise, a muscle-building regimen is recommended strongly. If lupus robs you of a percentage of strength and endurance, it makes sense to have a greater capacity on which to draw.

5. Stress—Although medical personnel debate whether or not stress can cause the onset of lupus, it generally is accepted that both physical and emotional stress are capable of producing flare-ups. There is a firm physiological basis for this statement. Stress increases the secretion of the hormones corticotropin and cortisol, and research in psychoneuroimmunology has identified pathways connecting the brain to the immune system (Berk et al. 1994). This same research also describes the positive effects of relaxation and laughter on interferon-gamma, an important immunoregulator, suggesting that patients' mood states play a role in the autoimmune process. Cohen et al. (1994) demonstrated that the immune system is responsive to basic Pavlovian conditioning and provided a summary of successful behavioral interventions. Daily meditation along with simple relaxation techniques, yoga, and biofeedback training can all prove useful in reducing stress and enhancing immune functioning.

NUTRITIONAL MANAGEMENT OF SLE

There are two avenues of approach with the nutritional management of SLE. These could be classified as (1) general nutrition and (2) autoimmune nutrition.

General Nutrition

People living with chronic illnesses have nutritional requirements well beyond those of the general public. The disease process places excessive demands on the entire system while interfering with the ability of the body to assimilate basic nutrients. It is difficult to nourish a chronically ill person with the best of diets. Add the fact that SLE patients frequently have gastric distress and variable appetites and the nutritional task becomes even more daunting. An early study by Cooke and Reading (1985) demonstrated the beneficial effects of nutritional supplementation of SLE patients. It is essential for those with lupus to take a regimen of a high-potency, easily assimilated, vitamin-mineral product such as Life Extension Mix.

Autoimmune Nutrition

In addition to general nutrition, there are specific nutritional treatments for the autoimmune disease group of disorders. The concept of autoimmunity is discussed further in the protocol entitled *Autoimmune Disease* and applies to SLE. Please refer to that protocol for additional nutritional information. SLE patients must also plan to avoid the most common serious complications of their disease. Certainly, the possible vascular involvement would weigh heavily in favor of a low-saturated fat diet, the benefit of which is shown in early research in animals with lupus-like disease (Corman 1985). Likewise, potential kidney problems suggest a diet relatively low in protein as well as low in salt (because kidney malfunctions lead to high blood pressure).

The effect of dietary modifications has been extensively studied in lupus mouse models. Calorie, protein, and especially fat restriction cause a significant reduction in immune-complex deposition in the kidney (immune-complexes are formed when the immune system locks on to the "foreign" tissue protein and are responsible for the organ destruction found in lupus); reduced proteinuria; and prolongation of the mice's life span. The addition of polyunsaturated fatty acids (PUFAs) such as fish oil or linseed oil was also related to decreased mice morbidity and mortality in animal models of lupus.

PUFAs such as eicosapetaenoic acid (EPA) and docosahexaenoic acid (DHA) competitively inhibit the inflammatory fatty acid known as arachidonic acid with a resultant decrease in inflammatory immune messengers. (Arachidonic acid is found in red meats.) Human studies support the effect of a PUFAs-enriched diet, clinically (Leiba et al. 2001). One study has shown a significant effect of flaxseed in preventing the renal dysfunction of SLE. This led the authors to conclude that flaxseed appears to be renoprotective in lupus nephritis, but a larger study will be needed to confirm this (Clark et al. 2001).

STEROID THERAPY SIDE EFFECTS

Many lupus patients have no choice in the use of steroid therapy: they must take these drugs or they will develop catastrophic organ involvement. Some side effects of steroids may be mitigated with the proper supplements. The most significant example is the loss of calcium leading to osteoporosis. Proper nutritional treatment of osteoporosis involves a delicate balance of minerals, far beyond simply taking calcium (*for a discussion of such treatments, please refer to the Osteoporosis protocol*).

Additionally, steroids may cause potassium levels to decrease. When this occurs, oral replacement is required. Because steroids can release clots of fat into the blood stream, nutritional supplements which break down fats are recommended (*for a complete description of how to deal with this problem, see the Thrombosis Prevention protocol*). Another possible result of steroid therapy is cognitive confusion and loss of concentration. If this occurs, there are many supplements available. Again, the reader is referred to another section, the *Age-Associated Mental Impairment Protocol*, for a listing of the treatments available. Finally, steroids may deplete vitamin B_6, vitamin D, and zinc. These substances require supplementation. Note that B-complex vitamins also are depleted by aspirin and indomethacin (Lupus Alert 1988), common anti-inflammatory medications.

SPECIFIC SYMPTOM TREATMENT

The complexity of SLE causes symptoms in many sites and in many ways. It is possible to treat some of these with supplements:

Osteoporosis. Besides being a side effect of steroid use, osteoporosis can occur as a direct result of lupus. Nutritional support for osteoporosis involves vitamins, minerals, and additional supplements to increase and/or stabilize bone density and bone mineral content and suppress bone resorption (*see the Osteoporosis protocol for specific recommendations*).

Pain. There are several supplements recommended for the chronic aching common in lupus. Two amino acids, *DL*-phenylalanine and tyrosine (500 mg taken 2 or 3 times a day), are capable of elevating brain endorphin levels. Endorphins are the body's natural pain killers, and raising their availability can reduce pain. Another substance used to limit pain is melatonin.

Arthritis. Because most lupus patients have some form of arthritic symptoms from mild to disabling, SLE may be treated with many of the same supplements used in the Arthritis Protocol. These substances include antioxidants, glucosamine, chondroitin, and essential fatty acids (particularly, gamma-linolenic acid or GLA) that help reduce inflammation. In addition to the recommendations for pain listed above, there are specific natural arthritic pain products such as ArthroPro and Natural Pain Relief for Arthritis that utilize agents used in European clinics as the primary treatment for joint inflammation.

Systemic Inflammation. Inflammation can be traced to destructive cell-signalling chemicals, known as cytokines, which contribute to many degenerative and autoimmune diseases.

1. Essential fatty acids such as those contained in perilla, flax, borage, or fish oil supplements are effective in inhibiting pro-inflammatory cytokines and inhibiting anti-inflammatory cytokines. Alexander et al. (1987) demonstrated a reduction in glomerulonephritis (kidney disease) and a significant rise in longevity in a fish oil supplemented group of lupus-prone animals, as compared to groups given either saturated fat or corn oil supplements. Robinson et al. (1985) stated that fish oil "had the most striking protective effect seen thus far in any animal model of inflammatory disease." These results were supported by Kelly et al. (1985), who showed that fish oil suppressed lupus in mice, delaying renal disease and prolonging survival.

2. Dehydroepiandrosterone (DHEA) is a hormone that the body may convert into both androgens and estrogens for various uses. DHEA has multiple interactions with the body's immune system and the excess or lack of this substance produces significant effects on an autoimmune disease such as SLE. In one study (Araghi-Niknam et al. 1998), supplemental dietary DHEA restored normal functioning to the deregulated cytokine (immune-modulating proteins) production in mice. Other research (Yang et. al. 1998) demonstrated that DHEA delayed the activity of a key inflammatory agent, interleukin-6 (IL-6), and prolonged the survival of mice with lupus-like disease. Similarly, Suzuki et al. (1995) showed that DHEA significantly increased production of IL-2 (an interleukin that moderates the system's inflammatory responsiveness), while reversing autoimmune disease in laboratory animals. An even broader statement of the importance of DHEA came from Jiang et al. (1998). These researchers concluded that DHEA restored IL-2 secretion, decreased the inflammatory agent interferon-gamma, and normalized IL-6 activity. In addition, they discovered that DHEA and antioxidant nutrients (vitamins E and C, curcumin,

alpha-lipoic acid, and others mentioned previously) have a synergistic effect upon one another, emphasizing the need for a complex nutritional approach.

3. An impressive study on the effects of DHEA on SLE was conducted by researchers at Stanford University Medical Center. The study group consisted of 50 females, 37 premenopausal and 13 postmenopausal, with mild to moderate SLE. Test subjects were treated with long-term therapy (up to 1 year) of 50–200 mg daily of oral DHEA: 34 patients (68%) completed 6 months of therapy, and 21 patients (42%) completed 12 months of therapy. The results showed that DHEA therapy was associated with a decrease in SLE disease activity as measured by the SLE Disease Activity Index Score, patient global assessment, and physician global assessment compared to baseline. Prednisone doses were concurrently reduced. These improvements were sustained over the entire treatment period. Mild acne was the most common side effect, affecting 54% of the study group. Researchers reported that efficacy was similar in both pre- and postmenopausal women and that DHEA was well tolerated and clinically beneficial in patients who maintained therapy.

4. Testosterone. This hormone appears to play a significant role in the body's autoimmune system. Kanda et al. (1996) studied the effects of testosterone on several inflammation-causing agents. They found that it reduced IL-6 and two immunoglobulins, IgG and IgM. In mice with lupus, Keisler et al. (1995) discovered low levels of testosterone and high levels of estradiol (estrogen), suggesting a causal relationship. When testosterone was given to these animals, longevity increased. This evidence indicates that hormone balances in SLE patients may be disrupted and that proper regulation may be therapeutic. This treatment is discussed in great detail in the *Male Hormone Modulation Therapy* protocol. Females must be more careful about using testosterone because there may be a more narrow therapeutic dosage range (*see Female Hormone Modulation Therapy* protocol).

Supplement Recommendations
Reducing Chronic Inflammation
Supplementation with omega-3 essential fatty acids from fish, flax, or perilla oils, along with borage oil, evening primrose oil, or black currant seed oil which contain the essential omega-6 fatty acid gamma-linoleic acid (GLA), can alleviate many symptoms of autoimmune disease through their anti-inflammatory activity. Docosahexaenoic acid (DHA) extracted

for electrolytes, it can give an indication of acid-base balance and degree of hydration.

Normal Range: 96–109 mmol/L
Critical Values: <80 or > 115 mmol/L

Carbon Dioxide: This test is used to assist in the evaluation of the pH and electrolyte status.

Normal Range: 20–32 mmol/L
Critical Values: <6 mmol/L

Calcium: This test is used to evaluate parathyroid function and calcium metabolism.

Normal Range: 8.5–10.6 mg/dL
Critical Values: <6.0 or > 13 mg/dL

Phosphorus: This test is used to measure serum phosphorus. An imbalance could indicate the possibility of any number of conditions.

Normal Range:
12–60 years: 2.5–4.5 mg/dL
>60 years male: 2.3–3.7 mg/dL
>60 years female: 2.8–4.1 mg/dL

Protein/Albumin/Globulin: This test is used to assist in the detection of many diseases that affect total blood protein or one single fraction of protein.

Normal range:
Total protein: 6.0–8.5 g/dL
Albumin: 3.5–5.5 g/dL
Globulin: 1.5–4.5 g/dL

Albumin/Globulin Ratio: This test is used to evaluate renal disease and other chronic disease.

Normal Range: 1.1–2.5

Bilirubin: This test is used to evaluate liver function.

Normal Ranges:
Total bilirubin: 0.1–1.2 mg/dL
Indirect bilirubin: 0.2–0.8 mg/dL
Direct bilirubin: 0.1–0.3 mg/dL

Alkaline Phosphatase: This test is used to detect and monitor liver and/or bone disease.

Optimal Range: 25–150 IU/L

LDH (Lactate Dehydrogenase): This test measures the intracellular enzyme LDH which, when present in the blood, can support the detection of injury or disease.

Normal Range: 100–250 U/L

AST (SGOT): This test is used to evaluate the possibility of coronary occlusive heart disease or liver disease.

Normal Range: 0–40 IU/L

ALT (SGPT): This test is used to identify liver disease and to distinguish between the liver and red blood cell hemolysis as the source of jaundice.

Normal Range: 0–40 IU/L

Iron: This test is used to evaluate many diseases including iron deficiency anemia and hemochromatosis.

Normal Range:
Male: 40–155 mg/dL
Female: 35–155 mg/dL
Optimal Range: 40–100 mg/dL

Cholesterol: This test is used to determine the risk of coronary heart disease (CHD) and hyperlipidemias.

Normal range: 100–199 mg/dL
Optimal Range: 180–200 mg/dL

Triglycerides: This test is used to identify the risk of developing coronary heart disease or if disorders of fat metabolism are suspected.

Normal Range: 0–199 mg/dL
Optimal Range: 40–100 mg/dL

HDL Cholesterol: This test measures alpha-lipoprotein and is used to predict heart disease.

Normal Range: 35–150 mg/dL
Optimal Range: 55–150 mg/dL

LDL Cholesterol: This test measures beta-lipoproteins and is used to predict heart disease.

Normal Range: 0–129 mg/dL
Optimal Range: <100 mg/dL

Total Cholesterol/HDL Ratio: This test is used to determine the risk for coronary heart disease.

Normal Range: 5:1 or less
Optimal Range: 3.1 or less

CBC (Complete Blood Count) with Platelets and Differential

This is a series of tests of the peripheral blood, which provides a variety of information about the blood components. This series includes the following tests:

Red blood cell count

Normal range:
Male: 4.1–5.6 million/mm^3
Female: 3.8–5.10 million/mm^3

Hemoglobin

Normal Range:
Male: 12.5–17.0 g/dL
Female: 11.5–15.0 g/dL
Critical Values: <5.0 g/dL or > 20 g/dL

Hematocrit

Normal Range:
Male: 36–50%
Female: 34–44%
Critical Values: <15% or >60%

Red Blood Cell Indices

- Mean Corpuscular Volume

  Normal Range: 80–98 mm^3

- Mean corpuscular Hemoglobin

  Normal Range: 27–34 pg

- Mean Corpuscular Hemoglobin Concentration

  Normal Range: 32–36 g/dL

- Red Blood Cell Distribution

  Normal Range: 11.7%–15.0%

- White Blood Cell Count

  Normal Range: 4000–10,500/mm^3
  Critical Values: <2500 or >30,000 mm^3

- Differential Count

  Normal Range: Reference Interval
  Polyneutrophils: 4000–7400/mm^3 1.8–7.8 × 10^{-3}/mcL
  Lymphocytes: 1400–4600/mm^3 0.7–4.5 × 10^{-3}/mcL
  Monocytes: 400–1300/mm^3 0.1–1.0 × 10^{-3}/mcL
  Eosinophils: 0–700/mm^3 0.0–0.4 × 10^{-3}/mcL
  Basophils: 0–300/mm^3 0.0–0.2 × 10^{-3}/mcL

- Platelet Count

  Normal Range: 140–415 × 10^{-3}/mcL
  Critical Values: <50,000 or > 1 million/mm^3

Coenzyme Q10

This test is used to measure serum levels of Coenzyme Q10. The body is capable of synthesizing Coenzyme Q10, however, deficiency clearly occurs, and can be seen in heart failure, cardiomyopathies, gingivitis, hypertension, Muscular Dystrophy, AIDS, and kidney problems. Low levels also appear more common in the elderly.

Cortisol

This test is used to identify adrenocortical insufficiency, Addison's disease, adrenocortical hypersecretion, Cushing's syndrome. Malfunction of the organs in the hypothalamic-pituitary-adrenal cortex axis will result in alteration of cortisol levels.

Normal Ranges:
a.m.: 4.3–22.4 mcg/dL
p.m.: 3.1–16.7 mcg/dL

Cortisol AM/PM

This test is to measure adrenal function. It is used to detect adrenal-cortical insufficiency/hypersecretion and Cushing's syndrome, and is useful in detecting the malfunction of the hypothalamic-pituitary axis.

Reference Interval
a.m.: 4.3–22.4 mcg/dL
p.m.: 3.1–16.7 mcg/dL

C-Peptide

This test is principally used in the evaluation of hypoglycemia. Individuals with insulin-secreting tumors have high levels of both C-peptide and endogenous insulin. Individuals with factitious hypoglycemia will have low C-peptide levels in the presence of elevated serum insulin. C-peptide is also useful in assessing residual beta-cell function in insulin-dependent diabetics, who may have antibodies that interfere with insulin assays. Further research has demonstrated the concentration of glucagon-stimulated C-peptide is a good discriminator between insulin-requiring and noninsulin-requiring diabetic individuals. The identification of islet cell tumor is supported by elevation of C-peptide.

Reference Interval: >16 years: 1.1–5.0 ng/mL

C-Reactive Protein (Cardiac) (High Sensitivity)

C-reactive protein (CRP) is a marker for systemic inflammation with linkage to blood vessel damage and vascular disease. This test is used to assess risk of cardiovascular and peripheral vascular disease.

Normal Ranges:

Relative Risks – Male

CRP (mg/L)	Future MI	Future Stroke
>2.11	2.9	1.9
1.15–2.10	2.6	1.9
0.56–1.14	1.7	1.7
<0.55	1.0	1.0

Relative Risks – Female

CRP (mg/L)	Future MI or Stroke
>7.30	5.5
3.80–7.30	3.5
1.50–3.70	2.7
<1.50	1.0

Cytokine Panel (IL-1b, IL-6, IL-8, TNF-α)

This panel is used to identify elevated levels of specific cytokines. Cytokines are critical early mediators of the inflammatory and overall immune response and as such, are believed to play an important role in the development of pathological conditions that result in chronic inflammation, septic shock, and hematopoietic defects. While inflammation is an important homeostatic mechanism that limits the effects of infectious agents, inflammation itself has the potential for inducing damage. The following tests are included in this panel: IL-1b, IL6, IL8, and TNF-α.

- *Interleukin-1β (IL-1β):* This test is used to identify elevated levels of interleukin-1β. IL-1β is a cytokine produced principally by mononuclear phagocytes but also by various other cell types including keratinocytes, epithelium, and cells of the CNS. Elevated levels of IL-1β have been implicated in sepsis, cachexia, rheumatoid arthritis, chronic myelogenous leukemia, asthma, psoriasis, inflammatory bowel disease, anorexia, AIDS, and graft-versus-host disease associated with bone marrow transplants. IL-1β is one of the key mediators of immunobiological responses to physical stress. A pilot study showed that higher levels of IL-1β were associated with anxiety/panic disorder. Higher than normal levels have also been associated with a significantly increased risk of myocardial infarction independent of cardiac levels of CRP.

Normal Ranges: <150 pg/mL

- *Interleukin-6 (IL-6):* This test is used to identify elevated levels of IL-6. IL-6 is a cytokine produced by many different cells including monocytes/macrophages, fibroblasts, endothelial cells, keratinocytes, mast cells, T cells, and many tumor cell lines. Elevated IL-6 serum or plasma levels may occur in different conditions including sepsis, autoimmune diseases, lymphomas, AIDS, alcoholic liver disease, tumor development, Alzheimer's disease, and in concert with infections or transplant rejection. Elevated levels of IL-6 may be associated with an increased risk of heart attack and stroke.

Normal Ranges: <29 pg/mL

- *Interleukin-8 (IL-8):* This test is used to identify elevated levels of IL-8. IL-8 is produced by stimulated monocytes, macrophages, fibroblasts, endothelial cells, keratinocytes, melanocytes, hepatocytes, chondrocytes, and a number of tumor cell lines. In many types of cells the synthesis of IL-8 is strongly stimulated by IL-1 and TNF-α. Elevated concentrations are observed in psoriasis, rheumatoid arthritis, chronic polyarthritis, tumor development, and Hepatitis C.

Normal Ranges: <80 pg/mL

- *Tumor necrosis factor alpha (TNF-α):* This test is used to identify elevated levels of TNF-α. A variety of cells are shown to produce TNF-α. TNF-α is a growth factor for fibroblasts and stimulates the synthesis of collagenase and prostaglandin E_2. Bone resorption can be induced by TNF-α because it activates osteoclasts. TNF-α enhances the proliferation of T cells after stimulation with IL-2. In the absence of IL-2, TNF-α induces the proliferation and differentiation of beta cells. TNF-α levels may be elevated in sepsis, cachexia, AIDS, Hepatitis C, transplant rejection, various infectious, and autoimmune diseases.

Normal Ranges: <25 pg/mL

D-Dimer

This test is a very specific confirmatory test for disseminated intravascular coagulation (DIC). This test is also used for the detection of deep vein thrombosis, acute myocardial infarction, and unstable angina. The Fragment D-Dimer assesses both thrombin and plasmin activity.

Reference Interval: 0.0–0.4 mcg/mL

Dehydroepiandrosterone (DHEA) Sulfate

This test is used to determine the cause of female infertility, amenorrhea or hirsutism, and aid in the evaluation of androgen excess, adrenocortical disease including congenital adrenal hyperplasia, and adrenal tumor.

Reference Interval (mcg/dL):

Age (years)	Male	Female
18–19	108–441	145–395
19–29	280–640	65–380
30–39	120–520	45–270
40–49	95–530	32–240
50–59	70–310	26–200
60–69	42–290	13–130
>69	28–175	17–90

Optimal Range Male: 400–500 mcg/dL
Optimal Range Female: 350–430 mcg/dL

Deoxypyridinoline (Dpd) Cross Link Test

This test can be used to assess bone resorption rates in healthy individuals and in those with enhanced risk of developing metabolic bone disease. Significantly high levels of Dpd are found in postmenopausal women due to estrogen deficiency, and in individuals with diseases that have high bone turnover rates. Dpd can be used to monitor anti-resorptive therapies (which may include bisphosphonates) in postmenopausal women and individuals diagnosed with osteoporosis.

Reference Interval:
Adults: 2.3–7.4 nmol Dpd/mmol creatinine

Dihydrotestosterone (DHT)

This test measures serum concentration of DHT and is closely related to that of testosterone. 5α-Dihydrotestosterone, the most potent naturally occurring androgen, is produced from testosterone through the action of steroid 5α-reductase. DHT is responsible for the development and maintenance of the male external genitalia and the prostate. It is also primarily responsible for the physical changes that occur during male sexual maturation. Elevated levels may indicate hypergonadism or hirsutism.

Reference Interval:
Adult Males: 25–99 ng/dL
Female:
Premenopausal: 2.4–36.8 ng/dL
Menopausal: 1–18.1 ng/dL

Epstein-Barr Virus (EBV) Acute Infection

This test is used to detect a suspected EBV infection (infectious mononucleosis). EBV is a herpes group virus, which is ubiquitous. It is the cause of classic infectious mononucleosis, and is causally implicated in the pathogenesis of Burkitt's lymphoma, some nasopharyngeal carcinomas, and rare hereditary lymphoproliferative disorders.

Reference Interval: Ranges are established by the laboratory

ESR Westergen Sedimentation Rate

The ESR is a nonspecific test used to detect illness associated with acute and chronic infection, autoimmune disorders, inflammation (collagen vascular diseases), advanced neoplasm, tissue necrosis, or infarction. Elevations in fibrinogen, alpha- and beta-globulins (acute phase reactants), and immunoglobulins increase the sedimentation rate of red cells through plasma. The test is important in the detection of temporal arteritis, and its management.

Reference Interval:

Male: 0–50 years: up to 15 mm/hour, 50 years and older: up to 20 mm/hour

Female: 0–50 years: up to 20 mm/hour, 50 years and older: up to 30 mm/hour

Estradiol

This test is used to assess hypothalamic and pituitary functions, and to evaluate menopausal status and sexual maturity. In males, it is helpful in the assessment of gynecomastia or feminization syndromes.

Reference Interval:

Male: <54 pg/mL

Optimal Range: 15–30 pg/mL

Menstruating female (day of cycle relative to LH peak):

Follicular (–12): 19–83 pg/mL

Follicular (–4): 64–183 pg/mL

Midcycle (–1): 150–528 pg/mL

Luteal (+2): 58–157 pg/mL

Luteal (+6): 60–211 pg/mL

Luteal (+12): 55–150 pg/mL

Postmenopausal (untreated): 0–31 pg/mL

Estriol

This test provides an objective assessment of placental function and fetal normality in high-risk pregnancies. Estriol is the major estrogen in the pregnant female.

> **Normal range:**
>
> **Male or nonpregnant female:** <2.0 mg/dL
>
> **Pregnant female:** Ranges are established by the laboratory

Estrogen Metabolite Ratio (Urine)

This test is used to evaluate estrogen metabolism in premenopausal and postmenopausal women, focusing on the critical balance between the body's two primary hydroxyestrones, 2-hydroxyestrone and 16α-hydroxyestrone. Measuring these primary estrogen metabolites allows practitioners to develop individualized therapy based on each woman's unique health risks. Estrogen is metabolized in two ways. Along one pathway, it is converted into a powerful metabolite, 16α-hydroxyestrone, which acts to stimulate target tissues. Levels of 16α-hydroxyestrone can rise in response to obesity, alcohol consumption, and exposure to toxic substances. High levels of this potent metabolite are linked to increased risk and poorer prognosis in conditions associated with estrogen excess, such as breast cancer and lupus. Alternately, the body can break down estrogen into a much weaker metabolite, called 2-hydroxyestrone, which binds weakly to cell receptors and may slow cell proliferation. However, excessive levels of 2-hydroxyestrone may increase the risk of developing conditions associated with estrogen deficiency, such as heart disease, depression, and osteoporosis.

> **Reference Interval:** Ranges are established by the laboratory

Estrogens, Total

Estrogen measurements are used to evaluate sexual maturity, menstrual problems, and fertility problems in females. This test is also used in the evaluation of males with gynecomastia or feminization syndromes. In pregnant women, it is used to indicate fetal-placental health. In individuals with estrogen-producing tumors, it can be used as a tumor marker.

> **Reference Interval:**
>
> **Male:** 40–115 pg/mL
>
> **Female cycle:**
>
> Day 1–10: 61–394 pg/mL
>
> Day 11–20: 122–437 pg/mL

Day 21–30: 156–350 pg/mL

Postmenopausal: <40 pg/mL

HMG treatment for ovulation induction: 400–800 pg/mL

Estrone

This test is used to evaluate postmenopausal bleeding due to peripheral conversion of androgenic steroids. Increased estrone levels may be associated with increased levels of circulating androgens and their subsequent peripheral conversion.

> **Reference Interval:**
>
> **Male:** 12–72 pg/mL
>
> **Female:**
>
> Follicular phase: 37–138 pg/mL
>
> Midcycle: 60–229 pg/mL
>
> Luteal phase: 50–114 pg/mL

Factor VIII Activity

This test is used to evaluate levels of coagulation factor VIII. A deficiency in factor VIII is known as hemophilia A. It is the most common of the hereditary bleeding disorders. Elevated levels are associated with a significantly increased risk of ischemic heart disease and to the development of the geriatric syndrome of frailty.

> **Reference Interval:** 50% to 150%
> (100% = approximately 10 mcg/L)

Fasting Glucose/Insulin

These two tests are used to determine elevated levels of glucose and insulin. Glucose and insulin are implicated in many age-related diseases, such as type 2 diabetes, hypertension, heart disease, and stroke, and are a hallmark of mammalian aging. **Please Note:** These tests require a fasting blood level; therefore, a 12-hour fast is required before the collection of a blood sample.

- *Glucose:* This test is used to detect diabetes mellitus and evaluate carbohydrate metabolism disorders including alcoholism. It is also used to evaluate acidosis, ketoacidosis, dehydration, coma, hypoglycemia, insulinoma, and neuroglycopenia.

> **Reference Interval:** 65–109 mg/dL
> (Optimal: 70–100 mg/dL)
> (Ideal levels may be under 86 mg/dL)

- *Insulin:* This test is primarily used to measure insulin in the evaluation of individuals with fasting hypoglycemia. Insulin levels tend to be inappropriately elevated in individuals with insulin-secreting tumors. Fasting hypoglycemia in association with markedly elevated serum insulin levels is considered the determining factor for insulinoma. Insulin is a protein hormone produced by the beta-cells of the pancreas. Insulin is an anabolic hormone that stimulates the uptake of glucose into fat and muscles and promotes the formation of glycogen. Insulin stimulates protein synthesis and inhibits protein degradation. Glucose, amino acids, and certain pancreatic and gastrointestinal hormones (e.g., glucagon, gastrin, secretin) stimulate the pancreas to secrete insulin. Insulin secretion is inhibited by hypoglycemia and somatostatin. In healthy individuals, insulin is secreted in a pulsatile fashion that is closely controlled by glucose levels. Insulin levels can be useful in predicting susceptibility to the development of type II diabetes, although C-peptide has largely supplanted insulin measurement for this role.

  Reference Interval: 6–27 mcIU/mL
  (Optimal: Under 5 mcIU/mL)

Female Panel Tests

This comprehensive panel is used to evaluate female health status. The following tests are included in this panel: Chemistry panel (CBC), Free Testosterone, Total Testosterone, DHEA-S, Estradiol, Progesterone, Homocysteine, and (cardiac) CRP. *Please Note:* This panel requires a fasting blood level; therefore, a 12-hour fast is required before the collection of a blood sample. For desired ranges, see specific tests by name.

Ferritin

This test is used to evaluate iron stores in the body and to determine iron deficiency anemia (hypochromic and microcytic anemias). This test can detect decreased levels found in iron deficiency anemia and increased levels found in iron overload. In hemochromatosis, both ferritin and iron saturation are increased.

  Reference Interval:
  Male: 22–322 ng/mL
  Female: 10–291 ng/mL

Fibrinogen, Quantitative

This test is used primarily for detecting suspected bleeding disorders or excessive bleeding, which could contribute to abnormal clotting. Fibrinogen is produced in the liver and is essential to the blood-clotting mechanism. It is an acute-phase reactant protein. Levels rise sharply during tissue inflammation or tissue necrosis. Elevated levels can be a predictor of increased risk of coronary artery or cerebrovascular disease. Decreased levels can indicate liver disease, malnutrition, disseminated intravascular coagulation (DIC), and numerous blood transfusions. (Individuals using oral contraceptives are found to have increased levels of fibrinogen.)

  Reference Interval: 215–519 mg/dL
  (Optimal: 215–300 mg/dL)

Fructosamine

This test is used to evaluate diabetic control. Fructosamine is indicated as an index of longer-term control rather than glucose levels. However, it reflects diabetic control over a shorter time period (2–3 weeks) than that of hemoglobin A (Hb A), which represents control over a 4–8 week time period. Fructosamine is found in the plasma of both normal and diabetic individuals. "Fructosamine" is the term used to describe glycated proteins (i.e., derivatives of the nonenzymatic reaction product of glucose and albumin). It has been advocated as an alternative test to Hb A for the monitoring of long-term diabetic control. Fructosamine and Hb A do not measure exactly the same thing. Fructosamine has a shorter half-life and appears to be more sensitive to short-term variations in glucose levels. Fructosamine is clearly superior in patients with abnormal hemoglobins because of the interference of abnormal hemoglobins in the anion-exchange chromatography methods for Hb A.

  Poorly controlled diabetic range: 228–563 mcmol/L

FSH and LH (Follicle-Stimulating Hormone and Luteinizing Hormone)

This test is used in the determination of menopause and is integral in the evaluation of suspected gonadal failure.

Normal range:	FSH
Adult male > 15 years:	1.4–18.1 mIU/mL
Optimal Range:	1.4–14 mIU/mL
Female:	
Follicular phase:	2.5–10.2 mIU/mL
Ovulatory phase:	3.4–33.4 mIU/mL
Luteal phase:	1.5–9.1 mIU/mL
Postmenopause:	23.0–116.3 mIU/mL

Normal Range:	LH
Adult Male:	
20–70 years:	1.5–9.3 mIU/mL
>70 years:	3.1–34.6 mIU/mL
Optimal Range:	0.5–9.3 mIU/mL
Female:	
Follicular phase:	1.9–12.5 mIU/mL
Ovulatory peak:	8.7–76.3 mIU/mL
Luteal phase:	0.5–16.9 mIU/mL
Postmenopause:	5.0–52.3 mIU/mL

Gamma Glutamyl Transpeptidase (GGT)

This test is a sensitive indicator of hepatobiliary disease (obstructive jaundice, intrahepatic cholestasis, pancreatitis). It is also used as an indicator of chronic and heavy alcohol abuse.

Normal Range:
Male and female: 0–65 IU/L

Glucose (Serum)

This test is used to detect diabetes mellitus. It is used to evaluate carbohydrate metabolism disorders including alcoholism. It is also used to evaluate acidosis, ketoacidosis, dehydration, coma, hypoglycemia, insulinoma, and neuroglycopenia. ***Please Note:*** This panel requires a fasting blood level; therefore, a 12-hour fast is required before the collection of a blood sample.

Reference Interval: 65–109 mg/dL
Optimal: Under 100 mg/dL
(Ideal may be under 86 mg/dL.)

HCG Beta Subunit, Pregnancy

This test is used to detect the beta subunit of human chorionic gonadotropin (HCG) and provides a sensitive, specific test for the detection of early pregnancy, ectopic pregnancy, or threatened abortion.

Reference Interval:
Negative: <10 mIU/mL
Borderline: 10–20 mIU/mL
Positive: >20 mIU/mL

HCG Beta Subunit, Quantitative (Cancer)

This test is used as a tumor marker for certain cancers. It is used to evaluate and monitor males with testicular tumors. This test is also used to determine the presence of HCG in individuals with gestational trophoblastic disease.

Reference Interval: Male and nonpregnant female: 99% have values <10 mIU/mL

Heavy Metals Profile I, Blood

This test is used to monitor exposure to arsenic, lead, and mercury.

Reference Interval:
Arsenic: 2–23 mcg/L
Lead

Environmental exposure (WHO): 0–19 mcg/dL
Occupational exposure, BEI® (sampling time is not critical): 30 mcg/dL
OSHA Lead Standard: 40 mcg/dL
USPHS Y2K goal: <25 mcg/dL

Mercury

Environmental exposure: 0.0–8.0 mcg/L
Individuals consuming large quantities of seafood may have values as high as 200.0 mcg/L
Occupational exposure, BEI®: inorganic mercury (sampling time is end of shift at end of work week): 15.0 mcg/L
Optimal range: As low as possible

Helicobactor (Campylobacter) Pylori, IGG

This test is used as an aid in the detection of *H. pylori* infection, to determine the cause of chronic type B gastritis, and ulcers of the stomach or duodenum.

Reference Interval:
Negative: <=0.8 U/mL
Indeterminate: 0.9–1.0 U/mL
Positive: >=1.1 U/mL

Hemoglobin A1C

This test is most frequently used to assess glucose control in insulin-dependent diabetic individuals whose glucose levels are very labile.

Normal Range (Adult): 4.5% to 5.7%

Hepatitis B Surface Antibody, Qualitative

This test is useful for evaluation of possible immunity in individuals who are at increased risk for exposure to hepatitis B.

Reference Interval: Negative

Hepatitis C Virus Antibody

This test is used to assess exposure to hepatitis C virus infection.

Reference Interval: Negative

Hepatitis Panel (A, B, C), Acute

This test is used as a comprehensive panel for detecting markers for HAV, HBV or HCV infections, and is used for all stages of infection.

Homocysteine

Homocysteine has been shown to be an independent risk factor for the premature development of coronary artery disease and thrombosis. This test is intended for use in screening individuals who may be at risk for heart disease and stroke. Studies have shown that even moderate levels of homocysteine pose an increased risk for arteriosclerosis compared with the lowest 20th percentile (<7.2 mcmol/L) of population controls.

Reference Interval:

Male: 6.3–15.0 mcmol/L

Female: 4.6–12.4 mcmol/L

Desirable: <7.2 mcmol/L

Hyperhomocysteinemia:

Borderline: 12–15 mcmol/L

Moderate: >15–30 mcmol/L

Intermediate: >30–100 mcmol/L

Severe: >100 mcmol/L

IL-6/IGF-1

This test is used to evaluate levels of Insulin-Like Growth Factor-1 (IGF-1) and Interkeukin-6 (IL-6). Research investigating DHEA-S levels found that IGF-I was positively correlated to DHEA-S levels and IL-6 levels were negatively correlated to DHEA-S levels.

- *Interleukin-6 (IL-6):* This test is used to identify elevated levels of IL-6. IL-6 is a cytokine produced by many different cells including monocytes/macrophages, fibroblasts, endothelial cells, keratinocytes, mast cells, T cells and many tumor cell lines. Elevated IL-6 serum or plasma levels may occur in different conditions including sepsis, autoimmune diseases, lymphomas, AIDS, alcoholic liver disease, tumor development, Alzheimer's disease, and in individuals with infections or transplant rejection. Elevated levels of IL-6 may be associated with an increased risk of heart attack and stroke.

Normal Ranges: <29 pg/mL

- *Insulin-Like Growth Factor 1 (IGF-1):* This test is used to determine acromegaly, in which somatomedin-C (Sm-C) and growth factor (GH) are increased. It is also used to evaluate hypopituitarism. Sm-C is a polypeptide hormone produced by the liver and other tissues, with effects on growth promoting activity and glucose metabolism (insulin-like activity). Sm-C is carried in blood bound to a carrier protein which prolongs its half-life. Its level is therefore more constant than that of growth hormone. Low values are measured with advanced age. Low values may indicate hypopituitarism, malnutrition, diabetes mellitus, Laron dwarfism, hypothyroidism, maternal deprivation syndrome, pubertal delay, cirrhosis, hepatoma, and some cases of short stature and normal GH response to pharmacologic tests. Low values may be found with nonfunctioning pituitary tumors, with constitutional delay of growth, and with anorexia nervosa. High values occur with adolescence, true precocious puberty, pregnancy, obesity, pituitary gigantism, acromegaly and diabetic retinopathy. Since Sm-C is decreased with malnutrition, its concentration provides an index with which to monitor therapy for food deprivation.

Reference Interval:

Females/Males (Age)	Range (ng/mL)
18	163–584
19	141–483
20	127–424
21–25	116–358
26–30	117–329
31–35	115–307
36–40	109–284
41–45	101–267
46–50	94–252
51–55	87–238
56–60	81–225
61–65	75–212
66–70	69–200
71–75	64–188
76–80	59–177
81–85	55–166

- *Insulin-like Growth Factor Binding Protein (IGFBP-3):* Elevated levels of this protein in hypertensive individuals (high blood pressure) have been associated with nine-fold increases in arteriosclerosis.

Insulin, Fasting

This test is used for insulin measurement in the evaluation of individuals with fasting hypoglycemia or hyperglycemia. High fasting insulin is a sign of insulin resistance and the start of type II diabetes or Syndrome X.

> **Reference Interval:** 6–27 mcIU/mL
>
> **Optimal:** Under 5 mcIU/mL

Interleukin-1 beta (IL-1b)

See Cytokine Panel.

Interleukin-6 (IL-6)

See Cytokine Panel.

Interleukin-8 (IL-8)

See Cytokine Panel.

Iron and Total Iron Binding (TIB)

This test is used in the detection of anemia. TIB levels are often used to monitor the course of individuals receiving hyperalimentation.

> **Normal range:**
>
> **Male:** 40–180 mg/dL
>
> **Female:** 50–170 mg/dL
>
> **Optimal Range:** 40–100 mg/dL
>
> **TIBC:** 250–420 mg/dL

Lipase

This test is used to diagnose pancreatitis or inflammatory bowel disease. An injured or diseased pancreas will produce abnormal amounts of this enzyme.

> **Normal Range:** 0–59U/L

Lipoprotein (a)

This test is used to measure excess small dense lipoprotein, which is a strong indicator for premature coronary disease and atherosclerotic vascular disease, and is associated with increased risk of cardiac death in individuals with acute coronary syndromes and coronary bypass procedures.

> **Normal Range:** 0–30 mg/dL
>
> **Desirable:** <20 mg/dL
>
> **Borderline High Risk:** 20–30 mg/dL
>
> **High Risk:** 31–50 mg/dL
>
> **Very High Risk:** >50 mg/dL

Magnesium

This test is used to evaluate magnesium levels. Decreased levels of magnesium have been associated with cardiac arrhythmias. Magnesium deficiency produces neuromuscular disorders causing weakness, tremors, tetany, and convulsions. Hypomagnesemia is associated with hypocalcemia, hypokalemia, long-term hyperalimentation, intravenous therapy, diabetes mellitus (especially during treatment of ketoacidosis), alcoholism, other types of malnutrition, malabsorption, hyperparathyroidism, dialysis, pregnancy, and hyperaldosteronism. Renal loss of magnesium occurs with *cis*-platinum therapy. Increased magnesium levels occur in renal failure. Marked increases may be found in individuals taking magnesium-containing antacids. Increased serum magnesium is found in Addison's disease and in pregnant woman with severe pre-eclampsia or eclampsia who are receiving magnesium sulfate as an anticonvulsant. Hypermagnesemia may occur in individuals using magnesium-containing cathartics. High magnesium levels are manifested by decreased reflexes, somnolence, and heart block.

> **Reference Interval:** 4.2–6.8 mg/dL

MALE HORMONE MODULATING PROFILE

This profile assesses the need for, or effectiveness of, hormone modulation. Included in this profile is the **Male Panel Test,** a comprehensive panel used to evaluate male health status. The following tests are included: Chemistry Panel/CBC, Free Testosterone, Total Testosterone, DHEA-S, PSA, Estradiol, Homocysteine, (cardiac) CRP, Progesterone, FSH, LH and TSH. *Please Note:* This panel requires a fasting blood level; therefore, a 12-hour fast is required before the collection of a blood sample. (For desired ranges, see specific tests by name.)

Osteocalcin

This is a blood test used to evaluate bone disease. Increased levels are found in bone diseases characterized by increased bone turnover, especially osteoporosis.

Parathyroid Hormone (PTH), Intact

This test is used in detecting parathyroid disease, detecting and monitoring other diseases of calcium homeostasis, and for monitoring individuals undergoing renal dialysis.

> **Normal range (adults older than 20 years):** 12–72 pg/mL

Pregnenolone

This test is used to determine ovarian failure, hirsutism, adrenal carcinoma, and Cushing's syndrome.

Normal range:
Male: 10–200 ng/dL
Female: 10–230 ng/dL

Progesterone

In females, this test is used to establish the presence of a functional corpus luteum or luteal cell function, confirm body temperature for occurrence of ovulation, obtain indication of day of ovulation, evaluate the functional state of corpus luteum in infertility, assess placental function during pregnancy, and evaluate ovarian function. In males this test is used to establish the presence of progesterone and 17-α-hydroxyprogesterone, considered weak androgens. Increased levels are found in congenital adrenal hyperplasia due to 21-hydroxylase, 17-hydroxylase, and 11-β-hydroxylase deficiency. Levels are decreased in primary or secondary hypogonadism.

Male:
Normal range: <0.3–1.2 ng/mL
Female:
Follicular: 0.2–14 ng/mL
Luteal: 3.3–25.6 ng/mL
Midluteal: 4.4–28.0 ng/mL
Postmenopausal: 0.0–0.7 ng/mL

Prolactin

This test is used to assess inappropriate lactation, and is also useful in the detection of prolactin-secreting pituitary tumors. Elevated prolactin is associated with anovulation and amenorrhea. Prolactin can also be elevated in hypothyroidism when TSH is high.

Males:
Normal range: 2.17–17.7 ng/mL
Females:
Normal range: 2.8–29.2 ng/mL
Nonpregnant: 2.8–29.2 ng/mL
Pregnant: 9.7–208.5 ng/mL
Postmenopausal: 1.8–20.3 ng/mL

Prostate Specific Antigen (PSA)

PSA is produced by normal, hyperplastic, and cancerous prostatic tissue. Serum PSA has been found to be the most sensitive marker for monitoring individuals with prostate cancer and to enhance efficacy in monitoring progression of disease and response to therapy.

Normal findings: 0–4.0 ng/mL
Optimal range: 0–2.6 ng/mL

PSA Free/Total Ratio Reflex

This test is used to measure the percentage of free PSA relative to the total amount of PSA in men. Serum PSA levels increase due to physical changes to prostate architecture due to trauma, infection, inflammation, and disease. Sensitivity of PSA levels to these changes serves as a basis for this test. A Higher percentage of free PSA is associated with a higher risk of prostate cancer.

Normal findings: 0–4.0 ng/mL

Free PSA (%)	50–64 years (%)	65–75 years (%)
0.00–10.00	56	55
10.01–15.00	24	35
15.01–20.00	17	23
20.01–25.00	10	20
>25	5	9

PT/PTT

Prothrombin time (PT) and partial thromboplastin time (PTT) tests are used to evaluate the extrinsic coagulation system. They may also aid in screening for congenital deficiencies of Factors II, V, VII, X and deficiencies of prothrombin, dysfibrinogenemia, and afibrinogenemia. PT and PTT tests enable evaluation of the effects of heparin and warfarin anticoagulant therapy, liver failure, disseminated intravascular coagulation (DIC), and vitamin K deficiency.

- *Prothrombin time (PT):* This test is used to evaluate the adequacy of the extrinsic system and common pathway in the clotting mechanism. PT is monitored to follow long-term anticoagulant therapy (e.g., warfarin, Coumadin®). Anticoagulant therapy that is properly monitored impedes thrombus formation without the threat of serious hemorrhage.

  Reference Interval: Ranges are established by the laboratory.

- *Partial Thromboplastin Time (PTT):* This test is used to evaluate the intrinsic coagulation system. It is also used to monitor heparin therapy, to aid in detecting classical hemophilia A, Christmas disease, and detection of congenital deficiencies of Factors II, V, VIII, IX, X, XI, and XII. PTT is used to screen for the presence of dysfibrinogenemia, DIC, liver failure, congenital hypofibrinogenemia, vitamin K deficiency, congenital deficiency of Fitzgerald factor, congenital deficiency of prekallikrein, high molecular weight kininogen, and circulatory anticoagulant.

Reference Interval: Ranges are established by the laboratory.

PT, PTT, Alpha-1-Antitrypsin, Thrombin, Antithrombin

This panel of tests is used to evaluate the extrinsic coagulation system. These tests may also aid in screening for congenital deficiencies of Factors II, V, VII, and X and deficiencies of prothrombin, dysfibrinogenemia, and afibrinogenemia. Levels of PT, PTT, thrombin and antithrombin are used to evaluate heparin effect, warfarin anticoagulant therapy, liver failure, DIC, and vitamin K deficiency. This test includes the following: PT, PTT, α-1-antitrypsin, thrombin and antithrombin. (See specific test descriptions.)

PT, PTT, D-Dimer

This panel of tests is used to evaluate the extrinsic coagulation system. These tests may also aid in screening for congenital deficiencies of factors II, V, VII, and X as well as deficiencies of prothrombin, dysfibrinogenemia, and afibrinogenemia. Levels of PT, PTT, and D-dimer are used to evaluate heparin effect, warfarin anticoagulant therapy, liver failure, DIC, and vitamin K deficiency. This test includes the following tests: PT, PTT, and D-dimer. (See specific test descriptions.)

PT, PTT, D-Dimer, Fibrinogen

This panel of tests is used to evaluate the extrinsic coagulation system. They may also aid in screening for congenital deficiencies of Factors II, V, VII, X as well as deficiencies of prothrombin, dysfibrinogenemia, and afibrinogenemia. Levels of PT, PTT, and D-dimer can determine heparin effect, warfarin anticoagulant therapy, liver failure, DIC and vitamin K deficiency. This test includes the following: PT, PTT, D-dimer, and fibrinogen. (See specific test descriptions.)

Rapid Plasma Reagent (RPR) Qualitative

This test is used to detect syphilis.

Reference Interval: Nonreactive

RBC Magnesium

This test is used to evaluate magnesium deficiency.

Reference Interval: 4.2–6.8 mg/dL

Reticulocyte Count

This test is used to evaluate erythropoietic activity, which increases in acute and chronic hemorrhage and in hemolytic anemias. It is also used to evaluate erythropoietic response to antianemic therapy.

Reference Interval: Reticulocytes are expressed as a percentage of the circulating red cell population. Normally, the reticulocyte cell count ranges from 1–2% and reflects the daily replacement of 0.8–1.0% of the circulating red cell population.

Reverse T3

This test is useful in evaluating thyroid function and metabolism, and to evaluate euthyroidic individuals with low T3 concentrations.

Reference Interval: Older than 15 years: 90–350 pg/mL

Rheumatoid Arthritis (RA) Factor

This test is used in the differential detection and prognosis of arthritic disorders. Rheumatoid factors are antibodies directed against the Fc fragment of IgG. These are usually IgM antibodies, but may be IgG or IgA. Rheumatoid factor is found in the serum of a majority of individuals with rheumatoid arthritis.

Reference Interval: Negative: <=10.0 IU/mL

Selenium

This test is used to monitor selenium deficiency and occupational exposure. Since selenium is a very important supplement for life extension, optimal levels are in the upper half of normal.

Reference Interval:
Environmental exposure: 79–326 mcg/L
Normal Range: 46–143 mcg/L

Sex Hormone Binding Globulin (SHBG)

This test is used to monitor SHBG levels, which are under the positive control of estrogens and thyroid hormones, and suppressed by androgens. Decreased levels will be found in hirsutism, virilization, obese postmenopausal women, and women with diffuse hair loss. Increased levels are present in hyperthyroidism, testicular feminization, cirrhosis, male hypogonadism, pregnancy, prepubertal children, and women using oral contraceptives.

Reference Interval:
Male (>18 years): 13–71 nmol/L
Female (>18 years): 18–114 nmol/L

Sex Hormone Profile—EPT

This test is used to evaluate hormone levels. The following tests are included in this panel: Estradiol, Free Testosterone, and Progesterone. (See specific test descriptions.)

Somatomedin-C (IGF-1)

Somatomedin-C is a screening test to identify individuals with growth hormone deficiency, pituitary insufficiency, and acromegaly.

Reference Interval:

Females/Males (Age, years)	Range (ng/mL)
18	163–584
19	141–483
20	127–424
21–25	116–358
26–30	117–329
31–35	115–307
36–40	109–284
41–45	101–267
46–50	94–252
51–55	87–238
56–60	81–225
61–65	75–212
66–70	69–200
71–75	64–188
76–80	59–177
81–85	55–166

T3 Uptake

This is a thyroid function test for the detection of hypothyroidism or hyperthyroidism.

Reference Interval: 24–39%

Testosterone, Free

This test is used to evaluate hirsutism and masculinization in women; to evaluate testicular function in clinical states where the testosterone binding proteins may be altered (obesity, cirrhosis, thyroid disorders). In women, the test evaluates hirsutism and masculinization.

Reference Intervals:

Male:

20–29 years:	9.3–26.5 pg/mL
30–39 years:	8.7–25.1 pg/mL
40–49 years:	6.8–21.5 pg/mL
50–59 years:	7.2–24.0 pg/mL
>60 years:	6.6–18.1 pg/mL
(Optimal: 15–26.5 pg/mL)	

Female:

20–59 years:	0.0–2.2 pg/mL
>60 years:	0.0–1.8 pg/mL

Testosterone, Free (with Total)

This test is used to evaluate hirsutism and masculinization in women and to evaluate testicular function in men in clinical states where the testosterone binding proteins may be altered (obesity, cirrhosis, thyroid disorders).

Reference Interval:

Free Testosterone:

Male: 5.00–21.00 ng/dL

Female: 0.10–0.85 ng/dL

Percentage of Total Testosterone:

Male: 1.0–2.7 ng/dL

Female: 0.5–1.8 ng/dL

Testosterone, Total

This test is used to evaluate gonadal and adrenal function. It is also helpful in diagnosing hypogonadism, hypopituitarism, Klinefelter's syndrome, and impotence.

Normal range:

Male: 241–827 ng/dL

Optimal Range: 500–827 ng/dL

Female Reference Interval: 14–76 ng/dL

Thrombin/Antithrombin III

These two tests are used to evaluate the intrinsic coagulation system. They are used to evaluate heparin effect, warfarin anticoagulant therapy, liver failure, and disseminated intravascular coagulation (DIC).

- *Thrombin:* This test is used to evaluate the fibrinogen-to-fibrin reaction. It is used to determine severe hypofibrinogenemia, dysfibrinogenemia, and the presence of heparin-like anticoagulants. Thrombin levels are used to confirm and monitor disseminated intravascular coagulation (DIC) and fibrinolysis. This test can also be used to monitor fibrinolytic therapy. The thrombin levels can be used to monitor therapy with heparin.

Reference Interval: <18.0%

- *Antithrombin III:* This test is used to evaluate the degree of hypercoagulation, fibrinogenolytic state, and the response to heparin. The hereditary deficiency of antithrombin III (autosomal dominant) is characterized by predisposition to thrombosis. Acquired deficiency is associated with severe cirrhosis, chronic liver failure, DIC, thrombolytic therapy, pulmonary embolism, nephrotic syndrome, or postsurgical state (especially liver transplant or partial hepatectomy). Decreased levels of antithrombin can be attributed to: a decline in antithrombin synthesis, excessive loss or consumption of antithrombin, or may be induced by drugs. Antithrombin III levels might also mark cases of suspected heparin failure, suspected DIC, or personal or familial history of thromboembolic disease. The test is indicated in the latter cases especially prior to heparinization, general or orthopedic surgery, prolonged bed rest, pregnancy, postpartum or postoperative state, or oral contraceptive use.

Reference Interval: 75% to 130% of normal

Thyroid Antithyroglobulin Antibody

This test is used to detect and confirm autoimmune thyroiditis and Hashimoto's thyroiditis.

Reference Interval: Negative

Thyroid Panel (TSH, T4, Free T3)

This panel is used to evaluate thyroid function. The combination of the serum T4 and T3 uptake (or Thyroid Hormone Binding Ratio, THBR) is an indirect assessment of thyroxine-binding globulin (TBG). TBG helps to determine whether an abnormal T4 value is due to alterations in serum thyroxine-binding globulin or to changes of thyroid hormone levels. Deviations of both tests in the same direction usually indicate that an abnormal T4 is due to abnormalities in thyroid hormone. Deviations of the two tests in opposite directions provide evidence that an abnormal T4 may relate to alterations in TBG. This panel consists of the following tests: Thyroid-Stimulating Hormone (TSH), Free Tri-iodothyronine (T3), and Thyroxine (T4).

- *Thyroid-Stimulating Hormone (TSH):* This test is used to identify primary hypothyroidism and to differentiate it from secondary (pituitary) and tertiary (hypothalamus) hypothyroidism.

Normal Ranges: 0.35–5.50 mIU/mL
Optimal Range: Under 2.1 mcIU/mL

- *Tri-Iodothyronine (T3), Free, Serum:* This test is used to evaluate thyroid function. It is primarily used to diagnose hyperthyroidism. It is also used to assess abnormal binding protein disorders and to monitor thyroid replacement and suppressive therapy.

Normal Ranges: 2.3–4.2 pg/mL

- *Thyroxine (T4):* This test is used to evaluate thyroid function. T4 is decreased in hypothyroidism and in the third stage of subacute thyroiditis. T4 is increased with hyperthyroidism, subacute thyroiditis in its first stage, and with thyrotoxicosis due to Hashimoto's disease. T4 is also used to diagnose toxicosis.

Normal Ranges: 4.5–12.0 mcg/dL

Thyroxine (T4)
See Thyroid Panel.

Thyroxine (T4) Free, Direct

This test is used to evaluate thyroid function in individuals who may have protein abnormalities that could affect total T4 levels. It is used to evaluate thyroid function and monitor replacement and suppressive therapy.

Normal Ranges: 4.5–12.0 mcg/dL

Tri-Iodothyronine (T3) Free
See Thyroid Panel.

Troponin 1

This test is used to detect cardiac injury, predict mortality in unstable cases of angina and serve as a marker for perioperative myocardial infarction.

Reference Interval: <1.0 ng/mL

Tumor Necrosis Factor Alpha (TNF-α) Blood Test
See Cytokine Panel.

Urinalysis, Routine

This test is used to detect abnormalities of urine and to identify and manage renal metabolic diseases, urinary tract infection, neoplasm, systemic diseases, and inflammatory or neoplastic disease.

Reference Interval: Ranges are established by the laboratory.

Vitamin D

This test is used to rule out vitamin D deficiency as a cause of bone disease. It can also be used to identify hypercalcemia.

Reference Interval: 8.9–46.7 ng/mL

HOW TO ORDER BLOOD TESTS

You can order blood tests by mail or by calling (800) 208-3444. All tests must be prepaid. As soon as you place your order, you will be sent a package with information regarding the location of the nearest blood-drawing stations, a Request for Phlebotomy form, and a Test Requisition form.

At your convenience, you can then take the Request for Phlebotomy form and Requisition to the designated blood-drawing station in your area. A phlebotomist will draw the appropriate specimens of your blood. You (or your physician) will be mailed your test results. These results will show if you have any abnormalities. If the results show abnormalities, you should make sure you show these results to your personal physician, who can determine if you have any serious problems and what you can do about them.

You can also request a free consultation with one of the Foundation's doctors to help interpret your test results to make certain that you stay in optimal ranges.

If longevity risk factors such as glucose, homocysteine, C-reactive protein, fibrinogen, or other tests are abnormal, slightly elevated or below normal, for example—you can take nutritional steps to reverse the trend. You can repeat the test in 45–60 days, and then chart your progress in improving your health and your chances of living longer in good health.

 PRODUCT AVAILABILITY

To order mail-order blood tests, call (800) 208-3444 or ask your physician.

Meningitis (Viral)

Meningitis means inflammation of the brain lining. Viral meningitis is the infection of the central nervous system by enteroviruses that can cause the infection. It is characterized by a severe headache, stiffness of the neck or back, fever, nausea, and malaise. The disease is typically severe and requires emergency medical care. Viral meningitis may occasionally progress to serious neurological confusion, particularly among infants infected before the age of 1 year.

According to the Meningitis Consensus Panel (Washington, D.C.) in May 1999: "The issue with viral meningitis is that there are no available treatments. As a consequence, patients suffer needlessly." Management of viral meningitis in the United States results in $1 billion in direct medical costs and an additional $200 million in indirect costs due to lost productivity. "Having meningitis once is a very scary thing, but to keep getting it, and not even have a clue as to why, is a living nightmare!" These comments from a patient with recurrent viral meningitis were reported by the Meningitis Foundation in 1999.

Mollaret's meningitis (recurrent) is characterized by repeated episodes of fever (up to 104°F), meningismus, and severe headache, which are separated by symptom-free intervals. Individual attacks are sudden, with signs and symptoms reaching maximum intensity within a few hours. Headache, neck pain, generalized muscle aches, and neck stiffness usually persist from 3–6 days, but may be present for up to 3 or more weeks. Following a number of recurrences, which can span a period of years, the disease suddenly disappears. The long-term health of the patient seems not to be adversely affected. However, transient neurologic abnormalities (seizures, diplopia, pathologic reflexes, cranial nerve paresis, hallucinations, and coma) occur in as many as 50% of cases.

CURRENT THERAPY

Mollaret's meningitis is a *syndrome* rather than a disease. As such, the syndrome of Mollaret's meningitis appears to have multiple etiologies. Presently, herpes simplex Type II and to a lesser extent Type I appear to be etiologic in most cases. Because of the rarity of this syndrome, there are no large clinical trials comparing one therapy against another. However, acyclovir (intravenous or oral) or valacyclovir (oral only) are worthy of consideration for both therapy and prophylaxis. A painkiller is generally administered during the first several days of an attack to reduce patient suffering from the severe headaches, stiffness, and overall body aches produced by the onset of the disease. There is currently no antiviral pharmaceutical for viral meningitis, although several are undergoing clinical trails and show promise for use in treatment.

ViroPharma Inc. is conducting a multicenter, double-blind, placebo-controlled, Phase IIIb clinical trial of oral formulation of *pleconaril* for treatment in adults. In preclinical studies, ViroPharma scientists have shown that pleconaril effectively inhibits the laboratory replication of 96% of the rhinoviruses and enteroviruses isolated from 332 human patients. The patient population from which these clinical samples were obtained exhibited the complete range of diseases caused by these viruses, including a number of fatal infections. Orally administered pleconaril also protected mice from lethal infection by enteroviruses in three distinct animal model systems and was effective even when therapy was initiated after infection in these models (Pevear et al. 1999).

Possible Causes

Although there is no simple answer to what causes recurrence, there are some theories. Stress and depression, reduced immune function, and even prolonged sun exposure have been implicated in causing a recurrent meningitis attack. Additionally, the Meningitis Foundation (1999) has cited chromosome defect/FMF, intracranial epidermoid cysts, herpes virus reactivation (systemic), allergic reaction, and chemical reaction as other possible causes of attack.

Points to Remember

- Mollaret's meningitis is usually a benign (but painful), self-limited, recurrent, and often febrile meningitis.

- Transient neurologic deficits (seizures, cranial nerve paresis, pathologic reflexes) occur in 50% of cases.

- Mollaret's meningitis may be caused by herpes simplex Type II; acyclovir may play a role in prophylaxis and therapy.

- Anecdotal patient information, as well as scientific evidence, suggests viral meningitis may be triggered by reduced immune system function, allergic response, stress and depression, as well as exposure to the sun. Persons who have recurrent meningitis should avoid becoming fatigued or stressed and should avoid excessive exposure to the sun.

ALTERNATIVE THERAPY

Nutritional and hormonal therapies to boost immune function, such as the recommended daily dose of Life Extension Mix, melatonin (300 mcg–6 mg taken at bedtime), DHEA (25–50 mg a day), vitamin C (6000 mg a day), and coenzyme Q_{10} (200 mg a day), are recommended.

For associated pain, consider using Inflacin. Inflacin is a topical pain relief, anti-inflammatory agent. In a double-blind, patient-randomized, placebo-controlled crossover clinical trial enrolling 30 participants, Inflacin was tested to evaluate its analgesic benefit when applying the topical cream to areas of the body affected by stiffness, soreness, and pain. These included hands, feet, knees, and shoulders and muscles of the neck, arms, legs, and back. Results of the study showed that Inflacin significantly reduced pain and stiffness after only one application. On the average, Inflacin reduced pain by 45% after 1 dose in the first 60 minutes of application (Keller 2002). DL-Phenylalanine and tyrosine may also be helpful to reduce chronic pain (refer to precautions before use) (see the Immune Enhancement protocol for other suggestions).

OVERLOOKED DRUGS

Cimetidine, sold under the brand name Tagamet, is used to suppress excess stomach acid production. A side benefit to cimetidine is that it inhibits T-suppressor cells from prematurely shutting off an immune attack against certain viruses. Clinical studies show that cimetidine dramatically shortens the duration of herpes simplex and herpes zoster outbreaks. Cimetidine can be purchased over-the-counter in drug stores, and those infected with viral meningitis may consider taking 200 mg of cimetidine three times a day and 400 mg at bedtime to duplicate successful studies.

Ribavirin is sold in the United States as a prescription drug under the name Rebetol. Ribavarin is a broad-spectrum antiviral drug, and it may be effective against certain viruses that cause meningitis. Suggested dose during viral attacks is 800 to 1200 mg a day taken in divided doses. Those with anemia may not be able to take ribavirin.

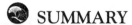 SUMMARY

Mollaret's meningitis is a poorly understood and rare disorder, the cause of which remains obscure. Typically, a physician's diagnosis of the disease is made by exclusion. The course of the disease, albeit protracted in some patients, is generally benign. Early recognition of this disorder and a patient's own self-care in maintaining optimum health may help reduce recurrence of the disease. However, sudden onset of viral meningitis can occur in a seemingly healthy person with few warning symptoms. The following supplements are recommended to help boost overall immunity and help with pain:

1. Take Life Extension Mix, 3 tablets 3 times a day.
2. Take 500 mcg–6 mg of melatonin daily at bedtime.
3. Take 25–50 mg of DHEA early in the day (see DHEA precautions in the DHEA Replacement Therapy protocol).
4. Take 6000 mg of vitamin C daily.
5. Take coenzyme Q_{10}, 200 mg daily.
6. Take DL-phenylalanine and tyrosine if needed for chronic pain. Typical doses are to start with 500 mg daily and gradually increase to 1500 mg daily (see the Phenylalanine and Tyrosine Dosing and Precautions protocol).
7. Consider cimetidine, 200 mg 3 times a day and 400 mg at bedtime.
8. Ask your doctor to prescribe ribavirin at the dose of 400 mg 2 to 3 times a day.
9. Apply Inflacin as need for pain.

FOR MORE INFORMATION

Contact the National Institute of Neurological Disorders and Stroke, (301) 496-5751.

PRODUCT AVAILABILITY

Life Extension Mix, melatonin, DHEA, vitamin C, coenzyme Q_{10}, Inflacin, DL- phenylalanine, and tyrosine are available by telephoning (800) 544-4440 or by ordering online at www.lef.org.

Migraine

According to the National Headache Foundation, one in four households in the United States, or 28 million people, are affected by migraine. Of that total, 11 million people have chronic migraine. Migraine most commonly strikes young adult women. The common characteristics are recurrent attacks of headache, with pain occurring most often on one side of the head, accompanied by various combinations of symptoms, such as nausea, vomiting, and sensitivity to light and sound. Migraines can occur at any time of day or night, but occur most frequently arising in the morning. A migraine episode can last from several hours to several days; it may migrate from one part of the head to another, and may extend into the neck and shoulders. Scalp tenderness often occurs during or after an attack.

Migraine is considered a hereditary disease. If both parents have migraine headaches, there is a 75% chance that the offspring will be a "migraineur"; if only one parent has migraine, the chance is as high as 50% that the offspring will be affected.

Migraine headaches are generally of two types: classic and common. Typically, migraine headaches are biased to one side of the head and often the pain is localized. A *Classic* migraine headache is characterized by an "aura" (light spots) or other sensations that are known by the migraineur to occur just prior to the migraine headache itself. A *Common* migraine headache is considered any migraine headache not preceded by an aura or other symptomatic warning to the patient. After a migraine attack, an individual may feel exhausted, listless, and irritable and have difficulty concentrating. Although migraine is not curable, with proper treatment, it is manageable.

During a migraine headache, blood vessels in the head go through a cycle of extreme constriction followed by rapid dilation. Nerve pathway changes and imbalances in brain chemistry may cause blood vessels to become inflamed. The actual interaction between the brain chemistry and blood vessel dilation is not clear, but scientists believe that migraine headaches are caused by alterations in the nerve pathways—specifically, the trigeminal nerve system that is a major pathway in the brain. The trigeminal nerve pathway carries nerve signals from the head and face to the brain. When a migraine headache is triggered, the trigeminal nerve releases neuropeptides, causing inflammation and dilation of the blood vessels. Subsequently, trigeminal nerve endings stimulate the release of more neuropeptides, and a vicious cycle begins.

Serotonin regulates pain messages via the trigeminal pathway. There is evidence that changed levels of serotonin (a neurotransmitter) may cause migraine headaches. Other common causes of migraine headaches include complicated combinations of "triggers" such as foods, food additives, medications, stress, flashing lights, loud sounds; changes in the weather, humidity, and altitude; and hormonal changes including hormone replacement therapy (HRT). Food products most commonly known to cause or increase the severity of a migraine include chocolates, meats preserved in nitrates (ham, etc.), pizza, aged cheese, alcohol, especially red wine and beer; caffeine (especially cutting back); nuts; fermented, pickled, or marinated foods; and foods prepared with monosodium glutamate (MSG).

Individuals with recurrent migraines are often encouraged by their physicians to keep a daily diary in order to identify dietary factors that may be related. The diary is a written record to determine the kinds of foods eaten, the weather conditions prior to the migraine, medications being taken (when and how much), and any other trigger factors that may exist prior to or at the beginning of migraine headache onset. It is designed to identify and quantify possible migraine triggers that precede the head pain. It is important to record the complete details of the symptoms such as the description and location of the pain and treatment used. It is very important that all medications be brought to the attention of the physician. The complexity of each individual's triggers can be extensive, so accurate entries in a diary must precede any therapeutic regimen. In many cases individual triggers may not cause migraine headaches; they may need to be in combination with other stimuli before a migraine headache will occur.

MIGRAINE TREATMENT AND MANAGEMENT

People who experience migraines should begin treatment by seeking a specialist in migraine, such as a neurologist who is able to detect the specific symptoms of migraine. Migraine symptoms are easily understood by the patient. Physicians knowledgeable about migraine may be able to help with a customized regimen of treatment. Each person who suffers from migraine is unique, so individual treatments are complex and varied—there is no single treatment method. Treatments for migraine include diet changes, stress management, proper sleep, hormone replacement therapy, supplements, and prescription drugs.

Preventive Therapy with Nonmigraine Medications

Certain medications most often prescribed for other conditions have been found to prevent or reduce the symptoms of migraine if taken regularly. These include tricyclic anidepressants (nortriptyline and doxepin); antihypertensive agents such as beta blockers (propranolol and timolol) and calcium channel blockers (verapamil); serotonin antagonists (methysergide); and antiseizure medications (divalproex sodium).

Depakote, a drug first used in the treatment of epilepsy, is one of the most effective treatments in preventing migraine. The United States Food and Drug Administration (USFDA) approved the use of Depakote as a prescribed treatment in the prevention of migraine.

Attack-Aborting Techniques

Generally, attack-aborting medications should be taken as early as possible once a migraine has begun. Certain agents in the general class of drugs known as cerebral vasoconstrictors are specifically designed for migraine. Such examples are Imitrex, Migranal, Zomig, Maxalt, and ergotamine derivatives. These preparations are available in a variety of preparations that include oral (the slowest acting), intranasal, subcutaneous injection, and rectal suppositories. There is also a class of drugs used for the relief of symptoms of nausea and vomiting associated with migraine, including metoclopramide (Reglan).

General Pain Management

General pain management includes the use of drugs to control pain once the migraine headache has started. These are generally classed as narcotic, non-narcotic, and nonsteroidal anti-inflammatory drugs (NSAIDs) such as naproxen, keto-rolac, and ibuprofen. Simple analgesics such as aspirin and acetaminophen are also used.

Dental Devices as a Preventive Measure

Many people who experience migraine clench the temporalis muscles on the side of the skull while they sleep, which may account for the pain they feel upon awakening. In 2001, the FDA granted marketing approval for the NTI Tension Suppression System (NTI-tss) neuromuscular suppression device for the prevention of medically diagnosed migraine pain and migraine associated tension-type headaches. This device is a small, removable matrix that a dentist custom fits to a patient's front teeth to be worn while sleeping. The intense clenching of the temporal muscles (which close and open the jaw) is suppressed to less than a third by eliminating contact of the back molar or canine teeth. By reducing this neuromuscular activity, migraine headache pain and associated tension-type headaches may be prevented or dramatically reduced.

In an 8-week trial conducted by the manufacturer, of patients who experienced at least two episodes of migraine monthly, 82% saw dramatic reductions in light and sound sensitivity, nausea, and the need for prescription medications such as Imitrex (www.headache-migraine.com).

Dr. Mark Friedman, a dentist practicing in New York, has developed a novel approach to treating migraines. He believes that migraines are caused when an inflammation above the last two upper molars causes swelling that presses on the maxillary nerve, triggering the migraine. He has created a machine that pumps cold water through plastic tubes, cooling a metal tip that is placed against the inflamed area. Applying the cold metal reduces the inflammation and seems to help prevent migraines. The dentist has also created an anti-inflammatory gel that patients can use at home to prevent the inflammation from ever starting or to help stop migraines after they have started. His findings have been published in the journal *Heart Disease*, but more research is needed before a solid recommendation can be made (Feig, 2002).

PREVENTIVE THERAPY WITH SUPPLEMENTS

Nondrug alternative therapies offer effective methods to prevent migraine. For most migraineurs, prevention therapy is successful and easily managed. Physicians skilled in migraine therapy are generally more aware of the synergistic effects of nondrug therapies.

Feverfew

Feverfew (*Tanacetum parthenium*) extracts are used widely in the United Kingdom and Germany. Feverfew works by inhibiting human blood aggregation and serotonin secretion. In a double-blind, placebo-controlled crossover study conducted in Israel, 57 patients were selected at random and divided into two groups. Both groups were treated with feverfew in the initial phase lasting two months. During the second and third phases, a double-blind, crossover study was conducted. The results showed that feverfew caused a significant reduction in pain intensity compared with placebo. Symptoms, such as vomiting, nausea, and sensitivity to noise and light, were also dramatically reduced (Palevitch et al. 1997).

An earlier randomized double-blind, placebo-controlled crossover study was conducted with 72 volunteers. At the completion of the trial, 59 patients had remained in the study; from their daily diaries and medical testing, it was found that "Treatment with feverfew was associated with a reduction in the mean number and severity of attacks [and a reduction in]. . . the degree of vomiting. . . . Scores also indicated a significant improvement with feverfew. There were no serious side effects" (Murphy et al. 1988).

Magnesium Supplementation

The role of magnesium in the pathogenesis of migraine has been studied extensively. The mechanism of action was presented in a Medline-excerpted abstract: "Magnesium concentration has an effect on. . . migraine-related receptors and neurotransmitters. . . . Evidence suggests that up to 50% of patients. . . have lowered levels of ionized magnesium. Infusion of magnesium results in rapid and sustained relief of. . . acute migraine in such patients." The study also found through two double-blind trials that oral magnesium supplementation may also reduce the frequency of migraine attacks. The report concluded, "Because of an excellent safety profile and low cost, and despite the lack of definitive studies, we feel that. . . oral magnesium supplementation can be recommended to a majority of migraine sufferers" (Mauskop et al. 1998).

Magnesium supplementation is used widely in Canada as a preventive regimen. At the Henry Ford Hospital, research on the pathogenesis of migraine found that magnesium may protect against migraine via a variety of mechanisms. The study concluded that "Magnesium deficiency and abnormal presynaptic calcium channels may be responsible for neuronal hyperexcitability between attacks" (Welch 1997).

Decreased serum and intracellular levels of magnesium have been reported in patients with migraine. It was also found that platelet levels of ionized magnesium were significantly lower in patients who have migraine headaches. In cases of juvenile migraine with low magnesium levels, it was found that a 20-day treatment with oral magnesium picolate seemed to normalize 90% of the patients. The data suggest that low brain magnesium may be related to migraine (Aloisi et al. 1997).

Riboflavin

Vitamin B_2 (riboflavin) is used as a prophylactic treatment for migraine. In a study conducted at the University of Liege (Belgium), Department of Neurology, it was postulated that since the brains of migraineurs were characterized by reduced mitochondrial phosphorylation, riboflavin could be used because of its potential to increase mitochondrial energy efficiency, and that a prophylactic effect may be realized. A group of 49 patients who have migraine were studied: 45 had common migraine and 4 had classic or "aura" migraine history. Patients were given 400 mg of riboflavin as a single oral dose for at least 3 months. Mean global improvement between the groups was 68.2%. It was concluded that high-dose riboflavin could be an effective, low-cost prophylactic treatment for migraine devoid of short-term side effects (Schoenen et al. 1994).

Further studies performed by Dr. Jean Schoenen (also at the University of Liege) reported that the combination of beta-blockers (which alter cortical information processing) and riboflavin may "increase clinical efficacy compared with monotherapy with either drug, without augmenting CNS side effects." His study in the journal *Headache* involved 26 migraineurs, the "majority" of whom showed improvement. The study is significant because the action of various drugs for migraine prophylaxis is poorly understood, but researchers have identified two principal functioning brain abnormalities: abnormal cortical information processing and decreased mitochondrial energy reserve. Therefore, a combined therapy using two drugs, each affecting one part of the problem, seems a logical approach (Sandor et al. 2000).

CoQ_{10}

According to researchers, the onset of migraine may occur due to mitochondrial dysfunction. CoQ_{10}, an essential element in the mitochondrial electron transport chain, may be an effective agent in preventing migraine. In a clinical trial conducted at the Cleveland Clinic Foundation, 31 patients showed a significant reduction in the average number of days with migraine after 3 months of treatment (7.34–2.95 days). Migraine frequency fell from 4.85 attacks at baseline to 2.81 at the study conclusion. The administered dose was 150 mg daily. No side effects were observed (Rosen 2002).

Butterbur Root

Butterbur root (*Petasites hybridus*) may be an effective preventive treatment for migraine due to its antispasmodic effects on vascular walls. In a double-blind test,

Myofascial Syndrome

Myofascial: from the Greek *myelos*, meaning marrow (muscle) and from the Latin *fascia* meaning bandage or band

Myofascial syndrome (MFS) is a painful musculoskeletal condition characterized by painful foci of muscle called trigger points (TrPs). MFS became better known based on the work of a well-known Washington, D.C. physician, the late Dr. Janet Travell. Dr. Travell was the White House physician for a number of presidents.

MFS has often been confused with fibromyalgia because they both involve muscle pain. The trigger points of MFS are different from the tender points of fibromyalgia in that they may be just about anywhere, whereas the tender points of fibromyalgia are in a specified pattern. When a physician presses on a tender point in patients with fibromyalgia, the patient describes exactly that—*tenderness*. When a physician pushes a trigger point in MFS, the trigger point elicits an involuntary "twitch" response. Additionally, the patient may report pain that radiates to an area away from the trigger point itself. This is what is considered "referred pain." The painful trigger point area is in the muscle or the junction of the muscle and fascia. Hence, myofascial pain is usually associated with a taut band, indicating a "ropey" thickening of the muscle tissue.

The fascia is a tough connective tissue that spreads throughout the body in a three-dimensional web from head to foot without interruption. The fascia surrounds every muscle, bone, nerve, blood vessel, and organ of the body, all the way down to the cellular level. Therefore, malfunction of the fascial system due to trauma, posture, or inflammation can create a "binding down" of the fascia, resulting in abnormal pressure on nerves, muscles, bones, or organs.

Much of the pain that accompanies MFS is due to inadequate blood flow to the trigger point area (ischemia) that inhibits the ability of the muscle to eliminate metabolic wastes, such as lactic acid and potassium. These accumulated metabolic byproducts combined with inadequate oxygen flow to the affected area then build up, stimulating nearby nerve endings that lead to trigger point pain.

DISTINGUISHING MYOFASCIAL SYNDROME FROM FIBROMYALGIA

What distinguishes MFS from fibromyalgia (FM) is that MFS is not usually associated with poor sleep or chronic fatigue, although some patients may have a little bit of both. The trigger points of MFS do not go away by getting the patient to sleep better. Since a patient can have both FM and MFS, treating the FM may improve things. However, persistent painful areas may be the result of MFS. For example, a patient may experience headaches and have classic FM. Following the FM protocol makes the patient feel much better, but the headache persists. Upon reexamination, the patient's physician finds the same mid-trapezoidal trigger points described above, greater on the right than the left. It turns out that the patient carries a heavy laptop every day on the right shoulder. When the trigger point is pressed upon very firmly, the patient develops neck pain that evolves into a migraine. Treating the trigger point and having the patient stop carrying the laptop for a while will result in resolution of the headaches. What has been described is, of course, the ideal diagnostic situation. Some patients may not develop the migraine right there in the office. However, any person who has unexplained headaches should have an evaluation for the presence of trigger points. The same is true for any persistent muscular pain that appears to be nondermatomal in origin.

Causative Factors

- Repetitive motions; excessive exercise; muscle strain due to overactivity
- Lack of activity (leg or arm in a sling)
- Nutritional deficiencies
- Nervous tension or stress
- Generalized fatigue
- Sudden trauma to muscles, ligaments, or tendons
- Hormonal changes (PMS or menopause)

Treatment

Mapping out the myofascial pain regions and their associated trigger points was attributed to the work of Dr. Travell. She developed a technique which is used to either inject a local anesthetic with a mild anti-inflammatory steroid solution into the trigger point or to break up the trigger point with a needle. The exact pathology of the trigger point is not entirely understood. What is clear is that treating the trigger point is responsible for resolving many types of pain patterns.

Janet Travell's work coincides with acupuncture points. The trigger points and associated pain radiation areas have been co-related by an acupuncture researcher. As it turns out, 87% of Dr. Travell's trigger points and their associated pain areas lie on acupuncture meridians and correlate with known acupuncture points. Additionally, acupuncturists describe a certain grabbing of the needle which is called taking Chi. This correlates with the twitch response described by Dr. Travell. When a trigger point is properly needled, there is a visible "grab" observed by the practitioner and a feeling of a grabbing or slight contraction around the needle experienced by the patient. Although new to Western medicine, Dr. Travell's work had already been discovered and utilized thousands of years before by the Chinese (Travell et al. 1983)!

The acupuncture points *He Gu* (the point near the wrist where the thumb and forefinger join) and *Yin Men* (on the back of the thigh) were found to increase blood flow and reduce MFS-related pain (Wang et al. 1998). Most studies, however, seem to indicate that although acupuncture is an effective short-term treatment of chronic pain due to MFS, there is only limited evidence that acupuncture will be effective in the long-term, and further human studies need to be conducted (Fargas-Babjak 2001; Irnich et al. 2001). One study on the use of amitriptyline in people with temporomandibular joint (TMJ) pain and MFS seemed to show that the beneficial effects of these pain treatments reduced over time, but the muscular pain was still manageable more than 1 year after treatment (Plesh et al. 2000). Amitriptyline is a tricyclic antidepressant drug with many side effects that preclude long-term use in most people.

For refractive cases of MFS, a homeopathic solution of traumeel and/or a mild narcotic called buprinorphine injected into the trigger point(s) may be employed. Dr. Travell's technique of injecting corticosteroids and/or local anesthetics into the trigger points appears to be effective in reducing muscle pain. Dr. Iwama and his colleagues at the Central Aizu General Hospital, Aizu, Japan conducted studies on 40 women with chronic lumbar, shoulder, or neck myofascial pain. Using Dr. Travell's technique each woman was given an injection of diluted anesthetic or a saline placebo and their pain levels were measured. In another portion of the study, 21 outpatient volunteers were given different dilutions of different anesthetics in each shoulder. Dr. Iwama concluded that the most suitable type of local anesthetic is lidocaine or mepivacaine and the most effective water-diluted concentration is 0.2–0.25% (Iwama et al. 2001).

Trigger points may require multiple treatments that necessitate excessive amounts of steroids over time. Some physicians feel that local anesthetics may irritate the muscle tissue, and multiple injections into the same trigger point may aggravate the problem.

Buprinorphine, when diluted and injected into the trigger points, may have a local pain-reducing action or in some way help to directly break up the trigger point. Additionally, buprinorphine is a mild narcotic analgesic that makes repetitive injections more tolerable for the patient. The dosage of traumeel is not critical since it is homeopathic. One to 2 ampules a session may be adequate, depending upon the number of trigger points and the volume of the solution. The proportion works out to 1 ampule per 10 cc of saline. Since buprinorphine has a systemic action and may produce drowsiness, no more than 2 ampules are usually used a session, again depending upon the volume used. Some patients, especially those who are obese, may tolerate more than 2 ampules a session. The dilution is 1/2–2 ampules (0.15–0.6 mg) per 20 cc of saline depending upon patient response and the number of trigger points treated per session. It is advised to begin with the lower concentrations.

The injections are usually only 2–4 cc per trigger point. Someone must drive the patient home after treatment because of the potential for sedation. For really difficult-to-treat trigger points, the Edegawa technique involves taking a 60-cc syringe filled with saline (salt water) and injecting it rapidly through an 18-gauge (large) needle. Anywhere from 20 cc up to the full 60 cc may be used for a particularly recalcitrant trigger point. It is believed that the rapid influx of saline pulls the muscle fibers apart where they cross the trigger point, resulting in a breakup of the trigger point itself.

If saline injections fail, traumeel and buprinorphine may be added to the saline. This combination is recommended at the outset due to the safety of the two preparations: the possible direct actions of both agents on the trigger point, and the systemic pain-killing properties of buprinorphine. After all, multiple injections of large volumes of fluids into the muscle tissue are painful. The dilution is 6 ampules of traumeel and 1–2 ampules of buprinorphine per 60 cc of saline. Each trigger point may require anywhere from 10–60 cc of fluid as previously described. The amount must be found empirically. No matter how many trigger points are treated, it is suggested that no more than 3 ampules a session of buprinorphine be used because of the potential for sedation. However, some patients, especially those who are obese, may require and tolerate more. There is no need to worry about addiction (*see the Pain protocol for more information*).

A Link to Depression and Anxiety

Many painful conditions, including headaches, migraines, TMJ pain, and muscle pain improve when the trigger points associated with myofascial syndrome are identified and treated. However, chronic pain may affect people emotionally, and many people with MFS experience depression or anxiety disorders. It may be beneficial to consult a mental health professional in addition to a regular physician (Glaros 2000) (*see the Depression and Anxiety and Stress protocols for additional information*).

Antidepressants are often prescribed for the treatment of MFS. At low doses, medications, such as tricyclic antidepressants relax muscles, improve sleep, and help in regulating neurotransmitter activity that contributes to the associated pain. At higher doses, they will help relieve depression, but have side effects that often preclude long-term use.

Reducing Pain and Associated Depression

The antidepressant supplement S-adenosylmethionine (SAMe) has been shown to be specifically effective as a therapy to reduce the chronic pain and depression associated with fibromyalgia (Jacobsen et al. 1991). SAMe is synthesized in the body from the amino acid methionine. An enzyme called methionine S-adenosyltransferase (MAT) catalyzes a reaction between methionine and ATP to form SAMe. SAMe has been tested for depression caused by a variety of diseases, including Parkinson's disease (PD), fibromyalgia, cancer, cardiovascular disease, and rheumatoid arthritis. Researchers have used SAMe successfully in conjunction with drug and alcohol withdrawal.

In a study reported in the *Scandinavian Journal of Rheumatology*, 44 fibromyalgia patients took 800 mg of SAMe for 6 weeks. Results showed that SAMe reduced pain at the tender points, as well as fatigue, morning stiffness, and resting pain (Jacobsen et al. 1991).

Buprenorphine is a mild narcotic with agonist and antagonist properties that has a very low addiction liability, if any, indicating it can be used for a long period of time without developing serious withdrawal symptoms. Buprenorphine is effective in conditions with multiple symptoms such as MFS because it acts rapidly on depression, reduces pain, and induces sleep (Cathelin et al. 1980).

Buprenorphine is available as an injectable, 0.3-mg ampule, a small dose even for injection. The dosage is variable. Because buprenophine is poorly absorbed orally, larger dosages must be used. When taken orally, the buprenophine liquid is withdrawn or shaken from the ampule and held under the tongue as long as possible. Compounding pharmacies can make up buprenorphine for sublingual use as a troche. Both forms, the ampules and troches, are expensive. For pain that prevents sleep, start with 2–6 ampules sublingually or 0.5–2 mg as a sublingual troche. For treating pain throughout the day that is associated with depression, begin with 2–6 ampules (or 0.5–2 mg as a sublingual troche) every 4–6 hours. As is common with most medications, begin with a low dose and increase slowly until the smallest dose that proves effective is reached. Do not be concerned about addiction.

Dietary Changes to Improve Symptoms

Patients with MFS are encouraged to employ proper basic nutrition and supplementation. Women with MFS have been found to have higher cholesterol levels than women without MFS, but no conclusive link has been made between blood lipid levels and MFS (Ozgocmen et al. 2000). The following dietary recommendations will improve overall health:

- Limit intake of stimulants (caffeine) and depressants (alcohol) because of their potential to disrupt neurological and metabolic function.

- Limit intake of refined sugars to avoid fluctuation of blood sugar levels, mood swings, lowered energy, and lowered immunity.

- Consume whole foods such as fruits and vegetables which contain phytochemicals and fiber. Fiber is helpful for maintaining digestive regularity. Eat more slowly, chewing food well.

- Increase intake of cold water fish which supply essential fatty acid building blocks (gamma linolenic acid, GLA; eicosapentaenoic acid, EPA) that are needed for cell membrane maintenance and function.

- Increase intake of probiotic cultures from food or supplements. (Probiotics are "healthy" bacteria that normally reside in the gastrointestinal tract. "Healthy" bacteria aid the proper digestion of food and prevent the absorption of ingested toxins.)

- Drink plenty of water (preferably purified) to ensure adequate fluid levels (Anon. 2001).

Amino Acid Supplementation

Phenylalanine is one of the 20 essential amino acids that must be obtained from the diet. It is a necessary precursor for neurotransmitter biosynthesis and may be helpful in relieving chronic pain. The amino acid tyrosine is synthesized in the body from phenylalanine. It is a precursor to the biosynthesis of the neurotransmitters epinephrine, norepinephrine, and dopamine. Tyrosine has been used as an antidepressant because it positively affects the neurotransmitters that are required to prevent depression. Supplementing with these two amino acids may be beneficial to people with MFS. Vitamins B_6 and C are cofactors in the bioconversion of these amino acids to their neurotransmitter receptors.

Exercise

With the help of a physical therapist or other health care professional, exercises can be designed for the person with MFS, which will avoid causing undue stress and pain to sensitive trigger points while improving physical fitness. In addition to promoting overall fitness, physical activity assists in maintaining flexibility and building muscle strength, helping to protect joints. Walking, bicycling, swimming, and some types of weight-bearing exercises are good examples of physical activity that may be appropriate. It is important to note that lack of exercise can lead to brittle bones and causes muscles to become smaller and weaker. In particular, people with MFS should avoid repetitive weight-bearing exercises involving the affected area. Gentle stretching of muscle groups should be done daily to their full range of motion within the limits of pain.

SUMMARY OF TREATMENT MODALITIES

- Trigger point therapy: myofascial release therapy, myotherapy, massotherapy spray, and stretch technique (stretching of the muscles with a vapocoolant spray, where a coolant is sprayed on the trigger point to lessen the pain and then the muscle is stretched). This is often done by a physical therapist.

- Trigger point injections: local anesthetics, such as lidocaine, injected directly into the trigger points. Trigger point injection has been shown to be one of the most effective treatment modalities to inactivate trigger points and provide prompt relief of symptoms (Alvarez et al. 2002).

- Dry needling: the use of a needle without injecting anything. TrP injections and dry needling mechanically disrupt the trigger point. The use of lidocaine is no more effective, but it reduces the soreness after injection. For MFS there is no role for injected steroids.

- Acupuncture is recommended as a treatment option for patients with associated musculoskeletal conditions (Kam et al. 2002).

- The application of ice packs will provide temporary relief by numbing the affected area.

- Chiropractic or osteopathic manipulation treatment

- Physical therapy (hands-on)

- Exercise

- Improved nutrition

- Elimination of stress; biofeedback; counseling for depression that may result from chronic pain

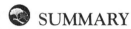 ## SUMMARY

Patients with unexplained persistent headaches or muscle pain should be examined for the presence of trigger points. Consult with a healthcare professional familiar with the various techniques used to relieve the pain associated with trigger points.

1. Make sure that both you and your physician find the source of the trigger points and seek ways to prevent recurrence. Look for repetitive injury as the cause before deciding that stress is the etiology. If stress is the etiology, it is most important to find ways of relieving it or the MFS pain will recur.

2. Consider phenylalanine and/or tyrosine, up to 1000 mg a day (see *Phenylalanine and Tyrosine Dosing and Precautions* protocol).

3. SAMe may be indicated for depression and trigger point pain associated with MFS. The suggested dose is 400–800 mg twice daily.

4. Supplementing with essential fatty acids will help maintain cell membrane integrity and relieve associated inflammation. A product called Super GLA/DHA is formulated with anti-inflammatory fatty acid GLA (gamma linolenic acid) along with DHA (docosahexaenoic acid) and EPA (eicosapentaenoic acid) extracted from fish oil. Six softgel capsules of Super GLA/DHA are recommended daily.

5. Follow good basic nutrition.

6. Supplement with a probiotic formula to help improve nutrient absorption and enhance immune system functioning. One 300-mg capsule of Life Flora daily is recommended.

7. Buprenorphine is a mild narcotic that can safely relieve multiple symptoms of MFS. Contact a compounding pharmacy to make a sublingual preparation. Buprenorphine must be prescribed by a physician.

8. Consider regular exercise under the guidance of a healthcare professional to maintain cardiovascular and musculoskeletal fitness.

 ### PRODUCT AVAILABILITY

DL-Phenylalanine, *L*-tyrosine, SAMe, Super GLA/DHA, and Life Flora are available by calling (800) 544-4440 or by ordering online at www.lef.org.

Nails

CAUSES OF NAIL DAMAGE

External Factors

Certain environmental factors may damage the nail. These include exposure to strong cleaning fluids, excessive submersion in water, and dryness caused by indoor heat. Brittleness may occur as a result of frequent use of nail polish remover. Nail biting and picking at the nail can also damage the nail and surrounding skin.

Internal Factors

There are various internal causes of nail abnormalities. Age, gender, the use of certain medications, and the presence of other physical symptoms determine whether a more serious medical condition exists.

Certain abnormalities can result from bacterial and fungal infections, kidney, liver, and thyroid disease, skin diseases, such as psoriasis, and injury resulting from trauma. It is important to consult a physician if the nail abnormalities are unexplained, persistent, or are associated with other symptoms.

One of the more common problems is fungal infection under the nail, caused by the fungus *Candida* growing in the nail beds, resulting in a painful swelling and pus secretion. Infected nails may turn white or yellow and separate from the surrounding skin. This condition is common among diabetics.

A treatment that sometimes is effective against fungal infections is a mixture of the antifungal agent ketoconazole in dimethylsulfoxide (DMSO). The DMSO carries the antifungal agent below the nail to do its work. Despite a lack of studies supporting this therapy, anecdotal and clinical reports have shown it to be useful in some cases. Nail fungus can also be treated with medicated creams and lotions often containing nystatin. Along with an antifungal cream, hydrocortisone (prescription-strength preferable) for nail infection may be used to relieve pain and itching. Keeping the nails dry will help to clear up the infection and prevent its return (*please refer to the Candida protocol*).

It is conceivable that some of the materials used in lengthening nails may cause problems for some women, resulting in an allergic response in the nails.

The only advice one could give would be avoidance of these materials on a trial basis.

Knox gelatin has been a popular home remedy for weak and brittle nails for years. It is derived from beef joint cartilage and is comprised of 85% protein. The anecdotal dosage is one packet taken per day mixed with water.

NUTRITIONAL CONSIDERATIONS

When nails do not grow properly or have abnormalities, the cause is often a nutritional deficiency stemming from an unbalanced diet, digestive problems, absorption problems, or eating disorders. The following list includes nutritional factors affecting the nails when there is a lack of vitamins, minerals, and trace elements in the diet.

- A lack of vitamin A and calcium causes dryness and brittleness.

- A vitamin B deficiency causes fragility of the horizontal and vertical ridges in the nail.

- A vitamin B_{12} deficiency leads to rounded and curved nails.

- A lack of protein, folic acid, and/or vitamin C causes hangnails.

- A lack of "friendly bacteria" (*Lactobacillus* sp.) leads to fungus under and around the nails.

- A deficiency of hydrochloric acid contributes to splitting nails.

- Low iron may cause concave or "spoon" nails and/or vertical ridges (*see Iron Deficiency*).

Iron Deficiency

Iron deficiency anemia affects 20% of women, 50% of pregnant women, and 3% of men. It can be caused by too little iron in the diet, poor bodily absorption of iron, heavy menstrual bleeding, or other loss of blood. In addition to pregnant or lactating women, children in rapid growth stages have an increased requirement for iron. People with a diet consisting of little or no meat or eggs for a sustained period may also suffer from iron deficiency. Symptoms of anemia are pallor, fatigue, weakness, shortness of breath, low blood pressure, decreased appetite, and brittle nails. Iron deficiency anemia can also cause a condition called koilonychia in which the fingernail is thin and concave, and has raised ridges. If these symptoms are present, dietary iron supplements should be taken.

CAUTION Have a blood test to measure ferritin levels in order to ensure that supplementing with iron is necessary prior to taking any iron supplements.

Zinc Deficiency

The inability to absorb adequate amounts of zinc has been linked to several dermatological disorders, including alopecia (hair loss), dermatitis, and nail weakness. Oral administration of zinc compounds appears to be effective in clearing up many of the dermatological manifestations associated with zinc deficiency (Pazzaglia et al. 1997).

L-Methionine

L-methionine, an antioxidant found in meat and dairy products, has also been found to be beneficial in strengthening nails. Supplemental *L*-methionine is especially recommended for people on a vegetarian diet. This antioxidant, mixed with juice or water, is most effectively utilized when taken with adequate magnesium.

CAUTION To prevent accumulation of harmful homocysteine, adequate folic acid and vitamins B_6 and B_{12} should be taken with *L*-methionine. Trimethylglycine (TMG) will also aid in this process.

Silicon

Silicon is an essential trace mineral that is vital to the health of bones, skin, and even arteries. Silicon helps facilitate the formation of collagen, which is necessary for the strength and healthy development of epithelial and skeletal connective tissue. The body requires 5–20 mg a day of silicon for healthy functioning.

Biotin

Biotin, a B-complex vitamin, has been shown in several studies to improve nail firmness, hardness, and thickness in test subjects with fragile and brittle fingernails (Hochman et al. 1993). After a 6-month treatment regimen consisting of oral administration of 2.5–10 mg of biotin, most test subjects show a marked improvement in the condition of their nails, often with complete clearing of nail fragility (Floersheim 1989; Bardazzi et al. 1993).

In a placebo-controlled, double-blind clinical study, 60 patients with reduced nail quality without a known biotin deficiency were treated for 6 months with a daily 2500 mcg dose of oral biotin. The changes in nail quality were documented by measuring the swelling behavior and water loss through the nail keratin after incubation with sodium hydroxide (NaOH), as well as by the clinical judgment of the investigator and the patients. All evaluation parameters showed improvement of nail quality (Anon. 1996).

Riboflavin

Vitamin B_2, or riboflavin, is an essential B vitamin that promotes healthy nails, skin, and hair. Most people take 75–200 mg a day.

Whey Protein

Whey protein has been used by athletes and body builders for years as a lean source of protein that helps build muscle mass. Protein is important to the body because it repairs and rebuilds cells, muscles, and bones. In recent years scientists have discovered that whey protein can boost immune function and raise cellular glutathione levels.

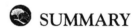 **SUMMARY**

The condition of our fingernails reflects our overall good health. Many factors contribute to the condition of nails, some of which are related to serious medical conditions. Studies repeatedly show that a diet that includes an adequate amount of essential nutrients is necessary to keep nails healthy. The following supplements are recommended:

1. Biosil, 6 drops orally a day (provides silica, a building block of nails).

2. Whey protein, 2 servings a day (provides approximately 40 grams of protein).

3. Riboflavin (vitamin B_2), 75–200 mg a day.

4. *L*-cysteine, 1500 mg a day.

5. Biotin, 2500–5000 mcg a day.

6. *L*-methionine, 500 mg a day, on an empty stomach; *L*-methionine should be taken with folic acid, 800 mcg; vitamin B_{12}, 300–600 mcg; and TMG, 1000 mg a day.

7. Life Flora will replace friendly intestinal bacteria to help prevent nail fungus, 1 capsule a day.

8. Zinc, one 30-mg capsule a day.

9. Take Iron Protein Plus if blood testing reveals iron deficiency anemia. Take 1 capsule a day or as recommended by your physician.

10. Knox gelatin, 1 packet daily mixed in water. The results will not be seen for a few months.

Note: *A multinutrient formula called Life Extension Mix provides optimal potencies of nutrients like biotin, zinc, riboflavin, and other health-protecting nutrients. Suggested dose is 3 tablets taken 3 times daily.*

 PRODUCT AVAILABILITY

Biosil, vitamin B$_2$, biotin, Enhanced Whey Protein, *L*-cysteine, *L*-methionine, Life Flora, folic acid, vitamin B$_{12}$, TMG, Iron Protein Plus, zinc, and Life Extension Mix can be ordered by calling (800) 544–4440 or by ordering online at www.lef.org. The DMSO/Ketoconizol mixture is available by prescription from the Medical Center Pharmacy, (800) 323–PILL.

Neuropathy and Diabetic Neuropathy

Neuropathy is a disturbance in the function of a nerve or particular group of nerves. The nerves affected are outside the brain and spinal cord and are known as *peripheral* nerves. Thus, neuropathy is often referred to as *peripheral neuropathy*. The nervous system is classified into two parts: the central nervous system (or CNS) and the peripheral nervous system (or PNS). The CNS is made up of the brain and the spinal cord. The PNS is composed of the nerves that branch off from the CNS. The peripheral nerves handle a diverse array of functions in the body.

When an individual has a peripheral neuropathy, nerves of the PNS have been damaged. Nerve damage can arise from a number of causes, such as disease, physical injury, poisoning, or malnutrition. Certain nerve cell axons, such as the ones in the PNS, are covered with a substance called *myelin*. The myelin sheath may be compared to the plastic coating on electrical wires: It is there both to protect the cells and to prevent interference with the signals being transmitted. Depending on the cause of damage, the nerve cell axon, its protective myelin sheath, or both may be injured or destroyed.

For example, in a very common form of neuropathy called *diabetic neuropathy*, there is a change in the microvascular network that supplies the nerve with nutrients. This lack of blood supply and nutrients causes the nerve to function abnormally. The disease of diabetes itself has an impact on the blood vessels of the whole body, causing problems in the kidneys and subsequent high blood pressure; in the eye, sometimes causing blindness; in the heart, causing angina or heart attack; and finally in the nerves, causing polyneuropathy.

In all neuropathy and neuropathic pain, there is abnormal conduction of nerve impulses from the input (usually peripheral in the extremities) to the spinal cord and brain. The pain of neuropathy is a result of the abnormal processing of nerve impulses that originate in these peripheral nerves. The terms *neuropathy* and *peripheral neuropathy* are often used interchangeably to describe the same process. Neuropathy can cause strange and extremely unpleasant sensations to arise in the affected area, including paresthesia (tingling or numbness), causalgia (burning sensations), and dysesthesia (unpleasant, burning, crawling, itchy, tingling or numb sensations)—or just plain pain.

Pain associated with neuropathy can be very intense and may be described as cutting, stabbing, crushing, burning, shooting, gnawing, or grinding. In some cases, a nonpainful stimulus (such as a feather drawn across the skin) may be perceived as excruciating, or pain may be felt even in the absence of a stimulus. If a problem with the motor nerve has continued over a length of time, muscle shrinkage (atrophy), or lack of muscle tone, may be noticeable. Autonomic nerve damage can also occur and is most noticeable when an individual stands upright and experiences difficulties such as lightheadedness or changes in blood pressure. Other indicators of autonomic nerve damage are lack of sweat, tears, and saliva; urinary retention; and impotence. In some cases, heart beat irregularities and respiratory problems can develop.

An example of peripheral neuropathy occurs in the disease of leprosy in which nerves are damaged as a result of bacterial infection and in Guillain-Barré syndrome when the neuropathy can arise as a result of complications from a viral infection. Lyme disease, AIDS, alcoholism, and trauma can also lead to neuropathic pain syndromes.

The complete classification of neuropathies is outside the scope of this protocol, but neuropathy can briefly be divided into several categories as follows:

1. *Sensorimotor neuropathies* are mainly characterized by sensory symptoms but also may have a minor component of motor nerve problems. Poisoning with heavy metals (e.g., lead, mercury, chromium, and arsenic), chemicals, or drugs are linked to this syndrome. Diabetes, Lyme disease, and malnutrition are also included in this category.

2. *Recurrent or relapsing polyneuropathy* consists of neuropathies that affect several nerves and may come and go, such as in the viral Guillain-Barré syndrome, porphyria, and chronic inflammatory demyelinating polyneuropathy.

3. *Mononeuropathy* nerve damage is limited to a single nerve or a few closely associated nerves. Mononeuropathy includes neuropathies related to physical injury to the nerve, such as carpal tunnel syndrome or sciatica.

4. *Mitochondrial neuropathy* focuses on mitochondria, organelles (structures within cells) responsible for handling a cell's energy requirements. If the mitochondria are damaged or destroyed, the cell's

energy requirements are not met and the cell can die. This includes nerve cells. The most well-known example of this is the case of Greg LaMond, an Olympic cyclist, who developed chronic fatigue syndrome and was found to have a mitochondrial neuropathy/myopathy (Rowbottom et al. 1998).

5. *Infections* stemming from certain viruses are associated with extremely painful sensory neuropathies. Shingles is a primary example of such a neuropathy. After a case of chickenpox, the varicella-zoster virus becomes inactive in sensory nerves. Years later, the virus may be reactivated. Once reactivated, it attacks and destroys nerve fibers. Infection with HIV is also associated with peripheral neuropathy, but the type of neuropathy that develops can vary. Some HIV-linked neuropathies are noted for myelin destruction rather than axonal degradation. Also, HIV infection is frequently accompanied by other infections, both bacterial and viral, that are associated with neuropathy.

6. *Physical injury* during sports and recreational activities are common causes of peripheral neuropathy. The common types of injuries in these situations occur from placing too much pressure on the nerve, exceeding the nerve's capacity to stretch, blocking adequate blood supply of oxygen and nutrients to the nerve, and tearing the nerve. Pain may not always be immediately noticeable, and the obvious signs of damage may take a while to develop. These injuries usually affect one nerve or a group of closely associated nerves. For example, a common injury encountered in contact sports such as football is the *burner*, or *stinger*, syndrome. Typically, overstretching the main nerves that span from the neck into the arm causes a stinger. Immediate symptoms are numbness, tingling, and pain that travel down the arm, lasting only a minute or two. A single incident of a stinger is not dangerous, but recurrences can eventually cause permanent motor and sensory loss.

7. *Toxin/drug-induced* peripheral neuropathy can be the result of contact with drugs, industrial chemicals, and environmental toxins. Neuropathy that is caused by drugs usually involves sensory nerves on both sides of the body, particularly in the hands and feet, and pain is a common symptom. Neuropathy is an unusual side effect of medications, but a few of the drugs that have been linked with peripheral neuropathy include Metronidazole, an antibiotic/antiprotozoal; phenytoin, an anticonvulsant; and Simvastatin, a common cholesterol-lowering medication of the HMG-Co-A reductase

inhibitor class. Anti-HIV retroviral (reverse transcriptase inhibitor drugs) medications frequently cause neuropathy. Isoniazid, a treatment for tuberculosis, induces a peripheral neuropathy due to its effect on vitamin B_6. This can easily be prevented by providing the patient with vitamin B_6 supplements prior to instituting chemotherapy with Isoniazid. (Certain industrial chemicals have been shown to be poisonous to nerves (neurotoxic) following work-related exposures. Chemicals such as acrylamide, allyl chloride, and carbon disulfide have all been strongly linked to development of peripheral neuropathy. Organic compounds, such as *N*-hexane and toluene, are also encountered in work-related settings, as well as in glue-sniffing and solvent abuse. Either route of exposure can produce a severe sensorimotor neuropathy that develops rapidly.)

Note: *Acrylamide was recently found to be present in small amounts in fried carbohydrate foods such as French fries. The impact of this is not yet known, but acrylamide is also carcinogenic.*

Heavy metals are the third group of toxins that cause peripheral neuropathy. Over time, lead and mercury can lead to sensorimotor neuropathies. Lead, arsenic, thallium, and mercury are not usually toxic in their elemental form but rather as components in organic or inorganic compounds. The types of metal-induced neuropathies vary widely (Chu et al. 1998). Arsenic poisoning may mimic Guillain-Barré syndrome (a viral illness). Although lead affects motor nerves more than sensory nerves, it can affect the sensory pathways as well—this may be due to lead-induced porphyria rather than the lead itself. Thallium produces painful sensorimotor neuropathy, and the effects of mercury are seen in both the CNS and PNS.

8. *Malnutrition and alcohol abuse* are another cause of neuropathy. The effects of alcohol abuse can be distinguished by burning sensations, stabbing pains, and numbness in the feet (sometimes in the hands). The level of alcohol consumption associated with this variety of peripheral neuropathy has been estimated as approximately 3 L of beer or 300 mL of liquor daily for 3 years. However, it is unclear whether alcohol alone is responsible for the neuropathic symptoms because chronic alcoholism is strongly associated with malnutrition. Malnutrition refers to an extreme lack of nutrients in the diet. It is unknown precisely which nutrient deficiencies cause peripheral neuropathies

Drugs and Toxins Causing Peripheral Neuropathy

Drug	Special features
Antibiotics	
Chloramphenicol	Distal, primarily sensory neuropathy, optic neuritis during prolonged high-dose use
Dapsone	Predominantly motor neuropathy
Dideoxycytidine, Dideoxyinosine, Dideoxythmidine	Painful sensory neuropathy
Ethambutol	Optic neuritis
Isoniazid	Distal axonal neuropathy, paresthesias are prominent. Prevented by vitamin B_6
Metronidazole	Distal sensory neuropathy
Nitrofurantoin	Distal sensorimotor neuropathy; occurs in renal failure
Suramin	Distal sensorimotor and demyelinating neuropathy
Antineoplastics	
Cisplatin	Sensory ataxia
Cytarabine	Sensorimotor neuropathy; rare
Misonidazole	Painful sensory neuropathy
Procarbazine	Distal paresthesias
Paclitaxel	Distal sensorimotor neuropathy
Vinca alkaloids: vincristine, vinblastine, vindesine, vinorelbine	Distal sensorimotor neuropathy
Antirheumatics	
Chloroquine	Neuromyopathy
Cholchicine	Mild sensory neuropathy, myopathy
Organic gold	Demyelinating sensorimotor neuropathy
Penicillamine	Demyelinating sensorimotor neuropathy
Other pharmaceuticals	
Amiodarone	Mild sensorimotor neuropathy
Disulfiram	Distal sensorimotor neuropathy
Ergots	Distal paresthesiae and dysesthesias
FK 506	Axonal neuropathy
Hydralazine	Prevented by vitamin B_6
Nitrous oxide	Associated with myelopathy
Perhexiline	Demyelinating neuropathy
Phenytoin	Mild distal sensory loss
Procainamide	Demyelinating neuropathy; rare
Pyridoxine	Sensory ataxia
Thalidomide	Painful axonal neuropathy, primarily sensory
L-tryptophan	Associated eosinophilia, fasciitis
Nonpharmaceutical toxic agents	
Acrylamide	Excessive sweating
Allyl chloride	Distal numbness
Arsenic	Elevated hair, urine, and fingernail levels
Buckthorn	Motor neuron syndrome causing bulbar and limb paralysis
Cadmium	Sensory neuronopathy
Propionitriles (e.g., dimethylaminopropionitrile)	Urinary hesitancy, sexual dysfunction
Ethylene oxide	Associated cognitive impairment
Hexacarbons (*n*-hexane, methyl *n*-butyl ketone)	Distal axonopathy
Lead	Predominantly motor; associated anemia
Mercury	Associated central nervous system manifestations
Methyl bromide	Calf-muscle tenderness
Organophosphorus esters	Diarrhea, sweating, fasciculations
Polychlorinated biphenyls	Acne, brown-pigmented nails
Thallium	Gastrointestinal symptoms, delayed alopecia
Trichlorethylene	Facial numbness
Vacor	Acute diabetes mellitus

in alcoholics and in famine and starvation victims, but it is suspected that the B vitamins have a significant role. For example, thiamin (vitamin B_1) deficiency is the cause of beriberi, a neuropathic disease characterized by heart failure and painful polyneuropathy of sensory nerves.

DIAGNOSIS

Clinical symptoms can indicate peripheral neuropathy, but an exact diagnosis requires a combination of medical history, medical tests, and possibly a process of exclusion. Certain symptoms can suggest a diagnosis, but more information is commonly needed. For example, painful, burning feet may be a symptom of alcohol abuse, diabetes, HIV infection, or an underlying malignant tumor, among other causes. Without further details, effective treatment would be difficult.

A clinical neurological examination evaluates the standard parameters such as reflexes, motor, and sensory modalities. This examination may be completely normal in early cases. By the time there is a loss of reflexes, the disease has progressed to an advanced state.

Early detection is essential to providing a treatment that can reverse the neuropathy. Therefore, ancillary testing that is more sensitive than a clinical examination is essential to confirm the diagnosis. There are several standard tests that are employed. The first and most common one is called nerve conduction velocity (NCV) test. NCV measures the precise electrical characteristics of nerve transmission.

The person's medical history may also provide clues as to the cause, because certain diseases and medications are linked to specific peripheral neuropathies. A medical history should also include information about diseases that run in the family because some peripheral neuropathies, such as Charcot-Marie-Tooth disease, are genetically linked. Information about hobbies, recreational activities, alcohol consumption, and workplace activities can uncover possible injuries or exposures to poisonous substances. Blood tests, such as those that check levels of glucose and creatinine to detect diabetes and kidney problems, should be performed. Levels of iron, thiamin (B_1), vitamin B_{12}, and other factors may be measured as well, to rule out deficiencies.

More specific tests, such as an assay for heavy metals or poisonous substances or hair analysis, may be helpful. Additional tests, such as an electromyograph that tests muscle reactions, can confirm that nerve damage has occurred and may also be able to indicate the nature of the damage. For example, some neuropathies are characterized by destruction of the myelin sheath covering peripheral nerves. This type of damage is shown by slowed nerve conduction. If the axon itself has suffered damage, the nerve conduction may be slowed, but it will also be diminished in strength. An electromyograph adds further information by measuring nerve conduction and muscle response, which determines whether the symptoms are due to a neuropathy or to a muscle disorder.

DIABETIC NEUROPATHY

The most important factor that contributes to the development of diabetic neuropathy is the blood sugar level. Tightly controlled blood sugar and insulin levels will often prevent the onset of diabetic polyneuropathy. Elevated blood sugar levels will of course add to free-radical generation and the production of what are termed glycosylated proteins that cause accelerated aging. Diabetic neuropathy is most frequently seen in developed countries. Neuropathy causes more hospitalizations than any other type of diabetic complication, and it is estimated that 50–70% of all amputations in the United States, not related to trauma, are due to diabetic neuropathy. Inadequate glycemic control is by far the most significant risk factor for developing diabetic neuropathy, the risk decreasing steadily and predictably as control becomes tighter, but other risk factors have also been identified including:

- Advanced age and increased duration of diabetes
- Greater height, due to greater neuronal length as well as greater pressures in the lower extremities
- High diastolic blood pressure
- Reduced HDL-cholesterol and elevated triglycerides, characteristic of diabetic hyperlipidemia, carry elevated risks of neuropathy

While the incidence of diabetic neuropathy in *newly* diagnosed diabetic patients is only about 7.5%, as many as 50% of those diagnosed 25 years ago are now symptomatic. Neuropathy is one of the most common diabetic complications, but it often remains asymptomatic, invisibly increasing the risks of developing sexual dysfunction, foot ulceration, and even cardiac arrhythmias. Although diabetic neuropathy can be subcategorized according to affected anatomy, polyneuropathy of the extremities involving the hands and feet is the most common finding (primarily with sensory symptoms) and usually with parasthesias in a glove-and-stocking distribution of the lower extremities. Because diabetes is such a prevalent disease in North America, a lot of the overall research in neuropathy has focused on the neuropathy of the diabetic.

As pointed out earlier, the nature of diabetes is such that the small blood vessels of the body are damaged due to high levels of blood sugar and blood insulin. Thus, damage is occurring to nerve endings long before the patient perceives any symptoms. Therefore, prevention is absolutely critical for diabetics. Alpha-lipoic acid, a powerful antioxidant, has been the subject of several studies. In the year 2000 in *Free Radical Biology and Medicine*, it was found that the *in vitro* addition of alpha-lipoic acid to human blood treated with high glucose concentrations markedly lowered oxidation and increased factors that would delay or inhibit the development of neuropathy in humans (Jain et al. 2000).

TREATMENT

Most of the research regarding the etiology and treatment of neuropathy has been done on diabetic neuropathy. Much of that research is done on rats that have been injected with Streptozotocin that induces an experimental form of diabetes for research purposes. Using this experimental model, it has been found that there are several possible mechanisms responsible for the induction of neuropathy. It is well-known that people with diabetes may develop vascular problems such as hypertension, eye problems, hardening of the arteries, and poor circulation. The nerve endings must be supplied with oxygen and nutrients like any other organ. In diabetic neuropathy, the so-called *vasa nervora* (small vessels that surround the tiny nerve endings) that supply the nerves themselves with oxygen and nutrients are damaged.

One predominant theory of neuropathy in diabetic rats involves abnormalities in what is called the *polyol pathway*. Polyol stands for polyhydroxy alcohols. While most of the cells in the body require insulin in order to transport glucose across the cell membrane, nerve cells are different. Membranes of nerve cells and their capillaries have insulin-independent glucose transport; that is, insulin is not required for glucose to pass into the cells. Since there is an excess of glucose in the bloodstream of diabetics, this glucose can easily be absorbed into nerve cells. In nerve cells, this glucose gets converted to sorbitol (a sugar alcohol) by an enzyme known as aldose reductase. The sorbitol cannot easily get out of the cell and consequently it accumulates, causing free-radical damage to nerves and blood vessels. This causes a decrease in an intracellular nutrient known as *myo-inositol* that is partly responsible for nerve conduction.

There is also an increase in free radicals such as peroxides and decreased nitric oxide production (a blood vessel-relaxing messenger), which, of course, leads to increased oxidative stress and the need for increased antioxidants. The amino acid taurine is also depleted (Hansen 2000). Terada et al. (1998) suggest that there is a close relationship between increased polyol pathway activity and carnitine deficiency in the development of diabetic neuropathy and that an aldose reductase inhibitor, a carnitine analog, and alpha-lipoic acid have therapeutic potential for the treatment of diabetic neuropathy (Terada et al. 1998).

Aldose Reductase Inhibitors

Aldose reductase is an enzyme that converts glucose to sorbitol. The accumulation of sorbitol causes a decrease in intracellular levels of myo-inositol and taurine, which eventually reduces the rate of cellular energy production. Aldose reductase inhibitors (ARIs) are drugs that act on a nerve exposed to high blood sugar. ARIs protect the nerve by preventing some of the chemical imbalances that are the result of elevated blood sugar. Three major laboratories are currently in Phase III testing of aldose reductase inhibitors; however, there are none currently available for clinical use (Hotta et al. 1990; Hibi 1997; Malik 2000).

A treatment with aldose reductase inhibitors (ARIs) should prevent the conversion of glucose to sorbitol, the subsequent depletion of myo-inositol and taurine, and thus help prevent the onset and progression of neuropathy. Sorbitol does not cross cell membranes and accumulates inside the cell, producing osmotic stress and a kind of intracellular edema. Marked sorbitol accumulation has been found in the lens of streptozotocin-induced diabetic rats, and ARIs prevented this accumulation and thus cataract formation. However, high accumulation has not been found in tissues of diabetic human subjects, and the therapeutic effects of reductase inhibitors have so far been disappointing. Clinical trials in humans have shown that these drugs have major side effects or no therapeutic effect. Even though the reduction of sorbitol by ARIs is possible, thereby increasing the production of the antioxidant glutathione, the clinical effects on human neuropathic states are not yet obvious.

Antiepileptic Drugs

Evidence from animal models of neuropathic pain suggests similarities between the pathophysiological phenomena observed in some epilepsy models and in neuropathic pain models. Anticonvulsants in the symptomatic management of neuropathic pain have been attempted. Positive results from laboratory and clinical trials further support such use. Carbamazepine was the first of this class of drugs to be studied in clinical

Preventing Cancer While Losing Weight

CLA is *not* just for fat loss. Studies show CLA may also help protect against many diseases including atherosclerosis and cancer.

In an article appearing in *The Journal of Nutrition*, significant cancer-preventing properties were shown when CLA was added to the diet (Ip et al. 1999a). The study revealed that CLA was a "potent cancer preventative agent in animal models." Specifically, it was determined that feeding CLA to female rats while they were young and still developing conferred lifelong protection from breast cancer. This preventive action was achieved by adding only enough CLA to equal 0.8% of the animal's total diet. This compares favorably with Life Extension's recommendation of 3000–4000 mg daily, which is approximately 1% of an average human's diet (Ip et al. 1999a).

In an earlier study in *Experimental Cell Research*, CLA was shown to prevent mammary cancer in rats if given before the onset of puberty (Ip et al. 1999b). Even more important, if CLA was ingested during the time of the "promotion" phase of cancer development, the rats were conferred substantial protection from further developing breast cancer. Another significant finding was that CLA appeared to actually inhibit the growth of normal mammary epithelial cell organoids and induced apoptosis or cell death in some of those same cells. The researchers concluded that this led to a reduction in the density of the developing mammary glands in rats and, therefore, the incidence of breast cancer was reduced (Ip et al. 1999b).

In the June 1999 issue of the journal *Carcinogenesis*, CLA was shown to reduce the size of breast tissue in the rat and thereby reduce the incidence of carcinogenesis (Banni et al. 1999). In another study reported in *Anticancer Research*, it was shown that CLA is also able to inhibit the growth of prostate cancer (Cesano et al. 1998). As reported in the article, CLA can be considered to be a powerful prostate cancer preventive as well as a partial treatment.

CLA may work via a similar mechanism to antidiabetic drugs such as Avandia and Actos to not only enhance insulin sensitivity, but to also protect against cancer. A report in the journal *Medical Hypothesis* pointed out that a number of human cancer cell lines express the PPAR-gamma transcription factor, and agonists for PPAR-gamma can promote apoptosis in these cell lines and impede their clonal expansion both *in vitro* and *in vivo*. CLA can activate PPAR-gamma in rat adipocytes, possibly explaining the antidiabetic effects of CLA in Zucker fatty rats. The report concluded by stating: "It is thus reasonable to

suspect that a portion of CLA's broad spectrum anticarcinogenic activity is mediated by PPAR-gamma activation in susceptible tumors" (McCarty 2000). **Note:** The term "PPAR-gamma" is an acronym for "peroxisome proliferator activator-receptors-gamma." A PPAR-gamma agonist such as Avandia, Actos, or CLA activates the PPAR-gamma receptor. This class of drug is being investigated as a potential adjuvant therapy against certain types of cancer.

Another finding that provides insight into the biochemical action of CLA is its ability to suppress arachidonic acid. Since arachidonic acid can produce inflammatory compounds that can aid cancer proliferation, this may be yet another explanation for the anticancer effects of CLA. The suggested amount required to obtain the overall cancer-preventing effects is only 3000–4000 mg a day.

Clearly, we can expect more research and more interest in this fascinating supplement that has already been proven to be a formidable foe against cancer and to be able to promote weight loss with the development of lean tissue.

How CLA Induces Fat Loss

The May 2002 issue of *The Journal of Nutrition* described a study conducted to ascertain the effects of CLA on calorie burning and fat storage in mice (Terpstra et al. 2002). CLA was shown to lower the amount of ingested food that was stored as body fat. CLA also increased the amount of fat excreted in the feces. Additionally, the study found that CLA induced a reduction in body fat mass on mice fed either a calorie-restricted or normal diet. The scientists defined the term "energy expenditure" as being the amount of food ingested minus the food retained in the body carcass and in the feces. CLA-fed mice showed a 74% increase in energy expenditure. The scientists thus concluded that the lower amount of ingested food stored on the body carcass was accounted for by this significant increase in energy expenditure (Terpstra et al. 2002).

This new finding corroborates a study conducted at Louisiana State University in which feeding male mice a CLA-enriched diet for 6 weeks resulted in 43%–88% lower body fat, especially in regard to abdominal fat. This occurred even if the mice were fed a high-fat diet. The effect was partly due to reduced calorie intake by CLA-supplemented mice and partly to a shift in their metabolism, including a higher metabolic rate (West et al. 1998).

In another study, performed at the University of Wisconsin-Madison, mice supplemented with only 0.5% of CLA showed up to 60% lower body fat and up to 14% increased lean body mass compared to controls. The researchers discovered that CLA-fed animals showed greater activity of enzymes involved in the delivery of fatty acids to the muscle cells and the utilization of fat for energy, while the enzymes facilitating fat deposition were inhibited (Terpstra et al. 2002).

The Safety of CLA

In a study conducted by the Nutrition Department of Kraft Foods, male rats were fed a diet of 1.5% CLA, which is 50 times higher than the estimated upper-range human intake. The animals were examined weekly for any signs of toxicity; no toxicity was found. After the end of the 36-week study, the animals were sacrificed and autopsied. Again, no abnormal pathology was found. The study confirmed that CLA supplementation is safe even at high doses. Nevertheless, high doses are not necessary for obtaining the benefits of CLA (Scimeca 1998).

A dose of three to four 1000-mg capsules of 76% CLA, taken in the morning or before lunch on an empty stomach, may be an effective part of an overall weight-loss program. Research studies indicate that it usually takes about 3 weeks before body fat loss occurs in response to CLA supplementation.

HOW GUARANA INDUCES FAT LOSS

Guarana is an herb that contains a form of caffeine called guaranine which is 2.5 times stronger than the caffeine found in coffee, tea, and soft drinks. What makes guaranine unique from the caffeine found in beverages is its slower release. That is because the guarana seed is fatty (even in powder form) and is not readily water-soluble. Therefore, the body does not quickly absorb it.

Since guaranine is released slowly, over a period as long as 6 hours, the energy boost that is experienced from guarana is not like that of coffee (a sudden rush and quick drop-off). Rather, the energy boost continues to escalate over hours.

While caffeine from beverages provides a short-lived energy burst that overheats and excites the body, guaranine has a cooling action that revitalizes and relaxes. This is because guarana contains other components that modify the activity of guaranine. The end result is more beneficial to the body than tea or coffee.

Guarana aids in a temporary, natural increase in body temperature and metabolic *thermogenesis* through nutritional stimulation of the body's beta-receptor pathway, which can induce the breakdown and release of stored body fat and thereby allow stored fats to be turned into energy. Thermogenesis refers to the body's production of heat. Heat production is a normal part of metabolic processes and can be enhanced by certain nutritional substances. Thermogenesis is both a source of heat and, when stimulated through appropriate dietary supplementation, a mechanism to increase metabolic rate. Stored body fat, if released and available for use, can provide the fuel for this increased metabolic rate.

Other active constituents of guarana are theobromine and theophylline, which are called xanthines (a class of thermogenic substances found in coffee, tea, and certain beans). They have some effect on increasing metabolic rate, suppressing appetite, and enhancing both physical and mental performance. They also act as muscle relaxants and possess diuretic properties.

Interestingly, caffeine accelerates the effectiveness of CLA, thus making CLA a more potent fat burner. Guarana has been shown to stimulate the migration of lipids so fat can be burned as energy. It is also an appetite suppressant.

Guarana also increases mental alertness, fights fatigue, and increases stamina and physical endurance. Guarana is taken daily as a health tonic by millions of Brazilians. In the United States, guarana holds GRAS-status (Generally Regarded as Safe). In 1989 a patent was filed on a guarana seed extract that was capable of inhibiting platelet aggregation in mammals. The patent described guarana's ability to prevent the formation of blood clots and to help in the breakdown of clots that had already been formed. Clinical evidence was presented in conjunction with the patent in 1989 and again in 1991 by a Brazilian research group demonstrating these anti-aggregation properties (Bydlowski et al. 1991).

Clinical Studies on Guarana

In a study reported in *The Journal of Human Nutrition Diet*), guarana extract induced weight loss for over 45 days in overweight patients taking a mixed herbal preparation containing yerbemate, guarana, and damiana (Andersen et al. 2001). Body weight reductions were 11.22 pounds in the guarana group compared to less than 1 pound in the group receiving placebo for 45 days.

Guarana extract and its fractions decreased platelet aggregation up to 37% of control values and decreased platelet thromboxane formation from arachidonic acid up to 78% of control values (Bydlowski et al. 1991). When platelets hyperaggregate and/or when excess thromboxane formation occurs, this can initiate an arterial blood clot, which results in a heart attack or ischemic stroke.

In a 1997 study in rats, guarana increased the physical activity of the rats as well as increased physical endurance under stress and increased memory with single doses as well as with chronic doses. Interestingly enough, this study revealed that whole guarana seed extract performed better and more effectively than a comparable dosage of caffeine or ginseng extract (Espinola et al. 1997).

Another Brazilian research group has studied the apparent effect of guarana to increase memory, which is thought to be linked to the essential oils found in the seed (Galduroz et al. 1996). Its antibacterial properties against *Escherichia coli* and *Salmonella* have been documented as well (da Fonseca et al. 1994).

A 1998 toxicology study with animals has shown that guarana is nontoxic at even high dosages of up to 2 grams/kg of body weight. This same study demonstrated the antioxidant properties of guarana, saying: "Guarana showed an antioxidant effect because, even at low concentrations (1.2 mcg/mL), it inhibited the process of lipid peroxidation" (Mattei et al. 1998).

A major advantage to taking guarana in an oil base capsule is its relatively slow release into the body. In a study reported in the journal *Pharmacology Biochemical Behavior* in November 1997, a comparison was made of the absorption of caffeine from coffee, cola, or capsules. Based on saliva caffeine concentrations, the absorption from capsules was about 40% slower than that of coffee or colas. These capsules were not oil-based, yet the rate of caffeine absorption was still significantly slower than coffee or cola (Liguori et al. 1997).

CLA + GUARANA

The effect of CLA on blocking excess absorption of serum glucose and fatty acids into adipocytes (fat cells) is remarkable. CLA induces a reduction in the size of adipocytes. One of the reasons that people gain weight as they age is that their adipocytes literally become fatter.

Another cause of increased body fat storage is the proliferation of adipocytes. Whereas CLA helps block the absorption of fat and sugar into adipocytes, CLA does not reduce the actual number of adipocytes present. Guarana has been shown to specifically reduce the number of adipocytes. When CLA was combined with guarana, there was a 50% reduction in adipocyte number (FASEB 2002).

In response to the FASEB (2002) study showing an added benefit when CLA is combined with guarana, a supplement has been formulated that contains potencies

of CLA and guarana that have demonstrated fat-loss effects in published studies (available from Life Extension Foundation). CLA is also available by itself as a supplement for those who are overly sensitive to caffeine.

Whereas many published studies document the fat-reducing effects of CLA, the fact that CLA may protect against cancer, vascular disease, and Type II diabetes makes it a preferred supplement for health-conscious people to use daily.

THE "FRIENDLY" FATS

There are fats that are healthy and fats that are dangerous. Hydrogenated fats are made by bubbling hydrogen gas with nickel as a catalyst to make the oil more solid at room temperature. This is how margarine and Crisco™ are made. During the process, many of the chemical bonds are broken and reformed into less healthy trans configurations.

Healthy fats have a distinct flavor and unfortunately tend to become rancid after a few weeks, even with refrigeration. The healthiest oils are cold-pressed to avoid the chemical changes that occur during heating. Healthy oils are made from olives, flax seed, borage seeds, and even hemp. Each has its own unique flavor.

Not long ago, low-fat diet gurus were trying to terrorize people into further reducing all fat consumption. Now that we have witnessed the epidemic of obesity that followed, we know better. Healthy fats help keep us slender! They also help protect against atherosclerosis, cancer, diabetes, autoimmune diseases, and various other degenerative disorders.

Through their impact on important metabolic enzymes, healthy fats increase the synthesis of beneficial prostaglandins E1 and E3 while decreasing the levels of inflammatory prostaglandin E2; they also modify cell membrane composition and fluidity. Hence, improved blood flow and tissue oxygenation, higher metabolic rate, improved insulin sensitivity, immune enhancement, more muscle and bone formation, better brain function, and faster nerve impulse conductance result, to mention just a few of the major benefits.

Thus, while in the 1970s and 1980s dietary fat was demonized and presented as being a problem, we are beginning to see various kinds of healthy fat as part of the solution.

Essential Fatty Acids

The omega-3 and omega-6 oils are called *essential fatty acids* because the body needs them to remain healthy.

The brain is composed almost entirely of essential fatty acids. Clinically, essential fatty acids (such as flax and borage oils) have a marked anti-inflammatory effect on the body.

Many times, scientific studies run counter to popular beliefs that are often spread via media commercials designed to sell a particular product. One such belief says that we should avoid all fats in order to lose weight. While this is true in the case of simple fats, the essential fatty acids found in high-quality oils are very healthy and may also promote weight loss.

An article in *The American Journal of Clinical Nutrition* described a study of dietary fish (Mori et. al. 1999). Overweight patients being treated for hypertension were randomly assigned to a daily fish meal (3.65 g of omega-3 fatty acids); a weight-loss regimen; the two regimens combined; or a control group for 16 weeks. Fasting triglycerides fell 29% with fish consumption and 26% with weight loss. The fish plus weight-loss regimen group showed the greatest improvement in lipids: triglycerides decreased by 38% and HDL(2) cholesterol increased by 24% compared with the control group. The authors concluded that adding a daily fish meal into a weight-loss regimen was more effective than either measure alone at improving glucose-insulin metabolism and dyslipidemia (Mori et. al. 1999).

The essential fatty acids found in fish oils are known to promote thermogenesis, the process by which foods are converted immediately to heat. In this way, the body burns off the calories instead of converting them into fats for storage (McCarty 1994). Another benefit of essential fatty acids is to make cell membranes more sensitive to the effects of insulin (Storlien et al. 1986, 1987, 1996; Borkman et al. 1993; Vessby et al. 1994; Pan et al. 1995). As discussed earlier in this protocol, insulin-resistance is a prime factor causing people to gain unwanted fat pounds as they age.

Eating fish is a good way to promote weight loss. Many people also choose to take essential fatty acid supplements that are high in DHA (docosahexaenoic acid) from fish oil extracts and GLA (gamma-linolenic acid) from borage oil. Other options include flax or perilla oil supplements that contain alpha linolenic acid (precursors to DHA and EPA). Consumption of these essential fatty acids confers a significant protective effect against chronic inflammation and vascular disease, a common problem in overweight people.

CHROMIUM

While thyroid hormone plays a definite role in weight management, both magnesium and chromium are also required to break down the cellular insulin resistance that causes higher blood sugar levels.

Overweight people usually experience insulin impairment that prevents the proper carbohydrates (sugars) from being metabolized by their muscle cells. Excessive serum glucose is converted into body fat unless this insulin resistance is broken down and the cells are able to regain youthful carbohydrate metabolism. Chromium has received widespread publicity for its ability to lower serum glucose levels by potentiating insulin sensitivity. Studies have shown that chromium supplementation results in a slight reduction in body fat and an increase in lean body mass. Niacin has been shown to improve the metabolic-enhancing effect of chromium.

In 1997, Austrian researchers conducted a study to assess the effects of chromium yeast and chromium picolinate on lean body mass during and after weight reduction with a very low-calorie diet: 36 obese nondiabetic patients undergoing an 8-week, very low-calorie diet followed by an 18-week maintenance period were evaluated. During the 26-week treatment period, study subjects received either placebo or chromium yeast (200 mcg/day) or chromium picolinate (200 mcg/day) in a double-blind manner. After 26 weeks, chromium picolinate-supplemented subjects showed increased lean body mass. Researchers reported chromium picolinate, but not chromium yeast, is able to increase lean body mass in obese patients in the maintenance period after a very low calorie diet without counteracting the weight loss achieved (Bahadori et al. 1997).

To improve the fat-reducing effects of dieting, a 200-mcg chromium capsule should be taken with every meal to facilitate youthful carbohydrate metabolism. The importance of taking a chromium capsule with each meal is illustrated in animal studies in which chromium was given throughout the day in order to lower serum glucose levels. When an individual consumes food, serum glucose levels rise significantly unless the cells are sensitized to insulin. Chromium will help sensitize your cells to insulin by helping to lower your blood sugar levels.

Do not take more than three 200-mcg chromium capsules a day. Always take antioxidant supplements such as vitamin E when taking chromium to protect against free-radical activity. At least 30 mg of niacin should be contained in each 200-mcg chromium capsule to facilitate its effects in the body.

MAGNESIUM

While chromium has received considerable media attention, the scientific literature shows that magnesium plays an even more important role in regulating carbohydrate metabolism. Magnesium is involved in a number of the enzymatic reactions required for cells to uptake and metabolize glucose. Magnesium deficiency causes insulin resistance and elevated blood sugar levels (Paolisso et al. 1990; Nadler et al. 1993, 1995; Lefebvre et al. 1994).

Approximately 80% of Americans are magnesium-deficient. When magnesium-deficient individuals go on a diet, they often become severely magnesium-deficient, which aggravates insulin resistance and contributes to the failure of the diet. For those individuals going on a calorie-restricted diet, it is suggested that 300–500 mg of supplemental magnesium be taken each day.

FIBER

Soluble fiber includes pectin, gum, and mucilage. Soluble fiber tends to form a gel when added to water. Soluble fiber is found in oat bran, barley, vegetables (carrots), and fruits (apples and oranges). Insoluble fiber is made from cellulose that is used primarily as structural material in plants. Insoluble fiber functions to increase the bulk of stools.

A study examined the use of fiber in a weight-loss program: 53 moderately overweight females (BMI >27.5 kg/m^2) on reduced energy intake (1200 kcal/day) were treated for 24 weeks with a fiber supplement on a random, double-blind, placebo-controlled basis. The fiber was administered as an initial dose of 6 grams and a maintenance dose of 4 grams. After treatment, mean weight loss in the fiber group was 8.0 kg (17.6 pounds) versus 5.8 kg (12.76 pounds) in the placebo group (Birketvedt et al. 2000).

A review of published studies on the effects of dietary fiber on hunger, satiety, energy intake, and body composition in healthy individuals found that under conditions of fixed energy intake, the majority of reports indicate that an increase in either soluble or insoluble fiber intake increases post-meal satiety (sensation of fullness) and decreases subsequent hunger. When energy intake is not restricted, mean values from published studies indicate that consumption of an additional 14 grams per day of fiber for more than 2 days is associated with a 10% decrease in energy intake and body weight loss of 1.9 kg over 3.8 months. The observed changes in energy intake and body weight occur both when the fiber is from naturally high-fiber foods and when it is from a fiber supplement. The authors concluded that increasing dietary fiber intake to at least the minimum recommended by the American Heart Association (25–30 grams per day) may help to decrease the currently high national prevalence of obesity (Howarth et al. 2001).

The best time to take fiber is with the highest-fat meal of the day. The objective is to have the fiber absorb some of the dietary fat to prevent it from absorbing into the bloodstream where it helps contribute to body fat accumulation. Do not take fiber at the same time you take beneficial fatty acids such as CLA, EPA/DHA, and GLA. The fiber can absorb these critically important fatty acids before they can reach your cells. Some people experience unpleasant gastrointestinal side effects when taking high doses of fiber. It is best to begin with a very low dose, increasing the dose slowly. Fiber supplements consisting of guar gum, pectins, and psyllium seed husks are available in capsule form and in powder that can be mixed in liquid and consumed immediately before eating a fatty meal.

STEVIA

Stevia is a South American herb (*Stevia rebaudiana*) that is known locally as "sweet herb" or "honey leaf." Stevioside extracted from this plant is 100–300 times sweeter than table sugar, yet it is not a carbohydrate. Stevia extract and powder can be used as a sweetener both in beverages and in cooking.

IMPLEMENTING A NATURAL WEIGHT LOSS PROGRAM

Taken together, everything presented so far provides a comprehensive approach to inducing fat-loss and achieving sustained weight control. Many of the weight-loss supplements outlined in *Step 1* of the following summary can be safely initiated without the need for hormone blood tests.

However, to optimize long-term weight management, we encourage the hormone blood profile as recommended in *Step 2* of the following summary. Too often, only partial weight loss results are achieved because imbalance of hormones such as testosterone, estrogen, and thyroid (T3) prevent the body from releasing more stored body fat.

Following is a summary of what should be done to implement a scientific-based weight loss program:

Step 1: Take the following dietary supplements to facilitate immediate weight loss:

Supplement	Dose
Avocado Sugar Extract (standardized D-mannoheptulose)	2 tablets after evening meal (Take 2 additional tablets if hunger returns before bedtime.)
CLA (76%) 1000 mg	3–5 capsules early in the day
or CLA with Guarana extract	3–5 capsules early in the day
Chromium (picolinate or polynicotinate)	200 mcg, 1 capsule with each meal
Super GLA/DHA (essential fatty acids)	6 capsules per day
Life Extension Mix (provides high doses of magnesium, zinc, and other important nutrients)	3 tablets, three times per day
Fiber (psyllium seed, guar, and pectin)	Start with 4 grams taken when high-fat meals are consumed. Do not take with CLA or Super GLA/DHA because fiber will bind to these important fatty acids before they can be absorbed into the bloodstream.

Step 2: Obtain the following blood tests from your physician or order them directly by calling (800) 208-3444.

1. Complete blood chemistry (includes serum glucose)

2. Fasting insulin

3. Free testosterone

4. Estradiol

5. Thyroid panel (T3, T4, TSH)

6. DHEA

7. PSA (for men)

8. Fasting insulin

(Be certain to *not* eat anything for 12 hours prior to having blood drawn.)

Step 3: Once the test results are received, initiate hormone modulation therapy as follows:

If there is any indication of thyroid deficiency, take an appropriate thyroid replacement medication (usually Cytomel). The starting dose of Cytomel is normally 12.5 mcg twice per day. Because calorie intake will normally be reduced in response to taking the avocado sugar extract, your thyroid gland may slow down and try to block fat loss by reducing thermogenesis. To guard against thyroid deficiency, have your blood tested or use the morning basal temperature test within 60 days of starting avocado sugar extract to be certain that you do not need a thyroid replacement drug.

If DHEA levels are low (they almost always are in people over age 35), then take the appropriate amount of DHEA (15–50 mg/day) to restore them to a youthful range. (Refer to *DHEA Replacement Therapy* protocol for precautions.)

For men, if free testosterone is in the low normal range or below normal, ask your physician to prescribe a transdermal cream to provide 5 mg per day of natural testosterone. If estradiol levels are high (over 30), use 0.5 mg of the drug Arimidex twice a week to block the aromatase enzyme that converts testosterone to estrogen. Before using testosterone, men should verify that they *do not have* prostate cancer by having a blood test for PSA and undergoing a digital rectal exam.

Once armed with a youthful hormone profile, along with supplements that help facilitate weight loss, you are in a position to determine how much body fat you want to lose. For instance, if you take the avocado sugar extract supplement every evening, your appetite will be reduced, fewer calories will be consumed, and you can expect to start losing about a pound a day. There may be social occasions when you do not want to curb your appetite because you want to eat a big meal. You may not want to take the avocado sugar extract during these occasions because it would not enable you to eat a lot of food.

If fasting insulin levels remain significantly above 5, you may need to take more avocado sugar extract tablets. Avocado sugar extract also decreases excess serum insulin that causes food to convert to body fat. By reducing high serum insulin, body fat can be released from storage (fat deposition) in your body. Obese people normally have high levels of fasting insulin (unless they are advanced Type II diabetics whose pancreatic beta cells no longer produce insulin). These insulin-dependent diabetics would not benefit from avocado sugar extract because they are not producing enough (or any) insulin to begin with.

Once on this program, you will find it easy to make healthy food choices such as including more fresh fruits and vegetables in your diet, avoiding high sugar snacks, and reducing total calorie intake.

Based on our research, this three step program is the only practical approach for the normal aging human to be rid of excess body fat over a continuous period. If you are seriously concerned about protecting yourself against multiple degenerative diseases and improving your appearance, we urge you to make the effort to have your blood tested, modulate your hormone profile accordingly, and take the supplements that can help you regain your youthful appearance. If you need a referral to a physician knowledgeable about hormone modulation, please call (800) 226-2370.

Precautions for Natural Weight Loss Protocol

Even when taking natural weight loss supplements, there are still some precautions that should be followed to guard against adverse side effects. For instance, if an individual has uncontrolled hypertension, CLA with guarana should not be taken. Instead, use the CLA product without guarana. Even though guarana tends to release slowly in the body, individuals who are hypersensitive to caffeine may want to use the CLA alone.

Avocado sugar extract may be used in several ways. The best way is to take two tablets after dinner and two additional tablets later in the evening if hunger returns before bedtime. Some people choose to take two tablets of avocado sugar extract 30–45 minutes after each meal and as needed to suppress inappropriate hunger (up to a maximum of eight tablets a day).

Some individuals should not take avocado sugar extract. It will not work for persons taking insulin. If you are an insulin-dependent diabetic, do not take avocado sugar extract. Also, those taking oral medications that stimulate insulin production (sulfonylureas) will receive no benefit from avocado sugar extract. Type II diabetics should only take this product under supervision of their physician who has read the specific instructions and warnings located on the Website (www.insulinreducer.com) or available by calling (866) 820-8090.

Avocado sugar extract should also be avoided by hospitalized or institutionalized patients and by persons who have loss of appetite, anorexia, HIV, or any form of catabolic (wasting) illness. Cancer patients may take this supplement provided they understand the precautions listed on www.insulinreducer.com or available by calling (866) 820-8090.

Reduced thyroid hormone output is a common response when less food is consumed. This response is nature's way of conserving body mass in response to what it perceives as a famine. If avocado sugar extract significantly reduces food consumption, check thyroid hormone status and ask your physician for Cytomel or Armour drug therapy if body temperature or blood tests indicate thyroid deficit. Refer to the *Thyroid Deficiency* protocol for details.

Chromium can induce the production of free radicals. Therefore, when taking a chromium supplement, be certain to simultaneously consume an antioxidant supplement.

SUMMARY

Obesity and weight loss remain controversial subjects. Scientists have identified underlying causes for age-associated weight gain. Yet the majority of overweight people and their physicians ignore these findings. The result is that most diet and exercise regimens fail.

The fact that conventional weight-loss methods do not work is confirmed by more Americans being obese and overweight than ever before. Yet never have so many people tried to reduce body fat.

While the long-term objective of any diet modification program is to maintain healthy body mass index (BMI below 25) with a reduced calorie intake, it is more important initially for obese individuals to shift the time of day when they consume the most calories. The instructions to overweight and obese individuals given earlier in the protocol will be repeated in order to achieve rapid and sustained fat loss:

1. Immediately after wakening: Eat a large breakfast. If you want a banana split, eat it for breakfast! Eat as much as you want of whatever you want. The reason we advocate a liberal breakfast is that you should follow this program for the rest of your life. If you are continuously deprived of the foods you like, at some point you may rebel and start eating at the wrong time of the day. Ideally, breakfast will consist of fresh fruit and whole grains, but if you need to consume high calorie foods, do it in the morning and not late in the day.

2. Late morning: Eat a snack equivalent in calories to a hamburger and potato fries. Healthier foods are recommended, but for the purposes of complying with this program, eat what you want at this time of the day instead of waiting until the evening when these calories readily convert to body fat.

3. Mid-afternoon: Have another snack equivalent to the calories obtained from a tuna salad sandwich on whole wheat bread and some fruit.

4. Dinner: No later than 6:30 p.m. have a modest dinner: fish or lean chicken-meat, potato, and several vegetable servings.

5. After dinner: Nothing goes in your mouth but *standardized avocado extract* pills and the water to swallow them!

6. Two avocado extract pills may be repeated if hunger returns later that evening.

It may take a week for some obese individuals to wake up hungry (as they are supposed to do) and not have the desire to eat after 6:30 p.m. After 45 days of following this program that alters the time of day when calories are consumed, an improvement in several metabolic parameters should become evident, including a reduction in fasting insulin levels. Enough fat loss should have occurred during this initial 45-day period to motivate the individual to reduce total calorie intake and begin to exercise. Using the standardized avocado extract pills makes restricting calorie intake much easier by cutting carbohydrate craving.

There are three important reasons to cut calorie intake throughout life:

1. The risk of degenerative disease declines dramatically in those who remain thin.

2. Reducing calorie intake slows and possibly reverses aging.

3. One of the most important aspects of one's appearance and self-esteem is to avoid the accumulation of unsightly body fat.

The appendices following this protocol provide information about conventional weight loss drugs, gastric surgery, the glycemic index, assessing insulin status, and other methods that have been promoted to be of help in shedding excess body fat.

For most people, the best weight-loss results will occur if they follow the three simple steps outlined in the preceding section, which were:

1. Supplement with *standardized avocado extract*, CLA, chromium, magnesium, fish oil.

2. Check hormone blood levels.

3. Take corrective action if there are any hormone imbalances such as asking your physician for a prescription for Cytomel if T3 levels are low; testosterone cream if testosterone levels are low; an aromatase inhibitor (such as Arimidex®) if estrogen levels are high (primarily for men), etc.

Combining the three steps listed above with a shift in calorie consumption to early in the day can produce profound body fat loss and sustained weight control.

 PRODUCT AVAILABILITY

Avocado sugar extract (d-mannoheptulose tablets), CLA with Guarana or CLA-only capsules, chromium caps, Life Extension Mix, Super GLA/DHA and other essential fatty acids, DHEA, magnesium, stevia, and fiber capsules and powders can be ordered by calling (800) 544-4440 or by ordering online at www.lef.org. Blood tests to ascertain hormone status, PSA, and other important parameters can be ordered by calling (800) 208-3444. Cytomel, Arimidex, and testosterone creams are prescription drugs. If you need referral to a physician knowledgeable about the hormone medications discussed in this protocol, call (800)226-2370 or log on to www.ledocs.com.

APPENDIX A

Weight Loss Drugs

Amphetamine and related sympathomimetic medications are thought to stimulate the release of norepinephrine and/or dopamine from storage sites in nerve terminals in the lateral hypothalamic feeding center, thereby producing a decrease in appetite.

Adrenergic drugs for weight loss include phentermine (Adipex, Fastin, Ionamin); diethylpropion (Tenuate, Tepanil); phendimetrazine (Adipost, Bontril, Plegine, Prelu-2); and benzphetamine (Didrex). These drugs are chemically related to amphetamine. Mazindol (Sanorex, Mazinor) is an isoindole thought to inhibit the reuptake of norepinephrine rather than to cause its release.

Adrenergic weight loss drugs are all classified as *controlled substances* by the U.S. Drug Enforcement Agency (DEA) due to their tendency to cause dependency and the risk of abuse. All of these drugs are approved by the U.S. Food and Drug Administration (FDA) for short-term use (about 12 weeks) (FDA 1992).

Sympathomimetic appetite suppressants stimulate the central nervous system and elevate blood pressure. Side effects of these drugs include dry mouth, anxiety, insomnia, dizziness and lightheadedness, headache, palpitations, and (rarely) increased blood pressure. Tolerance to the effects of medications in this class usually develops within a few weeks and rebound weight gain may occur after discontinued use of the medication.

Give a physician your complete medical history especially if you have high blood pressure, an overactive thyroid, glaucoma, diabetes, or emotional problems. Inform your physician if you think you are pregnant or if you are breast-feeding. Limit alcohol use. Alcohol can increase unwanted side effects of dizziness. Adipex and other stimulants that work via this mechanism are not recommended for use in children.

Also inform your physician about all medicines used (prescription and nonprescription), especially if you take high blood pressure medicine or MAO inhibitors (e.g., furazolidone, phenelzine, selegiline, tranylcypromine) or any other weight-loss medicine. Decongestants are commonly found in over-the-counter cough and cold medicines.

Orlistat (Xenical) is unique among current obesity drugs in that it does not act directly on the central nervous system. Orlistat inhibits an enzyme (pancreatic lipase) essential to fat digestion. In 2 years of clinical trials, orlistat has produced sustained weight loss similar to that of other single agents.

The most common side effects are intestinal symptoms, including cramping, gas, and diarrhea, particularly in patients who eat high-fat foods against the advice of their physician. It is possible that the desire to avoid these unpleasant side effects might encourage people to eat a diet that is lower in fat, thereby helping them to lose weight.

Sibutramine (Meridia) increases the levels of both serotonin and noradrenaline in areas of the brain that regulate food intake and body weight. It produces 1-year weight loss similar to that of other single agents and reduces some complications of obesity such as those involving blood glucose and lipids. Unlike some other anti-obesity drugs, sibutramine does not reduce blood pressure. The side effects may include dry mouth, lethargy, drowsiness, and insomnia

Obesity is associated with decreased human growth hormone levels. Growth hormone is released by the pituitary gland in response to exercise, deep sleep, hypoglycemia, and ingestion of protein. It stimulates the production of RNA (ribonucleic acid), mobilizes fat deposits, and is a central part of insulin metabolism (Fischbach 1996). Decreased levels of growth hormone are associated with obesity and corticosteroid use. Therapies that boost growth hormone can help facilitate weight loss. The cost of human growth hormone injections is cost-prohibitive for most people.

Most weight loss drugs have side effects that cause many people to discontinue using them before significant results are obtained.

APPENDIX B

Exercise and Diet

The goal of any weight-loss program is to attain better health through improved diet and exercise, in addition to restoring one's metabolic profile to fit that of a 21-year-old.

It is difficult for many overweight individuals to engage in exercise because excess body fat makes them too lethargic to contemplate a consistent exercise program. Additionally, some people just will not exercise. By properly modulating hormone levels, some individuals will feel revitalized enough to become physically active.

Restoring hormones to reflect more youthful profiles will produce some quick fat loss and alleviate depression. Feeling better and seeing real weight reduction can induce many people to improve their diet.

Those who remain hopelessly overweight may not be able to focus on proper diet or exercise, because neither was effective for them in the past. That is why it is so crucial to restore one's metabolic profile to a healthy, youthful level. For most people, this requires proper hormone balance. When there are hormone imbalances, such as too much fasting insulin and/or not enough testosterone, DHEA, thyroid, people gain weight. These age-related hormone imbalances often preclude sustained weight control, despite agonizing diet and exercise programs that are supposed to work!

APPENDIX C

The Glycemic Index

Much attention is being paid to avoiding foods that have a high glycemic index and glycemic load. The hypothesis is that since high glycemic foods increase production of insulin, avoiding them and eating only low glycemic foods will facilitate fat loss by reducing excess insulin. The problem with obese and severely overweight individuals relying on low glycemic diets is that they are already making too much insulin to achieve meaningful fat loss.

A review of published studies comparing the effects of consuming high as opposed to low glycemic diets on weight loss has yielded mixed results. Many studies indicate that it is healthier to eat lower glycemic index as opposed to high glycemic index foods, especially for diabetics.

A study in the July 2002 issue of the *American Journal of Clinical Nutrition* challenged the validity of many of the existing published studies showing increased weight loss and other health benefits associated with consuming low glycemic index foods (Pi-Sunyer 2002). The author's summary about glycemic index and disease follows:

"It has been suggested that foods with a high glycemic index are detrimental to health and that healthy people should be told to avoid these foods. This paper takes the position that not enough valid scientific data are available to launch a public health campaign to disseminate such a recommendation. . . . Presented herein are the reasons why it is premature to recommend that the general population avoid foods with a high glycemic index."

The purpose of this appendix is to provide the reader with the basis for why some people think consuming low glycemic foods is the solution for obesity. For severely overweight individuals, it is at best only a partial solution. This *Obesity* protocol has meticulously identified the need to correct multiple metabolic disorders in order to achieve significant and sustained fat loss. The failure to correct for even one metabolic imbalance (such as low T3) can render any fat loss program useless.

What Is the Glycemic Index?

Glycemic index refers to the rate blood glucose levels rise after eating food, in comparison with an equivalent amount of pure glucose (sugar) or white bread. Many people are sensitive to carbohydrates even though they have normal fasting glucose levels.

- Foods with high glycemic indices include corn flakes, instant potatoes, honey, pasta, bread, rice, and potatoes.

- Food with a low glycemic index include kidney beans, lentils, soy beans, peanuts, butter and haricot beans, blackeye and chick peas, apples, ice cream, milk, yogurt, and tomato soup.

Interestingly, ice cream has a fairly low glycemic index, a result of the fats that tend to slow blood sugar rises. This emphasizes the complexity of the subject of diet. Although ice cream is considered a low-glycemic index food, it is high in calories, carbohydrates, and fats.

Persons who have carbohydrate cravings and food addictions should be particularly aware of the glycemic index. Certain carbohydrates can cause a sudden elevation of glucose in the blood with a sudden rush of energy often accompanied by feelings of dizziness or lightheadedness followed by a "crash." In particular, children may become addicted to the energy rush from snacks and soda. The pattern is often continued into adulthood by substituting coffee and donuts (for breakfast) or by eating cakes and cookies (after dinner).

Get into the habit of stocking your refrigerator with oranges, grapefruit, apples, pears, and berries. These fruits have been shown to reduce disease risk as opposed to refined sugar snacks that cause excessive fat accumulation.

While people seeking to lose body fat try to avoid sucrose and fructose, too often the intense craving for sugar (induced by hyperinsulinemia) results in carbohydrate bingeing.

The food industry misleads the public into thinking that high-glycemic foods are healthy. For instance, orange juice is promoted as a source of folic acid, vitamin C, and calcium. The downside to orange juice is that it induces an acute influx of fructose into the bloodstream that then spikes serum insulin. When an orange is eaten, there is only a gradual release of sugar into the blood. However, once fruits or vegetables are juiced, they become catalysts for insulin overload because of their high concentration of rapidly absorbable sugar.

Carrots have a high-glycemic index, but since their glycemic load is very low, there is nothing wrong with eating carrots. However, once carrots are juiced, the sugar is concentrated into a form that instantly hits the bloodstream and provokes an insulin spike. The moral to this story is to eat high amounts of fruits and vegetables, but avoid their juice. A look at the calorie content of a glass of fruit or vegetable juice confirms their fat-inducing effects. For those persons who are concerned about obtaining adequate folic acid, vitamin C, alpha-carotene, etc., these nutrients can be obtained by eating whole fruits and vegetables and by taking supplements.

As can be seen in this section, foods that were once considered part of a healthy "low-fat diet" have a very high glycemic index and glycemic load. This means that ingesting too many of these types of foods could cause weight gain, even if you think you are eating a healthy diet.

As shown in Table 1, eating too many high sugar-content foods and beverages causes the release of excess insulin. When evaluating the insulin-elevating effects of foods, two measurements to consider are the "glycemic index" and "glycemic load." The "glycemic index" measures how fast a carbohydrate triggers a rise in circulating blood sugar. The "glycemic load" assesses the impact of carbohydrate consumption, but provides a fuller picture than does the glycemic index alone. Foods that are high in both of these measurements should be reduced.

Food Fraud

In spite of the term "low-fat" or "fat-free" appearing on more and more food labels, a record number of Americans are overweight. The problem is that "low

Pain (Chronic)

Chronic pain one is of the most costly health problems in North America. Estimated costs, including direct medical expenses, lost income, lost productivity, compensation payments, and legal charges, are approximately $90 billion a year. The following statistics are startling:

- 48 million Americans suffer from chronic pain.
- Over 21 million Americans routinely take prescription painkillers and also spend $3 billion on over-the-counter analgesics.
- Over 13 million Americans cannot perform routine activities because of pain.
- Fourteen percent of employees take time off from work because of pain.
- As many as 45 million Americans have chronic, severe headaches that can be disabling.
- Arthritis pain affects more than 40 million Americans each year.
- The majority of patients in intermediate or advanced stages of cancer suffer moderate to severe pain. (More than 1.2 million new cases of cancer are diagnosed each year in the United States, and more than 550,000 people die from the disease.)

According to the National Institutes of Health (Harris et al. 1999), lower back pain is one of the most significant health problems in the United States, with back pain being the most frequent cause of activity limitation in people younger than 45 years of age: 65–80% of all people have back pain at some time in their life.

Although pain is a major problem in this country, it is not treated compassionately or efficiently, and it is not just pain that is the problem. The side effects of chronic pain illnesses caused by a sedentary lifestyle, seclusion and depression, and, in some cases, addiction to pain killers can be just as devastating as the pain itself.

The premise of this protocol for pain management is to eradicate the underlying cause of chronic pain. Therefore, first consider the specific disorder that is causing your pain (for example, arthritis) and then refer to that specific protocol in this book.

All pain, whether chronic or acute, physical or emotional, is recognized, interpreted, and acted on by the brain. We may feel the pain in our toes when we stub them, but the recognition, interpretation, and reaction to the pain occur in the brain.

This is how it happens: sensory neurons (special nerves throughout the body) react to pressure, mechanical trauma, heat, cold, and other stimuli. They also respond to prostaglandins, histamine, and other chemicals released by injured or inflamed body tissue. Whether sensory neurons are stimulated depends on how powerful, prolonged, and widespread the heat, pressure, or other stimulus is. When sensory neurons are stimulated, the nerves fire, sending off messages that travel along the nervous system to the brain. In the brain, the pain information is rapidly evaluated, and orders are issued: "Yank your hand away from the hot stove!" or "Stop hitting your thumb with the hammer!"

ACUTE VERSUS CHRONIC PAIN

As a rule of thumb, physicians know how to treat acute pain quite well but are not as skilled at helping people who suffer from chronic pain because the cause of acute pain is often clear and easy to find, although the cause of chronic pain can baffle even teams of specialists.

Acute pain is the type of pain that tells you that something is harming or about to harm your body. Acute pain lets out a three-alarm warning when you accidentally put your hand on a hot stove; it makes you rush to the hospital when your appendix is about to rupture; or it forces you to leap to your feet when you sit on a thumbtack. Frequently, traumatic pain of this nature will respond to rest, ice, elevation of the affected part, and the judicious use of over-the-counter preparations or more natural agents such as homeopathic Arnica for tissue damage. Sometimes more potent medications are required, but only for a short period of time.

On the other hand, chronic pain may be a dull ache that never goes away like a vise squeezing our heads, a sword piercing our abdomens every time we move a certain way, a sharp knife stabbing our backs, or a hammer smashing our hips with every step. Chronic pain seems to have no reason to exist other than to vex us. Sometimes we can determine the causes of chronic pain: for example, cancer of the pancreas that has spread to the back, but often we are puzzled because the original condition has healed, and the pain should have vanished.

Modern medicine has devised many methods of attacking pain. Doctors have pain-killing medicines, sedatives, antidepressants, muscle relaxants, and anticonvulsants. They can inject substances into the body to "block" the nerves and prevent transmission of pain signals to the brain, and they often perform surgery—especially on persons with back pain, but none of these approaches is 100% successful and safe.

This protocol examines individual treatments, supplements, and other methods of pain relief on an individual basis. Indeed, most research involves taking one single, potentially therapeutic item and testing for its efficacy. However, particularly in the area of natural treatments, it is not a single item that does the job, but rather a synergy between different treatment modalities. This is true of all disease, but it is particularly true of chronic pain that can have so many precipitating factors and changing features.

The nature of pain is subjective and each person will perceive pain in his or her own particular way, sometimes as a result of prior experience and exposure to pain. To assume that one method will help your pain is probably naive. A combination of factors is much more likely to help. Pains that are muscular or skeletal in origin tend to respond well to treatments that relax muscles. These would include diverse modalities such as acupuncture, trans-electrical nerve stimulation (TENS), Reiki, therapeutic touch, all types of massage, hydrotherapy, self-hypnosis, yoga, Feldenkrais, and so forth. However, pains that are neurogenic in origin (when nerves have been damaged or cut) may respond less well to soft tissue techniques such as Reiki, therapeutic touch, and massage and more positively to acupuncture, nerve blocks, or treatment with opioid medications.

How should a person with a chronic pain condition approach healing using alternative or conventional methods? Many people with chronic pain conditions will be less than optimally nourished as a result of eating the standard American diet—consisting mostly of excess sugar, fat, and salt. Improving the diet as suggested in the section entitled Foods That Fight Pain would be a very good beginning. If chronic pain is due to an underlying condition of inflammation (such as in arthritis), then the supplements listed in this protocol that are anti-inflammatory will probably be beneficial. This is where essential fatty acids, ginger, borage oil, green tea, curcumin, and other anti-inflammatory mediators will be successful. These natural anti-inflammatories work best when combined with a healthy, natural-based diet.

If your pain is musculoskeletal in origin, it is essential to consider therapies such as biofeedback, massage, hypnosis, physiotherapy, acupuncture, magnetic therapy, and others. Exercise is an important part of any therapeutic regime, but in some cases it may exacerbate a pain condition. Over-the-counter preparations may be helpful in acute pain, but may not be strong enough for pain that is chronic. Prescription medications may be required in addition to other approaches. Whatever therapy you decide to use to help your pain condition, you must first discuss it with your primary healthcare provider.

Some people will opt to try one thing at a time, so that they can decide what impact each therapy is having on the condition. Other people will decide to use many modalities at once and are unconcerned with which particular one is beneficial. If your primary healthcare provider is supportive of alternative therapies, he or she will be able to advise you whether different modalities will be compatible with your current therapy. If, as is often the case, your primary provider is unaware of alternative therapies, then you may need to elect a complementary care provider to assist with your future plan for healing. This could be anyone from a knowledgeable friend to a therapeutic complementary care provider such as a massage therapist. Above all, you need someone who can support you in your journey toward wellness and relief from pain.

During the past few years, it has been recognized that despite extensive progress in the scientific understanding of pain in humans, serious mismanagement and under-medication in treating acute and chronic pain is a continuing problem. Weinstein, writing in the *Southern Medical Journal* in 2000, used a measure of physicians' attitudes, knowledge, and psychology to learn what contributes to pain management practices. Overall, a significant number of physicians in this survey revealed what the authors describe as opiophobia, or prejudice against the use of opioid analgesics (for example, morphine, oxycodone, Demerol, and so forth).

Physicians are strongly influenced by their perceptions of drug regulatory agencies, fearing censure or delicensure for over prescribing opioids. In this survey, over 50% of respondents believed, incorrectly, that addiction is a common result of legitimate prescriptions. They also believed that requests for increased prescriptions were a result of increasing tolerance or addiction to the analgesic rather than a result of unrelieved pain. A disturbingly high percentage of physicians showed negative psychological traits such as authoritarianism, intolerance of ambiguity, and reliance on technology regarding patients with chronic pain (Weinstein et al. 2000).

The under-treatment of pain has become such a serious issue that in 1999 Governor Gray Davis of California signed into law Assembly Bill 791. Under this law, pain is considered to be a fifth vital sign (CHSC 1999) along with pulse, temperature, blood pressure, and respiration rate. Section 1254.7 of Assembly Bill 791 requires that "pain be assessed and treated promptly, effectively, and for as long as pain persists" and that "as a condition of licensure, include pain as an item to be assessed at the same time as vital signs are taken." Nurses, physicians, and other healthcare workers must record the duration, frequency, and intensity of a patient's pain as a routine part of taking vital signs. It is believed that Assembly Bill 791 will help to raise the awareness to healthcare workers of the importance of this symptom. In the summer of 2000, the U.S. Congress passed a bill (signed by President Clinton) calling for a "Decade of Pain Control and Research" to begin on January 1, 2001 (Saner et al. 2000).

While the under-treatment of pain predominates at present, it is also important to not fall into the trap of thinking that we need more and more different kinds of medication for pain relief. Alarmingly, the International Society of Drug Bulletins (in its 2001 *Declaration on Therapeutic Advances in the Use of Medicines*) stated that 80% of new products approved for clinical use each year in developed countries provide no advantage over existing treatments. Only 2% of new drug treatments offer a real advance to patients and 5% provide minor benefits (ISDB 2001).

The perception of pain is a very individualized experience. No one person can have the experience of another person's pain. As a result, mind/body approaches are an integral part of any pain relief program. These approaches may include, but are not limited to, hypnosis, biofeedback, guided imagery, meditation, and yoga. Because of its very personal nature, the spiritual aspects of pain relief play an important role as well. Beliefs about oneself and maintenance of hope are very important in the production of any effective pain management process.

Because pain is under-treated, people often can become easily depressed, discouraged, and lose hope. These negative emotions tend to exacerbate the intensity and even the frequency of pain. Hope must always be available to a person with chronic pain, not only to avoid increasing pain perception, but also to provide a vision for the future increased comfort. By focusing on a number of different alternatives, hope can be kept in view. A person suffering pain should also try to find a good listener to communicate with while going through a chronic pain process. If depression does occur, it is important to seek help from a psychotherapist who can engender positive outcomes, as opposed to a therapist who focuses only on problems.

CONVENTIONAL PAIN TREATMENTS

Practically every home medicine cabinet has at least one nonprescription drug for pain, which has been purchased over the counter in a drugstore or supermarket. Nonprescription preparations are commonly taken with little regard for their possible side effects, but every medicine has potential side effects that can appear even if you take it only once. Even those that do not cause an immediate reaction can slowly but surely harm the body if taken over a long time or if mixed with the wrong medicines. A description of a few of the most popular pain medicines will follow.

Aspirin

Aspirin is an inexpensive drug that has helped countless people who have routine aches and pains, as well as others who have more serious ailments such as rheumatoid arthritis and osteoarthritis. However, this seemingly harmless pill has potential side effects when taken in high doses, including heartburn, nausea, vomiting, ringing in the ears, hearing loss, hives, and itching. A more serious side effect of taking high doses of aspirin is bleeding. Aspirin should be avoided by persons with ulcers, gout, asthma, liver, or kidney disease; pregnant women and women who are breast-feeding; and anyone who will soon undergo surgery or has a bleeding disorder.

CAUTION Do not take aspirin while taking Coumadin, except under the supervision of your physician (*refer to the Thrombosis Prevention protocol in this book for specific information about the precautions required when taking blood-thinning drugs*).

Aspirin can also cause problems when combined with certain substances. For example, taking aspirin and drinking alcohol increases the chances of gastrointestinal tract bleeding. Aspirin can also displace certain drugs from their binding sites on protein, altering their effectiveness. Drugs that should not be taken with aspirin include tolbutamide or chlorpropamide for diabetes; commonly used nonsteroidal anti-inflammatory medicines; methotrexate, which is used to depress the immune systems of rheumatoid arthritis patients; phenytoin, which is used to control epileptic seizures; and heparin, which is used to thin the blood in the treatment of blood clots.

Acetaminophen

Acetaminophen is an effective treatment for moderate pain and fever, but it is not effective against inflammation, swelling, or redness. Potential side effects include trembling, light-headedness, fatigue, itching, fever, sore throat, unexplained bruises or bleeding, blood in the urine, and pain in the side or lower back. Long-term use may cause anemia as well as liver and kidney damage. Acetaminophen causes massive free-radical damage to the liver that can be ameliorated with nutrients such as N-acetyl-cysteine (NAC). Anyone taking acetaminophen should take 600 mg of NAC, along with 2000 mg of vitamin C and 100–400 IU of vitamin E with each dose. In addition, do not consume alcohol while taking acetaminophen because the addition of even small amounts of alcohol seriously magnifies the production of free radicals, and liver damage can occur more easily.

Nonsteroidal Anti-Inflammatory Drugs (NSAIDs)

NSAIDs are used for joint pain, stiffness, swelling, and painful menstrual periods. Potential side effects include stomach pain, gastritis, peptic ulcers, gastrointestinal bleeding, headaches, nausea, dizziness, depression, drowsiness, ringing in the ears, vomiting, diarrhea, cramps, convulsions, blood in the urine and stool, chest tightness, rapid heartbeat, fainting, and chills. Ironically, these medicines can actually cause pain: the very thing they are taken to eliminate.

NSAIDs should not be taken by anyone who has asthma, bleeding problems, heart failure, elevated blood pressure, peptic ulcer disease, ulcerative colitis, and a number of other diseases. Long-term use can damage the eyes and ears and cause weight gain. NSAIDs are often used by people with arthritis, but paradoxically NSAIDs can increase arthritic inflammation due to their effect on the thickness of the intestinal lining (see the Arthritis protocol). Indocin (indomethacin) is a particular NSAID used for arthritis and other ailments. This powerful drug quells pain and inflammation but has potential side effects including nausea, vomiting, diarrhea, constipation, abdominal pain, gas, ulcers, rectal bleeding, headaches, dizziness, depression, fatigue, anxiety, insomnia, confusion, fainting, blurred vision, deafness, vaginal bleeding, asthma, weight gain, irregular heartbeat, high blood pressure, chest pain, and even coma.

Refer to the Thrombosis Prevention protocol in this book for specific information about the precautions required before combining aspirin or NSAIDs with other blood-thinning drugs.

Medications derived from opium (such as morphine), Demerol, and oxycodone require expert knowledge and careful monitoring but should not be dismissed as a form of treatment because of concerns about addiction. The vast majority of persons who have pain do not show addictive signs even when on high doses of opium derivatives. However, pain patients can be inadvertently labeled as addicts because of their need for repeated doses of these medications. The general bias against opium derivatives has led to considerable under-treatment of pain as described previously. It is not within the scope of this protocol to describe the uses of opium derivatives, but two are described below:

- Talwin is a synthetic, modestly addicting narcotic (opioid) that is prescribed for moderate pain. Talwin can cause nausea, vomiting, anorexia, diarrhea, dizziness, hallucinations, headaches, confusion, insomnia, fainting, sweating, chills, rash, lowered blood pressure, irregular heartbeat, and other problems.

- Percodan is a synthetic relative of codeine. It is a powerful painkiller available by prescription. Like many of the opiates, it has a potential for addiction and needs to be monitored carefully. Side effects of Percodan include dizziness, nausea, vomiting, constipation, and sedation.

Surgery can be an excellent means of curing many types of pain. For example, if pain is caused by a tumor pressing on a nerve or by a broken bone, surgery can often solve the problem—either by removing the growth or helping to "knit" the bone. However, surgery is not as effective as many surgeons claim.

Surgery is a questionable treatment for chronic pain because no one knows what the surgeon should do once the patient's body has been opened up on the operating table. If the patient has back pain, should the disc with a slight bulge be taken out? Maybe or maybe not.

Surgical residents operate on the 3F policy: find it; fix it; forget it. Their motto is "When in doubt, cut it out."

Any time that a patient has surgery, there is a risk of infection, excessive bleeding, shock, and even death. Also general anesthesia presents risks, including allergic reactions to anesthetic drugs, coma, and death. There is no such thing as risk-free surgery.

Neural Blockage

Neural blockage (a nerve block) is one of the most important tools for diagnosing and treating certain types of chronic pain. Physicians inject a local anesthetic or other drug to block nerve function in a specific area, thus temporarily stopping the pain message from flowing to the brain.

However, after ascertaining that the procedure works, many physicians will make the nerve block permanent by injecting alcohol or another drug that destroys the nerve's ability to function. Almost any nerve or nerve root can be found and blocked, producing at least temporary relief. But nerve blocks are not always the answer because in blocking the pain, the usefulness of the nerve is also blocked. For example, if a nerve that helps move a finger is blocked, that finger cannot be used.

Sclerotherapy

Sclerotherapy is a recognized orthopedic procedure that stimulates the body's own natural healing process to strengthen damaged joints and has a unique ability to stimulate damaged joints to produce new fibrous tissues. Osteopaths tend to use the term sclerotherapy, but it is also known as prolotherapy or proliferative therapy (by physicians), ligament reconstruction therapy, or fibro-osseous injection therapy by other physicians. The terms are often used interchangeably (ACOPMS 2002).

Sclerotherapy treatment requires the precise injection of a mildly irritating solution directly into the site of damage. The irritating solution causes a mild, controlled injury that, in turn, stimulates an inflammatory response. This inflammation triggers biochemicals that signal the beginning of the natural healing process.

This mild inflammatory response can encourage growth of new ligaments or tendon fibers. Additional treatments repeat the process, potentially resulting in a gradual buildup of tissue and strengthening of a weakened joint. The injected solution contains anesthetic agents and natural substances, which stimulate a healing response. Lidocaine and procaine are anesthetic agents frequently used to reduce pain at the injection site. The anesthetics are combined with natural substances that vary in composition and are tailored by the treating physician to meet each individual patient's needs. An often-used ingredient is 50% dextrose. Sometimes dextrose is not strong enough to achieve the desired result, and sodium morrhuate is used instead. Other substances that are used include sodium tetradecyl sulfate, phenol, and Sarapin (a nerve-soothing extract from the pitcher plant). None of these is a steroid (cortisone or its derivatives) (ACOPMS 2002).

Pain caused by sclerotherapy injections varies according to the structure being treated, choice of solution, skill of the administering physician, and individual pain tolerance levels. Generally, the pain passes quickly or can be treated successfully with a pain reliever such as Tylenol. Anti-inflammatory agents such as aspirin and ibuprofen (NSAIDs) should not be used. There may be mild swelling and stiffness associated with treatments.

Sclerotherapy can be used to treat dislocated joints, knee and shoulder pain, TMJ dysfunction, carpal tunnel syndrome, and disc problems at any level of the spine. Sclerotherapy affects only the area treated and does not cause problems in any other area of the body,

making it an attractive form of treatment for some people (Manchikanti et al. 2000). Treatment is usually administered at 1-, 2- or 3-week intervals, as determined by the treating physician. As with any medical treatment, the rate of success is dependent on several variables, including the type of solution used, the patient's medical history, the patient's ability to heal, and the presence of nutritional deficiencies that would affect healing. Patients who have lower back pain with hypermobility have reported an 85–95% remission of pain when sclerotherapy was used (ACOPMS 2002). (Another form of sclerotherapy is used for the cosmetic treatment of varicose veins. In the case of varicose veins, the solution used is hypertonic saline, Sotradecol, or sodium tetradecyl sulfate.)

Buprenorphine

Buprenorphine, a little-known pain medication, is a mild narcotic with agonist and antagonist properties that has a very low addiction liability, if any, indicating that it can be used for a long period of time without development of serious withdrawal symptoms. Buprenorphine is effective in conditions with multiple symptoms because it acts rapidly in depression, reduces pain, and induces sleep (Balint 2002).

Buprenorphine is available as an injectable 0.3-mg ampule, a small dose even for injection. The dosage is variable. Because buprenorphine is poorly absorbed orally, larger oral dosages must be used. When taken orally, buprenorphine liquid is withdrawn or shaken from the ampule and held under the tongue for as long as possible. Compounding pharmacies can make up buprenorphine for sublingual use as a troche. Both forms (the ampules and troches) are not inexpensive. For pain that prevents sleep, start with 2–6 ampules sublingually or 0.5–2 mg as a sublingual troche. For treating pain throughout the day that is associated with depression, begin with 2–6 ampules (or 0.5–2 mg as a sublingual troche) every 4–6 hours. As is common with most medications, begin with a low dose and increase slowly until the smallest dose that proves effective is reached.

HS-599 is a didehydroderivative of buprenorphine that promises to be a potent and safe new analgesic, preferentially acting at the spinal level.

ALTERNATIVE TREATMENTS

Some people find that boosting brain levels of endorphins can provide natural pain suppression. This approach is not an effective way of dealing with acute (short-term severe) pain, but it is the safest method of alleviating chronic (long-lasting) pain.

Early in the 1970s, researchers at the Johns Hopkins University School of Medicine wrestled with a baffling puzzle. They had just proven that morphine, a powerful pain-killing drug, fits perfectly into special receptors in brain cells just as a key fits into a lock. The brain receptors were just the right size and shape for the morphine keys, suggesting that the human brain had been designed to work with morphine, allowing it to unlock, enter, and control parts of the brain.

Why would the human brain have evolved receptors specifically designed for morphine? After all, morphine is made by plants, not by the human body. Morphine is not supposed to be in humans and it rarely gets there. Most of us go through life without ever taking morphine.

Researchers theorized that if there were receptors for morphine in the brain, then there had to be morphine or a morphine-like substance somewhere in the body, but what was it, where was it, and what did it do?

The puzzle was solved when the first components of the human body's natural, morphine-like substances were discovered. They were called endorphins (endogenous morphine), and, like the drug, they are powerful painkillers that can alter mood. In fact, studies have proven that an endorphin called beta-endorphin is approximately 50 times more potent than morphine at quelling pain. Morphine was once the most powerful pain killer known (Li et al. 1977).

Endorphins are part of the natural pain-control network in the human body. They work by interfering with pain messages traveling through the nervous system. Endorphins cut off the pain message, stopping it dead in its tracks. Unfortunately, we cannot use endorphins themselves as painkillers. Taking endorphin pills or injecting endorphins into the body is inefficient, costly, impractical, and potentially dangerous.

Supplements That Fight Pain

Fortunately, we do not have to take endorphins to experience their pain-killing benefits. Instead, we can use natural substances that protect or boost the endorphins in our bodies, allowing their levels to rise to higher, more powerful levels. A brief description will follow of some of the supplements to consider if you suffer from chronic pain.

Tyrosine

Tyrosine is a nonessential amino acid that is manufactured by the body or absorbed from food. The body uses tyrosine to make the neurotransmitters dopamine, norepinephrine, and epinephrine, all of which play a role in elevating mood and keeping us alert (Gibson et al. 1977).

A suggested dose of tyrosine is 500 mg taken 2–3 times daily.

Phenylalanine

Phenylalanine, like other amino acids, comes in *D* and *L* (right and left) forms. The difference between the forms is like the difference between your hands. They are identical, but are opposite, mirror images of each other. The left-handed form is known as *L*-phenylalanine (LPA). This is the form in which phenylalanine is normally found in foods. The right-handed form is known as *D*-phenylalanine (DPA). DPA is the form that protects endorphins in our bodies and helps us to fight pain and depression (Beckmann et al. 1977; Cheng et al. 1979). A mixture of the two forms, which has been used to fight pain since 1978, is known as *DL*-phenylalanine (DLPA).

Phenylalanine protects our endorphins. It has helped many people overcome pain, as well as the depression that often accompanies chronic pain. In the original study of the effects of phenylalanine on pain, three of 10 patients reported significant relief. Phenylalanine has also been proven to be effective against painful inflammation. According to Russell et al. (2000), phenylalanine may work by up-regulating what is called the "endogenous analgesia system" (EAS), a neural pathway that occurs in a part of the spinal column. When stimulated by chronic pain or therapeutic measures such as opiates or acupuncture, the EAS suppresses activation of pain-receptive nerves in the spinal column and thereby alleviates pain (Russell et al. 2000).

Phenylalanine is not a drug, and it does not work directly against pain. Instead, it acts as an *endorphin shield*, battling pain indirectly by helping the body's built-in pain control system grow more powerful.

Phenylalanine was first tested against pain in a 1978 study at the Chicago Medical School. Researchers began by timing how long laboratory mice would remain on a hot plate before jumping off. Then they injected hundreds of mice with phenylalanine and again watched to see how long the mice would remain on the heated surface before scurrying off.

The amino acid blocked pain in 70% of the mice, allowing them to stay on the hot surface longer. The pain blocking action actually grew stronger with time. Standard medicines tend to become less effective over time as the body grows accustomed to them, but phenylalanine was actually more effective on the ninth day than it was on the first. Plus, there was more good news. Phenylalanine worked with other medicines, making them stronger, and did all this without any apparent side effects.

Excited by these surprisingly positive results, the Chicago scientists tested phenylalanine on humans. The results were astounding. All 10 patients studied who had been suffering from long-standing chronic pain (people who had not been helped by modern medicine) found pain relief with this simple amino acid (Ehrenpreis et al. 1978). Phenylalanine relieved chronic pain that had not been helped by conventional methods. There were no harmful side effects, and no one became addicted (as can be the case with powerful pain medicines). Also, no one developed a tolerance to phenylalanine, requiring larger and larger doses to get the same effect, as is often the case with conventional pain drugs.

Additional research supported these early promising results. In one landmark study, 43 patients suffering from various types of severe pain were given 250 mg of phenylalanine 4 times a day. Some of the patients reported marked relief within 1 week. But by the end of the fourth week, 75% of the patients reported that their pain had been relieved (Balagot et al. 1983).

In Great Britain, a double-blind, controlled study was undertaken to determine whether the amino acid really worked or whether the pain relief reported in other studies was caused by the so-called placebo effect. It is well-known that the power of belief can act as a medicine. Thus, when patients are given pills that contain no medicine but are told that the pills contain powerful drugs, many patients will get better. The participants in this study were adults suffering from long-standing, intractable pain of varied causes that had not been cured by conventional drugs or physical therapy. Despite the fact that lower doses of the substance were given and a 50% reduction in pain was required to qualify as improvement, more than 30% of the participants experienced significant relief. Phenylalanine outperformed the placebo, showing that it is, indeed, a powerful medicine (Budd 1983).

There are some people, however, who cannot use phenylalanine. This includes those born with a genetic deficiency called phenylketonuria (PKU) that prevents them from metabolizing phenylalanine, those with preexisting high blood pressure (phenylalanine can elevate blood pressure in people who are already hypertensive), and people with cancer (phenylalanine can promote cancer cell division).

Although phenylalanine is a powerful painkiller, it does not begin to work as rapidly as aspirin and other pain medications. This is because the amino acid helps to increase the body's supply of endorphins, rather than attacking pain directly. Strengthening the body's natural pain-control mechanisms is a very effective strategy, but it takes time to begin working. For headaches and other acute pain, people naturally prefer the almost instant pain relief they get from aspirin and other conventional medications.

What about chronic pain that does not respond to standard medicines, physical therapy, or surgery? Phenylalanine has ample time to begin working in such cases, so why is it not used more? The reason is because phenylalanine is not profitable for drug companies. It is a simple amino acid that cannot be patented. Thus, most physicians know that phenylalanine is an amino acid but have never heard about its powerful analgesic properties because no drug companies promote it.

The suggested dose of phenylalanine is 500 mg taken 2–3 times daily.

Glucosamine

Glucosamine is found in fish, meat, and other foods. This amino acid compound is particularly helpful in treating arthritis pain because it stimulates connective tissue, encouraging it to repair itself. Glucosamine is chondro-protective which means that it protects the chondrocytes that are found in large quantities in the joints.

Glucosamine is made in the body from glucose (sugar) and an amino acid called glutamine. Glucosamine serves as a building block of mucopolysaccharides (MPS) which are important for the development of cartilage, bone, ligaments, nails, hair, and skin. We can also get glucosamine from supplements.

As we get older or when we are injured, the body produces less glucosamine. This is surprising. One would think that the body would produce more glucosamine in order to repair the injury. Unfortunately, even small injuries that are not repaired can lead to greater damage and pain. Taking glucosamine gives the body the material it needs to help repair damaged cartilage. It often works best when taken with the fatty acids GLA, DHA, and EPA; chondroitin sulfate; manganese; and vitamins C and E.

Many studies have shown glucosamine to be a potent natural remedy for osteoarthritis that seems to affect so many of us as we age. It also opposes degeneration of the substance of the joints that occurs in arthritis. Several studies conducted at research centers in Europe have shown that supplemental glucosamine reduces joint pain, tenderness, and swelling, making joints that had been frozen with pain and inflammation usable again (Vajaradul 1981).

Glucosamine does not work as fast as some standard pain medications, but it does so without the serious side effects associated with drugs. In fact, many European physicians give glucosamine to their osteoarthritis patients as a first-line treatment, turning to drugs only in cases where the amino acid is not effective. Currently, over 5 million Americans take glucosamine or glucosamine and chondroitin combinations (Maher 2001).

Glucosamine appears to be even more effective in the form of glucosamine sulfate. Like glucosamine, sulfate is a component of joint cartilage. The sulfate also appears to strengthen the healing effects of glucosamine. Here are some of the studies on glucosamine sulfate.

A group of 20 patients with osteoarthritis of the knee was given either 500 mg of glucosamine sulfate 3 times a day, or a placebo. Within 6–8 weeks, subjects receiving glucosamine sulfate experienced significant reductions in pain, joint tenderness, and swelling. There were no reported side effects (Pujalte et al. 1980).

A randomized, placebo-controlled, double-blind study was carried out with 202 patients for 3 years. Some were given glucosamine sulfate, 1500 mg, once a day. The researchers wanted to see if long-term treatment with glucosamine could alter the progression of osteoarthritis in the knee. Based on the various tests that were carried out, there was a significant improvement of 20–25% in the glucosamine group. The authors concluded that long-term use with glucosamine slowed progression of the disease, possibly determining disease modification (Pavelka et al. 2002).

A group of 80 osteoarthritis patients experiencing pain, movement restriction, and swelling was given either glucosamine sulfate or a placebo: 73% of subjects receiving glucosamine sulfate experienced an improvement in symptoms within 3 weeks. What is more, when those who received glucosamine sulfate were biopsied and their cartilage was examined under an electron microscope, it looked much healthier than the cartilage taken from the placebo group (Drovanti et al. 1980).

Glucosamine sulfate was compared to ibuprofen in a double-blind study involving 40 patients with osteoarthritis of the knee. As expected, the ibuprofen worked faster. But, by the eighth week, subjects taking glucosamine sulfate were doing better than subjects taking ibuprofen, with significantly fewer complaints (Lopes Vaz 1982). In two other studies, one with 200 patients and another with 178, similar results were noted. The researchers in one of the studies noted that glucosamine was more effective because it curbed the pathogenic mechanisms of osteoarthritis (Muller-Fassbender et al. 1994; Gui et al. 1998). If taking glucosamine sulfate, follow the directions on the bottle. (This approach is explored in more detail in the *Arthritis protocol*.)

Chondroitin Sulfate

Chondroitin sulfate provides building materials for cartilage that is so often damaged in arthritis. Chondroitin sulfate slows the free radicals that attack the cartilage in joints. It also increases the flow of blood to joints, thus allowing antioxidants and other healing substances produced by the body to protect and repair body tissue. When arthritis patients were given injections of chondroitin sulfate, joint pain diminished significantly, and mobility and function returned.

Chondroitin sulfate is found in shark cartilage. A summary of two studies in which shark cartilage was used on arthritis patients follows:

- Shark cartilage capsules were given to six osteoarthritis patients who had not found relief with conventional anti-inflammatory medications. By the fourth week, the patients reported less pain and inflammation and greater joint mobility (Orcasita 1989).
- Either cartilage extracts or a placebo were given to 147 patients who had osteoarthritis in another long-term, double-blind study. After 5 years, average pain scores had fallen by 85% in the cartilage group, compared with only 5% in those receiving the placebo. The cartilage group also had less joint deterioration and took significantly less time off from work (Rejholec 1987).

The suggested dosage of shark cartilage for arthritis patients is 2000–3000 mg daily. However, most people take a combination supplement that provides 400–500 mg each of both chondroitin and glucosamine sulfate. Typical daily doses are 2–8 capsules daily.

Melatonin

Melatonin is a hormone with potential as a therapy for treatment of diseases with pain and abnormal immune response. The effects and mechanisms of melatonin on inflammation and immuno-regulation have been studied systematically (Maestroni 2001). Melatonin showed significant analgesic effects in animal studies. Melatonin was also shown to enhance the pain-suppressing effects of analgesics (Cuzzocrea et al. 2002).

Further studies showed that melatonin could enhance the functions of T and B lymphocytes and macrophages *in vitro* and in adjuvant (assistive) arthritis treatment. In animal studies, melatonin was shown to inhibit swelling (Bilici et al. 2002).

These factors suggest that melatonin possesses marked anti-inflammatory, immunoregulatory, and analgesic effects that may be related to the system of opiate modulation.

CAUTION Use melatonin cautiously when treating autoimmune diseases such as rheumatoid arthritis. Some scientists speculate that melatonin could worsen the severity of autoimmune diseases.

For nighttime pain relief, 3–10 mg of melatonin should be taken before bedtime. Melatonin should not be used during the day.

Refer to the *Migraine protocol* for more information on melatonin's pain-relieving properties. Also refer to the *Fibromyalgia protocol* if this condition is an underlying cause of your pain.

Vitamins That Fight Pain

Vitamins and antioxidants can help to reduce pain in many people. Just like many things in life, the oxygen we breathe is both good and bad. On the one hand, oxygen is a nutrient gobbled up by every cell in the body, and without it, we would quickly die. On the other hand, oxygen is a highly reactive substance that can do quite a bit of damage. We know what oxygen can do to metal: oxygen causes metal to rust. Uncontrolled, oxygen can do something equally dangerous to our body cells and tissues.

Oxygen occurs in different packages. The oxygen we breathe is composed of two oxygen molecules attached to each other, but other highly toxic single oxygen molecules called singlet oxygen also occur in the body and can cause trouble. These oxidants (including all reactive oxygen species) are created as byproducts of bodily functions, but they may also be inhaled or taken in when we are exposed to drugs, pesticides, certain foods, cigarette smoke, and air pollution. If not carefully controlled by antioxidants, oxidants would travel through the body, "rusting" substances in cells and tissues.

As more and more "rust spots" appear, the body's ability to function, heal itself, and fend off disease begins to falter. Eventually the immune system, circulatory system, and nervous system weaken.

Certain oxidants called free radicals are unstable molecules. Seeking to balance themselves, free radicals take electrons from other molecules. By setting up a chain reaction of electron stealing, free radicals can cause irreparable damage to the body.

There is much to learn about oxidants: we have not yet figured out all of the ways oxidants harm the body. But many researchers believe that oxidation is a major cause of many of the diseases associated with aging, including arthritis, and we know that oxidation can harm already damaged arthritic joints, as well as their surrounding tissue, making swelling and pain increasingly worse.

The body maintains its own antioxidant "police force" to control oxidants. SOD, catalase, and glutathione peroxidase are three of our natural "oxidant policemen." Unfortunately, our built-in antioxidant militia is not always proficient in protecting us, especially as we age or are subjected to various chemical substances. That is when antioxidant supplements, including vitamins, can be helpful.

Plant antioxidants, the best antioxidants, occur naturally in plants. Potent antioxidants such as tocotrienols have to be extracted from palm oil, while others such as lycopene can be obtained from tomato paste or juice. People often consume supplements that are a variety of plant antioxidants including beta-carotene, alpha-carotene, zeaxanthin, and lutein.

Vitamin B₁ (Thiamin)

Vitamin B_1 (thiamin) is a vitamin that is an overlooked source of pain relief. Vitamin B_1 is particularly helpful for patients with neuritis, shooting pains in the legs related to chronic liver disease or alcoholism, and diabetic neuropathy (nerve disease caused by diabetes), as well as nerve and joint pains associated with a B_1 deficiency.

In a study of the efficacy of B_1, the vitamin was given to 133 people who had headaches, joint pain, nerve pain, or neuritis (pain caused by inflammation of the nerves). None of the patients had found relief with conventional pain pills or physical therapy, but when given 1–2 grams of B_1 once or twice daily, patients reported that 78% of headaches improved, 71% of spine or joint pain improved, and more than 62% of patients with neuralgia reported relief (Quirin 1986).

Start with 25 mg of B_1 twice a day. Studies have shown that in order to get the best effect from water-soluble vitamins (for example, vitamins B and C), they should be taken at least twice a day. B_1 can be found in almonds, whole-grain wheat and oats, nuts, and beans.

Vitamin B₃

Vitamin B_3 is nicotionic acid, a derivative is niacinamide. Vitamin B_3 is a potent antiarthritis supplement. In certain people, it may reduce pain and increase mobility and is considered to be a useful agent for pancreatic cancer treatment (Kawa et al. 1997a).

Vitamin D

In tumor-bearing mice given a vitamin D analogue (EB 1089) 3 times weekly for 4–6 weeks, tumor growth was significantly inhibited in the absence of hypercalcemia (Colston et al. 1997).

Vitamin D was also shown to inhibit cell growth in pancreatic cancer lines by up-regulating cyclin-dependent kinase inhibitors (p21 and p27) (Kawa et al. 1997b).

Zugmaier et al. (1996) reported that vitamin D analogues together with retinoids were shown to inhibit the growth of human pancreatic cancer cells.

A study by Kawa et al. (1996) also reported that a new vitamin D3 analogue, 22-oxa-1,25-dihydroxyvitamin D3 (22-oxa-calcitriol), was tested and found to markedly inhibit the proliferation (three of nine cell lines) and cause a G1 phase cell cycle arrest in pancreatic cancer cells.

Green Tea

A review article on green tea stated that "pancreatic cancer studies hint at an inverse association in two of three studies" (Bushman 1998).

Black and green tea extracts and components of these extracts were examined *in vitro* for their effect on tumor cell growth. Results showed inhibition (approximately 90%) of cell growth in pancreatic tumor cells by black and green tea extracts (0.02%). Black and green tea extracts also decreased the expression of the K-ras gene (Lyn-Cook et al. 1999).

An article in the journal *Pancreas* described two experiments in which green tea extract was tested in hamsters with pancreatic cancer. In the first experiment, pancreatic cancer was induced by a drug. Fewer of the green tea extract-treated hamsters had pancreatic cancers (54% versus 33%) and the average number of tumors was less (1 versus 0.5 per hamster). In the second experiment, pancreatic cancers were transplanted onto the back of hamsters. Tumor growth was similar in both groups until 11 weeks after transplantation, when inhibition of tumor growth became apparent in the green tea extract group. At 13 weeks, the average tumor volume in the green tea extract group was significantly smaller than that in the control group. These results demonstrated that green tea extract has an inhibitory effect on the process of pancreatic carcinogenesis and on tumor promotion of transplanted pancreatic cancer (Hiura et al. 1997).

Quercetin

Quercetin, a bioflavonoid found in many vegetables, has been studied for use in many types of cancer, including breast, bladder, and colon cancer. Its use in pancreatic cancer has yet to be examined, but many of the cancer pathogenesis mechanisms are similar (Lamson et al. 2000).

Quercetin was also found to down-regulate the expression of mutant p53 protein in human breast cancer lines to nearly undetectable levels (Avila et al. 1994).

In addition, quercetin has been found to arrest the expression of p21-ras oncogenes in colon cancer cell lines (Ranelletti et al. 2000).

A study reported in the Japanese journal *Cancer Research* found that quercetin was a potent inhibitor of cyclooxygenase-2 (COX-2) transcription in human colon cancer cells (Mutoh et al. 2000).

Selenium

A study in the journal *Carcinogenesis* tested the effects of beta-carotene and selenium on mice with pancreatic tumors induced by azaserine. Beta-carotene and selenium were found to have inhibitory effects on pancreatic cancer growth (Appel et al. 1996).

Also, a diet high in selenium was found to significantly reduce the number of drug-induced pancreatic cancers in female Syrian golden hamsters (Kise et al. 1990).

Mistletoe

In a Phase I/II study, the effect of mistletoe (Eurixor) treatment was evaluated in 16 patients with pancreatic cancer. Mistletoe was administered twice a week by subcutaneous injection. Apart from one anaphylactic reaction, which necessitated suspension of treatment for a few days, no severe side effects were observed. Eight patients (50%) showed a CT-verified status of "no change" (according to the World Health Organization criteria) for at least 8 weeks. Median survival time in all patients was 5.6 months (range = 1.5-26.5 months). All except two patients claimed that mistletoe had a positive effect on their quality of life, with an obvious decline only during the last weeks of life. These results indicate that mistletoe can stabilize quality of life and therefore may help patients to maintain adequate life quality in their few remaining months (Friess et al. 1996).

Another study described a patient with inoperable cancer of the pancreas who developed marked eosinophilia during treatment (on day 22) with injections of *Viscum album* (mistletoe). Furthermore, histology performed on day 28 revealed accumulation of eosinophils in the pancreas. Although the overall clinical

- Green tea extract, five 350-mg capsules with each meal (3 meals a day). Each capsule should be standardized to provide a minimum of 100 mg of epigallocatechin gallate (EGCG). It is the EGCG fraction of green tea that has shown the most active anticancer effects. These are available in decaffeinated form for those who are sensitive to caffeine or who want to take the less stimulating decaffeinated green tea extract capsules in their evening dose. (Green tea is also a potent antioxidant.)

- Silibinin, two 250-mg capsules 3 times a day.

Step Four: Maintaining Optimal Fatty Acid Balance

Rationale:

Several studies show that gamma linolenic acid (GLA) inhibits pancreatic cancer cell growth. Fish oil concentrate high in EPA and DHA has been shown to reverse weight loss (cachexia), reduce levels of growth-promoting prostaglandin E2, and inhibit ras oncogene expression.

How To Implement:

- Consume an encapsulated borage oil supplement that provides a minimum of 1500 mg of gamma-linolenic acid (GLA) each day.

- Consume a fish oil concentrate that provides 3200 mg of EPA and 2400 mg of DHA each day.

Step Five: Inducing Cancer Cell Differentiation and Apoptosis

Rationale:

Cancer cells fail to properly differentiate and undergo normal apoptotic processes (programmed cell death). Vitamin A and vitamin D drug analogs are suggested, but oncologists do not always prescribe them. Accutane (13-cis-retinoic acid) is an example of a vitamin A drug that could benefit many pancreatic cancer patients.

How To Implement:

- If Accutane will not be prescribed, supplement with 100,000–300,000 IU of emulsified vitamin A liquid drops (refer to *Appendix A: Vitamin A Precautions*).

- If a vitamin D analog drug is not available, supplement with 6000 IU of vitamin D3 (monthly blood tests are necessary to guard against hypercalcemia and kidney damage).

Step Six: Pancreatic Enzyme Therapy

Rationale:

A pilot study published in June 1999 indicated that aggressive nutritional therapy with large doses of pancreatic enzymes dramatically prolonged survival of pancreatic cancer patients (Gonzalez et al. 1999). This approach is currently being evaluated in a large-scale study, funded by the National Institutes of Health's National Center for Complementary and Alternative Medicine with collaboration from the National Cancer Institute. A key component of this program is the ingestion of large quantities of pork pancreas enzymes throughout the day.

How To Implement:

- You can enroll as a patient of Dr. Nicholas Gonzalez who practices in New York City. For information, contact Michelle Gabay, R.N., at (212) 305-9468 or visit the Gonzalez Web site at http://www.dr-gonzalez.com/.

- If you cannot enroll as a patient of Dr. Gonalez, consider taking a minimum of five 425-mg pork pancreas enzyme capsules 6 times a day. Take pancreatic enzymes with meals and in-between meals around the clock. Some patients wake up at night to take more enzymes. After the first several months, the dose of pancreatic enzymes is usually reduced significantly. Some patients take the equivalent of over 100 pork pancreas enzyme capsules a day (under the supervision of Dr. Gonzalez).

Step Seven: Keep in Touch with The Life Extension Foundation

Rationale:

Many new therapies are being developed that could dramatically improve the odds of a pancreatic cancer patient achieving long-term survival. These new approaches include agents that inhibit 5-lipoxygenase (5-LOX), an overlooked enzymatic pathway involved in pancreatic cell progression. There are also new agents being developed to suppress the expression of nuclear factor-kappa beta, a cell signaling component that enables cancer cells to develop rapid resistance to conventional therapies. Perillyl alcohol also appears very promising and is expected to be readily available soon.

How To Implement:

Check the website www.lefcancer.org or call (800) 544-4440 to subscribe to *Life Extension Magazine*.

Note: *Pancreatic cancer patients are encouraged to refer to the following protocol chapters in this book:*

1. Cancer Chemotherapy

2. Cancer Treatment: The Critical Factors

3. Cancer Adjuvant Therapies

4. Cancer Surgery

5. Cancer Clinics

Pancreatic cancer patients may choose to maintain a diet suitable for diabetics that restricts simple carbohydrates (such as sugar and grains) and emphasizes complex carbohydrates and proteins. Protein supplements and essential fatty acids (i.e., borage and fish oils) will help by shifting the carbohydrate-protein-fat ratio.

CONVENTIONAL EXPERTISE

Some of the most advanced clinical applications of the experimental therapies to treat pancreatic cancer are being conducted at:

University of Virginia Department of Medicine

Charlottesville, Virginia

Contact: Dvorit Samid, M.D., (804) 243-6747

Rush-Presbyterian-St. Luke's Medical Center

Section of Medical Oncology

Chicago, Illinois

Contact: K.N. Anderson, M.D., (312) 942-5906

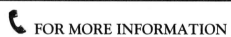 **FOR MORE INFORMATION**

Call the Life Extension Foundation at (800) 544-4440. Please visit our website at www.lef.org

 PRODUCT AVAILABILITY

High potency soy, curcumin, silibinin, green tea extracts, Kyolic garlic, concentrated borage oil (source of GLA), fish oil (source of EPA and DHA), liquid emulsified vitamin A drops, quercetin, selenium, Kyolic garlic caplets, vitamin D3 caps, and pork pancreas enzymes are available by calling (800) 544-4440 or by ordering online at www.lef.org

STAYING INFORMED

The information published in this protocol is only as current as the day the manuscript was sent to the printer. This protocol raises many issues that are subject to change as new data emerge. Furthermore, cancer is still a disease with unacceptably high mortality rates, and none of our suggested regimens can guarantee a cure.

The Life Extension Foundation is constantly uncovering information to provide to cancer patients. A special website has been established for the purpose of updating patients on new findings that directly pertain to the published cancer protocols. Whenever Life Extension discovers information that may benefit cancer patients it will be posted on the website www.lefcancer.org

Before utilizing the cancer protocols in this book, we suggest that you check www.lefcancer.org to see if any substantive changes have been made to the recommendations described in this protocol. Based on the sheer number of newly published findings, there could be significant alterations to the information you have just read.

Alternatively, call 1-800-226-2370 and ask a Health Advisor if your topic of interest has been updated on the website - www.lefcancer.org

DISCLAIMER

This information (and any accompanying printed material) is not intended to replace the attention or advice of a physician or other health care professional. Anyone who wishes to embark on any dietary, drug, exercise, or other lifestyle change intended to prevent or treat a specific disease or condition should first consult with and seek clearance from a qualified health care professional.

The information published in the protocols is only as current as the day the manuscript was sent to the printer. This protocol raises many issues that are subject to change as new data emerge. None of our suggested protocol regimens can guarantee a cure.

Parathyroid (Hyperparathyroidism)

The primary function of the parathyroid glands is to regulate calcium within the blood. The parathyroid glands also control how much calcium is in the bones, and therefore how strong and dense the bones are. Calcium is the primary element which causes muscles to contract. Calcium levels are also very important to the normal conduction of electrical currents along nerves.

Knowing the major functions of calcium helps explain why people can get a tingling sensation in their fingers or cramps in the muscles of their hands when calcium levels drop too low. Additionally, too high a calcium level can cause a person to feel run down, sleep poorly, and cause irritability. Too high a calcium blood level can even cause a decrease in memory. More than half of patients with hyperparathyroidism (high blood calcium) state that they feel fine. However, after treatment, more than 85% of these patients say they feel "much better."

The parathyroid glands are sometimes confused with thyroid glands, but they have no related function. The thyroid gland regulates the body's metabolism and has no effect on calcium levels, while the parathyroid glands regulate calcium levels and have no effect on the metabolism.

An overactive parathyroid gland often mandates surgery, but as you will read in this protocol, some types of parathyroid disorders can be corrected with the proper use of dietary supplements.

NORMAL PARATHYROID ACTIVITY

The four to six parathyroid glands are quite small, and receive a large supply of blood. This assists them in monitoring the calcium level in the blood 24 hours a day. As the blood flow filters through the parathyroid glands, the glands detect the amount of calcium in the blood. Depending on calcium levels, they react by making more or less parathyroid hormone (PTH).

If calcium levels in the blood are too low, the cells of the parathyroids react and make more parathyroid hormone. Once the parathyroid hormone is released into the blood, it circulates to act in a number of places to increase the amount of calcium in the blood (such as removing calcium from bones). When the calcium level in the blood is too high, the parathyroids make less parathyroid hormone, allowing calcium levels to naturally decrease.

PRODUCING CALCIUM IN THE BLOOD

Parathyroid hormone (PTH) has a strong effect on bone cells, causing them to release calcium into the bloodstream. Under the presence of too much parathyroid hormone, however, the bones will continue to release their calcium into the blood at a rate which is too high, resulting in bones that have too little calcium and in serum calcium overload. This results in conditions medically defined as osteopenia and osteoporosis. When bones are subjected to high levels of parathyroid hormones over several years, they become brittle and prone to fractures.

Additionally, parathyroid hormones can act to increase blood levels of calcium by their influence on the intestines. The presence of the parathyroid hormone causes the lining of the intestine to become more efficient at absorbing calcium normally found in our diet.

HYPERPARATHYROIDISM: OVERACTIVITY

Too much PTH secretion is the primary disease of parathyroid glands. This condition is called hyperparathyroidism (excess hormone production). It occurs when one or more of the parathyroid glands function improperly, making excess hormones regardless of the level of calcium.

The most common cause of hyperparathyroidism is the development of a benign tumor in one or more of the parathyroid glands. Enlargement of one parathyroid gland is called a parathyroid adenoma and accounts for about 90% of all primary hyperparathyroid disease. Hyperparathyroidism inflicts damage to the body because it causes an abnormally high level of calcium in the blood, which slowly destroys the tissues by accelerating the calcification process.

Parathyroid adenomas are typically much bigger (about the size of a walnut) than the normal pea-sized parathyroid. Approximately 10% of all patients with primary hyperparathyroidism will have an enlargement of all parathyroid glands, called parathyroid hyperplasia. This condition is much less common than hyperparathyroidism, but the end results are identical on the tissues of the body.

Signs and Symptoms

Patients with persistently elevated calcium levels due to overproduction of parathyroid hormones can have complaints of bone pain. In the severe form, bones can give up so much of their calcium that they become brittle and break (osteoporosis and osteopenia). This problem is even more of a concern in older patients. Bones can also have small hemorrhages within their center that will cause "bone pain."

Other associated symptoms of hyperparathyroidism are the development of gastric ulcers and pancreatitis. High levels of calcium in the blood (hypercalcemia) can be dangerous to a number of organs, including the lining of the stomach and the pancreas, causing both of these organs to become inflamed and painful (ulcers and acute pancreatitis). The heart and vascular system may also be vulnerable to chronic calcium overload. Another common presentation for persistently elevated calcium levels is the development of kidney stones. Because the major function of the kidneys is to filter and clean the blood, they will be constantly exposed to high levels of calcium in patients with hyperparathyroidism.

The constant filtering of large amounts of calcium will cause the collection of calcium within the renal tubules, leading to kidney stones. In extreme cases the entire kidney can become calcified and even take on the characteristics of bone because of the deposition of so much calcium within the tissues. Not only is this painful because of the presence of kidney stones; in severe cases it can cause kidney failure.

The incidence of these problems depends primarily on the duration of the disease and its severity. Everybody will lose bone density, which is progressive. Pancreatitis and ulcers are much more rare. After diagnosis, almost 80% of patients claim to feel better (sleep better, etc.) 3 months after treatment.

Other Causes of Excess Calcium

There are several causes of hypercalcemia which should be considered in the initial diagnosis:

- Hypothyroidism causes increased bone turnover which results in mildly elevated serum calcium in about 20% of cases.

- Immobilization is a rare cause of hypercalcemia in adults.

- Benzothiadiazines (thiazides) cause a transient increase in blood calcium which reverts to normal after about a week. Thiazides can cause hypercalcemia in patients with high rates of bone turnover (i.e., hyperparathyroid patients).

- Vitamin A intoxication is a rare cause of hypercalcemia.

DIAGNOSIS

Hyperparathyroidism is relatively easy to detect because the parathyroid glands will be making an inappropriately large amount of PTH in the presence of elevated serum calcium. Another way to confirm the diagnosis is by measuring the amount of calcium in the urine over a 24-hour period of time. If the kidneys are functioning normally, they will filter much of this calcium in an attempt to rid the body of calcium, leading to an abnormally large amount of calcium in the urine. Measuring calcium in the urine, however, is an indirect measure of parathyroid activity and is only accurate 25–35% of the time.

The most accurate and definitive way to diagnose primary hyperparathyroidism is by testing for elevated PTH in the presence of elevated serum calcium. A standard blood-chemistry test can reveal elevated calcium levels caused by hyperparathyroid disease. If your blood test is high in calcium and parathyroid hormones, it may be an indication of hyperparathyroidism. People who do not have regular blood tests usually find out they have hyperparathyroidism when a bone suddenly breaks, a kidney stone develops, or when their kidneys fail altogether.

There are other diagnostic procedures (MRI, CT scans, sonography) to determine if excess parathyroid hormone is caused by a tumor or by a vitamin D_3 or calcium deficiency.

Several additional lab tests may be ordered to examine some of the conditions associated with hypercalcemia. These would include:

- Thyroid and adrenal function tests that may include measurements of thyroid-stimulating hormone (TSH), and A.M. and P.M. cortisol levels

- Measurements of serum magnesium

- A comprehensive hormone profile, including measurements of estrogen and progesterone

CONVENTIONAL TREATMENT OPTIONS

Surgical Parathyroidectomy

Since the mid-1920s, the standard treatment for primary hyperparathyroidism has been to surgically remove the gland (or glands) overproducing hormones. Remember: this is a hormone problem, so the goal is to remove the source of the excess hormone. The patient is put to sleep under general anesthesia, an incision is made in the neck, and the thyroid gland is mobilized to allow the surgeon to identify the four to six parathyroid glands which reside moderately deep in the neck behind the thyroid. Patients are typically hospitalized overnight and occasionally as long as 1–2 days. The incision must be of sufficient length to allow the surgeon adequate exposure of the numerous important structures in the neck, and thus it is typically 3–4 inches long.

Because of the numerous small nerves and other important structures within the neck, this operation can be technically challenging and is usually performed only by experienced endocrine surgeons or surgeons with extensive head and neck operative experience. During this operation, the surgeon identifies all four parathyroid glands and removes whichever ones are enlarged. Approximately 90% of the time, there is one large gland (an adenoma) and three normal glands. In this situation, the one large gland would be removed, leaving the three normal ones to function in a normal fashion indefinitely.

Interestingly, if the surgeon finds all four glands to be enlarged (hyperplasia), he or she typically takes out three or three and a half of these glands, leaving some parathyroid tissue behind to function normally in the future. Done successfully, this procedure has a cure rate of about 95%.

Although most people with hyperparathyroidism say they feel well when the diagnosis is made, the majority of these will actually say they feel better after the problem has been cured. This can only be known retrospectively when patients are allowed to comment on how they feel several months after the operation. Many patients who thought they were asymptomatic preoperatively will claim to sleep better at night, will be less irritable, and will find that they remember things much more easily than they could when their calcium levels were high. Some physicians elect not to refer their patients for a surgical procedure if they have a mild form of primary hyperparathyroidism.

Conventional Drug Treatments

Bisphosphonates

Healthy bone tissue is constantly being broken down and then restored. This occurs so that old bone can be replaced by new bone. Bisphosphonates are analogues of pyrophosphate which concentrate in areas of increased bone turnover and inhibit bone resorption. As a result, the breakdown of bone tissue occurs more slowly than the laying down of new bone. This action helps to preserve the density and strength of the bone. Bisphosphonates include etidronate (Didronel), pamidronate (Aredia), and alendronate (Fosamax).

Some physicians have begun using bisphosphonates (especially Fosomax) to increase bone calcium rather than referring a patient for surgical hyperparathy-

roidectomy. Fosamax is an effective drug, but must be used appropriately. It is *not* a replacement for removal of an over-active parathyroid gland. The mechanism of action of bisphosonates does not cure the underlying problem of overproduced PTH. Experts in the field believe that after a parathyroid is surgically removed, Fosomax may have a role in trying to build bone density and replace the calcium that the parathyroid hormone removed.

Calcitonin

Calcitonin is a parathyroid hormone that acts to decrease the release of skeletal calcium, phosphorus, and hydroxyproline. Administration of glucocorticoids in combination with synthetic calcitonin (Calcimar, Cibacalcin, Miacalcin) may augment or prolong the action of calcitonin. Calcitonin therapy is of limited efficacy.

Plicamycin

Plicamycin (Mithramycin) is a natural substance isolated from *Streptomyces plicatus* that inhibits DNA synthesis. It's main use is to treat hypercalcemia of malignancy of the testes. The exact mechanism responsible for its effects on calcium is unknown. Because of plicamycin's extreme toxicity, it is considered only in cases of hypercalcemia in association with advanced neoplasms.

Gallium nitrate

Gallium nitrate (Ganite) inhibits bone resorption and alters the structure of bone crystals. It is prescribed for hypercalcemia in relation to certain cancers. Gallium nitrate is highly toxic to the kidneys (nephrotoxic).

Glucocorticoids

Glucocorticoids (cortisol, hydrocortisone) increase urinary calcium excretion and decrease intestinal calcium absorption when given in pharmacologic doses (e.g., 40–200 mg prednisone daily in divided doses). Glucocorticoids are mainly prescribed to inhibit inflammation in a variety of autoimmune disorders and also to treat deficiency of natural steroid hormones.

Phosphorus

Low phosphorus levels are associated with primary hyperparathyroidism. Hypophosphatemia decreases the rate of calcium uptake into bone, increases intestinal calcium absorption, and directly and indirectly stimulates bone breakdown.

Raising the serum inorganic phosphate concentration above the normal level does decrease serum calcium levels, sometimes strikingly. Intravenous phosphate is one of the most dramatically effective treatments available for severe hypercalcemia. However, its toxicity is so dangerous that it is used rarely and only in severely hypercalcemic patients with cardiac or renal failure.

Estrogen-Replacement Therapy

Synthetic estrogens may be indicated in postmenopausal women with hyperparathyroidism. Estrogen-replacement therapy may potentially be an alternative form of therapy to surgery in elderly women with primary hyperparathyroidism. In one study, estrogen-replacement therapy (ERT) appeared as effective as parathyroidectomy (combined with either calcitriol or calcium supplements) for the treatment of osteoporosis in elderly postmenopausal women showing primary hyperparathyroidism symptoms. According to the researchers: "Although hormone replacement therapy has little effect on serum calcium levels, it suppresses bone turnover, reduces urinary calcium excretion, and increases bone mineral density throughout the skeleton in postmenopausal women with mild primary hyperparathyroidism. This therapy is thus an important management option for these patients" (Grey et al. 1996).

Later that same year, the Department of Endocrinology at St. George Hospital (Sydney, Australia) reported ERT appeared to be as effective as parathyroidectomy (combined with either calcitriol or calcium supplements) for the treatment of osteoporosis in elderly postmenopausal women presenting with primary hyperparathyroidism (PHPT) (Diamond et al. 1996).

The concern with using estrogen drugs is that several well-controlled human studies show that they increased the risk of breast cancer and cardiovascular disease. Therefore, the use of estrogen drugs to mitigate the effects of primary hyperparathyroidism should be limited to elderly women who are too debilitated to tolerate surgical removal of the affected parathyroid glands.

An alternative to synthetic estrogen to combat bone loss may lie in soy-derived natural estrogens. The main ingredients in soy, the isoflavones genestein and daidzin, bind loosely with estrogen receptors and may positively affect bone health.

A 6-month study on 66 postmenopausal women was conducted at the University of Illinois at Urbana-Champaign to investigate bone density and bone mineral content in response to soy therapy (Potter et al. 1998). In this study, postmenopausal women received on a daily basis either phytoestrogens derived from soy protein or milk-derived protein (that contained no phytoestrogens). The results showed significant increases in bone density and bone mineral content for the lumbar spine in the women receiving the phytoestrogens derived from soy protein diets compared to the control diet. Increases in other skeletal areas also were noted in the women on the soy diets. Dr. J. W. Erdman, Jr., the lead scientist, concluded that soy isoflavones show real potential for maintaining bone health.

Kenneth D. Setchell, Ph.D., of Children's Hospital and Medical Center (Cincinnati, OH), confirmed the estrogenic activity of the principal soy isoflavones daidzin, genistein, and glycitein. Setchell (1997) conducted research on the chemical structure and metabolism of soy phytoestrogens and concluded that consuming modest amounts of soy protein results in relatively high blood concentrations of phytoestrogens and that this could have a significant hormonal effect in many individuals. Theoretically, there are enough phytoestrogens in the newer soy extracts for many women to derive effective estrogen replacement therapy.

WHEN SURGERY CAN BE AVOIDED

Although primary hyperparathyroidism normally mandates surgery to remove one or more parathyroid glands that have developed benign tumors, secondary hyperparathyroidism can be caused by a dietary calcium or vitamin D deficiency. To rule out secondary hyperparathyroidism, a good first step is to supplement with 1000 IU of vitamin D_3 every day, along with 2000 mg of elemental calcium. This much calcium and vitamin D_3 will act as a signal to your parathyroid glands to stop producing so much parathyroid hormone. When your bloodstream is loaded with calcium, your parathyroid glands will no longer have to pull it from your bones to guarantee proper calcium metabolism. Many people undergo surgery to remove one or more parathyroid glands when, in fact, all they may need to do is take calcium and vitamin D_3. This amount of daily vitamin D_3 supplementation was confirmed to be safe in the *American Journal of Clinical Nutrition* in May 1999 (Vieth 1999).

Numerous studies demonstrate and report that glucocorticoid-induced osteoporosis is associated with the development of secondary hyperparathyroidism. Supplementation of calcium and vitamin D has been shown to be an effective method for prevention and treatment.

Magnesium

A decrease in plasma magnesium stimulates parathyroid secretion, and magnesium may exert a direct inhibitory effect on the gland (Ganong 1995).

Magnesium is a mineral that is commonly paired with calcium due to their opposing effects. While calcium serves to contract muscles, magnesium loosens. Thus, excess calcium causes constipation and muscle cramping, while excess magnesium causes diarrhea. The appropriate daily dose of magnesium can be determined by increasing the amount until loose stools occur, and then reducing to maintain normal consistency of stools.

Hemodialysis Considerations

In treating hemodialysis patients who have uremic hyperparathyroidism, the addition of the drug calcitonin to vitamin D_3 therapy may inhibit bone resorption and increase bone mineral density. Dialysis patients often suffer from uncontrolled serum phosphate levels that preclude successful treatment with vitamin D_3. Blood phosphate levels should be carefully monitored in dialysis patients.

Calcium-alpha-ketoglutarate is known as a highly effective phosphate binder in hemodialysis patients. Also, alpha-ketoglutarate has been shown to improve metabolic alterations. A study investigated the effect of long-term phosphate-binding therapy with calcium-alpha-ketoglutarate to determine whether phosphate accumulation is the main reason for secondary hyperparathyroidism in kidney dialysis patients. Calcium ketoglutarate was prescribed to 14 patients in a mean dosage of 4.5 grams a day (which provided 975 mg of elemental calcium) for a period of 36 months. Serum phosphate levels continuously dropped, whereas serum calcium levels increased to normal levels. Intact parathyroid hormone levels continuously normalized in all patients. The present data show that long-term treatment with calcium-alpha-ketoglutarate normalizes secondary hyperparathyroidism by simultaneously binding phosphate and correcting the calcium/phosphate ratio in serum without vitamin D treatment (Zimmerman et al. 1996).

🌑 SUMMARY

Too much parathyroid hormone is clinically defined as hyperparathyroidism. The excess parathyroid hormone pulls calcium from the bones which overloads the blood system with excessive amounts of calcium. Many long-term degenerative diseases have been linked to this type of calcium imbalance.

A standard blood-chemistry test can reveal elevated calcium levels caused by hyperparathyroid disease. Only a PTH (parathyroid hormone) blood test can effectively diagnose hyperparathyroidism. If your blood test is high in calcium and parathyroid hormone, it may be an indication of hyperparathyroidism.

Surgery is necessary when there is a parathyroid tumor that causes the overproduction of PTH. This is called primary hyperparathyroidism. Surgery is the often the only option in treating this condition.

When overproduction of PTH is caused by a calcium deficiency, this is classified as secondary hyperparathyroidism. The first step in countering secondary parathyroidism is to take 1000 IU of vitamin D_3 every day, along with 2000 mg of elemental calcium. This much calcium and vitamin D_3 will act as a signal to your parathyroid glands to stop producing so much parathyroid hormone.

A serum magnesium deficiency can stimulate the parathyroid glands to secrete more PTH, thus removing too much calcium from the bones. Consuming 500–1500 elemental mg of magnesium a day can help maintain optimal serum magnesium status.

Soy phytoestrogens have been shown to increase bone density and bone mineral content in postmenopausal women. One caplet morning and night of Mega Soy Extract (135 mg) is recommended.

Elderly postmenopausal women with primary hyperparathyroidism who are not candidates for surgery may consider estrogen-replacement therapy combined with either calcitriol or calcium supplements for the treatment of osteoporosis. The use of a bisphosphonate drug would also mitigate against calcium depletion from the bones.

PRODUCT AVAILABILITY

Calcium Citrate w/D_3 capsules, Magnesium Citrate capsules, Bone Assure (encapsulated calcium-magnesium-vitamin D_3 and bone protecting nutrients), and Mega Soy Extract can be ordered by telephoning (800) 544-4440 or by ordering online at www.lef.org.

Group therapy also may be effective in treating phobias. In Lyon, France, 55 patients with social phobias received cognitive and group therapy. The patients were evaluated after six months and twelve months. Researchers found that the patients showed statistically significant improvement (Fanget 1999).

Reducing Cortisol Levels Naturally

KH3 is a European drug that mitigates the effects of the overproduction of cortisol, the adrenal hormone that can occur with anxiety and stress. The overproduction of cortisol has been shown to damage the immune system, arteries, and brain cells, and it may cause premature aging. The recommended dosage of KH3 is 1–2 tablets taken on an empty stomach in the morning and afternoon. KH3 should not be taken by people allergic to procaine (the active ingredient in the medication). It is contraindicated for patients taking sulfa drugs and should not be used by children or pregnant or lactating women.

In addition to KH3, the hormones melatonin and dehydroepiandrosterone (DHEA) may also reduce and protect against the effects of cortisol. In a group of people with major depression, low levels of nocturnal melatonin were associated with hypersecretion of cortisol (Chazot et al. 1985). The recommended dose range of melatonin is from 300 mcg–6 mg taken approximately 30 minutes before bedtime. DHEA is a steroidal hormone that declines with aging and has been shown in studies to increase perceived physical and psychological well-being in both men and women (Morales et al. 1994). In a 1996 study on children with depression, abnormally low DHEA levels were found along with abnormally high cortisol levels. This study also suggests that the adverse effects of low DHEA levels may be found in people of all ages (Goodyer et al. 1996) (*prior to taking DHEA, refer to the DHEA Replacement Therapy protocol*).

NATURAL THERAPIES

Natural therapies may be effective in treating phobias and other anxiety disorders. These alternative techniques may be employed individually or in conjunction with conventional treatments.

Inositol

Inositol is a natural substance derived mainly from cereals and legumes that can influence certain biological activities in the body. Inositol has been found to be effective in the treatment of panic attacks and OCD by helping to reverse desensitization of serotonin receptors. In an eight-week study, patients were given 12 grams of inositol daily for four weeks and then placebo for another four weeks. Researchers found that while taking inositol, panic attacks decreased from ten a week to three a week compared to a decrease from ten a week to six a week in the placebo group. The researchers concluded that because inositol is a natural substance found in the diet, it is safe and potentially therapeutic in the treatment of panic disorder (Benjamin et al. 1995). In OCD patients, inositol has shown therapeutic benefit at doses of 18 grams a day. Improvements were noted at six weeks during a double-blind, placebo-controlled study (Fux et al. 1996). The improvements noted in this study on inositol were comparable to the effectiveness of the SSRIs, fluoxetine (Prozac), and fluvoxamine (Luvox) (Koponen et al. 1997). Longer treatment with inositol may yield better results.

L-Theanine

Theanine, an amino acid derived almost solely from green tea, readily crosses the blood-brain barrier of humans and exerts subtle changes in biochemistry, increasing concentration and focusing thought. *L*-theanine increases GABA, which creates a relaxed feeling and a sense of well-being. In volunteers who were given 50–200 mg of theanine orally, alpha waves of the brain were recorded 40 minutes later. Researchers found that the theanine had a relaxing effect, without causing drowsiness in the subjects (Juneja et al. 1999). A study on spontaneously hypertensive rats showed theanine lowered blood pressure (Yokogoshi et al. 1995).

Adapton

The active ingredient in Adapton is *Garum amoricum* extract, a class of unique polypeptides, that act as precursors to endorphins and other neurotransmitters and exert a regulatory effect on the nervous system, thereby improving the body's ability to adapt to mental and physical stress. Adapton is widely used in Europe and Japan for the treatment of stress, anxiety, and depression. Because it is an extract of a deep sea fish, the garum, Adapton is a naturally occurring substance. It functions at the cellular level to increase energy efficiency, resulting in improved concentration, mood, and sleep and promoting a general sense of well-being.

Adapton contains an omega-3 essential fatty acid that enhances certain prostaglandins and prostacyclin, the chemical mediators that regulate major biological functions. These polypeptides are believed to contribute to the stress-relieving effects of Adapton. For people who suffer from acute panic attacks, the addition of a 10-mg dose of the cardiovascular medication propranolol can produce immediate results. Propranolol is a beta-adrenergic blocker that inhibits the overproduction of adrenaline during a panic attack. The low dose of propranolol required to produce this effect is well-tolerated by the majority of patients.

Lifestyle Stress Reducers

People who perform meditation exercises take an active role in their treatment, teaching themselves how to quiet or clear the mind. Several clinical studies have shown that during meditation the body is altered in ways that are beneficial for people who experience anxiety (Dillbeck 1977; Kabat-Zinn et al. 1992; Miller et al. 1995). For example, the rate of metabolism drops, and the blood pressure decreases. Meditation may be performed daily, several times a week, or just before a situation that might provoke anxiety.

In addition, Canadian researchers report that regular exercise may help many people who suffer from psychiatric disorders, including phobias (Asmundson et al. 1994). Researchers Gregg A. Tkachuk and Garry L. Martin of the Department of Psychology at the University of Manitoba examined studies of anxiety disorder and exercise dating back to 1981. They found that strength training, running, walking, and other forms of aerobic exercise help to alleviate mild to moderate depression and also may help to treat other mental disorders, including anxiety and substance abuse. In their study, which was reported in *Professional Psychology: Research and Practice*, these researchers stated: "There is now considerable evidence that regular exercise is a viable, cost-effective, but underused treatment for mild to moderate depression that compares favorably to individual psychotherapy, group psychotherapy, and cognitive therapy" (Gregg et al. 1999). In one study cited by the researchers, people who ran, walked, or performed strengthening exercises three times a week for 20–60 minutes were significantly less depressed after five weeks. What is more, their gains lasted for up to a year (Greist et al. 1979; Doyne et al. 1987).

The Canadian researchers also reported that exercise is more effective than placebos at reducing symptoms of panic. In one study of 46 people with moderate to severe panic disorder, those who ran three times a week for ten weeks and those who took antianxiety medications felt better than people who took placebo medicines. The investigators noted, however, that treatment with the drug chlomipramine was a faster, more effective treatment than exercise in patients with panic disorder (Broocks et al. 1998).

Studies included in the Canadian review also showed that exercise may help to treat symptoms of schizophrenia, a psychiatric disorder marked by delusions, confusion, and emotional turmoil. However, more studies are needed to confirm these findings, the researchers noted.

In 1999, Fox conducted a review of the literature on costs of mental health and stated in his conclusionary remarks that there is now sufficient evidence for the use of exercise in the treatment of clinical depression. He also stated that aerobic and resistance exercise enhances mood states, and there is also some evidence to support its use for cognitive function. This shows that "moderate regular exercise should be considered a viable means of treating depression, anxiety and improving mental well-being in the general public" (Fox 1999).

In the meantime, the researchers said, exercise may be an important component of treatment for body image problems, substance abuse problems, and somatic disorders in which mental symptoms manifest as physical pain. Exercise, they said, is an effective short-term treatment for reduction of destructive behavior and for increasing work performance in people with developmental disabilities, such as attention deficit disorder, which is marked by an inability to concentrate and hyperactivity.

Exactly how exercise helps to lessen depression and other psychiatric disorders is not fully understood. Improvements may result from a combination of factors, including release of brain chemicals called endorphins. Endorphins produce calming, soothing effects. In addition, exercise may provide a distraction from negative emotions such as sadness and hopelessness, two hallmarks of depression. Exercise may also help to buffer the effects of stress.

⬤ SUMMARY

Natural therapies for phobias and anxiety disorders may be employed individually or in conjunction with conventional treatments.

1. Cortisol is an adrenal hormone that is oversecreted during times of anxiety and stress. Prolonged hypersecretion of cortisol negatively affects the immune system and contributes to atherosclerosis and premature aging. The following supplements may help to reduce cortisol levels:

   - KH3, 1–2 tablets daily on an empty stomach.
   - Melatonin, 300 mcg–3 mg at bedtime
   - DHEA, 15–25 mg daily for women and 50 mg daily for men (*refer to DHEA Replacement Therapy protocol for complete information and contraindications*).

2. Inositol may diminish panic attacks by resensitizing serotonin receptors. Begin with 4 grams daily in divided doses. Increase gradually up to 12 grams daily as needed.

3. *L*-theanine increases GABA to create a relaxed feeling and a sense of well-being, 100–400 mg a day.

4. Adapton may help to reduce anxiety and stress by improving neurotransmitter function. The recommended dosage of Adapton is 4 capsules taken in the morning on an empty stomach for 15 days. Thereafter, the dose is reduced to 2 capsules each morning. If complete relief of the symptoms occurs, Adapton may be discontinued and restarted if the symptoms return. There is no toxicity associated with the daily use of Adapton. Some patients use 2–3 capsules of Adapton every other day and still report relief of their symptoms.

5. Exercise helps to alleviate depression and reduce symptoms of panic and anxiety.

6. Meditation helps to clear the mind of anxious or disturbing thoughts.

Those who are unable to adequately suppress phobias may have to rely on prescription drugs, many of which produce undesirable side effects. The use of a low-dose beta-blocker like propranolol does not pose a side effect risk for most people. As little as 10 mg of propranolol can be effective.

Refer to the *Anxiety and Stress protocol* for additional suggestions.

 FOR MORE INFORMATION

Contact the National Mental Health Association, (800) 969-6642.

 PRODUCT AVAILABILITY

L-theanine, DHEA, melatonin, Adapton, and inositol are available from the Life Extension Foundation by calling (800) 544-4440 or by ordering online at www.lef.org. Ask for a listing of offshore companies that sell KH3 to American citizens by mail for personal use.

Polymyalgia Rheumatica

Polymyalgia rheumatica (PMR) is a systemic rheumatic inflammatory disorder characterized by severe aching and stiffness in the neck, shoulder girdle, and pelvic girdle. A person with PMR may also have a headache. The pain is usually more severe when the person gets up in the morning. Although PMR is classified as a rheumatic disease, its exact cause remains unknown.

UNDERLYING FACTORS

Polymyalgia means "many muscle pains." *Rheumatica* (related to rheumatism) means "changing" or "in flux." The etiology of PMR is as yet unknown, but it is associated with temporal arteritis, inflammatory conditions (rheumatoid arthritis, systemic lupus erythematosus), occasionally cancer, and other degenerative diseases.

The disease rarely occurs in persons under the age of 50, and it affects twice as many women as men. PMR is at least 10 times more prevalent in persons over 80 than in persons of age 50–59 and predominantly affects the Caucasian population (Beers et al. 1997; Labbe et al. 1998).

PMR may be classified as an autoimmune disease, meaning the body's own immune system attacks healthy tissues analogous to the way it normally would attack viruses, bacteria, and foreign proteins. Simply stated, in PMR an autoimmune aspect would indicate that the body is attacking itself.

Another theory is that autoimmune diseases can start when a virus with a protein coat invades certain cells. Cells in the body already contain receptors on their surfaces that resemble the proteins in the viral protein coat. Therefore, antibodies designed to attack the virus also attack receptors on the cells and kill them. Even when the virus infection is no longer present, the circulating antibodies continue destroying normal cells with the receptor on their surface.

Although stress likely does not cause autoimmune reactions, it may be a factor. Stress can cause the hypothalamus and pituitary to release hormones that promote inflammation. Stress hormones are useful in a traumatic situation, but they are very damaging in autoimmunity. Anxiety can also worsen autoimmune conditions and has been linked to release of a hormone-like substance called the corticotropin-releasing factor (present in excess in tissues affected by rheumatoid arthritis (Bunch 1999). In this regard, PMR may be viewed as a classic psychoneuroimmunological syndrome (*for more information, refer to the protocols on Autoimmune Diseases and Inflammation: Chronic*).

ARTERIAL INFLAMMATION

Polymyalgia rheumatica (PMR) is closely linked with giant cell arteritis, which is also called temporal arteritis. Giant cell arteritis primarily affects the medium-sized muscular arteries, such as those that pass over the temples in the scalp. The temporal arteries become inflamed, subjecting them to damage. In giant cell arteritis, the most common symptom is a severe headache on one or both sides of the head. The ophthalmic arteries are affected in nearly half of all patients, sometimes resulting in partial loss of vision or even sudden blindness. Because of the risk of blindness, early diagnosis of giant cell arteritis is essential.

A diagnostic temporal artery biopsy is recommended in all patients suspected of having giant cell arteritis. In a temporal artery biopsy, a small tissue sample is taken from a temporal artery and tested for abnormality. Blood testing for the presence of an elevated erythrocyte sedimentation rate is also part of the diagnostic process. Patients can have PMR, giant cell arteritis or both, representing a spectrum of the severity and manifestation of these two similar processes (Beers et al. 1997; Egland 2001; Matsen 2002).

SYMPTOMS OF POLYMYALGIA RHEUMATICA AND GIANT CELL ARTERITIS

The major symptom associated with PMR is pain or aching, usually in the large muscle groups, especially those around the shoulders and hips. Other symptoms include stiffness in the morning upon rising or after resting, weakness and fatigue, a general feeling of illness, occasional low-grade fevers, and weight loss. Unfortunately, there are many other diseases that are easily confused with PMR (e.g. rheumatoid arthritis, infections, fibromyalgia, inflammation of blood vessels or vasculitis, cancer). Because of the difficulty of arriving at a diagnosis, a number of tests are usually needed as described below to rule out other conditions.

In giant cell arteritis, inflammation causes arteries to thicken, reducing blood flow. The symptoms of giant cell arteritis are atypical, mild-to-severe headaches, scalp tenderness, fatigue, a general feeling of illness, jaw or facial soreness, weight loss, night sweats, and vision changes or distortions. Classically, the arteries are lumpy and tender.

DIAGNOSIS

Because there are so many illnesses that mimic PMR, the possibility of other illnesses such as hypothyroidism, malignancy, infection, and inflammatory arthritis must be ruled out. Although there is no specific single diagnostic test for PMR or giant cell arteritis, there are tests used by health professionals as part of obtaining a diagnosis.

To establish a diagnosis for PMR, the following tests are considered:

- A physical exam and interview regarding the patient's symptoms and medical history.
- An ESR (erythrocyte sedimentation rate) blood test. (Inflammation in the body usually results in an elevated ESR. A high ESR, >40 mm/hour, is known to be common in PMR patients. The ESR has been shown to be a good predictor of relapse of PMR and can be repeated to monitor the patient's progress during treatment.)
- A complete blood count (CBC) testing. (Patients with PMR may also have mild anemia.)
- A high-sensitivity C-reactive protein (CRP) test. (Inflammation in the body often causes an elevated CRP. CRP is a more sensitive indicator of current activity.)
- A rheumatoid factor (RA) test. (The RA test checks for rheumatoid arthritis, an autoimmune disease causing inflammation.)
- An antinuclear antibody (ANA) test. (This test checks for lupus and is considered the prototypical test for autoimmune disease causing inflammation.)
- A thyroid-stimulating hormone (TSH) test. (This test checks for hypothyroidism.)

To illustrate the difficulty in diagnosing PMR, in a study of 117 patients, approximately one-fifth of all PMR patients had a normal ESR (more common in males). Therefore, absence of the characteristically abnormal laboratory finding of elevated ESR may result in a delay of proper diagnosis and treatment (Helfgott et al. 1996). Some physicians confirm the diagnosis of PMR by using a trial of low-dose corticosteroid medication, the standard treatment for PMR (Cecil et al. 1992). Persons with PMR are likely to experience significant relief of their symptoms within 2–4 days after starting corticosteroid treatment. Although symptom relief in response to corticosteroid treatment reinforces a diagnosis, using corticosteroids to confirm a diagnosis of PMR is not without concern. Most patients require corticosteroid therapy for 2–3 years and experience one or more treatment complications (Meskimen et al. 2000).

To establish a diagnosis for giant cell arteritis, the following tests are considered:

- A physical exam and interview about the patient's symptoms and medical history
- An erythrocyte sedimentation rate (ESR) test and high-sensitivity C-reactive protein (CRP)
- A temporal artery biopsy. (It is often necessary to obtain a temporal artery biopsy to confirm the diagnosis of giant cell arteritis.) Although a biopsy is the most definitive test available, it may not be necessary if the patient's physical symptoms and ESR rate and CRP levels are strongly suggestive of giant cell arteritis.

WARNING If there are visual disturbances indicative of temporal arteritis (TA), the patient must have immediate diagnosis and often treatment with corticosteroids to help reduce the risk of blindness (Matsen 2002).

The Role of Inflammation

Inflammation, marked by swelling and pain, is a defense mechanism that the body uses to protect itself against injury to tissue or cells. One cause of pain in inflammation is the stimulation of nerve endings by inflammatory chemicals. Inflammatory cytokines are one of the destructive cell-signaling chemicals known to increase with advancing age leading to degenerative and autoimmune diseases (Van der Meide et al. 1996; Licinio et al. 1999).

An article in the *Cleveland Clinic Journal of Medicine* discussed the involvement of inflammatory actions occurring in the arterial wall and circulation of PMR and giant cell arteritis patients (Goronzy et al. 2002). The proinflammatory cytokine interleukin-6 (IL-6) was shown to be a marker in measuring the severity of the disease and monitoring its progress. Also noted was the role of IFN-gamma as a key regulator in determining the direction and nature of the inflammatory response. The scientists concluded that targeting IFN-gamma may eventually emerge as the prime target for novel therapeutic approaches (Goronzy et al. 2002).

In rheumatoid arthritis, excess levels of cytokines, such as IL-6, interleukin-1b (IL-1[b]), leukotriene-B(4) (LTB[4]), and tumor necrosis factor-alpha (TNF-alpha), are known to cause or contribute to the inflammatory syndrome (Deon et al. 2001). In PMR, there is an increase in IL-6 serum levels. Another inflammatory marker, C-reactive protein (at levels over 1.3 mg/L), may be present in PMR, also indicating that an inflammatory event is occurring.

Sleep Deprivation

On June 22, 2002, at the annual meeting of the Endocrine Society (San Francisco), researchers reported that sleep deprivation markedly increases inflammatory cytokines. This finding helps explain why pain flare-ups occur in a variety of disorders in response to lack of sleep. According to the researchers, even a modest lack of sleep adversely affected cytokine and hormone levels. In this carefully controlled study, two potent proinflammatory markers were affected. Sleep deprivation caused a 40–60% average increase in the inflammatory marker IL-6 in men and women, although a 20–30% increase in TNF-alpha was shown in men alone (Vgontzas et al. 1999; 2001).

PRESCRIPTION DRUG THERAPY

Synthetic Corticosteroids

Natural corticosteroids are substances produced by the adrenal glands (located adjacent to the kidneys) with potent anti-inflammatory properties for conditions such as arthritis, colitis, asthma, bronchitis, certain skin rashes, and allergic or inflammatory conditions of the nose and eyes. Synthetic corticosteroid drugs are often used to treat PMR (and more importantly, giant cell arteritis). They help reduce inflammation, aching, and stiffness.

Synthetic corticosteroids act quickly, sometimes within hours. There are many forms of synthetic corticosteroids, but prednisone is the form most often used (Li et al. 2000; Matsen 2002). Low doses of prednisone (10–20 mg daily) are used for PMR and high doses (initially 40–60 mg daily) are used for giant cell arteritis (Goodwin 1992; Hunder 1997). (Prednisone or the equivalent doses of other glucocorticosteroids may be increased for giant cell arteritis up to 100 mg daily.)

Treatment (and dosing) with synthetic adrenal corticosteroids must be carefully monitored because many PMR patients will be treated for a minimum of 2 years (Myklebust et al. 2001). Glucocorticoids consist of synthetic corticosteroids and include hydrocortisone and dexamethasone. Because corticosteroids and glucocortocoids have toxic metabolic side effects, efforts have been made to find alternative treatments to reduce exposure to these drugs (Meskimen et al. 2000).

If patients respond to corticosteroid treatment, the initial dose should be continued until the ESR normalizes (usually in approximately 4 weeks). Then a slow steroid taper is initiated. The approach varies but generally involves decreasing the dosage by 1–2.5 mg each day every 4 weeks (Evans et al. 1998). If symptoms should recur (not uncommon), they are treated by returning to the initial dose.

In patients who fail to respond or who have unacceptable side effects from corticosteroids, azathioprine (immunosuppressant), methotrexate (antineoplastic, antirheumatic), and dapsone (sulfone, antibacterial) have been used, although evidence of efficacy is sparse (Beers et al. 1997). Additionally, studies to assess the concurrent use of methotrexate and corticosteroids as a steroid-sparing strategy have produced mixed results (Ferraccioli et al. 1996; van der Veen et al. 1996; Labbe et al. 1998).

However, concomitant therapy with corticosteroids and dapsone, azathioprine, cyclosporine, antimalarial drugs, methotrexate, cyclophosphamide, or gold salts was not found to reduce corticosteroid toxicity and still maintain therapeutic effectiveness (Ferraccioli et al. 1996; Hefgott et al. 1996; Beers et al. 1997; Evans et al. 1998). Although immunosuppressive drugs do suppress inflammation and may allow corticosteroid doses to be reduced, they have major side effects. Patients must be fully informed of the benefits versus the risks. Drugs in this category should be administered only under supervision of a specialist (Beers et al. 1997).

A study looked at glucocorticoid treatment in recently diagnosed PMR patients who had not been previously treated with glucocorticoids. The researchers evaluated the relationship between adrenal hormone levels, IL-6, and other acute phase reactants in 41 PMR patients and healthy sex and age-matched controls. After 12 months of glucocorticoid treatment, inflammatory mediators such as IL-6 were reduced and remained stable after glucocorticoids were tapered. This study suggests the beneficial mechanisms by which glucocorticoid drugs effectively treat these syndromes (Cutolo et al. 2002).

Adverse Effects of Corticosteroid Therapy

PMR is characterized by highly variable relapses that require increasing the dose of corticosteroids over time, which is associated with a higher rate of adverse reactions. These adverse reactions often preclude successful long-term treatment.

In one study, the course of the disease was evaluated in 78 PMR patients who were observed for a mean of 28 months. Giant cell arteritis was histologically confirmed in 20 out of 71 patients (28%). Of the 70 patients who were observed for more than 6 months, 18 (26%) experienced a relapse, which required escalation of corticosteroid dosages. After 24 months, 36% of the patients had been in remission without treatment for an average period of 9.3 months. Therapy-associated complications arose in 21 of 64 patients (34%) who were observed for more than 9 months. Most common was steroid-induced diabetes mellitus or aggravation of an already known diabetic metabolic condition (33%) (Ehlert et al. 1997).

The most severe adverse reaction was osteoporotic vertebral fracture that was reported in three patients. Additional complications of corticosteroid therapy were various frequencies of arterial hypertension; cataract; glaucoma; subjectively disturbing weight gain; and hypokalemia. Overall, the researchers' data confirmed that the usually favorable course of PMR is modified by relapses and by complications of corticosteroid therapy (Ehlert et al. 1997). Therefore, the researchers tended to reduce steroids or to use immunosuppressants at an early stage of PMR, especially in high-risk cases such as patients with inadequately controlled diabetes mellitus or manifest osteoporosis.

If using oral steroids, adequate intake of minerals to maintain bone density, such as magnesium and calcium, and vitamins D and K are necessary to protect against bone depletion. Persons with PMR on steroid therapy should also consider bisphosphonate drug therapy (refer to the Osteoporosis protocol for complete information about preventing bone loss and fractures).

NSAIDs

Attempts have been made to treat PMR with high doses of nonsteroidal anti-inflammatory drugs (NSAIDs). Adequate control of symptoms is occasionally achieved with these agents. However, most patients do not respond satisfactorily to NSAIDs (Goodwin 1992; Salvarani et al. 1996; Beers et al. 1997; Hunder 1997; Labbe et al. 1998). Yet, some doctors still consider them as a treatment option. Besides relieving pain, NSAIDs also reduce inflammation. In conditions such as early or mild PMR, NSAIDs are usually taken daily, often for a long time. Unfortunately, long-term use can cause stomach irritation and other significant side effects.

NSAIDs are thought to be effective because they reduce prostaglandins (hormone-like fatty acids). Unfortunately, because prostaglandins are also present in the stomach, using high doses of NSAIDs can cause stomach irritation.

NSAIDs function to suppress the cyclooxygenase (COX) enzymes. There are two forms of the COX enzyme: COX-1, a good enzyme that protects the stomach lining and intestine, and COX-2, a bad enzyme involved in inflammation. However, NSAIDs do not discriminate in their attack on these enzymes. Therefore, resultant stomach problems can include nausea or vomiting. Long-term use of NSAIDS can lead to gastric erosion and ulcers (Garcia Rodriguez et al. 1992; Langman et al. 1994; Henry et al. 1996).

Taking NSAIDs with food or immediately after a meal may help keep stomach problems at a minimum. Even if taking these precautions, some persons will need to take other steps to control their adverse reaction to NSAIDs. In Germany, doctors prescribe a special soy extract called polyenylphosphatidylcholine (PPC) to protect against NSAID-induced gastric toxicity. This product is available as a dietary supplement in the United States. The recommendation for high-dose NSAID users is 1800 mg a day of PPC. If you are taking NSAIDS, consult your physician immediately with any adverse symptoms.

Some of the more popular over-the-counter NSAIDs include aspirin, ibuprofen (Advil, Motrin), and naproxen (Aleve). Examples of the many NSAIDs that require prescriptions are indomethacin (Indocin), celecoxib (Celebrex), diclofenac (Voltaren), etodolac (Lodine), and rofecoxib (Vioxx). Please note that while some of these NSAIDS claim to only suppress the COX-2 enzyme, they also have been shown and must be assumed to inhibit beneficial COX-1.

Pentoxifylline

Pentoxifylline (PTX) (generic name for Trental) is a low-cost prescription medication approved by the FDA to treat peripheral vascular disease. Numerous studies show that pentoxifylline (PTX) is also a potent inhibitor of TNF-alpha, IL-1(b), IL-6, and other proinflammatory cytokines (Neuner et al. 1994; Noel et al. 2000; Pollice et al. 2001; Ventura et al. 2001). The standard dose is 1200 mg daily to improve circulation. To suppress proinflammatory cytokines, a lower dose of 400 mg twice a day can be used.

In numerous studies, PTX has shown to be an effective inhibitor of proinflammatory cytokines in inflammatory conditions as diverse as psoriasis, lupus, pancreatitis, fibrosis due to radiation therapy, leprosy, asthma, and kidney failure. PTX may be obtained from any pharmacy with a physician's prescription (see the Inflammation: Chronic protocol for more information on studies involving PTX).

CAUTION   Persons who have a risk of bleeding (such as a recent stroke), Parkinson's disease, infections, or people with asthmatic, liver, or kidney conditions are advised to be

extract lycopene was the most effective nutrient shown to protect against the development of prostate cancer. This study, started in 1982, followed 578 men for 13 years. Lycopene strongly reduced prostate cancer risk and more importantly, lowered the risk for aggressive cancer. This study confirmed many previous studies showing that lycopene can help prevent pancreatic, prostate, and a host of other cancers. A surprising finding revealed at the April 12, 1999, meeting of the American Association of Cancer Research showed that 30 mg of lycopene supplements a day slowed the growth of existing prostate cancer and lowered serum PSA readings by 20%!

Men with high intake of vitamin E were 35% as likely to develop colorectal adenomas as men with low vitamin E intake (Tseng et al. 1996). (Adenomas are neoplastic lesions that are considered precursors to colon cancer.) In a related study in the February 1999 issue of *Diseases of the Colon and Rectum* (Whelan et al. 1999), the use of multivitamins, vitamin E, and calcium supplements was found to be associated with a lower incidence of recurrent adenomas in 448 patients with previous neoplasia who underwent follow-up colonoscopy. This study found a protective effect against the recurrence of precancerous adenomas when any vitamin supplement was used. On this same subject, a report in the *American Journal of Epidemiology* (Tseng et al. 1996) showed that women with high folate intake were 40% less likely to develop adenomas of the colon than women with low folate intake.

But what if you already have cancer? Again, the research shows a prolongation of lifespan with proper supplementation.

In a study in *Cancer Letters* (Evangelou et al. 1997), animals with malignant tumors given high doses of vitamins C and E and selenium manifested a significant prolongation of the mean survival time. Complete remission of tumors developed in 16.8% of the animals. Low-dose administration of these vitamins failed to exert any beneficial effect on mean survival time of the animals. Results indicated that high doses (mega doses) of vitamins C and E in combination with other carefully selected antioxidants are probably needed in order to achieve sufficient prevention and treatment of malignant diseases. This study indicated that low-potency supplements are of little value.

Vitamin E succinate was shown to inhibit growth and induced apoptotic cell death of estrogen receptor-negative human breast cancer cells in a study in *Cancer Research* (Turley et al. 1997). These findings suggest that vitamin E succinate may be of clinical use in the treatment and possible prevention of human breast cancers.

The research clearly shows the risk of contracting cancer is reduced in those who supplement with adequate amounts of nutrients, such as selenium, folate, carotenoids, vitamins, and other plant extracts.

Reducing Mortality

One of the most compelling reports that high-potency supplements extend lifespan in humans was by Losonczy et al. in the August 1996 issue of the *American Journal of Clinical Nutrition*. This study involved 11,178 elderly people, who participated in a trial to establish the effects of vitamin supplements on mortality. The study showed that the use of vitamin E reduced the risk of death from all causes by 34%. Effects were strongest for coronary artery disease, where vitamin E resulted in a 63% reduction in death from heart attack. In addition, the use of vitamin E resulted in a 59% reduction in cancer mortality. When the effects of vitamins C and E were combined, overall mortality was reduced by 42% (compared to 34% for vitamin E alone) (Losonczy et al. 1996). These results provided significant evidence about the value of vitamin supplementation, yet the media failed to report on it. What made this study so credible was that:

- It compared people who took low-potency "one-a-day" multiple vitamins to those who took higher-potency vitamins C and E supplements. Previous studies measuring the life expectancy of the "one-a-day" crowd did not show significant benefits, thereby causing most doctors to conclude there is no value in vitamin supplementation. In this new report, those taking "one-a-day" multivitamins did not do any better than people taking nothing at all, which supports the Life Extension Foundation's position that higher doses of antioxidants are required to reduce the risk of heart disease and cancer than those found in conventional supplements.

- It lasted 9 years! Most studies that attempt to evaluate the benefits of vitamin supplementation are for shorter time periods. It should be noted, however, that the famous *Harvard Nurses' Health Study* found that vitamin E reduced coronary artery disease mortality by more than 40% after only 2 years!

- It included 11,178 people, a larger group than most previous studies.

Controlling Aging

The National Academy of Sciences published three reports showing that the effects of aging may be partially reversible with a combination of acetyl-*L*-carnitine and lipoic acid (Hagen et al. 2002). One of these studies showed that supplementation with these two nutrients resulted in a partial reversal of the decline of mitochondrial membrane function while consumption of oxygen significantly increased. This study demonstrated that the combination of acetyl-*L*-carnitine and lipoic acid improved ambulatory activity, with a significantly greater degree of improvement in the old rats compared to the young ones. Human aging is characterized by lethargy, infirmity, and weakness. There is now evidence that supplementation with two over-the-counter supplements can produce a measurable antiaging effect.

The second study published by the National Academy of Sciences showed that supplementation with acetyl-*L*-carnitine and lipoic acid resulted in improved memory in old rats. Electron microscopic studies in the hippocampus region of the brain showed that acetyl-*L*-carnitine and lipoic acid reversed age-associated mitochondrial structural decay. In the third National Academy of Sciences study, scientists tested acetyl-*L*-carnitine and lipoic acid to see if an enzyme used by the mitochondria as biologic fuel could be restored in old rats. After 7 weeks of supplementation with acetyl-*L*-carnitine and lipoic acid, levels of this enzyme (carnitine acetyl-transferase) were significantly restored in the aged rats. Supplementation also inhibited free radical-induced lipid peroxidation, which enhanced the activity of the energy-producing enzyme in the mitochondria. The scientists concluded that feeding old rats acetyl-*L*-carnitine and lipoic acid can ameliorate oxidative damage, along with mitochondrial dysfunction.

Hormone Replacement

Proper hormone replacement can produce an immediate improvement in the quality of life and also prevent many diseases. DHEA is one of several important hormones whose production in the body diminishes rapidly as people age past year 35. There now exists a wide body of evidence that supplementation with DHEA can prevent many degenerative diseases, while improving feelings of well-being and alleviating depression.

In the October 1996 issue of the journal *Drugs and Aging*, an overview of published studies by Watson et al. (1996) on DHEA revealed the following:

- In both humans and animals, the decline of DHEA production with aging is associated with immune depression, increased mortality, increased risk of several different cancers, loss of sleep, and decreased feelings of well-being.

- DHEA replacement in aged mice significantly normalized immune function to youthful levels.

- DHEA replacement has shown a favorable effect on osteoclasts and lymphoid cells, an effect that may delay osteoporosis.

- Low levels of DHEA inhibit energy metabolism, thus increasing the risk of heart disease and diabetes mellitus.

- Studies conducted on humans show essentially no toxicity at doses that restore DHEA to youthful levels.

- DHEA deficiency may expedite the development of some diseases that are common in the elderly.

Since this overview was published in 1996, hundreds of additional studies have substantiated DHEA's role as an antiaging hormone-replacement supplement. In a study published in *Biological Psychiatry* (Wolkowitz et al. 1997), DHEA was tested on middle-aged and elderly patients with major depression. DHEA was administered for 4 weeks in doses ranging from 30–90 mg a day. This level of dosing elevated DHEA serum levels to those observed in younger people. Depression ratings, as well as aspects of memory performance, significantly improved. This data suggested that DHEA may have antidepressant and promemory effects and corresponded with previous human studies in which DHEA supplementation (50 mg a day) significantly elevated mood in elderly people.

For specific information on antiaging hormone replacement, *refer to the Male Hormone Modulation Therapy, Female Hormone Replacement Therapy, and DHEA Replacement Therapy protocols*.

THE LIFE EXTENSION FOUNDATION'S PREVENTION PROTOCOL

If you are healthy now and want to stay that way, the Life Extension Foundation has designed protocols that incorporate the best-documented disease-preventing nutrients and hormones.

The Foundation's Prevention protocols consist of the 12 most important supplements for the average person to take every day to reduce risk of contracting the degenerative diseases of aging.

Note: *The Prevention protocol is for healthy people. Those seeking to treat an existing disease may refer to the many specific disease prevention protocols contained in this book.*

The following recommendations are listed in order of importance:

Recommendation 1:

Life Extension Mix (Multivitamin-Mineral-Herbal-Amino Acid Formula)

Suggested dosage: 3 tablets with breakfast; 3 tablets with lunch; 3 tablets with dinner. (Also available in capsule and powder form.)

Life Extension Mix™ contains 90 unique vegetable, fruit, and herbal extracts along with high-potency amino acids, vitamins, minerals, and special antioxidants. The Life Extension Mix formula is fortified with botanical extracts that protect against aberrant cell proliferation via physiological processes separate from traditional antioxidants. Consumption of these types of plants is being recommended based on research emanating from the most prestigious medical centers in the world.

D-glucarate is a botanical extract found in grapefruit, apples, oranges, broccoli, and brussels sprouts. D-glucarate effectively supports a necessary detoxification process that helps to remove DNA toxins from the body. For its potential risk reduction benefit, 200 mg of D-glucarate are included in the daily dose of Life Extension Mix.

Ellagic acid is a detoxifying agent found in raspberries, strawberries, and other fruit. Ellagic acid has demonstrated DNA-protecting properties, including the ability to bind to toxins and neutralize them. Studies have also shown that ellagic acid may protect against chromosome damage, promote wound healing, and reduce the effects of chemically induced hepatic structural degeneration. Studies show that people who consume fruits that are high in ellagic acid have lower rates of common disorders. Raspberry extract (130 mg) is included in Life Extension Mix to provide 38.5% ellagic acid.

Apigenin and luteolin are flavonoids found in such foods as parsley, artichoke, basil, celery, and other foods. Both substances have shown the ability to inhibit DNA oxidative damage. In a study on antioxidant potency, apigenin proved more effective than vitamin C in reducing DNA oxidative damage. When measured against 27 citrus flavonoids, luteolin exhibited the most anti-proliferative activities against aberrant cell colonies. The labiatae extract (300 mg) in Life Extension Mix provides 10 to 18 mg of apigenin and 1.5 to 4 mg of luteolin.

Life Extension Mix has also been fortified with high doses of antioxidants for optimal protection against free radicals; broccoli extract (sulforaphane) and citrus bioflavonoids to protect against disorders related to aberrant cell propagation; biotin to help regulate glucose levels and improve the appearance of hair and nails; and bioavailable chromium, a mineral that is required to maintain optimal blood sugar levels.

Life Extension Mix supplies all of the most powerful antioxidants, including vitamin C, E, and lycopene, which are known to help protect against cellular DNA damage and help prevent the oxidation of LDL cholesterol that contributes to the buildup of fatty deposits in the endothelial lining.

In a study published in the *Lancet,* researchers at Cambridge University in England looked at serum vitamin C and how long people lived. Of the 19,000 people studied, those who had the lowest levels of vitamin C were twice as likely to die compared to those with the highest serum vitamin C levels (Khaw et al. 2001).

One of the most compelling reports that high-potency supplements extend life span in humans was published in the August 1996 issue of the *American Journal of Clinical Nutrition.* This study involved 11,178 elderly people who participated in a trial to establish the effects of vitamin supplements on mortality. This study showed that the use of vitamin E reduced the risk of death from all causes by 34%. Effects were strongest for coronary artery disease, where vitamin E resulted in a 63% reduction in death from heart attack. In addition, the use of vitamin E resulted in a 59% reduction in cancer mortality. When the effects of vitamin C and E were compared, overall mortality was reduced by 42% (compared to 34% for vitamin E alone) (Losonczy et al. 1996).

Life Extension Mix saves time and money by combining the most popular nutrient supplements into one product, eliminating the need to buy and keep track of separate bottles of B-complex, vitamins C and E, mineral supplements, and much more that would be required to achieve the same effects. Life Extension Mix is the cornerstone of a comprehensive supplement program because it provides so many well-studied nutrients. If you are on a budget, the Life Extension Mix provides the best "cost-per-milligram" value.

The Life Extension Foundation mandates that the ingredients in the Life Extension Mix come only from pharmaceutical-grade suppliers such as Roche and Nutrition 21. These premium companies charge more for their vitamins and trace elements, but the purity of these substances greatly exceeds that of the lower cost generic versions that are so prevalent in the vitamin industry.

Life Extension Mix (9 tablets) provides:

Vegetable-Fruit Complex

Broccoli concentrate	500 mg
(1.5 mg sulforaphane, 25 mg d-glucarate)	
Raspberry extract (38.5% ellagic acid)	130 mg
Alpha carotene	89 mcg
Beta-carotene (natural *D. Salina*)	5000 IU
Bromelain	15 mg
Calcium D-glucarate	200 mg
Labiatae extract (10–18 mg apigenin & apigenin	300 mg
glucoside/1.5–4.0 mg luteolin)	
Lutein Complex (marigold)	300 mg
(15.4 mg lutein/75 mcg zeaxanthin)	
Milk thistle extract (85% silymarin)	100 mg
Lycopene (tomato extract)	3 mg
Citrus Bioflavonoids (470 mg hesperidin/140 mg	1300 mg
naringin & 10 mg naringenin 7-B-Rutioside)	
Acerola juice powder	300 mg
Bilberry (25% anthocyanidin)	30 mg
Grapeseed extract (Leucoselect®)	25 mg
(95% proanthocyanidin)	
Grape extract (Biovin®) (84–93% proanthocyanidin	25 mg
index/46% polyphenol/500 ppm resveratrol)	
Ginger extract (5% gingerols)	200 mg

Water-Soluble Vitamins and Enzymatic Activators

Vitamin C as: ascorbic acid (Roche), calcium,	2605 mg
magnesium & niacinamide, ascorbate, acerola	
juice powder	
Folic acid	800 mcg
Biotin	3000 mcg
Trimethylglycine (TMG)	100 mg
Vitamin B_1 (thiamine HCL)(Roche)	125 mg
Vitamin B_2 (riboflavin) (Roche)	50 mg
Supplying: Riboflavin 5-phosphate	2 mg
Vitamin B_3 (niacinamide) (Roche)	100 mg
Vitamin B_3 (niacin) (Roche)	75 mg
Vitamin B_5 (calcium pantothenate)(Roche)	600 mg
Pantothene	5 mg
Vitamin B_6 (pyridoxine HCL) (Roche)	100 mg
Pyridoxal 5-phosphate	2.5 mg
Vitamin B_{12} (cyanocobalamin)	250 mcg
Vitamin B_{12} (hydroxyl cobalamin)	250 mcg
Vitamin B_{12} (ion exchange resin)	100 mcg
PABA (para-aminobenzoic acid)	200 mg

Fat-Soluble Vitamins

Vitamin A (acetate)	5000 IU
Vitamin D_3 (cholecalciferol)	400 IU
Ascorbyl Palmitate (fat-soluble vitamin C)	250 mg
Vitamin E (natural d-alpha tocopherol succinate)	400 IU

Amino Acid Complex

N-acetyl-cysteine	600 mg
Taurine	500 mg
L-Lysine	500 mg

Mineral Complex

Selenium (from Se-Methylselenocysteine)	100 mcg
Selenium (from selenomethionine—Nutrition 21)	50 mcg
Selenium (from sodium selenate)	50 mcg
Zinc (methionate) (OptiZinc)	20 mg
Zinc succinate	15 mg
Boron (as boron citrate/asparatate/glycinate)	3 mg
Calcium	227 mg
Copper (amino acid chelate)	1 mg
Chromium polynicotinate	200 mcg
Potassium aspartate (11.4 mg elemental)	50 mg
Potassium chloride (26 mg elemental)	49 mg
Molybdenum (sodium molybdate)	125 mcg
Manganese gluconate	3 mg
Iodine (potassium iodide)	75 mcg
Magnesium oxide (260.96 mg elemental)	400 mg
Magnesium citrate (15.66 mg elemental)	100 mg
Magnesium aspartate (19.62 mg elemental)	100 mg
Magnesium glycinate (11.74 mg elemental)	100 mg
Magnesium taurinate (7.83 mg elemental)	100 mg
Magnesium arginate (5.87 mg elemental)	100 mg
Magnesium ascorbate (3.40 mg elemental)	57.69 mg

Cholinergic Complex

Choline (from bitartrate)	117.5 mg
Phosphatidylcholine	150 mg
Inositol	250 mg

Secondary Antioxidants

Dilaurylthiodipropionate	25 mg
Thiodiproprionic acid	25 mg

Recommendation 2:
Life Extension Super Booster

Suggested dosage: 1 softgel per day with a meal.

The benefits of some nutrients are so well documented that people often want to take even higher amounts than provided by the Life Extension Mix. The Life Extension Super Booster contains many important nutrients that cannot fit into the tightly packed Life Extension Mix formula.

Just one capsule of Life Extension Super Booster provides critically important nutrients such as gamma tocopherol that are lacking in multi-nutrient formulas. Scientists have shown that people supplementing with the alpha tocopherol form of vitamin E should also consume gamma tocopherol. The reason is that alpha tocopherol displaces gamma tocopherol in the body, which may result in a lack of protection against some free radicals.

Alpha and gamma tocopherols complement each other, since it appears they work on different physiologic functions. Numerous published studies show that gamma tocopherol and the tocotrienols are more effective than alpha tocopherol.

Since gamma tocopherol and the tocotrienols come in an oil base, they cannot be included in the Life Extension Mix multi-nutrient formula (which contains only dry powders). Because of the importance of obtaining the gamma fraction of vitamin E, most members who take Life Extension Mix also take one capsule of Life Extension Booster or the Gamma E Tocopherol/Tocotrienols formula.

In order to reduce the cost and inconvenience of taking many different pills, the Super Life Extension Booster has been formulated to provide important nutrients not found in Life Extension Mix. Instead of having to take many different capsules, members can now obtain vitamin K, ginkgo extract, gamma tocopherol, chlorophyllin, tocotrienols and many other nutrients in just one capsule.

Here are all the ingredients contained in just one capsule of Life Extension Super Booster:

Gamma Tocopherol	210 mg
Gamma Tocotrienol	35.5 mg
Delta Tocopherol	78.4 mg
Delta Tocotrienol	9.3 mg
Alpha Tocopherol	66.3 mg
Alpha Tocotrienol	18.5 mg
Beta Tocopherol	3.5 mg
Lycopene extract	10 mg
Lutein extract	2.2 mg
Methyl-selenocysteine	100 mcg
Selenomethionine	50 mcg
Sodium Selenate	50 mcg
Folic Acid	800 mcg
Vitamin B_{12}	500 mcg
Ascorbic acid	90 mg
Ascorbyl Palmitate	50 mg
Chlorophyllin	100 mg
Ginkgo extract	120 mg
Vitamin K_1	9 mg
Vitamin K_2	1 mg

Since most of these ingredients are fat-soluble, Life Extension Super Booster should be taken with the heaviest meal of the day. Since the largest meal of the day often contains the most dietary mutagens, it is appropriate to consume the chlorophyllin contained in Life Extension Super Booster at this time.

Life Extension Super Booster not only contains pharmaceutical-quality ingredients, but also pharmaceutical potency. This means that the potencies of the ingredients provide the benefits indicated in published studies.

CAUTION Those taking Coumadin or other anticoagulant drugs cannot take Super Booster because of the vitamin K. Those with Wilson's disease should not take chlorophyllin supplements. The previous Life Extension Booster formula (without vitamin K and chlorophyllin is still available).

Recommendation 3:
Coenzyme Q10

Suggested dosage: 60 to 300 mg per day with a meal.

Coenzyme Q10 is incorporated into the mitochondria of cells throughout the body where it facilitates and regulates the oxidation of fats and sugars into energy. Aging humans produce only 50% of the CoQ10 that young adults do. This finding makes CoQ10 one of the most important nutrients for people over 30.

About 95% of cellular energy is produced in the mitochondria. The mitochondria are the cells' "energy powerhouses" and many maladies have been referred to as "mitochondrial disorders." A growing body of scientific research links a deficiency of CoQ10 to age-related mitochondrial disorders.

The coenzyme Q10 offered by the Life Extension Buyers Club is dissolved in rice-bran oil capsules for optimal assimilation. These CoQ10 rice-bran oil capsules are fortified with a standardized tocotrienol extract to provide additional antioxidant protection, especially to the brain.

The Life Extension Foundation was the first organization (in 1983) to introduce CoQ10 to the American public. Since that time, many new scientific studies on CoQ10 document the multiple health benefits of this versatile nutrient.

The heart is often adversely affected by a CoQ10 deficiency, but increasing evidence indicates that the brain is the organ most likely to suffer from an inadequate supply of CoQ10. Since cells need CoQ10 for energy production, the result of a CoQ10 deficit can be seen in a greater incidence of age-associated disorders.

Life Extension was first to offer CoQ10 in softgel oil-based capsules. When CoQ10 is taken orally, it is absorbed through the lymphatic canals and distributed to cells throughout the body. CoQ10 should be taken with some form of fat, since absorption through the lymphatic canals is greatly enhanced in the presence of dietary fat.

Life Extension's Super CoQ10 is in an oil base to enhance its assimilation into the bloodstream. Because CoQ10 is a relatively expensive supplement, we recommend that it be taken as a separate oil-based capsule so that it is effectively absorbed.

Life Extension's coenzyme Q10 comes exclusively from the finest Japanese pharmaceutical-grade supplier. Life Extension was the first to fortify its CoQ10 softgels with palm-oil tocotrienols. Tocotrienols are especially effective in protecting brain cells against oxidative damage. Studies indicate that tocotrienols may provide enormous health benefits, but their high cost keeps many consumers from being able to afford them.

The tocotrienols found in Life Extension's CoQ10 are extracted from palm oil. Why palm oil tocotrienol? Published studies indicate that tocotrienols extracted from palm oil are much more effective than rice-bran oil tocotrienols. Palm oil tocotrienols cost more, but they provide benefits that rice-bran tocotrienols don't. The dominant fraction in tocotrienols is gamma tocotrienol. This gamma fraction of vitamin E protects against some free radicals better that the alpha fraction. Published studies indicate that those supplementing with vitamin E should obtain both the alpha and gamma fraction.

While Super CoQ10 provides some palm-oil tocotrienols, an even greater concentration of tocotrienols can be found in the Gamma E Tocopherol/Tocotrienol and Life Extension Super Booster formulas. By taking Gamma E Tocopherol/Tocotrienol and/or Life Extension Super Booster plus Super CoQ10, Foundation members receive an abundant potency of these unique forms of vitamin E.

Life Extension's Super CoQ10 is available in 30-mg and 100-mg softgel capsules in which the CoQ10 is dissolved in tocotrienol-rich rice bran oil. (There are also 300-mg CoQ10 softgel caps available that are dissolved in perilla oil, but contain no tocotrienols.)

Recommendation 4:
ChronoForte

Suggested dosage: 3 capsules, two times per day.

During the 1980s, excess free radical activity was thought to be a primary culprit behind premature aging. Health conscious people supplemented with lots of antioxidants (such as vitamin E) to guard against free radical damage to cells. Scientific studies have since identified multiple factors, in addition to free radicals, that are associated with aging and premature death.

ChronoForte was formulated in 1999 to address newly discovered functional alterations that induce so much suffering as humans age. ChronoForte has been continuously updated since then to provide even greater protection against adverse functional alterations.

Nettle Leaf Extract. A major cause of structural and immune system breakdown is a chronic inflammatory cascade of events that attacks virtually every cell in the body. Tumor necrosis factor-alpha (TNF-a) and interleukin-1B (IL-1B) are dangerous inflammatory cytokines that can cause joint damage, cardiovascular events, and immune system dysfunction.

During aging, particularly in overweight individuals, TNF-a activity increases, causing a rise in the levels of plasminogen activator inhibitor-1, one of the body's blood clotting agents (Samad et al. 1999; Yamamoto et al. 2002).

Increased levels of IL-1B were recently found to predict death or myocardial infarction independently of high-sensitivity C-reactive protein and standard risk factors in patients with coronary artery disease (JACC 2002). ChronoForte contains a European pharmaceutical-grade extract of nettle leaf to help maintain healthy levels of TNF-a, IL-1B, and 1L-6.

Benfotiamine. Aging people often suffer from destructive fluctuations of blood glucose that can lead to the development of a host of life-threatening conditions. Newer studies reveal that even high normal levels of blood glucose (86–109 mg/dL) can damage the endothelial lining (Bjornholt et al. 1999; Hammes et al. 2003).

Elevated glucose is associated with many age-associated processes. Until recently, there was little physicians could do to prevent the complications of excess blood glucose. Exciting research indicates that a nutritional supplement, benfotiamine, a lipid soluble B_1 derivative, can block three of the four major pathways leading to glucose-induced tissue damage.

The study reported that administration of benfotiamine might prevent or delay the development of hyperglycemia-induced complications. A potent dose of benfotiamine is included in the ChronoForte formula.

Acetyl-L-Carnitine and Lipoic Acid. The National Academy of Sciences published three reports showing remarkable effects when a combination of acetyl-L-carnitine and lipoic acid was given to old rats. One of these studies showed that supplementation with these two nutrients resulted in a partial reversal of the decline of mitochondrial membrane function while consumption of oxygen significantly increased (Hagen et al. 2002).

This study demonstrated that the combination of acetyl-L-carnitine and lipoic acid improved ambulatory activity with a significantly greater degree of improvement in the old rats compared to the young ones. Human aging is characterized by lethargy, infirmity, and weakness. There is now evidence that supplementation with two over-the-counter supplements can produce a beneficial effect.

The second study published by the National Academy of Sciences showed that supplementation with acetyl-L-carnitine and lipoic acid resulted in improved memory in old rats. Electron microscopic studies in the hippocampus region of the brain showed that acetyl-L-carnitine and lipoic acid reversed age-associated mitochondrial structural decay (Liu et al. 2002a).

In the third National Academy of Sciences study, scientists tested acetyl-L-carnitine and lipoic acid to see if an enzyme used by the mitochondria as biologic fuel could be restored in old rats (Liu 2002b). After seven weeks of supplementation with acetyl-L-carnitine and lipoic acid, levels of this enzyme (carnitine acetyltransferase) were significantly restored in the aged rats. Supplementation also inhibited free radical-induced lipid peroxidation, which enhanced the activity of the energy-producing enzyme in the mitochondria. The scientists concluded that feeding old rats acetyl-L-carnitine and lipoic acid can ameliorate oxidative damage, along with mitochondrial dysfunction. High potency acetyl-L-carnitine and alpha lipoic acid are part of the ChronoForte formula.

Carnosine. Aging causes irreversible damage to the body's proteins. The underlying mechanism behind this damage is glycation. A simple definition of glycation is the cross-linking of proteins and sugars to form nonfunctioning structures in the body. The process of glycation can be superficially seen as unsightly wrinkled skin. Glycation is also an underlying cause of age-related calamities including neurologic, vascular, and ocular disorders. Carnosine is a multifunctional dipeptide that interferes with the glycation process. When compared to the anti-glycating drug, aminoguanidine, carnosine has been shown to inhibit glycation earlier in the process.

Carnosine levels are reduced with age. Muscle levels decline 63% from age 10 to age 70, which may account for the normal age-related decline in muscle mass and function (Stuerenburg et al. 1999). Since carnosine acts as a pH buffer, it can keep on protecting muscle cell membranes from oxidation under the acidic conditions of muscular exertion. Carnosine enables the heart muscle to contract more efficiently through enhancement of calcium response in heart myocytes (Zaloga et al. 1997). Long-lived cells such as nerve cells (neurons) and muscle cells (myocytes) contain high levels of carnosine. Muscle levels of carnosine correlate with the maximum life spans of animals. ChronoForte provides a potent dose of carnosine.

Water-Soluble Quercetin. Quercetin belongs to a class of plant pigments known as flavonoids. Quercetin is present in varying amounts in vegetables and fruits such as apples, onions, and tea and is one of the best researched of the flavonoids. Quercetin has demonstrated inflammation suppression, antihistamine, and potent antioxidant properties. Its most relevant brain-health effect is its anticoagulant activity (Pignatelli et al. 2001).

In response to stress, blood in the brain becomes more prone to clotting, especially among the aged (Yamamoto et al. 2002; Breteler 2000). Clotting causes ischemia, which is responsible for the majority of cases of vascular dementia. Quercetin promotes a healthy blood flow. The brain-enhancing effects of quercetin may also owe to its ability to block an enzyme that leads to the accumulation of sorbitol. The carbohydrate sorbitol has been linked age-associated nerve problems. Quercetin helps to promote the normal function of healthy neural tissue.

The problem with quercetin supplements is that they don't absorb well into the bloodstream. ChronoForte contains a water-soluble quercetin that enables easy facilitation, absorption and utilization of this important flavonoid.

The ChronoForte Formula. Based on the accumulating body of research showing how the catastrophic consequences of aging manifest, ChronoForte has been re-formulated to provide a convenient and economical way of obtaining the following nutrients in each daily dose:

Acetyl-L-carnitine HCL	2000 mg
Nettle leaf extract	1000 mg
Carnosine	1000 mg
Biotin	3000 mcg
Alpha lipoic acid	300 mg
Benfotiamine	150 mg
Quercetin (water soluble)	150 mg
Zinc	15 mg

Six capsules a day of ChronoForte must be taken in order to benefit from carnosine. The reason for this is that the body automatically metabolizes lower amounts of carnosine into an inert substance, but the body cannot neutralize the amount of carnosine (1000 mg) contained in six capsules of ChronoForte.

Recommendation 5:
Cognitex

Suggested dosage: 3 capsules early in the day.

Many factors conspire to rob us of mental acuity as we age. But scientists have discovered natural agents with the potential to slow or even reverse this once inevitable decline.

Since 1982, Life Extension has offered the multi-nutrient Cognitex formula to protect and enhance neurological function. Over the years, Cognitex has been improved in accordance with the latest research on the underlying causes of brain aging.

The active ingredients in Cognitex attack the presumptive causes of age-related brain decline at the source. To inhibit the neuroinflammatory enzymes COX-2 and 5-LOX, Cognitex contains pharmaceutical extracts of Nexrutine® and 5-Loxin. Water-soluble quercetin helps improve cerebral blood flow. Phosphatidylserine maintains neuronal membrane integrity and guards against cortisol toxicity. Alpha-glycerylphosphorylcholine (GPC) helps boost acetylcholine, a critical neurotransmitter. Vinpocetine enhances circulation and oxygenation to brain cells, improves neural electrical conductivity, and protects against neuron-destroying excitotoxicity.

Cognitex is available with or without pregnenolone, a hormone that may be especially beneficial to the brain. (Those with existing steroid hormone-sensitive cancers should not take pregnenolone.)

Just three softgel capsules of Cognitex contain pharmaceutical-grade potencies of the following nutrients:

Glycerylphosphorylcholine (GPC)	600 mg
Nexrutine®	500 mg
Quercetin (water-soluble)	125 mg
Phosphatidylserine (PS)	100 mg
5-Loxin	50 mg
Pregnenolone	50 mg
Vinpocetine	15 mg

There are 90 capsules in each bottle meaning that a bottle will last a healthy person one month.

Brain aging is a leading cause of disease, disability, and death in the elderly. The quest to slow brain aging —heralded by loss of ability in thinking, remembering, and reasoning—is the reason most people contact the Life Extension Foundation. The antioxidants found in the Life Extension Mix and the Life Extension Booster protect against free radical damage to brain cells. The Cognitex formula contains nutrients that help maintain healthy cognitive function via additional mechanisms.

Recommendation 6:
Essential Fatty Acids

Suggested dosage: Depends on type of oil used (fish, flax, perilla, borage, etc.)

If you search the medical databases, you will find that just about every physical and mental disorder affecting mankind can be related to the body's essential fatty acid status. This makes sense based on the fact that our cell membranes require essential fatty acids to maintain their function and structure. The vitality and viability of our cells is totally dependent on healthy membrane function.

The typical American diet is loaded with dangerous omega-6 and *trans* fats, while deficient in beneficial omega-3 fatty acids. According to an article published in the *Lancet*, men who consume the most *trans* fatty acids have twice the risk of developing heart disease compared to their counterparts who consumed the least (Oomen et al. 2001). The American Heart Association published a study of 11,323 heart attack survivors showing that those who took a 1000-mg fish oil supplement every day were 45% less likely to be dead at the end of 3.5 years (Kris-Etherton 2002).

On May 27, 2003, The White House urged health agencies of government to encourage Americans to increase their consumption of foods rich in omega-3 fatty acids and decrease their intake of *trans* fatty acids.

Based on overwhelming documentation that greater consumption of omega-3 fatty acids confers enormous benefits, a health claim petition has been filed with the FDA seeking the right to convey this information on the labels of omega-3 dietary supplements.

Most people associate omega-3 fatty acids with a reduced cardiovascular risk. Increasing evidence, however, about the crucial role that DHA plays in maintaining neuronal membrane structure has caused people of all ages (including pregnant women) to consider adding fish, flax, or perilla oil to their daily regimen.

The most important essential fatty acids to supplement with are GLA (gamma linolenic acid), DHA (docosahexaenoic acid) and EPA (eicosapentaenoic acid).

Some people choose to take flax or perilla oil, which are rich in alpha linolenic acid. In a healthy body, alpha linolenic acid is enzymatically transformed into DHA and EPA. Some people are deficient in the enzyme (delta-6-desaturase) needed to convert alpha-linolenic acid into DHA and EPA. This is one reason why fish oil, which directly provides DHA and EPA, is becoming a more popular way of obtaining life-sustaining omega-3 fatty acids.

GLA can be obtained from several sources, but borage oil provides the highest concentration of this inflammation-suppressing prostaglandin E1 precursor.

Typical doses of essential fatty acid supplements are six capsules a day of Super GLA/DHA; or six capsules a day of perilla oil and three capsules of Mega GLA.

Six softgels of Super GLA/DHA supplies:

Borage (*Borago officinalis*) seed oil providing	4000 mg
GLA (gamma-linolenic acid)	920 mg
Marine lipid concentrate providing	2000 mg
DHA (docosahexaenoic acid)	1000 mg

Recommendation 7 (for women):
Bone Assure

Suggested dosage: 6 capsules per day (at dinner or before bedtime).

Osteoporosis is a common consequence of aging and can cause disabling fractures (most commonly hip fractures) or even death. Since osteoporosis has no symptoms in its early stages, prevention is critical. Living bone is never at rest metabolically; its "walls" or matrix and mineral stores are being remodeled constantly, and minerals like calcium play crucial metabolic and structural roles.

Doctors often recommend calcium supplements, but weak bones and joints are associated with deficiencies of a wide range of nutrients, including magnesium, vitamin D_3, manganese, and zinc. In order for calcium to prevent bone loss, adequate amounts of vitamin D_3 and certain trace minerals must be available so that calcium, magnesium, and phosphorus will be incorporated into the bone matrix. The Bone Assure formula provides the nutrients that have been shown to prevent bone loss and/or rebuild bone mass.

Bone Assure is in capsule form to ensure that it breaks down fully in the digestive tract (unlike calcium tablets). The capsules burst open within 5 minutes of swallowing, making the minerals and vitamin D_3 immediately available for absorption.

The daily dose of 6 capsules of Bone Assure contains:

Calcium (from bis-glycinate) supplying elemental calcium	1000 mg
Magnesium oxide supplying elemental magnesium	320 mg
Zinc citrate	35 mg
supplying elemental zinc	12 mg
Manganese citrate	10 mg
supplying elemental manganese	3 mg
Boron (from amino acid chelate)	2 mg
Copper sulfate	3.7 mg
supplying elemental copper	1.5 mg
Oat straw (10:1 – silica source)	40 mg
Vitamin D_3	400 IU
Folic acid	200 mcg
TMG (trimethylglycine/betaine)	100 mg
Vitamin B_6	15 mg

Recommendation 7 (for men):
Natural Prostate Formula (Saw Palmetto, Nettle, Pygeum, and Lycopene Extracts)

Suggested dosage: 1 capsule with breakfast and 1 capsule at bedtime.

Prostate enlargement (BPH) is an inevitable consequence of aging for most men. Natural Prostate Formula contains the three most potent herbs to alleviate prostate discomfort, plus lycopene and boron to help protect against the formation of aberrant cell colonies.

Saw palmetto extract inhibits the binding of DHT (dihydrotestosterone) to prostate cell receptor sites. Saw palmetto also acts as an alpha-adrenergic receptor inhibitor, reducing urinary urgency and inflammatory action in the prostate gland.

Nettle root extract (*Urtica dioica*) helps suppress the effects of estrogen and sex hormone-binding globulins by stopping them from binding to prostate cells. Pygeum inhibits inflammatory processes and has been shown to alleviate prostate discomfort.

Natural Prostate Formula provides the identical herbal extracts successfully used by European doctors for decades.

Each capsule of Natural Prostate Formula contains:

Saw Palmetto CO2 extract (*Serenoa repens*) (berries)	160 mg
Free fatty acids & sterols	136 mg
(85–95% from saw palmetto extract)	
Stinging Nettle extract (*Urtica dioica*) (root)	120 mg
Pygeum extract (*Pygeum africanum*) (bark)	50 mg
Sterols (from Pygeum extract)	6.5 mg
Lycopene (from tomato extract)	5 mg
Boron (from boron citrate, glycinate, and aspartate)	1.5 mg
Rosemary extract (*Rosmarinus officinalis*)	400 mcg

Recommendation 8:

Restoring Youthful Hormone Balance—DHEA

Taking lots of vitamins will not make you feel better if you suffer from a hormone imbalance. Youthful hormone balance is critical to maintaining health in all women and men over age 40.

Aging men and women are invariably DHEA deficient. Many men over age 40 often have too much estrogen and too little free testosterone. Aging women need to balance their progesterone and estrogen (using safe natural estrogen supplements and drugs) levels. Thyroid deficiency is an epidemic problem, especially for women.

The proper blood tests can provide the data needed to design an individualized hormone modulation program. Life Extension offers special blood test panels designed to help provide the information needed to safely achieve youthful hormone balance.

You can read about restoring optimal hormone levels in the chapters entitled *DHEA Replacement*, *Male Hormone Modulation*, *Female Hormone Modulation*, and *Thyroid Deficiency*.

DHEA supplements are available in 15 and 25-mg strengths. Men usually need 50–75 mg of DHEA each morning, while women typically take 15–50 mg.

Based on the results of blood tests, some people will need natural hormone prescription drugs. Foundation members can discuss their hormone status with one of our staff physicians at no charge.

Recommendation 9:

SAMe (S-Adenosyl Methionine)

Suggested dosage: 200 mg to 1600 mg per day.

The unique biological properties of SAMe make it a critical component of a health maintenance program. SAMe is the most effective facilitator of youthful methylation. Published research shows that methylation defects create a variety of age-related disorders including neuronal and hepatic dysfunction. Enhancing youthful methylation facilitates healthy enzymatic life processes throughout the body.

Not only can SAMe enhance mood and alleviate melancholy, but it can also protect the joint linings from structural degradation. Since aging people often suffer joint discomfort and immobilization, SAMe addresses multiple problems people face as they grow older.

An agency of the U.S. Department of Health and Human Services conducted a meticulous evaluation of SAMe in the year 2002. Their findings show the efficacy of SAMe in helping maintain stable mood and healthy joint structure, without any side effects (AHRQ 2002).

This U.S. government report concluded that SAMe is 80% more effective in relieving osteoarthritis pain than placebo. This report also verified that SAMe was as effective as nonsteroidal anti-inflammatory (NSAIDs) drugs in treating osteoarthritis. The significance of this finding is that NSAIDs are associated with serious side effects, whereas SAMe provides benefits throughout the body.

SAMe should be taken with cofactors vitamin B_{12} and folic acid. If you take the Life Extension Mix and/or the Life Extension Booster, you will get these cofactors.

Not all SAMe supplements are created equal. SAMe is an unstable molecule that requires special processing to ensure stability. Analysis of several popular brands of SAMe revealed many of them did not contain what was claimed on the label.

Recommendation 10:

Indole-3-Carbinol/Resveratrol Capsules

Suggested dosage: Two capsules a day for those under 121 pounds; three capsules a day for those weighing between 120–180, four capsules per day for those weighing over 180 pounds.

Multiple agencies of the Federal government are advocating that Americans consume more fruits and vegetables for a healthier life style. Indole-3-carbinal and resveratrol are two important vegetable/fruit extracts.

Indole-3-carbinol (I3C) is a plant compound from cruciferous vegetables such as cabbage and brussels sprouts. It has been shown to function via multiple mechanisms to inhibit the development of aberrant cell colonies. I3C has been shown to:

- Protect the genomic structure of DNA
- Convert dangerous estrogens (16-alpha-hydroxyestrone) that cause the development of aberrant cell colonies to safer forms of estrogen (2-hydroxyestrone) that prevent the development of aberrant cells.
- Block estrogen receptor sites on the membranes of breast and other cells
- Restore p21 suppressor gene function
- Induce apoptosis of aberrant cells
- Protect cells against the genotoxic effects of pesticides and other environmental pollutants including dioxin
- Slow the propagation of aberrant breast and prostate cells

Resveratrol is an extract from red grapes and other plants that scientists are very excited about. A tremendous number of studies published in 2003 indicate that resveratrol provides multi-faceted benefits. Resveratrol is available in a standardized whole grape extract designed to provide many of the benefits attributed to red wine, without the ethanol.

Most people find it hard to consume enough I3C-containing vegetables every day. That is why I3C is becoming such as popular dietary supplement. For most people, just two to three capsules a day provide the amount of I3C needed to derive optimal protection against the development of aberrant cell colonies. I3C is now available with a standardized resveratrol extract to provide even greater health benefits without having to take additional pills.

Each capsule of Indole-3-Carbinol/Resveratrol contains:

Resveratrol (from 70 mg of Regrape X™)	7 mg
Naturally occurring polyphenols from organic red grapes	31 mg
Quercetin17	40 mg
Indole-3-carbinol (I3C)	200 mg

Recommendation 11:
Aspirin

Suggested dosage: 1 tablet per day with a heavy meal.

A chronic inflammatory cascade characterizes many of the problems associated with aging including brain cell degeneration, aortic stenosis, and sudden death heart attack. Low-dose aspirin helps to inhibit chronic inflammatory conditions that are known to result in lethal events. A particularly dangerous agent in the blood called C-reactive protein causes inflammation of the interior arterial wall that can result in acute blockage of a coronary or cerebral artery. Aspirin reduces blood levels of the dangerous C-reactive protein.

The most common cause of disability and death in the United States is an abnormal clot that develops inside an artery to cause a heart attack (blocked blood vessel in the heart) or a stroke (blocked blood vessel in the brain). Aspirin has an immediate and lasting effect on blood platelets, making them less likely to clump together and form a catastrophic clot in arteries. The low dose of aspirin (81 mg) provided by the Healthprin™ tablet has been shown to be beneficial to reduce the risk of heart attacks, strokes, and transient ischemic attacks (little strokes).

More than 50 randomized trials have documented the safety and effectiveness of aspirin as a cardiovascular drug. Low-dose aspirin is advised by legions of physicians as well as a 70-member panel convened by the American College of Chest Physicians, which recommended aspirin for all people over 50 with one risk factor and no conditions that make aspirin use inadvisable. This translates into the majority of people over 50, since risk factors include male gender, high blood pressure, elevated cholesterol, diabetes, cigarette smoking, lack of exercise, and family history of heart attack or stroke.

In fact, aspirin is commonly considered a "miracle" drug and a recent report stated that it is expected to have many undiscovered health benefits.

While there are many nutrients that can reduce the risk of an abnormal blood clot forming inside a blood vessel, it is still beneficial for most older people to take aspirin in the low dose provided by the Healthprin tablet, which minimizes stomach irritation. We also recommend that it be taken with a heavy meal to further decrease the possibility of stomach irritation.

Recommendation 12:
Melatonin

Suggested dosage: 300 mcg to 6 mg at bedtime.

Melatonin is a hormone secreted at night by the pineal gland that regulates multiple body processes. Not only does melatonin help induce drowsiness in most people, but it plays a crucial role in regulating the complex function of the immune system and guarding against aberrant cell propagation.

Melatonin is one of the body's most prolific natural antioxidants and is especially effective in protecting neurons against damaging free radicals.

Like so many other hormones, the secretion of melatonin declines with age as the pineal gland calcifies. The good news is that melatonin is a very low-cost supplement that provides broad-spectrum health benefits.

The typical dose is to take 3 milligrams of melatonin at bedtime, but for some people, much lower doses of melatonin (300 mcg to 1 mg) help them sleep better. Conversely, some people take 6 mg to 10 mg of melatonin for better sleep. Because of the wide range of individual variability, melatonin is available in capsules containing 300 mcg, 500 mcg, 750 mcg, 1 mg, 3 mg, 5 mg, and 10 mg. It is also available in dissolve-in-the-mouth and time-release versions.

● SUMMARY

The concept of taking action now to maintain youthful health is based on published scientific studies showing that the diseases of aging may be prevented or at least can be postponed.

New members often write to the Foundation for evaluation lists of the supplements they are taking. Many of these health-conscious people are under-dosing or overdosing on nutrient supplements. In many cases, people are missing just a few critical nutrients or hormones that would greatly enhance the effectiveness of their personal life extension program.

Foundation members are pleasantly surprised to find that they can drop many of the expensive supplements they are currently using and replace them with lower-priced and more complete disease-preventing formulations by following the step-by-step disease prevention program outlined above.

The following supplements are the most important in preventing the common diseases of aging:

1. Life Extension Mix as a cornerstone in a comprehensive supplement program (available in tablets, capsules, or powder).

2. Life Extension Super Booster containing the essential gamma fraction of vitamin E and tocotrienols along with plant extracts.

3. Coenzyme Q10 oil-filled softgel caps to improve cellular energy in the heart and brain.

4. ChronoForte, containing carnosine, a potent anti-glycation agent, antioxidant, and metal chelator.

5. Cognitex and ginkgo to slow brain aging and enhance cognition.

6. Essential Fatty Acids serve as building blocks for nerve cells and cell membranes and help prevent a host of physical disorders.

7. Natural Prostate Formula for men to protect against prostate miseries; Bone Assure for women to prevent bone loss due to osteoporosis.

8. Restoring youthful hormone balance to stave off the diseases of old age that affect both men and women. (*Refer to specific Male or Female Hormone Modulation protocol, and the DHEA Replacement protocol.*)

9. SAMe to enhance youthful methylation and protect against neuronal, hepatic, and joint degeneration.

10. I3C/Resveratrol capsules to protect against aberrant cell growth.

11. Melatonin at bedtime to induce drowsiness and provide broad-spectrum antioxidant protection.

12. Low-dose aspirin (for most people) to help prevent dangerous blot clots and reduce chronic inflammation.

 PRODUCT AVAILABILITY

Life Extension Mix, Life Extension Super Booster, Coenzyme Q10, Cognitex, *ginkgo biloba*, Natural Prostate Formula, Bone Assure, ChronoForte, DHEA, SAMe, I3C/Resveratrol capsules, Healthprin, melatonin, and Super GLA/DHA can be ordered by telephoning (800) 544-4440 or by ordering online at www.lef.org.

Prostate Cancer

INTRODUCTION TO DR. STRUM'S PROSTATE CANCER UPDATE

When I was diagnosed with advanced prostate cancer in September 1991, I thought my life, as I had envisioned it, was over. Instead, I have found a whole new universe of living and, in doing so, have come to terms with my own mortality.

Transformation is what is possible when we are faced with a life-threatening illness. When the unthinkable happens to us and we are faced with our mortality, we have an opportunity to transform our lives.

Acceptance of our situation is the first milestone we must pass before we can truly begin the process of healing. For me this translates into doing everything I can to understand the entire process of my illness and what I can do to become well. While I do not blame myself for my diagnosis, it has been valuable for me to take an introspective look at my life in relation to the kinds of stressors or environmental exposures that may have played a role. Sometimes it is not until we are on the reef that we realize it is there.

Fortunately for us, the cancer patient today has many more resources available than there were just a few years ago. What follows by Dr. Stephen Strum is an update of the treatment of prostate cancer. I have known Steve for over 10 years. He is one of the precious few who have brought a new and compassionate dimension to the patient/physician relationship.

Frederick Mills
Prostate Cancer Survivor
Founding Member of Educational Council
    for Prostate Cancer Patients

PROSTATE CANCER UPDATE 2003

Stephen B. Strum, M.D., F.A.C.P.

GENERAL INTRODUCTION

In this, the year 2003 edition of *Disease Prevention and Treatment*, I will discuss prostate cancer (PC), using the metaphor of a military incursion—needing to have a focused, strategic approach, deployed in a systematic, problem-solving manner. The purpose of such a metaphor is to bring to the student of this disease a different perspective that will hopefully provide new insights that will lead to victories in our battles against this disease. The reason for such a departure from the conventional formal discussion of PC is that this latter academic approach is not being translated into winning strategies for the man with PC. The battle is being lost because we, the generals, are not translating what has been published in medical journals and discussed at national meetings into real-time preventive, diagnostic, evaluatory, and treatment tactics. Medical pragmatism—the art of being practical and using common sense—is not being practiced.

The battle to prevent this disease, to diagnose it earlier, and to treat it effectively is also not occurring at the proper pace largely because men are not taking an active role in winning this war. As we are learning in our war against terrorism, you defeat the enemy by recognizing their presence early (not late), preventing their buildup, learning their location, and eradicating them with the proper weaponry. There are too many men, already diagnosed with PC, who are not taking an active role in their own recovery. Many believe that because they are consulting a professional with a medical degree (who may also command a generous salary), all or part of this equates with getting the very best advice and treatment. Wrong. In today's world of rapid pace, where medicine is practiced with 15-minute office visits and where physicians are too busy to read and translate much of what is being published, the patient and his partner must not take a passive role and assume that all that can be done is being done.

My recommendations, therefore, either to patients with PC or to their loved ones, will be those of a counselor or guide, offering practical advice based on 20 years of working on the front lines of PC management. I do not hesitate in telling you that for the vast majority of men diagnosed with PC, a successful outcome can be realized. But the principles you are about to learn must become part and parcel of the strategic approach used by the patient/partner/physician (PPP) team. The patient and his partner have the most to gain as well as the most to lose when encountering PC. They must expend serious energy to win this particular war. In doing so, they learn the art of battle; they are brought closer together and evolve in their lives; and other intertwined health issues are brought to light and healed. This is the beauty of such an approach. Are you willing to invest in the time to help yourself? Are you worth it?

THE *2003 DISEASE PREVENTION AND TREATMENT* EDITION

The most important take-home lesson that I can relate to you within the pages that follow relates to

Table 1: *Comparison of a Military Campaign with Prostate Cancer Strategy*

Winning a Military Campaign	Defeating Prostate Cancer (PC)
1 Preventing War	1 Preventing PC
2 Basic Military Training	2 Getting Help to Understand Biological Principles
3 Military Information (Intel)	3 The Importance of the Medical Record
4 Early Recognition of Enemy Activity	4 Early Diagnosis of PC
5 Assessment of the Enemy	5 Risk Assessment of the PC Patient
6 Knowing Pros and Cons of Weaponry	6 Understanding Pros and Cons of Treatment Options
7 Understanding Enemy Vulnerability	7 Learning Principles Underlying Tumor Growth
8 Stopping Supply Lines to the Enemy	8 Antiangiogenesis Treatments, Dietary Changes
9 Stabilizing Key Arenas of Conflict	9 Focus on Bone Integrity, Biomarkers, etc.
10 Supporting the Troops	10 Supportive Care of the Patient
11 Boosting Morale of Troops	11 Fostering a Will to Live, Empowering the Patient

your ability to use concepts. It is through the use of concepts—the structural framework of our thinking—that we intelligently plan a strategy of success.

As stated in the introduction, defeating PC is a military campaign. Winning a military campaign, or a war against PC, involves concepts such as prevention, basic training, military intelligence (Intel), early recognition of enemy activity, assessment of the strength of the enemy, an understanding of the pros and cons of the weapons in our arsenal, stabilization of key areas of conflict, stopping supply lines to the enemy, supporting our troops, and other issues common to a military arena (*see Table 1*). A strategy for success, be it in a military war or a war against PC, simply involves adding factual information to a sound conceptual framework.

Please refer to the glossary on page 1444 following this chapter to better understand unfamiliar terms that are used throughout the text.

The approaches used in a winning strategy, whether for a military campaign or a medical battle, are superimposable. That which occurs in the life of a cell is reflected in society as well.[1] Cellular battles are but a microcosm of what takes place on a more macromolecular level within the individual, his community, his country, the planet, and the universe. This is reflected repeatedly throughout the entire history of man.

1. PREVENTING WAR: PREVENTING PC

Most students of either campaign will maintain that prevention is the key to being truly victorious. There is no argument there. However, the desire to understand the principles and importance of preventive tactics does not appear to be a top priority for most

people until the harsh reality of war or cancer is present. For example, the appreciation of terrorism in America was not brought home until September 11, 2001. This appreciation of the enemy may take the form of seeing the reality of cancer up close and personal when a father, brother, or other family member is diagnosed with PC or another malignancy. Otherwise, the motivation to learn and utilize prevention tactics does not seem to be part of human reality for the vast majority of us. What can we do to foster an appreciation of the value of preventing PC?

Hereditary PC: Risk Factors

Out of every 100 men diagnosed with PC, approximately 5 will have hereditary PC (HPC).[2] HPC is presently defined by any one of the following three criteria:

- Three successive generations with members having PC

- Three first-degree relatives, for example, a father and two brothers, three brothers, or a father and two sons with PC

- Two relatives with PC diagnosed before age 55[3]

It is not surprising that the incidence of hereditary breast cancer is also about 5% of the total population of breast cancer patients—the same incidence as that of HPC.[4]

Genetic Transmission from Father to Son and Father to Daughter

HPC is transmitted by a gene from father to son and from father to daughter and then to her son. When HPC is present, nearly half the male offspring will have PC, and many of these will develop PC before

Table 9: *Correlation of Patient Age, Total PSA, and Free PSA Percentage with the Probability of Having PC.*

		Percentage of Free PSA			
		6.0–6.9%	7.0–14.9%	15.0–25%	>25%
Patient Age	Total PSA	Probability of Prostate Cancer (%)			
50–59	2.5–4.0	84	23	10	2
60–70	2.5–4.0	94	47	25	6
71 and older	2.5–4.0	96	57	33	9
50–59	4.1–10.0	87	28	12	3
60–70	4.1–10.0	95	52	29	7
71 and older	4.1–10.0	97	62	38	11

Table 10: *Stability of PSA Over 10 Years of Testing in Dr. Stephen Strum.*

These PSA values were obtained over a 10-year span. They show minimal changes which are consistent with the known literature on minute increases in PSA in the healthy prostate. The PSA slope in such situations is essentially flat. Earlier PSA levels dating back to 1987 were in the 0.7–0.8 range, but unfortunately these records were lost by Dr. Strum's former primary physician. (Always keep a backup of your medical records!)

Date	11/2/92	3/5/94	5/1/94	4/2/95	5/17/96	4/13/97	1/26/98	2/19/98	5/14/99
PSA	0.75	0.83	0.83	1.0	0.82	0.7	0.75	0.83	0.6

Date	8/4/99	9/6/00	8/31/01	9/4/02
PSA	0.73	0.571	0.66	0.75

Hybritech, Bayer, etc., which is being run in the same laboratory facility.

PSAV and PSADT determinations are most valid when the PSA testing interval selected for the analysis is approximately 6 months or more. However, what is important to stress in this context is the PSA trend or slope over time. *Serial PSA values showing a progressive increase in PSA should always raise concern that a biological process is occurring. It is the rapidity of such an increase that will suggest if this is a malignant or a benign process.*[139]

The PSA increases over time associated with a healthy prostate are tiny. They amount to average increases of less than 0.1 ng/mL a year (range 0.055–0.128) of PSA in the blood.[140–142] Therefore, the use of PSAV thresholds of greater than 0.75 ng/mL a year is quite generous in raising concern about the presence of PC. Table 10 shows my PSA values over the course of 10 years.

The PSA trend or slope (also referred to as PSA kinetics or dynamics) is a far more important biological expression than any one PSA absolute value. Such kinetic values express active changes in the status of the PC patient over the dimension of time. *Realizing that aberrations in laboratory testing do occur should mandate that, when a major change is found in a laboratory test result, repeat testing for validation purposes should be required until a definite trend is clearly seen.* Too often, patients with PC are ready to make major changes in their evaluation or management based on one or two PSA changes. This also applies to other biomarkers such as PAP (prostatic acid phosphatase), CGA (chromogranin A), CEA (carcinoembryonic antigen), and NSE (neuron-specific enolase), which the physician may be using to monitor the PC patient.

> TRENDS ARE IMPORTANT IN BOTH THE EVALUATION AND MANAGEMENT OF ANY ILLNESS—INCLUDING PROSTATE CANCER.

What Does This Mean for Patients?

In prior paragraphs, it was emphasized that first-time PSA levels of less than 2.0 are uncommonly associated with PC and that, in such patients, PSA testing can be done every 2–3 years. Patients with first-time values of PSA that are less than 4.0 ng/mL but at least 2.0 ng/mL *should not be regarded* as having a PSA within the normal range. The guidelines for a normal first-time PSA are up to 1.9 ng/mL.

It was also pointed out that the PSA and its derivatives, such as PSA velocity, PSA doubling time, PSAD (total gland and for transition zone), and free PSA percentage, are instrumental in our understanding of biological reality. It is akin to the story of the three blind men feeling different parts of one elephant and describing three entirely different animals. What is needed in the elephant story, in the management of PC and other health issues, in a military campaign, and in the management of any world challenge, is an integrative way of thinking, which fosters unified concepts and embodies principles of synergy and harmony.

We also presented new findings on the free PSA percentage; it can be done on PSA levels as low as 2.0. This finding, coupled with the information on first-time PSA readings being significant when the PSA is found to be 2.0 or higher, should lead to an earlier diagnosis of PC and greater probability of cure.

Additional reading on the subjects of free PSA, PSADT, and PSAV can be found in the *Primer* published by Life Extension Media and available either by telephoning (866) 820-7457 or on the Life Extension website at www.lefprostate.org. Software on free PSA percentage versus the diagnosis of PC, correction for PSA results if ejaculation has occurred within 48 hours of PSA testing, and calculators for PSAV and PSADT can be found on the PCRI (Prostate Cancer Research Institute) website at www.pcri.org. This software, PC Tools I and PC Tools II, was developed by Glenn Tisman, M.D., a medical oncologist in Whittier, California, who specializes only in PC.

5. RISK ASSESSMENT OF THE PC PATIENT

Once a diagnosis of PC is established by means of tissue biopsy and microscopic findings showing PC, the foundation of the medical record should have further information added to it to allow for an even greater understanding of the patient's true status. In this context, status refers to the actual extent of disease, or stage of disease. Is the PC really confined to the prostate gland or does it penetrate the capsule of the prostate or perhaps invade local surrounding tissues such as the seminal vesicles and nearby lymph nodes? Are there any clues that the PC has spread or metastasized to more distant lymph nodes or bone?

The orientation of most specialists will be toward recommending a local therapy to eradicate PC within the gland. This is the essence of the reasoning behind the surgical removal of the prostate—RP. The other approaches toward treating PC with curative intent may be slightly more regional, but most are still designed to primarily treat the prostate gland. For example, external beam radiation therapy (EBRT) will include not only the prostate gland itself, but also a margin around the gland to kill any tumor cells that may be in this area trying to escape and spread to more distant sites. The same is true for the iceballs created by cryosurgery.[143] *The critical concept here is that local measures treat local disease.* The determination of the true **extent** or stage of the disease is one of the critical variables in the strategy of successful treatment of PC. For example, if the disease is present outside the prostate gland in tissues such as the seminal vesicle or nearby regional lymph nodes (the obturator or internal iliac lymph nodes), an RP will have a significantly diminished chance in curing the patient with PC. The same is true for RT or cryosurgery. *For such therapies to have a great chance of cure, the cancer must be within the scope of the scalpel, within the boundaries of the radiation ports of therapy, and within the periphery of the iceball(s) created by cryosurgery.*

An additional limiting factor for radiation therapy and cryosurgery is the **amount** of PC. The tumor volume has a bearing on the ability of RT or cryosurgery to destroy the entire tumor mass.[78,144,145] This second variable in the equation may relate to the penetrating ability of the radiation particle used (photon < proton < neutron)[146–148] or to the understanding that the core of a large tumor has a diminished oxygen supply (a hypoxic center) that confers resistance (called radioresistance) to the treatment.[149,150] This actually may not be as critical a factor in cryosurgery as it is in RT. These aspects of RT are discussed and illustrated in detail in the *Primer*. The reader is recommended to review pages 90–127 of the *Primer* to better understand these concepts.

A third variable, one under-discussed with the patient for obvious reasons, is the variability in skill of the physician, regardless of the specialty. Some physicians are talented artists, while others are average in skill and still others are below average.

Unfortunately, all physicians quote the outstanding literature on a particular treatment but very few present to the patient their own scorecard of performance statistics.

There are additional variables relating to diagnosis and staging. The number of these biological observations is increasing as we learn more and more about the cancer process. Some of these variables include the following:

- Baseline PSA and PAP

- Gleason score read by a recognized expert in PC

- Clinical stage based on DRE

- Gland volume—the volume of the prostate gland in cubic centimeters or grams

- Core percentage involvement—the percentage of biopsy cores involved with PC

- DNA status

- PSAD

- AUA symptom index score and uroflowmetry

- TGF-b1 and IL-6sR

Baseline PSA and Baseline PAP Are Keystones in Our Understanding of PC

The *Primer* goes into great depth on the importance of the baseline PSA and PAP. Let me make a few salient points. The PSA is a blessing. There are no other common malignancies that forecast their development through such a simple and inexpensive blood test as the PSA. But there are limitations to the PSA, as there are with everything in life.

Everything in life is a two-edged sword.

One major limitation of the PSA is that it is a laboratory test, which makes it subject to error and to conditions that elevate the PSA and possibly result in false alarms. However, one can state safely that a healthy prostate is one not subject to progressive or persistent elevations of PSA. In such situations, if PC is not the underlying cause, then prostatitis or BPH is the cause. These conditions significantly affect the quality of life of many men. Many scientists involved with PC research also believe that prostatitis may be a precursor to PC.[151,152]

In regard to the laboratory errors that may occur with PSA; these may occur with all tests. The rule of thumb is that if a test shows a reading at any time that is of concern, the test should be repeated and then repeated again after a short period of time to confirm whatever trend now seems apparent. It is this persistent *trend* that is so important in declaring the presence of biological conditions that should concern us.

PSA Leak Is Relatively Low in Undifferentiated PC

Another aspect of the PSA that may be misleading is in the setting of patients with a low PSA level that is associated with a high Gleason score, for example, (4,3) or higher. The problem here is that high Gleason score lesions, having a significant component of Gleason grade 4 or 5 PC, do not secrete as much PSA into the blood as lower grade lesions. This is called the PSA leak. Table 11 shows the PSA leak as a function of average (weighted) Gleason grade.

Here is where the Gleason score is very important in elaborating on the significance we give the PSA during the initial and subsequent evaluations of the patient. I have seen patients present with Gleason scores of 9 and 10 with low levels of PSA and yet they had large tumor volumes reflecting PC that was outside the prostate gland and not amenable to cure with local therapy.

A Microsoft Excel software program for tumor volume (which can be found on the PCRI home page at www.pcri.org) shows the above relationships clearly. The program requires the b (baseline) PSA, gland volume, and Gleason score. The PSA leak is calculated from the weighted Gleason grade. The outputs of this program give you benign PSA, PC-related PSA, and *calculated* tumor volume. Additional integrated programs give you probability of organ-confined disease, probability of cure with RP, and likelihood of freedom from biochemical relapse at 20 months after RT.

Gleason Score Versus Gleason Grade

The Gleason score is composed of two grades: the primary grade and the secondary grade. The primary grade is the preponderant glandular pattern of PC as seen under the microscope. By definition, it composes a minimum of 51% of the picture and possibly as much as 95% of the picture. In contrast, the secondary grade must represent at least 5% and as much as 49% of the glandular architectural pattern.

The most common Gleason score seen in biopsies obtained during contemporary times is (3,3). Gleason scores of (4,4), (4,5), (5,4), and (5,5) make up about17% of all PC cases.[153] The Gleason score of 7 is a special situation that has significant implications depending on whether the 7 is a (3,4) or a (4,3). This distinction is based solely on the amount of Gleason grade 4 PC that is present. As previously stated, a (3,4) could have as little as 5% Gleason grade 4 disease or as much as 49%. In contrast, a Gleason score of (4,3) must, by definition, have at least 51% Gleason grade 4 disease and possibly as much as 95% (since there must be at least 5% of Gleason grade 3 PC in a (4,3) lesion). A major difference in prognosis has been found for patients with a Gleason score of (3,4) versus (4,3) located within the RP specimen.[154–156] The new Partin Tables for 2001 have different readings of risk assessment for Gleason score (3,4) versus (4,3) on the diagnostic biopsy specimen.[157] This distinction is easily seen when using the PC Tools II software program developed by Dr. Glenn Tisman (available on the PCRI website at www.pcri.org).

Table 11: *PSA Leak Versus Weighted Gleason Grade.*

The weighted Gleason grade is applicable when there are multiple core biopsies showing various Gleason scores. In such a setting, an average weighted Gleason score is determined. Half of that number would be the weighted Gleason grade. If all biopsy cores indicate (3,3), it makes no difference; the average weighted Gleason grade would, of course, be 3. In this table, an undifferentiated PC with a Gleason score of 10 would have an average Gleason grade of 5 (bolded) and a PSA leak of only 0.93, or approximately 1 (both bolded). In contrast, the most common Gleason score (3,3) having a weighted Gleason grade of 3 would have a PSA leak that is 4.26, or approximately 4 times higher. That means that for each cubic centimeter of PC, the Gleason score 10 lesion is leaking one-fourth the amount of PSA into the serum.

Gleason Grade (weighted)	PSA Leak (rounded off)	PSA Leak (exact)
5	1	**0.93**
4.5	1.5	1.36
4	2	1.99
3.5	3	2.92
3	**4**	**4.26**
2.5	6	6.23
2	10	9.12
1.5	15	13.33
1	20	19.49

Source: After Aihara et al.(1994)[127]

In the hands of expert pathologists, focused only on PC pathology, the Gleason score identification is one of the most important biological determinants of prognosis. I have suggested that the Gleason score be embellished with what I call the Gleason differential: a quantification of the amount (in percent) of Gleason grade 4 or 5 in the pathology specimen. Therefore, a patient with a Gleason score of 7 that is (4,3) might have 95% Gleason grade 4 and only 5% Gleason grade 3 to give the following Gleason differential: GS(4,3)[95/5]. In contrast, he might only have 51% Gleason grade 4 or a Gleason differential of GS (4,3)[51/49]. Evaluations of the *diagnostic biopsy* material that quantitate the amount of Gleason grade 4 or 5 disease may allow for a further enhancement in the prognosis of PC.

These variables are part of the equation to determine extent and amount of PC as well as the ability to deliver specific kinds of therapy with greater or lesser probability of disease progression after completion of such therapy. Pending this kind of input, the astute physician, empowered patient, and partner can determine what other tests should be considered or discarded. Additionally, with this *foundational* information at hand, the healthcare team can use history to develop a risk assessment for the patient that relates to outcome: What is the probability that your treatment will be successful? Again, the latter presumes that the therapist delivering the treatment is as talented as the physicians involved in the studies that were the basis for the risk assessment.

Cross One Bridge at a Time

A common path that patients and partners as well as physicians take after a diagnosis of PC is to immediately make the choice of a treatment option the main focus. Too often, a patient goes from a diagnosis to a bone scan, often a CT scan, and then to the discussion of treatment options. The medical detective work of assessing the patient's risk for organ-confined disease versus nonorgan-confined disease is just not done routinely.

The risk assessments involved with PC take the form of multiple inputs into a statistical evaluation in which the output has more statistical significance than any single input. In such a scenario, the whole is greater than the sum of its parts. These assessments are termed algorithms, nomograms, neural nets, etc.[154,158–160] They look at data in terms of searching for meaningful variables and then combine these variables to provide a closer sense of the truth about a particular patient based on how other patients with the same variables fared in a large series of patients. This is the essence of what we call the Partin Tables.

Partin et al. looked at the findings of radical prostatectomy (RP) and noted whether or not the pathologic findings showed the PC to reflect OCD, and whether there was evidence of capsular penetration (CP), seminal vesicle (SV) or lymph node (LN) involvement.[104,157,161] Statistical analysis was done to determine which presurgical findings would equate with a high probability of these RP findings upon pathological review of the surgical specimens. This is the essence of many of the tools we use to assess risk for the hypothetical patient. Everyone is unique in his or her biology, but a general statement of risk can still be presented to the patient.

Unfortunately, despite the availability of this tool and many others similar to it, perhaps only 5–10% of physicians go through the discipline of doing the

Partin Table and/or other algorithmic calculations. Sitting down and inputting medical variables of known significance and doing the homework involved in the risk assessment of the PC patient is a very crucial step in a logical, rational approach to this disease. Not only the patient but also the physician should be crossing one bridge at a time. When this is done, the PPP team reaches a superior understanding of the disease process and attains a greater sense of what is likely to be the reality for a particular patient.

Appendix F in the *Primer* goes into great depth about these diagnostic and staging variables. The reader is referred to *Appendix F* for further information. In addition, the May 2001 issue of the *PCRI Insights* newsletter contains a comprehensive review of risk assessment algorithms by Glenn Tisman, M.D. This issue can be obtained online at www.pcri.org or by calling the PCRI at (310) 743-2110. The software section on the PCRI website also has risk assessment computer programs that can be downloaded without charge.

What does all this lead to? It leads to a more accurate assessment of the patient's true status. Knowing where the PC may have spread gives direction to the PPP team to perform certain tests to exclude disease at those site(s). For example, if the algorithms show a high risk for lymph node disease, the staging process should include the monoclonal antibody scan called ProstaScint. However, if the risk is negligible for lymph node involvement, this study could be excluded. The same approach is used to evaluate disease at the different stations of involvement. Is there disease in the capsule of the prostate, the seminal vesicles, the lymph nodes, or the bones? If one finds a high probability of disease confined to the prostate, then local therapies such as RP, RT (3D conformal radiation, IMRT, seed implantation, HDR, or a combination of these radiation approaches), or cryosurgery can be used with a greater probability of success. However, there are caveats that relate to the successful use of these therapies as well.

What Does This Mean for Patients?

Algorithms involve human experiences of men who have gone before you. Take advantage of the information that others have provided you. Obtaining data from the algorithms is critical homework that must involve you and your medical coaches. Assessing your risk for PC spread to particular sites and evaluating those sites with special testing is an essential part of the successful management of the man with PC. Remember, if man does not learn from history, he is forced to repeat it.

6. KNOWING PROS AND CONS OF WEAPONRY: UNDERSTANDING PROS AND CONS OF TREATMENT OPTIONS

In winning a military battle, an understanding of the appropriate strategy for the situation at hand is critical for success. Military tactics, including the weapons used, must be matched intelligently to the circumstances that are present. The same is true for the management of PC and other illnesses. The most important aspect of this match is the realization that a local treatment will have its greatest chance of being curative if the biological expressions of disease suggest that it is likely that only local disease is present. Therefore, obtaining as many insights as possible into what constitutes a high probability of OCD is warranted.

The preceding sections have laid the groundwork, the reconnaissance so to speak, for the gathering of that information. The medical strategist takes these variables into account and builds a case for or against local therapy. The major algorithms such as the Partin 2001 Tables[157] and the nomograms from Kattan et al.,[162–164] D'Amico et al.,[76,158] Narayan et al.,[73] Bluestein et al.,[165] Gilliland et al.,[166] Lerner et al.,[167] Pisansky et al.,[168] and others[72,109,154,159,160,169–180] should be used. These only take minutes to do and there is little to lose in seeing if a consensus is present for organ-confined disease.

If an assumption is made that a patient has a high probability of organ-confined disease and that there are no medical issues or financial issues that preclude any particular choice of local procedure to cure PC, the $64,000 question is this: "What procedure has the best track record?" Certainly, given the many publications on this subject over the last few years, one would have to state that overall there is no striking difference in success rates between any of the local therapies for PC—RP, RT of any type, or cryosurgery.[181–183] The longest follow-up period after definitive local therapy relates to RP. However, it appears unlikely that the 10- and 11-year data following RT are going to suddenly deteriorate or that the 15-year data after RP are going to change. The follow-up data after cryosurgery are at most 10 years old with most of the modern-day approaches to this technique beginning in 1992 with the work of Onik and Cohen et al.[184,185] The cryosurgery literature is more difficult to evaluate because in the last 10 years there have been major technological advances. These include the following:

- The use of temperature monitoring using thermo-couples[143,186,187]

- The use of double and triple freezing techniques[143,186]

- The use of Argon gas[188–190] instead of liquid nitrogen to induce the freezing necessary for creation of the iceball

- The recent use of templates to guide the placement of the cryosurgery probes, similar to those used in brachytherapy[191]

The fine points of RP, RT, and cryosurgery are extensively dealt with in the *Primer* (now available through amazon.com, Barnes & Noble, Borders, and the Life Extension Foundation at (866) 820-7457).

The issue then is which of these local therapies, if any, does the patient choose. Assuming that the patient at risk is not a candidate for watchful waiting, any of these therapies might be a perfectly reasonable strategy to eradicate organ-confined or regionally confined PC. My recommendations to patients on this matter are based on the following differential factors:

- Age

- Overall medical status after a detailed examination

- Patient priorities

- Patient access to experts in the selected modality of therapy

- Financial and insurance issues

- Lower urinary tract symptoms (LUTS) at the time of diagnosis

- Prostate gland volume

- History of scar formation (keloids) after any prior surgery

- Baseline PAP

- Baseline plasma TGF-b1, IL-6, and IL-6 soluble receptor levels

- PSA response to ADT (androgen deprivation therapy) after 3 months of therapy

In essence, a combined modality analysis of sorts is being employed. This involves variables that have not been interactively evaluated as part of an effort to define the best local therapy for an individual patient. Hopefully, a true nomogram or artificial neural net (ANN) looking at such additional variables can validate their significance for such an analysis.

Some of these issues have been discussed in prior sections. A short review of each of these topics is justifiable for this section.

Age

Traditionally, patients beyond age 70 are excluded as being candidates for RP. I believe that this decision should be individualized based on the patient's health, youthfulness for his age, and the other listed factors rather than using age as an arbitrary reason for excluding a patient. I have evaluated some men in their 50s who are much older in appearance and in biological status than their stated age. I have seen others in their late 70s who appear to be in their early 60s and who are healthier on examination than men in their 60s.

Overall Medical Status after Detailed Examination

This has been alluded to in the section on medical record-keeping and the use of summary and/or surveillance forms. Patients being considered for any invasive procedure should have a thorough physical examination. Factors that place them at much higher risk for morbidity after RP, RT, or cryosurgery should be candidly discussed with the patient and his partner.[192] Cardiovascular disease, Type II diabetes, kidney disease, hypertension, and neurodegenerative diseases should be red flags that an invasive procedure may be associated with greater adverse effects.[192,193] The evaluation of the patient's cardiac status with triglyceride/HDL ratios[194,195] as well as the conventional LDL and total cholesterol levels, the use of hypersensitive C-reactive protein,[196–198] and homocysteine levels are reasonable to do in this setting (*discussions of these topics can be found in several other protocols in this volume*).

The use of fasting insulin levels and the ratio of AA to EPA may be an excellent screening tool to evaluate the overall health of a patient considering any of these procedures.[199–202] In addition to a very thorough internal medicine history and physical examination, the studies that I have found particularly revealing include a stress echocardiogram with calculation of the ejection fraction and electron beam tomography with coronary artery calcium scoring.[196]

A significant factor in patients having problems with RP, RT, or cryosurgery is small vessel disease due to diabetes or hypertension. Diabetic patients represent a great challenge because of the prolonged delay in return of urinary function after any local therapy. Tissue healing is not optimal in such a setting.

Patient Priorities

The patient's inclinations toward a particular therapy are often a product of decades of programming that will not be undone in a course of weeks or even months. Some men are adamant about having surgery, while others are exactly the opposite. Some feel that RT is the choice for them, while others are more comfortable with freezing. The poet Robert Frost may have encountered this same problem and reflected upon it in "Fire and Ice:"[203]

Fire and Ice

Some say the world will end in fire,
Some say in ice.
From what I've tasted of desire
I hold with those who favor fire.
But if I had to perish twice,
I think I know enough of hate
To say that for destruction ice
Is also great
And would suffice.

There are those patients who cannot decide between fire (RT), ice (cryosurgery), or surgery and who instead pursue objectified ongoing observation. But as my father used to tell me, "That's what makes horse racing."

Patient Access to Experts in the Selected Modality of Therapy

I have no issues with any decision that a patient and his partner make if it has reasonable backing with biological data and the ability to involve physicians with gifted technical skills. Patients should interact with their fellow patients at support groups, asking about the details of experiences with local physicians in these fields. Patients and their partners should explore the Internet, looking for any listings of physicians considered to be outstanding in their skills.

Moreover, patients and their partners should have a formal consultation with the physician(s) that they are considering to see if there is rapport between all three parties and to witness the interaction of the physician with other patients in his or her medical office. The physician should be asked for names of patients who are willing to be telephoned by you and/ or your partner. These should be patients who have undergone the procedure within the last year or two. Obtaining three such names would be appropriate— perhaps one that had the procedure 6 months ago, another who had the procedure 12 months ago, and a third who had it 1 1/2–2 years ago. You should not be embarrassed to ask the physician about his success rate or about the incidence rates of complications his patients have experienced. These should be his figures and not those cited in someone else's series of patients.

Financial and Insurance Issues

The choices being made are quality-of-life decisions that also can affect quantity of life. Some patients may elect to stay within their medical insurance plans and feel that this is adequate for them.

Lower Urinary Tract Symptoms (LUTS) at the Time of Diagnosis

LUTS will often adversely affect the quality of life of a patient undergoing RT of any kind or cryosurgery. The physiological interaction is likely related to radiation urethritis due to RT or thermal (cold) injury to the urethra from cryosurgery.

LUTS can be quantified with the AUA symptom index score.[84,204] Patients should consider scores of 10 and higher as a relative negative risk factor in choosing RT or cryosurgery as a local therapy. A more powerful argument can be made for baseline AUA scores of 15 to 20 and higher. A relatively recent study used a combined modality assessment to determine what findings are most significant for predicting bladder outflow obstruction. A combination of an AUA symptom index of greater than 20, a prostate gland volume of 40 grams or more, and a urine flow of 10 mL or less per second, when present, predicted for obstruction 100% of the time.[86] Urine flow rate was determined using uroflowmetry.

The prophylactic and long-term use of alpha blockers (Flomax, Cardura, or Hytrin) to reduce LUTS prior to, during, and after brachytherapy has been reported to reduce the time to return to baseline urinary function.[84]

Prostate Gland Volume

Often, but not invariably, men with LUTS will have prostate gland enlargement due to BPH. The large gland volume is another confounding factor affecting potential radiation or cryotherapy-related injury to the urethra, rectum, and bladder. Options for the patient in such a situation include the use of ADT to reduce the gland size prior to local therapy. Usually, within 3 months of starting ADT, the gland volume will be reduced by as much as 40%. After 6 months of ADT, the gland volume may be reduced 60% or more from baseline. The proper use of ADT with monitoring of the serum testosterone using the goal of less than 20 ng/dL may be a factor in why some men have dramatic reductions in gland size with ADT and others do not. The use of three-drug ADT involving an anti-androgen plus Proscar or possibly another 5-alpha reductase inhibitor Avodart (dutasteride) in conjunction with an LHRH-agonist like Lupron, Zoladex, or Trelstar LA has provided me with excellent results in both prostate cancer reduction and prostate gland volume reduction.

In men who are reluctant to receive ADT and/or do not have a dramatic response to alpha-1-blockers, choosing an RP is an excellent way to eliminate LUTS and restore urinary function to a high level. The urologist is essentially providing the patient with a new urethra, without the adverse effect of compression of the urethra by an enlarged prostate. Urinary flow in such patients is restored to that of a young man. This presumes that the operating urologist is skilled in the RP procedure and has an impeccable track record with a complication rate for gross incontinence at less than 2%, but total continence rates in the order of 92–95% with no need for protective pads of any kind, and anastomotic stricture rates that are less than 5%.

History of Scar Formation (Keloids) after Any Prior Surgery

If we could identify patients most likely to develop complications, we could direct them to other therapeutic strategies. An investigation that comes close to this was done by Park et al.[205] This study correlates the probability of developing a narrowing or stricture after RP to a patient history of excessive scar formation from the actual RP or evidence of such scarring in prior surgical procedures. This study spanned a 5-year period and involved 753 radical retropubic prostatectomies performed by a single surgeon. The overall incidence of stricture at the anastomosis or connection of the bladder neck and distal urethra (anastomotic stricture) was 4.8%. The only significant finding that predicted the development of such a stricture was the maximal width of the abdominal scar resulting from the skin incision made at the time of RP.

In other words, the patient's reaction to surgery at a skin level was reflected in the tissue healing at the site of union (anastomosis) between the bladder neck and membranous urethra joined together after the excision of the prostate and prostatic urethra (*see Figure 5*). Men with a maximal scar of greater than 10 millimeters (mm) were 8 times more likely to develop strictures than men with smaller scars. The percentage of men who required protective pads 1 year following radical retropubic prostatectomy in the stricture group was 46.2%, while the figure for those without a stricture was 12.5%.

The authors of this study speculated that prior history of excessive scar formation may have implications in the adverse outcomes of other surgical procedures such as coronary bypass grafts, angioplasties, bile duct operations, etc. This is highly provocative, and the potential implication is that a history of excessive scar

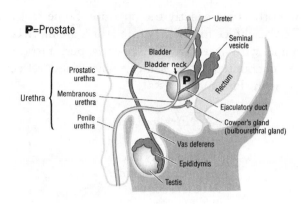

Figure 5. **The Anatomy of the Prostate in Relation to the Bladder Neck and Components of the Urethra.** During a radical prostatectomy (RP), the prostate and its prostatic urethra are excised and an anastomosis is made between the bladder neck tissue and the membranous urethra. (Modified from Figure 8 in *A Primer on Prostate Cancer, The Empowered Patient's Guide* by Strum, S.B. and Pogliano, D., Life Extension Media, 2002).

formation after any of the latter procedures may be a warning for those men considering a RP as a possible choice of local therapy.

Baseline PAP

The importance of the baseline PAP blood level has been published in three major papers.[74,75,206] These papers are referenced in detail in the *Primer*. The routine use of the PAP as part of our understanding of the biology of PC, its relation to the tumor cell population, and the probability of disease progression after RP or RT (with or without seed implantation) appears to be justified.

Baseline Plasma TGF-b1, IL-6, and IL-6 Soluble Receptor Levels

Molecular biomarkers relate the mechanisms of biologic behavior, function, and cell-to-cell interaction that add to the profile of the PC cell population. This has been known for PAP and PSA as well as CGA (chromogranin A) and NSE (neuron-specific enolase). Many physicians, however, are not aware of the functionality of biomarkers. For example, PSA has major activity as an enzyme—a kallikrein-like serine protease to be exact. PSA is a normal component of the seminal fluid component of the ejaculate and helps to keep the ejaculate liquid. However, as stated earlier, everything in life is a two-edged sword.

PSA produced from malignant prostate cells functions to break down specific proteins. These glycoproteins are found within the basement membrane of the microscopic glandular architecture. Simply, they are the ground

Table 12: *Plasma TGF-b1, IL-6, and IL-6 Soluble Receptor Pre-RP and Post-RP.*

This battery of laboratory tests done on plasma can predict the findings at RP and also the patient's post-operative course. Modified from Shariat, S.F., Shalev, M., Menesses-Diaz, A. et al. *J. Clin. Oncol.*; 19: 2856–64, 2001.

Preoperative Test Findings			Positive (+) or Negative (−) Correlations at RP				
TGF-b1	IL-6	IL-6sR	ECE	SV	GS	LTvol	LN
®	--	--	−	−	+	+	−
--	«	«	+	+	−	−	−
--	--	--	+	+	+	+	+
Postoperative Test Findings			Correlations with Clinical Course Postoperatively				
−	−	−	Nonprogression of PC post-RP				
«	−	−	**Progression of PC post-RP**				

Key: ® not significantly elevated; -- significantly elevated; ⁻ significantly decreased; « no significant change; ECE = extracapsular extension; SV = seminal vesicle involvement; LN = lymph node involvement; GS = Gleason score at RP (+ = higher; − = lower); LTvol = local tumor volume (cancer within prostate gland).

substance to which the basal cells of the prostate glands are anchored. PSA degrades these proteins (fibronectin and laminin) and facilitates invasion by the PC cells. Thus, PSA made by the PC cell population is not only a biomarker of disease activity, but also a functional protein that is important to the survival of the cancer cell. Reducing PSA is therefore not only a good sign that a therapy is working, but also that one is reducing a substance that facilitates spread of the disease.[207] In another publication, PSA was shown to suppress T-cell mediated immunity.[208] This functional activity of PSA may be mediated by TGF-b1 production from the prostate cell.[209]

That cell products that we identify as biomarkers may have function appears to be the case for virtually every cell product identified. They have function as well as form. Another enzyme produced by both benign and malignant prostate cells is uPA. uPA was discussed earlier in this review (*see the section on General Preventive Measures*). uPA is stimulated by IGF-1 and inhibited by GLA and EPA. uPA is believed to play a key mechanistic role in PC invasion and metastasis.[210]

TGF-b1 is a growth factor produced by the prostate cell as well as by cells of the bone matrix. Interleukin-6 (IL-6) is a cell product, or cytokine, that is made essentially by the primary tumor as well as by osteoblasts. IL-6 facilitates bone resorption by acting on IL-6 receptors located on the osteoclast and osteoclast precursor cells. This incredible cascade was illustrated in Figure 1 of this chapter. Studies recently published by Shariat et al. show a very strong positive correlation between higher plasma levels of pre-RP TGF-b1 and findings at RP of ECE (extracapsular extension), seminal vesicle involvement, and lymph node involvement.[211] In this study, preoperative plasma TGF-b1 median levels of approximately 15 ng/mL was significantly associated with lymph node and bone metastases. Healthy noncancer controls and men with RP findings not indicating extra-prostatic involvement had median levels of TGF-b1 of 4.7–4.8 ng/mL.

In a subsequent study involving 302 men with clinically localized PC, the same investigators evaluated preoperative and postoperative plasma TGF-b1 levels, and also IL-6 and its soluble receptor (IL-6sR), to determine correlations with disease progression. Of the study participants, 88.8% of the men had PSA progression-free survival at 3 years and 85.1% remained progression-free at 5 years post-RP. Cancer progression occurred in 43 of the 302 men (14%), with average postoperative follow-up of 50.7 months. Of the 43 men with PC progression, 19 were categorized as having nonaggressive progression postoperatively because they had complete responses to salvage RT or because their PSA doubling times postoperatively were equal to or greater than 10 months.

The remaining 24 men had aggressive progression because of positive lymph nodes found at RP (n = 6), because of positive metastatic workup on bone or ProstaScint scan (n = 6), because their PSA doubling times were less than 10 months (n = 23), or because they failed to respond to salvage RT (n = 14). What Shariat and colleagues found were significantly higher pre- and postoperative TGF-b1 levels and higher preoperative IL-6 and IL-6sR levels in men with "aggressive progression" versus those with "nonaggressive progression." These findings are summarized in Table 12.

This laboratory testing is allowing us to use the biology of the patient's tumor cell and host interaction to declare the probabilities of organ-confined disease versus nonorgan-confined disease. These findings are nicely in keeping with the Lerner algorithm from the Mayo Clinic in Rochester, MN. In that large-scale study, 904 men with apparently pathologically organ-confined PC were found to have PSA recurrences within 5 years based on the RP Gleason score, baseline PSA, and whether or not the PC at surgery had a normal DNA amount (diploidy) or abnormal amount (aneuploidy). Even in the best of circumstances, with baseline PSA values of less than 10 ng/mL, a Gleason score at RP of 6, and diploidy, the data still show a biochemical failure rate of 15% within the first 5 years. If the RP specimen was aneuploid, this increases the failure probability to 30%. It would be of interest to see whether the TGF-b1 status of the patient is independent of the ploidy status. Evolving algorithms using these kinds of inputs will clarify our recommendations to patients and their partners.

PSA Response to ADT after 3 Months of Therapy

Michael Zelefsky of Memorial Sloan Kettering (New York City), a radiation oncologist, published a paper about the predictive value of the PSA after 3 months of ADT.[212] The purpose of his study was to identify prognostic variables that predict for improved biochemical and local control outcomes in patients with localized PC who had been treated up-front with ADT, which was then followed by three-dimensional conformal radiotherapy (3D-CRT).

Between 1969–1995, 213 patients with apparently localized PC were treated with 3 months of ADT before 3D-CRT. The ADT consisted of leuprolide acetate and flutamide (ADT_2). The purpose of ADT was to reduce the preradiotherapy target volume in order to decrease the dose delivered to adjacent normal tissues and minimize the risk of morbidity from high dose RT. The median pretreatment PSA level was 13.3 ng/mL (range of 1–360 ng/mL). The median 3D-CRT dose was 73.6 Gy (range of 64.8–81 Gy), and the median follow-up time was 3 years (range of 1–7 years).

The significant predictors for improved outcome identified by multivariate analysis included a pretreatment PSA level less than or equal to 10.0 ng/mL (p < 0.001), an ADT-induced preradiotherapy PSA nadir of less than or equal to 0.5 ng/mL (p < 0.001), and a clinical stage less than or equal to T2c (p < 0.04). The 5-year PSA relapse-free survival rates were 93%, 60%, and 40% for patients with pretreatment PSA levels less than or equal to 10 ng/mL, 10–20 ng/mL, and greater than 20 ng/mL, respectively (p < 0.001). *Patients with preradiotherapy nadir levels after 3 months of ADT_2 that were less than or equal to 0.5 ng/mL experienced a 5-year PSA relapse-free survival rate of 74%, as compared with 40% for patients with higher nadir levels (p < 0.001).* The incidence of a positive

biopsy among 34 patients pretreated with ADT was 12%, as compared with 39% for 117 patients treated with 3D-CRT alone who underwent a biopsy (p < 0.001).

Zelefsky and colleagues concluded that, in settings of PC treated with ADT_2 and high dose 3D-CRT, pretreatment PSA, preradiotherapy PSA nadir response, and clinical stage are important predictors of biochemical outcome. Patients with PSA nadir levels greater than 0.5 ng/mL after 3 months of ADT_2 are more likely to develop biochemical failure after radiotherapy and may benefit from more aggressive therapies. A summary of these findings is shown in Table 13.

What Zelefsky et al. have done is to use the biological response of the tumor to indirectly gain insight into the tumor biology in order to help assess the probability of successful outcomes with radiation therapy. A low probability of success should prompt the PPP team to discuss different treatment strategies.

The reduction of PSA to a lowest point or nadir is the same principle used in our study on intermittent androgen deprivation (IAD) to identify men with a high probability of PC that most likely reflects a homogeneous tumor cell population of androgen-dependent cancer cells.[213] In our study, we used an ultrasensitive PSA and required a threshold of less than 0.05, 10 times more than the threshold of acceptability in the Zelefsky study. *It is quite conceivable that the use of the PSA nadir is identifying a number of biological events that would equate with a better prognosis or response to therapy in general.*

For example, the ability to drop the PSA to very low levels suggests that androgen-independent PC (AIPC) is not present. If it were, the efficacy of

Table 13: *Relationship of Pretreatment PSA Levels and 5-Year Relapse-Free Survival in PC Patients Treated with ADT_2 and High-Dose 3D-CRT According to Zelefsky et al.[212]*

Prognostic Finding	Five-year Relapse-Free Survival
PSA £ 10	93%
PSA > 10 £ 20	60%
PSA > 20	40%
PSA nadir £ 0.5 after 3 m*	74%
PSA nadir >0.5 after 3 m*	40%

*After 3 months of neoadjuvant androgen deprivation with Flutamide, 250 mg every 8 hours, plus Lupron, 7.5 mg i.m. monthly. This is the PSA value after a full 3 months of ADT, i.e., the PSA taken just prior to starting the fourth injection of Lupron.

androgen deprivation would not decrease the PSA to the very low levels determined with an ultrasensitive PSA assay such as the Tosoh or DPC Immulite Third Generation assay. AIPC represents PC that has undergone mutation. It is associated with more aggressive PC that is also more likely to have left the prostate. If so, then RT would be less effective in preventing biochemical recurrence manifested by a persistently rising PSA after RT is completed. This *may* be one of the operative factors in the Zelefsky study.

Additionally, resistance factors to RT may have also developed in a setting of mutated tumor. This might be related to an increased amount of the anti-apoptosis protein bcl-2, which confers radiation resistance. It could also be attributed to elevated levels of mutated p53.[214–216] Lastly, in a study by Rakozy et al. on the use of up-front (neoadjuvant) androgen deprivation with RT, it was shown that levels of mutated p53 in PC tissue biopsied from patients failing RT were significantly increased in patients who had not received neoadjuvant ADT compared to those who did receive ADT (82% versus 38%, respectively).[217] bcl-2 and *mutated* p53 are adverse biochemical findings because they protect the cancer cell from undergoing apoptosis.

PSA also reflects tumor volume. RT is a volume-dependent modality. It is also reasonable to consider that the PSA threshold of 0.5 or less after 3 months of ADT_2 required in the study reflects a significantly diminished tumor cell volume. This would enhance the efficacy of any form of RT because the target volume is smaller. ADT also decreases angiogenesis by reducing VEGF.[218] A major stimulus to increase VEGF and angiogenesis occurs in the centers of large tumors where oxygen tensions are low and cells cannot extract as much oxygen. This is called tumor hypoxia, and its occurrence is associated with resistance to radiation. *If ADT is decreasing the size of the tumor, the probability of tumor hypoxia is less and also the ability of the tumor to nourish itself or spread via new blood vessel growth (angiogenesis) is less, again due to the effect of ADT.*[218] Therefore, the Zelefsky publication is a landmark paper because it stimulates much thinking as to what explanation exists for its findings. It should also prompt others to test the many hypotheses that are implicit in this study.

All of the biological events above are pertinent to translating the findings of the patient's clinical situation into a real-time medical strategy. They should direct the team to select a particular tactic(s) pending the biological feedback obtained because, in biological reality, all of these tests are reflections of the tumor-host interaction. Therefore, in all six steps discussed so far, we are investigating biological indicators—medical gauges or LEDs—to help us obtain true information about the enemy and how our soldiers will likely fare in a particular medical-military tactic. This is the essence of Lewis Thomas's *The Lives of a Cell*, the foundation of Eastern philosophy that the microcosm reflects the macrocosm (and vice versa) and the truth behind optimizing outcomes for any issue vital to life.

Hormone Therapy in Advanced PC

Hormone therapy may be used in advanced PC (Stage 3) or cancer that spreads beyond the prostate (Stage 4; metastasis often to the bones). Hormone therapies such as anti-androgens and estrogens (e.g., ethinylestradiol) are used to reduce testosterone levels (androgen ablation therapy). Hormone analogues are also used as anti-androgens, i.e., to interfere with the action of androgen.

A number of selective somatostatin analogues have been developed for clinical use in the treatment of PC. Somatostatin was first found in hypothalamic extracts and identified as a hormone that inhibited secretion of growth hormone. Somatostatins are regulatory hormones produced by neuroendocrine, inflammatory, and immune cells in the central nervous system and in most major peripheral organs. Somatostatin can act as an endocrine hormone; can participate in paracrine/autocrine regulation; or can act as a neurotransmitter. And when activated, many tumor cells produce somatostatin (Abrahamsson et al. undated).

Changes in PSA levels are commonly used to monitor response to PC therapy. A PSA value that declines by more than 50% is considered to indicate an objective clinical response to therapy in hormone-refractory disease. Often, measurement of another marker, chromogranin A (CgA), is required to accurately monitor response to treatment and to identify some patients with advanced disease who do not have elevated serum PSA (Deftos et al. 1996).

A study reported in the *Journal of Urology* evaluated whether a combination therapy of ethinylestradiol and somatostatin analogue can reintroduce objective clinical responses in patients with metastatic androgen ablation refractory prostate cancer. The test subjects (10 patients with stage D3 PC disease and bone metastases) had disease progression despite an initial response to combined androgen blockade and subsequent failure to anti-androgen withdrawal. The combined androgen blockade was discontinued and the patients were given 1 mg of oral ethinylestradiol daily and 73.9 mg of intramuscular lanreotide acetate (a somatostatin analogue) every 4 weeks. Serum PSA,

CgA, the Eastern Cooperative Oncology Group (ECOG) Performance Status, and bone pain scores were monitored (median, 18 months; range, 10–24 months).

Although the number of patients in the study group was small, results were encouraging when combination therapy was used: 90% of the patients experienced an objective clinical response and an improvement in symptoms. In 9 of 10 subjects, PSA decreased greater than 50% and in 3 subjects PSA normalized (less than 4 ng/mL). All subjects had significant improvement in bone pain (median duration 17.5 months) and ECOG Performance Status (median duration 18 months) without major treatment-related side effects. There was also a statistically significant decrease in serum CgA during administration and at the response to therapy (median 38.4%, range 28.6% to 64.9%) that was not increased at relapse. Although two patients died secondary to prostate cancer, all of the other patients were without disease progression (Di Silverio et al. 2003).

Note: *The ECOG Performance Status is used to assess disease progression, to assess how the disease affects the patient's daily activities, and to determine appropriate treatment and prognosis. The Status has Grades 0 to 5: 0, fully active, no physical restrictions; 1, physical restrictions, but ambulatory and able to do light work; 2, ambulatory, can care for self, active more than 50% of waking hours, but unable to perform any work activity; 3, self-care is limited, in bed or chair more than 50% of waking hours; 4, completely disabled, no self-care, confined to bed or chair; 5, deceased.*

7. UNDERSTANDING ENEMY VULNERABILITY: LEARNING PRINCIPLES UNDERLYING TUMOR GROWTH

To understand the weakness and vulnerability of an enemy in military battle, one must first try to understand his apparent strengths. The analogy of the tumor or cancer cell being the societal equivalent to a terrorist is a strong one. What we learned and are still learning from September 11, 2001, is that we did not understand the strengths of the enemy. Hence, we were not successful in deterring a successful incursion by the terrorists on September 11. If we do not learn from this historical event, we will see history repeated. The same remarks about cancer are true.

What are the characteristics of malignancy that justify a metaphor with terrorists? First of all, both arenas often share common terminology. Some comparable words include "disorderly," "inflammatory," "primitive," "network," "radical," "invasive," "instability," "hits," "cells," "resistance," "surveillance," "eradication," "preemptive," "checkpoints" and "survival."

Every cancer, including prostate cancer, is a *disordered* and abnormal cell growth. Cancer cells have lost the ability to *network* and communicate in the way that normal cells do, and they no longer function as intended in the overall framework of body chemistry. Such cells take on a demeanor of juvenile delinquents, with no respect for parental direction. Attempts to restrict disruptive or nonproductive behavior are ignored. Such disruptive cells are usually censored and expelled by regulatory monitors—guardians of the genome, proteins such as p53, p21, and p27, which normally identify and biologically excise such *maladapted* cells. In malignant conditions, these regulatory proteins lose control for largely unknown reasons.

In one study involving the development of malignancy of the esophagus, antibodies to p53 were found in 4 of 36 (11%) premalignant lesions of the esophagus and in 10 of 33 (30%) of those with cancer of the esophagus. In two of the esophageal cancer patients, the p53 antibodies were detected prior to a clinical diagnosis of cancer.[219] Therefore, the cellular counterparts of terrorists are finding a way past one of the surveillance mechanisms (p53) that usually stand guard to detect DNA damage and halt the machinery of the cell cycle in G1 or G2 when DNA defects are found (*see Figure 3*). In a later section, another mechanism that tumor cells and viruses use to get past the surveillance system will be discussed.

The development of malignancy results from a combination of *hits* on the cell—repeated *insults*. Initial factors that lead to cancer production (carcinogenesis) are shown in Figure 6. Ongoing promotional and progression events eventually lead to premalignant changes such as prostatic intraepithelial neoplasia (PIN), then to noninvasive cancer, and finally to invasive cancer. If not diagnosed early and eradicated, metastatic cancer may eventually develop.

Malignant tumors develop multiple genetic abnormalities that accumulate progressively in individual cells during the course of tumor evolution. For example, abnormalities involving p53 generally occur early in the development of invasive breast cancers.[220] What biological situation(s) or conditions allow p53 or other DNA repair proteins, the guardians at the gate, to become mutated enough to allow such expressions? If we know what steps are involved in this process(es), we can avoid or reduce them and prevent initiation or promotional events.

Table 19: *Commonly Reported Acute and Chronic ADS Symptoms.*

These are possible findings that may occur in men receiving ADT. Many of these issues can be prevented, lessened, or resolved as part of the supportive care directed to the PC patient. This improves the therapeutic index of ADT. The PC patient and his partner, as a result, have an improved quality and quantity of life.

System or Tissue Affected	Symptom Onset and Details	
	Acute (Symptoms in < 2 Months)	**Chronic** (Symptoms in > 6 Months)
Sexual	Decrease in libido; decrease in erectile ability	Penile shrinkage; testicular atrophy
Psycho-social	Mood "swings;" easy crying	Depression; hostility
Endocrine	Hot flashes; poor blood sugar control in patients with diabetes	Gynecomastia (breast enlargement)
Musculo-skeletal	Loss of energy, feeling weak; aches and pains in joints and muscles	Decrease in strength and endurance; muscle atrophy; chronic fatigue-like symptoms; osteoporosis
Skin and nails	Increased dryness	Thinning of skin; nails brittle and break easily
Body mass		Weight increase due to increased body fat; blood pressure control more difficult
Central nervous system	Decrease in short-term memory	Alzheimer's-like symptoms (severe short-term memory difficulties, inability to concentrate, etc.)
Hematologic	Anemia unrelated to blood loss, iron deficiency or bone marrow involvement	Chronic anemia
Urinary	Decrease or increase in urinary symptoms	
Lipids		Increase in LDL cholesterol and/or triglyceride levels

therefore a metabolite of testosterone and is five times more potent than testosterone in stimulating cell growth. In addition to this, Proscar also down-regulates the expression of the androgen receptor. Therefore, it should not be surprising that ADT_3, as described previously, would have the greatest potential for side effects due to androgen deprivation, but would also have a higher probability to have a greater anti-tumor effect on the PC cell population for the very same reason. If we were to routinely add the use of an alpha-1-blocker such as Hytrin or Cardura, we should have even greater effects against the PC population due to a decrease in microvessel density, down-regulation of bcl-2, and enhanced apoptosis (as discussed in the section on LUTS and shown in Table 17).

In fact, the designation ADT_4 could indicate the addition of a piperazinyl quinazoline compound of the alpha-1-blocker class to the standard ADT_3 regimen of LHRH-A, antiandrogen, and 5-alpha-reductase inhibitor.

As emphasized earlier, *there is a spectrum of side effects that may be seen with the use of ADT.* These untoward effects are highly variable from man to man. Some men have no significant clinical symptomatology associated with the use of ADT, while others state they cannot function with a reasonable quality of life. The supportive care of the patient by the physician in using ADT is vital to the acceptability of this very important modality used in the treatment of prostate cancer. We

Androgen deprivation with four agents or ADT_4 would involve the routine use of an agent of the quinazoline class of alpha-1-blockers such as Hytrin or Cardura. These agents will not only improve urinary flow, but also act to enhance the effects of ADT_3. Therefore, the typical ADT_4 regimen would include:

- LHRH-agonist: Lupron, Zoladex, Trelstar LA, or Viadur
- Antiandrogen: Eulexin, Casodex, or Nilandron
- 5-alpha-reductase inhibitor: Proscar or Avodart
- Alpha-1-blocker: Hytrin or Cardura

can improve the therapeutic index of ADT by finding solutions to the problems that may occur as part of the androgen deprivation syndrome, or ADS.

Signs and symptoms that are part of the spectrum of ADS are shown in Table 19. These are divided into systems or tissues affected and the nature and onset of the symptoms, that is, acute and chronic. Again, it is of vital importance to understand that there is significant variability from patient to patient regarding frequency of occurrence and timing of all such findings.

To assess the significance of common ADS symptoms, we evaluated 177 hormone-naïve PC patients consecutively treated with an LHRH-agonist and an antiandrogen between 1994–1997. We asked patients to grade the frequency and severity of ADS as absent

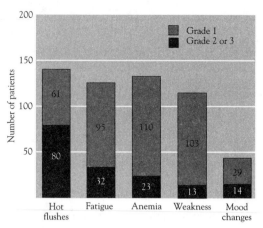

Figure 10. **Signs or Symptoms Relating to Most Common *Acute* Symptoms that May Be Seen in ADS.** Of the common side effects seen with ADT involving Grade 2 or 3 symptom intensity, hot flushes were most common at 45.1% (80/177) and fatigue was next at 18% (32/177). Although anemia occurred in 75% of the patients evaluated, it was found to be of Grade 2 to 3 intensity in only 23/177 or 12.9% of patients.

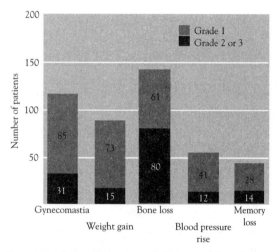

Figure 11. **Signs or Symptoms Relating to Most Common *Chronic* Symptoms that May Be Seen in ADS.** Of all findings that may occur in the chronic setting of androgen deprivation therapy, bone loss was most significant occurring in 45.1% of the patients studied.

(Grade 0), occasional (Grade 1), frequent or bothersome (Grade 2), or requiring drug therapy (Grade 3). Other than loss of libido and impotence, Figures 10 and 11 depict the most commonly reported acute and chronic symptoms. Only Grade 1, 2, or 3 findings are shown.

Several patient-related and treatment-related factors were found to influence the incidence and severity of ADS symptoms (*see Figures 12–14*). Figure 12 depicts hot flashes with respect to age, Figure 13 relates the intensity of anemia to the specific drugs used in ADT, and Figure 14 shows the effect of ADT duration on incidence of bone loss.

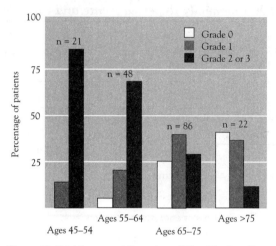

Figure 12. **Incidence and Severity of Hot Flushes Occurring in Younger Men on ADT.** Hot flushes were of significantly greater incidence and severity in patients less than 65 years of age. This most likely relates to the stronger stimulation by the hypothalamus on the pituitary to make LH in the absence of testosterone. The LH surges are believed to cause the severe hot flushes (flashes).

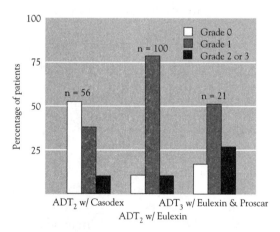

Figure 13. **Incidence and Intensity of Anemia Resulting from Androgen Deprivation May Relate to Intensity of ADT.** More intense anemia was observed with ADT_2 using Eulexin or in ADT_3 with the addition of Proscar. This strongly suggests that the degree of anemia may relate to the depth of androgen deprivation on a tissue level. Androgen receptors have been detected in the bone marrow. It therefore appears that three-drug ADT more profoundly affects androgen deprivation in this respect than two-drug ADT and that Eulexin has stronger anti-androgen effects than Casodex when using ADT_2.

Finally, the incidence and the intensity of bone loss are affected by the duration of ADT. This assumes that the patient on ADT is not receiving concomitant therapies to prevent bone resorption, e.g., a bisphosphonate plus a bone supplement in conjunction with an exercise program. The mechanism of progressive bone loss during ADT relates to the fact that androgens are known inhibitors of osteoclast function. During ADT, this inhibition is lost and osteoclasts are activated, allowing

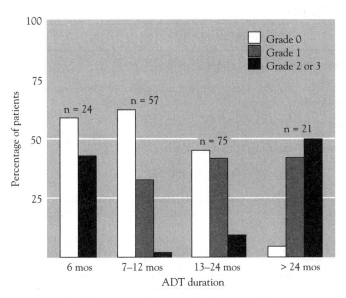

Figure 14. ADT Duration Affects the Incidence and Severity of Bone Loss. Symptoms and/or signs of bone loss invariably occur with the chronic administration of ADT. Of interest is that clinically significant bone loss is found also within the first 6 months of ADT and can affect the patient's quality of life. This often requires therapeutic intervention. It is suggested that all patients with PC, including those not receiving ADT, should understand the importance of bone integrity and the need to evaluate the bone mineral density and resorption status of the bones. PC patients should be actively treated with a combination of a bisphosphonate compound plus bone supplement and exercises. (Read the *Primer* for detailed information about bone integrity.)

for promotion of bone loss (resorption). Testosterone, therefore, is an anabolic steroid for bone, muscle and other tissues. The deprivation of androgens pushes the balance towards catabolism or breakdown. The data for this are shown in Figure 14.

Clearly, a comprehensive care plan that takes the overall health of the PC patient into account must look at the impact of each and every ADS-related finding. Prevention of the undesirable consequences of ADT equates with a higher therapeutic index, which in turn means a higher quality of life for the PC survivor. Therefore, the intelligent use of ADT, as with any therapy, should take into account the

• Therapeutic purpose of ADT

• Nature of ADT (neoadjuvant, intermittent, or continuous treatment)

• Age and overall general health of the patient

• Degree of tolerance by the patient of the various ADT side effects

• Prevention or resolution of any signs and symptoms of ADS

• Net picture of pros versus cons

For example, the duration of neoadjuvant ADT rarely exceeds 1 year in patients who are candidates for potentially curative local therapies with RT or cryosurgery. Therefore, such patients have the potential risk for the typical acute ADS symptoms, but they will not experience chronic ADS symptoms to any significant extent. Patients who may be involved in this scenario include those with large-volume PC within the prostate with extracapsular extension (ECE). Such patients fare better when ADT is used up-front (neoadjuvant therapy), prior to the RT or cryosurgery, to decrease both the cancer volume as well as the gland volume. In the *Primer*, Physician's Note #5 relays such a story in the case of patient GB. The patient completed IMRT over 3 years ago and his PSA remains flat at 0.4 ng/mL.

Even with a highly responsive physician who is knowledgeable about ADS, acute ADS-related symptoms invariably compromise the lifestyles of healthy and active prostate cancer patients. This mandates that certain changes be made in the patient's diet, exercise, and work habits during ADT.

Chronic ADS symptoms are much more prevalent in PC patients treated with ADT than are currently recognized, and some are nearly inevitable in patients treated for longer than 1 year. For such patients, specific treatment strategies must be implemented to minimize or prevent the development of chronic ADS. Left untreated, chronic ADS is progressive with ongoing ADT and often leads to other medical complications. Useful preventive or active strategies against acute ADS-related symptoms are shown in Table 20, and chronic ADS-related symptoms in Table 21.

In the past, patients who were not candidates for local therapy were typically treated with continuous androgen blockade. Armed with our current knowledge about the signs and symptoms of acute and chronic ADS, we prevent or correct these findings with one or more of the therapies listed in Tables 20 and 21.

Another approach that avoids symptomatology attributable to chronic ADT is through the use of intermittent androgen deprivation (IAD). Depending on the required duration of ADT, individually determined for patients, IAD may be a reasonable alternative approach. This is an example of how therapy should be individualized to the patient's biological constitution. (A discussion of IAD with graphs indicating outcomes using ADT_2 versus ADT_3 can be found in the *Primer*.)

Supporting the patient through measures such as some of those discussed relates to the fine-tuning that is characteristic of outstanding medical care. This is the essence of holistic medicine. There are other

Table 20: *Preventive and Active Treatments for Acute ADS-Related Symptoms*

Acute ADS-Related Symptom	Treatment Strategy
Hot flashes	Soy, genistein, Megace, Depo-Provera,[1] DES,[2] or venlafaxine (Effexor)[1]
Aches and pains in joints and muscles	Acetaminophen, ibuprofen, Fosamax,[1] Actonel,[1] Aredia,[1] or Zometa,[1] plus bone supplement, resistive exercise (weights, Bowflex), walking
Fatigue and feeling weak	Walking, muscle stretching
Memory difficulties	Ginkgo biloba,[3] Eldepryl, memory exercises, DMAE,[3] Cognitex[3]
Mood and emotional swings	Patience (may improve), Depo-Provera[1]
Symptomatic anemia (shortness of breath, chest pain, dizziness, severe weakness)	Injections of recombinant human erythropoietin (Procrit[1], Aranesp[1]); iron supplementation only if documented iron deficiency via low ferritin or elevated serum transferrin receptor (> 28.3)
Increased urinary frequency	Hytrin,[1] Cardura,[1] Flomax,[1] patience
Impotence and loss of libido	Viagra,[1] Muse,[1] (alprostadil intraurethral pellet) or Caverject,[1] or combinations of these.

[1]Physician's prescription is required to obtain medication.

[2]Not recommended in this setting due to toxicity.

[3]Available from health food suppliers, such as Life Extension Foundation.

Table 21: *Preventive and Active Treatments for Chronic ADS-Related Symptoms*

Chronic ADS-Related Symptom(s)	Treatment Strategy
Loss of muscle bulk and strength; worse in pectoral, biceps, and quadriceps	Exercise with light weights; Bowflex
Weight gain and fat redistribution	Sears's *Omega Rx Zone* approach; regular exercise
Chronic fatigue syndrome	Walking, regular exercise, avoid inactivity
Penile atrophy	Viagra[1] and other similar agents
Gynecomastia	Breast radiation to prevent; liposuction or surgery to treat severe established cases
Osteoporosis	Fosamax,[1] Actonel,[1] Aredia,[1] or Zometa[1] plus bone supplement; synthetic vitamin D (Rocaltrol[1]); aerobics, walking, resistive exercises
Alzheimer's-like symptoms	Ginkgo biloba,[3] DMAE;[3] see Life Extension Foundation protocols in this book for Alzheimer's disease; reading and other mind-stimulating activities
Increased serum cholesterol and triglyceride levels	Sears's *Omega Rx Zone* approach; if no help, Lipitor,[1] Pravacol,[1] Zocor,[1] Mevacor[1] (may require supplemental CoQ_{10}[3])

[1]Physician's prescription is required to obtain medication.

[2]Not recommended in this setting due to toxicity.

[3]Available from health food suppliers, e.g., Life Extension Foundation.

issues of supportive care that relate to the settings of pre- and postoperative care for a patient undergoing RP, cryosurgery, RT, and even watchful waiting. Some of these issues and possible resolution therapies worthy of your review and subsequent discussion with your physician are outlined in Table 22.

(7) Supportive Care for PC Patients Undergoing Chemotherapy: A comprehensive review of this topic is a book in itself and such a treatise is being considered. Due to limitations of space and time, this topic is not discussed at this time. The reader is advised to log on to the *Prostate Chemotherapy* protocol that can be accessed at www.lefprostate.org

11. BOOSTING MORALE OF THE TROOPS: FOSTERING A WILL TO LIVE, EMPOWERING THE PATIENT

The previous 10 sections have presented strategic issues that need to be addressed in our battle with

Table 22: *Some Considerations for Supportive Care Involved in Radical Prostatectomy, Radiation Therapy, Cryosurgery, and Watchful Waiting.*

Suggestions that can be discussed with your physician(s) to prevent adverse effects of any of the major therapies for PC (note that ADT and its supportive care were discussed in earlier sections).

PC-Related Complication	Strategy for Resolution of Adverse Effects
Radical Prostatectomy	
Need for blood transfusions	Pre- or perioperative use of Procrit[1] or Aranesp[1] and iron (only if biochemically indicated)
Incontinence	Kegel exercises (National Association for Continence at www.nafc.org); penile clamp, artificial urinary sphincter, urinary sling procedure
Impotence	Use of Viagra[1], Muse[1], combination therapy, injections of PGE$_1$, visual aids
Penile atrophy	Viagra[1] and other similar new agents; PGE$_1$
Anastomotic stricture	Avoidance of surgery if history of exuberant scar formation (keloids); use of Pentoxifyllene[1] and vitamin E[3]
Radiation Therapy (Any Kind)	
Urinary obstructive symptoms	Pre-RT use of ADT to reduce gland volume plus use of Cardura[1] or Hytrin[1]; for post-RT problems, use of Hytrin[1] or Cardura[1] and, if severe, supra-pubic tube; possibly transurethral laser surgery if scar tissue
Radiation injury to rectum (proctitis)	Rowasa[1] suppositories, SOD[3] (Orgotein[1] or superoxide dismutase[3]), vitamin E[3], Pentoxifyllene[1], Sears' *Omega Rx Zone* approach[3]
Radiation injury to bladder (cystitis)	Rowasa[1] suppositories, SOD[3] (Orgotein[1] or superoxide dismutase[3]), vitamin E[3], Pentoxifyllene[1], Sears' *Omega Rx Zone* approach[3]; avoid spicy foods, alcohol, coffee; use of Prelief[3]; trial of Elmiron[1]
Impotence	Use of Viagra[1], Muse[1], combination therapy, injections of PGE$_1$, visual aids
Incontinence	Kegel exercises (National Association for Continence at www.nafc.org); penile clamp
Cryosurgery	
Urinary obstructive symptoms	ADT prior to cryosurgery to reduce gland volume; post-cryosurgery use of supra-pubic tube; Cardura[1], Hytrin[1]
Incontinence	Kegel exercises (National Association for Continence at www.nafc.org); penile clamp, supra-pubic tube
Impotence	Use of Viagra[1], Muse[1], combination therapy, injections of PGE$_1$, visual aids
Watchful Waiting (Objectified Ongoing Observations)	
Progressive disease that is clinically out of control	Interval testing and physical examination (DRE); graphing trends in PSA dynamics (velocity, doubling time); Sears' *Omega Rx Zone* approach[3]; modified citrus pectin[3], dietary supplements[3]

[1]Doctors prescription is required to obtain medication.

[3]Available from health food suppliers, e.g., Life Extension Foundation.

prostate cancer. And, make no mistake, it is a battle—but one that can be won. There is much to be gained, by many people in viewing this medical confrontation using a military metaphor. Such tactical thinking undoubtedly plays a pivotal role in achieving an optimal outcome for any life-endangering encounters.

However, all the good science and all the outstanding medicine in the world will not achieve its true goal of healing without the presence of spirit. This may not seem relevant to the man feeling the immediate threat of prostate cancer because of its philosophical orientation. But, I assure you, over the course of your journey, at some important crossroad in your life, it will be seen as the take-home lesson for all that has been written here. Your spirit, your will to live fully, is the crust of the holistic pie of life. Without this *esprit*, it is unlikely that you would have accepted the challenge of reading this chapter.

> *Out of the night that covers me, black as the Pit from pole to pole,*
> *I thank whatever gods may be for my unconquerable soul.*
> – from *Invictus* by William Ernest Henley

The basis for any victory must therefore involve morale—a state of spirit of a person or group as exhibited by confidence, cheerfulness, discipline, and willingness to perform assigned tasks. Morale, as defined in this fashion, and in the context of a war against prostate cancer, is embodied in acts reflecting empowerment of the patient and his partner.

Empowerment in this context becomes a process by which people assert control over factors that affect their health. This comes as a result of sharing resources and collaboration, which in turn lead to a more complete understanding of all aspects of a health issue.[308] My perspective developed through thousands of patient encounters each year with prostate cancer is that the empowered patient is better able to decide on treatments, and better able to choose physicians to guide him on his medical journey. The empowered patient is less anxious and more secure about his clinical course.[309] Empowerment, by its very nature, links people with resources.[310]

The empowered patient will explore options, look for new trials, participate in adjunctive or complementary therapies to enhance treatment outcomes, and be interactive in support groups. The empowered patient will take a politically active stance to increase funding, research, and awareness of the disease. The empowered patient is the purveyor of his medical records. The empowered patient views the physician as co-navigator, companion, and friend on his medical journey. An empowered patient expects bidirectional communication with his medical team to be the rule and not the exception.

In the process of opening channels of learning to the patient, we foster his empowerment and that of his partner, and that in turn encourages further learning. This extension of the physician as educator to the patient at a time of need is a manifestation of love. From this love comes wisdom in many walks of life.

> *How do you choose to learn love?*
> *How do you choose to learn authentic empowerment—*
> *through doubt and fear, or through wisdom?*
> – Gary Zukav

Those of you with prostate cancer are focused on your lives—your life is in jeopardy and what you took for granted before is no longer guaranteed to be there in the years to come. But

> *Out of crisis comes opportunity.*
> – Old Chinese saying

or

> *A smooth sea never made a skilled mariner.*
> – English proverb

During this crisis of prostate cancer, you will be provided multiple opportunities to overcome many obstacles. This is part of the lesson of life, of living, and of evolving. Remember that there are many out there without prostate cancer who will live their lives, day after day, without the appreciation to see the beauty of a tree or a sunrise; to say I love you; to smell the flowers; to marvel at the innocence of children; and to appreciate the uniqueness of your humanity. But this journey you are on should not be just an appreciation of life at a time of crisis, which is conveniently forgotten once the crisis is over. There are lessons here, crucial to your well-being and to that of your family, friends, community, and to all life forms.

> *Life is the ultimate prize and it takes on ultimate value*
> *when suddenly we discover how tentative and fragile it can be.*
> *The essential art of living is to recognize and savor its*
> *preciousness when it is free of imminent threat or jeopardy.*
> – Norman Cousins

Louis Armstrong said: "It's a wonderful world." The creation is *wonder-full*. We are part of that creation. We are also the caretakers of this wonderful world. Prostate cancer should change your life; it should make you aware of this creation—not just the natural wonders, but the wonder of you and your fellow humankind—all are linked together in a system longing for balance and communication. This is the essence of health for all biological systems. This is the heart of all that has been discussed in this chapter and throughout this book.

> *Our humanity lies in our human unity.*
> – Strum

This statement is not a political one. It is a sociobiological expression of what should be the underlying theme of virtually all life forms. On a biological level we are multicelled organisms that seek to achieve and maintain high levels of communication to remain in balance. It is a restatement of yin and yang. On every level of existence, from that of cellular interactions to the complexity of the individual human being to societies and governments, the call is the same: communication and balance. Without this, our health declines. Without this, our world dies.

My vision is for an empowered patient, who now enters the new millennium with an ability to use technological enhancements that provide the patient/physician team with far-reaching insights into the natural history and treatment of disease. At the same time, this empowerment embraces human unity—humanity—a realization that we are all in this together. The empowered patient shares his newfound understanding with others. He leaves the world of "I" and enters the world of "we."

● SUMMARY

The objective of this chapter on prostate cancer has been to provide specific and critical data that are an integral part of the comprehensive care of a patient with prostate cancer. The use of military metaphor has not been used simply as a literary tool, but more as a unique perspective—a different way of looking at things—that may yield new approaches in thinking about what tactics we could employ in our war against cancer. What may surprise the reader is the enormity of published information that is not routinely incorporated into the prevention and active treatment of prostate cancer. Much of this involves an understanding of what encourages tumor growth and what enhances its rate of growth and its ability to metastasize. The reader is encouraged *not* to look for a paragraph or two that summarizes all of what has been presented here; this is not realistic. Instead, read one section at a time and ask yourself: "Is this applicable to my situation?" If so, then take this information to your physician(s) and provide him with the appropriate references. Providing information in this manner improves your situation and that of all patients under the care of such physicians.

The first part of this chapter dealt with prevention. This is of importance not only to family members (and others) concerned about contracting prostate cancer, but also to patients seeking to slow disease progression and enhance the odds of a successful long-term outcome. As was discussed, many of the lifestyle changes that reduce prostate cancer risk also interfere with existing cancer cell proliferation.

Understanding the biological principles of the disease is crucial to understanding why such meticulous attention should be paid to keeping an accurate medical record of all test results, lifestyle changes and therapeutic interventions. The medical record provides a basis for determining the status of the disease and what therapeutic modalities should be considered if adequate control of the disease has not been achieved.

By precisely assessing all of the measurable individual risk factors, a prostate cancer patient can better decide on the treatment options that offer the greatest opportunity for long-term control or cure, while minimizing potential side effects.

The knowledge base of how prostate cancer cells propagate and what can be done to interfere with these processes is colossal. This is good news for a prostate cancer patient who seeks a comprehensive scientific approach to eradicating his disease. Contrast this with a pancreatic cancer patient, who has little hope of survival beyond 12 months.

Prostate cancer can easily be diagnosed at an early curable stage. Recurrence of existing disease can also be readily monitored. This is different from other cancers, in which a patient often waits for a dreaded physical symptom before learning the cancer has occurred or recurred. The bottom line is that a prostate cancer patient can exert a tremendous amount of control over his disease. What has been written here provides a systematic guide to taking advantage of the many technologies available today.

The Life Extension Foundation has identified an extensive array of integrated prostate cancer therapies based on published scientific findings and the clinical experience of practicing oncologists. While this protocol provides information in a practical format, the cooperation of the attending physician is crucial.

WHERE TO GO FROM HERE

While this chapter on prostate cancer provides an abundant quantity of life-saving guidance, many patients will need additional information to address their particular type and stage of disease. A special website has been established (www.lefprostate.org) to provide comprehensive updates, along with information specific to different stages and treatment options. The following reports were posted on this website as of the writing of this protocol:

1. Prostate Cancer: Early-Stage

2. Prostate Cancer: Late-Stage

3. Prostate Cancer: Chemotherapy

4. Prostate Cancer: Adjuvant Therapy

5. Prostate Cancer: PSA Parameters and Heredity

6. Prostate Enlargement: Benign Prostate Hypertrophy

For specific information about implementing some of the adjuvant drug therapies discussed in this chapter, refer to the *Cancer Treatment: The Critical Factors* protocol in this book. Please remember that everything that is read should be done so with the conscious thought of how this could apply to the current situation.

Those who have prostate cancer are urged to log on to www.lefprostate.org to read in-depth discussions that pertain to their stage of the disease and the different therapeutic modalities to consider.

1. Nutritional Aspects of Prostate Cancer

   • Vitamins, minerals, and supplements that prevent PC or decrease mortality

      • Selenium and vitamin E
      • Genistein
      • Vitamin D
      • Minerals
      • Green tea
      • Lycopenes

   • Caloric restriction and reduction of carbohydrate intake

   • The eicosanoid pathway in relation to cancer promotion versus prevention

2. Early-Stage Prostate Cancer

   • Biology of prostate cancer

      • Staging
      • PSA dynamics (PSA velocity and doubling time)
      • Gleason score and the PSA leak
      • Clinical stage

   • Risk assessment and algorithms
   • Ingredients for successful outcomes

3. Androgen Deprivation Therapy (ADT)

   • Biology of ADT and its rationale
   • Combination ADT (ADT_2 and ADT_3)
   • Biomarkers to assess ADT efficacy
   • Side effects of ADT: the androgen deprivation syndrome (ADS)

4. Late-Stage Prostate Cancer

   • Androgen-independent prostate cancer (AIPC)
   • Androgen receptor mutation (ARM)
   • Antiandrogen withdrawal (AAW)

   • Effective therapies for AIPC

      • Ketoconazole
      • Estrogens (including PC SPES)

5. Chemotherapy for Prostate Cancer

   • Principles of chemotherapy
   • Supportive care of the patient

      • Bone marrow support
      • Nausea and vomiting avoidance

   • High-response chemotherapy regimens

      • Anthracyclines, for example, Adriamycin and Mitoxantrone
      • Cytoxan
      • Vinca agents, for example, Velban and Navelbine
      • VePesid or VP-16 regimens
      • Taxanes, for example, Taxotere and Taxol
      • Carboplatin
      • 5-Fluorouracil

   • Small cell prostate cancer

6. Hereditary Aspects of Prostate Cancer

GLOSSARY OF TERMS

3DCRT (3-DIMENSIONAL CONFORMAL RADIATION THERAPY): An approach to radiation treatment planning that focuses on directing the radiation energy to the tumor target while sparing surrounding normal tissues.

5-ALPHA REDUCTASE (5-AR): The enzyme that converts testosterone to dihydrotestosterone (DHT).

ADENOCARCINOMA: A form of cancer that develops from a malignant abnormality in the cells comprising a glandular organ, such as the prostate. Almost all prostate cancers are adenocarcinomas.

ADVANCED PROSTATE CANCER: Prostate cancer that is no longer organ-confined; systemic prostate cancer, sometimes with metastases to lymph nodes, seminal vesicles, bone, or vital organs of the body such as liver and/or lungs. Advanced prostate cancer is treated with systemic therapies currently in use such as androgen deprivation and chemotherapy.

AGONIST: A chemical substance, such as a drug, capable of combining with a receptor on a cell and initiating a reaction or activity. In PC, the LHRH agonist is also called LHRH-A. The most commonly used LHRH-As are Lupron and Zoladex. Either of these agents interacts with the LHRH receptor and forms a complex that results in a decrease in the release of LH over a period of 2 weeks and hence a lowering in serum testosterone.

ALGORITHM: In prostate cancer, one of a group of systems whereby the human experiences of a number of patients are statistically or numerically analyzed to produce data that can be generalized to predict the probable disease status of patients who have not yet been treated and therefore have no empirical data of their own on which to base judgments regarding their disease status. Examples include the Partin Tables, Narayan Stage, and Kattan Nomograms.

ALPHA-1 BLOCKERS: Oral medications prescribed to improve urine flow by relaxing periurethral smooth muscle tissue; those of the quinazoline class (Hytrin and Cardura) have been shown to be synergistic with Proscar in causing programmed cell death in prostate cells, both benign and malignant.

ALPHA-TOCOPHEROL ISOMER: A component of vitamin E.

AMERICAN UROLOGICAL ASSOCIATION (AUA) SYMPTOM INDEX SCORE: A series of subjective questions used by physicians to evaluate the extent of existing lower urinary tract symptoms.

ANASTOMOSIS: In prostate cancer, the surgical connection made between the bladder neck and the remaining urethra after the prostate is removed.

ANASTOMOTIC STRICTURE: In prostate cancer, a narrowing at the site of the anastomosis between the bladder neck and urethra after radical prostatectomy.

ANDROGEN: A hormone produced primarily by the testicles, but also in the cortex of the adrenal glands, that is responsible for male characteristics and the development and function of the male sexual organs and also affects muscle and bone mass, emotional stability, cognitive function, skin and hair, and so forth.

ANDROGEN-DEPENDENT PC (ADPC): Prostate cancer cells that depend on androgens for continued growth and vitality.

ANDROGEN DEPRIVATION SYNDROME (ADS): A constellation of symptoms directly or indirectly due to the drop in testosterone that occurs following surgical castration or the suppression of testicular and adrenal androgens by the use of medications.

ANDROGEN DEPRIVATION THERAPY (ADT): A prostate cancer treatment that is based on blocking the amount of available androgen to the prostate cancer cell.

ANDROGEN-INDEPENDENT PC (AIPC): Prostate cancer cells that do not depend on androgen for growth.

ANDROGEN RECEPTOR: A structural entity that is essentially a docking site for androgen to communicate with the cell and affect cell function. The substance interacting with the receptor is called a ligand. The interaction of ligand and receptor is a major mode of biochemical communication in all life forms.

ANEUPLOID: Having an abnormal number of sets of chromosomes.

ANEUPLOID: Cells that have an abnormal number of sets of chromosomes. Aneuploid cancer cells tend not to respond as well to androgen deprivation therapy.

ANGIOGENESIS: Relating to the formation of blood vessels.

ANTAGONIST: A chemical that acts within the body to reduce the physiological activity of another chemical substance.

ANTIGEN: A substance that elicits a cellular-level immune response or causes the formation of an antibody.

APOPTOSIS: Programmed cell death due to an alteration in a critical substance or chemical necessary for cell viability. For example, the lack of male hormones causes apoptosis of androgen-dependent prostate cancer cells.

ARACHIDONIC ACID (AA): An omega-6 fatty acid that is known to generate free radicals and is considered an unfavorable eicosanoid. AA is metabolized via enzymes of the COX and LOX family to generate prostaglandins, thromboxanes, leukotrienes, hydroxylated fatty acids, lipoxins, and 5-HETE compounds that are implicated in cancer, inflammatory disease, immune dysfunction, and degenerative disorders. Organ meats and egg yolk are rich in AA.

ARTIFICIAL NEURAL NET (ANN): An approach to analyzing data that uses statistical analysis of historical data to produce systems that can predict probabilities of future outcomes based on inputted variables.

BASELINE PSA: The PSA level before a new treatment has begun; used to establish the efficacy of a therapy based on response of the PSA to treatment.

BENIGN: Not malignant; noncancerous.

BENIGN PROSTATE HYPERPLASIA OR HYPERTROPHY (BPH): A noncancerous condition of the prostate that results in the growth of both glandular and stromal (supporting connective) tissue, enlarging the prostate and potentially leading to obstructive symptoms relating to urine flow (*see American Urological Association Symptom Index Score*).

BILATERAL: Both sides; for example, a bilateral nerve-sparing radical prostatectomy is one in which the nerves on both sides of the prostate are left intact.

BIOMARKER: An indicator of biological activity of cells or tissues that can be used as a means to monitor a state of health or disease. PSA is one of the most useful biomarkers in medicine.

BIOPSY: Sampling of tissue from a specific part of the body in order to check for abnormalities such as cancer.

BISPHOSPHONATES: A class of compounds that stops bone loss (resorption) by actions directed against the osteoclast.

BONE SCAN: An imaging technique using a radioactive isotope that is selectively taken up by bone tissue to identify abnormal or cancerous growths within bone such as metastases.

BRACHYTHERAPY: A form of radiation therapy in which radioactive seeds or wires are used to deliver the radiation dose close to the site of a tumor. Seeds can be permanently implanted or radioactive wires can be temporarily introduced and then withdrawn after the radiation dose is delivered.

CANCER: The growth of abnormal cells in the body in an uncontrolled and disordered manner, invading surrounding tissues and sometimes spreading to distant sites within the body via the bloodstream and/or lymphatic system.

CARCINOEMBRYONIC ANTIGEN (CEA): A biomarker of prostate cancer that may be expressed in prostate cancer variants associated with higher Gleason scores, for example, Gleason scores 8–10 may indicate that androgen-independent cells are present.

CASODEX: Brand name of an antiandrogen medication that functions by occupying and therefore blocking the androgen receptor, thus preventing natural androgens from stimulating cell growth.

CAT or CT SCAN (COMPUTERIZED AXIAL TOMOGRAPHY): An imaging method used to identify abnormalities by combining images from multiple X-rays under the control of a computer to produce cross-sectional or three-dimensional pictures of internal structures.

CBC (COMPLETE BLOOD COUNT): Complete blood workup including white blood count, hematocrit, and platelet count.

cc (CUBIC CENTIMETERS): Used as a measurement of prostate gland volume or amount of prostate cancer; cubic centimeters are equivalent to grams (g) in determinations of prostate gland volume.

cGy (centiGray): A unit of measurement of radiation dose; 1 cGy equals the energy absorbed from ionizing radiation equal to 1 joule (a unit of energy) per kilogram.

CHEMOTHERAPY: The use of pharmaceuticals or other chemicals to kill cancer cells. In many cases these agents may also damage normal cells in the process of killing cancer cells, resulting in various adverse side effects.

CHROMOGRANIN A (CGA): A biomarker of prostate cancer that may be expressed in prostate cancer variants associated with higher Gleason scores, that is, Gleason scores 8–10. Progressive increases of CGA in the blood indicate an aggressive clone of prostate cancer is present that exhibits an increased tendency to metastasize to lymph nodes, liver, and lungs. CGA is produced by the neuroendocrine cells associated with androgen independent PC.

CLINICAL STAGE: The TNM (tumor, nodes, metastases) system of classification for communicating extent of disease in a specific patient based on all available information. This system has largely replaced the older Whitmore-Jewett staging classification system.

CORE INVOLVEMENT: Expressed as a percentage; indicates the amount of biopsy cores involved by prostate cancer divided by the total number of cores that have been sampled. If 12 cores of tissue were obtained and 6 showed PC, then the percentage core involvement would be 50%.

COX-2 (CYCLOOXYGENASE 2): The enzyme that converts arachidonic acid to prostaglandin E_2. Inhibition of COX-2 is now an important approach to reducing the production of unfavorable eicosanoids implicated in the cause and progression of malignancy and inflammatory disorders.

CRYOPROBES: The hollow probes used to freeze tissue during a cryosurgery procedure.

CRYOSURGERY: The use of liquid nitrogen or argon gas circulated through cryoprobes to freeze and kill tissue, including any cancerous tissue.

DEDIFFERENTIATION: Relatively more primitive in appearance and function than well-differentiated cells that, by contrast, are mature and able to function properly. As the disease progresses, cancer cells become more dedifferentiated (i.e., primitive) than normal cells, losing the characteristics that normal cells possess.

DEXA SCAN: An imaging procedure used to evaluate bone mineral density and evaluate the status of bone integrity as regards a diagnosis of osteopenia or osteoporosis. The DEXA may understate the true extent of abnormality by attributing unrelated conditions such as arthritis and vascular calcifications to normal bone density.

DIAGNOSIS: The evaluation of signs, symptoms, and tests to determine physical and biological causes of these signs and symptoms and evaluate whether a specific disease or disorder is involved.

DIGITAL RECTAL EXAMINATION (DRE): The use by a physician of a lubricated and gloved finger inserted into the rectum to feel for abnormalities of the prostate and rectum.

DIHYDROTESTOSTERONE (DHT): A male hormone five times more potent than testosterone; DHT is converted from testosterone within the prostate and in other tissues by the enzyme 5-alpha-reductase.

DIPLOID: Cells having one complete set of 46 normally paired chromosomes, that is, a normal amount of DNA. Diploid cancer cells grow relatively slowly and usually respond well to androgen deprivation therapy.

DNA (DEOXYRIBONUCLEIC ACID): The basic biologically active chemical that defines the physical development and growth of nearly all living organisms; a complex protein that is the carrier of genetic information.

DOWNREGULATING (DOWNREGULATION): Turning off a mechanism of action in the body at the biochemical level.

DUTASTERIDE (AVODART): A 5-alpha-reductase inhibitor that prevents the conversion of testosterone to the five times more potent dihydrotestosterone (DHT). Unlike Proscar, which blocks only 5-alpha reductase Type II, dutasteride also blocks 5-alpha reductase Type I.

EICOSANOIDS: Hormones made within the cell membrane of every living cell in the body controlling every physiological function. Eicosanoids have opposing actions operating as a check-and-balance system. Therefore, a balance of these opposing actions is essential for optimal health.

EICOSAPENTENOIC ACID (EPA): An omega-3 fatty acid that has been shown to inhibit the formation of AA by inhibiting the enzyme delta-5 desaturase, which converts DGLA to AA.

EJACULATION: The release of semen through the penis during orgasm.

ENDOCRINE GLAND: Any of various glands producing hormonal secretions that pass directly into the bloodstream. Examples of endocrine glands include the thyroid, parathyroids, anterior and posterior pituitary, pancreas, adrenals, pineal, and gonads.

ENDORECTAL MRI: Magnetic resonance imaging of the prostate using a probe inserted into the rectum.

ENZYME: Any of a group of chemical substances that are produced by living cells and cause particular chemical reactions to happen while not being changed themselves.

EPITHELIAL CELL: A cell type in the prostate gland that lines the ducts and functionally secretes substances such as PSA into the bloodstream or into the duct openings or lumens.

EULEXIN: The brand name of an antiandrogen that blocks the androgen receptor and prevents testosterone and/or DHT from stimulating cell growth.

EXTERNAL BEAM RADIATION THERAPY (EBRT): A form of radiation therapy in which the radiation is delivered by a machine directed at the area to be radiated as opposed to radiation given within the target tissue, such as brachytherapy.

EXTRACAPSULAR EXTENSION: A disease status in prostate cancer in which the cancer has penetrated the outer shell or capsule of the prostate and extends into the periprostatic tissue.

FINASTERIDE (PROSCAR): An inhibitor of the 5-alpha-reductase Type II enzyme, which converts testosterone to the five times more potent dihydrotestosterone (DHT); used to treat BPH and PC.

FOLLICLE STIMULATING HORMONE (FSH): A hormone produced in the pituitary gland that, in males, stimulates cells (Sertoli cells) in the testicles to make sperm; may be a factor in prostate cancer growth because FSH receptors have been identified on prostate cancer cells.

FREE PSA: PSA unbound to any major protein; free PSA relates to benign prostate growth. The percentage of free PSA is one indicator of whether or not prostate cancer is likely present.

FREE RADICALS: Substances that damage cell membranes and disrupt the integrity of the cell; reactive oxygen species (ROS).

GAMMA-LINOLENIC ACID (GLA): One of the building blocks of eicosanoids that is metabolized to DGLA. The pathway that is taken after metabolism to DGLA is either toward AA and the unfavorable eicosanoids or toward the production of good eicosanoids such as PGA1 and PGA2.

GAMMA-TOCOPHEROL ISOMER: A component of vitamin E.

GLAND: A structure or organ that produces a substance that may be used in another part of the body.

GLAND VOLUME: The volume of the prostate gland in cubic centimeters or grams. (Both units of measurement, cubic centimeters and grams, yield the same result.)

GLEASON GRADE: After Donald Gleason, M.D. who developed the Gleason grading system as a tool to profile the aggressiveness of prostate cancer. A number from 1 to 5 that describes one of the two most predominant tissue patterns seen in the microscopic analysis of glandular architecture. The primary grade is the most predominant pattern, comprising 51% to 95% of the specimen, while the secondary grade comprises 5–49%.

GLEASON SCORE (GS): The two Gleason grades, represented as (primary grade, secondary grade). An example of a high Gleason score would be (4,4) or (5,4) compared to a Gleason score of (3,3), the most common Gleason score at the time of diagnosis of PC.

GLYCEMIC INDEX (GI): A measurement of the rate of carbohydrate entry into the bloodstream.

GLYCEMIC LOAD (GL): The amount of insulin-stimulating carbohydrate multiplied by the glycemic index of the carbohydrate.

HDR: See **High-Dose Rate Brachytherapy**

HEREDITARY: Traits inherited from one's parents and from earlier generations via their DNA.

HIGH-DOSE RATE (HDR) BRACHYTHERAPY: Involves inserting iridium wires into the prostate gland through hollow plastic needles that are placed under transrectal ultrasound guidance. Once the radiation dose is delivered, the wires are withdrawn from the prostate.

HORMONE: Substances that are produced in the body that act as messengers, communicating information between cells. Usually peptides or steroids, they are produced by one tissue and delivered via the bloodstream to another tissue to affect physiological activity such as growth or metabolism.

HYPERINSULINEMIA: A state of high insulin levels in the blood that can be caused by disproportionate consumption of simple or complex carbohydrates in the diet in proportion to dietary proteins and fats.

HYPOXIC CENTER: The center of a prostate cancer tumor in which a state of lower oxygen tension exists. This stimulates VEGF, a substance that stimulates the blood vessel growth necessary for the nourishment of the tumor.

IMAGING: A radiology technique or method allowing a physician to see something that would not ordinarily be visible. Imaging studies include X-ray examinations, CT scans, bone or other nuclear medicine scans, and MRI and ProstaScint studies.

INTENSITY MODULATED RADIATION THERAPY (IMRT): An approach to external beam radiation therapy delivery using sophisticated computer planning to specify the tumor target dose and the amount of radiation allowable to nearby tissues and to modulate the intensity of the radiation as the delivery system rotates around the patient, thus minimizing damage to normal tissues.

INTERFERON: A molecule that is active against viruses and cancer cells.

INTERLEUKIN-6 (IL-6): A cell product made by the primary tumor as well as by osteoblasts that facilitates bone resorption and promotes osteopenia and osteoporosis by stimulating mature osteoclasts to break down bone.

INTERFERON-SIGNALING PATHWAY (ISP): One of the defensive pathways that healthy cells use against the development of malignancy and invasion by viruses involving the interaction of interferon, which is produced in response to an invader.

KATTAN NOMOGRAMS: Various algorithms named after Michael Kattan that present probabilities of response to therapies, such as radical prostatectomy, external beam RT, and seed implantation based on a combination of biological inputs such as PSA, Gleason score, and clinical stage.

KELOID: Excessive scar tissue at the site of a surgery or an internal procedure. A history of this type of scar tissue formation may indicate the probability of the development of anastomotic stricture after radical prostatectomy.

LACTIC DEHYDROGENASE (LDH): Elevated levels of this substance are associated with high Gleason score prostate cancer. LDH used to be routinely included in the standard chemistry panel and was considered an excellent overall tumor marker. For reasons unclear, LDH has been omitted from the standard panel.

LHRH ANTAGONIST: An agent that blocks the LHRH receptor by pure antagonism without the initial release of LH, which is responsible for causing a testosterone surge seen with LHRH agonists; Abarelix (Plenaxis) is an example of an LHRH antagonist.

LIGAND: A protein or an enzyme that combines with its appropriate binding site or receptor. The interaction of a ligand and its receptor initiates a biochemical reaction leading to the synthesis of other substances, often proteins, hormones, or enzymes. Almost all reactions in the human body involve ligands interacting with their appropriate receptors.

LNCaP: One of the many prostate cancer cell lines. LNCaP is an androgen-dependent cell line.

LOWER URINARY TRACT SYMPTOMS (LUTS): Urinary difficulties including slow stream, urinary urgency, difficulty in starting urination, and incomplete emptying of the bladder. These symptoms are quantified in the AUA Symptom Index or Score.

LUPRON: Brand name of one of the drugs acting as an LHRH agonist.

LUTEINIZING HORMONE (LH): A pituitary hormone that stimulates the Leydig cells within the testicles to produce testosterone.

LUTEINIZING HORMONE-RELEASING HORMONE (LHRH): Hormone from the hypothalamus that interacts with the LHRH receptor in the pituitary to release LH which in turn stimulates Leydig cells in the testicles to make testosterone.

LYMPH NODES: Small glands occurring throughout the body that filter out bacteria and other toxins, including cancer cells. During the process of metastasis, they are one of the first sites of involvement when the cancer leaves the primary site of origin.

MAGNETIC RESONANCE: Absorption of specific frequencies of radio and microwave radiation by atoms placed in a strong magnetic field.

MAGNETIC RESONANCE IMAGING (MRI): Use of magnetic resonance with atoms in the body tissues to produce distinct cross-sectional or three-dimensional images of internal structures.

MALIGNANCY: A growth or tumor composed of cancerous cells.

MALIGNANT: Cancerous; tending to become progressively worse and to result in death; having the invasive and metastatic (spreading) properties of cancer.

METASTASIS (pl. METASTASES): Secondary tumor formed as a result of a cancer cell or cells from the primary tumor site traveling to a new site and growing there.

MICROVESSEL DENSITY: An objectified measurement of angiogenesis.

mL (MILLILITER): Unit of volume equal to one-thousandth of a liter.

NARAYAN STAGE: Part of the algorithm developed by Perry Narayan that assesses if the microscopic findings of prostate cancer were limited to one side of the prostate (Narayan B1) or both sides (Narayan B2).

NERVE-SPARING: A technique used in radical prostatectomy in which the erectile nerves are left intact by the surgeon.

NEURON-SPECIFIC ENOLASE (NSE): A biomarker of prostate cancer that may be expressed in prostate cancer variants associated with higher Gleason scores, that is, Gleason scores 8–10.

ng (NANOGRAM): Unit of measurement that is one-billionth of a gram.

NOMOGRAM: A graphic representation, often used in analyzing data, consisting of several lines marked off to scale. Specific variables such as PSA, Gleason score, clinical stage, etc. are given point values. The sum of all the points equates with the prognostic outcome.

OBJECTIFIED ONGOING OBSERVATION: A more appropriate term than *watchful waiting* that indicates that a patient not undergoing a definitive procedure using surgery or radiation or other treatments will be objectively monitoring his biological status in a consistent ongoing fashion.

ONCOGENES: Genes relating to tumor growth.

ONCOLOGY: The branch of medical science dealing with tumors. Oncologists study cancer and treat patients who are afflicted with cancer.

ONCOLYTIC VIRUS: A virus that can kill tumor cells having defects in the interferon-signaling pathway or by other mechanisms.

ORGAN: A group of tissues that work in concert to carry out a specific set of functions in the body.

ORGAN-CONFINED DISEASE: Prostate cancer that is apparently confined to the prostate as determined either by clinical findings or, in the case of radical prostatectomy, by pathological findings; prostate cancer that has not penetrated the prostate capsule.

OSTEOBLAST: A cell type within bone that promotes bone formation.

OSTEOCLAST: A cell type within bone that promotes breakdown of bone or bone resorption.

OSTEOPENIA: A condition of bone that indicates that an imbalance between bone formation and resorption is compromising bone integrity. Osteopenia indicates that the degree of bone loss is more than 1 standard deviation from the WHO definition of normal, but not more than 2.5 standard deviation below that level.

OSTEOPOROSIS: A reduction in bone mineral density that is more that 2.5 standard deviation below the normal level defined by the WHO.

PARTIN TABLES: Tables constructed based on results of the PSA, clinical stage, and Gleason score and associating those values with the findings at radical prostatectomy. Data involving thousands of men with PC used to predict the probability that the prostate cancer has penetrated the capsule, spread to the seminal vesicles or lymph nodes, or has remained confined to the prostate. The tables were developed by a group of scientists at the Brady Institute for Urology at Johns Hopkins Medical Center.

PATHOLOGICAL STAGE: The extent of disease as determined by a pathologist's microscopic analysis of tissue removed at the time of surgery.

PERIPROSTATIC: Pertaining to the soft tissues immediately adjacent to the prostate gland.

PLOIDY: DNA analysis to establish whether normal or abnormal numbers of pairs of chromosomes are present in a cell.

PROCTITIS: Inflammation of the rectum; may be an adverse effect of radiation therapy used to treat prostate cancer.

PROSCAR: Brand name of finasteride, a 5-alpha-reductase inhibitor that blocks the conversion of testosterone to DHT.

PROSTAGLANDIN: An eicosanoid isolated from the prostate gland that acts locally, metabolizes rapidly, and has a hormone-like effect, stimulating target cells into action.

PROSTAGLANDIN E$_2$ (PGE$_2$): A major metabolite of arachidonic acid, known to stimulate vascular endothelial growth factor (VEGF) and hence, angiogenesis.

PROSTASCINT: A monoclonal antibody (mAb) tagged with a radioactive isotope that is used to detect prostate cancer, particularly within lymph nodes. The ProstaScint mAb is directed against the prostate-specific membrane antigen (PSMA). PSMA is associated with androgen-independent PC. A few centers are using the ProstaScint scan to identify PC in the prostate gland.

PROSTATE: The gland surrounding the urethra and immediately below the bladder in males.

PROSTATE CANCER: Adenocarcinoma of the prostate gland.

PROSTATECTOMY: Surgical removal of part or all of the prostate gland. If the entire gland is removed, a radical prostatectomy has been performed. Transurethal resection of the prostate (TURP), performed to improve urinary difficulties, is an example of removal of part of the gland.

PROSTATE-SPECIFIC ANTIGEN (PSA): A protein secreted by the normal epithelial cells of the prostate gland as well as by prostate cancer cells if they are present. Elevated PSA levels in the blood can be due to benign or malignant causes. After diagnosis of prostate cancer, this biomarker is typically used to monitor disease progression and/or response to therapy.

PROSTATIC ACID PHOSPHATASE (PAP): An enzyme or biomarker secreted by prostate cells that is associated with a higher probability of disease outside the prostate when pretreatment levels are 3.0 or higher. PAP elevations connote that the disease is not organ-confined disease.

PROSTATIC INTRAEPITHELIAL NEOPLASIA (PIN): A pathologically identifiable condition believed to be a possible precursor of prostate cancer; broken down into high-grade PIN or PIN 2 and PIN 3 versus low grade PIN or PIN 1. High grade PIN is associated with having PC.

PROSTATITIS: Infection or inflammation of the prostate gland that can be treated with medication and/or prostate massage.

PSA ASSAY: The means by which a blood sample is analyzed to determine its PSA content. Various assays can result in different in readings from the same sample; therefore, it is wise to use the same assay for each subsequent PSA test. Very sensitive assays that measure PSA down to two or three decimal points are called hypersensitive or ultrasensitive PSA assays. These assays play a major role in early detection of relapse after radical prostatectomy or in the assessment of the tumor cell population in response to ADT.

PSA DENSITY (PSAD): The amount of PSA (expressed in nanograms) for each cubic centimeter of prostate volume; the serum PSA value divided by an accurate gland volume determination.

PSA DOUBLING TIME: The length of time in months that it takes for the PSA to double in amount.

PSA LEAK: The secretion of PSA from the cells into the blood. Low levels of serum PSA are often associated with higher Gleason scores, as an expression of less PSA leak because more aggressive prostate cancers lose the ability to secrete PSA. Thus, PSA is an unreliable marker of disease progression in high Gleason score prostate cancer, e.g., Gleason scores 8–10.

PSA RECURRENCE (PSAR): Elevated PSA following treatment of prostate cancer, signaling that cancer cells are still present and that monitoring for disease progression is indicated.

PSA RELAPSE-FREE SURVIVAL: Survival of the patient that relates to no evidence of a progressively rising PSA.

PSA TREND: The slope that a series of PSA readings over time would exhibit on a graph.

PSA VELOCITY: A statement of how fast the PSA is accelerating; the rate of change in PSA calculated per year of time.

PYRILINKS-D (Dpd): Deoxypyridinoline, or Dpd, is a laboratory test to monitor the biologic endpoint of bone resorption activity obtained by analysis of the second-voided urine of the day.

QCT SCAN: Quantitative CT bone densitometry; a superior way to evaluate bone density compared to the DEXA scan because it is uninfluenced by unrelated conditions such as arthritic changes and/or vascular calcifications. (Telephone numbers that may be helpful in finding QCT sites near you: Mindways, (877) 646-3929 (www.qct.com), or Image Analysis, (800) 548-4849 (www.image-analysis.com).)

RADIATION THERAPY (RT): The use of X-rays and other forms of radiation to destroy malignant cells and tissue.

RADICAL PROSTATECTOMY (RP): Surgical removal of the entire prostate gland and seminal vesicles.

RECEPTOR: A docking site on the cell membrane in the cell cytoplasm or in the nucleus that interacts with a ligand. All cells have multiple receptors.

RECURRENCE: The reappearance of disease manifested by clinically based findings, either upon physical examination or by the results of laboratory findings such as a rising PSA.

RESORPTION: Loss of bone caused by an imbalance in the dynamics of bone formation by osteoblasts or bone loss due to breakdown of the bone by osteoclasts.

RISK ASSESSMENT: An analysis of probabilities related to a specific patient's case, obtained by analyzing medical variables of known significance and used to derive an overall impression of how different disease management options would impact an optimal or suboptimal outcome for the patient.

SCREENING: Evaluation of populations of people who have no symptoms of the disease for which they are being evaluated in an effort to diagnose disease in its early stages.

SEED IMPLANTATION (SI): A treatment for prostate cancer in which radioactive seeds encased in titanium shells are permanently implanted into the prostate gland.

SELENOMETHIONINE: A substance that shows an inhibitory effect on certain prostate cancer cell lines that appear to be independent of androgen receptor or PSA pathways.

SEMINAL VESICLES: Glandular structures located above and behind the prostate that secrete and store seminal fluid. Seminal fluid is one component of ejaculate.

STAGE: See **CLINICAL STAGE, PATHOLOGICAL STAGE.**

SYSTEMIC: Throughout the whole body; in prostate cancer, cancer that is no longer organ-confined.

TESTOSTERONE (T): The male hormone or androgen that comprises most of the androgens in a man's body. Chiefly produced by the testicles, testosterone is essential to virtually every male function from the brain to toenails.

THERAPEUTIC INDEX (TI): Treatment benefit divided by treatment side effects.

THERMOCOUPLES: In relation to prostate cancer, devices used during cryosurgery to monitor the temperature achieved by cryoprobes, thus helping to improve the therapeutic index of the procedure.

TRANSFORMING GROWTH FACTOR BETA-1 (TGF-b1): A growth factor produced by prostate cells, as well as by cells of the bone matrix. Elevated plasma levels of TGF-b1 obtained at baseline are associated with distant disease involving bone and/or lymph nodes.

TRANSRECTAL: Through the rectum (as in transrectal ultrasound of the prostate).

TRANSRECTAL ULTRASOUND OF THE PROSTATE (TRUSP OR TRUS): A method that uses the echoes of ultrasound waves to image the prostate by inserting an ultrasound probe into the rectum.

TRANSURETHRAL: Through the urethra. See **Transurethral Resection of the Prostate.**

TRANSURETHRAL RESECTION OF THE PROSTATE (TURP): A surgical procedure to remove prostate tissue obstructing the urethra.

T SCORE: A designation used in evaluation of bone mineral density that relates the patient's bone density to that found in a population of healthy women of approximately 30 years of age. The T score is in contrast to the Z score, which relates the patient's bone density to a pooled population of an age similar to the patient. The T score is the desired test result. (No T score levels have been ascertained for men as of the end of 2002.)

TUMOR: An excessive growth of cells caused by uncontrolled and disorderly cell replacement that can be either benign or malignant.

TUMOR VOLUME: The amount of tumor measured in cubic centimeters.

ULTRASENSITIVE PSA ASSAY: PSA assays that are able to measure very small amounts of PSA in the blood sample, reliable to the hundredth or even the thousandth of a nanogram per milliliter of blood. Tosoh and DPC Immulite Third Generation assays are examples of ultrasensitive PSA assays.

UPREGULATING (UPREGULATION): Turning on or increasing a mechanism of action at the biochemical level in the body.

UROKINASE-TYPE PLASMINOGEN ACTIVATOR (uPA): A substance believed to play a role in prostate cancer invasion and metastasis that is stimulated by IGF-1 and inhibited by GLA and EPA.

UROLOGIST: A surgically trained physician who specializes in disorders of the genitourinary system.

VASCULAR ENDOTHELIAL GROWTH FACTOR (VEGF): A substance known to stimulate blood vessel growth or angiogenesis and hence to stimulate PC growth.

VIADUR: Brand name of an LHRH agonist that is implanted under the skin and releases medication over the course of one year.

VITAMIN E SUCCINATE: Substance that inhibits the growth of prostate cancer cells of certain cell lines by suppressing androgen receptor expression and PSA expression.

WATCHFUL WAITING: Objective ongoing observation and regular monitoring of a patient with prostate cancer without actual treatment or invasive therapies.

ZOLADEX: Brand name of one of the LHRH-agonists.

Z SCORE: A designation of bone mineral density that relates the patient's bone density to that of a pooled population of similar age. See T Score.

SUGGESTED READING

Those seeking additional information may order a copy of *A Primer on Prostate Cancer, the Empowered Patient's Guide*. The *Primer* reflects the synergistic efforts of Stephen B. Strum, a medical oncologist involved with PC since 1983, and Donna Pogliano, a partner of a PC warrior. The *Primer* is in full color with many graphic images, clinical vignettes, and a comprehensive appendix replete with material that is the essence of top-of-the-line health care as it relates to PC. The *Primer* is a working manual and companion tool to this protocol. The *Primer* is to be regarded as required reading for those serious at winning the war against PC. It is your basic field guide—but much more so. The *Primer* is available through Life Extension at (866) 820-7457 or on the Life Extension website at www.lefprostate.org. You may fax an order to the United States at (954) 761-9199. The *Primer* is also available through amazon.com, the Prostate Cancer Research Institute, Us Too!, the Educational Council for the Prostate Cancer Patient, Barnes & Noble, and Borders.

ADDITIONAL READING

Books About PC

Patrick Walsh, M.D., Janet Farrar Worthington.
Dr. Patrick Walsh's Guide to Surviving Prostate Cancer

Sheldon Marks, M.D.
Prostate & Cancer. A Family Guide to Diagnosis, Treatment & Survival

Medical Journals Focused on PC

Urology

Journal of Urology

Prostate

Prostate Cancer and Prostatic Diseases

PC Newsletters

Prostate Cancer Research Institute's *PCRI Insights*

Dr. Snuffy Myers's *Prostate Forum*

ECPCP's (Education Center for Prostate Cancer Patients) *Prostate Exchange*

PAACT's (Patient Advocates for Advanced Cancer Treatments) *Cancer Communication*

Internet Websites

PCRI (www.pcri.org)

Don Cooley (http://www.cooleyville.com/cancer/)

Robert Young (http://www.phoenix5.org)

PubMed
(http://www.ncbi.nlm.nih.gov/entrez/query.fcgi)

Internet-Based Tools (Software)

PC Tools I and II (www.pcri.org)

Kattan Nomograms
(http://www.mskcc.org/mskcc/html/10088.cfm)

 PRODUCT AVAILABILITY

High potency genistein extracts, lycopene, gamma-E tocopherol, curcumin, selenium, silymarin, Life Extension Booster, Mega EPA/DHA, Mega EPA, Super GLA/DHA, Vitamin E Succinate (natural), Mega GLH, Super Max EPH, PectaSol, vitamin D_3, Tri Boron, Bone Up, Bone Assure, vitamin K, Calcium Citrate w/vitamin D_3, and other supplements discussed in this protocol can be ordered by telephoning (800) 544-4440 or by ordering online www.lef.org.

STAYING INFORMED

The information published in these protocols is only as current as the day the book was sent to the printer. This protocol raises many issues that are subject to change as new data emerge. Furthermore, cancer is still a disease with unacceptably high mortality rates, and none of our suggested treatment regimens can guarantee a cure.

The Life Extension Foundation is constantly uncovering information to provide cancer patients with more ammunition to battle their disease. A special website has been established for the purpose of updating patients on new findings that directly pertain to the cancer protocols published in this book. Whenever Life Extension discovers information that points to a better way of treating cancer, it will be posted on the website www.lefcancer.org.

Before utilizing the cancer protocols in this book, we suggest that you log on to www.lefcancer.org to see if any substantive changes have been made to the therapeutic recommendations described in this protocol. Based on the sheer number of newly published findings, there may be significant alterations to the information you have just read.

Doctors recommend staying at the lowest dose that relieves your symptoms. Inositol hexanicotinate, which does not cause flushing, should be taken daily at doses of 1500–4000 mg in 3 or 4 divided doses. Be aware that niacin is destroyed by excessive sugar, alcohol, sulfa drugs, and the antibiotic chloramphenicol.

CAUTION Niacin has been known to cause liver enlargement and elevation of liver enzymes in high doses. If you have liver disease, do not take high doses of niacin without medical supervision. Taking methylation-enhancing supplements, such as folic acid, vitamin B_{12}, and trimethylglycine (TMG), can mitigate niacin's toxic effect to the liver.

Magnesium and Calcium

Adequate calcium and magnesium are essential to maintain relaxation of the smooth muscle of the small arteries affected by Raynaud's syndrome. In addition, the requirement for magnesium increases with psychological or physical stress, which in turn is associated with Raynaud's syndrome episodes (Adee 1993; Golf et al. 1998).

Essential Fatty Acids

Gamma-linolenic acid (GLA) is an omega-6 essential fatty acid found in evening primrose, borage, or black currant oils. GLA has been shown to reduce inflammation in people with rheumatoid arthritis and osteoarthritis. Because it is the precursor for prostaglandin E1, GLA is involved in smooth muscle relaxation. One study found that taking evening primrose oil dramatically decreased the number of Raynaud's syndrome attacks, and blood tests showed some antiplatelet (blood thinning) activity (Belch et al. 1985). Because of its functions, GLA may also enhance micro-capillary circulation.

Omega-3 essential fatty acids found in flax, perilla, and fish oils have been shown to lower serum triglycerides (fats) and decrease platelet aggregation (thin the blood). Fish oils containing DHA and EPA inhibit arachidonic acid metabolism, elevated levels of which can lead to increased systemic inflammation. Research has shown that fish oil is useful in the treatment of autoimmune diseases, like those associated with Raynaud's syndrome (Candela et al. 1994).

In this same study, it was also found that a higher percentage of patients given fish oils reported clinical improvement in a variety of symptoms, including Raynaud's symptoms, in comparison to a control group. A significant decrease in laboratory values that reflect autoimmune disturbances (cryocrit and rheumatoid factor) was also observed (Candela et al.

1994). Another clinical study found that ingesting fish oil increased the median time (especially in those patients with primary Raynaud's) before the onset after exposure to cold. Moreover, fish oil improved tolerance to cold exposure, as evidenced by significantly increased blood pressures in the fingers. Almost half of the patients in the fish oil group did not exhibit Raynaud's in response to cold water baths (DiGiacomo et al. 1989).

The proper balance of omega-6 and omega-3 fatty acids can help reduce systemic inflammation that contributes to a multitude of autoimmune and degenerative diseases.

Other Vitamins

There are many nutrients that improve circulation and thus may benefit the Raynaud's syndrome patient. A convenient way of including these supplements in one's everyday program is to take a formula such as *Life Extension Mix with Niacin* that provides high potencies of vitamins C, E, and niacin along with dozens of other nutrients, such as magnesium.

Antiplatelet Agents

Platelets clump together to form clots, inhibiting circulation; antiplatelet agents prevent this. Dipyridamole is a prescription drug that has antiplatelet effects. Low-dose aspirin is also a highly effective antiplatelet agent. Most people take one low-dose aspirin tablet (81 mg) a day, while others need one whole aspirin (325 mg) each day. *Ginkgo biloba* is a well-tolerated plant extract and has been proven to stimulate circulation in the small blood vessels and to have antiplatelet effects (Koltringer et al. 1993; DeFeudis et al. 2000). A typical dose is 120 mg a day of a standardized ginkgo extract. If you are taking anticoagulants, please discuss taking ginkgo with your physician. A template bleeding test can help determine the optimal dose of aspirin and other antiplatelet nutrients and drugs.

Pentoxifylline

Pentoxifylline (PTX), first marketed under the name of Trental, was first used in Europe in 1972 and long ago came off patent (meaning it is not cost-prohibitive). PTX is prescribed to improve the flow properties of blood by decreasing its viscosity. It works by improving red blood cell flexibility, decreasing platelet aggregation, and reducing fibrinogen levels (Manrique et al. 1987; di Minno et al. 1992; de la Cruz et al. 1993; Gara 1993; Gaur et al. 1993). PTX has fallen out of favor, because no drug company has the economic incentive to market it to physicians.

PTX functions via multiple mechanisms of action that can reduce the risk of diseases related to Raynaud's syndrome. An important function of PTX is that it suppresses proinflammatory cytokines that can damage the blood vessels. Refer to the PTX precautions at the end of this protocol before asking your physician to prescribe it. A dose of 400 mg twice a day has shown efficacy, even though patients with certain conditions take 400 mg 3 times a day.

New Drugs

Several pharmacological therapies are being studied for effectiveness on Raynaud's syndrome, including iloprost (a stable prostacyclin), piracetam, Ketanserin (S2-serotonergic antagonist), and dazoxiben (thromboxane synthetase inhibitor). Although prostaglandin E1 and prostacyclin have been successfully used to treat Raynaud's syndrome, they are unstable and require intravenous administration (reserved for emergencies).

Another route to increasing the levels of these beneficial molecules is to stimulate the body's own production, using evening primrose oil (see below). Piracetam is a drug used in Europe whose therapeutic efficacy has been experimentally established. It has a unique dual mode of action: inhibition of platelet function by inhibition of thromboxane synthetase; or antagonism of thromboxane and increasing cell membrane deformability along with decreasing plasma concentrations of clotting factors. Piracetam appears to be devoid of adverse effects at the recommended dose (Moriau et al. 1993). Nitroglycerine dilates blood vessels but must be used sparingly. It can be used in some cases as cream for topical application.

⬤ SUMMARY

Raynaud's syndrome is caused by spasms in the blood vessels supplying the fingers and toes. These spasms are brought on by cold or stress. Although symptoms are usually mild, they can have serious consequences, such as tissue death or gangrene, if not tended to. The best treatment for Raynaud's syndrome is prevention through behavioral strategies, including keeping yourself warm at all times, protecting your hands from becoming cold, and avoiding precipitating factors (such as stress and activities that expose you to cold weather and substances). Given the association of Raynaud's syndrome with serious diseases, consult a physician upon developing the symptoms.

1. Prevent attacks by adopting the behavioral strategies outlined above to keep warm and protect your hands from the cold. Reduce stress and avoid precipitating substances and activities.

2. Respond immediately to every attack with motion and moist heat.

3. Use biofeedback to train your blood vessels to relax.

4. The prescription drug pentoxifylline may help improve circulation. Suggested dose is 400 mg every 12 hours. See pentoxifylline precautions at the end of this protocol.

5. The following dietary supplements should be considered on a daily basis:

   - 400 IU of vitamin E (alpha tocopheryl) along with 200 mg of gamma tocopherol.
   - 2500 mg of vitamin C.
   - The lowest dose of niacin that relieves Raynaud's symptoms. A dose of 750 mg daily or less is often effective. If the niacin "flush" is not tolerable, take 1500–4000 mg of inositol hexanicotinate, which does not cause flushing. Take in 3 divided doses.
   - 1000 mg of elemental magnesium along with 1000 mg of elemental calcium.

Note: *Many of the nutrients listed above [except the calcium and gamma tocopherol] can be obtained by taking 3 tablets, 3 times a day, of the Life Extension Mix with Niacin multinutrient formula. This product supplies 89 different nutrients, many having antiplatelet properties.*

   - 900 mg daily of gamma linolenic acid (GLA) from borage oil, 1000 mg of DHA, and 400 mg EPA from fish oil. Six capsules of Super GLA/DHA provide these potencies.
   - 120 mg of *ginkgo biloba* extract once daily.
   - One low-dose aspirin tablet (81 mg) a day with the heaviest meal. Some people need to take an entire aspirin tablet (325 mg).

Consult your physician regarding any progression in your condition, alterations in your health, and any infections or injuries in affected areas to prevent serious consequences.

PENTOXIFYLLINE (PTX) PRECAUTIONS

PTX should not be used in those with bleeding disorders, such as those with recent cerebral or retinal hemorrhage

(*Physicians Desk Reference* (PDR) 2001). Patients taking Coumadin should have more frequent monitoring of prothrombin time. Those who have other types of bleeding should receive frequent physician examinations. Furthermore, evaluating the individual patient's coagulation status to see what effect PTX has on the template bleeding time is recommended. This is an inexpensive test that relates the biological effect of PTX (or aspirin or nonsteroidal anti-inflammatory agents) on the function of platelets. All of these agents affect platelet aggregation, and this effect can be manifested in a prolonged template bleeding time.

According to two studies, PTX should be avoided by Parkinson's patients (Godwin-Austen et al. 1980; Serrano-Duenas 2001). It is important to note that the body does use tumor necrosis factor-alpha (TNF-alpha) to acutely fight infections. If patients are showing any sign of infectious disease, drugs such as Enbrel (that inhibit the effects of TNF-alpha) are temporarily discontinued.

A new FDA advisory states that patients should be tested and treated for inactive, or latent, tuberculosis prior to therapy with another TNF-alpha inhibiting therapy (infliximab). Since PTX, fish oil, and nettle directly suppress TNF-alpha, perhaps these agents should be temporarily discontinued during the time when one has an active infection.

 PRODUCT AVAILABILITY

Super GLA/DHA, Life Extension Mix, calcium citrate capsules, vitamin E, gamma tocopherol, ginkgo extract, varying strength niacin capsules, inositol hexanicotinate (No-Flush Niacin), magnesium capsules, evening primrose oil, Healthprin tablets (aspirin), and other supplements discussed in this protocol are available from the Life Extension Buyers' Club by calling (800) 544-4440 or by ordering on-line at www.lef.org. Pentoxifylline and conventional therapies, such as calcium-channel blockers, described in this protocol are prescription drugs.

Retinopathy

Diabetic retinopathy (DR), the leading cause of visual disability and blindness among adults in the developed world, may affect as many as 20 million people. Early detection and treatment are keys to preventing the vision loss and blindness associated with the disease. Unfortunately, only about half of those with diabetes have proper eye examinations on a yearly basis. It is very important that diabetics have a dilated eye exam each year.

Retinopathy damages the retina by destroying the capillaries (minuscule blood vessels connecting arteries and veins) that provide blood to the retina, the light-sensitive nerve tissue that sends visual images to the brain. With the onset of retinopathy, these vessels weaken or bulge with microaneurysms that may hemorrhage, leaking blood or fluid into surrounding tissue. When new blood vessels grow on the retina (and into the vitreous), they can cause blurred vision and even temporary blindness. The real danger lies in the scar tissue that ultimately forms, detaching the retina from the back of the eye and often causing permanent loss of vision.

Chronically elevated blood insulin and glucose levels induce retinopathy. Fortunately, research shows that even after having long-term diabetes, lowering glucose has a positive effect on slowing the progression of retinopathy. A study took place involving 834 people who were over the age of 30 when they developed diabetes and who were approximately 65 at the start of the study. A glycohemoglobin test was performed at the start of the study, along with two follow-ups, 4 and 10 years later, which included a physical and eye exam. Glycohemoglobin (also known as hemoglobin A1C) is the best measurement of long-term glucose control. A high glycohemoglobin number correlates with uncontrolled diabetes.

In noninsulin treated participants, those that had the highest glyohemoglobin levels at the start of the study had nearly a threefold greater chance of having developed retinopathy after 10 years than those with the lowest levels. In participants who already showed proof of retinopathy at the start of the study, the presence of elevated glycohemoglobin resulted in a fourfold greater risk of retinopathy progression and a fourteenfold greater risk of proliferative retinopathy.

In those people on insulin with the highest levels of glycohemoglobin, there was a 90% increased risk of developing retinopathy than those in the lowest levels. The researchers concluded that controlling hyperglycemia even later on in the course of diabetes will result in a significant decrease in the incidence and progression of retinopathy and in the development of visual loss (Klein et al. 1994). Published studies show that controlling excess serum insulin is also important in preventing retinopathy (Raccah et al. 1998; Boehm et al. 2002; Leslie et al. 2002).

There are additional precautions that can be taken to guard against the development of retinopathies. Deficiency of vitamin B_6, for instance, is a proven cause of the disease. In order to rule out a nutritional deficiency as the cause of retinopathy, a 10-week program is suggested that incorporates a high-potency B-complex vitamin formula along with other supplements that will be described in this protocol.

AN INTERESTING STUDY IN RATS

A newborn rat model of retinopathy was used to test the hypothesis that a lack of the antioxidant superoxide dismutase (SOD) contributes to retinal damage. The study concluded that delivery of SOD to the retina via long-circulating liposomes was beneficial and suggested the potential value of the restoration or supplementation of antioxidants in retinal tissue as a therapeutic strategy (Niesman et al. 1997). It is difficult to provide SOD directly to the retina, but adequate supplementation with nutrients, such as zinc, copper, and manganese, provide the minerals needed for the formation of SOD in the cells.

ANTIOXIDANT LENS AND VITREOUS ACTIVITY

Another study investigated antioxidant activity in the lens and vitreous of diabetic and nondiabetic subjects. Researchers found significantly decreased glutathione peroxidase activity and lower ascorbic acid levels in the lenses of diabetic patients, especially in the presence of retinal damage. (Ascorbic acid is known to exert important antioxidant functions in the eye compartment.) This study indicated that oxidative damage is involved in the onset of diabetic eye complications, in which the decrease in free radical scavengers was shown to be associated with the oxidation of vitreous and lens proteins (Altomare et al. 1997).

DECREASED RETINAL ANTIOXIDANT ACTIVITY IN DIABETICS

Activities of enzymes that protect the retina from reactive oxygen species were investigated in diabetic rats known to have developed retinopathy. Diabetes significantly decreased the activities of glutathione reductase and glutathione peroxidase in the retina. Activities of two other important antioxidant defense enzymes—superoxide dismutase and catalase—were also decreased (by more than 25%) in the retinas of diabetic rats (Kowluru et al. 1997).

The study showed that diabetes is associated with significant impairment of the antioxidant defense system and that antioxidant supplementation can help alleviate the subnormal activities of antioxidant defense enzymes. Administration of supplemental vitamins C and E for 2 months prevented the diabetes-induced impairment of the antioxidant defense system in the retina (Kowluru et al. 1997). Another study found no protective effect from antioxidant nutrients for diabetic retinopathy and concluded that further research is necessary to confirm associations of nutrient antioxidant intake and the disease (Mayer-Davis et al. 1998).

RETINOPATHY OF PREMATURITY

A study assessed retinopathy in 60 oxygen-treated, premature infants and their mothers. All 60 infants showed signs of acute oxidative stress. The concentrations of methionine-cysteine in the plasma, as well as blood selenium levels, were significantly lower in the premature infants who had moderate retinopathy than they were in the oxygen-treated premature infants without retinopathy. The mothers of the premature infants with retinopathy showed the same pattern of deficiencies as their babies. Vitamin E treatment of premature infants seemed to have a positive effect against the development of retinopathy of prematurity (Papp et al. 1997).

The close correlation between the antioxidant capacity of the mothers and babies suggests that supplementation with sulfur-containing amino acids (methionine, cysteine) and folic acid during pregnancy might improve the antioxidant capacity of premature infants. An antioxidant cocktail of selenium plus vitamin E given to high-risk mothers (high risk factors include advanced age, smoking, and pregnancy-induced hypertension) before delivery might be useful in the prevention of retinopathy in premature infants (Papp et al. 1997).

THE ROLE OF *L*-CARNITINE

Other research examined the effect of propionyl-*L*-carnitine (an analogue of *L*-carnitine) on retinopathy in rats with laboratory-induced diabetes. Findings pointed to a potential therapeutic value of propionyl-*L*-carnitine for diabetic retinopathy (Hotta et al. 1996). Until propionyl-*L*-carnitine becomes commercially available, taking 2000 mg a day of acetyl-*L*-carnitine should be considered by those with retinopathy. (*L*-carnitine is a natural substance that is found in meat. It is related to the B vitamins.)

GLYCATION

Glycation of proteins has been shown to play a prominent role in the development of many diseases related to diabetes, including atherosclerosis, cataract formation, and retinopathy. Oxidation induced by glycation can wreak havoc on the eye. Protein glycation occurs when sugar molecules inappropriately bind to protein molecules, forming cross-links that distort the proteins and consequently render them useless. High blood sugar also increases glycation activity, which may also explain the various kinds of tissue damage that characterize advanced diabetes. Diligently controlling blood sugar is a major means of preventing or at least slowing the onset and progression of diabetic retinopathy. Glycation appears to increase oxidative processes, which may explain why both glycation and oxidation simultaneously increase with age.

Strategies for the prevention of diabetic complications should therefore aim to prevent both the effects of glycation and oxidative stress.

A drug called aminoguanidine has been used successfully to protect against glycation (Guillausseau 1994). Compounds produced through metabolism of sugars bind preferentially to aminoguanidine rather than to lysine proteins. Thus, aminoguanidine is able to inhibit advanced glycation end-product (AGE) formation and can help prevent the harmful development of collagen cross-links and changes in the proliferation of mesangial cells.

Aminoguanidine used in the dose of 300 mg a day can specifically inhibit glycation, as can the nutrients keto-glutarate and pyruvate. Studies have shown aminoguanidine to be useful in slowing complications of diabetes, such as retinopathy. (Aminoguanidine can also inhibit the formation of atherosclerotic plaques.)

Carnosine is a naturally occurring antiglycation agent found in red meat. In the lens of the eye, protein cross-linking is part of cataract formation. Carnosine eye drops have been shown to delay vision senescence in humans, being effective in 100% of cases of primary senile cataract and 80% of cases of mature senile cataract (Wang et al. 2000). The most widely used antiglycating therapy is to consume orally 1000 mg a day of supplemental carnosine.

A DRUG THAT MAY REVERSE GLYCATION

One promising advanced glycation end product (AGE) breaker is ALT-711 (3-phenacyl-4,5-dimethylthiazolium chloride). ALT-711 is being developed by the Alteon Corporation to reverse the degenerative effects on soft tissues from diseases, such as diabetes and cardiovascular disease. It is currently in Phase II trials. ALT-711 inserts itself into AGE cross-links, separates and cleaves the linked molecules, and releases the proteins. The safety of ALT-711 and its efficacy in reversing age-related cardiovascular damage has been confirmed in animals and in Phase I and Phase IIa clinical trials. Alteon is planning a Phase IIb clinical trial. The randomized, double-blind, placebo-controlled, clinical study will test the effects of multiple doses of ALT-711 in improving isolated systolic hypertension. The trial will be set up in 42 clinical sites and involve several hundred patients.

CAROTENOIDS AND THE RETINA

Countless studies demonstrate an association between consumption of carotenoids with lowered risk of cancer and cardiovascular disease. Carotenoids, especially lutein and zeaxanthin, have also been found to help preserve eye health. Lutein is a pigment found in dark, green, leafy vegetables, including spinach, kale, broccoli, collard greens, etc. Zeaxanthin is found in fruits and vegetables with yellow hues, such as corn, peaches, persimmons, mangoes, etc. They are often lumped together when discussed or studied because they are structurally very similar, found in many of the same foods, and both are present in the retina. Lutein and zeaxanthin have been found to positively affect macular pigment density and to help prevent age-related macular degeneration (AMD).

Although there are several hundred carotenoids to be found in fruits and vegetables, only lutein and zeaxanthin are found in the retina (Schalch 1992; Yeum et al. 1999). Compared to other antioxidant concentrations found in the eye, German researchers found that lutein and zeaxanthin did not break down nearly as fast as lycopene and beta-carotene when exposed to free radical or UV light induced oxidative stress (Siems et al. 1999). The authors suggest that perhaps the slow degradation of lutein and zeaxanthin may explain the strong presence of these carotenoids in the retina. Also, the quick breakdown of lycopene and beta-carotene may suggest why these carotenoids are lacking in the same retinal tissues.

Researchers have also found that lutein and zeaxanthin are more highly concentrated in the center of the macula. There, the amounts of lutein and zeaxanthin are much greater than their concentrations in the peripheral region. At the Baylor College of Medicine in Houston, scientific investigators demonstrated, using retinas from human donor eyes, that the concentration of lutein and zeaxanthin was 70% higher in rod outer segment (ROS) membranes where the concentration of long-chain polyunsaturated fatty acids and susceptibility to oxidation is highest, than in residual membranes (Rapp et al. 2000). The fact that lutein and zeaxanthin are particularly concentrated in these parts of the eye suggests that they may act as a shield or filter that helps to absorb harmful UVB light and dangerous free-radical molecules, both of which threaten the retinal tissue (Moeller et al. 2000; Bernstein et al. 2001).

THE IMPORTANCE OF ADEQUATE VITAMIN STATUS

Vitamin B_{12}. (Cyanocobalamin, or hydroxycobalamin, a naturally occurring form) is critical for several functions, such as folate metabolism, myelin synthesis, and the normal development of red blood cells. A lack of this vitamin may leave the optic nerve more susceptible to damage. Studies have suggested that marginal vitamin deficiency plays an indirect but important role in the development of diabetic complications (Anon. 1990).

Vitamin E. One study showed that reducing lipid peroxidation stress of the erythrocyte membrane using vitamin E (alpha-tocopherol nicotinate) therapy may be useful in slowing deterioration of microangiopathy in Type II diabetes mellitus. The dose used in the study was 300 mg 3 times a day, after meals, for 3 months (Chung et al. 1998). In the August 1999 issue of the journal Diabetes Care, Dr. George L. King and his colleagues reported that vitamin E supplements normalized blood-flow to the retina and kidneys. Following a 4-month clinical trial in which subjects were given doses of vitamin E that were 60 times the recommended daily allowance, kidney function improved and blood flow to the retina was increased almost to the normal rate. Dr. King is recommending a large follow-up clinical trial (Bursell et al. 1999).

Another study evaluated the use of antioxidants as a prophylactic for eye disorders, such as macular degeneration, cataracts, retinopathy of prematurity, and cystic macular edema. The study points to the positive role of antioxidants in both experimental research and clinical observations (KaLuzny 1996).

Green Tea. Green tea is another potent antioxidant that could be of use in the treatment of retinopathy. The active compounds in green tea are chiefly catechins. Powerful polyphenolic antioxidants, catechins are astringent, water-soluble compounds that can be easily oxidized. They are a subgroup of flavonoids, weak phytoestrogenic compounds widely available in vegetables, fruit, tea, coffee, chocolate, and wine. The antioxidant potential of both green and black teas, as measured by the Phenol Antioxidant Index, was found to be significantly higher than that of grape juice and red wines. Green tea also has anti-angiogenic properties, indicating that it could be used for the prevention and possibly even the treatment of degenerative eye disorders, such as diabetic retinopathy, that also depend on the development of new blood vessels (Zigman et al. 1999; Thiagarajan et al. 2001).

Silibinin. An *in vitro* study showed that silibinin (milk thistle extract) can normalize the degree of ribosylation and the sodium pump activity even in the presence of abnormally high glucose levels (Di Giulio et al. 1999). A similar protective effect of silibinin against ribosylation was found in the retina (Gorio et al. 1997). Thus silibinin may be able to decrease the extent of diabetic neuropathy and retinopathy, two extremely serious complications of diabetes. Considering that silibinin has also been shown to protect the kidneys, another organ seriously damaged by glycation (kidney failure is a frequent cause of death in diabetics), silibinin should be seriously explored as an adjunct treatment in diabetes.

CONCLUSION

Retinopathy is a major cause of blindness among adults in the developed world. Risk factors are diabetes (especially with elevated blood glucose levels), vitamin deficiency, and old age. In retinopathy, the retina of the eye is damaged when retinal capillaries bulge or burst, leaking blood or fluid into the surrounding tissue. New capillaries that grow on the retina (and into the vitreous) cause blurred vision or blindness. Permanent blindness can result from retinal detachment caused by scar tissue. Prevention requires annual dilated eye exams and proper vitamin and nutrient intake. Researchers conclude that improved levels of antioxidants in pregnant women could help prevent retinopathy in their premature infants.

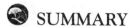 **SUMMARY**

1. Long-term antioxidant protection of the eyes can be provided by taking 3 tablets 3 times a day, of Life Extension Mix and 1 capsule a day of the Life Extension Booster formula. These two supplements provide the alpha and gamma forms of vitamin E, lutein, minerals for the formation of superoxide dismutase (SOD), such as zinc, manganese, and copper along with potent B complex vitamins. Some people may also want to take additional vitamin B_6 (up to an additional 250 mg).

2. Carnosine is an antiglycating agent that helps protect against the damaging effects of glycation. As an oral supplement, two 500-mg capsules daily are recommended. As an eyedrop, carnosine may help prevent protein cross-linking in the retina. One to two drops daily of carnosine eyedrops are recommended. Those with any kind of eye problem may want to apply 1–2 drops several times a day.

3. Zeaxanthin and lutein may help filter harmful UVB light and quench free radicals that harm the retina. Suggested dose from diet or supplements is 5 mg a day of zeaxanthin and 15–20 mg a day of lutein.

4. Silibinin may help slow the extent of diabetic retinopathy; 250–500 mg a day is suggested.

5. Green tea extract is a powerful antioxidant that has shown promise in the treatment of degenerative eye disease; 600–700 mg of a 95% polyphenol extract is suggested.

6. Taking 2000 mg a day of acetyl-*L*-carnitine should be considered by those who have retinopathy, particularly if on a vegetarian diet.

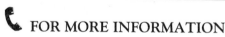 **FOR MORE INFORMATION**

Contact the National Eye Health Education Program of the National Institutes of Health, (301) 496-5248.

 PRODUCT AVAILABILITY

Life Extension Mix, Life Extension Booster, Super Carnosine, Brite Eyes II (carnosine drops), Super Zeaxanthin with Lutein, vitamin E, green tea extract, Gamma E Tocopherol/Tocotrienols, Silibinin Plus, vitamin B_6, ornithine alpha-ketoglutarate, calcium pyruvate and acetyl-*L*-carnitine can be ordered by calling (800) 544-4440 or by ordering online at www.lef.org. Ask for a list of European suppliers of aminoguanidine.

Scleroderma (Systemic Sclerosis)

Scleroderma: from the Greek words *sklēro-*, meaning hardness, and *derma*, meaning skin

Scleroderma, also known as systemic sclerosis, is a chronic, progressive, disabling autoimmune connective tissue disorder with various complex symptoms. A highly individualized disease, its involvement may range from very mild symptoms to life-threatening complications. Fourteen million people worldwide, 150,000 in the United States, suffer from scleroderma. It affects four times more women than men, with symptoms usually occurring between the ages of 35–65. Scleroderma is not contagious, cancerous, or considered malignant in any way. The 5-year fatality rate of those with the severe form (about 60,000) has been estimated at 50–70%. The cause of scleroderma is unknown, although it is known that the disease process in scleroderma involves an overproduction of collagen. This protocol will briefly survey the most recent information regarding the symptoms, the hypothetical causes, and conventional and integrated medical treatments for scleroderma.

A potentially life-threatening condition, scleroderma must be managed by a knowledgeable physician. Because it is fairly rare, one should seek out specialists in the types of symptoms caused by scleroderma—that is, dermatologists (skin), rheumatologists (joints and connective tissue), and dentists—who have specific experience with the disease. Although there is no known treatment that can stop or slow the progression of scleroderma, many physicians feel that early medical intervention yields better results and positively affects the course of the disease. Given the ineffectiveness of conventional treatments, many physicians take the position that patients might as well try any alternative treatments that could be of benefit and will not hurt them. It is imperative that your physician knows all therapies you are using, and that you be an active self-advocate, asking for specific information, educating yourself about your disease, and seeking support.

DEFINITIONS

Localized Scleroderma

Considered the mild form of scleroderma, localized disease predominantly affects the skin. Although it may affect muscles and joints, it does not affect organs. It is very rare for localized disease to become systemic; if this occurs, the initial diagnosis was likely mistaken. Two common types are the following:

- **Linear scleroderma** is characterized by a line of hardened skin affecting the underlying tissues (muscles, bones). It usually occurs on the arms, legs, and forehead on one side of the body and is common in children.
- **Morphea** is characterized by patches of yellowish or ivory-colored rigid, dry skin that become hard, slightly depressed oval plaques. It usually occurs on the trunk, although it may be widespread (generalized morphea).

Systemic Scleroderma

The systemic disease occurs throughout the body, affecting internal organs. It is progressive and can be life-threatening because it affects the connective tissue of the lung, kidney, heart, and other organs as well as blood vessels, muscles, and joints. The skin thickening for which the disease is named is symmetrical on both sides of the body, usually beginning on the fingertips and moving up the arms. Legs and thighs also are affected. Some common medical terms associated with systemic scleroderma are as follows:

- **CREST** stands for calcinosis (small, movable, nontender calcium lumps under the skin). CREST may occur alone or in combination with any autoimmune disease. There is no way to predict if or when it will progress to diffuse scleroderma.
- **Limited scleroderma** occurs on the hands and possibly on the face and neck.
- **Diffuse scleroderma** is defined as skin tightening above the wrists or elbows. Early thickening and hardening of the skin, sometimes preceded by itching, are present in 95% of patients, although skin involvement may not be prominent. More widespread disease can lead to severe organ damage.

DISEASE SYMPTOMS

The diagnosis of scleroderma is a clinical one based on symptoms rather than tests. However, skin or kidney biopsies can be done to look for signs of the disease, and other investigations can be carried out to evaluate the function of different organ systems. Blood tests commonly reveal certain antibodies, which may have informative value beyond simply confirming the diagnosis. For example, although antinuclear antibodies are some common findings in many autoimmune diseases (90%

red pepper (capsicum) to stimulate salivation and tears. The red pepper is best added to food or drink to increase watery secretions.

19. The late John Christopher, M.D., herbalist and founder of the School of Natural Healing, suggested holding grape juice in the mouth and "chewing" and swishing the liquid to increase saliva secretion. Individuals with "dry mouth syndrome" often report an excellent response from this simple, low-cost therapy.

20. Acupuncture has helped many SS patients successfully cope with the symptoms of dry mouth. In a Swedish study of oral diseases, 70 patients between ages 33–82 with dry mouth showed significant increases in salivary flow after 6 months of acupuncture treatment (Blom et al. 2000).

21. SS patients should see a dentist regularly (3 times a year) to closely monitor changes in tooth structure.

Tips for Treating Nasal and Throat Dryness

1. Potassium iodide helps promote nasal and throat secretions. A dose of 225 mcg a day is regarded as safe and without significant side effects.

2. Pilocarpine, a cholinergic, can be used orally (to stimulate salivary secretion) or topically (in the nose) to promote moistness (Vivino et al. 1999). Dr. Steven Carsons cautions that because the range is narrow between efficacy and toxicity, pilocarpine must be used under close medical supervision.

3. Cevimeline (EVOXAC), another cholinergic, can be used orally (30 mg 3 times daily) to stimulate mucous and salivary glands. Cevimeline, available by prescription, can cause nausea, sweating, headaches, frequent urination, visual disturbances, and diarrhea (Fife et al. 2002).

4. Guaifenesin, the main ingredient in many expectorants, increases respiratory tract fluid, loosening phlegm and mucus. Guaifenesin is available in a concentrated form by prescription.

5. A humidifier assists in keeping air moist.

6. Try to breathe through the nose, rather than open-mouth breathing. A soft cervical collar, used while sleeping, may prevent open-mouth breathing by supporting the jaw. Sleep in a cool bedroom (Carsons 1998).

7. Vitamin E is an excellent lubricant, with some patients reporting a better response when applied around the rim of the nose rather than deep into the nasal chamber.

8. Saline and Aloe (a product provided by Naturade) relieves dry nasal membranes and nosebleeds. This product is considered safe and gentle enough for continued usage.

9. Lily Bulb formula (Bai He Gu Jin Tang, a Chinese therapeutic) has been used for dry throat and nose. The dosage is 3 tablets 3–4 times daily, taken between meals. Lily Bulb may be purchased from Health Concerns, (800) 233-9355.

10. Clearing the throat repeatedly can be irritating. If throat clearing cannot be avoided, use an "h" sound or hum to lessen trauma to the vocal cords (Carsons 1998).

Tips for Treating Skin and Vaginal Dryness

1. Avoid antibacterial soaps or abrasive cleansers.

2. Select soaps with added moisturizers or oils.

3. Bathe no more than once daily. If tub baths are used, soak in tepid bath water for 10–15 minutes to rehydrate the skin. Upon emerging from either a tub or shower, do not dry skin completely. Leave a film of moisture and then moisturize with a cream.

4. Emollients with urea, lactate, or salicylic aid assist in sloughing off dead skin, allowing a healthier, softer skin to emerge.

5. Water-based vaginal lubricants may help relieve dryness and discomfort. Sustained use of lubricants can, however, disrupt the normal mucosa of the vagina, making lubricants inappropriate for long-term application. Women needing a daily vaginal lubricant may find vitamin E suppositories helpful. During the first month of use, insert the suppository into the vagina once daily; after several months, 1 suppository 1–3 times a week may suffice.

⬤ SUMMARY

1. Essential fatty acids found in several fish and vegetable oils will also help reduce inflammation. Super GLA/DHA, a balanced formula derived from marine lipid concentrate and borage oil (providing 920 mg of GLA, 1000 mg of DHA, and 400 mg of EPA), is an excellent anti-inflammatory choice. Use 6 capsules daily. Use 2–4 grams of evening primrose oil each day (with meals) to halt lacrimal and salivary atrophy and normalize the immune response.

2. Restoring DHEA to optimal levels appears to modulate the immune and inflammatory responses.

Tests should be performed to determine DHEA level before treatment and during DHEA supplementation. Most studies in humans used 50 mg daily of DHEA with few side effects noted. DHEA is contraindicated in individuals with either prostate or estrogen-related cancers.

3. To help fight fatigue, supplement with coenzyme Q_{10} (50 mg 2 or 3 times daily), L-carnitine (1000–2000 mg daily), green barley, and trifala (one 490-mg capsule, taken 1 hour before meals). Trifala, an Ayurvedic herbal complex containing *Emblica offinalis*, *Terminalia belerica*, and *Terminalia chebula*, is regarded as a systemic balancer. Trifala can be purchased from Bazaar of India, (800) 261-7662.

4. Vitamin C, 3000 mg taken daily in divided doses, protects against inflammation and infection and reduces dental caries. Chewable vitamin C should be avoided because of acid damage to tooth enamel.

5. Goldenseal (*H. canadensis*) has antibacterial activity against streptococcal bacteria. Thirty drops of goldenseal dissolved in 2 oz of warm water and swished about in the mouth may reduce inflammation and infection, killing opportunistic organisms.

6. Deficiencies of vitamin A can cause abnormal dryness. Beta-carotene (a nontoxic form of vitamin A) in a dose of 25,000–50,000 IU may increase the integrity of mucous membranes and protect against bacterial and viral assaults. Viva Drops, a vitamin A product available through LEF, is helpful against dry or irritated eyes. Place 2 or more drops in each eye and blink. Repeat as necessary.

7. Some SS patients report a loss of taste and smell that may respond to zinc supplementation. A dose of 30–60 mg daily for men and 30–45 mg daily for women may also improve T-helper and suppressor ratios.

8. Pancreatic enzymes taken between meals assist in breaking up circulating immune complexes and reducing inflammation. Use 2–4 tablets 3 times daily.

9. Thymus fractions may help produce a population of mature T-cells capable of distinguishing foreign antigens from self tissue. Patients with seriously compromised immune function often use 3 doses a day until blood tests remain normal for 3–6 months. Use the thymic protein sublingually, retaining for 3 minutes to allow for maximum absorption. Assays to determine immune competency should, however, precede supplementation.

10. Life Flora capsules are available containing 3 billion freeze-dried organisms (*B. longum*, *B. bifidum*, *L. acidophilus*, *S. faecium*, and *L. casei*). Use 6 capsules daily (between meals) for an initial GI loading; thereafter use 1–4 capsules daily for maintenance of healthy GI bacteria. Life Flora is best utilized with NutraFlora (FOS) Powder. One to four tsp daily are suggested for the treatment of chronic disease states that could be exacerbated by a deficiency of friendly bacteria or an overgrowth of harmful GI organisms. A maintenance dose is 1/2–1 tsp daily.

11. A diet favoring alkaline foods such as fruits and vegetables has a stimulating effect on the parasympathetic nervous system and reduces both oral and systemic acidity.

12. Try to reduce stressful situations in your life. Emotional factors play a role in the course of many diseases, including autoimmune conditions.

 PRODUCT AVAILABILITY

Super GLA/DHA, DHEA, Beta Carotene, CoQ10, Digest RC, evening primrose oil, Gamma E Tocopherol/Tocotrienol, goldenseal, Jarrow's EPS (*L. acidophilus*), L-carnitine, Life Extension Mix (capsules, tablets, or powder), Life Flora, Liquid Emulsified Vitamin A, NutriFlora (FOS Powder), Optizinc, ProBoost Thymic Protein A, Super Digestive Enzymes, vitamin B2 powder, vitamin C capsules, vitamin E succinate, Viva Drops, and Wobenzyme N are available by calling (800) 544-4440 or by ordering online at www.lef.org.

Skin Aging

INTRODUCTION

Skin is the largest organ of the human body, weighing approximately 10 pounds and covering an area of about 16 square feet. We generally take skin for granted and tend not to take very good care of it. Our skin is responsible for protecting our internal organs from the toxic external world. Our skin protects us from heat, cold, and physical injuries. It also provides us with sensory information about the nature of the external world and is our first defense against invasion by bacteria, viruses, and other toxic elements. The skin is also an excretory organ, removing toxins from the body via perspiration.

Although there are many diseases that can affect the skin, the most common problems that we *all* have are the effects of our exposure to ultraviolet (UV) radiation from the sun over time. Having a healthy tan has, in the past, been a sign of good health. In the last 10 years, with the changes in the ozone layer in the upper atmosphere, it is clear that the effects of UV radiation from the sun are much more dangerous than originally thought. There are many causes for the accumulated cellular damage in the skin that we call aging. Among these are the oxidative processes and related free radical damage that result from UV sunlight, smog, toxins, cigarette smoke, X-rays, drugs, and other stressors. Young skin is also exposed to these potentially damaging changes, but when we are young, there is sufficient cellular energy (ATP) for DNA repair and cell renewal. Enzymes that provide antioxidant activity such as SOD and catalase are readily available. As we age, there is increased wear and tear, while at the same time the energy for cell repair and renewal is diminished and the antioxidant enzymes are less available.

Specific diseases that affect the skin will not be covered in this protocol, but will rather be listed under the disease category itself (e.g., *Acne*). This protocol will primarily deal with the effects of aging on the skin.

Health-conscious Americans are concerned about the damage that sunlight inflicts on the skin. Protecting against the effects of ultraviolet radiation is a multi-million dollar industry. Creams, lotions, cosmetic products, and protectants are to be found everywhere, resulting in con-

fusion for the consumer regarding what products are really helpful. Cosmetic companies may seize upon an idea, put that ingredient into a cream or lotion without much research, and then advertise it to an unsuspecting public. This protocol will only use evidence from peer-reviewed journals.

The Anatomy of Our Skin

Our skin consists of two main layers: the dermis and epidermis. The dermis is the inner layer of skin that contains nerve fibers, fat cells, blood vessels, sweat and oil glands, and hair follicles. The dermis also contains collagen and elastin, two proteins that are responsible for the structure and elasticity of the skin itself. These proteins are subject to the process of aging. The sweat and oil glands in the dermis protect the outer layer of skin with a thin coating of oil and perspiration.

The epidermis is the outermost layer of our skin. New cells generated by the dermis continually replace this layer. Removal of the epidermis, as in a scrape or burn, reveals an unprotected sensitive dermis underneath. The epidermis also contains melanocytes or pigment cells. These cells produce melanin, which determines the shade of your skin (a heritable factor).

SKIN AND FREE RADICALS

Scientists now believe that the free radical theory of disease also applies to the aging of the skin. Free radicals are unstable small molecules generated by an oxygen environment which require stabilization by the body's antioxidant system. Free radicals occur throughout every cell in our body simply by virtue of the fact that oxygen is our principal metabolic fuel. Strong sunlight readily generates free radicals in the skin. Our hands, face, neck, and arms are the areas usually chronically exposed to light. These parts of the body, particularly the face, are where aging of the skin shows up.

The skin protein collagen is particularly susceptible to free radical damage, and when this damage occurs, it causes the collagen protein molecules to break down and then link back up again in a different way; this is known as cross-linking. Collagen cross-linking causes the normally mobile collagen to become stiff and less mobile. Sunlight also causes the messenger molecules present in skin cells to become active and create inflammatory products. Fisher et al. (1977) have shown that the multiple small exposures to ultraviolet irradiation lead to sustained elevations of enzymes that degrade skin collagen and contribute to photo-aging.

Skin cancer typically occurs in skin that is photo-aged. Wrinkles, laxity, uneven pigmentation, brown

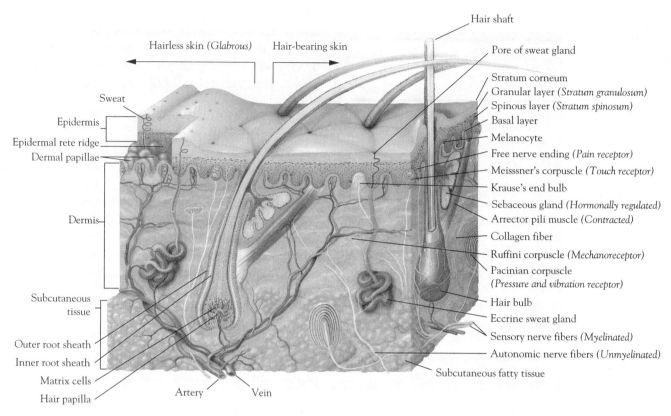

Anatomy of the skin. (Anatomical Chart Company 2002®, Lippincott Williams & Wilkins)

spots, and a leathery appearance characterize photo-aged skin. In contrast, chronologically aged skin that has been protected from the sun is thin and has reduced elasticity, but is otherwise smooth and unblemished.

The following factors can accelerate skin aging:

- sun exposure
- first- or secondhand cigarette smoke
- environmental toxins
- poor diet
- excess alcohol consumption
- stress
- harsh soaps or detergent-based moisturizers
- sleep deprivation

One way of mitigating the effects of these skin-damaging foes is to increase levels of protective anti-oxidants through a diet rich in fruits and vegetables or by direct topical application.

Critics used to claim there was no evidence that topically based products affected skin aging. Over the years, a remarkable number of published studies have proven these skeptics wrong! Science clearly substantiates the role that free radicals play in causing skin aging and the fact that topically applied antioxidants confer significant protection and can even partially reverse some aspects of skin aging. Indeed, various animal and human studies have proven that low molecular weight antioxidants, especially vitamins C and E, as well as alpha-lipoic acid exert protective effects against free radical damage (oxidative stress) (Podda et al. 2001).

In a double-blind study, a topical vitamin C complex was applied to one half of the face and a placebo gel to the opposite side. Clinical evaluation of wrinkling, pigmentation, inflammation, and hydration was performed prior to the study at weeks 4, 8, and 12. The results showed a statistically significant improvement of the vitamin C-treated side, with decreased photoaging scores of the cheeks and the perioral area. The peri-orbital area improved in both the vitamin C and placebo-gel group, probably indicating improved hydration. The overall facial improvement of the vitamin C side was statistically significant. Biopsies showed increased collagen formation in the vitamin C group. This study showed that topically applied vitamin C results in clinically visible and statistically significant improvement in wrinkling when used for 12 weeks. This clinical improvement correlated with biopsy evidence of new collagen formation (Fitzpatrick et al. 2002).

In response, cosmetic companies have increased the percentages of active ingredients with the goal of replicating the antiaging effects revealed in the published studies. The problem of increasing the level of active ingredients is that the wrong layers of the skin can be overly saturated resulting in irritation and reduced efficacy.

The first step in resolving this problem is to encase the active ingredients so that they can be absorbed through the top layer into the lower layers of the skin where they are most active. The second step is to design a delayed release system so that the active ingredients can be released over an extended amount of time.

Other Factors

In spite of the effect of sunlight on the skin, there are other factors that affect skin health that occur regardless of our exposure to sun rays. Dryness, loss of tone and fullness, diminished immune responses, and reduced ability to repair damage are all factors that contribute to the aging process.

There are many types of skin tones and qualities. Men tend to have thicker skin than women due to the dominant hormone testosterone. However, in later years, the lack of estrogen in women and testosterone in men tend to cause changes in both genders.

Each individual will have a different skin, with different oil production, color, and texture. Clearly, people with dry, white skin should use only mild cleansers and never use grainy cleansing products. Moisturizers and oil-based make-ups will also be required. On the other hand, those with an oily, darker skin can use mild liquid cleansers and an oil-blotting foundation. Generally, the use of sunscreens is reasonable as long as it does not create a false sense of security. Do not go out for longer periods of time in the sun just because you're wearing a sunscreen.

Skin damage occurs when the membrane covering of the skin cell is damaged by free radicals. Free radicals make the membrane more permeable, allowing the cells to dehydrate (lose water). The membrane of the cell is what is called a lipid bilayer: two layers of fat end-on-end. Enzymes are activated when the skin is traumatized or exposed to sun. Enzymes break down the lipid bilayer and cause inflammation. Thus, any antioxidants must be fat-soluble to protect this layer.

Chronic inflammation is an underlying cause of common degenerative diseases. One study found that pro-oxidative factors that accelerate skin aging might activate a self-maintained micro-inflammatory process that interferes with skin elasticity and thickness. This study stated that topical antioxidants decrease this inflammatory cascade and thus afford protection to the skin structures (Giacomoni et al. 2000).

The effect of exposure to even ambient UV irradiation increases the risk for long-term, detrimental effects characterized by wrinkles and loss of skin tone and resilience. Photo-aged skin displays prominent alterations in the cellular component and the extracellular matrix of the connective tissue. UV exposure results in an accumulation of disorganized elastin and a severe loss of collagens, the major structural proteins of the dermal connective tissue. The unifying pathogenic agents for these changes are UV-generated free radicals. As well as causing permanent gene mutations, free radicals activate signal transduction pathways that are related to growth, differentiation, senescence, and connective tissue degradation (Scharfetter-kochanek et al. 2000).

WHAT IS GOOD FOR YOUR SKIN?

When most people think about good things that they can do for their skin, they usually think about things they will put on their skin rather than what they will put inside themselves to make their skin healthier. Although topical application of certain products is essential, equally important is the nourishment of the skin from the inside. Everything from essential fatty acids, antioxidants, and other supplements to the food that we eat is critical in maintaining healthy skin that ages slowly.

The Outside Story

The first preventive measure you can take is to reduce the amount of UV light that you are exposed to. This can be done either by avoiding the sun completely or more practically by wearing at least an SPF15 sunblock. One danger with using a sun block is that it tends to make people feel like they can go out in the sun more! So they end up with the same amount of UV radiation because they are simply out in the sun longer. For areas that are more exposed, such as the nose and cheekbones, a sun-blocking titanium oxide would probably be best.

Considerable interest has been generated about combining antioxidants with sunscreens to provide enhanced protection against UV rays. Two of the best-known antioxidants are vitamins C and E, both of which have been shown to be effective in different models of photodamage. In a study done on swine skin, vitamin C provided additive protection against acute UVB damage (sunburn cell formation) when combined with a UVB sunscreen. When a combination of vitamins E and C were used, very good protection from a UVB insult occurred. Vitamin C, however, was significantly better than vitamin E at protecting against a UVA-mediated phototoxic insult in this animal model (Darr et al. 1996).

When it comes to makeup and skin care products, people with oily skin should clearly avoid products that have oil in their formula. Those with dry skin need products that have essential oils combined in the formula. Cleansing the skin by washing once daily without astringent products is probably a good idea as well. Facial masks can help hydrate skin, but can be harmful if they cause irritation. They should never be used more than once a week.

Antioxidants

Although antioxidants are well-known for their beneficial effects inside the body when taken orally, in the case of skin, there are a number of antioxidants that are helpful when applied topically (Podda et al. 2001).

Human studies have demonstrated pronounced protective effects of antioxidants when applied topically before UV radiation exposure. With respect to UVB-induced skin damage, the photoprotective effects of antioxidants are significant. Topical application of such combinations may result in a sustained antioxidant capacity of the skin, possibly due to antioxidant synergisms. Free radicals are culprits behind UVA-induced skin alterations, thus indicating a basis for topical antioxidant administration. In a human study, topical application of antioxidants resulted in diminished severity of UVA-induced sun damage. Thus, regular application of skin care products containing antioxidants may be of the utmost benefit in efficiently preparing skin against exogenous oxidative stressors occurring during daily life. Sunscreen agents may also benefit from combination with antioxidants resulting in increased safety and efficacy of such photoprotective products (Dreher et al. 2001).

Vitamin C Esters. Vitamin C ester is vitamin C with a fatty acid attached to it. It is fat-soluble and rapidly penetrates the skin, being much better absorbed than vitamin C alone. Products containing vitamin C ester, such as ascorbyl palmitate, will be helpful in reducing and preventing skin damage (Yamamoto et al. 2002).

Vitamin C does more than inhibit skin-damaging free radical activity. It is also required for collagen synthesis, which declines markedly in aging skin. As humans age, they suffer diminished microcapillary circulation within the skin, thereby depriving skin cells of the supply of vitamin C it needs for youthful collagen synthesis. The topical application of vitamin C in a skin-penetrating medium can enhance the availability of vitamin C for collagen production. Vitamin C regenerates vitamin E in the skin. An antioxidant like vitamin E can only suppress a limited number of free radicals before it runs out of electrons to donate. Vitamin C regenerates vitamin E and enables vitamin E to provide sustained antioxidant protection in the skin's elastin fibers. Vitamin C also plays a vital role in skin repair. When skin is injured, its vitamin C content is used up rapidly in the scavenging of free radicals, and in synthesizing collagen to speed healing.

A randomized double-blind controlled study was conducted on human volunteers to determine the efficacy of topical vitamin C application in treating mild to moderate photodamage of facial skin. Methods of evaluating efficacy included an objective computer-assisted image analysis of skin surface topography, subjective clinical and photographic appearance and patient self-appraisal questionnaires. Topical vitamin C was applied to one side of each patient's face and a control vehicle on the other side for 3 months.

The results using the optical image analysis demonstrated that compared to the placebo-vehicle, the vitamin C-treated side of the face showed a statistically significant 71% combined score improvement. Clinical assessment parameters demonstrated significant improvement with vitamin C treatment compared to the placebo vehicle for fine wrinkling, tactile roughness, coarse rhytids, skin tone, sallowness, and overall features. Patient questionnaire results demonstrated statistically significant improvement overall, with the vitamin C treatment 84.2% greater than control. Photographic assessment demonstrated significant improvement with vitamin C treatment (57.9% greater than the improvement in the control group). This 3-month study using topical vitamin C provided objective and subjective assessment of the improvement in photodamaged facial skin (Traikovich et al. 1999).

Alpha-Lipoic Acid. Alpha-lipoic acid is an antioxidant that has been found to be extremely important in the management of Type II diabetes. It appears to be able to increase the beneficial effects of other antioxidants and is both water and fat-soluble. Alpha-lipoic acid is also found in the mitochondria, the powerhouses of the cell itself. Thus, it can augment the metabolic processes of the cells, and in addition, it turns off an inflammatory messenger known as nuclear factor kappa beta (NFKB), which turns on inflammation.

Note: *NFKB is a transcription factor. Transcription factors are messengers found inside the cell, which carry information from the cytoplasm to the nucleus. There they may activate or inhibit the production of certain proteins or enzymes, which then carry out a particular cell function. Such a function might be increased inflammatory factors.*

Another factor known as AP-1 may either damage or heal skin depending upon how it is activated. If it is activated by sunlight, it produces free radicals; but if it is activated by alpha lipoic acid, then it turns on enzymes that digest only the damaged collagen. As we age, proteins can become glycated. Glycation is a process where a glucose molecule is attached to the protein and is commonly measured in the body by estimating the blood levels of glycosylated hemoglobin (Hba1c). Alpha-lipoic acid can decrease glycation, decrease pore size, and activate AP-1. Often the result of this is a decrease in facial lines when applied topically.

A concern amongst dermatologists is whether agents that are proven effective in fighting skin aging can be consistently delivered to the specific layers of the skin where they are known to induce their biological effect. The advent of liposome delivery technology has enabled scientists to increase the efficacy of topical anti-aging agents by delivering them into the inner layers of the skin.

A patented liposome delivery system trademarked *QuSomes®* (meaning "quick liposomes")was discovered in late 2000. This technology represents a substantial enhancement in conventional liposome vehicles. QuSomes not only delivers active skin-protecting ingredients faster into the lower layers of the skin, but these liposomes are also designed to protect the active ingredient from deterioration. With the unique QuSome delivery system, the solubility of the active anti-aging agents is preserved, thereby enabling them to reside longer in the areas of the skin where they exert their greatest biological effects. The availability of QuSomes enables nutrients like alpha lipoic acid to be reliably delivered to the inner layers of the skin. This makes alpha lipoic acid an exciting new weapon in the battle against the ravages of time.

Alpha- and Beta-Hydroxy Acids (Glycolic Acid and Salicylic Acid). Alpha-hydroxy acids have been around for about 20 years and make a marked improvement in skin quality by their exfoliative action. Exfoliation removes dead skin cells from the surface. In the late 1980s, the media reported on the age-reversal properties of glycolic acid, an alpha- hydroxy fruit acid that functioned to slough dead skin cells off the surface so that more youthful appearing fresh cells would be visible. The effect of the topical application of these fruit acids was the disappearance of fine lines and wrinkles and a fresher looking tone to the skin.

Importantly, several years before this announcement, a researcher named Carmen Fusco had added an alpha-hydroxy fruit acid (lactic acid) to a skin cream formula called Rejuvenex. This formula became the first anti aging cream in history to incorporate an alpha-hydroxy fruit acid as an active ingredient.

A physician, Dr. Benjamin S. Frank, first developed Rejuvenex in the 1970s. He believed that nutritition played a major role in preventing disease. Dr. Frank proposed that aging was partially a result of decreased energy production in the cell's mitochondria. He felt that in the presence of reduced mitochondrial function, cells become defective and lack the energy needed to effectively repair DNA. Published scientific studies have since validated Dr. Frank's theory about cell energy depletion and aging.

One of Dr. Frank's most famous hypotheses was that the topical application of RNA improved cell energy metabolism and therefore the health and appearance of the skin.

Much has been discovered about skin aging since Dr. Frank began experimenting with RNA-based face creams at his New York City medical office. His premature death did not deter the further development of his skin-saving cream. His assistant, Carmen Fusco, continued the research, producing a cream with the nutrients and antioxidants noted for their anti-aging properties.

Hydroxys are not just an exfoliant, but also a stimulator of collagen production and cell growth (Kim et al. 1998). In animals they have been found to reduce tumor incidence (Hong et al. 2001). Psoriasis, a common debilitating skin condition with increased epidermal production, also responds to hydroxy acids and even more so with topical steroid added, according to Kostarelos et al. (2000). The authors concluded from this double-blind study:

> The present clinical study demonstrates for the first time that the effective and well tolerated therapeutic efficacy of glycolic acid scalp lotions is enhanced when used in conjunction with a 0.1% betamethasone scalp application against scalp psoriasis. This potential offers the practising dermatologist novel treatment modes against severe skin conditions by combining topical corticosteroid with exfoliative agent therapy.

DMAE (Dimethylaminoethanol). One of the major problems of advanced aging is the sagging of tissues caused by the destruction of the skin's underlying support structure (primarily collagen and elastin). While much of this structural deterioration may be preventable by lifestyle changes and proper use of oral and topical agents, it is difficult to reverse this unsightly collapse of facial tissues. In a study published in *Skin Research Technologies*, DMAE was shown to produce a firming effect on the skin (Uhoda 2002). This mechanism may be due to the fact that DMAE functions as a cell membrane stabilizer. Based on clinical reports, DMAE may be the first topical agent that can help firm sagging skin.

Other Antioxidants and Topical Treatments. Tixier et al. (1984) found that the antioxidant pycnogenol (Pine Bark extract) can bind to elastin (one of the skin proteins) and prevent its degradation by elastase in a rabbit model. Another study indicates that oral supplementation of pycnogenol (PBE) reduces erythema in the skin (Saliou et al. 2001).

Vitamin A analogs such as tretinoin and tazarotene creams are also available for topical treatment of photo-damaged skin (Nyirady et al. 2001).

Vitamin A and its retinoid analogs stimulate skin cell renewal by increasing the rate of mitotic cell division (Ridge et al. 1988; Chapellier et al. 2002; Koussoulakos et al. 1990). One mechanism by which vitamin A induces this phenomenon is to act as a signaling agent to stimulate the binding of epidermal growth factor to skin cells (Chapellier et al. 2002).

A characteristic of sun-damaged skin is the degradation of the supporting structure of skin caused by reduced collagen synthesis. A study involving 72 individuals of varying age groups was done to see if the topical application of natural vitamin A could improve function in both natural aged, sun-protected, and photo-aged skin. In one of the study groups consisting of individuals 80+ years of age, topical application of vitamin A for 7 days increased fibroblast growth and collagen synthesis, while reducing levels of a collagen degrading skin enzyme (metalloproteinase).

The overall findings indicated that naturally aged, sun-protected and photo-aged skin share important molecular features including connective tissue damage, elevated metalloproteinase levels, and reduced collagen production. Topical vitamin A treatment reduced matrix metalloproteinase expression and stimulated collagen synthesis in naturally aged and sun-protected skin, as it does in photo-aged skin (Varani et al. 2000). Vitamin A drugs (Retin-A) have shown more profound acute effects in reversing both photo damaged and naturally aged skin, but some people find it irritating to the skin (Varani et al. 1998).

Studies show that the upper layer of the skin (epidermis) can be easily loaded with natural vitamin A by topical application. Besides being a precursor for retinoic acid, vitamin A also has a free-radical scavenging potential. Vitamin A absorbs ultraviolet light to help protect the most delicate areas of the skin against damaging free-radical attack (Sorg et al. 2001). Natural vitamin A thus functions via several pathways to guard against normal and sun-induced skin aging.

Other studies indicated that natural vitamin A (retinyl palmitate), had some of the cell renewal properties that were once attributed solely to retinoic acid drugs.

Going Beyond Antioxidants

While free radicals have been implicated in much of the damage that occurs to aging skin, there are other injurious factors that result in unsightly structural and functional deterioration.

For instance, aging skin cells suffer from metabolic imbalances that preclude them from performing youthful repair functions. The groundbreaking work of Benjamin S. Frank, M.D,. showed that RNA improved cellular energy and the ability of the skin's cells to use oxygen. This improved metabolism enhances the movement of young cells to the surface of the skin where they replace old cells.

Another benefit from topically applied RNA is to repair early skin cell damage. Clinical trials by Dr. S.J. Jellinek in the 1970s demonstrated how creams containing RNA/DNA caused a visible lifting and tightening of the skin, with the wrinkles appearing to be less visible in a three-week period. Although this was a small-scale study, it was nonetheless a double blind test. Very few commercial products provide the potency of RNA and DNA used in these studies.

Keeping the Skin Moist

Replacing moisture lost to aging is a prime reason why women use face creams. Most commercial face creams are oil-based and work by blocking the release of water from the skin. As people grow older, however, they cannot rely on oil-based preparations to block the release of moisture. That is because aged skin loses the ability to attract moisture in the first place and fundamentally becomes dehydrated. At this point, aged skin needs to be replenished with its natural moisturizer complex in order to attract and retain water.

The most advanced moisturizer is Ceraphyl GA-D, which functions by reducing the excessive drying in the upper layers of the skin. Drs. Stig Friberg and David W. Osborne showed that Ceraphyl GA-D inhibits transepidermal water loss by preventing the lipids (fats) from crystallizing. This mechanism is central to preventing dry, thin, leathery, dull, wrinkled skin. Ceraphyl GA-D also seems to increase the effectiveness of sunscreens and enhance the receptiveness of skin cells to antioxidants such as vitamins A, C, and E.

Hyaluronic acid helps the skin retain its youthful moisture via a different mechanism than Ceraphyl GA-D. Hyaluronic acid maintains the integrity of the connective tissue because it is a source of manganese and glucosomine. Injectable hyaluronic acid may one day replace injectable collagen, but this important skin-preserving nutrient is available without a prescription today in over-the-counter skin creams.

The ability of skin to hold moisture is directly related to its sodium pyrrilidone carboxylic acid (NaPCA) content. NaPCA is one of the skin's most important natural moisturizers. Old skin, however, contains only about half the NaPCA as young skin. NaPCA facilitates the moistening by pulling water into the skin from the air. Optimal protection against age-accelerating dehydration is best obtained by the topical application of NaPCA, hyaluronic acid, lactic acid, urea, Ceraphyl GA-D and squalene every day.

Botox (Botulinum Toxin)

Botox is quite literally a very dilute solution of the botulinum toxin Type A produced by the botulism species of bacteria. For about 10 years now, very dilute preparations of this toxin have been injected into humans to improve facial appearance (Becker-Wegerich et al. 2001). Botox partially blocks the nerve to the injected muscle. It usually takes about 3–5 days to notice the effects of Botox, and the effect lasts 4–6 months. Botox injections are best done on the upper third of the face. Forehead lines, furrows between the eyebrows, and lines around the eyes ("crow's feet") respond favorably to Botox. Frown lines (below the mouth) and chin creases may also be improved with a Botox injection, but the response varies. The cost of a Botox injection is about $400 and includes up to 35 units of Botox. If Botox migrates to the wrong muscle, side effects such as drooping of the eyelid or unevenness of the eyebrows may develop. Botox is purely cosmetic and has no actual healing effect on the skin itself.

The Inside Story

Nourishing the skin with topical ingredients is important, but in addition it is essential that you feed your skin nourishing food and drink. The effects of aging can be seen directly by looking at skin, not something possible for most organs in the body, which are hidden from view. The following are general considerations for nutritional optimization of skin function:

1. As much as possible, remove all processed foods from your diet. There are two reasons for this. First, processed foods tend to contain high levels of sodium, sugar, fat, and other undesirables, such as color and preservatives. Second, processed foods usually contain less nutrition than whole foods. Strange as it may seem, "enriched bread" has had 60% of its minerals removed along with most of the fiber. Some nutrients have been added back, but only some. The nutrient density of processed foods is very low and leaves much to be desired.

2. Eat foods that are natural and whole, such as whole grains, fresh or frozen vegetables, fruits, nuts and seeds, and so forth. Your plate should contain mainly fruits, vegetables, and grains with a small amount of protein, such as fish or poultry, added.

3. Drink plenty of water: 8 glasses a day are recommended. (Some of our water requirements can come from fruits and vegetables.)

4. Do not fry foods or barbecue them for long periods of time.

5. Use alcohol only in moderation: one drink a day, for example.

6. Eat foods that are high in antioxidants. These foods are highly colored, such as cantaloupe, spinach, berries, and cruciferous vegetables (cauliflower, cabbage, and sprouts).

7. Remove sugar and saturated fats. Use a sweetener if you like.

8. Take a good multivitamin with an added antioxidant formula, particularly mixed carotenes, vitamin C, vitamin E, selenium, and zinc. Add some vitamin A, the "skin vitamin," together with supplements of RNA and B vitamins (for coenzymes) and the minerals zinc, copper, and manganese. These provide even more intensive protection against damaging free radicals. The increased cellular energy helps the skin repair, renew, and revitalize itself.

Foods rich in nucleic acids (RNA), such as sardines, salmon, tuna, shellfish, lentils, and beans, help improve cell energy through a "salvage pathway" (see *Life Extension Magazine August 1997*, 5–8).

Foods rich in antioxidants and other phytochemicals, such as fruits, vegetables, and green tea, help protect against oxidative damage and free radical attack of all body cells including the skin.

Aging causes a progressive decline in our ability to internally synthesize the essential fatty acids (EFAs) required by the skin to maintain a youthful, moist appearance. The most important oils to supplement are the omega-3s that can make the skin smoother, softer, and more radiant-looking. When skin is properly nourished, it shows less of the effects of aging. The oral ingestion of fish, flax, or perilla oil provides abundant quantities of the omega-3 fatty acids that are so beneficial to the health and appearance of the skin. Also, if there is a tendency to develop eczema (a common skin condition), oil of evening primrose or borage oil are essential nutrients to be supplemented.

Avoidance of more than modest exposure to the sun's UV light is critically important to protect the skin against the oxidizing effects of solar radiation.

UV rays are categorized by wavelengths: UVA, UVB, and UVC.

The ozone layer filters out the UVC and many of the UVB rays, but the ozone layer is not the same as it used to be and seems to have little or no effect on UVA rays which make up 90% or more of the sun's radiation that reaches the earth. Indeed, it is exposure to UVA that causes most of the photo-aging damage: the premature wrinkles, loss of elasticity, hyperpigmentation, and a dry, dull, leathery texture.

UVB, which is most intense from 10 A.M.–2 P.M., can cause sunburns and basal-cell cancers of the skin as well as increase the risk of melanomas. Yet sunscreens, which are geared to filter out UVB, seem to have no effect on the incidence of melanoma. Of interest are studies showing that people who are continuously exposed to the sun—farmers and fisherman, for example—seem to be less at risk for melanoma than a vacationer, especially a fair-skinned sunbather who exposes his or her skin to intense sun for a few days or a week.

A Word about Vitamin D

Recent publications regarding the adequacy of vitamin D in the general population have been alarming. It appears as though not only are people not getting enough of this vitamin, but that even in the summer months the amount is suboptimal in some population groups in the northern latitudes (i.e., above the 35th parallel) (Viethl et al 2001). Most of our vitamin D comes from sunlight, specifically the UVB fraction. Lack of sun exposure will, in time, inevitably lead to suboptimal levels of vitamin D (Tangpricha et al. 2002). The supplemented form of vitamin D found in milk is insufficient to bring levels to normal (Trang et al. 1998). Milk is fortified with vitamin D_2, not vitamin D_3, which is the active component. Vitamin D_2 is also the form of vitamin D that is likely to lead to toxicity if taken in large quantities. What is the answer? First, if you live above the 35th parallel, make sure you obtain at least 400 IU a day of vitamin D_3 in supplement form. Some doctors are advising much higher amounts of vitamin D_3 to protect against cancer. Because this is such as inexpensive vitamin, doses up to 1400 IU daily should be considered without the need for blood tests to guard against vitamin D toxicity. Some research indicates that much higher amounts of supplemental vitamin D_3 are safe and desirable.

Thyroid Function

Like most hormones in our body, as we age, less and less thyroid hormone is available. Glands, which produce these hormones, become sluggish or irregular. The thyroid gland is no exception. Often physicians will see patients who are not only overweight, but who also have dry, flaky, sluggish skin. A thyroid profile in the blood will often show a low or borderline-low thyroid function. Nutrients and foods which support the thyroid such as sea vegetables, seafood, fish, and iodized sea salt, or prescription thyroid preparations such as Armour or Cytomel, when necessary, can reverse this form of skin aging.

Hormones and Skin

DHEA and Melatonin

The sleep hormone (melatonin) and the anti-stress hormone (DHEA) are both found in human skin. Both are converted to other entities with important jobs to do. DHEA is converted into estrogen- and androgen-type metabolites found only in skin (Labrie et al. 2000). Melatonin is synthesized in skin. In low concentrations it can stimulate cell growth. This type of on-site, organ-specific production of hormones is called *intracrine biosynthesis*. Intracrine biosynthesis allows different organs to manufacture the substances they need without flooding the entire body with growth factors.

Estrogen's skin-enhancing effects are well-known (Dunn et al. 1997; Shah et al. 2001). It provokes collagen and a moisture factor known as *hyaluronic acid*. Aging decreases both estrogen and collagen. Enzymes that convert DHEA to estrogen also decline. Not surprisingly, women who take synthetic estrogen have scientifically proven thicker skin. Women who take both estrogen and testosterone have really thick skin (48% thicker than women who don't take either hormone) (Brincat et al. 1983). DHEA is converted to both estrogen and testosterone, providing the benefits of both hormones.

Although the exact roles of DHEA and melatonin in human skin are still under scrutiny, researchers have identified several mechanisms through which these hormones protect against aging, maintain the health of skin, and affect how sunlight reacts with skin cells.

Skin is such a specialized organ that it has its own immune system. It has been proposed that faulty skin immunity affects the entire immune system. Sunlight can penetrate deep into skin and alter immunity directly, or it can cause changes in dermis and epidermis that provoke immune changes. Sunlight affects hormones. It decreases melatonin, norepinephrine, and acetylcholine, and increases cortisol, serotonin, GABA, and dopamine.

and diabetes mellitus, all of which may be autoimmune in nature.

Euthyroid sick syndrome is hypothyroidism, associated with a severe systemic illness, that causes decreased peripheral conversion of T4 to T3, an increased conversion of T3 to the inactive reverse T3, and decreased binding of thyroid hormones. Conditions commonly associated with this syndrome include fasting, starvation, protein-calorie malnutrition, general surgical trauma, myocardial infarction, chronic renal failure, diabetic ketoacidosis, anorexia nervosa, cirrhosis, thermal injury, and sepsis. Once the underlying cause is treated, the condition is usually resolved.

Treatment for hyperthyroidism, which includes administering radioactive iodine and surgical removal of the thyroid gland, may also result in hypothyroidism.

In many undeveloped countries, where there is a chronic lack of iodine in the diet, goitrous hypothyroidism resulting from an underactive thyroid gland is common. Hypothyroidism resulting from a lack of dietary iodine has disappeared in the United States.

Drugs that may produce hypothyroidism as an adverse reaction include amiodarone (Cordarone), colchicine (Colsalide), fluoxetine (Prozac), interferon-alfa (Alferon N, Intron A, Roferon A), lithium (Eskalith, Lithobid), methimazole (Tapazole), potassium iodide, KI (Pima, SSKI), and propylthiouracil.

Risk Factors

Smoking
Smoking has also been identified as a risk factor for hypothyroidism, but the reason for the association is unknown (Nystrom et al. 1993).

Lead
Hypothyroidism may also be caused by occupational exposure to lead (Lasisz et al. 1992).

Homocysteine
A recent study measured the plasma homocysteine levels in 50 hypothyroid and 46 hyperthyroid patients. They found that plasma homocysteine concentrations increased in hypothyroidism and decreased in hyperthyroidism. They also found that restoration of the euthyroid state (by drug treatment) decreased both homocysteine and creatinine in hypothyroid patients and increased both homocysteine and creatinine in hyperthyroid patients. Folate levels were found to be lower in the hypothyroid group when compared with the hyperthyroid group. They proposed that a higher creatinine clearance in hyperthyroidism could partially explain the changes in homocysteine. A similar study found the same relationship between homocysteine

and hypothyroidism, but the authors believed it was due to decreased hepatic levels of enzymes involved in the remethylation pathway of homocysteine (Nedrebo et al. 1998; Hussein 1999; Catargi et al. 1999; Diekman et al. 2001).

DIAGNOSIS

Overt hypothyroidism is easy to diagnose by a simple blood test. Low levels of T3 and T4 are signs that you do not have enough thyroid hormones. An elevated TSH is a sign of thyroid deficiency. When your TSH is high, it means the pituitary gland is trying to make the thyroid gland produce more hormones. Patients with euthyroid sick syndrome, however, have a normal TSH.

Hashimoto's thyroiditis is diagnosed by high titers of antithyroid (antimicrosomal) antibodies. High titers of antibody against thyroglobulin (TG) and thyroid peroxidase (TPO) are present in most patients.

If, however, someone is suffering from the classic symptoms of thyroid deficiency but has normal test results, the thyroid slowdown could be slight or age-related and is not easily detected by a blood test. Thyroid deficiency often mimics many symptoms associated with old age. One way to determine a thyroid deficiency is to have your physician test for a substance called transthyretrin (also known as prealbumin). Thyroid hormone is carried through the bloodstream and brain by transthyretrin. Even when all other hormones are normal, a low level of transthyretrin could mean that you are not producing enough thyroid hormones and that it is not being delivered to the cells.

Another sensitive laboratory test to measure thyroid deficiency is the TRH (thyrotropin-releasing hormone) stimulation test. It can show whether a patient is suffering from an underactive thyroid even when routine thyroid tests reveal nothing. The patient's level of TSH is measured through a blood test, then the patient is given an injection of TRH (a harmless synthetic hormone, modeled after the TRH secreted by the hypothalamus gland in the brain); 25 minutes later blood is drawn and the TSH is measured again. If the measures from the second TSH blood test are high (above 15), then the patient's thyroid is underactive.

The TRH injection stimulates the brain's pituitary gland, which produces TSH and regulates the thyroid. If the thyroid is under-functioning, the pituitary gland will secrete excess TSH.

Barnes Basal Temperature Test

Another way of detecting a possible thyroid deficiency is to take your basal body temperature. Place a thermometer at your bedside, and as soon as you wake up before you step out of bed, place the thermometer under your arm for at least 3 minutes. If you are T3 deficient, you will find your basal temperature to be below 97.8°F (normal throughout the day is 98.6°F). If your first-thing-in-the-morning temperature is consistently low, it likely means that your basal (resting) metabolic rate is also low.

Record the time, date, and temperature every morning for 2 weeks to show your doctor. In addition to following up with blood tests, your doctor can determine the potency of your deep tendon reflexes, especially the time it takes your Achilles tendon to recover after first elicitation.

CONVENTIONAL TREATMENTS

Synthroid

Conventional treatment calls for the oral replacement of deficient thyroid hormones. A synthetic form of T4 (Synthroid, Levothroid, Levothyroxine) is most often administered. Treatment, especially in older people, begins with low doses of thyroid hormone because serious side effects may occur with too large a dose. The dose is gradually increased until TSH levels in the blood return to normal. The medication must usually be taken for life.

Synthroid is the third most popular drug prescribed in the United States, being taken by 8 million people. The drug was introduced in 1955 without FDA approval. Recently the safety, stability, and efficacy of this drug have come under fire. In April 2001 the FDA denied Abbott Laboratory's request that Synthroid be allowed to bypass a new drug application and be declared "generally recognized as safe and effective." Instead the FDA stated that Synthroid "had a history of problems with potency and stability" and required Abbott to file the necessary application and study results by August 14, 2001, for official review and approval. Final review and approval was granted by the FDA in July 2002. A condition of approval was that Abbott is required to "develop an analytical method for the determination of impurities and degradation products in the drug substance and the drug product" by July 31, 2003.

Several studies have questioned the effectiveness of levothyroxine and other synthetic T4 drugs for various treatments of thyroid disorders. One study evaluating its ability to suppress the number of nodules in patients with multinodular euthyroid goiter showed limited effectiveness in reduction of nodules. This study also indicated it was ineffective for body weight reduction in obese patients (Imbrogno et al. 2001).

For some patients, hypothyroidism symptoms persist despite standard thyroxine replacement therapy. Thyroxine therapy was no more effective than placebo in improving cognitive function and psychological well-being in patients with symptoms of hypothyroidism, despite thyroid function tests falling well within the reference range (Pollock et al. 2001; Walsh et al. 2001).

Unithroid

Unithroid (levothyroxine), previously known as Thyrox, was approved by the FDA on August 22, 2000, as the first FDA-approved levothyroxine (synthetic T4) drug on the market. Many physicians are recommending that their patients switch from other non-FDA-approved drugs (such as Synthroid) to Unithroid.

Levoxyl

On May 25, 2001, Levoxyl received FDA approval as the second levothyroxine drug. Many patients prefer Levoxyl because of its lower price.

INNOVATIVE DRUG STRATEGIES

Armour Thyroid

Armour thyroid (Thyrar), Nathroid, and Westhroid are prescription medications that contain desiccated thyroid derived from the thyroid gland of the pig. Natural thyroid extracts have been used since 1892 and were approved by the FDA in 1939. Armour thyroid and most other natural glandular preparations are made to standards approved by the United States Pharmacopoeia (U.S.P.), which ensures that its potency is accurately stated on the label.

Natural thyroid extracts were largely replaced in clinical medicine by levothyroxine (Synthroid). Most physicians are reluctant to prescribe natural glandulars because they are told that they are impure and inconsistent from dose to dose. If your physician requires more information on natural glandulars, contact the Broda O. Barnes Research Foundation listed in the summary.

An article in the *New England Journal of Medicine* described a study in which patients with hypothyroidism showed greater improvements in mood and brain function if they received treatment with Armour thyroid rather than Synthroid (thyroxine). The authors also detected biochemical evidence that thyroid hormone action was greater after treatment with Armour thyroid. The patients who were on Armour thyroid had significantly higher serum concentrations of sex hormone-binding globulin; having higher concentrations of sex hormone-binding globulin is not a favorable event (Bunevicius et al. 1999).

Cytomel

Liothyronine (Cytomel, Triostat) is a synthetic form of T3 that was approved by the FDA in 1954. It is preferred over Synthroid (synthetic T4) by many doctors because it does not require conversion in the body (T4 must be converted to T3, the metabolically active form). For this reason, the Life Extension Foundation recommends Cytomel instead of synthetic T4 medication.

The standard dose of Cytomel is 25 mcg orally once daily, increasing by 12.5 mcg every 1–2 weeks if required. Approximately 15–37.5 mcg of Cytomel is equal to 60 mg of desiccated thyroid.

An article in the *New England Journal of Medicine* reports on the results of research comparing the effects of thyroxine alone with those of thyroxine plus triiodothyronine (Cytomel) in 33 patients with hypothyroidism. The combination group scored higher on six of the 17 tests of cognitive performance and assessments of mood. The authors stated: "Treatment with thyroxine plus triiodothyronine improved the quality of life for most patients" (Bunevicius et al. 1999). Gupta et al. (2001) showed a link between low serum T3 levels and patient mortality in elderly hospitalized patients.

Thyrolar

Liotrix (Thyrolar) is a mixture of synthetic T4 and T3 in a 4:1 ratio by weight used to treat hypothyroidism. The standard dose is initially 30 mg orally per day, with an increased dose every 2–3 weeks if clinical response indicates. Most patients will require 60–120 mg per day. Approximately 60 mg of Thyrolar is equal to 60 mg of desiccated thyroid.

DRUG SIDE EFFECTS AND INTERACTIONS

Because the various thyroid drugs have similar actions, the side effects, contraindications, and drug interactions are almost identical for each.

Adverse reactions to thyroid medications include many of the signs of hyperthyroidism, including:

- Heat intolerance, fever, diaphoresis (sweating)
- Headache, insomnia, irritability, tremor
- Menstrual irregularity, amenorrhea
- Palpitations, angina, atrial fibrillation, heart failure, sinus tachycardia
- Nausea and vomiting, diarrhea, anorexia, weight loss
- Alopecia (hair loss)

Thyroid medications interact with several classes of medications:

- Cholestyramine (colestipol) decreases the efficacy of thyroid preparation. The doses should be separated by 4–6 hours.
- Estrogens can produce a decrease in thyroid agent effectiveness secondary to increased thyroid-binding globulins.
- Anticoagulant effect of anticoagulant drugs is increased.
- Beta-blockers may have decreased effectiveness.
- Digoxin clearance decreases with hypothyroidism; when corrected with thyroid hormone, clearance returns to normal.
- Theophylline's clearance is decreased with hypothyroidism; when corrected with thyroid hormone, clearance returns to normal.

Thyroid medications are contraindicated in:

- Cardiac disease, acute myocardial infarction
- Hyperthyroidism, thyrotoxicosis
- Hypoadrenalism
- Tartrazine sensitivity (a food coloring, FD&C Yellow No. 5)

Absorption of thyroid medications is impaired by:

- Iron sulfate
- Calcium pills (Tums and Os-Cal)
- Aluminum hydroxide antacids
- Phenytoin (Dilantin), carbamazepine (Tegretol), rifampin, cholestyramine, sucralfate

NATURAL SUPPLEMENTS

Natural supplements for thyroid problems include vitamin A; vitamin B complex; B_{12}; and the vitamins C, and E; as well as coenzyme Q_{10}; and especially the minerals magnesium, manganese, selenium, and zinc, all of which can be found in ample amounts in the Life Extension Mix. Deficiencies of any of these minerals can prevent the conversion of T4 to T3 and should be corrected. Sufficient protein iodine and especially the amino acid tyrosine are necessary to make T4 in the thyroid gland.

Treatment of autoimmune hypothyroidism (Hashimoto's) and euthyroid sick syndrome is based upon the underlying disorder (*refer to the Autoimmune, Arthritis, and other relevant protocols for more information*).

Iodine

Thyroid hormones are made by adding iodine molecules. Hence, a dietary deficiency of iodine can be a cause of hypothyroidism. Iodine is found in kelp and other seaweeds and seafood. It is also available in iodized salt. Those who suffer from autoimmune thyroid disease, such as Hashimoto's thyroiditis or Graves' disease, may want to avoid taking extra iodine because this disorder is not due to iodine deficiency and will not be of much help. For some it may irritate the thyroid and make matters worse.

Tyrosine

Tyrosine is a precursor of thyroid hormone and the neurotransmitters dopamine, norepinephrine, and epinephrine. A deficiency of tyrosine leads to hypothyroidism and low adrenal function. The recommended daily amount of tyrosine is about 1 gram per day for adults (Marz 1997).

Selenium

Selenium assists in removing toxins from the body through the enzyme glutathione peroxidase. Selenium is readily available in many foods, such as asparagus, grains, garlic, and mushrooms. Many agricultural areas, however, are extremely deficient in selenium. Research has linked selenium with thyroid function. One study found that the combination of both iodine and selenium deficiency was particularly toxic to the thyroid gland (Contempre et al. 1995).

A recent study in Belgium used selenium (20–60 mcg per day) to treat 18 children with congenital hypothyroidism. Supplementation with selenium caused a 74% increase in plasma selenium and normalized the levels of TSH. The authors concluded that selenium improves the thyroid hormone feedback system and improves the conversion of T4 to active T3 (Chanoine et al. 2001).

Another article described the use of selenium in three cases of hypothyroidism in children. After only 4 weeks of supplementation, they saw a marked improvement of all clinical symptoms and a return to normal metabolism (Pizzulli et al. 2000).

A double-blind, placebo-controlled study of 36 elderly subjects conducted in Italy found a linear correlation between selenium levels and T4 (as well as the ratio of T3:T4). Reduced conversion of T4 to T3 causes an overt hypothyroid condition that is common in the elderly. The main result of the study was a significant improvement in selenium levels and a decrease in the T4 levels in selenium-treated subjects (Olivieri et al. 1995).

Dehydroepiandrosterone (DHEA)

DHEA, a hormone that enhances the body's metabolic functioning, may also be deficient in individuals with hypothyroidism (Tagawa et al. 2000). A DHEA blood test should be administered to achieve optimal dosing (*see the DHEA-Pregnenolone Precautions in the DHEA Replacement Therapy protocol for more detailed information*).

Thyroid & *L*-Tyrosine Complex

Thyroid & *L*-Tyrosine Complex by Enzymatic Therapy combines thyroid tissue, the amino acid tyrosine, and synergistic trace minerals that must be present for endocrine gland functions, especially the thyroid. The thyroid gland needs iodine and *L*-tyrosine to produce hormones that control the body's metabolism. The trace minerals manganese, zinc, copper, and molybdenum included in the formula are involved with specific enzymes linked to endocrine glandular processes.

Soy

The effect of soy on thyroid function is currently a controversial topic. Some believe that soy increases metabolic rate and thyroid function. Several recent articles, however, have noted problems with people taking soy supplements.

One study identified the mechanism of soy's effect on thyroid function. Genistein and daidzein, the isoflavones in soy, inhibited thyroid peroxidase by acting as alternative substrates (Divi et al. 1997).

Soy-based infant formulas have been associated with an increased incidence of autoimmune thyroid disease and diabetes when compared with breast-fed infants (Fort et al. 1986; Fort et al. 1990).

Soy supplements should be avoided by hypothyroid patients because they increase the amount of thyroxine needed to attain clinical effect (Bell et al. 2001; Jabbar et al. 2001).

DIETARY RECOMMENDATIONS

Some foods contain goitrogenic substances that prevent the utilization of iodine. Goitrogens are found in sweet potato, cabbage, cauliflower, turnips, rutabaga, rapeseed oil (canola), cassava, pine nuts, mustard, millet, soybeans, and peanuts. The actual content of goitrogens in these foods, however, is quite low, and cooking inactivates them.

THE PROBLEM WITH CURRENT REFERENCE RANGES

How to best diagnose thyroid deficiency has been a long-standing medical controversy. Conventional doctors rely on thyroid blood tests, whereas alternative physicians look for signs and symptoms of thyroid deficiency. An article in *The Lancet* revealed surprising findings about reference ranges that may alter the way physicians assess individual thyroid status.

Before *The Lancet* article is discussed, the reader should be reminded of the serious consequences of a thyroid hormone deficiency. Aging people encounter a variety of ailments that doctors often attribute to problems other than thyroid deficiency. Some of the most noticeable symptoms caused by low thyroid are poor concentration, memory disturbances, cold hands and feet, accumulation of excess body fat, difficulty in losing weight, menstrual problems, dry skin, thin hair, and low energy levels. Some specific disorders related to thyroid deficiency include depression, elevated cholesterol, migraine headaches, hypertension, and infertility (Stanosz 1992; Saito et al. 1994; Vierhapper 1997; Michalopoulou et al. 1998; Pop et al. 1998; Lincoln et al. 1999; Krassas 2000; Hagen et al. 2001; Spierings 2001).

Broda O. Barnes was a physician-scientist who dedicated more than 50 years of his life to researching, teaching about, and treating thyroid and related endocrine dysfunctions. In his book entitled *Hypothyroidism: The Unsuspected Illness*, Dr. Barnes described more than 47 symptoms that may be related to poor thyroid function. During his many years of research and practice, Dr. Barnes condemned conventional doctors who ignored obvious clinical manifestations of thyroid deficiency. According to Dr. Barnes: "The development and use of thyroid function blood tests left many patients with clinical symptoms of hypothyroidism undiagnosed and untreated."

In lieu of blood tests, Dr. Barnes advocated that patients measure their temperature upon awakening. If the temperature is consistently below normal ranges, this is indicative of a thyroid deficiency. The Barnes Basal Temperature test, which appears earlier in this protocol, provides specific instructions on how best to measure your body temperature in order to assess thyroid hormone status.

Dr. Barnes believed that 40% of the adult population suffered from thyroid deficiency. Based on the percentage of adults now taking prescription drugs to treat depression, elevated cholesterol and high blood pressure, Dr. Barnes' observations about the epidemic of thyroid deficiency may now have been validated.

The Lancet is one of the most prestigious scientific journals in the world. It often reports new medical findings that defy conventional wisdom. According to the August 3, 2002, issue of *The Lancet,* the problem with thyroid blood tests may be caused by inadequate laboratory reference ranges that fail to reflect what the optimal level of thyroid hormone should be in a particular individual (Dayan et al. 2002).

The Life Extension Foundation has discussed the issue of faulty laboratory reference ranges for many years. The problem is that for many blood tests, the laboratories provide a wide range that represents "average" populations, rather than what the optimal level should be to maintain good health.

Back in the 1960s, for instance, the upper reference range for cholesterol extended up to 300 (mg/dL). This number was based on a statistical calculation indicating that it was "normal" to have total cholesterol levels as high as 300. At that time, it was also "normal" for men to suffer fatal heart attacks at relatively young ages. As greater knowledge accumulated about the risk of heart attack and high cholesterol, the upper limit of the reference range gradually dropped to the point where it is now 200 (mg/dL) (ADVANCEDATA).

The same situation occurred with homocysteine reference ranges. Up until recently, it was considered normal to have a homocysteine blood reading as high as 15 (mcmoles/L) (Mahanonda et al. 2001). Most reference ranges now provide a chart showing that homocysteine levels above 7 increase risk of heart attack and stroke (Robinson et al. 1995).

It is not just blood laboratory reference ranges that fail to provide physicians and patients with optimal numbers. For example, when your blood pressure is checked, a diastolic number up to 90 (mmHg) is considered normal. Yet a diastolic blood pressure reading greater than 85 is associated with an increased stroke risk. A high percentage of people over age 60 have diastolic readings greater than 85, and this is the age group most vulnerable to stroke (Hansson et al. 1998). So when your doctor checks your blood pressure and says it is normal, your response should be that "normal" is not good enough because it is also normal for people over age 60 to suffer a stroke. Instead, you should ask your doctor what is the "optimal" range. In the case of diastolic blood pressure, taking steps to keep it at 85 or below could greatly reduce long-term vascular damage. It is important to note that midlife hypertension predisposes people to stroke later in life, so keeping blood pressure readings in optimal ranges is important at any age.

Scientists are now examining epidemiological data related to thyroid hormone reference ranges, and their findings indicate that it may be time to change the way laboratories report their TSH results.

THE THYROID STIMULATING HORMONE (TSH) TEST

The standard blood test used to determine thyroid gland hormone output is the TSH test. When there is a deficiency in thyroid hormone, the pituitary gland releases more TSH to signal the thyroid gland to produce more hormones.

When the TSH test is in normal range, doctors usually assume that the thyroid gland is secreting enough thyroid hormone. The question raised by *The Lancet* authors, however, is whether today's reference range for TSH reflects optimal thyroid hormone status.

The TSH reference range used by many laboratories is between 0.2–5.5 (mU/L). A greater TSH number is indicative of a thyroid hormone deficiency. That is because the pituitary is over-releasing TSH based on lack of thyroid hormone in the blood. Any reading more than 5.5 alerts a doctor to a thyroid gland problem and that thyroid hormone therapy may be warranted.

The trouble is that the TSH reference range is so broad that most doctors will look at a TSH reading as low as 0.2 and think it is as normal as a 5.5 reading. The difference between 0.2–5.5, however, is an astounding 27-fold. It would seem almost absurd to think that a person could be in an optimal state of thyroid health anywhere along this 27-fold parameter, that is, TSH readings between 0.2–5.5.

A review of published findings about TSH levels reveals that readings of more than 2.0 may be indicative of adverse health problems related to insufficient thyroid hormone output. One study showed that individuals with TSH values of more than 2.0 have an increased risk of developing overt hypothyroid disease over the next 20 years (Vanderpump et al. 1995). Other studies show that TSH values greater than 1.9 indicate abnormal pathologies of the thyroid, specifically autoimmune attacks on the thyroid gland itself that can result in significant impairment (Hak et al. 2000).

More ominous was a study showing that TSH values of more than 4.0 increase the prevalence of heart disease, after correcting for other known risk factors (Hak et al. 2000). Another study showed that administration of thyroid hormone lowered cholesterol in patients with TSH ranges of 2.0–4.0, but had no effect in lowering cholesterol in patients whose TSH range was between 0.2–1.9 (Michalopoulou et al. 1998). This study indicates that in people with elevated cholesterol, TSH values of more than 1.9 could indicate that a thyroid deficiency is the culprit causing excess production of cholesterol, whereas TSH levels below 2.0 would indicate no deficiency in thyroid hormone status.

Doctors routinely prescribe cholesterol-lowering drugs to patients without properly evaluating their thyroid status. Based on the evidence presented to date, it might make sense for doctors to first attempt to correct a thyroid deficiency (based on a TSH value over 1.9) instead of first resorting to cholesterol-lowering drugs.

In a study to evaluate psychological well-being, impairment was found in patients with thyroid abnormalities who were nonetheless within "normal" TSH reference ranges (Pollock et al. 2001).

Defying the Reference Ranges

The authors of *The Lancet* study stated that "the emerging epidemiological data begin to suggest that TSH concentrations above 2.0 (mU/L) may be associated with adverse effects." The authors prepared a chart based on previously published studies that provide guidance when interpreting the results from TSH blood tests. Here are three highlights from their chart that may be useful in ascertaining what your TSH values really mean:

1. TSH greater than 2.0: Increased 20-year risk of hypothyroidism and increased risk of thyroid autoimmune disease (Vanderpump et al. 1995)
2. TSH greater than 4.0: Greater risk of heart disease (Hak et al. 2000)
3. TSH between 2.0–4.0: Cholesterol levels decline in response to thyroxine (T4) therapy (Michalopoulou et al. 1998)

Despite presenting these intriguing findings, *The Lancet* authors stated that more studies were needed to define optimal TSH level as between 0.2–2.0 instead of between 0.2–5.5. For a health-conscious person, however, this type of precise information provides an opportunity to correct a medical condition that has been unresponsive to mainstream therapies or possibly to prevent disorders from developing in the first place.

This means if you have depression, heart disease, high cholesterol, chronic fatigue, poor mental performance, or any of the many other symptoms associated with thyroid deficiency, you may want to ask your doctor to "defy the reference ranges" and try different thyroid replacement therapeutic approaches.

Measuring Thyroid Hormone Levels

TSH is just one blood test that doctors use to assess thyroid status. Other blood tests measure the actual amount of thyroid hormone found in the blood.

The primary hormone secreted by the thyroid gland is called thyroxine (T4). The T4 is then converted in the peripheral tissues into metabolically active triiodothyronine (T3). Doctors often test for TSH and T4 together, but this may not accurately reflect thyroid deficiency in tissues throughout the body. One study found that psychological well-being could be improved if T3 (e.g., the drug Cytomel) were added to T4 (e.g., the drug Synthroid) therapy, while maintaining thyroid function broadly within the standard reference ranges (Bunevicius et al. 1999; Walsh et al. 2001). What this means is that even when TSH and T4 blood tests are within normal ranges, a person can still be deficient in peripheral T3 and benefit from Cytomel therapy.

Because T3 is the metabolically active form of thyroid hormone, some physicians use it exclusively in lieu of T4 drugs like Synthroid. The FDA's recent notice to ban synthetic T4 drugs like Synthroid because of inconsistent potencies helps to validate a statement made by Broda Barnes more than 50 years ago: "Patients taking thyroid replacement therapy have much better improvement of symptoms with natural desiccated thyroid hormone rather than synthetic thyroid hormones."

Although the FDA has found many problems in T4 drugs, the T3 drug Cytomel has produced consistent clinical results and is not a subject of the FDA's proposed ban. Dr. Barnes fought the drug companies against synthetic T4 drugs for years and recommended desiccated thyroid (Armour) drugs as the therapy of choice for most patients.

An article in the *New England Journal of Medicine* described a study in which patients with hypothyroidism showed greater improvements in mood and brain function if they received treatment with Armour thyroid rather than Synthroid (thyroxine). The authors also detected biochemical evidence that thyroid hormone action was greater after treatment with Armour thyroid (Toft 1999).

Thyroid deficiency occurs when the thyroid gland under-produces the hormones thyroxine (T4) and triiodothyronine (T3) needed to regulate the body's metabolic rate. In some individuals, the thyroid does not properly convert T4 to T3, the metabolically active form. Supplementation with synthetic or animal-derived thyroid hormone is necessary to return hormone levels to normal.

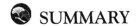 **SUMMARY**

Synthetic hormone supplementation, prescribed by a physician, includes synthetic T4 (Synthroid, Unithroid, and Levoxyl), synthetic T3 (Cytomel), and a combination of synthetic T3 and T4 (Thyrolar).

Natural glandulars (by prescription), such as Armour Desiccated Thyroid Hormone, Nathroid, and Westhroid, derived from the thyroid gland of the pig, contain T4 and T3, and most closely resemble natural human thyroid hormone.

Suggested supplements and their dosages follow:

1. Iodine, 1 mg per day

2. Selenium, 200–600 mcg per day

3. Tyrosine, 500–1000 mg per day

4. Melatonin, 300 mcg–6 mg at bedtime

5. DHEA, 25 mg 1–3 times per day (*refer to DHEA Replacement Therapy protocol*)

6. CoQ$_{10}$, 100–200 mg daily

7. Life Extension Mix for vitamin A, vitamin B complex, magnesium, manganese, selenium, and zinc, to be taken as directed

8. Thyroid & *L*-Tyrosine Complex, 2 capsules 3 times daily

 FOR MORE INFORMATION

Contact the Thyroid Foundation of America, (800) 832-8321. For more information on natural glandulars or the basal body temperature test, contact the Broda O. Barnes, M.D. Research Foundation, P.O. Box 98, Trembly, CT 06611, (203) 261-2101.

 PRODUCT AVAILABILITY

Life Extension Mix, Coenzyme Q$_{10}$, selenium, melatonin, *L*-tyrosine, and Thyroid & *L*-Tyrosine Complex by Enzymatic Therapy are available by calling (800) 544-4440 or by ordering online at www.lef.org.

Tinnitus

Tinnitus: from the Latin word *tinnire* meaning to ring

Tinnitus is a subjective disorder characterized as chronic ringing, roaring, buzzing, humming, chirping, or hissing in the ears in the *absence* of environmental noise (ATA 2002). Symptoms of tinnitus are frequently found in elderly persons and are often associated with hearing loss related to the aging process (presbycusis). Although the cause is usually unknown, tinnitus can be a symptom of almost any ear disorder, including infection (otitis media), a blocked ear canal (ear wax) or eustachian tube, otosclerosis (overgrowth of bone in the middle ear), labyrinthitis, and Meuniere's disease. Even blast injury from explosions has been known to cause symptoms of tinnitus. Additionally, adverse side effects from some drugs (e.g., aspirin and antibiotics) cause tinnitus symptoms.

Sometimes tinnitus is called "head noise." In tinnitus, the acoustic nerve transmits impulses to the brain that are not the result of vibrations produced by sound waves. Instead the impulses are the result of stimuli that originate inside the head or within the ear. In healthy ears, thousands of auditory cells maintain an electrical charge. There are microscopic hairs on the surface of each auditory cell that move in relation to the pressure of sound waves. Movement of the hairs discharges electrical charges through the hearing nerve to the brain. The brain interprets these electrical signals as sound. If the hairs are damaged, they move erratically and are in a constant state of irritation. As a result, the auditory cells cannot hold their charge and random electrical impulses flow to the brain as noise (MFMER 2001).

In most persons, the noise of tinnitus is present continuously, even if the person is not always aware of it. Tinnitus can change in nature or intensity. Tolerance of tinnitus varies from person to person and is largely determined by personality. Many people accept tinnitus without significant distress, but for some the noise is almost intolerable (ATA 2002).

Tinnitus affects 35–50 million persons in the United States, with 12 million people being severely affected (ATA 2002). Tinnitus may disappear independently or it can disappear when an underlying problem is successfully treated. In cases of chronic tinnitus for which there is no treatable underlying problem, a variety of therapies and suggestions may help to provide substantial relief for persons who suffer from the symptoms.

DIAGNOSIS

See a physician to discuss your symptoms: when they began, their severity, and what seems to make them worse. Be sure to include information about any health conditions you have (e.g., high blood pressure) and what medicines you take. First, any accumulation of earwax or an infection will be eliminated as a possible cause. The physican will also attempt to hear the noise you describe using a stethoscope. If noise can be heard from a vascular condition, you have *objective* tinnitus. However, if damage to the inner ear is causing your tinnitus, you will be the only person who can hear the noise (*subjective* tinnitus) (MFMER 2001). Your physician may refer you to other specialists such as an otolaryngologist or audiologist in an attempt to learn more about the cause of your tinnitus.

TREATMENT

The treatment of tinnitus depends on the cause. As noted earlier, if the tinnitus is caused from a health condition, there may be steps your physician can take to eliminate or reduce the noise: removing earwax, treating an ear infection, correcting a vascular condition, changing or discontinuing a medicine, or recommending a hearing aid (MFMER 2001). If tinnitus is caused by age-related hearing loss or damage to your ears from exposure to excessive noise, there is no treatment to reduce the noise (MFMER 2001; NIH 2001). Instead, treatment consists largely of managing the condition. Not every suggested treatment works for everyone, so you may need to try several to find one that will help. It is important to avoid anything that could make your tinnitus worsen, including smoking, alcohol, and loud noises. If you are a construction worker, an airport worker, a hunter, or are often exposed to loud noise at home or at work, you should wear ear plugs or special ear protection (muffs) to protect your hearing (NIH 2001).

Lifestyle Changes

Sometimes symptoms of tinnitus improve with time. However, many people must learn to make adjustments to their lifestyle (coping skills) (MFMER 2001; NIH 2001). Try some of these techniques to help reduce the severity of tinnitus and to increase your tolerance of it:

- *Avoid irritants.* Tinnitus can be aggravated by loud noises, nicotine, caffeine, tonic water containing quinine (used to treat malaria), alcohol, and excessive doses of aspirin. Nicotine and caffeine constrict blood vessels, increasing the force of blood through veins and arteries. Alcohol also increases the force of blood by increasing the speed of blood flow.

- *Mask or cover up noise.* A fan or soft music can help mask the noise of tinnitus. Tinnitus maskers are devices that are similar to hearing aids in appearance, but they produce a pleasant sound. Listening to recordings of soothing music or sounds such as ocean waves may help cover the unwanted noise, especially while sleeping. There are some electronic sound devices that provide several relaxing sounds to facilitate sleep by masking tinnitus.

- *Use a hearing aid.* If you have tinnitus that is accompanied by a loss of hearing, a hearing aid can amplify outside sounds and possibly make tinnitus noise less noticeable.

- *Reduce stress.* Stress seems to make tinnitus worse. Learn how to relax when the noise in your ears is frustrating. Practicing stress management (relaxation therapy, biofeedback, or exercise) may provide some relief. Engaging in regular exercise may also provide relief by increasing blood circulation to the head.

- *Reduce use of salt.* This can increase the buildup of fluid in the ear.

Dietary Supplements

Ginkgo Biloba
A plant extract used to reduce the symptoms of cognitive deficits such as decreased memory function, poor concentration, and reduced alertness, ginkgo biloba has been shown to have positive results in the treatment of tinnitus and dizziness in the scientific literature (Stange et al. 1975; Jung et al. 1998). Studies have shown that 120–240 mg a day of pharmaceutical-grade ginkgo biloba extract can alleviate tinnitus, although some earlier studies failed to show benefits (Burschka et al. 2001). The therapeutic effect of ginkgo biloba is attributed to several active constituents with vasoactive and free-radical-scavenging properties.

In a study conducted in Denmark, tinnitus and dizziness were reduced after a treatment of 4–6 weeks with ginkgo biloba. Researchers also noted that there were minimal side effects in patients who followed the recommended dosage (Soholm 1998).

Another controlled study showed that ginkgo extract caused a statistically significant decrease in behavioral manifestation in the animal model of tinnitus (Jastreboff et al. 1997). In human studies, it was shown in patients who had cerebrovascular insufficiency (a common condition associated with normal aging) that ginkgo extract produced a significant improvement in the symptoms of vertigo, tinnitus, headache, and forgetfulness (Holstein 2001; Morgenstern et al. 2002).

Melatonin
Rosenberg et al. (1998) evaluated a treatment for subjective tinnitus at the Ear Research Foundation in Sarasota, Florida. Patients were given 3 mg of melatonin nightly for 30 days. In patients with difficulty sleeping due to the symptoms of tinnitus, an overall improvement was seen in 46% of the study group as opposed to 20% in the group given placebo. The researchers also concluded that patients with bilateral (two-sided) tinnitus showed significant improvement over those with unilateral (one-sided) tinnitus. Because of the minimal side effects associated with melatonin, it is considered a safe alternative treatment for chronic tinnitus (Rosenberg et al. 1998).

B Vitamins
According to Michael Seidman, M.D. (Tinnitus Center in Bloomfield, Michigan), there are specific nutrients that have been suggested to benefit persons with tinnitus. B-complex supplements lead this category because deficiencies in the B vitamins have been shown to result in tinnitus. The B vitamin complex stabilizes nerves and appears to have a beneficial effect on some tinnitus patients. However, only anecdotal evidence is available on this therapy.

Some patients say vitamin B_1 (thiamine) supplemented at 100–500 mg daily has provided them with relief from symptoms. Vitamin B_3 (niacin) is the subject of numerous anecdotal reports that purport it to help reduce symptoms. Dr. Seidman usually recommends a starting dosage of 50 mg twice a day of niacin, up to a maximum of 500 mg twice a day, but he believes that if there is no improvement within 3–4 months, it is unlikely to occur.

There may also be some correlation between the decline in vitamin B_{12} levels and the increasing prevalence of tinnitus in the elderly. A study by Shemesh et al. (1993) showed that there was a high prevalence (47%) of vitamin B_{12} deficiency in patients with chronic tinnitus. This deficiency was more widespread and severe in the tinnitus group that was associated with noise exposure, suggesting a relationship between vitamin B_{12} deficiency and dysfunction of the auditory pathway. Supplemental cobalamin was found to provide some relief in several patients with severe tinnitus.

exaggerated proliferation of fibroblast cells, leading to scarring and scar contraction. Conversely, in ligament injuries such as the medial collateral ligament (MCL) of the knee, a certain level of fibrous tissue must form in order for the ligament to heal. The release of IL-6 promotes MCL collagen synthesis leading to fibrous tissue formation (Hankenson et al. 2000). It has been suggested that IL-6 levels should be monitored in skeletal joints, aiming for a certain optimal level that promotes enough influx of inflammatory cells to encourage healing, but not so much as to damage healing tissue with excessive scarring (Skutek et al. 2001; Swartz et al. 2001). (*See the Chronic Inflammation protocol for recommendations on reducing the effects of inflammation.*)

IL-10 is a cytokine that inhibits the inflammatory response. Some of the most interesting work involving IL-10 relates to fetal healing. The human fetus has the ability to heal without scarring and, according to some researchers, IL-10 is "necessary for scarless wound repair to occur" (Liechty et al. 2000). Hyaluronon (hyaluronic acid) is a glycosaminoglycan found in lubricating fluids (synovial fluid, cartilage, blood vessels, skin) and is also present in high concentrations in the fetal environment (cord blood). It is theorized that fetal fibroblasts may mute the inflammatory response to inflammatory cytokines due to the high levels of IL-10, hyaluronon, and other substances in the fetal environment (Kennedy et al. 2000).

NUTRITIONAL SUPPLEMENTS

Research has shown that certain nutrients such as aloe vera, arginine, glutamine, zinc, copper, and vitamin C play key roles in wound healing (Vaxman et al. 1990; Worwag et al. 1999). The typical Western diet is deficient in these nutrients. Under normal conditions, the 5 grams a day of arginine found in the typical Western diet would be marginally sufficient to maintain tissue health. Research has demonstrated, however, that in patients undergoing gall bladder surgery, supplementing 15 grams of arginine for 3 days prior to surgery significantly reduced nitrogen excretion (evidence that the patients were using, not excreting, amino acids in order to heal) when compared with patients receiving conventional nutritional support. In patients undergoing surgery for gastrointestinal cancer, supplementation with 25 grams of arginine a day for 7 days improved their nitrogen balance as measured 5–7 days after surgery and led to more rapid recovery and discharge from the hospital (Daly et al. 1995).

In a study of women being treated for venous leg ulcers, it was revealed that the women had suboptimal dietary intake of energy-providing food sources and key wound-healing nutrients such as vitamin C and zinc even though they had well-organized food habits (Wissing et al. 1997). Research on other nutritional supplements has demonstrated encouraging results. Some of these studies will be presented in the paragraphs that follow.

Centella

Also known as Gotu kola, centella comes from the *Centella asiatica* plant. According to legend, elephants use this plant as a food source and owe their longevity to its age-defying properties. (Scientists would likely claim that the elephants' lifespan falls as expected on the curve relating size, metabolic oxygen utilization, and lifespan in various species.) Centella has been found to induce levels of antioxidants in wounds and newly formed tissue, including superoxide dismutase, glutathione peroxidase, vitamin E, and vitamin C. Centella improves collagen formation and angiogenesis (Shukla et al. 1999a). A review article of centella noted the most beneficial effects to date involved the stimulation and mutation of scar tissue by production of Type I collagen and an inhibition of the inflammatory reaction. This article reviewed seven other articles about centella, stating "*Centella asiatica* has been documented to aid wound healing in a large number of scientific reports" (Shukla 1999b; Widgerow et al. 2000).

Aloe Vera

Aloe vera is a plant well-known for centuries to have healing properties. Aloe contains the major carbohydrate fraction, acemannan, which also has antiviral properties. Aloe can be applied topically to wounds and taken internally for both skin wounds and gastrointestinal ulcers (Chithraet al. 1998). Aloe's mode of action may be through modulating macrophage function in the wound, enabling an immune response that ingests and destroys foreign pathogens (Zhang et al. 1996). It has been suggested that aloe works as a free radical scavenger and improves blood flow to the wound (Heggers et al. 1997). The healing of dermal wounds in rats has been consistently found to improve with aloe in several studies.

Aloe vera contains up to 200 different substances beneficial to the human body. These substances include enzymes, glycoproteins, growth factors, vitamins, and minerals. Long-chain sugars, or mucopolysaccharides (especially acemannan), have been of particular interest for their remarkable properties. Aloe vera is commonly considered a general tonic for increasing well-being and longevity. It provides the micronutrients required for protein synthesis. Its many components work together to reduce inflammation and pain, promote healing, and stop infection. Some of these components cause cells to divide and multiply; some stimulate the growth of white blood cells. Aloe vera also enhances cell wall permeability, increasing cell access to nutrients and facilitating the removal of toxins from the cells. Aloe vera can be used on the skin and can also be taken internally as a juice (2 ounces of concentrate in a 6-ounce beverage).

Arginine

Injury significantly increases the need for the amino acid arginine, which is essential for a variety of metabolic functions. Animal studies have demonstrated that, following surgical trauma, dietary supplementation with arginine results in an increase in nitrogen retention and increased body weight, both of which are essential for successful recovery (Sitren et al. 1977; Minuskin et al. 1981; Chyun et al. 1984; Jeevanandam et al. 1997; Mane et al. 2001). In a clinical study published in a major medical journal, arginine supplementation significantly increased the amount of reparative collagen synthesized at the site of a "standard wound" (an incision 5 cm long and 1 mm in diameter, into which a catheter was inserted) made in healthy volunteers. The same study found marked enhancement of the activity and efficacy of peripheral T-lymphocytes (white blood cells in the bloodstream) (Kirk et al. 1993).

Other animal and human studies have demonstrated that arginine stimulates the cell-mediated immune response and protects against bacterial challenges (Gurbuz et al. 1998). In animals, dietary supplementation with arginine increases the weight of the thymus, the master gland of the immune system, and reduces shrinkage of the thymus following trauma and in normally aging animals. The benefits of arginine for thymic function have also been demonstrated. Its ability to restore thymic endocrine function is evidenced by increased blood levels of thymulin, one of the hormones secreted by the thymus gland. Clinical studies have shown improved immune function in cancer patients fed arginine. Arginine's ability to improve wound healing and immune-system function is thought to be related to its stimulation of the release of growth hormone. Growth hormone plays a critical role in modulating the immune system and is essential for muscle growth and development. That growth hormone secretion diminishes progressively with advancing age is one of the primary reasons for the decline in immune-system function and muscular strength as we grow older. To accelerate wound healing, the Life Extension Foundation recommends 10–22 grams of supplemental arginine daily.

Glutamine

The amino acid glutamine is an important substrate for rapidly proliferating cells, including lymphocytes (white blood cells). It is also the major amino acid lost during muscle protein catabolism in the initial response to injury. An article documented beneficial effects from supplying burn patients with glutamine and arginine in amounts 2–7 times those found in the normal diet of healthy persons (De-Souza et al.1998). The Foundation recommends 2000 mg of glutamine daily.

Zinc

Zinc plays a well-documented role in wound healing. Although zinc is present in the body in only a small quantity, it is found in many tissues, including bone, skin, muscle, and organs. It is a component of DNA, RNA, and numerous enzyme systems that participate in tissue growth and healing. Zinc is crucial for protein synthesis and is a key part of the thymulin molecule which enables T-lymphocytes to mature.

A study involving zinc supplementation in inflammatory bowel disease illustrated the importance of taking adequate supplementation, but not too much. In this study, excess amounts of zinc caused tissue injury and impaired wound healing (Cario et al. 2000). However, relative zinc deficiencies, especially in the elderly, are common in the United States (Andrews et al. 1999).

CAUTION Zinc should be taken at least 2 hours after copper or the antibiotic tetracycline.

Copper

A German physician first observed the role of copper in healing, noting that broken bones seemed to heal faster when patients were given a copper salt during convalescence. Since then, the role of copper in the biosynthesis of bone and connective tissue has been well established, although its mechanism of action is only partially known (Tenaud et al. 1999). Copper supplementation has enhanced bone healing. It works with vitamin C to create strong collagen, and it creates cross-links in collagen and elastin that give strength to proteins.

Note: *The Life Extension Foundation does not recommend high-dose copper as a long-term dietary supplement because of the preponderance of evidence that long-term copper supplementation generates too much free-radical activity throughout the body. On the other hand, therapeutic, short-term supplementation of copper (8 mg daily) to enhance wound healing at* *localized injury sites is appropriate. Copper supplementation as early as possible after serious burns has been demonstrated to replenish the copper depletion that is so typical of burn victims.*

Superoxide Dismutase (SOD)

Copper also plays a critical role in the synthesis of a natural antioxidant called copper/zinc superoxide dismutase (SOD). In the initial phase of wound healing, immune cells are rushed to the wound site to protect against harmful invaders. They actually use free radicals to fight bacteria and to dispose of dead tissue. Once the free radicals have accomplished their job, however, they must be neutralized so the actual healing process can begin. SOD and other antioxidants such as vitamins C and D stop the free-radical oxidation process and promote the healing and repair process itself. Injury can deplete SOD and other antioxidants. In certain antioxidants depletion levels as high as 70% have been reported following injury (Ballmer et al. 1994). SOD should be supplemented to encourage new tissue to grow, to enhance collagen, and to reduce swelling. Wounds treated with SOD have been shown to heal better and more quickly (Niwa 1989; Misaki et al. 1990; Eldad et al. 1998). Current research indicates that SOD taken orally is destroyed in the digestive tract. A lipid-encapsulated injectable form of SOD (LIPSOD) and a sublingually administered form currently show the most promise for direct supplementation.

Vitamin C

Vitamin C is crucial for the proper function of the enzyme protocollagen hydroxylase which produces collagen, the primary constituent of the granulation tissue that heals a wound and the key component in blood vessel walls. A published review stated that vitamin C plays a variety of roles in the prevention and treatment of cancer, including stimulating the immune system and enhancing wound healing (Head 1998). Wound healing requires more vitamin C than diet alone can easily provide. It must be replenished daily because it is water soluble. Any excess is excreted rather than stored. Three tablets of Life Extension Mix 3 times a day provide the vitamin C and other nutrients needed for wound healing. For instance, vitamin A is important for tissue synthesis and enhances resistance to infection. B vitamins are needed for cell proliferation and for the replacement and maturation of red blood cells lost through bleeding. One response to a wound is a higher rate of metabolism. This leads to higher energy-level requirements in order to heal a wound, and to increased requirements for thiamine, niacin, and riboflavin.

In a topical solution, vitamin C has shown to be very effective in encouraging healing of the cornea in the wounded eye (Gonul et al. 2001).

Vitamin B$_5$

Pantothenic acid (vitamin B$_5$) improves healing by encouraging the migration of cells into the wounded area, thus establishing epithelialization (Weimann et al. 1999). At the same time that new cells are migrating into the wounded area, cell division is increased and protein synthesis is increased, improving the efficiency of the healing process. Vitamin B$_5$ also helps prevent an excess of inflammatory response in the wound and has been shown to improve surgical wound healing (Kapp et al. 1991).

Vitamin B$_5$ has been demonstrated to speed up wound healing, increase protein synthesis, and multiply the number of repair cells available at the wound site (Aprahamian et al. 1985). Vitamin B$_5$ seems to have the most benefit early on in wound repair, actually increasing the distance that repair cells can travel.

Vitamins B$_5$ and C in Combination

French researchers examined combined supplementation with vitamins B$_5$ and C before the removal of tattoos. One week prior to surgery, some patients were administered 200 mg of vitamin B$_5$ and 1 gram of vitamin C. Scars of all patients were measured 75 days after surgery. The scars of those who had been supplemented with vitamins B$_5$ and C were stronger and thicker and had more color. Researchers concluded that the vitamins had "recruited" more minerals to the wound areas (Vaxman et al. 1995). These "recruited" minerals included copper, magnesium, and manganese, all proven to enhance wound repair. Vitamins B$_5$ and C also kept iron from the wound areas, thus enhancing the healing process. The same group of researchers found that supplementation with vitamins B$_5$ and C strengthens the healing of wounds incidental to colon surgery.

Bromelain

Bromelain is found in pineapple and contains a proteolytic enzyme with the ability to break down or dissolve proteins. This mechanism of action can be helpful in chronic wounds or wounds having too much scar tissue. According to the *PDR for Nutritional Supplements* (2001, p. 72), bromelain speeds up healing time after surgical procedures, shows positive effects in the treatment of athletic injuries, and in at least one study has reduced swelling and pain from injuries of the musculoskeletal system. It has also been found to have antitumor properties (Maurer 2001). Bromelain is commonly taken as a digestive aid to enhance absorption of proteins.

Curcumin

Curcumin is an extract of the spice turmeric, known to have antioxidant properties and other health benefits. In Indian medicine, curcumin is used to reduce inflammation and treat wounds and skin ulcers. Topical application of curcumin encourages wound remodeling via effects on transforming growth factor-beta (TGF-b). It also improves reepitheliazation (new skin formation) and migration of cells such as myofibroblasts, fibroblasts, and macrophages, necessary for healing at the wound site. In animal studies, curcumin has shown effectiveness in both topical and oral solutions (Sidhu et al. 1999).

OTHER SUBSTANCES OF INTREST IN WOUND HEALING

Although major studies have not been done with the following substances, they are of interest and have been used in wound healing. Some of them have particular interest for the aging person.

Topical Estrogen

Compared to youthful skin, in aging skin complications are more likely to develop, such as the progression of a wound to a chronic nonhealing state. This is related to an increased amount of elastase in the wound. Elastase is an enzyme that breaks down elastic proteins and is upregulated in impaired wound healing states. In a study by Ashcroft et al. (1999) involving 36 patients over the age of 70, half male and half female, topical estrogen was found to decrease delays in wound healing in both the male and female patients. Wound size, collagen levels, and fibronectin levels all improved with topical estrogen, indicating improved wound healing. In this study, estrogen was delivered to the wound site for 24 hours as a patch routinely used in female estrogen replacement therapy (Ashcroft et al. 1999). Fibronectin levels have been found to be deficient in chronic wounds of the aged, such as venous ulcers in humans or laboratory wounds in aged animals (Herrick et al. 1997).

Dilantin (Phenytoin)

Dilantin is a drug commonly used to treat epilepsy and seizure disorders. One of the known complications of Dilantin is gingival overgrowth (overgrowth of tissue at the gum margins in the mouth), suggesting that Dilantin might have an ability to alter and improve healing in chronic wounds by the same mechanism of encouraging tissue growth. Although no studies have been reported in the United States, Dilantin has been reviewed in Great Britain and suggested for this use (Talas et al. 1999). In another study, topical Dilantin was compared with glucose analogs (honey) in patients with chronic leg ulcers over a 4-week period and showed superiority (Oluwatosin et al. 2000). Honey has been recognized as an agent to improve wound healing for some time. In the United States, topical agents of glucose analogs are commonly used for chronic wounds.

FRACTURE HEALING

Bone fracture, or a break in a bone, is a very common wound. Almost all persons experience a bone fracture at some time in their lives. Because of the tensile strength needed in bone, particularly the long bones that support the weight of the skeleton, this type of wound generally takes longer to heal than soft tissue wounds. Bones that do not support as much weight, such as the clavicle, take about 6 weeks to heal after a fracture, but structural bones (such as the femur) that support skeletal weight can take 3–5 months to heal. Weight-supporting bones must be well stabilized (or immobilized) in order to heal. They must remain immobile in a splint or a cast while new bone forms. New bone formation, called callus, is evident on an x-ray about 10 days after the fracture has occurred. At this stage, the new bone is soft and flexible. Over weeks to months, replacement with hard bony tissue occurs and the bone is able to function again and support weight.

The same events of inflammation, proliferation, and remodeling that occur in soft tissue injury also occur with fractures, although these stages are spread over a longer time period.

The same therapeutic and supplement recommendations also apply to bone injury, although there is a particular importance for copper and zinc. Copper supplementation is important in fracture healing and in the early formation of collagen in the wound.

Copper, 8 mg daily, provides adequate supplementation and should be taken for 6 weeks for a fracture of a non-weight-bearing bone. It should be taken for 2–3 months for a major weight-bearing bone. Because copper is also a pro-oxidant, supplementation should be stopped after this period of time.

Zinc should be taken at a dose of 90 mg daily (as recommended earlier for healing of other wounds). Zinc's enhancement of fracture healing may be related to its effects on increasing IGF-1 and TGF-beta, both of which are growth factors discussed previously.

In an animal study, rats were divided into groups: one control and one supplemented with vitamin C. All had fractured tibias. After examination at four 5-day intervals, "It was seen that the vitamin C-supplemented group went through the stages of fracture healing faster compared with the control group" (Yilmaz et al. 2001).

Glucosamine and chondroitin should also be supplemented to encourage cartilage formation and repair if the fracture has extended along an articular (joint) surface and there is likely cartilage injury also.

Growth factors have been studied with respect to fracture healing. At the present time, most of this work is in the research stage, although even now synthetic bone grafts impregnated with growth factors such as IGF-1 are available (Schmidmaier et al. 2001; Spiroet al. 2001). Administration of IGF-1 has been found to enhance bone fracture healing, but so far the evidence for using TGF-beta has been conflicting (Tielinen et al. 2001). To date, the use of fibroblast growth factor (FGF) has also been discouraging (Nakajima et al. 2001).

Another growth factor important in bone healing is osteogenic protein-1 or OP-1. A study of OP-1 to enhance fracture healing is in its infancy, but preliminary results are encouraging (Blokhuis et al. 2001). As shown in animal studies, parathormone (parathyroid hormone) also has promise in enhancing fracture strength and early callus formation (Andreassen et al. 2001), although in humans, parathormone is being used primarily to treat osteoporosis and in fractures associated with osteoporosis. Several new drugs stimulating bone healing are being tested, and most of these exert their effects via various growth factors, especially IGF-1, TGF-b, and FGF. In the future, stem cells may be used to improve bone healing (Moutsatsos et al. 2001).

Adequate dietary intake of protein is important. In an animal model, three groups were studied: controls (20% protein), malnourished animals (6% protein), and renourished animals (6% protein, but fed a 20% diet in the postfracture period). The researchers found that in renourished animals, the cross-sectional area of the fracture callus (the bony deposit that forms around broken ends of bones during healing) was greater than in those in the malnourished and well-nourished animals. They concluded: "Protein deprivation has a profound detrimental effect on fracture healing" (Day et al. 2001). In general, the diet should contain an adequate amount of protein for healing of all wounds and proteins should definitely be supplemented. Glutamine and arginine, amino acids mentioned earlier in this article, should definitely be supplemented.

Smoking is especially harmful when the body is trying to provide substrates for adequate wound healing. Smoking has been shown to "adversely affect bone mineral density, lumbar disk disease, the rate of hip fractures, and the dynamics of bone and wound healing" (Porter et al. 2001).

For fractures complicated by a nonunion (the ends of the fractured bone do not rejoin), work has been done for over 20 years using various types of electrical stimulation on the bone ends to encourage union of the fracture site.

For additional information on accelerating healing of bone fractures, the reader is encouraged to refer to the protocol on *Osteoporosis*. Bone healing rates may be enhanced by following some of the recommendations for preventing and reversing age-associated bone loss, such as supplementing with the nutrients calcium, magnesium, boron, vitamin D_3, and vitamin K; hormones such as DHEA and topical natural progesterone; and even a physician-prescribed bis-phosphonate drug such as Actonel.

⬤ SUMMARY

First, the type of wound, its cause, and its severity must be determined. Serious wounds must be evaluated and treated by a healthcare professional to prevent infection or development of serious complications. If there is any indication that the wound is not healing and has become infected, consult a healthcare professional immediately.

Next, the stage of healing of the wound should be identified. Then, follow the four principles of basic wound care: debride and cleanse, maintain a moist environment, prevent further injury, and provide supportive dietary nutrients for healing.

1. Arginine and glutamine are two essential amino acids that are required for protein synthesis. Take 10–22 grams daily of arginine and 2000 mg daily of glutamine.

2. Zinc and copper have been documented to promote wound healing. These minerals should be taken at least 2 hours apart to avoid antagonistic effects. Take 8 mg of copper daily for a limited time only during healing; take 90 mg of zinc.

3. Life Extension Mix provides vitamin C, vitamin E, vitamin B_5, and other essential nutrients to support and enhance wound healing: 9 tablets daily.

4. Additional vitamin C may be supplemented several times daily to promote collagen formation and provide additional antioxidant protection. Consult with a healthcare provider for serious wounds.

5. Aloe vera has numerous healing properties in both oral and topical applications. As a juice, 2 ounces of aloe concentrate may be mixed with a 6-ounce beverage. Topical aloe vera creams may be applied several times daily.

6. The digestive enzyme bromelain may help promote healing, reduce pain, and prevent scar tissue formation by helping to break down protein: one 500-mg tablet with meals.

7. Curcumin may help promote new skin growth in both oral and topical solutions. Take one 900-mg capsule daily. A compounding pharmacy should be consulted for topical applications.

8. For skeletal fractures, glucosamine and chondroitin may promote healing. Four 1000-mg combination capsules, taken twice daily, are suggested. Several other nutrients mentioned for wound healing are also recommended for fracture healing.

9. Taken orally, centella may improve collagen formation and reduce the effects of inflammation: one 500-mg capsule daily, or applied as an ointment, 1–2 applications daily.

10. In people with adequate levels of HGH and IGF-1, wounds heal faster than in those with low levels. HGH supplementation should not be started during the catabolic period of critical illness because it increases the risk of mortality. However, people on an HGH antiaging protocol heal faster than others of their age. If HGH is not affordable, consider supplementing with 75–100 mg of DHEA during the healing process. Refer to the *DHEA Replacement protocol* for details.

11. For chronic or serious wounds, consider alternative treatments such as hyperbaric oxygen therapy, whirlpool therapy, ultrasound treatment, electrical stimulation, magnetic therapy, and therapeutic touch.

12. For wounds and fractures that do not heal as expected, it might be beneficial to seek help from a university orthopedic or plastic surgery section using local application of growth factors and new drugs that affect growth factors. For nonunion bone fractures, electrical stimulation is an option available at university hospitals as well as other institutions.

To learn what you can do to reduce the risk of medically induced complications, refer to the Foundation's *Anesthesia and Surgical Precautions protocol.*

 PRODUCT AVAILABILITY

Cold-pressed, whole-leaf aloe vera juice concentrate; topical aloe vera ointment; arginine powder, tablets, and capsules; glutamine powder and capsules; vitamin B$_5$ powder and capsules; curcumin with bioperine; bromelain; zinc; copper; vitamin C; glucosamine-chondroitin caps; DHEA; and Life Extension Mix may be ordered by phoning (800) 544-4440 or by ordering online at www.lef.org.

Appendix A
Avoiding Vitamin A Toxicity

Based upon hundreds of published studies, the Life Extension Foundation has recommended vitamin A analog drugs to cancer patients. For the many cancer patients who cannot gain access to vitamin A analogs because the FDA classifies them as "unapproved new drugs," the Foundation has recommended the use of water-soluble vitamin A liquid drops.

The dosage range of vitamin A liquid drops that cancer patients have been using is 100,000–300,000 IU a day. The Foundation has cautioned that these high doses could produce toxicity if taken over extended periods of time, yet cancer patients often are forced to risk some degree of toxicity to obtain an effective dose of vitamin A.

VITAMIN A AND BONE

Reports of increased bone fracture risk are a concern when higher potency vitamin A supplements are taken over the long-term (Michaelsson et al. 2003). One study showed bone mineral density was reduced by 10 percent in those taking more than 5000 IU of vitamin A from both dietary sources and supplements. This study showed that compared to lower intakes of vitamin A, those taking more than 5000 IU of vitamin A had a 2.1 time higher risk of hip fracture.

One reason people take vitamin A supplements is to reduce cancer risk. What these bone density/fracture studies fail to ascertain is whether the same people taking higher doses of vitamin A had lower incidences of cancer. These studies also fail to establish whether the study participants were taking adequate amounts of bone-protecting nutrients such as manganese, zinc, copper, vitamin K, and magnesium. It could be that people consuming lots of vitamin A-fortified milk and eating vitamin A-rich organ meats had deficiencies of other nutrients critical to bone maintenance. One of these nutrients is folic acid, which lowers homocysteine levels. Excess homocysteine participates in degenerative bone degradation.

From a practical standpoint, a healthy person is left with some unanswered questions. A plethora of published studies associates low vitamin A intake with increased cancer risk (see Reference list for

Appendix A). Guarding against vitamin A deficiency is thus a critical component of a cancer prevention program. It would therefore appear practical to supplement with 5000 IU a day of vitamin A, but perhaps higher doses are not needed. In fact, taking higher doses of vitamin A over an extended time period without other bone-protecting nutrients would appear to increase fracture risk. Refer to the *Osteoporosis protocol* for complete details about the steps you can take to protect against the loss of bone mineral density and subsequent risk of fracture.

Concerns for Cancer Patients

Cancer patients often take high potencies of vitamin A drugs, such as Vesanoid (all-trans retinoic acid), Accutane (13-cis-retinoic acid) or vitamin A supplements. These vitamin A drugs have potent anti-proliferative, differentiation-inducing, and apoptosis-promoting effects against cancer cells.

Retinoic acid (a potent vitamin A drug) has been shown to suppress osteoblast activity (bone-building cells) and promote formation of osteoclasts (cells that remove old bone) *in vitro* (test tube studies).

Depletion of bone mineral density is of concern to cancer patients, since some cancer drugs also cause bone mineral depletion. Some cancers have a proclivity to metastasize to bone, and weakened bones may be more vulnerable to cancer cell adhesion and infiltration. Beta-carotene does not induce any loss of bone density, but it fails to exert the same potent effects against existing cancer cells as vitamin A drugs.

Cancer patients taking high potencies of vitamin A drugs or supplements should pay particular attention to the "Maintaining Bone Density" section of the protocol entitled *Cancer: The Critical Factors*. This section describes the steps that cancer patients should take to maintain bone integrity.

Anyone taking very high doses of vitamin A for cancer or any other reason should do so under the care of a physician and should be on the lookout for symptoms of vitamin A toxicity. The following are common symptoms of vitamin A overdose that should be watched for in cancer patients taking high doses of any vitamin A product:

- Headache
- Dizziness
- Blurred vision
- Joint pain
- Dry lips
- Scaly, dry skin
- Excessive hair loss

Blood tests showing elevated liver enzymes may be a sign of a vitamin A overdose. If any of these symptoms appear, discontinue using vitamin A until the symptoms disappear, and then resume vitamin A therapy at a much lower dosage. The cancer patient faces a dilemma in attempting to use the maximum dose of vitamin A to fight his or her cancer, while trying to avoid vitamin A toxicity.

The thyroid gland works with the liver to produce a vitamin A binding protein called transthyretin. This keeps vitamin A bound in the blood and only releases it to the body when needed. When there is no thyroid gland, the lack of transthyretin makes high doses of vitamin A potentially toxic because there is no control mechanism to hold the vitamin A in a biologically unavailable form. *Therefore, those with thyroid cancer should avoid vitamin A.*

Appendix B: Supplement Partners

I n nature nothing acts in isolation. Connections and synergistic cooperation abound throughout all systems. Yet, some in our medically driven culture tend to think that one cure applies to each cause—perhaps even that there is one supplement for one cause and another for some other cause. However, nature does not work that way, and neither should we. Balance is important when considering supplementation. Although synergistic supplement formulas are available, it is important for consumers to know why certain supplements have specific ingredients, but not other ingredients. The table below lists some of the supplement combinations that are synergistic. A short explanation is included. Some of these combinations are only in the research stages (labeled *in vitro* or in laboratory studies), whereas others are well known and refer to use in humans (labeled *in vivo* or in a living organism). In many cases in which the antioxidant vitamins are involved, there is an ongoing shuttle process where once a vitamin is oxidized (carrying excess oxygen as a result of depotentizing a free radical), it is then regenerated (is reduced or has the excess oxygen removed) by another vitamin that is ready to accept its oxygen—and so on, like a bucket brigade.

Combined Substances	Beneficial Effect(s)	Synergy	Reference
Vitamin C + Vitamin E	Water-soluble antioxidant/antiviral Fat-soluble antioxidant	In the retina and in other highly oxidant tissues, vitamin C must be present to help regenerate the vitamin E oxidized by ultraviolet (UV) radiation. Regeneration of vitamin E may also be helped by lipoic acid—another antioxidant.	Stoyanovsky et al. 1995
Vitamin C + Coenzyme Q_{10} + Vitamin E	Antioxidant Antioxidant/energy molecule Antioxidant	Both vitamin C and reduced coenzyme Q_{10} interact with vitamin E to regenerate the antioxidant properties of vitamin E.	Beyer 1994
Vitamin C + Vitamin E	Antioxidant Antioxidant	Ascorbic acid acts as a synergistic antioxidant in conjunction with vitamin E; ascorbic acid is in the water-soluble areas and vitamin E in the lipid (fat) areas of the cell.	Sato et al. 1990
Vitamin A + Vitamin D	Skin, night vision, growth, cell differentiation Calcium metabolism	In human brain cancer cells, vitamins A and D act synergistically to inhibit cell growth *in vitro*.	Stio et al. 2001
Vitamin A + Zinc	Skin, night vision, growth, cell differentiation Enzyme cofactor for skin, prostate	Zinc potentiates the effect of vitamin A in restoring night vision in night-blind pregnant women with low initial serum zinc concentrations.	Christian et al. 2001
Lycopene + Vitamin E, glabridin, rosmarinic acid, carnosinic acid, garlic	Antioxidant, especially in prostate tissue Antioxidants	Lycopene acts synergistically as an antioxidant against low-density lipoprotein (LDL) oxidation, with several natural antioxidants such as vitamin E, the flavonoid glabridin, the phenolics rosmarinic acid and carnosinic acid, and garlic (*in vitro* and *in vivo* human studies).	Fuhrman et al. 2000
Vitamin E + Aspirin	Antioxidant Nonsteroidal anti-inflammatory drug (NSAID)	Coadministration of vitamin E renders the inflammatory enzyme COX-2 more sensitive to inhibition by aspirin (*in vitro* cell culture).	Abate et al. 2000

Combined Substances	Beneficial Effect(s)	Synergy	Reference
Catechin + Quercetin	Bioflavonoids acting as antioxidants	When present together *in vitro* (also in red wine *in vivo*), catechin and quercetin strongly inhibit platelet aggregation and adhesion to collagen.	Pignatelli et al. 2000
Vitamin C + Soy isoflavones	Antioxidant Usually act as weak estrogens; thought to be cancer protective	Increasing levels of genistein, daidzein, and equol (soy isoflavones) inhibited LDL oxidation; this inhibitory effect was further enhanced in the presence of ascorbic acid (*in vitro*). (Some consider LDL oxidation to be a partner in the formation of plaque and hardening of the arteries.)	Hwang et al. 2000
Vitamin A + Vitamin D$_3$	Skin, night vision, cellular growth and differentiation Calcium and phosphorus metabolism	Human-derived leukemia cells were found to differentiate into more mature (and stable) cells in the presence of vitamins A and D$_3$, together much more so than alone, thus making them less "cancerous."	Taimi et al. 1991
L-Carnitine + Coenzyme Q$_{10}$	Enhances fatty acid transport across cell membranes; improves cognitive function Antioxidant and energy-generating molecule	*L*-carnitine and CoQ$_{10}$ exert a stronger protection against damage by the cancer drug doxorubicin and induce a greater utilization of fatty acids as compared with the effects of each compound alone (*in vitro*).	Conte et al. 1990
Chromium + Niacin	Mineral that improves glucose tolerance Often used in high doses to lower cholesterol; one of the B vitamins in B-complex	A combination of these caused a significant decrease in fasting and total glucose in normal, elderly humans.	Urberg et al. 1987
Vitamin E + Selenium	Antioxidant Mineral involved in antioxidant pathways, protects against certain types of heart disease and cancer	Vitamin E potentiates the anti-tumor action of high-dose selenium by a mechanism different from upregulating the glutathione pathway (animal study).	Horvath et al. 1983
Vitamin C + Vitamin E	Antioxidant Antioxidant	Optimum combination of vitamins C and E might substantially enhance the detoxifying ability of the liver through upregulation of hydroxylation enzymes (study in guinea pigs).	Ginter et al. 1982
Folic acid + Trimethyglycine or betaine (TMG)	Prevents neural tube defects in developing human embryo; lowers homocysteine levels together with vitamins B$_6$ and B$_{12}$ Donates methyl groups to help in detoxifying homocysteine; aids in proper liver function and cellular replication; helps in other detoxification reactions	Although taking folic acid, either in a B-complex form or by itself, will in most cases lower homocysteine to healthy levels, clinical experience has shown that the addition of TMG will enhance this process and is essential in certain people. Folate, TMG, SAMe, and choline are all "methyl donors," critical in oxidation/reduction, detoxification, and DNA repair. Taking folic acid without ensuring adequate B$_{12}$ intake might lead to anemia and serious neurological damage.	McGregor 2002 Wilcken et al. 1983 Reynolds 2002 Tomczyk et al. 2001

Combined Substances	Beneficial Effect(s)	Synergy	Reference
Glucosamine sulfate + Chondroitin sulfate and manganese ascorbate	Helps to form cartilage building blocks in arthritic joints Chondroitin facilitates the entry of glucosamine into inflamed joints; both retard cartilage degeneration	Studies of each supplement separately have yielded good results. However, together they enhance each other's activity.	Lippiello 2000
L-cysteine; N-acetyl cysteine; glutathione + Vitamin C	Critical amino acids required for antioxidant pathways Antioxidant and antioxidant regenerator	For these amino acid supplements to function effectively as antioxidants, adequate vitamin C must be taken to ensure they are kept in their reduced form.	Nowak et al. 2000 Sprince et al. 1975
Calcium + Magnesium	Bone metabolism, muscle contraction Found in dark green leafy vegetables; a critical mineral in smooth muscle relaxation	Although the actions of these two minerals are somewhat opposite, they work in tandem to contract and relax muscles. Because people are often magnesium-deficient, it is important that magnesium be taken whenever extra calcium is consumed.	Gourgoulianis et al. 2001 Gordon 1976
Vitamin B_{12} + Vitamin B_9 (folic acid)	Deficiencies lead to pernicious anemia; involved in blood formation and energy production Formation of amino acids; central to all rapidly dividing cells	These two B vitamins work in tandem to reduce a toxic cardiovascular amino acid known as homocysteine. Taking folic acid without ensuring adequate B_{12} intake might lead to anemia and serious neurological damage.	Clarke et al. 2002
Evening primrose oil (EPO) + Zinc; vitamin C; chromium	One of the omega-6 essential fatty acids; often deficient in North American diet; anti-inflammatory and immune-enhancing Cofactors required for the body to properly use EPO	The conversion of the active component of EPO (DGLA) to anti-inflammatory prostaglandins requires vitamin C and the minerals zinc and chromium in adequate amounts.	Belch et al. 2000 Hansen et al. 1983
Unsaturated oil products (primrose oil; fish oils; CLA, etc.) + Antioxidants (usually vitamin E as mixed tocopherols in the case of oils)	Presence of these oils in the diet or by supplementation ensures a balance of anti-inflammation, muscle relaxation, and immune enhancement	Consuming supplements that contain unsaturated oils requires an adequate supply of antioxidants to ensure that the oils are protected from oxidation.	Grau et al. 2001
Lycopene + Lutein	Especially important in the health of the prostate gland in males over the age of 40; found in tomatoes; better absorbed if cooked Found in green leafy vegetables; helps build macular pigment density, a critical factor in the health of the macula and the retina (Macular pigment density is related to clarity of the lens of the eye.)	Mixtures of carotenoids are more effective than the single compounds. This synergistic effect is most pronounced when lycopene or lutein are present. The superior protection of mixtures might be related to specific positioning of different carotenoids in cell membranes because cell membranes have both a fat and water layer.	Stahl 1998

Combined Substances	Beneficial Effect(s)	Synergy	Reference
Bioflavonoids, e.g., quercetin, rutin (This group includes anthocyanins, flavins, flavonols, flavones, flavonones, quercetin, carotenoids, lutein, and resveratrol.) + Vitamin C	Enhances the potency of vitamin C; strengthens capillaries Maintains healthy collagen; antioxidant	In general, these antioxidants tend to work together, with vitamin C often providing the replenishment of hydrogen to oxidized quercetin, rutin, etc.	Kandaswami 1993
Vitamin K$_3$ + Methotrexate	Blood coagulation; immune system upregulator; found in green leafy vegetables An anticancer and anti-arthritic drug. **Note:** Methotrexate depletes folic acid.	K$_3$ added to methotrexate resulted in *in vivo* synergy in a rat study, a finding that might extend to humans.	Gold 1986

Appendix C

Why Pharmaceutical Grade Supplements Are Critical

A growing concern among physicians and consumers is whether dietary supplements contain all of the active ingredients listed on the label. This apprehension is based on well-publicized analyses of commercial supplements showing considerable variation in ingredient quality and quantity.

The Life Extension Buyers Club learned a long time ago that there were few ingredient suppliers who can be trusted to consistently deliver pharmaceutical-grade ingredients. That is why the Buyers Club mandates extraordinary quality-control measures in order to guard against the counterfeiting that has become so prevalent in the supplement industry.

An example of misleading products can be found in the prostate-protection formulas now offered by dozens of companies. One of the key ingredients in these products is *pygeum*, which functions by several mechanisms to prevent and alleviate the effects of benign prostate enlargement. The scientific literature clearly states that 100 mg a day of *pygeum* is required to produce a biological effect, yet some companies are putting in only 10 mg of *pygeum* and claiming this small amount will produce a benefit. To make matters worse, the high cost of *pygeum* extract has motivated unscrupulous suppliers to dilute *pygeum* with sterols from other plants.

The Life Extension Buyers Club restricts its *pygeum* purchases to Indena, the premium producer of *pygeum* (and other botanical extracts). Rather than trust the certificate of analysis that comes with every batch of Indena's *pygeum*, the Buyers Club assays the material to verify that it meets pharmaceutical-grade standards.

Companies offering low-cost ingredients constantly solicit Life Extension Buyers Club's business. An assay of the ingredients from these discount companies, however, using HPLC (high performance liquid chromatography) or mass spectrophotometry (mass spec), often reveals inconsistencies. This is why Life Extension restricts its purchases of ingredients to nutrient suppliers that take extra steps in their manufacturing process to ensure the active ingredients are of pharmaceutical quality and potency.

Some companies that sell finished dietary supplements attempt to verify ingredient authenticity by using a low-cost method known as the "melting point." The problem with using the melting point test is that counterfeiters can find substances that melt at the same temperature as the real ingredient, thus enabling them to pass on an inactive agent as the legitimate ingredient. The quantitative analysis (HPLC/mass spec) mandated by the Buyers Club verifies not only the potency, but also the purity. If impurities are detected, the quantitative analysis can often identify them.

A COMPANY THAT REFUSED TO DO BUSINESS WITH LIFE EXTENSION

A deceptive practice that occurs in the ingredient industry is to submit samples that meet pharmaceutical standards, but not deliver the same high quality material for use in the finished dietary supplement. That is why Life Extension has active ingredients assayed before they go into the bottle.

One company that desperately wanted Life Extension's business guaranteed their quality would meet pharmaceutical standards. This company provided all kinds of impressive documentation and ingredient samples showing they were capable of meeting the Buyers Club's exacting requirements. When Life Extension told the company that acceptance of any shipments would be contingent on the ingredients passing a quantitative analysis (mass spectrophotometry / HPLC) test, the company said they would prefer not to enter into a business relationship.

THE IMPORTANCE OF PURITY

The Chinese have done the American vitamin consumer a tremendous favor. For decades, European and Japanese companies maintained a virtual monopoly that forced supplement users in the United States to pay inflated prices. The Federal Trade Commission (FTC) even brought an antitrust case against these companies that resulted in them disgorging huge amounts of their profits.

Free markets, however, do not need a government watchdog to protect against price fixing. The outrageous profits generated by the European-Japanese monopoly motivated the Chinese to copy just about every dietary supplement and sell them at sharply reduced prices.